PEDIATRIC EMERGENCY MEDICINE

A Comprehensive Study Guide

Second Edition

NOTICE

Medicine is an ever-changing science. As new research and clinical experience broaden our knowledge, changes in treatment and drug therapy are required. The editors and the publisher of this work have checked with sources believed to be reliable in their efforts to provide information that is complete and generally in accord with the standards accepted at the time of publication. However, in view of the possibility of human error or changes in medical sciences, neither the editors nor the publisher nor any other party who has been involved in the preparation or publication of this work warrants that the information contained herein is in every respect accurate or complete, and they are not responsible for any errors or omissions or for the results obtained from use of such information. Readers are encouraged to confirm the information contained herein with other sources. For example and in particular, readers are advised to check the product information sheet included in the package of each drug they plan to administer to be certain that the information contained in this book is accurate and that changes have not been made in the recommended dose or in the contraindications for administration. This recommendation is of particular importance in connection with new or infrequently used drugs.

PEDIATRIC EMERGENCY MEDICINE

A Comprehensive Study Guide
Second Edition

American College

of Emergency

Physicians

Edited by

Gary R. Strange, MD, FACEP
Chairman
Department of Emergency Medicine
University of Illinois at Chicago
Chicago, IL

William R. Ahrens, MD
Associate Professor of Clinical Emergency Medicine
Director, Pediatric Emergency Medicine
University of Illinois at Chicago
Chicago, IL

Steven Lelyveld, MD, FACEP, FAAP
Associate Professor of Clinical Pediatrics and Medicine
Chief, Section of Pediatric Emergency Medicine
Pritzker School of Medicine
University of Chicago
Chicago, IL

Robert W. Schafermeyer, MD, FACEP, FAAP
Chairman
Department of Emergency Medicine
Carolinas Medical Center
Charlotte, NC

McGraw-Hill
Medical Publishing Division

*New York   Chicago   San Francisco   Lisbon
London   Madrid   Mexico City
Milan   New Delhi   San Juan   Seoul
Singapore   Sydney   Toronto*

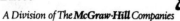

McGraw-Hill

A Division of The McGraw·Hill Companies

Pediatric Emergency Medicine: A Comprehensive Study Guide, Second Edition

1234567890 DOCDOC 098765432

ISBN 0-07-136979-1
This book was set in Times Roman by Atlis Graphics.
The editors were Andrea Seils and Regina Y. Brown.
The developmental editor was Michelle Watt.
The production supervisor was Philip Galea.
The index was prepared by Jerry Ralya.
R. R. Donnelley and Sons Company was printer and binder.
This book was printed on acid-free paper.

Library of Congress Cataloging-in-Publication Data
Pediatric emergency medicine: a comprehensive study guide / edited by
Gary R. Strange
 . . . [et al.]. — 2nd ed.
     p. ; cm.
   Includes bibliographical references and index.
   ISBN 0-07-136979-1
   1. Pediatric emergencies—Handbooks, manuals, etc. I. Strange, Gary R., 1947-
   [DNLM: 1. Emergencies—Child—Handbook. 2. Emergencies—Infant—Handbook.
   3. Pediatrics—Handbooks. WS 39 P3713 2002]
 RJ370.P4523 2002
 618.92′0025—dc21   2001045261

To those who have worked so long and hard to allow me to develop as a person, a physician, and academician—my parents, Elmer and Onas Strange, who gave me the confidence and enthusiasm to try; countless teachers who inspired and had the patience to redirect; and to my wife, Sarah, and daughters, Jackie and Betsy, who have remained supportive and helpful throughout seemingly never-ending projects.

Gary R. Strange

To my wife, my parents, and my teachers.

William R. Ahrens

To my parents, Mark and Adelaide Lelyveld, whose hard work, encouragement, and support started me on this path; to my wife, Betsy McCormick, and daughter, Katie, whose patience and understanding made the completion of this task possible.

Steven Lelyveld

To those physicians who have helped me develop professionally and learn how to provide quality patient care to children in time of need; to my parents, Virginia and William, as well as my brothers and sisters, Richard, Donna, Mary Ann, and Michael, who provided love and support as I pursued my career in medicine; and to my loving wife Ann and our children, Christina, David, Matthew, and Joseph, for their love and support while I pursued my many educational efforts.

Robert W. Schafermeyer

CONTENTS

CONTRIBUTORS

Thomas J. Abramo, MD [2, 121]
Emergency Center
Children's Medical Center of Dallas
Dallas, TX

Thomas J. Abrunzo [67, 68]

William R. Ahrens, MD [9, 46, 52]
Associate Professor of Clinical Emergency Medicine
University of Illinois at Chicago
Chicago, IL

Steven E. Aks, DO, FACEP, FACMT [82, 89, 91, 92, 95, 104]
Dept. of Emergency Medicine
Mercy Hospital and Medical Center
Chicago, IL

Yona Amatai, MD [97]
Section of Clinical Toxicology
Cook County Hospital
Chicago, IL

Tanya R. Anderson, MD [119]
Assistant Professor of Psychiatry
University of Illinois
Chicago, IL

Grace Arteaga [5]

Joilo Barbosa, MD [33,35]
Dept. of Emergency Medicine
Emory University
Atlanta, GA

Roger Barkin, MD [61]
Division of Emergency Medicine
University of Colorado Health Sciences Center
Denver, CO

Brian A. Bates, MD [6, 8]
Methodist Children's Hospital of South Texas
San Antonio, TX

Elizabeth E. Baumann, MD [54, 55, 56]
Instructor in Pediatrics
Section of Endocrinology
Dept. Pediatrics
University of Chicago
Chicago, IL

Kenneth Bizovi, MD [84]
Dept. of Emergency Medicine
Oregon Health Science University
Portland, OR

Ira J. Blumen, MD [116, 117, 121]
Division of Emergency Medicine
University of Chicago
Chicago, IL

Mary Jo A. Bowman, MD [110, 111, 112]
8700 Diley Road
Canal Winchester, OH

Kathleen Brown, MD [26, 27, 28, 29, 30, 31]
Dept. of Emergency Medicine
Upstate Medical University
Syracuse, NY

Richard M. Cantor, MD [25]
Central NY Poison Control Center
Dept. of Emergency Medicine
SUNY University Hospital
Syracuse, NY

Andrea Carlson, MD [105]
Dept. of Emergency Medicine
Christ Hospital and Medical Center
Oak Lawn, IL

The numbers in brackets following the contributor name refer to chapter(s) authored or co-authored by the contributor.

Stephen A. Colucciello, MD [16, 17]
Dept. of Emergency Medicine
Carolinas Medical Center
Medical Education Bldg.
Charlotte, NC

D. Mark Courtney [17]
Division of E.M.
Northwestern Memorial Hospital
Chicago, IL

Michael Cowan, MD [2]
Children's Medical Center of Dallas
Emergency Center
Dallas, TX

Ronald A. Dieckmann, MD [120]
Pediatric Emergency Medicine
San Francisco General Hospital
San Francisco, CA

Valerie A. Dobiesz, MD [18]
Associate Professor of Clinical Emergency Medicine
University of Illinois
Chicago, IL

Timothy Erickson, MD [79, 81, 93, 98, 100, 102, 106, 110, 111, 112]
Associate Professor of Emergency Medicine
Dept. of Emergency Medicine
University of Illinois
Chicago, IL

Susan Fuchs, MD [36, 37, 38, 39, 40, 41, 42, 43, 44, 45]
Division of Pediatric Emergency Medicine
Children's Memorial Hospital
Chicago, IL

Marianne Gausche-Hill, FACEP, FAAP [59, 60]
Dept. of Emergency Medicine
UCLA School of Medicine
Harbor-UCLA Medical Center
Torrance, CA

Michael J. Gerardi, MD [10, 24]
Pediatric Emergency Services
St. Barnabas Medical Center
Livingston, NJ

Jill Glick, MD [118]
Medical Director Child Protective Services
University of Chicago
Chicago, IL

Collin S. Goto, MD [6, 7]
Children's Hospital and Health Center
San Diego, CA

Michael Green, MD [96]
Dept. of Emergency Medicine
Mercy Hospital and Medical Center
Chicago, IL

Russell H. Greenfield, MD [18, 19, 21, 22]
Carolinas Integrative Health
Charlotte, NC

Geetha Gurrala, MD [70]
Attending Physician
Department of Emergency Medicine
University of Illinois at Chicago
Chicago, IL

Leon Gussow, MD [80, 108]
Dept. of Emergency Medicine
Cook County Hospital
Chicago, IL

Suchinta Hakim, MD [46]
Dept. of Emergency Medicine
Hinsdale Hospital
Hinsdale, IL

Brenda N. Hayakawa, MD [75]
Emergency Dept.
Foothill Presbyterian Hospital
San Dimas Community Hospital
Arcadia, CA

Bruce E. Herman, MD [110, 111, 112]
ED, Primary Children's Medical Center
Salt Lake City, UT

Daniel Hryhorczuk, MD [97]
Dept. of Environmental and Occupational Medicine
University of Illinois
Chicago, IL

Will Ignatoff [106]
Dept. of Emergency Medicine
University of Illinois at Chicago
Chicago, IL

David M. Jaffe, MD, FAAP, FACEP [12]
Dept. of Pediatrics
Washington University School of Medicine
St. Louis Children's Hospital
St. Louis, MO

Shabnam Jain, MD [48, 49]
Assistant Professor of Pediatrics
Emory University School of Medicine
Attending Physician
Emergency Department,
    Children's Healthcare of Atlanta at Egleston
Atlanta, GA

Alan E. Jones, MD [16]
Dept. of Emergency Medicine
Carolinas Medical Center
Medical Education Bldg.
Charlotte, NC

Susan A. Kecskes, MD [57]
Director, Pediatric Intensive Care Unit
Dept. of Pediatrics
University of Illinois at Chicago
Chicago, IL

Katherine M. Konzen, MD [69]
Dept. of Pediatric Emergency Medicine
Children's Hospital MC 5088
San Diego, CA

Jane E. Kramer, MD [71, 72, 73, 74]
Associate Professor of Pediatrics
Director, Section of Pediatric Emergency
    Medicine
Department of Pediatrics
Rush Medical College
Chicago, Illinois

Ann Krantz [90]
Division of Occupational Medicine
Cook County Hospital
Chicago, IL

John D. Lantos, MD [123]
Associate Professor of Pediatrics and Medicine
Associate Director, Center for Clinical Medical Ethics
Co-Director, Robert Wood Johnson Clinical Scholars
    Program
Chief, Section of General Pediatrics
The University of Chicago
Chicago, IL

Jerrold B. Leikin, MD [83, 85, 92, 103]
Department of Occupational Medicine & Clinical
    Toxicology
Rush North
Glencoe, IL

Steven Lelyveld, MD FACEP, FAAP [47, 50, 122]
Associate Professor of Clinical Pediatrics and Medicine
Chief, Section of Pediatric Emergency Medicine
Pritzker School of Medicine
University of Chicago
Chicago, IL

Marshall Lewis, MD [58]
Dept. Pediatrics
University of Illinois Hospital
Chicago, IL

Jordan D. Lipton, MD, FACEP [23]
Carolinas Emergency Physicians
Department of Emergency Medicine
Mercy Hospital South
Charlotte, NC

Wendy Ann Lucid, MD [13, 14, 15]
Good Samaritan & Phoenix Hospitals
Phoenix, AZ

John Marcinak, MD [47]
Section of Infectious Disease
Dept. of Pediatrics
University of Illinois
Chicago, IL

Diana Mayer, MD [76, 77, 78]
Dept. of Pediatrics
University of Illinois
Chicago, IL

Bonnie McManus, MD [88, 94]
Hinsdale, IL

Rustin Morse, MD [5]
Phoenix, AZ

Mark Mycyk, MD [90, 97]
Section of Clinical Toxicology
Dept. of Emergency Medicine
University of Illinois
Chicago, IL

Thomas T. Mydler, MD [7]
Children's Medical Center of Dallas
Dallas, TX

Margaret Paik, MD [58]
Dept. of Pediatrics
University of Chicago
Chicago, IL

Frank P. Paloucek, PharmD, DABAT [107]
Director, Residency Programs
Clinical Associate Professor in Pharmacy Practice
Dept. of Pharmacy Practice
College of Pharmacy University of Illinois
   at Chicago
Chicago, IL

Barbara Pawel, MD [114]
Section of Emergency Medicine
Philadelphia, PA

Nattasorn Plipat, MD [46]
Pediatric Infectious Diseases Fellow
Division of Infectious Diseases, Box #20
Children's Memorial Hospital
Chicago, IL

Elizabeth C. Powell [51]
Children's Memorial Hospital
Chicago, IL

Heather M. Prendergast, MD [119]
Assistant Professor of Emergency Medicine
University of Illinois
Chicago, IL

Patricia Primm, MD [4]
Children's Medical Center of Dallas
Emergency Center
Dallas, TX

Kimberly S. Quayle, MD [11]
Division of Pediatric Emergency Medicine
St. Louis Children's Hospital
One Children's Place
St. Louis, MO

Veena Ramaiah, MD [118]
Dept. of Pediatrics
Division of Pediatric Emergency Medicine
University of Chicago Children's Hospital
Chicago, IL

Rebecca R. Reamy [4]
MUSC Children's Hospital
Pediatric Emergency/Critical Care
Charleston, SC

Sally L. Reynolds [51]
Children's Memorial Hospital
Chicago, IL

Timothy J. Rittenberry, MD, FACEP [19, 96, 99]
Dept. of Emergency Medicine
Illinois Masonic Medical Center
Chicago, IL

Jaime Rivas [99]

Howard Rodenberg, MD [121]
Medical Director, Volusia County EMS
Adjunct Professor of Human Factors,
Embry-Riddle Aeronautical University
C/O Advanced Medical Direction
Daytona Beach, FL

Simon Ros, MD [113]
Department of Pediatrics
Loyola University Medical Center
Maywood, IL

Julia A. Rosekrans, MD [62, 63, 64, 65, 66]
Mayo Medical Center
Rochester, MN

Robert L. Rosenfield, MD [54, 55, 56]
Division of Pediatric Endocrinology
The University of Chicago
Chicago, IL

Alfred Sacchetti [24]
Department of Emergency Medicine
Our Lady of Lourdes Medical Center
Voorhees, NJ

John P. Santamaria [67, 68]
USF School of Medicine
Tampa, FL

Robert W. Schafermeyer, MD, FACEP, FAAP
  [120]
Chairman
Department of Emergency Medicine
Carolinas Medical Center
Charlotte, NC

Susan M. Scott, MD [1, 3]
Assistant Professor
Children's Medical Center of Dallas
Emergency Center
Dallas, TX

Ghazala Q. Sharieff, MD, FACEP [69]
Orange Park, FL

Kimberly Sing, MD [105]
Madison, WI

Jonathan Singer, MD [53]
Dept. of Emergency Medicine
Wright State University
Kettering, OH

Tulika Singh, MD [52]
Depts. of Pediatrics and Emergency Medicine
University of Illinois
Chicago, IL

Edward P. Sloan, MD, MPH [21, 22]
Dept. of Emergency Medicine
University of Illinois at Chicago
Chicago, IL

David F. Soglin, MD [71, 72, 73, 74]
Chairman, Pediatric Emergency Medicine
Cook County Children's Hospital
Dept. of Pediatrics
Chicago, IL

Gary R. Strange, MD FACEP [47, 49, 50, 76, 77, 78,
  84, 113, 114, 115]
Chairman
Dept. of Emergency Medicine
University of Illinois at Chicago
Chicago, IL

Todd B. Taylor, MD [13, 14, 15]
Good Samaritan & Phoenix Hospitals
Phoenix, AZ

Frank Thorp, MD [54]

William C. Toepper [33, 34, 35]
Dept. of Emergency Medicine
Illinois Masonic Medical Center
Chicago, IL

David A. Townes, MD [109]
Division of Emergency Medicine
University of Washington
Seattle, WA

Timothy Turnbull, MD [87]
Atlanta, GA

Dennis T. Uehara, MD [20]
Chairman
Dept. of Emergency Medicine
Rockford Memorial Hospital
Rockford, IL

Michael VanRooyen, MD [70]
Department of Emergency Medicine
John Hopkins University
Baltimore, MD

Robert A. Wiebe, MD [1, 3]
Children's Medical Center of Dallas
Emergency Center
Dallas, TX

Kelly D. Young, MD [32]
Harbor-UCLA Medical Center
Dept. of Emergency Medicine
Torrance, CA

Michele Zell-Kanter [86, 98, 101]
Division of Occupational Medicine
Cook County Hospital
Chicago, IL

PREFACE

THE CURRENT WORK HAS BEEN DEVELOPED as a resource for clinicians who regularly provide pediatric emergency care as well as for those who only occasionally are called upon to care for a sick or injured child.

Many pediatric emergencies occur with relatively low overall frequency, often too infrequently to allow practitioners to develop experience with the specialized diagnostic and management skills required. Therefore, we have attempted to present readable and rapidly accessible clinical reference material designed to assist practitioners in the management of both common and less frequently occurring conditions.

We have devoted our efforts to developing both a clinical reference and a review tool for the pediatrician, the emergency physician, the family physician, and the primary care provider. We feel that the result is a concise overview of the field of pediatric emergency medicine that will be useful to practitioners, fellows, and educators involved in teaching pediatrics.

One impetus for the development of the first edition of this work was the 1993 report of the Institute of Medicine (IOM) on emergency medical services for children. The IOM report highlighted training issues for pediatricians, family physicians and other pediatric primary care providers, citing insufficient attention to both the recognition and management of emergencies and to the appropriate use of EMS systems. In addition, training programs in emergency medicine were assessed as not adequately addressing the pediatric aspects of patient care and system development.

In the developmental years of emergency medicine, the major foci were cardiac and trauma care. Work by Pantridge and others had demonstrated that rapid treatment of cardiac emergencies could improve survival. The landmark report entitled "Accidental Death and Disability: The Neglected Disease of Modern Society" brought attention to the need for raising the level of trauma care. As the specialty matured, attention was extended to include other subsets of emergency care, including pediatric emergency medicine.

One of the first moves in the development of the pediatric aspect of the specialty of emergency medicine was the development of specialized continuing education courses in pediatrics. Under the auspices of the American Heart Association, the Pediatric Advanced Life Support Course was developed. Additionally, joint efforts by the American Academy of Pediatrics and the American College of Emergency Physicians resulted in the Advanced Pediatric Life Support Course.

Beginning in the 1980s, joint pediatric and emergency medicine residency programs were developed and pediatric emergency medicine fellowships have continued to grow. Subspecialty certification for pediatric emergency medicine, under the auspices of the American Board of Pediatrics and the American Board of Emergency Medicine, has been available since 1992. This process has continued to produce board-certified subspecialists in pediatric emergency medicine who now play a major role in defining the subspecialty and providing direction and leadership. Research in the area of pediatric emergency medicine has also grown, allowing us to base more and more of our recommendations on sound evidence.

We are very proud of the authors who have worked with us on this book. Whenever possible, we have recruited practicing pediatric emergency physicians to author our chapters. For some highly specialized topics, we have recruited appropriate specialists to discuss the topics. We feel that this approach has resulted in an extremely practical as well as authoritative approach to the material. Throughout, we have striven to maintain clear concise style that can be easily understood and readily adopted by the on-line practitioner. The extensive pediatric emergency medicine background of the authors and editors has also helped to assure that the content of the field has been appropriately defined, neither omitting important pediatric concerns nor falling prey to over-inclusiveness.

It is difficult to single out parts of this work as most exemplary of the quality and value—we have been pleased with the outcome of each and every chapter. With trauma continuing to be the number one killer of our children, we were especially attuned to developing an excellent trauma section. It includes an excellent overview of the evaluation and management of the multiple trauma patient and an authoritative review of spinal cord injury. Given the great improvements in the management of the airway, we have separated out the material on "crash induction" and created a full chapter on rapid sequence intubation. A new chapter on conscious sedation and pain control has also been added to reflect the major advances in this area. The cardiovascular emergencies section provide an in-depth discussion of pediatric heart disease, with an expanded section on congenital heart disease. The dermatology section provides an extensive review of both common and life-threatening problems. The toxicology section is really a text within a text, with 30 chapters covering general principles, the specific management of toxins commonly encountered in pediatrics and less common toxins, with special implications in the pediatric patient. The psychosocial aspects of pediatric emergency medicine are dealt with in specific chapters on psychiatric emergencies, child maltreatment and dealth of a child, as well as being discussed throughout the book as they pertain to specific clincial problems.

We are proud to present this book to the practitioners of pediatric emergency medicine. We hope that it will be useful as a tool in the provision of quality pediatric emergency care for all our children.

We are pleased to acknowledge the many contributions of individuals who have assisted us along the way.

At McGraw-Hill, we have enjoyed wonderful support and encouragement from Andrea Seils and Regina Y. Brown.

At University of Illinois, the support of Bailet Wright has allowed us to move through the publication process smoothly and mostly on time.

At the University of Chicago, Ms. Eula Davis provided support in many ways, not the least of which has been many hours tracking down authors and chapters during the review process.

At Carolinas Medical Center, the excellent efforts of Janice Furtney kept the authors on schedule and the review process on the move. The support of John Marx, M.D., is highly appreciated.

At University of Texas Southwestern, we are grateful for the help of Lynn Heise, Secretarial Assistant to Robert A. Wiebe, M.D., in assimilating the materials for the Resuscitation Section of the text.

GARY R. STRANGE

1

Introduction

Robert A. Wiebe
Susan M. Scott

HIGH-YIELD FACTS

- Pediatric cardiopulmonary arrest usually results from the deterioration of an underlying medical problem.
- Up to 80 percent of pediatric arrests result from respiratory compromise.
- After 1 year of age, trauma is a leading cause of death in children.
- Despite some advances in the technique of pediatric cardiopulmonary resuscitation, the prognosis for a patient in full arrest remains dismal.

By providing artificial circulation and ventilation until natural function is restored, cardiopulmonary resuscitation (CPR) attempts to deliver nutrients, especially oxygen and glucose, to vital organs. Ultimately, the goal is to restore life and preserve normal function.

When CPR became the standard of care in the treatment of cardiac arrest, techniques used in adult resuscitation were applied to the resuscitation of the child. It is now well recognized that pediatric cardiopulmonary arrest and resuscitation is different from that of adults in its etiology, anatomy, and physiology. Emotional aspects also differ. The establishment of separate techniques and protocols for pediatric basic and advanced life support has acknowledged these differences.

One major difference between adult and pediatric resuscitation is the pathology of the event. Cardiac arrest in the adult is usually a primary event that results from a sudden dysrhythmia. Hypoxia and acidosis occur sud-

denly secondary to the cardiac event. In contrast, the pediatric cardiac arrest is usually the end result of pulmonary or circulatory embarrassment that results from deterioration of an underlying medical problem. Decreased tissue perfusion, hypoxia, and acidosis generally precede cardiac arrest. The antecedent period of deterioration results in significant end organ damage and makes the restoration of spontaneous circulation difficult. The combination of prearrest end organ damage and the damage that occurs during asystole has important implications for prognosis.

EPIDEMIOLOGY

There are no nationwide statistics to indicate the incidence of cardiac arrest in the pediatric population. It is estimated that 16,000 children die each year in the United States from unexpected cardiopulmonary arrest. Studies that address the epidemiology and outcome of pediatric cardiac arrest have demonstrated inconsistent but generally dismal results. Inconsistent patient inclusion criteria, outcome definitions, small sample sizes, and retrospective data collection make comparison of large studies by meta-analysis impossible. Sirbaugh and colleagues estimated that there are 19.7 cardiac arrests per 100,000 individuals under the age of 17. Reports reveal that almost 10 percent of ambulance runs involve children less than 19 years of age and of these 1 percent involve a cardiac arrest. Studies report that from 45 to 70 percent of pediatric cardiac arrests occur in infants less than 1 year of age. There is no reported gender difference until adolescence, when trauma becomes a leading cause of death and males predominate. Young and Seidel, in a collective review of 44 studies with a total of 3094 pediatric arrests, described 56 percent under 1 year of age; 62 percent were males. Out-of-hospital cardiac arrests were witnessed in 31 percent of cases and bystander CPR given 30 percent of the time. One important factor influencing the incidence of pediatric cardiac arrest is the presence of underlying disease. Zaritsky estimated that 87 percent of children resuscitated have an underlying disorder such as cancer, prematurity, or chromosomal abnormality.

The specific causes of pediatric cardiopulmonary arrest are more diverse than in adults. Studies estimate that 43 to 80 percent of pediatric cardiopulmonary arrests are secondary to respiratory compromise. When cardiac arrest occurs in children, it is usually the result of respiratory failure or shock that progresses from hypoxia-induced bradycardia to pulseless electrical activity and asystole. Most studies report that ventricular tachydysrhythmia occurs in less than 10 percent of pediatric arrests. In infants and young children most cardiac arrests are of respiratory origin (Table 1-1). Common causes of arrest include bronchiolitis, asthma, and upper airway obstruction. Although sudden infant death syndrome has decreased 40 percent in the past decade, largely due to supine positioning during sleep, it still remains a significant cause of arrest in infants. In older children, asthma continues to increase as a cause of cardiovascular collapse. Several studies have demonstrated the relationship between seizures and unexpected pediatric arrests. Mortality associated with asthma and epilepsy could probably be significantly reduced by effective and consistent pharmacologic management.

Myocarditis is a common cause of cardiac arrest in all pediatric age groups. Hypertrophic cardiomyopathy is not uncommon in adolescents and should be considered when a previously healthy asymptomatic child has a sudden catastrophic event. Intraabdominal hemorrhage from gastrointestinal tract bleeding and ruptured ectopic pregnancy contributes significantly to mortality statistics in adolescents. Toxic ingestions of tricyclic antidepressants, multiple drug ingestions, and use of street drugs are common among adolescents. Other causes of cardiac arrest include congenital heart disease, infectious and central nervous system disorders, and other congenital anomalies. After 1 year of age, trauma becomes a leading cause of pediatric death.

Table 1-1. Epidemiology of Cardiopulmonary Arrest in Children

Age	Etiology
Less than 1 year	Respiratory disease
	Pneumonia
	Bronchiolitis
	Upper airway obstruction
	Central nervous system disease
	Seizures
	Meningitis
	Hydrocephalus
	Cardiac disease
	Congenital heart disease
	Cardiomyophathies
	Myocarditis
	Sepsis and shock
	Sudden infant death syndrome
	Congenital anomalies
	Metabolic disease
1 to 2 years	Injuries
	Drownings
	Falls
	Electrical shock
	Pedestrian/bike/motor vehicle crashes
	Congenital anomalies
	Malignancies
	Homicide
	Cardiac disease
	Asthma
Adolescence	Injuries
	Asthma
	Suicide, toxic ingestions
	Homicide
	Cardiac disease
	Hypertrophic cardiomyopathy

PROGNOSIS

Many recent studies have evaluated the outcome of pediatric cardiopulmonary arrest (Table 1-2). These reports are difficult to interpret since they vary with respect to the population reviewed, whether the arrest occurred in or out of the hospital, the presence of prehospital CPR, and the etiology of the arrest itself. Morbidity, mortality, and survival rates quoted are often not differentiated according to the type of arrest or the quality of survival. A comprehensive literature review by Young and Seidel demonstrated that patients with cardiac arrest had a hospital discharge rate of 13 percent after cardiac arrest. In those assessed for neurologic outcome, 62 percent had a good outcome. Patients with only respiratory arrest had a 75 percent hospital discharge rate with 88 percent of those assessed having a good neurologic outcome. Survival to discharge was 8.4 percent for patients with out-of-hospital cardiac arrest and 24 percent for patients who had an arrest while in the hospital.

The difference in survival rates is likely due to the prompt recognition and treatment of arrests for hospitalized patients as well as the lack of prompt advanced life support in the prehospital setting. In a study of 300 con-

Table 1-2. Recent Outcome Studies of Pediatric CPR

Author	Series Size	Population	Outcome
Hazinski et al, 1994	30	Out of hospital	23% Admitted 0% Discharged
Mogayzel et al, 1995	157	Out of hospital	25% Return of pulse 9.5% Discharged
Ronco et al, 1995	63	Out of hospital	29% Admitted 9.5% Discharged
Dieckmann et al, 1995	65	Out of hospital	5% Admitted 3% Discharged
Hickey et al, 1995	95		26% Discharged
Kusima et al, 1995	34	Out of hospital	14.7% Discharged
Schindler et al, 1995	101	Out of hospital	15% Discharged
Sirbaugh et al, 1999	300	Out of hospital	11% Return of pulse 2% Admitted 0% Discharged
Bhende et al, 1995	40	In/out of hospital	35% Admitted 5% Discharged
Schwenzer et al, 1993	42	Inpatient	49% Discharged
Pickert et al, 1994	92	Inpatient	10% Alive at 1 year

secutive out-of-hospital pediatric arrests by Sirbaugh and colleagues, only 6 survived to hospital discharge. Of the survivors, only one was considered free of neurological deficits.

Predictors of successful outcome after pediatric CPR have been evaluated. Isolated respiratory arrests have a much better resuscitation success rate, long-term survival, and neurologic outcome than cardiac arrests. Other outcome indicators include the initial pH, duration of the resuscitation, and the number of doses of epinephrine used during the resuscitation. Fiser reported a statistically significant difference in overall outcome between patients presenting with a blood pH <7.0 and those with an initial pH >7.0. The lower pH was thought to indicate a longer duration of hypoxia and ischemia. Several studies have demonstrated that response to epinephrine administration is related to outcome. Schindler and coworkers found no survivors among children who required >2 doses of epinephrine during resuscitation. This may indirectly reflect the severity of the hypoxia, ischemia, and acidosis which render the heart refractory to treatment. The study by Nicholls reported a long-term survival rate of 60 percent in resuscitations that lasted <15 minutes when compared to those that lasted longer. Gillis found no survivors in resuscitations lasting >15

minutes and Zaritsky found no survivors in children with cardiac arrest who had compressions for >10 minutes.

It is clear that children who suffer a cardiac arrest have a grim prognosis. Future efforts to improve outcome in pediatric CPR should be directed toward preventive care, early recognition of shock and respiratory failure, improved prehospital care, and increased public knowledge of basic life support skills.

BIBLIOGRAPHY

Dieckmann RA, Vardis R: High-dose epinephrine in pediatric out-of-hospital cardiopulmonary arrest. *Pediatrics* 95: 901–013, 1995.

Fiser DH, Wrape V: Outcome of cardiopulmonary resuscitation in children. *Pediatr Emerg Care* 3:235, 1987.

Gillis J, Dickson D, Rieder M, et al: Results of inpatient pediatric resuscitation. *Crit Care Med* 14:469, 1986.

Hazinski MF, Chahine AA, Holcomb GW, et al: Outcome of cardiovascular collapse in pediatric blunt trauma. *Ann Emerg Med* 23:1229–1235, 1994.

Hickey RW, Cohen DM, Strausbaugh S, et al: Pediatric patients requiring CPR in the pre-hospital setting. *Ann Emerg Med* 25:495–501, 1995.

Kuisma M, Suominen P, Korpela R: Pediatric out-of-hospital cardiac arrests: epidemiology and outcome. *Resuscitation* 30:141–150, 1995.

Mogayzel C, Quan L, Graves JR, et al: Out-of-hospital ventricular fibrillation in children and adolescents: causes and outcomes. *Ann Emerg Med* 25:484–491, 1995.

Nicolls DG, Kettrick RG, Swedlow DB, et al: Factors influencing outcome of cardiopulmonary resuscitation in children. *Pediatr Emerg Care* 2:1, 1986.

Pickert CB, Torres A, Firestone J, et al: Outcome of in-hospital pediatric cardiopulmonary arrest (abstract). *Crit Care Med* 22:A161, 1994.

Ronco R, King W, Donley DK, et al: Outcome and cost at a children's hospital following resuscitation for out-of-hospital cardiopulmonary arrest. *Arch Pediatr Adolesc Med* 149:210–214, 1995.

Schindler MB, Bohn D, Cox PN, et al: Outcome of out-of-hospital cardiac or respiratory arrest in children. *N Engl J Med* 335:1473–1479, 1995.

Schwenzer KJ, Smith WT, Durbin CG, et al: Selective application of cardiopulmonary resuscitation improves survival rates. *Anesth Analg* 76:478–484, 1993.

Sirbaugh PE, Pepe PE, Shook JE, et al: Outcome of out-of-hospital pediatric cardiopulmonary arrest. *Ann Emerg Med* 33:174–184, 1999.

Young KD, Seidel JS: Pediatric cardiopulmonary resuscitation a collective review. *Ann Emerg Med* 33:195–205, 1999.

Zaritsky A, Outcome of pediatric cardiopulmonary resuscitation. *Crit Care Med* 21:325–327, 1993.

2

Respiratory Failure

Thomas J. Abramo
Michael Cowan

HIGH-YIELD FACTS

- Respiratory failure is the most common cause of cardiopulmonary arrest in children. In most cases respiratory distress precedes respiratory failure, but the time from respiratory distress to failure may be very short.
- Gastric distension may compromise diaphragmatic movement and impede effective ventilation.
- Past medical history may have an important role in determining the etiology of respiratory distress. Examples are prematurity, bronchopulmonary dysplasia, bronchiolitis, asthma, and heart disease.
- Accessory muscles of respiration have an order in their recruitment that dictates the degree of distress, as follows: subcostal muscles < intercostals < substernal < supraclavicular < nasal flaring < head bobbing.
- Pulse oximetry can be used as a noninvasive measure for respiratory compromise but in moderate-severe distress does not replace the arterial blood gas.
- Diagnosis of respiratory failure is based on clinical judgment and is related to the work of breathing, fatigue of the patient, and level of consciousness.
- Indications for assisted ventilation/intubation are as follows:
  - Apnea
  - Inadequate respiratory effort
  - Pending failure
  - To reduce the work of breathing (SIRS, sepsis)
  - Airway protection (ingestion, altered mental status)
  - For controlled ventilation (increased intracranial pressure).
- The formula for the correct endotracheal tube size is as follows:
  - Uncuffed tube size = (16 + age [years])/4 = internal diameter of endotracheal tube
  - Patient's fifth digit
  - Cuffed tube size = (12 + age [years])/4 = internal diameter of endotracheal tube
  - Depth of placement can be calculated by taking the internal diameter and multiplying by 3.
- End-tidal CO_2 measurement can detect proper placement of the endotracheal tube, endotracheal tube dislodgement, and ventilatory changes/compromise.
- A laryngeal mask airway can be safely utilized by a properly trained individual for the management of the difficult pediatric airway.

Respiratory failure is the most common cause of cardiac arrest in the pediatric population. It occurs when the exchange of oxygen and carbon dioxide across the alveolar-capillary network becomes inadequate to sustain life. Respiratory failure can result from primary disease of the upper or lower airway, or it may be the end result of disease involving other organ systems. In most cases, respiratory failure is preceded by a period of respiratory distress, characterized clinically by the expenditure of an inordinate amount of energy in breathing, and by laboratory parameters that indicate impaired exchange of oxygen and carbon dioxide. The emergency physician must recognize and treat respiratory distress before respiratory failure occurs.

ANATOMY AND PHYSIOLOGY

Certain anatomic and physiologic characteristics render the infant and young child particularly vulnerable to severe respiratory disease and can make it difficult to assess the degree of compromise in a patient with respiratory distress. Young infants may be obligate nose breathers, and any degree of obstruction of the nasal passages can produce respiratory difficulty. The upper airway of infants and young children is relatively narrow and therefore susceptible to obstruction from congenital anomalies, foreign bodies, and infections, such as croup and bacterial tracheitis.

The chest wall is highly elastic and collapsible, and the chest musculature is poorly developed. The major muscle of respiration is the diaphragm, which must generate significant negative intrathoracic pressure to expand the underdeveloped lungs. The limitation of diaphragmatic movement by gastric distention, increased residual capacity from air trapping from asthma, bronchiolitis, or foreign body obstruction can result in reduction of tidal volume, which may produce respiratory failure. The relatively smaller lower airways are especially vulnerable to mucus plugging and ventilation-perfusion mismatch associated with common diseases of the lower airways, such as asthma and bronchiolitis.

The actual area available for gas exchange in infants and young children is relatively limited. Alveolar space doubles by 18 months of age and triples by 3 years of age. The limited ability to recruit additional alveoli makes the infant dependent on increasing the respiratory rate to augment minute ventilation and eliminate carbon dioxide. Tachypnea, therefore, is a universal finding in infants and young children in respiratory distress. The combination of increased muscle exertion and the need to sustain a rapid respiratory rate can result in progressive muscle fatigue and respiratory failure. This is especially true in young infants, who have a limited metabolic reserve.

HISTORY

Most commonly, a patient in respiratory distress will present to the emergency department with a history of difficulty breathing. Parents may note coughing, rapid noisy breathing, or a change in behavior. Feeding problems are often a sign of respiratory compromise in infants. In older children, wheezing or decreased physical activity may be presenting complaints.

The past medical history is essential in determining the etiology of the acute problem. Infants with a history of significant prematurity may have bronchopulmonary dysplasia, a syndrome characterized by varying degrees of hypoxia, hypercarbia, reactive airway disease, and a heightened susceptibility to respiratory infections. Infants with a history of sweating during bottle-feedings may have undiagnosed congestive heart failure. For patients with a history of asthma, information regarding the frequency and severity of past exacerbations is important in determining both the acute treatment and disposition. A patient with a history of a chronic cough or a history of recurrent pneumonia may have an underlying disorder, such as reactive airway disease, cystic fibrosis, or a retained foreign body.

Respiratory symptoms can also be due to systemic disorders. Effortless tachypnea and hyperpnea accompany disorders such as diabetic ketoacidosis and sepsis, as an attempt to compensate for metabolic acidosis.

PHYSICAL EXAMINATION

Simply observing the patient yields a wealth of information regarding the degree of respiratory distress. Mental status is the first and foremost factor to evaluate. Infants and young children with mild respiratory difficulty will have normal mental status. Patients with more severe disease become irritable or anxious and can appear restless and unable to assume a comfortable position. Older patients in extreme distress are usually unable to lie supine and may exhibit head-bobbing. Young infants in severe distress will appear anxious, will often not make eye contact, and usually will not smile. If feeding is attempted, they will refuse the bottle, since the work of breathing precludes the exertion of sucking. Incipient respiratory failure is heralded by extreme agitation, and finally by lethargy or somnolence. Cyanosis is an ominous finding.

Observing the patient's chest will add to the assessment of the degree of respiratory distress. Patients with significant respiratory difficulty will virtually always be tachypneic. However, because respiratory rate is age dependent and can be influenced by underlying medical conditions, it must be viewed in the context of the overall clinical picture. Visual inspection of the chest wall may reveal retractions, which signify the use of accessory muscles of respiration. Retractions are seen in the supraclavicular and subcostal areas. In more severe cases, nasal flaring is seen. Retractions imply a significant degree of respiratory distress and must never be overlooked.

Listening to grossly audible breath sounds will help to localize the pathology. Stridor is generally heard on inspiration, but with severe obstruction, it can be present on both inspiration and expiration. Stridor suggests upper airway pathology, such as croup, epiglottitis, or foreign body obstruction. Grossly audible wheezing usually indicates obstruction of the lower airways. Lower airway disease resulting in alveolar collapse can also be associated with grunting, which is caused by premature closure of the glottis during expiration. Grunting increases airway pressure and can help prevent further alveolar collapse and thus preserve functional residual capacity. Grunting is most often seen in infants and always indicates severe respiratory distress, whether from primary lung disease or a systemic illness, such as sepsis.

Auscultation of the chest supplements the information gained from observation of the patient. The first factor to assess is air exchange. Upper airway obstruction predominantly affects the inhalation of air, whereas lower airway obstruction predominantly affects exhalation. Patients who appear to be struggling to breathe and have limited air exchange appreciated on auscultation are in imminent danger of respiratory failure. For patients with adequate air exchange, breath sounds are evaluated for specific findings such as wheezing, rales, rhonchi, or localized areas of diminution. For patients with isolated tachypnea and no positive auscultatory findings suggestive of airway disease, a metabolic process, such as sepsis or metabolic acidosis, is possible.

LABORATORY STUDIES

Laboratory studies are useful in assessing the degree of respiratory compromise. The advent of a reliable measurement of oxygen saturation via percutaneous pulse oximetry has made it possible to evaluate a patient's blood oxygen-carrying status quickly and painlessly. Pulse oximetry is especially useful in infants, in whom the physical examination may be difficult and an arterial blood gas difficult to obtain. However, pulse oximetry provides only limited information regarding overall pulmonary physiology. The slope of the oxygen-hemoglobin dissociation curve is such that patients with marginal oxygen saturations may have significant hypoxemia. The pulse oximeter does not measure the arterial carbon dioxide tension or acid-base status, and therefore careful clinical correlation is necessary in many situations, such as asthma and bronchiolitis, in which CO_2 retention and respiratory acidosis are possible. Pulse oximetry is also unreliable for patients with low perfusion states, carbon monoxide toxicity, and methemoglobinemia.

For patients with moderate to severe respiratory distress, pulse oximetry cannot replace the information obtained by an arterial blood gas. Strictly defined, respiratory failure is arterial oxygen tension (Pa_{O_2}) < 60 mmHg despite supplemental inhaled oxygen of 60 percent or arterial carbon dioxide tension (Pa_{CO_2}) > 60 mmHg.

However, absolute values of arterial oxygen and carbon dioxide tension must be viewed in the context of the clinical situation, as well as the patient's baseline pulmonary status. A patient may not meet strict criteria for respiratory failure but may develop muscle fatigue such that the work of breathing cannot be sustained despite blood gas values that appear adequate. Conversely, a patient with severe underlying lung disease, such as bronchopulmonary dysplasia or cystic fibrosis, may be well adjusted to chronic hypercarbia; in this case the clinical assessment of the work of breathing supplants the laboratory data. In most children with severe lung disease, parents are aware of baseline information that can aid the physician in interpreting percutaneous oxygen saturation and the arterial blood gas values.

INDICATIONS FOR ASSISTED VENTILATION

In the event that respiratory failure occurs, assisted ventilation is indicated. The most common indication for assisted ventilation in a pediatric patient in respiratory distress is progressive muscle fatigue. In this situation, laboratory parameters will often reveal hypoxemia refractory to supplemental oxygen and a rising Pa_{CO_2}.

Other indications for assisted ventilation are apnea, inadequate respiratory effort, and conditions in which it is desirable to reduce the work of breathing, such as refractory shock or increased intracranial pressure that requires controlled ventilation. For patients with altered mental status, when the ability to maintain an adequate airway is in question, assisted ventilation is also indicated, although pulmonary function may be normal.

ESTABLISHING AN AIRWAY

The first step in providing assisted ventilation is to gain control of the airway. Because of anatomic differences, the pediatric airway can be more difficult to manage than that of the adult. The large, prominent occiput of the young infant can force the head into flexion when the patient is on a flat surface, and the airway can become occluded. The oral cavity of the infant and young child is small, and the tongue is relatively large. Therefore visualization of the epiglottis is difficult. The epiglottis itself is relatively larger and is less rigid than in adults. The vocal cords lie more anteriorly, and the anterior attachment is relatively more caudal. The relationship between the ligamentous and cartilaginous portion of the cords is inconsistent during development. This can cause the shape and direction of the cords to change and make the pediatric vocal cords difficult to recognize. Up to the age of about 8 years, the subglottic ring or the cricoid cartilage is the narrowest part of the airway. Therefore, an endotracheal tube that traverses the cords may be unable to pass the narrower cricoid cartilage.

Ventilatory assistance begins with establishing a patent airway. Remove secretions or vomitus with suctioning. If a cervical spine injury is possible, stabilize the head and neck. Open the airway with a jaw thrust maneuver, by placing two or three fingers under the angle of the mandible and lifting the jaw upward and outward. If a cervical injury is not a consideration, place the child in the sniffing position, with the head slightly extended and the neck slightly flexed, to remove the tongue from the posterior oropharynx. Do not overextend the head, as this may cause airway obstruction.

An oropharyngeal airway can bypass obstruction from a posteriorly displaced tongue, which is especially common in obtunded or unconscious patients. The appropriate oral airway spans the distance from the central incisors to the angle of the mandible. Oral airways are inappropriate for conscious patients, in whom they can produce vomiting. In awake or somnolent patients, a nasopharyngeal airway is useful for bypassing the tongue. The diameter of the nasopharyngeal airway should approximate that of the patient's nostril.

VENTILATION

Initial ventilation is usually provided by the bag-valve-mask (BVM) technique. Skillful bagging will usually provide adequate oxygenation and ventilation until an artificial airway can be inserted. Bagging with supplemental oxygen always precedes attempts at intubation.

A transparent mask should fit snugly from the bridge of the nose to the prominence of the symphysis of the mandible. Circular masks with seals are more effective in infants and small children than triangular masks that attempt to duplicate the shape of the face. The mask is held in place with the thumb and forefinger of the hand, while the remaining fingers lift the jaw to maintain a patent airway and establish a seal. Care is taken not to put excessive pressure on the eyes.

Two types of bags are commonly available, the anesthesia bag and the self-inflating bag. The anesthesia bag is collapsible and refills by the constant inflow of oxygen. If the seal of the mask on the face is not tight, the bag will not refill adequately. When used correctly, anesthesia bags deliver a very high concentration of oxygen, avoid excessive airway pressure, and ensure a tight seal. However, the anesthesia bag requires expertise to use.

The self-inflating bag requires less training to use and in most instances is capable of providing adequate ventilation when used by both hospital and prehospital personnel. To deliver an inspired oxygen content of 60 to 90 percent, it must come equipped with a reservoir and be used with an oxygen flow rate of 10 to 15 L/min. Self-inflating bags usually have a pop-off valve to regulate maximum inspiratory pressure. In resuscitations, the valve may need to be bypassed since some patients require high inspiratory pressures to provide adequate oxygenation and ventilation. For patients with normal lung compliance, the valve can prevent complications of barotrauma, such as pneumothorax. Self-inflating bags come in three sizes: 250 mL for neonates, 450 mL for infants and young children, and 1000 mL for adults. Infants are ventilated at a rate of 20 to 30 breaths/min and older children at 16 to 20 breaths/min. If the technique is adequate, the chest expands with each assisted breath and breath sounds are heard bilaterally.

During assisted ventilation air is forced into the stomach, and gastric distention becomes a problem. Gastric inflation can be reduced by prolonging inspiratory time and using lower ventilatory rates to ensure an adequate exhalation phase. Prolonged BVM ventilation can produce gastric distention. When severe, gastric distention can impede ventilation by compromising tidal volume and inducing regurgitation and aspiration of gastric contents. Nasogastric suction alleviates gastric distention, evacuates the gastric contents, and is usually necessary in children receiving assisted ventilation. Gentle cricoid pressure, the Sellick maneuver, can reduce gastric distention and prevent aspiration until a nasogastric tube is placed.

ADVANCED AIRWAY MANAGEMENT

In most situations that require BVM ventilation, insertion of an endotracheal tube is necessary to establish an adequate airway and allow optimal management. Successful intubation of the trachea depends on adequate preparation of personnel, medications, and equipment.

Preoxygenation displaces nitrogen from the lungs and provides a physiologic reservoir of oxygen that protects the patient from anoxic injury during the process of intubation. In spontaneously breathing patients, 3 to 5 minutes of 100 percent O_2 delivered by a non-rebreather mask provides the patient with 3 to 4 minutes of adequate oxygenation even in the face of apnea. For patients receiving assisted ventilation, minimizing the time of bagging is important in reducing the possibility of gastric distention and aspiration during intubation. In this situation, several breaths with 100 percent O_2 provides an adequate reservoir of oxygen. The Sellick maneuver may be used to prevent gastric distention and emesis.

After preoxygenation, place the head in the sniffing position to align the oral, pharyngeal, and laryngeal vectors. A towel placed under the shoulders may assist in alignment. The mouth is opened, and any debris removed from the airway by suctioning. The laryngoscope blade is inserted into the right corner of the mouth, and the tongue is swept to the left. For infants and young children, a straight blade is preferred (Table 2-1). The epiglottis is elevated, and the endotracheal tube is inserted between the vocal cords. During laryngoscopy, the Sellick maneuver is performed to reduce the risk of aspiration. This maneuver can also aid in visualizing the anteriorly displaced vocal cords of infants and small children. During intubation, heart rate and oxygen saturation are continuously monitored.

With a well-positioned endotracheal tube of the proper size (Table 2-1), an audible air leak is heard when ventilation is applied at a pressure of 15 to 20 cmH$_2$O. If no air leak is audible, the tube is too tight. Conversely, if the air leak is too large, it will impair ventilation since insufficient tidal volume is generated. Cuffed endotracheal tube sizes are available for the young infant or child under certain conditions requiring high inspiratory pressure such as respiratory failure from status asthmaticus or acute respiratory distress syndrome. The proper monitoring of the cuff pressure has been shown to have the same complication rates as uncuffed endotracheal tubes in studies.

Correct endotracheal tube placement is confirmed clinically by observing adequate chest wall expansion and auscultating bilateral breath sounds. Asymmetric breath sounds imply that the tube is too far down the trachea and has lodged in either the right or left mainstem bronchus. The anatomic vectors are such that the right mainstem bronchus is more likely to be intubated, and breath sounds are heard louder on the right side. In young infants, however, the airway vectors are such that intubation of the left mainstem bronchus may occur. This situation is corrected by slowly withdrawing the tube until equal breath sounds are heard. If unilateral breath sounds persist despite withdrawal of the tube, a pneumothorax is possible.

Congenital conditions can create potentially difficult intubations. The Pierre Robin syndrome is characterized by a relatively large tongue, mandibular hypoplasia, and a cleft or high arched palate. Down's syndrome is also associated with a large tongue and mandibular hypoplasia, as well as a short neck and instability of the cervi-

Table 2-1. Endotracheal Tube Size and Length and Size of Laryngoscope Blades by Age[a,b]

Age	Size (mm)	Type
Endotracheal Tubes		
Newborn	3.0	Uncuffed
Newborn–6 months	3.5	Uncuffed
6–18 mo	3.5–4.0	Uncuffed
18 mo–3 yr	4.0–4.5	Uncuffed
3–5 yr	4.5	Uncuffed
5–6 yr	5.0	Uncuffed
6–8 yr	5.5–6.0	Uncuffed
8–10 yr	6.0	Cuffed
10–12 yr	6.0–6.5	Cuffed
12–14 yr	6.5–7.0	Cuffed
Laryngoscope Blades		
<2.5 kg	0	Straight
0–3 mo	1.0	Straight
3 mo–3 yr	1.5	Straight
3 yr–12 yr	2.0	Straight or curved
Adolescent	3.0	Straight or curved

[a]Uncuffed tracheal tube size (mm) = (16 + age [years])/4 = internal diameter of endotracheal tube or patient's fifth digit.
[b]Cuffed tube size (mm) = (12 + age [years])/4 = internal diameter of cuffed endotracheal tube. Depth can be calculated by taking the internal diameter and multiplying by 3.

cal spine. Turner's syndrome is associated with cervical spine instability and mandibular or maxillary hypoplasia. Arthrogryposis multiplex congenita is associated with a high arched palate, mandibular or maxillary hypoplasia, and restricted mandibular movement.

Infections that obstruct the upper airway often cause difficult intubations. Severe croup, epiglottitis, and bacterial tracheitis can distort normal anatomic landmarks and make visualization of the vocal cords difficult. In such cases, chest compressions during laryngoscopy can force air out of the trachea through the larynx, where bubbles can be seen. The endotracheal tube is inserted through the bubbles. Bacterial tracheitis can cause a fragile tracheal membrane that obstructs the endotracheal tube. If this occurs, a surgical airway is necessary. When extreme difficulty is anticipated, it is prudent to perform the intubation in the operating room, where a surgical airway can be created if endotracheal intubation is unsuccessful.

The laryngeal mask airway (LMA) is a tube with a deflatable mask-like projection at the distal end. The LMA is an alternative to the endotracheal tube for a patient with a difficult airway. The LMA is passed through the pharynx and advanced until resistance is felt when the mask is over the epiglottis/tracheal opening. The inflation of the cuff occludes the hypopharynx but leaves the distal end open over the glottic opening, providing a clear secure airway. The LMA has been demonstrated in numerous studies as a successful airway management tool in the hospital and in out-of-hospital settings. Numerous studies have shown that the LMA is effective in pediatrics, but proper training and supervision is required to master correct LMA placement. LMA is contraindicated in the infant or child with a gag response or with the potential for excessive patient movement. There is a risk of aspiration that must be considered when using LMA.

Capnometry is the measurement and numerical display of the carbon dioxide level appearing at the airway, and capnography is the measurement and graphic display of the carbon dioxide level appearing at the airway. End-tidal CO_2 is the partial pressure of CO_2 at the end of an exhaled breath. This can be measured by colorimetry and is useful in confirming a tracheal as opposed to esophageal intubation. In an esophageal intubation, the colorimeter fails to detect the presence of carbon dioxide, which is normally present in expired air.

A chest radiograph will confirm optimal tube placement, which is signified by the tip being midway between the carina and vocal cords.

MECHANICAL VENTILATION

It is occasionally necessary to provide mechanical ventilation for intubated patients in the emergency department while awaiting transport or intensive care unit admission. Although a thorough discussion of ventilators is beyond the scope of this chapter, a few facts regarding the use of these machines are important.

The two major types of mechanical ventilators are pressure and volume ventilators. Both assist the patient by delivering compressed gases with positive pressure; however, they differ in the method that terminates the inspiratory phase of the breathing cycle.

A volume ventilator delivers a preset volume of gas during each mechanical inspiration. This type of ventilator compensates for all changes in resistance and is therefore useful for patients with decreased lung compliance. The danger of volume ventilators is that they generate high airway pressures that can result in barotrauma. Currently they are used for children and older infants. The usual tidal volume in an infant or child is 12 to 15 mL/kg. The rate depends on the patient's age and the clinical condition.

Pressure ventilators terminate inspiration when a preset pressure is reached and therefore avoid excessive inflating pressures. With pressure ventilators, it is possible to control the inspiratory time, and exhalation is allowed when the preset pressure is reached. They do not compensate for changes in lung compliance, and they deliver a variable amount of gas with each breath. Currently pressure ventilators are used mainly in neonates and young infants. The inspiratory pressure used is the lowest pressure that attains adequate chest expansion and ventilation. This is best determined by observing a manometer while the patient is being bagged.

Both volume and pressure ventilators have the ability to provide positive end-expiratory pressure (PEEP), which is added to prevent alveolar collapse during exhalation and to preserve functional residual capacity. This can alleviate ventilation-perfusion mismatch and consequent hypoxemia and is especially important in situations in which there is decreased lung compliance. The major side effect of excessive PEEP is decreased venous return to the right side of the heart and decreased cardiac output. In the emergency department setting, PEEP is usually set at 3 to 5 cmH$_2$O.

Despite the widespread availability of pulse oximetry and end-tidal CO_2 monitoring, most patients on ventilators will require serial arterial blood gases until the optimal parameters for ventilating the patient are determined.

BIBLIOGRAPHY

Berry AM, Brimacombe JR, Verghese C: The laryngeal mask airway in emergency medicine, neonatal resuscitation and intensive care medicine. *Int Anesthesiol Clin* 36:91–109, 1998.

Cardoso MM, Banner MJ, Melker RJ, et al: Portable devices used to detect endotracheal intubation during emergency situations: A review. *Crit Care Med* 26:957–964, 1998.

Gausche M, Lewis RJ, Stratton SJ, et al: A prospective randomized study of the effect of out of hospital pediatric endotracheal intubation on survival and neurological outcome. *JAMA* 283:783–790, 2000.

Richman PB, Nashed AH: The epidemiology of cardiac arrest in children and young adults: Special considerations for ED management. *Am J Emerg Med* 17:264–270, 1999.

Saugstad OD: Practical aspects of resuscitating asphyxiated neonates and infants. *Eur J Pediatr* 157(suppl):S11–S15, 1998.

Ward KR, Yearly DM: End-tidal carbon dioxide monitoring in emergency medicine, clinical applications. *Acad Emerg Med* 5:637–646, 1998.

3

Shock

Susan M. Scott
Robert A. Wiebe

HIGH-YIELD FACTS

- Shock in children is the endpoint of many disease processes including sepsis, trauma, gastroenteritis, anaphylaxis, and cardiac dysfunction.
- Early recognition, aggressive intervention, and continual reassessment are the keys to successful treatment of shock in children.
- Tachycardia is the earliest and most sensitive sign of shock in children. Tachycardia can also be caused by anxiety, pain, and fever.
- Hypotension may be a late sign of decompensated shock and should be considered an ominous sign.
- Resuscitation of the child in shock should always begin with establishment and maintenance of adequate oxygenation and ventilation. Endotracheal intubation and assisted ventilation may be necessary.
- Isotonic fluids (normal saline, lactated Ringer's, albumin) in 20 mL/kg boluses should be used in the acute resuscitation of the child in shock. Solutions containing glucose should be used only in response to hypoglycemia.
- Reassessment (heart rate, capillary refill, peripheral pulses, mental status) should follow every bolus. Continual reassessment and monitoring is essential throughout the treatment of the child in shock.

Shock is a physiologic condition in which there is insufficient delivery of vital nutrients to the tissues and inadequate removal of the waste products of cellular metabolism. Aberrations in oxygen delivery and utilization result in tissue hypoxia and anaerobic metabolism, which alters acid-base status and can ultimately cause cell dysfunction and death. The clinical manifestations of shock result from both the metabolic consequences of cell dysfunction and the compensatory mechanisms activated to preserve metabolic integrity.

Shock may be compensated, decompensated, or irreversible. In compensated shock, tissue perfusion is maintained and cardiac output is adequate, although blood flow may be maldistributed. In decompensated shock, compensatory mechanisms are unable to maintain organ perfusion, and alterations occur in metabolism that can result in severe metabolic derangement. In irreversible shock, cell damage is so extreme that cell death occurs, precipitating a devastating physiologic cascade that is refractory even to the most aggressive treatment.

Clinically, shock is categorized as hypovolemic, septic, distributive, and cardiogenic. While these categories have specific etiologies and varies in presentation, there is considerable overlap clinically and biochemically, especially in the more advanced stages. Recognition and aggressive management of shock in its early stages may avoid the cascade from tissue hypoxia and hypoperfusion to multiple organ failure and death.

PATHOPHYSIOLOGY

Shock affects all organ systems. Cardiac output, blood pressure, and tissue perfusion are affected due to alterations in the cardiovascular system, including myocardial dysfunction and loss of vascular tone. The work of breathing is increased, leading to muscle fatigue and respiratory distress. Decreased renal perfusion results in oliguria, and in severe cases renal failure may occur. Shunting of blood away from the splanchnic circulation to the brain and heart leaves the intestine vulnerable to ischemic injury. Clumping of neutrophils and platelets and fibrin deposition impair microcirculatory flow. Activation of the coagulation cascade can produce disseminated intravascular coagulation. Hypoxia, hypercarbia, and hypoperfusion of the brain can lead to alteration in mental status.

Many of the systemic manifestations of shock result from chemical mediators that are released in response to hypoxia and tissue ischemia. These mediators affect myocardial function, pulmonary and systemic vasomotor tone, vascular integrity, and platelet function. In a certain sense, shock behaves as an acute systemic inflammatory disease.

Many specific inflammatory cell mediators have been described. Eicosanoids are substances derived from the metabolism of arachidonic acid and are released from macrophages and the endothelium. They include leukotrienes, thromboxanes, prostaglandins, and platelet activating factor (PAF). Leukotrienes increase capillary permeability, inhibit platelet activation, contribute to myocardial depression, and are potent systemic and pulmonary vasoconstrictors and vasodilators. Thromboxanes enhance platelet aggregation and are systemic and pulmonary vasoconstrictors. Prostaglandins cause both vasoconstriction and vasodilation and stimulate smooth muscle in the bronchial tree and intestinal tract. PAF is released from the endothelium, leukocytes, monocytes, and platelets, and increases systemic and pulmonary vascular permeability, causes systemic and pulmonary vasoconstriction and vasodilation, and enhances platelet aggregation and leukocyte activation. Myocardial depressant substances are also produced. Cytokines produced by macrophages and other cells are the principal mediators of septic shock. Activation of the complement system leads to release of C3A and C5A, which cause neutrophil activation, increased vascular permeability, and hypotension. Endothelial-derived substances are capable of producing both vasoconstriction and vasodilation.

HYPOVOLEMIC SHOCK

Hypovolemic shock results from a decrease in circulating intravascular volume. Common causes in pediatric patients include fluid and electrolyte losses from gastroenteritis, acute hemorrhage following trauma, and fluid loss secondary to severe burns.

The decreased intravascular volume associated with hypovolemic shock results in decreased cardiac preload, decreased stroke volume, and, ultimately, decreased cardiac output and impaired peripheral perfusion. Secretion of endogenous catecholamines increases heart rate, myocardial contractility, and systemic vascular resistance. Neuroendocrine factors increase the kidney's retention of water and sodium. If there is delayed or inadequate volume replacement or blood loss continues, compensatory mechanisms fail and decompensated shock occurs with circulatory failure and multiorgan dysfunction.

SEPTIC SHOCK

Sepsis is an inflammatory response to invading microorganisms and the toxins they produce, resulting in clinical, metabolic, and hemodynamic dysfunction. The

American College of Chest Physicians and The Society of Critical Care Medicine standardized the definition of the *systemic inflammatory response syndrome* (SIRS) seen in response to infection. This response is manifested by derangement in temperature, heart rate, respiratory rate, and white blood cell count, and if the inflammatory response continues, hypotension and organ dysfunction. It was also recognized that this inflammatory response can occur in response to other clinical insults, including trauma.

There are two clinical stages of septic shock. The early, or hyperdynamic phase, is characterized by a normal or high cardiac output. Blood pressure may be normal or there may be a widened pulse pressure. Systemic vascular resistance is decreased, the pulses are bounding, and the extremities are pink and warm. The patient usually has a normal mental status, but is tachypneic. The late or decompensated phase is similar to other types of shock, with signs of cardiac dysfunction and poor peripheral perfusion. Mental status is usually impaired, and the extremities are cool with diminished or absent pulses. Hypotension may be present and is considered an ominous sign. At this stage, septic shock is indistinguishable from other types of shock.

DISTRIBUTIVE SHOCK

Distributive shock is characterized by the maldistribution of normal intravascular volume. This maldistribution can result in tissue hypoxia, with cell damage and dysfunction. Causes of distributive shock include anaphylaxis, neurogenic or spinal shock, and certain drug toxicities.

Anaphylactic shock is characterized by hypotension secondary to profound vasodilation and increased vascular permeability. It may be accompanied by acute angioedema of the upper airway, bronchoconstriction, pulmonary edema, or urticaria. Anaphylaxis is initiated by the interaction of an antigen with cell bound IgE. This interaction activates the complement system and various cells, including basophils, mast cells, and eosinophils that release mediators such as histamine, leukotrienes, PAF, and prostaglandins. All of these substances produce arterial and venous vasodilation. Increased capillary permeability results in the loss of intravascular fluid into the interstitium. This loss of intravascular fluid impairs cardiac preload and exacerbates hypotension.

Neurogenic shock is characterized by hypotension secondary to a total loss of sympathetic cardiovascular tone. The loss of vasomotor tone results in pooling of blood in the vascular bed. Etiologies of neurogenic shock include total transection of the spinal cord, brain stem injuries, and, rarely, isolated intracranial injuries.

CARDIOGENIC SHOCK

Cardiogenic shock results when the heart fails to deliver sufficient nutrients to the rest of the body as a result of primary cardiac dysfunction. In adults the most common cause of cardiogenic shock is acute myocardial infarction, but this is rare in the pediatric age group. In infants and children, cardiogenic shock more commonly results from dysrhythmias, such as supraventricular tachycardia, or congenital heart lesions that obstruct the left ventricular outflow tract. Impaired cardiac function may also occur after cardiac surgery, with ingestion of certain drugs, and in the late stages of septic shock.

Whatever the cause, inadequate output provokes compensatory mechanisms similar to those seen in other forms of shock. Some responses, such as an increase in endogenous catecholamines that increases systemic vascular resistance, can increase cardiac work and oxygen consumption and may contribute to cardiac dysfunction.

RECOGNITION

Recognition of shock in its early stages is of paramount importance so that interventions aimed at arresting the disease process and averting the cascade of irreversible shock can be implemented. In infants and young children, the early phases of shock are notoriously difficult to detect, in part because compensatory mechanisms are able to preserve blood flow to vital organs until late in the disease process.

History

The history of the present illness can provide information that may increase the index of suspicion for shock. Profuse vomiting or diarrhea, polyuria, or trauma-related blood loss suggest intravascular volume depletion and potentially hypovolemic shock. Septic shock is usually associated with a febrile illness and is especially common in young infants and immunosuppressed patients. Cardiogenic shock is often preceded by symptoms of congestive heart failure, but can present in a fulminant form in young infants with undiagnosed congenital heart

disease, especially hypoplastic left heart and coarctation of the aorta. Anaphylactic shock may be accompanied by a history of exposure to a known antigen, but should be suspected in a hypotensive patient with any manifestation of an acute allergic reaction. Neurogenic shock is possible in any patient with an acute spinal cord injury, but it should be diagnosed with great caution in the presence of head trauma and altered mental status, where hemorrhage is the most likely cause of shock.

Physical Examination

A careful physical examination is the key to the early diagnosis of shock. In the late stages of the disease, when the patient is obtunded with marked decreases in peripheral perfusion and diminished or absent pulses, the situation is obvious and the challenge is to determine the etiology. In the early phases, the problem is much less evident. Vital signs in infants and children are often harder to interpret than those of adults. A crying or frightened infant or child is often tachypneic and tachycardic. Fever is much too common to be helpful in most cases. Blood pressure is often maintained by profound peripheral vasoconstriction until late in the course of the illness, when it falls precipitously. A high index of suspicion and repeated examinations are needed to reveal the subtle signs of early shock.

The first factor to assess is the patient's vital signs. Tachycardia is the most sensitive sign of circulatory compromise in children. Persistent tachycardia in a calm, afebrile child indicates a metabolic abnormality. Young infants and children rely on tachycardia as the primary compensatory mechanism to maintain cardiac output, and a markedly increased heart rate accompanies most cases of shock. Tachypnea is also present in most cases of shock as the patient attempts to compensate for the metabolic acidosis caused by anaerobic metabolism. Blood pressure may be normal due to increased systemic vascular resistance, until this compensatory mechanism fails and hypotension occurs. Hypotension is a late sign of decompensated shock and is an ominous sign. Peripheral pulses may be diminished in comparison to central pulses. Capillary refill may be prolonged to greater than 2 seconds and the extremities may feel cool or appear mottled. In the early phase of septic shock the opposite may be true, with bounding pulses and warm extremities. Irritability or lethargy can imply central nervous system dysfunction secondary to hypoperfusion; therefore, shock must always be considered a possibility in the patient with an altered level of consciousness. The diagnosis of shock can be extremely difficult and all data available need to be carefully and repeatedly considered in order to reach the correct diagnosis.

Laboratory Data

Laboratory data can be helpful in diagnosing shock, but do not replace the clinical evaluation. In cases of hemorrhagic shock, decreased hemoglobin and hematocrit can confirm the presence of blood loss, but shortly after the hemorrhage these parameters are usually normal or only slightly decreased, and are not reliable indicators of the degree of hemorrhage. An elevated white blood cell count can support the presence of a bacterial infection in a patient with suspected septic shock, but is neither sensitive nor specific enough to verify the diagnosis. Neutropenia in a child suspected to be in septic shock suggests an overwhelming bacterial infection. Thrombocytopenia suggests the possibility of disseminated intravascular coagulation.

Elevation of the blood urea nitrogen and serum creatinine imply prerenal azotemia, secondary to hypoperfusion of the kidney. Evaluation of serum electrolytes may reveal an anion gap acidosis, which can result from a byproduct of anaerobic metabolism, lactate. If a metabolic acidosis is present, a toxicology screen is needed to exclude drug-related causes. Blood sugar should be measured to rule out hypoglycemia, which is common in shock, and to exclude the possibility of diabetic ketoacidosis. Hypocalcemia is common in shock and can negatively affect many physiologic functions.

Arterial blood gas is a sensitive measure of the overall metabolic state of the patient. While respiratory alkalosis is common in the early stages of shock, the presence of metabolic acidosis implies significantly impaired perfusion and a fairly advanced state of disease. The adequacy of ventilatory function and oxygenation, which can be especially important for patients with underlying cardiopulmonary disease, can also be ascertained.

TREATMENT

The primary goal for the management of the patient in shock is the restoration of perfusion and oxygenation, especially to the brain, heart, and kidneys. Regardless of the etiology of the shock, tissue oxygenation and perfusion can be reestablished by addressing four therapeutic variables:

- Ventilation and oxygenation
- Cardiac output and adequacy of circulating blood volume

- Oxygen-carrying capacity (hemoglobin)
- Underlying conditions

Ventilation and Oxygenation

Since shock is ultimately a failure of tissue oxygenation, the first step in management is to provide adequate oxygen delivery. Airway maintenance, ventilatory support, and 100 percent oxygen are all critical. Maintenance of the airway and adequate oxygenation and ventilation are often neglected during the acute phase of resuscitation as the clinician focuses on vascular access and fluid administration. Assessment of the adequacy of airway and ventilation should be performed while administering 100 percent oxygen. Blood gas analysis is the best method of monitoring adequacy of ventilation and should be performed early in the resuscitation.

Intubation and assisted ventilation is indicated in cases of fulminant shock and when acidosis or hypotension is not quickly corrected by volume resuscitation. This is particularly important in managing septic and cardiogenic shock. Early intubation will protect the airway and ventilatory support will decrease the work of breathing and improve metabolic balance. Appropriate use of sedation and paralysis should be a part of controlled intubation in managing shock.

Cardiac Output and Fluid Resuscitation

Without adequate cardiac output, oxygen cannot be carried from the alveoli to vital tissues. Fluid resuscitation and pressor agents are the two principal methods used to increase cardiac output and restore perfusion to vital organs.

Initial treatment must include rapid fluid replacement to establish effective intravascular volume. Since the only contraindication to aggressive fluid management is congestive heart failure, an assessment to rule out cardiogenic shock should precede fluid resuscitation. In hypovolemic shock of any cause, fluid resuscitation begins with the infusion of isotonic crystalloid, either lactated Ringer's solution or normal saline. For patients in whom peripheral intravenous access is difficult, fluids are administered by intraosseous or central venous routes. The initial fluid bolus is 20 mL/kg, which in an unstable patient is administered as quickly as possible. The hemodynamic status is then reassessed by evaluating heart rate, peripheral perfusion, and mental status. If improvement is not seen an additional 20 mL/kg is administered and the patient is reassessed. Cardiogenic shock must be reconsidered if there is no improvement after volume resuscitation. Special attention is directed to auscultating the lungs and heart and assessing liver size. The vast majority of patients in hypovolemic shock will respond to 40 mL/kg if ongoing fluid losses have been stopped. If an additional 20 mL/kg is required, the patient is a candidate for invasive monitoring and a cause of shock other than simple hypovolemia must be considered.

Septic shock causes increased capillary permeability, which results in leakage of intravascular fluid into the interstitium. Thus the goal of fluid resuscitation in septic shock is not only to restore intravascular volume but also to preserve it in the intravascular space. Whether the hydrating solution used should be crystalloid or colloid is controversial. Administration of crystalloid may lead to the development of pulmonary edema by lowering intravascular oncotic pressure and encouraging capillary leakage. Colloid may better maintain oncotic pressure, but may eventually leak into the interstitium due to the significant loss of vascular integrity. The resuscitation of septic shock may require the use of both crystalloid and colloid to restore adequate perfusion.

In recent years, there has been interest in the use of hypertonic saline in the resuscitation of patients in hemorrhagic shock. Experimental and clinical evidence suggests the use of hypertonic saline may be helpful in the patient with closed head injury and shock. These solutions reduce brain water, decrease intracranial pressure, and increase blood pressure. Studies in children have supported this hypothesis.

Patients with distributive shock, such as anaphylaxis, may have profound hypovolemia relative to their vascular space. Rapid administration of crystalloids has been shown to significantly improve survival.

Pressor Agents

When patients with hypovolemic, septic, or distributive shock have not shown improvement with 40 mL/kg of isotonic fluids, the patient is a candidate for invasive monitoring. If monitoring demonstrates adequate fluid replacement but perfusion remains poor, pressor agents must be considered.

Several drugs are available for use as adjunctive agents in the treatment of shock when fluid resuscitation alone is not sufficient to stabilize the cardiovascular system. Inotropic agents increase myocardial contractility, while chronotropic agents increase heart rate. Most pressors possess both characteristics and, in addition, may have other effects on specific parts of the vascular bed, often in a dose-dependent fashion. Drugs with vasoactive prop-

erties usually act by stimulating or blocking one or more adrenergic receptors. Table 3-1 reviews the tissue effects produced by stimulation of these adrenergic receptors.

The most widely used group of pressor agents are the sympathomimetic amines. They activate adenyl cyclase resulting in cyclic AMP synthesis, activation of protein kinases, phosphorylation of intracellular proteins, and an increase in intracellular calcium. These drugs include the endogenous catecholamines, epinephrine, norepinephrine, and dopamine, and the synthetic catecholamines, dobutamine and isoproterenol. Pressors may improve blood pressure, but at the expense of increasing vascular resistance and decreasing blood flow. The use of pressor agents in the management of shock should only be attempted after aggressive efforts have been made to improve cardiac output by fluid administration and alveolar oxygenation has been maximized.

The choice of pressors for managing shock remains controversial. Considerations in selecting a drug include the underlying disease process, the condition of the myocardium, the state of the vascular bed, and the use of concurrent agents. Table 3-2 provides a summary of pressor agents commonly used to manage pediatric patients in shock. In children with cardiomyopathies or severe septic shock, very high doses of pressor agents may be needed to achieve the appropriate pharmacologic effect.

Epinephrine is produced in the adrenal medulla and is secreted during times of stress. At lower doses it has a predominantly inotropic effect, with little chronotropic or vasoactive activity. Thus there is an increase in stroke volume and cardiac index, with little effect on heart rate. As the dose increases, alpha effects begin to predominate, causing increased vascular resistance due to in-

Table 3-1. Adrenergic Receptors

Receptors	Tissue Effect
Alpha (α)	Peripheral vasoconstriction
	Dilation of the iris
	Intestinal smooth muscle relaxation
	Increased bladder and intestinal sphincter tone
Beta-1 (β_1)	Increased heart rate
	Improved myocardial contractility
Beta-2 (β_2)	Peripheral vasodilation
	Bronchodilation
	Bladder, uterine, and intestinal smooth muscle relaxation

Table 3-2. Inotropic Agents

Agents	Dose	Clinical Effects and Considerations
Dobutamine	2–20 μg/kg/min	Enhances myocardial contractility
		Useful in cardiac decompensation in shock states
Dopamine	2–20 μg/kg/min	Low dose (4–5 μg/kg/min) enhances renal blood flow
		α-Effect in higher doses
		Enhances myocardial contractility as dose is increased
		Poor response often seen in septic shock
Epinephrine	0.05–1.0 μg/kg/min	Low dose: β-effect
		High dose: α-effect
		Useful in combination with low-dose dopamine
Norepinephrine	0.05–1.0 μg/kg/min	Profound α-effect
		Refractory hypotension
Amrinone	0.75–4.0 mg/kg load	In adjunct with catecholamines
	5–20 μg/kg/min	Enhances myocardial function
Milrinone	50–75 μg/kg load	In adjunct with catecholamines
	0.5–1.0 μg/kg/min	Enhances myocardial function

tense vasoconstriction. Epinephrine is used in shock with hypotension and poor perfusion. Some prefer its use in septic shock because of the possible depletion of endogenous catecholamines that may occur in sepsis. It has also been shown to increase renal blood flow when used with low-dose dopamine.

Norepinephrine is produced in the adrenal medulla and sympathetic postsynaptic receptors. It produces profound vasoconstriction due to its alpha effect. It is used primarily in profound hypotension refractory to volume expansion and other vasoactive agents. Its profound effect on systemic vascular resistance has been helpful in the treatment of septic shock.

Dopamine is an endogenous catecholamine with cardiac β-adrenergic effects, peripheral α-adrenergic effects, and renal dopaminergic effects. Low-dose dopamine causes vasodilation of the afferent renal arteries, resulting in increased renal blood flow and increased glomerular filtration. In moderate doses, the effect is primarily inotropic and in high doses the α-effect predominates and there is peripheral vasoconstriction. Poor response to dopamine has been seen in septic shock and is thought to be due to a decrease in sensitivity of the β-receptors and a decrease in dopamine β-hydroxylase activity. This decrease in enzyme activity decreases the metabolism of dopamine to the more active compounds, epinephrine and norepinephrine. Common adverse effects of dopamine include hypoperfusion of the myocardium with resulting ischemia and tachydysrhythmias. The optimal use of dopamine may ultimately be in low

doses to enhance renal perfusion in combination with other vasopressors.

Dobutamine is a synthetic catecholamine with β_1 cardiac and β_2 peripheral effects that result in enhanced myocardial contractility and decreased systemic vascular resistance. Dobutamine is useful in the treatment of myocardial dysfunction associated with shock, since it enhances myocardial contractility, decreases afterload, and increases preload. Higher doses may have significant chronotropic effects and dysrhythmic potential.

Isoproterenol is a synthetic catecholamine with β_1 and β_2 activity. It increases heart rate and myocardial contractility and decreases systemic vascular resistance. Isoproterenol is used primarily in the treatment of bradycardia and hypotension associated with heart block that is refractory to epinephrine and atropine. It is associated with myocardial ischemia and tachydysrhythmias.

Another useful class of inotropic agents is the phosphodiesterase inhibitors. These agents enhance myocardial contractility by preventing the metabolism of cyclic AMP. As levels of cyclic AMP increase there is intracellular calcium influx and enhanced myocardial contractility. There is also a concomitant decrease in systemic vascular resistance. Other beneficial characteristics include a lower tendency to cause tachycardia and tachydysrhythmias and no increase in myocardial oxygen consumption.

Amrinone and milrinone are the phosphodiesterase inhibitors most commonly used in pediatrics. They are primarily used in volume-resuscitated patients, as an adjunct to the sympathomimetics in an effort to improve myocardial function. Due to a significant effect on systemic vascular resistance, they are used with caution in patients with hypotension.

Hemoglobin Replacement

Most pediatric patients in shock do not require blood replacement. However, the intravascular space must have sufficient oxygen-carrying capacity to meet tissue oxygen demands and assessment of hemoglobin concentration is an important part of shock management. When hemorrhage is the cause of shock, early administration of packed red blood cells is indicated. Blood replacement must be considered after 60 mL/kg of isotonic fluid has been administered with no improvement. However, volume support must not be delayed while awaiting arrival of blood products. Blood from a universal donor, type O, is used when immediate replacement is needed to prevent death. Type-specific blood, which is generally available in less than 10 minutes, is preferred when the demand is somewhat less urgent and fully cross-matched blood is used when the condition of the patient permits a delay of 30 minutes or more.

With acute hemorrhage from trauma or other causes, the intravascular space may not have had time to equilibrate from blood loss and hemoglobin levels may be falsely elevated. Blood replacement must be started on clinical grounds and not based on hemoglobin concentration. When providing rapid blood replacement, it is important to provide warmed blood and to watch closely for acidemia, hypocalcemia, hyperkalemia, and hypothermia.

When managing a child in shock with chronic anemia, blood should be given with caution. Unless there are ongoing losses, no more than 5 to 10 mL/kg should be given over a 4-hour period in order to avoid congestive heart failure.

Management of Underlying Conditions

Early recognition and treatment of the underlying condition is an important part of comprehensive shock management. The patient with septic shock needs appropriate antibiotics without delay. Diagnostic studies, such as lumbar puncture, should be deferred until the patient is stable. When managing a patient with hypovolemic shock, attention must be directed to assessing ongoing losses from hemorrhage or from the gastrointestinal tract. Cardiogenic shock may require pharmacologic therapy to reduce afterload or surgical intervention to correct a life-threatening obstruction (see Chapters 32 and 33). Anaphylactic shock will require epinephrine, elimination of the cause, and antihistamines. Steroids may prevent or lessen delayed reactions.

BIBLIOGRAPHY

Checchia P: Current concepts in the recognition and management of pediatric cardiogenic shock and congestive heart failure. *Emerg Med Rep* 5:41–59, 2000.

Choi P, Yip G, Quinonez L: Crystalloids vs. colloids in fluid resuscitation: A systematic review. *Crit Care Med* 27:200–210, 1999.

Lindsay C, Barton P, Lawless S: Pharmacokinetics and pharmacodynamics of milrinone lactate in pediatric patients with septic shock. *J Pediatr* 132:329–334, 1998.

Perkin RM, Levin DL: Current concepts in the recognition and management of pediatric hypovolemic and septic shock. *Emerg Med Rep* 4:95–113, 1999.

Simma B, Burger R, Falk M: A prospective, randomized and controlled study of fluid management in children with severe head injury: Lactated Ringer's solution versus hypertonic saline. *Crit Care Med* 26:1265–1270, 1998.

4

Cardiopulmonary Resuscitation

Patricia A. Primm
Rebecca R. Reamy

HIGH-YIELD FACTS

- Primary cardiac arrest is rare in children. The usual course begins with respiratory arrest and culminates in profound bradycardia or asystole and cardiovascular collapse.

- It is vitally important to quickly restore ventilation in pediatric patients who have suffered an arrest. Children over 8 years of age follow the same sequence as adults (i.e., call emergency medical services before providing rescue breathing).

- An automated external defibrillator (AED) can be used in children 8 years of age or older in an out-of-hospital setting.

- There is a lack of evidence for the use of these adult advanced CPR techniques in pediatrics: interposed abdominal compression CPR, active compression–decompression CPR, vest CPR, open-chest CPR, and extracorporeal life support.

- Intraosseous access may be used in all children over 6 years of age; there is no upper age limit.

- Epinephrine is the most important agent used in pediatric resuscitation. It is the drug of choice for asystole and bradycardia, both with and without a pulse.

- Use of high-dose epinephrine (HDE) for pulseless arrest is de-emphasized in pediatrics. HDE can have adverse effects including increased myocardial oxygen demand, hyperadrenergic state, tachycardia, hypertension, and myocardial necrosis.

- Infants and young children have high glucose requirements but minimal glycogen stores and often become hypoglycemic during periods of stress.

- Supraventricular tachycardia (SVT) is the most common tachydysrhythmia, and may cause cardiovascular instability during infancy.

- Maintain normal ventilation without hyperventilation. Hyperventilation reduces cerebral blood flow and can cause cerebral ischemia.

Pediatric cardiopulmonary resuscitation (CPR) differs from adult resuscitation in both etiology and treatment priorities. Primary cardiac arrest is rare in children. The usual course begins with respiratory arrest and culminates in profound bradycardia or asystole and cardiovascular collapse. Inevitably, by the time asystole occurs, the brain, kidneys, and gastrointestinal tract have sustained severe damage. Survival in children after cardiac arrest is dismal and most who do survive have significant neurological impairment (see Chapter 1).

PEDIATRIC BASIC LIFE SUPPORT

Pediatric basic life support (PBLS) is the process that provides oxygenation and ventilation to reverse cardiac arrest. Prompt and proper PBLS is extremely important in infants and children because the etiology of arrest is primarily respiratory.

The Sequence

The basic CPR technique described here assumes that one rescuer is present in a nonhospital setting. The sequence of the resuscitation differs if more than one provider is present or if the setting is more specialized. The following sequence is used for the delivery of PBLS to children up to 8 years of age:

- Determine unresponsiveness
- Open the airway
- Provide rescue breathing
- Assess pulse
- Perform chest compressions for 1 min
- Notify emergency medical services (EMS)

- Resume rescue breathing and chest compressions
- Reassess pulse

This sequence differs from adult basic life support in the timing of EMS notification, which is delayed until rescue breathing is initiated. It is vitally important to quickly restore ventilation in pediatric patients who have suffered an arrest. For children over 8 years of age, follow the same sequence as for adults (i.e., call EMS before providing rescue breathing).

Determine Unresponsiveness

Quickly determine the level of consciousness by tapping the child and speaking loudly. Shout for help if you are alone. Do not move a victim who may have sustained head or neck trauma, as this may aggravate a spinal cord injury. In such cases, immobilize the cervical spine to prevent neck movement. If available, an assistant can maintain in-line traction while CPR is performed.

Open the Airway

The establishment of an adequate airway is essential for successful resuscitation. In some cases, opening the airway will in itself result in the resumption of spontaneous respirations. Infants and small children are especially vulnerable to obstruction of the airway from collapse of the relatively large tongue against the posterior pharynx.

Open the airway using the head-tilt chin-lift maneuver (Fig. 4-1A). If a neck injury is possible, do not use the head-tilt, since this can cause untoward motion of the cervical spine. Instead use the jaw-thrust maneuver with in-line cervical stabilization (Fig. 4-1B).

Provide Rescue Breathing

After assuring a patent airway, check for the presence of spontaneous respirations by looking for chest excursion, listening for exhaled air, and feeling for airflow at the victim's mouth. If no spontaneous respirations are pres-ent, begin rescue breathing. In an infant, the rescuer places his mouth or mouth-to-mask device over the infant's nose and mouth. Mouth-to-nose breathing is an acceptable alternative to mouth-to-nose and mouth or mouth-to-mouth breathing if the rescuer is unable to cover the infant's nose and mouth. In a child larger than an infant, the rescuer makes a mouth-to-mouth seal, pinching shut the victim's nose with the thumb and forefinger of the same hand used to maintain the head tilt. Provide two slow (1 to 1.5 seconds) breaths to the

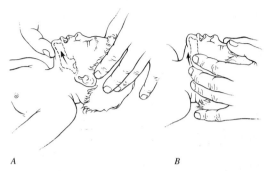

A   B

Fig. 4-1. *A.* The head-tilt chin-lift maneuver. To open the airway, place one hand on the patient's forehead and tilt the head back into a neutral or slightly extended position. Use the index finger of the other hand to lift the patient's mandible upward and outward. *B.* The jaw-thrust maneuver. To open the airway while maintaining cervical spine stabilization, place two or three fingers under each side of the lower jaw angle and lift the jaw upward and outward. Maintain the neck in a neutral position manually to prevent craniocervical motion.

victim, pausing to take a breath in between the two rescue breaths. The correct volume for each breath is that which causes the chest to rise. If air does not flow freely, either the airway is obstructed or more pressure or volume is required to inflate the lungs. If the airway is obstructed, reposition the head-tilt chin-lift and attempt another rescue breath. If rescue breathing again fails to expand the chest, suspect airway obstruction from a foreign body. If there is adequate chest wall excursion, begin ventilation of the patient at a rate of 20 breaths/min.

Foreign Body Aspiration

Foreign body aspiration is likely in infants and children who have experienced a sudden onset of respiratory distress associated with coughing, gagging, or stridor. Do not intervene as long as the child has spontaneous coughing, adequate ventilation, and can speak. Intervene if the cough becomes ineffective, there is increasing respiratory difficulty, or the victim loses consciousness.

Airway Foreign Body in an Infant

In the conscious or unconscious infant with airway obstruction from a foreign body, use a combination of back blows and chest thrusts to clear the obstruction. Hold the infant face down over the rescuer's forearm, supported on the rescuer's thigh, with the infant's head lower than the trunk. Deliver five back blows between the infant's scapulae, using the heel of the hand. After the back blows, turn the infant face up, and deliver five chest thrusts over the mid-sternum. Remove the foreign body if it is visualized. Blind finger sweeps are not advisable. If the infant is unconscious, attempt rescue breathing. If the airway remains obstructed, repeat back blows, chest thrusts, and rescue breathing until the object is removed.

Foreign Body in the Airway of a Child

In the conscious child whose airway is obstructed by a foreign body, perform a series of five Heimlich maneuvers. These consist of sub-diaphragmatic abdominal thrusts. Stand behind the victim, with the rescuer's arms under the victim's axillae and wrapped around the child's chest. Place the thumb side of one fist against the child's abdomen, above the umbilicus and below the xiphoid, and grasp it with the other hand. Administer five quick upward thrusts as separate, distinct maneuvers.

Place the unconscious child on his back on a flat surface and straddle his hips. Place the heel of one hand above the umbilicus and below the xiphoid, and grasp it with the other hand. Administer a quick upward thrust and repeat five times, if necessary. Remove the foreign body if it is visualized. If necessary, initiate rescue breathing. If the airway remains obstructed, administer five additional abdominal thrusts.

Assess the Pulse

After opening the airway and initiating rescue breathing, palpate for a pulse. In infants, feel for a pulse over the brachial or femoral arteries, since the infant's short, thick neck makes it difficult to feel a carotid pulse. In children, palpate for a carotid pulse. Take only a few seconds to palpate a pulse. If no pulse is appreciated, initiate chest compressions in coordination with rescue breathing. Use the 5:1 ratio in pediatric arrest regardless of whether one or two rescuers are involved.

Chest Compressions

Chest compressions are performed to establish some circulation to vital organs until a perfusing rhythm is restored. Perform CPR where the patient is found.

To perform chest compressions, place the patient on a firm, flat surface. In infants, the area of compression is the lower third of the sternum or one finger width below the intermammary line. Using two fingers, the rescuer compresses the chest to a depth of one-third to one-half the depth of the chest, which corresponds to a depth of one-half to one inch (Fig. 4-2A). The 2-thumb-

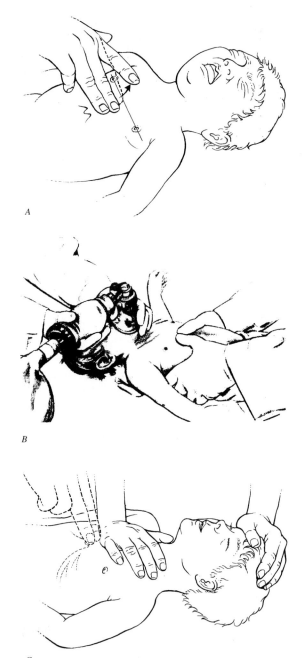

A

B

C

Fig. 4-2. *A.* Proper finger position for chest compressions in infants less than 1 year of age: use two fingers to perform compressions one finger width below the intermammary line. *B.* Proper technique for two-thumb encircling hands technique over lower third of sternum. *C.* Proper finger position for chest compressions in children from 1 to 8 years of age: use the heel of one hand to perform compressions two finger widths above xiphoid.

encircling hands technique of chest compression is preferred for chest compressions in infants performed by health care providers when two rescuers are available.

In children receiving chest compressions, place the heel of the hand two finger widths above the lower edge of the xiphoid (Fig. 4-2C). Compress the chest one-third to one-half of its anterior-posterior diameter, or 1 to 1.5 inches. Allow the chest to return to a resting position between compressions, but do not remove the hand. The rate of compressions is 100 per minute for victims of all ages. After every fifth compression, allow a 1- to 1.5-second pause for ventilation.

After 20 cycles of compression and ventilation (approximately 1 minute) and every few minutes thereafter, reassess the patient for the development of a pulse or spontaneous respirations.

Notify Emergency Medical Services

Activate the EMS system after 1 min of rescue support in children up to 8 years of age. If the rescuer is unable to activate the system, continue CPR until help arrives or the rescuer becomes exhausted.

Automatic External Defibrillators

An automated external defibrillator (AED) can be used in children 8 years of age and older in the out-of-hospital setting. Limited data suggest that these devices are accurate in differentiating between shockable and nonshockable rhythms for adolescents. In children older than 8 years of age, the median weight should be ≥ 25 kg, so a 150-J biphasic shock would deliver no more than 6 J/kg to a child of average size. A monophasic AED with escalating shocks would initially deliver 8 J/kg (a 200-J initial shock), and this could increase to 14 J/kg if a 360-J dose is delivered to a 25-kg child. The potential for harm from energy levels much greater than the recommended upper limit of 4 J/kg is of great concern. Defibrillators with adjustable energy dose are recommended for in-hospital use in areas that routinely care for infants and children.

Complications of Basic Life Support

Complications of basic life support in pediatric patients are similar to those in adults. These include gastric distension, lung contusion, pneumothorax, fractured ribs, liver laceration, and damage to other organs. Gastric distension can result in respiratory compromise, as upward pressure on the diaphragm decreases tidal volume. In children, intraabdominal organs are not as well protected by the bony

thorax as in adults, which, at least theoretically, makes them more susceptible to injury. For pediatric patients, there is a lack of evidence to support the use of advanced CPR adjuncts, such as interposed abdominal compression CPR, active compression-decompression CPR, vest CPR, open chest CPR, and extracorporeal life support.

PEDIATRIC ADVANCED LIFE SUPPORT

Pediatric advanced life support (PALS) refers to the resuscitation and stabilization of infants and children through the use of invasive means that range from simple intravenous fluids to full artificial cardiopulmonary support. The chapter on respiratory failure includes a discussion of airway management and artificial ventilation. This chapter will focus on resuscitation and support of the cardiovascular system during cardiac arrest (Fig. 4-3).

Oxygen

The vast majority of patients who require CPR will need to have an airway secured by tracheal intubation (see Chapter 5). Deliver 100 percent oxygen to the patient during ventilation with a bag-valve-mask and after intubation. Since most pediatric patients suffer hypoxic-ischemic arrests, administration of oxygen is the first and most essential measure during pediatric resuscitation. It should supersede attempts to deliver intravenous medication and, except in extremely rare circumstances, defibrillation or cardioversion. The majority of pediatric patients who survive cardiopulmonary arrest with good neurologic outcome will do so by ventilation with 100 percent oxygen alone.

Delivery of Fluids and Medications

The delivery of fluids and medications is an essential aspect of PALS and is somewhat more complicated than in an adult resuscitation. It is often difficult to obtain peripheral venous access in an infant or young child, especially when the patient is dehydrated or in full cardiopulmonary collapse. An alternative route to deliver medications is via the endotracheal tube, where absorption of medications takes place across the vast capillary surface of the lower airways. The tracheal route, however, is restricted to lipid-soluble drugs, such as epinephrine, atropine, lidocaine, and naloxone. In addition, recent studies have cast doubt on the reliability of absorption of tracheally administered epinephrine in the arrest situation. Since epinephrine is the primary pharmacologic adjunct used in PALS, it is essential to obtain intravenous access in a timely fashion during a pediatric

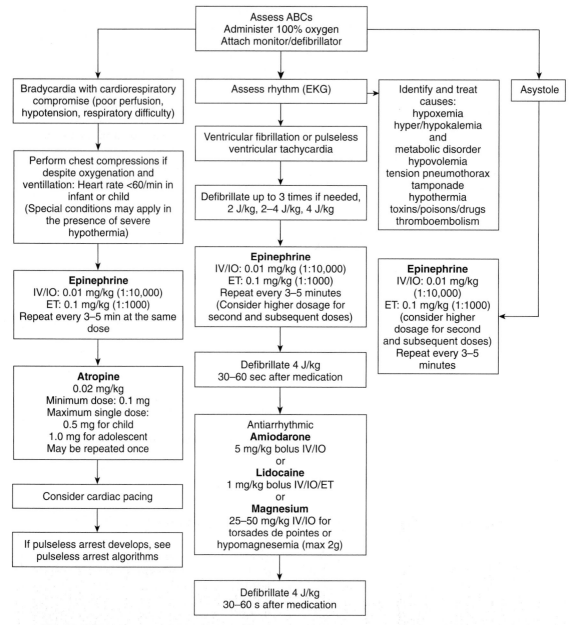

Fig. 4-3. CPR decision tree. ABCs, airway, breathing, circulation; ET, endotracheal; IO, intraosseous; IV, intravenous.

resuscitation. If venous access is impossible or must be delayed, deliver medications via the tracheal route.

Venous Access

In the event that peripheral venous access is not immediately available, establish access by cannulating a central vein or inserting an intraosseous catheter. A protocol that places a time limit on attempts to establish a peripheral line prior to placing a central venous catheter or intraosseous line can hasten the attainment of venous access.

In infants and small children, the preferred sites for central venous catheterization are the right internal jugular and femoral veins. In emergent situations, catheterization of the subclavian vein is associated with a high rate of complications. If a femoral venous catheter is used, insert the tip to a level above the diaphragm.

Intraosseous (IO) lines are increasingly popular in the management of critically ill pediatric patients. They are relatively easy to place and appropriate for virtually every drug required in an acute resuscitation. The venous sinusoids of the bone marrow do not collapse in the presence of advanced shock or full cardiopulmonary arrest. In long bones, the marrow sinusoids ultimately drain into the systemic venous system. The age range for intraosseous access extends to all victims including children over 6 years of age; there is no upper age limit. The optimal site of insertion for an IO line is the proximal tibia. Alternatively, the distal tibia or distal femur can be used.

Contraindications to the use of an IO line include osteogenesis imperfecta and osteopetrosis. Because of the risk of extravasation, an ipsilateral fracture is also a contraindication. Reported complications of IO insertion include iatrogenic fracture, tissue necrosis from extravasation of fluid and medication and compartment syndrome, also from extravasation. Osteomyelitis has also been reported. Fat embolism may occur, but does not appear to be clinically significant. The technique for inserting an IO line is described in Chapter 10.

Fluid Resuscitation

It is essential to re-establish effective intravascular volume for patients with cardiovascular collapse secondary to severe dehydration or massive acute blood loss. Attain volume expansion by administering isotonic crystalloid in the form of normal saline or Ringer's lactate. In certain situations, colloid solutions such as 5 percent albumin may be used.

For children in cardiopulmonary arrest who do not respond to oxygenation and ventilation, administer a fluid bolus of 10 to 20 mL/kg to provide sufficient circulating volume and aid in the restoration of a perfusing rhythm. For a more detailed discussion of fluid therapy, see Chapter 3.

Pharmacologic Therapy

The pharmacology of advanced life support in infants and children differs in important ways from that of adults. This reflects the fact that the usual pediatric arrest results from an asphyxial process, while the adult classically suffers a primarily cardiac process. Thus, while the emphasis in adult arrest is to provide rapid defibrillation and manage acute arrhythmias, in pediatric patients both defibrillation and pharmacologic therapy are adjuncts to adequate oxygenation and ventilation (Table 4-1).

Epinephrine

Epinephrine is the most important agent used in pediatric resuscitation. It is the drug of choice for asystole and bradycardia both with and without a pulse, which are the most common dysrhythmias encountered in pediatric resuscitation.

Epinephrine is an endogenous catecholamine with both β- and α-adrenergic stimulating properties. In an arrest situation, α-mediated vasoconstriction probably plays the most important role, by increasing aortic diastolic pressure and coronary perfusion. Epinephrine also increases myocardial contractility and ventricular irritability, although in pediatric arrests this is not as important as it is in adults. High-dose epinephrine (HDE) for pulseless arrest is de-emphasized in pediatrics. Large multicenter adult studies, well-controlled animal studies, and uncontrolled retrospective pediatric data show no benefit from HDE. HDE can have adverse effects including increased myocardial oxygen demand, a hyperadrenergic state, tachycardia, hypertension, and myocardial necrosis.

The initial dose of epinephrine recommended for asystolic or pulseless arrest is 0.01 mg/kg of 1:10,000 solution administered intravenously or intraosseously. The same dose is recommended for second and subsequent doses in unresponsive asystolic and pulseless arrest, but higher doses of epinephrine (0.1 to 0.2 mg/kg) by any intravascular route may be considered. Subsequent doses are administered at 3- to 5-minute intervals. Doses as high as 0.2 mg/kg may be effective.

In the event that intravenous or intraosseous access is delayed, administer epinephrine tracheally at a dose of 0.1 mg/kg of a 1:1000 solution. Dilute the epinephrine in 2 to 3 mL of normal saline and administer the solution via the endotracheal tube. Follow with several positive pressure breaths. This higher recommended dose reflects the erratic absorption of epinephrine from the lungs.

If a perfusing rhythm is restored, use an epinephrine infusion to maintain blood pressure until cardiovascular stability is achieved. Especially in infants, epinephrine is preferable to dopamine. At low doses (<0.3 μg/kg/min) β-adrenergic action predominates. At higher doses, α-mediated vasoconstriction predominates.

Atropine Sulfate

Atropine sulfate is a parasympatholytic drug that accelerates sinus and atrial pacemakers and increases atrioventricular (AV) conduction. It is less useful in the treatment of bradycardia in pediatric patients than in adults, in whom bradycardia is often secondary to myocardial infarction and AV block. In infants and children, epinephrine is the primary pharmacologic therapy for symp-

Table 4-1. Drugs Used in Pediatric Advanced Life Support

Drug	Dose	Remarks
Adenosine	0.1 mg/kg Repeat dose: 0.2 mg/kg Maximum single dose: 12 mg	Rapid IV/IO bolus Rapid flush to central circulation Monitor ECG during dose
Amiodarone	5 mg/kg	Rapid IV bolus Maximum dose 15 mg/kg/day Hypotension may occur Consider for VF pulseless VT

Atropine sulfate	0.2 mg/kg
	Minimum dose: 0.1 mg
	Maximum single dose: 0.5 mg in child,
	    1.0 mg in adolescent
		IV/IO/ET
		Tachycardia and pupil dilation may occur
		    but not fixed dilated pupils

Calcium chloride 10%	20 mg/kg; may be increased	Slowly IV for K, Mg, calcium channel blocker toxicity

Epinephrine
    For bradycardia
	IV/IO: 0.01 mg/kg (1:10,000)
	    ET: 0.1 mg/kg (1:1000)
		Be aware of effective dose of preservatives
		    administered (if preservatives are present
		    in epinephrine preparation) when high
		    doses are used

For asystolic or
    pulseless arrest
	All doses IV/IO: 0.01 mg/kg (1:10,000)
	    ET: 0.1 mg/kg (1:1000)
	Doses as high as 0.2 mg/kg may be
	    effective
		Tachyarrhythmia, hypertension may occur

Glucose	0.5–1.0 g/kg 1–2 mL/kg D50W 2–4 mL/kg D25W	IV/IO
Lidocaine	1 mg/kg per dose	Rapid bolus IV, ET
Magnesium	25–50 mg/kg Maximum 2 g/dose	Use for torsades, hypomagnesemia
Naloxone	<20 kg: 0.1 mg/kg >20 kg: 2.0 mg	For total reversal of narcotic effect Use repeat doses

Sodium bicarbonate	1 mEq/kg per dose or 0.3 × kg × base
	    deficit
		Infuse slowly and only if ventilation is
		    adequate

Abbreviations: IV, intravenous route; IO, intraosseous route; ET, endotracheal route.

Drug	Dose, μg/kg/min	Dilution in 100 mL D5W, mg/kg	IV Infusion Rate, μg/kg/min
Dopamine	2–20	6	1 mL/h = 1
Dobutamine	2–20	6	1 mL/h = 1
Epinephrine	0.1–1.0	0.6	1 mL/h = 0.1
Lidocaine	20–50	6	1 mL/h = 1

tomatic bradycardia, except in the unusual setting of AV block bradycardia, where atropine is the drug of choice. Atropine is also indicated for vagally induced bradycardia during intubation. It is often administered prophylactically, prior to intubation.

The recommended dose of atropine is 0.02 mg/kg with a minimum dose of 0.1 mg in infants and a maximum dose of 0.5 mg in a child or 1 mg in an adolescent. The minimum recommended dose reflects the propensity for atropine to cause a paradoxical bradycardia if not given in a vagolytic dose. The endotracheal dose is the same as the intravenous and intraosseous dose.

Sodium Bicarbonate

Sodium bicarbonate has been used as a buffer for the treatment of the metabolic acidosis that usually accompanies arrest states. In adults with cardiac arrest, metabolic acidosis results from the abrupt cessation of cardiac activity, while in the pediatric patient metabolic acidosis usually results from an ongoing asphyxial process and precedes cardiac arrest. Currently, there are no data to support the routine use of sodium bicarbonate in an arrest situation. The exception to this is in hyperkalemic arrest, where sodium bicarbonate may alter cellular physiology in a beneficial way. For patients resuscitated from cardiac arrest with ongoing metabolic acidosis, the role for therapy with sodium bicarbonate remains under investigation.

Complications of therapy with sodium bicarbonate include hypernatremia, hyperosmolality, and metabolic alkalosis, which can impede delivery of oxygen to the tissues by shifting the oxygen-hemoglobin dissociation curve to the left.

Calcium

Calcium is necessary in myocardial excitation-contraction coupling and has a positive inotropic effect, but it may impair cardiac relaxation. Ionized hypocalcemia is common in prolonged arrests; however, the administration of calcium has not been shown to improve the outcome. Likewise, calcium has been found ineffective in the treatment of pulseless electrical activity. Calcium is not recommended for the routine management of cardiopulmonary arrest in children, but is indicated for documented hypocalcemia, hyperkalemia, hypermagnesemia, and in calcium channel blocker overdose. Calcium chloride provides greater bioavailability than calcium gluconate. The recommended dose is 20 mg/kg of a 10 percent solution.

Glucose

Infants and young children have high glucose requirements but minimal glycogen stores and often become hypoglycemic during periods of stress. Therefore, monitor blood glucose carefully during resuscitation. In hypoglycemic patients, the dose of glucose is 0.5 to 1.0 g/kg, which can be provided by 2 to 4 mL/kg of 25 percent solution.

Amiodarone

Amiodarone can be used for both supraventricular and ventricular arrhythmias. Consider it for refractory ventricular fibrillation (VF) persisting despite three shocks.

Amiodarone has been used in children in the postoperative period, where it is effective for ectopic atrial or junctional tachycardia. It is also effective for ventricular tachycardia (VT) in postoperative patients or children with underlying heart disease.

There are no prospective randomized trials of amiodarone in pediatric cardiac arrest. It has been added as a drug to consider in pediatric arrest due to evidence extrapolated from adult prospective clinical trials. In these trials, amiodarone was associated with a significant increase in the rate of admission to the hospital, but not survival rate, in adult patients with shock-refractory VF/pulseless VT.

Lidocaine

Lidocaine suppresses ventricular ectopy and raises the threshold for ventricular fibrillation. It is indicated in ventricular tachycardia associated with a pulse, where it may be administered prior to synchronized cardioversion. Lidocaine is also indicated for the treatment of pulseless ventricular tachycardia and ventricular fibrillation. In each of these situations, defibrillation takes precedence over the administration of lidocaine. Evidence continues to accumulate that pediatric VF may be more common than previously suspected. The dose of lidocaine is 1 mg/kg. It can be administered as a continuous infusion at a rate of 20 to 50 μg/kg/min. Excessive plasma concentrations of lidocaine can cause disorientation, muscle twitching, and seizures.

Bretylium

There is no published data supporting the use of bretylium in the pediatric age group. It is no longer included in the treatment of VF or pulseless VT.

Transcutaneous Pacing

Noninvasive transcutaneous pacing may be useful in children with profound symptomatic bradycardia refractory to basic and advanced life support. It requires an external pacing unit and two adhesive-backed electrodes. The negative electrode is placed over the heart on the anterior chest with the positive electrode behind the heart on the patient's back. Alternatively, the negative electrode may be placed near the apex of the heart and the positive electrode on the right side of the anterior chest under the clavicle. If the child weighs <15 kg, small or medium electrodes are recommended. Both output and sensitivity will need adjustment. The pacemaker must function so that every paced impulse results in ventricular depolarization, or capture.

Defibrillation

Defibrillation is the unsynchronized depolarization of the myocardium. It is the primary treatment of VF and pulseless VT. Defibrillation is not useful for asystole, which is the most common rhythm encountered in pediatric arrests.

In children weighing <10 kg, use pediatric paddles. Use adult paddles for all other children. The paddle-chest interface can be an electrode cream or paste, or self-adhesive defibrillation pads. Avoid the use of alcohol pads, which can result in severe burns. Bare paddles are ineffective. Place one paddle over the right side of the upper chest and the other over the apex of the heart. The initial defibrillation is at 2 J/kg. If that is unsuccessful, defibrillate the patient twice more in rapid succession at 4 J/kg. If a perfusing rhythm is not restored, administer epinephrine and defibrillate again at 4 J/kg. If that does not succeed, administer amiodarone or lidocaine, and defibrillate at 4 J/kg (Fig. 4-3).

Management of Pulseless Electrical Activity

Cardiopulmonary collapse with organized electrical activity but no palpable pulse is termed *pulseless electrical activity* (PEA). Manage it in the same manner as asystole (Fig. 4-3). Always consider treatable causes of PEA, such as tension pneumothorax, acidosis, pericardial tamponade, hypovolemia, hypoxemia, hypothermia, hyperkalemia, metabolic disorders, and drug toxicity.

Management of Supraventricular Tachycardia

Supraventricular tachycardia (SVT) is the most common tachydysrhythmia causing cardiovascular instability dur-

ing infancy. Usually due to a reentrant mechanism, SVT produces heart rates from 220 to 300 with no beat-to-beat variability in infants. In older children with SVT, heart rates are lower. In general, the electrocardiogram reveals a narrow QRS complex without discernible P waves. Occasionally it is difficult to distinguish SVT from sinus tachycardia. When the electrical impulse is aberrantly conducted, the QRS complex can be wide and SVT becomes difficult to distinguish from VT (Table 4-2).

The child in shock or severe congestive heart failure from SVT requires immediate synchronized cardioversion. The initial dose is 0.5 to 1 J/kg. If SVT persists, increase the dose to 1 to 2 J/kg. If vascular access is readily available, use adenosine to treat the infant in cardiogenic shock due to SVT before performing cardioversion. However, do not delay cardioversion while attempting IV access.

Adenosine is an endogenous nucleoside that interrupts the reentrant pathway. It has a half-life of 10 seconds and must be administered at a proximal site such as the antecubital or external jugular vein. It is administered in a dose of 0.1 mg/kg. If the initial dose is unsuccessful, double the dose. The maximum dose is 12 mg.

Patients with stable SVT may respond to vagal maneuvers (such as carotid massage) or induction of the diving reflex by placing an ice bag over the face. Do not use ocular massage in children. If vagal maneuvers are unsuccessful, adenosine is the drug of choice. Verapamil is discouraged for use in children because it has been associated with profound hypotension and death.

Cerebral Resuscitation

Since survivors of pediatric cardiorespiratory arrest often have significant neurological impairment, a major goal is resuscitation of the brain as well as the heart. Some brain cells are damaged during the primary insult, but a cascade of processes follow arrest and can lead to further loss of brain cells over the hours following the

Table 4-2. Differentiating Types of Tachycardia

	Sinus Tachycardia	Supraventricular Tachycardia	Ventricular Tachycardia
Rate	Usually <220	Usually >220	120–400
QRS complex	Narrow	Usually narrow	Wide
Beat-to-beat variability	Yes	No	No
P waves	Yes (although they may be difficult to see)	No	No

arrest. At the cellular level, ion pump failure causes influxes of calcium, sodium, and chloride ions and leads to intracellular swelling. Free radicals are also believed to cause membrane damage during reoxygenation.

The following postresuscitation interventions improve neurological outcomes:

- Maintain normal ventilation without hyperventilation. Hyperventilation reduces cerebral blood flow and can cause cerebral ischemia. It should not be used routinely.
- Monitor temperature and treat hyperthermia but allow mild hypothermia. Some evidence suggests that mild hypothermia reduces damage from an ischemic insult, especially when the hypothermia precedes the insult. This protective effect of hypothermia on the brain and organs is under investigation. Hyperthermia increases oxygen demand and should be corrected.
- Manage postischemic myocardial dysfunction.
- Maintain normal glucose levels. Both hyperglycemia and hypoglycemia can have detrimental effects.

BIBLIOGRAPHY

American Heart Association: Guidelines 2000 for cardiopulmonary resuscitation and emergency cardiovascular care. *Curr Emerg Cardiovasc Care* 11(3):3, 2000.

American Heart Association: Pediatric basic life support. *Circulation* 102(suppl I):I-253, 2000.

American Heart Association: Pediatric advanced life support. *Circulation* 102(suppl I):I-291, 2000.

5

Rapid Sequence Intubation

Rustin B. Morse
Grace Arteaga

HIGH-YIELD FACTS

- Rapid sequence intubation (RSI) involves the use of pharmaceuticals to rapidly achieve intubation and to minimize the adverse effects of endotracheal intubation (ETI).
- RSI is the safest and most effective method of establishing a definitive airway in a pediatric patient.
- At the very least, RSI involves the use of preoxygenation (ideally without the use of bag-mask ventilation) followed by rapid sedation, paralysis, cricoid pressure, and ETI with confirmation of tube placement.
- Adjunctive premedications, including lidocaine and fentanyl, may be used to reduce intracranial pressure (ICP) or pain.
- Etomidate or midazolam can be used to sedate any patient requiring RSI.
- Rocuronium can be used to paralyze any patient requiring RSI. The vast majority of patients can also be paralyzed with succinylcholine.
- Atropine should be used in all patients <5 years of age and for those receiving succinylcholine or ketamine.

Physicians practicing pediatric emergency medicine need to be able to accurately assess a patient's airway and respiratory status. Maintaining a patent airway and ensuring adequate gas exchange are essential components of the management of severely ill children. Endotracheal intubation (ETI) is indicated in the following circumstances:

- A child is unable to maintain a patent airway.
- Respiratory failure is present or is imminent.
- The work of breathing is physiologically unsustainable.
- An intracranial event requires mechanical ventilation.

Electing to intubate a patient in the emergency department is not without some risk. Failure to obtain control of the airway is obviously the ultimate problem, but aspiration of gastric contents and trauma to the oropharynx or airway can also occur. Transient hypoxemia, cardiovascular instability, and increased intracranial pressure (ICP) are physiologic responses to the insertion of a laryngoscope blade and endotracheal tube (ETT) into the airway and can complicate RSI.

Rapid sequence intubation (RSI) is a process designed to aid in the successful ETI of a patient while minimizing these potential adverse consequences. RSI involves the use of pharmaceutical agents to rapidly induce unconsciousness and paralysis, as well as the possible use of agents to prevent the physiologic responses of ETI such as pain, cardiac instability, and increased ICP. Ideally, RSI also utilizes preoxygenation with minimal or no positive pressure ventilation and cricoid pressure (Sellick maneuver) to minimize the risk of aspiration. RSI is preferred over other emergency forms of definitive airway control including nasotracheal intubation, ETI without paralysis, and surgical airway management.

RSI should be considered for all patients requiring definitive airway control in the emergency department. The management of patients requiring emergency ETI is more challenging than management of that same patient electively undergoing ETI in the operating room. Past medical history and the immediate history leading up to the patient's current state is often scant or absent. Patients must be assumed to have a full stomach, and therefore are at risk for aspiration. Most patients are under physiologic stress that may adversely affect their oxygen reserve and shorten the time required to become hypoxic during an attempt at ETI. Patients presenting in cardiac arrest or flaccid paralysis may be intubated without many of the pharmaceutical aids described in RSI, but consideration should be given to preoxygenating such patients using bag-mask ventilation (BMV) and minimizing the risk of aspiration by using cricoid pressure. Most other patients will require sedation and paralysis.

RSI should not be undertaken if the physician is not comfortable with his or her ability to successfully intubate the patient or to effectively maintain a patent airway and adequate air exchange via BMV if intubation should be difficult. Situations that may add to the difficulty of ETI and BMV include major facial or laryngeal trauma, upper airway obstruction, and anatomic congenital airway abnormalities (Table 5-1). Physicians practicing pediatric emergency medicine need to be well versed in advanced airway techniques including the use of laryngeal mask airways (LMAs) and needle cricothyroidotomy. Use of these adjunctive airway techniques may be life saving in the event a patient cannot be successfully intubated or ventilated via BMV and is in respiratory failure.

EMERGENCY DEPARTMENT STAFF TRAINING

Emergency department staff members who care for children need to have the following skills:

- Adeptness at estimating the weight of pediatric patients

- Dosing and drawing up medications on a per-kilogram basis in an expeditious fashion

- Using airway equipment of many different sizes

- Ability to remain calm when faced with a critically ill child

Since true pediatric airway emergencies are relatively uncommon even in emergency departments dedicated solely to pediatric care, the use of "mock codes" may ensure that staff members are prepared to function smoothly during a pediatric emergency. RSI involves preparation and equipment assembly, premedication and preoxygenation, rapid sedation and paralysis, the application of cricoid pressure, successful intubation, and confirmation of proper tube placement (Table 5-2). Many of the steps prior to ETI can be performed simultaneously by different members of the resuscitation team. As with any high-stress situation in the emergency depart-

Table 5-1. Congenital Anatomical Features Associated With a Difficult Airway

Macroglossia [trisomy 21 (Down's syndrome)]
Micrognathia (Pierre Robin syndrome)
Midface hypoplasia (Apert's or Crouzon's syndrome)
Cleft lip
Cleft palate
Subglottic stenosis
Tonsillar hypertrophy

Table 5-2. RSI Time Course

−5 minutes	Focused history and physical examination
	Provide 100% oxygen; avoid BMV
	Place patient on monitors
	Draw up medication doses
	Assemble airway equipment
−3 minutes	Premedicate (optional)
−1 minute	Give sedative and paralytic
	Apply cricoid pressure
0 minutes	Perform intubation
+1 minute	Confirm placement of endotracheal tube
	Secure endotracheal tube
	Release cricoid pressure

ment, it is important to have a clearly identified leader assigning roles and overseeing the proper sequence of actions in the room. An orderly environment aids significantly in the staff members' ability to remain calm and focus on the task at hand.

INITIAL ASSESSMENT

Prior to intubation a brief history and physical examination is performed when possible. The history focuses on:

- Allergies to medications

- Current medications the patient is taking

- Medical problems that may influence resuscitative efforts

- Circumstances which led up to the patient's current situation

The physical examination focuses on findings that may impede intubation. These include:

- Facial trauma

- Congenital facial anomalies

- Tonsillar hypertrophy

- Limited cervical spine mobility

- Evidence of medical illnesses that might potentially make muscle tone or positioning important in maintaining airway patency. A short neck, small mandible, high arched or cleft palate, or macroglossia should alert the physician to the possibility of a difficult airway.

PREPARATION AND EQUIPMENT ASSEMBLY

As with most procedures, proper preparation for RSI will significantly facilitate successful completion. All critically ill patients need to have their cardiac rhythm and pulse oximetry continuously monitored. Once the decision to intubate a patient is made, the patient's weight is estimated and airway equipment is prepared. Use of a length-based tape (Broselow tape) can be very helpful in estimating the patient's weight and helps ensure appropriate doses of medication and proper size of airway equipment. Color coded crash carts corresponding with the colors on the Broselow tape measure provide emergency departments with guidelines to ensure that they are properly stocked with pediatric airway equipment.

Although BMV is avoided when possible, a bag and mask need to be available in the event that a patient requires assisted ventilation prior to insertion of an ETT or in the event that ETI is unsuccessful. Emergency physicians often have to choose between self-inflating bags and anesthesia flow-dependent bags. Self-inflating bags are readily available and require less training to establish proficiency than anesthesia flow-dependent bags. Anesthesia flow-dependent bags require a continuous high flow of oxygen and a virtually perfect mask-to-mouth seal in order to inflate the bag and provide adequate patient ventilation. Physicians should become familiar with the equipment in their emergency department and ensure that masks of varying sizes are readily available.

Laryngoscopic blade selection is often based on personal preference. Straight laryngoscopic blades (e.g., Miller) are often used in infants because their smaller size makes placing the blade in the mouth of a child easier, and the lack of a curve in the blade often makes visualization of the cephalad vocal cords easier. For patients more than 2 years old, curved laryngoscopic blades (e.g., Macintosh) are most commonly used. The physician should assemble the blade and ensure that the light is strong and properly secured. Various sizes of both types of laryngoscopic blades must be available.

Proper ETT size can be estimated using:

- The Broselow tape measure
- The size of the child's nares
- The size of the child's fifth fingernail
- The formula (16+ age in years)/4

Children <8 years of age are intubated using uncuffed ETTs, as their funnel-shaped airway provides enough resistance to prevent air leakage. Cuffed ETTs are checked for balloon integrity prior to use. The ETT of the size most likely to be appropriate as well as ETTs one-half size larger and one-half size smaller are also made available, as well as appropriate size stylets. The ETT may be lubricated with sterile lubricant or 1 percent viscous lidocaine. A tube holder or tape to secure the ETT is prepared.

Suction equipment is readied, consisting of at least one ridged catheter and a flexible catheter capable of being inserted into the ETT. As emesis is not uncommon during ETI attempts, it is prudent to have a second ridged catheter readily available in case the first one becomes occluded with gastric contents.

The following equipment should be available to aid in the management of a difficult airway:

- McGill forceps
- Laryngeal mask airways (LMAs)
- Needle cricothyroidotomy kits
- Surgical cricothyroidotomy kits

It should be noted that surgical cricothyroidotomy in a pediatric patient is significantly more difficult than it is in an adult patient and is associated with more complications including bleeding and airway damage. Surgical cricothyroidotomy is therefore reserved for the gravest of circumstances, when all else has failed to secure the airway.

PREINTUBATION THERAPY

Children have a higher metabolic oxygen demand than adults and are therefore prone to desaturating more rapidly during ETI attempts. Preoxygenation of children fills their lungs with 100 percent oxygen by displacing nitrogen (nitrogen washout) and allows them to tolerate a longer period of apnea during laryngoscopy. If possible, BMV is not initiated in a breathing child as this will distend the stomach and increase the risk of emesis and aspiration. During the preparation of equipment and medications, patients with adequate respirations are placed on 100 percent O_2 via a tight nonrebreathing mask. If ventilation is inadequate to preoxygenate effectively via a face mask, and BMV is begun, cricoid pressure is initiated and maintained until ETT placement is confirmed.

Atropine is an adjunctive medication used to decrease airway secretions and it has vagolytic action that may prevent bradycardia sometimes associated with ETI. Its use should be considered standard for patients less than 5 years of age and in any pediatric patient who is to receive succinylcholine or ketamine. To achieve maximum effect, atropine is ideally given 3 to 5 minutes before ETI (Table 5-3).

For patients with head injury or when increased ICP is possible, the use of intravenous lidocaine prior to in-

Table 5-3. Adjunctive Premedications

Medication	IV Dose	Indications
Atropine	0.02 mg/kg Min: 0.1 mg Max: 0.5 mg in child 1 mg in adolescent	Age <5 years Required if ketamine or succinylcholine are used
Lidocaine	1–3 mg/kg	Head injury Suspected elevated ICP
Fentanyl	2–5 μg/kg	Head injury Suspected elevated ICP Pain control

sertion of the laryngoscope may modulate the increase in ICP noted with ETI. To be most effective, lidocaine has to be given 5 minutes before laryngoscopy. Lidocaine has no sedating properties, and the use of lidocaine remains somewhat controversial.

SEDATION

Patients who are intubated and paralyzed almost invariably require sedation, and if possible sedation should be achieved prior to intubation. The physician has many options when choosing a sedative agent. The patient's hemodynamic and neurological status, as well as the illness or injury that has led to the need for RSI, are important factors in determining the appropriate drug. Common agents used to induce rapid sedation for RSI are listed in Table 5-4.

Midazolam is a time-tested, short-acting benzodiazepine with anticonvulsant and amnestic properties. It has minimal effects on the cardiovascular system and can be used in any patient undergoing RSI. One shortcoming is the fact that midazolam is slower acting than other sedative agents used in RSI and is therefore opti-

mally administered a few minutes before paralysis. The dose for sedation for RSI is considerably higher than the dose used to sedate a child for a procedure such as a spinal tap. While midazolam is considered to minimally affect blood pressure, it is capable of producing hypotension in a hypovolemic or physiologically stressed patient. Midazolam is not an analgesic.

Etomidate is a rapid-acting sedative hypnotic that has the benefit of not causing cardiovascular instability or respiratory depression. In addition, etomidate decreases ICP and is therefore neuroprotective. It has a duration of action of about 5 minutes. Etomidate may cause vomiting, and myoclonic activity can occur if the patient is not paralyzed. In addition, it may suppress the synthesis of cortisol after just one dose. However, the endocrinologic side effects of etomidate can be easily treated with corticosteroids. Because it can produce rapid unconsciousness while decreasing intracranial pressure and is neuroprotective with minimal hemodynamic effects, etomidate is an excellent choice as a sedative for use in a hypovolemic trauma patient with head injury.

Thiopental is a rapid-acting sedative with anticonvulsant properties and is commonly used for patients with head injury or status epilepticus. Thiopental reduces ICP

Table 5-4. Sedative Agents for Use in Rapid Sequence Intubation

Sedatives	IV Dose (mg/kg)	Onset (min)	Effects On	
			BP	ICP
Midazolam	0.2–0.4	1–2	Minimal	Minimal
Etomidate	0.2–0.4	<1	Minimal/increase	Decrease
Thiopental	2–5	<1	Decrease	Decrease
Ketamine	1–2	1	Minimal/increase	Increase
Propofol	2–3	<1	Decrease	Decrease

and cerebral metabolic demands, making it a sedative to consider along with etomidate and possibly propofol in patients with head injury. Side effects include vasodilation and myocardial depression. Hypotension due to these effects is most often noted in hypovolemic patients, and the patient's volume status needs to be considered if thiopental is used. In addition to its cardiovascular effects, thiopental causes histamine-related bronchospasm and therefore should be used cautiously if at all for patients with reactive airway disease.

Propofol is a short-acting sedative that is a relatively new agent for use in RSI, though it has been used as an induction agent for years by anesthesiologists. The onset of action is probably faster than that of thiopental, and it may be more prone to causing hypotension and myocardial depression. Respiratory depression is minimal.

Fentanyl is an opioid agonist with a rapid onset of action, and it has the advantage of providing both sedation and analgesia with minimal cardiovascular side effects. The combined sedative and analgesic effects of fentanyl may provide a neuroprotective effect during intubation by blunting the effects of laryngoscopy. The primary use of fentanyl is probably as a continuous infusion once the patient is intubated and transferred to the intensive care unit. It takes much higher doses of fentanyl (>5 µg/kg) to produce intubating conditions than to provide pain relief (1 to 2 µg/kg).

Ketamine is a dissociative agent with sedative and analgesic properties. Ketamine acts as a sympathomimetic agent and therefore it not only stabilizes blood pressure and causes bronchodilation, but it also increases ICP. The clinical relevance of the increase in ICP induced by ketamine remains unclear, but this drawback has limited its use in head-injured patients. At this time the predominant indication for ketamine in RSI is for patients with status asthmaticus who require intubation. Ketamine requires the use of adjunctive pharmaceuticals to address the side effects of increased secretions and emergence reactions. Secretions are commonly reduced through the use of atropine or glycopyrrolate, and emergence reactions, which are more common in older children and adults, are treated prophylactically with a benzodiazepine such as midazolam.

PARALYSIS

A brief review of the physiology of nerve conduction and muscle movement will help clarify some of the differences among the paralytic agents currently used for RSI. Normally, an action potential travels down a nerve fiber and triggers the release of acetylcholine into the neuromuscular junction. Acetylcholine then binds to a nicotinic receptor on the muscle fiber, and through the opening of ion channels triggers a biochemical cascade that leads to the coupling of actin and myosin, and ultimately muscle contraction. In a nonparalyzed patient, movement is terminated after the bound acetylcholine molecule is hydrolyzed by the enzyme acetylcholinesterase. Paralytic agents are classified as either depolarizing or nondepolarizing agents. Nondepolarizing agents such as vecuronium, rocuronium, and rapacuronium attach themselves to the nicotinic receptor and competitively block acetylcholine from stimulating the receptor and triggering muscle movement. Their paralytic action ends when they diffuse away from the nicotinic receptor and are metabolized by the liver. A depolarizing agent such as succinylcholine binds to the nicotinic receptor and triggers the opening of ion channels. Initially the binding of succinylcholine to the nicotinic receptors mimics acetylcholine, leading to fasciculations. The paralytic property of succinylcholine stems from its prolonged attachment to the nicotinic receptor, which leads to prolonged depolarization of the muscle fiber, rendering it unresponsive to further acetylcholine stimulation. Over time the patient regains spontaneous movement as plasma cholinesterase produced by the liver metabolizes succinylcholine, and repolarization of the muscle fiber occurs.

Succinylcholine

Succinylcholine is a fast-acting paralytic agent with a short duration of action that is used extensively in RSI. There are side effects associated with succinylcholine, some of which preclude its use in certain clinical scenarios (Table 5-5).

In the process of inducing paralysis, succinylcholine causes transient uncontrolled muscle fasciculations, which can lead to variable degrees of muscle pain after recovery. Fasciculations can be avoided by giving a low dose of a nondepolarizing paralytic agent a few minutes prior to administering succinylcholine. This should be considered for patients >5 years of age. The defasciculating dose of medication is usually $\frac{1}{10}$ the paralyzing dose of any nondepolarizing agent (e.g., 0.1 mg/kg of rocuronium is used instead of the usual 1 mg/kg paralytic dose). For practical purposes, most RSI scenarios in the emergency department will not allow sufficient time to block the fasciculations associated with succinylcholine.

Table 5-5. Use of Succinylcholine in RSI

Contraindications
Muscular dystrophy
Neuromuscular disease
Significant burn/trauma that occurred at least 48 hours
   prior and within the previous 10 days
Personal or family history of malignant hyperthermia
Preexisting hyperkalemia

Considerations
Defasciculate if >5 years of age
Premedicate with atropine in children
Must use atropine prior to a second dose
Treat malignant hyperthermia with dantrolene

In addition to its effect on skeletal muscle, succinylcholine can cause stimulation of sympathetic and parasympathetic nicotinic receptors. In older children and adolescents, this can lead to hypertension and tachycardia. In younger children and infants, the parasympathetic response predominates and can lead to bradyarrhythmias or asystole. Premedication with atropine can minimize parasympathetic stimulation.

While succinylcholine is known to cause a clinically insignificant increase in serum potassium (0.5 to 1 mEq/L) in normal patients, there are certain situations in which serious hyperkalemia can result. In certain clinical conditions, muscle fibers develop an abundance of nicotinic receptors outside of the neuromuscular junction. Stimulation of these receptors can produce an exaggerated increase in serum potassium, which may cause significant arrhythmias or even cardiac arrest. Conditions in which this is of concern include:

- Significant crush injuries
- Severe trauma
- Burns
- Diseases causing significant muscle atrophy, such as spinal cord injury or myopathy

In general, extrajunctional nicotinic receptors do not develop until 2 to 3 days after an injury, but they may remain present for a prolonged period. Therefore, while use of succinylcholine would not be expected to cause hyperkalemia in a patient who presents immediately after being struck by a motor vehicle, it is possible that hyperkalemia might result from its use in a patient who sustained significant burns 2 weeks earlier. In extremely rare instances, patients who receive succinylcholine may develop malignant hyperthermia. An inherited condition, malignant hyperthermia is characterized by a rapid increase in the patient's body temperature and can be fatal if not identified and treated rapidly. Dantrolene sodium is the initial emergent treatment of choice for malignant hyperthermia.

Succinylcholine can increase intracranial and intraocular pressure. Its use should be avoided in patients with open globe injuries and it should be used with caution in patients with suspected increased ICP.

Nondepolarizing Agents

Of the nondepolarizing agents commonly used in RSI, vecuronium has the longest onset of action and produces the longest duration of paralysis. Rocuronium is about $\frac{1}{10}$ as potent as vecuronium, is faster acting, and produces a shorter duration of paralysis. Because of this, rocuronium is becoming a popular nondepolarizing agent in RSI. When rocuronium is used in conjunction with a rapid-acting sedative, it produces intubating conditions in <1 minute. Rocuronium can be used to paralyze any patient who needs to undergo RSI. Its rapid onset of action and relative lack of contraindications make rocuronium a strong candidate as the paralytic agent of choice for RSI. Rapacuronium is a new short-acting nondepolarizing agent with rapid onset. It is the first nondepolarizing agent to have an onset of action and duration of paralysis similar to succinylcholine (Table 5-6). To date, data on rapacuronium are conflicting. Future studies will determine its role in RSI.

Table 5-6. Paralytic Agents

Medication	IV Dose (mg/kg)	Time to Intubating Conditions (min)	Recovery (min)
Vecuronium	0.1–0.2	1–2	At least 20
Rocuronium	1–1.2	<1	At least 20
Rapacuronium	1.5–2	<1	5–7
Succinylcholine	1–2	<1	3–10

Controversy continues regarding the ideal paralytic agent to use for RSI in children. Succinylcholine reliably produces complete muscle paralysis in a short time and has a short duration of action, which is desirable in the event that the patient cannot be successfully intubated or ventilated by BMV. Succinylcholine has been used for many years and, while it has significant side effects and contraindications, these have been well studied. However, rocuronium produces intubating conditions virtually as rapidly as succinylcholine, with fewer side effects and contraindications. This may make it the most desirable paralytic agent for use in RSI. Further study and clinical experience should help clarify this situation.

CRICOID PRESSURE

The Sellick maneuver consists of the application of pressure with the thumb and index finger on the cricoid cartilage, with simultaneous dorsal and cephalad force against the sixth cervical vertebra. This maneuver occludes the esophagus and prevents passive regurgitation of stomach contents. In infant cadavers, this has been shown to effectively occlude the esophagus, even with a nasogastric tube present. Several points regarding this procedure are important. During RSI a trained individual, who is not participating in any other aspect of patient care, needs to be responsible for performing cricoid pressure. It is important to apply cricoid pressure when sedation and paralysis is initiated and to continue cricoid pressure until successful intubation is confirmed. In the event that BMV is deemed necessary, cricoid pressure should be provided even if this occurs prior to sedation and paralysis. The person performing intubation should communicate with the person providing cricoid pressure. If too much pressure is applied, the airway can also be inadvertently compressed.

ENDOTRACHEAL INTUBATION

After appropriate preparation is complete, the head is placed in the sniffing position to align the oral, pharyngeal, and laryngeal vectors. A towel placed under the shoulders may assist in alignment. The mouth is opened and the oropharynx is visualized. Any secretions or debris are removed by suctioning. The laryngoscope blade is inserted into the right corner of the mouth and the tongue is swept to the left. When using a straight blade, as is preferred for infants and young children, the epiglot-

Table 5-7. Endotracheal Tube and Laryngoscope Sizes for Pediatric Patients

Age	Tube Size[a]
Endotracheal Tubes	
Newborn	3.0 uncuffed
Newborn–6 months	3.5 uncuffed
6–18 Months	3.5–4.0 uncuffed
18 Months–3 Years	4.0–4.5 uncuffed
3–5 Years	4.5 uncuffed
5–6 Years	5.0 uncuffed
6–8 Years	5.5–6.0 uncuffed
8–10 Years	6.0 cuffed
10–12 Years	6.0–6.5 cuffed
12–14 Years	6.5–7.0 cuffed

Age	Blade Size
Laryngoscopes	
Premature (<2.5 kg)	0 straight
0–3 Months	1.0 straight
3 Months–3 years	1.5 straight
3–12 Years	2.0 straight or curved
Adolescents	3.0 straight or curved

[a]Appropriate depth of insertion can be estimated by multiplying the tube size by 3.

tis is elevated and the ETT is inserted between the vocal cords. The Sellick maneuver is initiated before insertion of the laryngoscope and maintained throughout the procedure in order to reduce the risk of vomiting and aspiration. The Sellick maneuver may also aid in visualization of the anteriorly situated vocal cords of infants and small children. The heart rate and oxygen saturation are monitored continuously during ETI.

With a well-positioned ETT of proper size (Table 5-7), an audible air leak is heard when ventilation is applied at a pressure of 15 to 20 cmH$_2$O. If no air leak is audible, the tube is too tight, and conversely if the air leak is too great, it will impair ventilation.

CONFIRMATION OF ETT PLACEMENT

Once an ETT has been placed, it is important to maintain cricoid pressure until it has been confirmed that the ETT is properly placed in the airway. Physical examination findings, including the bilateral presence of breath sounds with good chest rise, and the absence of breath sounds in the epigastric region, help confirm correct tube placement. Disposable colorimetric carbon dioxide detectors provide a quick and accurate means of determining that the ETT is in the airway. These small, lightweight plastic devices are positioned between the ETT and the resuscitation bag. If the ETT is in the airway, exhaled CO_2 changes the paper indicator from purple to yellow after several manual breaths. A lack of this color change suggests an esophageal intubation. It is important to note that while the detection of expired CO_2 confirms placement of the ETT in the airway, it does not assure proper position of the tube within the trachea. A chest radiograph will confirm that the ETT has not been inadvertently positioned in either mainstem bronchus. Once ETT placement is confirmed and the balloon is inflated (if using a cuffed ETT), cricoid pressure may be released and the tube secured.

Physicians need to be prepared for intubation in situations in which intravenous access is not available. Should such a scenario arise, one can use 4 mg/kg of succinylcholine or 2 mg/kg of rocuronium intramuscularly to induce paralysis. The paralytic effects will have a delayed onset due to the slower absorption of the medication. Appropriate sedative mediation must also be used.

It is important to mention that trauma patients need to have their cervical spine stabilized during ETI. One person on the resuscitation team should be responsible for holding the head in a neutral position during attempts at ETI performed while the cervical spine collar is off. Once the ETT is in place, the cervical collar should be replaced. Should emesis ensue, the patient as a unit should be log-rolled to minimize spinal movement.

SPECIAL SITUATIONS

Table 5-8 provides premedication and sedation suggestions. Many alternative premedications and sedatives are acceptable. The choice of pharmaceuticals is often based on personal experience, institutional formularies, and the given clinical scenario. When choosing medications for RSI, one needs to consider the time required for preparation of medications, and the clinician should recognize that in some cases the time to successful ETI may be inversely correlated to the number of pharmaceutical preparations required.

SUMMARY

Rapid sequence intubation should be considered for all patients requiring ETI in the emergency room. The procedure should take less than 5 minutes to complete and is the safest and most effective way of obtaining a definitive airway. Preoxygenation is an important component of RSI. Vomiting and aspiration are potential complications that are more likely when BMV is used. Avoidance of BMV and use of cricoid pressure can reduce the frequency of these problems. Atropine should be used in all patients under 5 years of age. The use of etomidate as a

Table 5-8. RSI Options for Special Clinical Situations

Scenario	Premedication	Sedation
Head injury or elevated ICP		
Normal BP	Lidocaine	Etomidate, thiopental, midazolam
	Consider fentanyl	
Decreased BP	Lidocaine	Etomidate, midazolam, low dose thiopental
	Consider fentanyl	
No head injury or elevated ICP		
Normal BP		Etomidate, thiopental, midazolam, ketamine
Decreased BP		Etomidate, ketamine, midazolam
Status epilepticus		Thiopental, midazolam
Status asthmaticus	Atropine	Ketamine
	Midazolam	
Any patient <5 years old	Atropine	
Ketamine used	Atropine	
	Midazolam	

sedative and rocuronium as a paralytic agent is acceptable in almost any situation. Experienced physicians may choose from a number of different premedications, sedatives, and paralytic agents, based on the clinical scenario.

BIBLIOGRAPHY

Cook DR: Can succinylcholine be abandoned? *Anesth Analg* 90:S24-28, 2000.

Doobinin KA, Nakagawa TA: Emergency department use of neuromuscular blocking agents in children. *Pediatr Emerg Care* 16:441–447, 2000.

Gerardi MJ, Sacchetti AD, Cantor RM, et al: Rapid-sequence intubation of the pediatric patient. *Ann Emerg Med* 28:55–74, 1996.

Martin LD, Bratton SL, O'Rourke PP: Clinical uses and controversies of neuromuscular blocking agents in infants and children. *Pediatr Crit Care* 27:1358–1368, 1999.

McAllister JD, Gnauck KA: Rapid sequence intubation of the pediatric patient. *Pediatr Clin North Am* 46:1249–1284, 1999.

Sokolove PE, Price DD, Okada P: The safety of etomidate for emergency rapid sequence intubation of pediatric patients. *Pediatr Emerg Care* 16:18–21, 2000.

Yamamoto LG, Yim GK, Britten AG: Rapid sequence anesthesia induction for emergency intubation. *Pediatr Emerg Care* 6:200–213, 1990.

6

Resuscitation of the Newly Born Infant

Collin S. Goto
Brian A. Bates

HIGH-YIELD FACTS

- Most newly born infants will respond to adequate stimulation and warming. Very few will require advanced life support.

- Chest compressions are only initiated if there is no pulse or if the heart rate remains <60 beats/min after adequate assisted ventilation for 30 seconds.

- Only isotonic crystalloid or packed red blood cells should be used for initial volume resuscitation. Albumin-containing solutions are no longer recommended.

- The dose of epinephrine for the newly born infant should be 0.1 to 0.3 mL/kg of 1:10,000 solution. Higher doses of epinephrine are *not* recommended.

- When meconium-stained amniotic fluid is present, the mouth, nose, and pharynx should be suctioned as soon as the head is delivered. Intratracheal suctioning should only be performed if after delivery the infant has absent or depressed respirations, decreased muscle tone, or a heart rate <100 beats/min.

- The best site to palpate for pulses in the newly born infant is the umbilicus.

- The umbilical vein is the best site for intravenous access.

- The ratio of chest compressions to ventilations in the newly born infant should be 3:1, with 90 compressions and 30 ventilations per minute.

- The recommended technique for chest compression in the newly born infant is the 2-thumb-encircling hands technique.

- Epinephrine is indicated for asystole or a heart rate <60 beats/min after 30 seconds of adequate ventilation and chest compressions.

At least 6 percent of the 3.5 million newly born infants delivered each year in the United States will require some form of life support. This percentage dramatically increases to >80% for newly born infants weighing <1500 g. While the ideal environment for neonatal resuscitation is the delivery room, it is inevitable that the emergency department physician will be confronted with a woman in labor in whom delivery cannot be delayed until she is transported to the obstetric unit. Therefore expertise in the special requirements of the newly born infant is an integral part of emergency department practice (Fig. 6-1).

PHYSIOLOGY OF THE NEWLY BORN INFANT

Many complex changes occur in the cardiovascular and respiratory systems at the moment of birth that allow gas exchange to be transferred from the placenta to the lungs. Amniotic fluid filling the lungs is expelled and ventilation and perfusion of the lungs is established. The stimuli responsible for the first fetal breath include decreased PaO_2 and pH and increased $PaCO_2$ due to interruption of the placental blood flow. Decreased body temperature and tactile stimulation are also contributing factors. The pressure required to inflate the airless lungs is high, ranging up to 40 cmH$_2$O for 0.5- to 1.0-second intervals.

Termination of placental blood flow and the onset of respirations trigger a redistribution of blood flow. Pulmonary artery pressure decreases and systemic blood pressure increases. Blood that had bypassed the fetal lungs through the ductus arteriosus is distributed to the pulmonary circulation. The ductus itself begins to close, stimulated in large part by the rising PaO_2. Within days the pattern of the mature circulation is established.

HISTORY

Even during a precipitous delivery, it is essential to obtain a brief summary of the medical history of the mother as well as the history of the current pregnancy and labor. Pertinent information from the mother includes the date

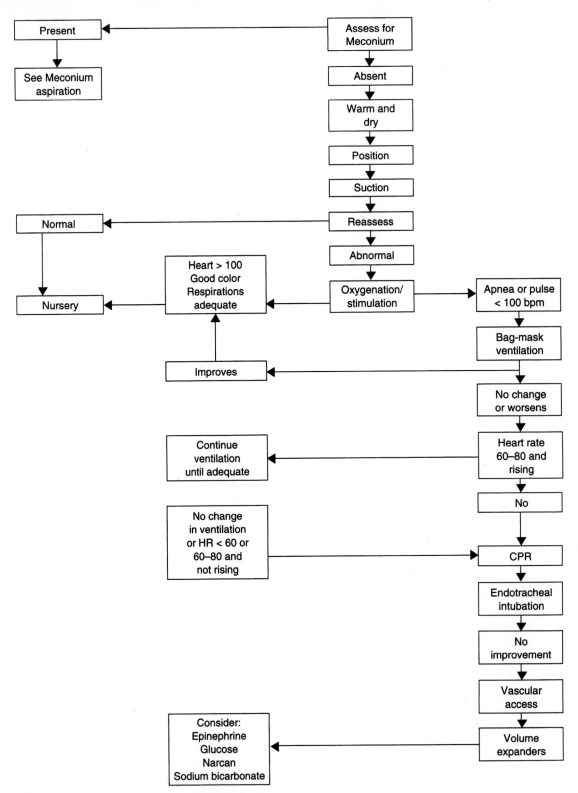

Fig. 6-1. Summary of neonatal resuscitation.

of her last menstrual period, which is essential for estimating the gestational age of the baby, and the number of previous pregnancies and living children. Any history of diabetes or hypertension should be elicited, since both medical conditions are associated with increased perinatal morbidity. A history of drug abuse alerts the physician to the possibility of narcotic-induced respiratory depression in the newly born infant, or to the potential development of a withdrawal syndrome.

A complete description of the labor should be obtained since a difficult labor or delivery may result in fetal distress and the need for aggressive intervention. Prolonged rupture of membranes, foul-smelling amniotic fluid, and maternal fever are indications of a potentially septic newborn. Meconium-stained amniotic fluid increases the risk of meconium aspiration syndrome. Vaginal bleeding associated with placenta previa or abruptio placentae can result in a shocky, asphyxiated newborn. Lack of prenatal care often implies a high-risk delivery.

ASSESSMENT OF THE NEWLY BORN INFANT

The emergency physician should be prepared to assess and manage the newly born infant. Appropriate supplies and equipment are listed in Table 6-1. The Apgar score is used to assess the overall status of the newly born infant (Table 6-2). For the purposes of resuscitation, the most important aspects of the score are heart rate, respiratory effort, and color.

The heart rate is evaluated by auscultating the chest or counting the umbilical pulse. Bradycardia is virtually always due to hypoxia and should quickly improve as the newly born infant develops effective ventilation. Color can be somewhat difficult to evaluate. Virtually all newly born infants have peripheral cyanosis, which can be distinguished from central cyanosis by assessing the tongue, which should be pink.

The muscle tone is an indication of the degree of intrauterine ischemia. An extremely hypotonic newly born infant has usually suffered prolonged hypoxia. The degree of reflex irritability is usually assessed during nasal suctioning.

Resuscitative efforts may be guided by the 1-minute Apgar score, but resuscitation should not be delayed while obtaining the score. Neonates with a 1-minute Apgar score of ≥7 require little or no resuscitation beyond gentle stimulation, drying, and suctioning of the mouth and nose. If the newly born infant has a 1-minute Apgar score of 4 to 6, mild to moderate asphyxia has occurred. Vigorous stimulation, supplemental oxygen, and other resuscitative efforts may be necessary, depending on the change in respiratory status and heart rate. If the Apgar score is ≤3, the newly born infant has been subjected to moderate to severe asphyxia, and aggressive resuscitation is initiated. All infants should be observed closely for deterioration.

RESUSCITATION

Positioning of the Newly Born Infant

The newly born infant is placed on its the back or side in a radiant warmer. The newly born infant has a relatively large tongue that can cause obstruction of the airway.

Table 6-1. Supplies for Neonatal Resuscitation

Resuscitation Tray (Sterile)	Resuscitation Equipment
Bulb syringe	Radiant warmer
DeLee suction trap	Wall suction with manometer
Endotracheal tubes (2.0, 2.5, 3.0, 3.5, and 4.0 mm)	Oxygen source with flow meter
Suction catheters (6, 8, 10, and 12F)	Resuscitation bag (250–500 mL) with manometer
Endotracheal tube stylet	Laryngoscope
Umbilical catheter (3.5, 5F)	Laryngoscope blades (Miller 0 and 1)
Syringes (5, 10, and 20 mL)	Charts with proper drug doses and equipment sizes for various sized neonates.
	Warmed linens
Three-way stopcock	
Feeding tubes (5, 8F)	
Towels	
Umbilical cord clamps	
Scissors	

Table 6-2. The Apgar Score

Parameter	0	1	2
Color	Blue, pale	Body pink, extremities blue	Totally pink
Muscle tone	None, limp	Slight flexion	Active, good flexion
Heart rate	0	<100	>100
Respiration	Absent	Slow, irregular	Strong, regular
Reflex irritability (response to nasal catheter)	None	Some grimace	Good grimace, crying

To calculate Apgar score, add numbers for all parameters together.

Placing the head in the sniffing position with a towel under the shoulders can help move the tongue away from the posterior oropharynx and open the airway. Care is taken to avoid hyperextension of the neck, since this may also cause airway obstruction.

Suctioning

After positioning the head, the newly born infant's mouth and nose are suctioned to remove amniotic fluid and mucus. A bulb syringe or DeLee suction trap is usually adequate for this purpose. If wall suction is used, pressure should not exceed 100 mmHg (136 cmH$_2$O). Deep suctioning can cause laryngospasm and bradycardia due to vagal stimulation, so the heart rate should be monitored during the procedure. Suctioning should be performed for 5-second intervals and is discontinued if severe bradycardia develops.

Tactile Stimulation

Most newly born infants with mild to moderate cardiorespiratory depression respond well to tactile stimulation, as evidenced by an increased heart rate and the development of more concerted respiratory efforts. Vigorous drying is often sufficient. Other more aggressive methods of stimulation include rubbing the infant's back and gently flicking or slapping the soles of the feet.

Thermoregulation

The process of delivery puts the newly born infant at great risk for hypothermia. A relatively large body surface area makes the newly born infant particularly vulnerable to rapid cooling as amniotic fluid evaporates. Hypothermia results in increased oxygen consumption, hypoglycemia, and if it is severe, respiratory and metabolic acidosis. Premature and asphyxiated newborns are especially vulnerable to the deleterious effects of hypothermia.

Heat loss is prevented by placing the newly born infant under a radiant warmer and quickly wiping the amniotic fluid from the skin to minimize evaporative heat loss. The newly born infant's body is then wrapped in warm blankets and the large surface area of the head is covered with a cap. However, close monitoring of the infant's temperature should continue and hyperthermia should be avoided.

Oxygen

Hypoxia is presumed to be present in any infant with even mild cardiorespiratory depression at delivery. Oxygen can be administered to infants with mild bradycardia and respiratory depression by holding the tube close to the infant's face, with a flow rate of 5 L/min. Oxygen can also be delivered by placing a mask connected to an anesthesia bag over the nose and mouth. Some self-inflating bags may not deliver sufficient oxygen unless squeezed. Once cardiopulmonary stability has been established, oxygen may be discontinued, but there is no contraindication to short-term oxygen administration for any newly born infant at this time. Recent work has shown that most newborns are adequately-resuscitated with room air; further work will clarify potential oxygen toxicity.

Bag-Valve-Mask Ventilation

Indications for initiating assisted ventilation with a bag-valve-mask device are apnea (or gasping respirations) and bradycardia (heart rate <100 beats/min) that do not respond to tactile stimulation and supplemental oxygen. Central cyanosis unresponsive to supplemental oxygen is also an indication for assisted ventilation.

Ventilations are performed with a tight fitting mask with a cushioned seal. If a self-inflating bag is used, the pop-off valve is bypassed since the initial pressures required to inflate the lungs can be as high as 40 cmH$_2$O. Subsequent breaths usually require lower pressures. A pressure manometer is useful to gauge the minimum inspiratory pressure required to produce adequate chest expansion so that excessive airway pressures can be avoided. Bag-valve-mask resuscitation of the asphyxiated newly born infant has traditionally utilized 100% oxygen. While this is still current practice, there is evidence that the majority of asphyxiated patients will respond to ventilation with room air.

The initial rate of assisted ventilation is 40 to 60 breaths/min. After 15 to 30 seconds of assisted breaths, the infant is reassessed. If resuscitation has been successful, improvement will be indicated by an increase in heart rate to >100 beats/min, the infant will begin to establish spontaneous respirations, and muscle tone and color will generally improve, although peripheral cyanosis may persist. If improvement is not apparent and the heart rate remains between 60 and 100 beats/min, assisted ventilation is continued. If the heart rate is <60 beats/min despite at least 30 seconds of assisted ventilation, begin chest compressions and intubate the infant.

Endotracheal Intubation

If there is an inadequate response to assisted ventilation, endotracheal intubation is indicated. Other indications for intubation are a requirement for endotracheal suctioning, a need for prolonged positive pressure ventilation, and extreme prematurity.

The size of the endotracheal tube depends on the patient's weight (3.5 mm internal diameter for a 3- to 4-kg newly born infant, 3.0 mm for a 2-kg newly born infant, and 2.5 mm for a 1-kg premature infant). Intubation is performed with a no. 0 or 1 straight blade. Proper tube positioning is assessed by adequate chest expansion, equal bilateral breath sounds on auscultation, and improvement in heart rate, muscle tone, and color. In addition, an exhaled CO_2 monitor may be used to verify endotracheal tube placement, but the physician should be aware that data about sensitivity and specificity of exhaled CO_2 detectors in reflecting tracheal tube position are limited in newly born infants.

In newly born infants, it is common to inadvertently intubate either of the mainstem bronchi, in which case breath sounds are heard preferentially over one hemithorax. If this occurs the tube is pulled back carefully until bilateral breath sounds are appreciated.

Particular attention should be paid to potential complications of positive pressure ventilation. Pneumothorax should be promptly decompressed by needle or tube thoracostomy. Gastric distention is promptly decompressed by nasogastric tube insertion.

Chest Compressions

Since newly born infants have limited ability to increase myocardial contractility and stroke volume, they are far more dependent than adults on heart rate to sustain adequate cardiac output. In addition, there are data to suggest that chest compressions are more effective at providing circulation in infants than in adults. Indications for chest compressions in neonates are absent pulse at any time and a heart rate <60 beats/min despite adequate assisted ventilation for 30 seconds.

There are two techniques for providing chest compressions in neonates and infants:

- In the two-finger technique, the ring and middle fingers are placed on the sternum just below the nipple line and the chest is compressed to a depth of one-third of the anterior-posterior diameter of the heart.

- In the preferred technique, the hands are wrapped around the chest and both thumbs are placed over the lower third of the sternum, again just below the nipple line. The chest is compressed to the same depth as in the two-finger technique.

Compression of the xiphoid is avoided due to the potential for injury to abdominal organs. The ratio of chest compressions to ventilations is 3:1 with 90 compressions and 30 ventilations per minute. Adequacy of chest compressions is assessed by the generation of palpable umbilical artery pulses.

It is extremely important to remember that in the vast majority of depressed neonates, bradycardia is secondary to hypoxia. Ventilation with 100 percent oxygen is continued during chest compressions. Reassessment of the infant's heart rate should be done every 30 seconds and compressions continued until the heart rate is sustained at >60 beats/min.

Vascular Access

In a newly born infant who does not respond to assisted ventilation and chest compressions, it is necessary to obtain vascular access in order to deliver medication and fluids. The preferred site of access is the umbilical vein, which is easily located and cannulated. The vein is distinguished from the umbilical arteries by the fact that it is solitary, while the arteries are paired. The vein also has a thin, distensible wall, while each artery has a narrow lumen lined with a muscular layer that constricts when the umbilical cord is cut. To insert an umbilical vein catheter, the umbilical cord is trimmed with a scalpel to 1 cm above the skin. The umbilical stump is encircled with a ligature that is secured tightly enough to prevent excessive bleeding. A 3.5 or 5F umbilical catheter is inserted just below the skin, and effective cannulation is assured by the free flow of blood on aspiration. Deep insertion of the catheter is avoided because this can result in the infusion of hypertonic fluids into the liver. The catheter is sutured in place to avoid inadvertent dislodgment and hemorrhage.

Pharmacologic Agents

Epinephrine

Epinephrine is the most important drug used in infant resuscitation. Indications for its use are asystole and a heart rate that remains ≤60 despite effective ventilation with 100 percent oxygen and chest compressions for more than 30 seconds. The dose of epinephrine is 0.1 to 0.3 mL/kg (0.01 to 0.03 mg/kg) of 1:10,000 solution given intravenously, but the drug can also be given intratracheally. Despite indications that a higher dose of epinephrine must be administered intratracheally to achieve adequate blood levels, there is insufficient evidence to recommend this in newly born infants, and currently the same dose is recommended for intravenous and intratracheal administration. Epinephrine is given every 3 to 5 minutes. An intratracheal dose can be diluted to 1 to 2 mL with normal saline.

Sodium Bicarbonate

Sodium bicarbonate buffers hydrogen ion and reverses metabolic acidosis, but may cause hyperosmolarity and increased intracellular acidosis. An intravenous dose of 1 to 2 mEq/kg of 0.5 mEq/mL solution may be considered in cases of prolonged resuscitation only after adequate ventilation and perfusion are established.

Naloxone Hydrochloride

Naloxone is a direct narcotic antagonist. It is indicated to reverse respiratory depression in the newly born infant that results from administration of narcotics to the mother within 4 hours of delivery. Since the duration of action of naloxone is longer than that of narcotics, infants treated with naloxone must be observed closely for recurrent respiratory depression. In infants of narcotic-addicted mothers, naloxone can induce a severe drug withdrawal syndrome.

The dose of naloxone is 0.1 mg/kg given intravenously, intratracheally, intramuscularly, or subcutaneously. The standard form of 0.4 mg/mL should be utilized.

Glucose

Hypoglycemia commonly occurs in infants born to diabetic mothers and in premature infants. Glycogen stores are low and glucose needs are high in premature and other stressed neonates, therefore rapid blood glucose determination should be made in all such situations. Signs of hypoglycemia include jitteriness, hypotonia, hypertonia, seizures, and coma.

Hypoglycemia in the newly born infant is defined as blood glucose <40 to 50 mg/dL. If the infant is symptomatic due to hypoglycemia, intravenous glucose administration is necessary. In contrast to older children and adults, a 2- to 4-mL/kg bolus of a 10 percent glucose solution should be used to correct hypoglycemia. Higher concentrations may lead to hyperosmolarity and possibly intraventricular hemorrhage, particularly in premature infants. Intravenous glucose is continued as an infusion to deliver 6 to 8 mg/kg of glucose/min until the infant is stabilized and can tolerate oral feedings.

Volume Expanders

Volume expansion is indicated to restore circulating blood volume. Conditions that can produce acute blood loss in the newly born infant are placenta previa, abruptio placentae, and twin-twin transfusion. Significant blood loss can also occur if the umbilical cord is clamped prematurely, resulting in interruption of placental flow.

The detection of acute anemia in the newly born infant can be extremely difficult and a high level of suspicion is necessary to make the diagnosis before cardiovascular collapse occurs. Profound vasoconstriction may cause the infant to appear pale despite adequate oxygenation and peripheral pulses may be diminished.

The average term newly born infant's hemoglobin is 16.8 gm/dL. Hemoglobin levels are lower for premature infants, with the average for a 34-week infant being 15 g/dL and that for a 28-week infant being only 14.5 g/dL. In the setting of placental disruption, the initial hemoglobin may be normal. Nevertheless, volume resuscitation is initiated and levels are rechecked periodically.

Volume resuscitation is accomplished with 10-mL/kg infusions of normal saline or Ringer's lactate administered over 5 to 10 minutes. Packed red blood cells, crossmatched with maternal and neonatal blood may be necessary. Uncrossmatched O-negative blood is administered to the severely anemic infant when there is not enough time to wait for a full type and crossmatch.

Special Situations

Meconium

Approximately 12 percent of deliveries are complicated by the presence of meconium in the amniotic fluid. Meconium is especially likely if there is fetal distress or asphyxia. The aspiration of meconium can cause airway obstruction, hyperinflation, air leaks, and severe pneumonitis. Profound hypoxia and, in severe cases, persistence of the fetal circulation can result. Meconium aspiration syndrome is more likely if the material is thick and particulate.

If meconium is present in the amniotic fluid, the infant's oropharynx is suctioned as the head is delivered, prior to delivery of the body and clamping of the cord. If after delivery the infant has absent or depressed respirations, a heart rate of <100 beats/min, and poor muscle tone, direct tracheal suctioning should be performed. Under laryngoscopic visualization, the trachea is intubated with an endotracheal tube connected to a meconium aspirator and wall suction. Suction is applied as the tube is slowly withdrawn. The process is repeated until the trachea is free of meconium. In the event that the infant becomes severely bradycardic, clinical judgment is used to determine when suctioning is discontinued and positive pressure ventilation is instituted. The vigorous newly born infant with meconium-stained fluid usually does not require tracheal suctioning.

Prematurity

A newly born infant is considered premature if born before completing 37 weeks of gestation. The premature newly born infant presents a complex set of problems that require special consideration and management. Birth asphyxia is more likely in preterm labor. The immature lungs are deficient in surfactant, which leads to decreased lung compliance, atelectasis, and the respiratory distress syndrome of prematurity. The premature infant has decreased muscle mass and metabolic reserve and tires easily from the work of breathing. The underdeveloped chest wall is extremely compliant, creating a mechanical disadvantage due to paradoxical chest wall motion. The premature nervous system is immature, resulting in apnea and periodic breathing. The subependymal germinal matrix of the brain is extremely fragile and intracranial hemorrhage is common, especially when the neonate is subjected to hypoxia or rapid changes in blood pressure or osmolarity. The epidermis is thin and the body surface relatively large, predisposing to hypothermia.

The determination of viability has become very complex as new technologies have evolved. Unfortunately, the emergency physician is not usually in a position to consider long-term viability or quality of life prior to acting. Whenever an infant is born with a pulse and spontaneous respirations, initial resuscitative efforts should be initiated. The decision to discontinue support should be based on the infant's response to resuscitation and in consultation with a neonatologist.

Diaphragmatic Hernia

The combination of a scaphoid abdomen, cyanosis, and respiratory distress suggests a diaphragmatic hernia. Diaphragmatic hernias occur most commonly on the left side (Bochdalek type). The presence of abdominal contents in the left hemithorax results in varying degrees of hypoplasia of the left lung. Right lung hypoplasia can also occur due to displacement of the heart and mediastinum into the right chest. Breath sounds are diminished or absent on the left, and heart sounds can be heard in the right chest.

In the presence of a diaphragmatic hernia, bag-valve-mask ventilation is contraindicated, since this can fill the stomach and bowel with gas and further compromise respiratory status. The infant is intubated and the lungs expanded and ventilated. A nasogastric tube is placed to deflate the stomach. Early transport to a tertiary care facility with pediatric surgery and neonatal intensive care capabilities is imperative. Many of these infants will require extracorporeal membrane oxygenation or high-frequency ventilation due to their severe lung disease.

Infant of a Diabetic Mother

Diabetes occurs in 3 to 4 percent of pregnancies and remains a significant cause of perinatal morbidity and mortality. High maternal blood glucose results in high fetal insulin levels, which can lead to fetal macrosomia, functional immaturity, and a host of other problems. These include birth asphyxia, hyaline membrane disease, polycythemia and hyperviscosity syndrome, renal vein thrombosis, and hyperbilirubinemia. Associated congenital malformations include congenital heart disease, the caudal regression syndrome, and small left colon syndrome. Associated metabolic abnormalities include hypocalcemia and severe hypoglycemia.

Gastroschisis and Omphalocele

These congenital malformations occur when there is herniation of the abdominal contents through the umbilical ring. Herniation usually involves only the intestines, but in severe cases can involve other abdominal organs. An omphalocele is covered by a thin layer of peritoneum, while a gastroschisis is not.

The protruding organs should not be forced back into the abdominal cavity. They are covered with a sterile saline-soaked dressing and a sterile plastic bag to prevent evaporation and desiccation. Intravenous volume resuscitation may be indicated. After the infant is stabilized, a nasogastric tube is placed. Urgent pediatric surgical consultation and transfer to a tertiary pediatric facility with neonatal intensive care capabilities is indicated.

BIBLIOGRAPHY

American Heart Association in Collaboration with the International Liaison Committee on Resuscitation: Guidelines 2000 for cardiopulmonary resuscitation and emergency cardiovascular care: An international consensus on science. Part II: Neonatal resuscitation. *Circulation* 102(suppl I):I-343, 2000.

Finer NN, Horbar JD, Carpenter JH: Cardiopulmonary resuscitation in the very low birth weight infant: The Vermont Oxford Network Experience. *Pediatrics* 104:428-434, 1999.

Saugstad OD, Rootwelt T, Aalen O: Resuscitation of asphyxiated newborn infants with room air or oxygen: An international controlled trial: The resair 2 study. *Pediatrics* 102:130–133, 1998.

Thibeault DW, Haney B: Lung volume, pulmonary vasculature and factors affecting survival in congenital diaphragmatic hernia. *Pediatrics* 101:289–295, 1998.

Vento M, Asanel M, Jastar J, et al: Resuscitation with room air instead of 100% oxygen prevents oxidative stress in moderately asphyxiated term neonates. *Pediatrics* 107(4):642-647, 2001.

Wiswell TE, Gannon CM, Jacob J, et al: Delivery room management of the apparently vigorous meconium-stained neonate: Results of the multicenter, international collaborative trial. *Pediatrics* 105:1–7, 2000.

7

Sudden Infant Death Syndrome and Apparent Life-Threatening Events

Collin S. Goto
Thomas T. Mydler

HIGH-YIELD FACTS

- SIDS remains the most common cause of infant death beyond the neonatal period, with a peak incidence between 2 and 4 months of age.
- Prone sleeping is associated with an increased incidence of SIDS. The SIDS rate in the United States has decreased significantly since the initiation of the Back to Sleep campaign.
- An apparent life-threatening event (ALTE) is characterized by apnea, decreased mental status, color change, alteration in muscle tone, or choking.
- Common causes of ALTE include gastroesophageal reflux and apnea secondary to respiratory infections. Other important causes of ALTE include seizures, meningitis, sepsis, occult trauma, arrhythmias, and metabolic defects.
- Infants with a true life-threatening event should be admitted to the hospital for further monitoring and evaluation.

SUDDEN INFANT DEATH SYNDROME

Sudden infant death syndrome (SIDS) is defined as the sudden death of an infant <1 year of age, which remains unexplained after a thorough case investigation, including a complete autopsy, examination of the death scene, and review of the clinical history. Every emergency department physician should be prepared to manage the infant who presents with SIDS or an apparent life-threatening event (ALTE). It is equally important that the

physician give a thorough, well-informed, and compassionate explanation of the situation to the parents, who will undoubtedly be anxious and distressed.

Epidemiology and Pathophysiology

SIDS remains the most common cause of infant death beyond the neonatal period. The peak incidence is between 2 and 4 months of age and it is more common in males and during the winter months. The rate of SIDS is highest among American Indians and blacks, intermediate among Hispanics and whites, and lowest among Asians.

Multiple risk factors have been associated with SIDS (Table 7-1) but the exact etiology is not yet completely understood. There is postmortem evidence that certain victims of SIDS have an abnormality of the arcuate nucleus, an area of the brain stem that regulates the hypercapneic ventilatory response, chemosensitivity, blood pressure, and arousal responses to noxious stimuli. It is likely that there is a complex interaction between an infant's underlying ability to maintain cardiorespiratory stability and the various environmental risk factors, that ultimately leads to SIDS.

Prone sleeping is the environmental risk factor with the greatest potential for modification. Protective reflexes, such as swallowing to clear the airway of noxious stimuli, and arousal responses to the laryngeal chemoreceptor reflex and the baroreceptor reflex are diminished in the prone compared to the supine sleeping position. It is important to note that the SIDS rate in the United States has decreased by >40 percent since the 1992 recommendation by the American Academy of Pediatrics that infants be placed to sleep on their backs (supine) and the initiation of the Back to Sleep campaign in 1994. Other modifiable risk factors include asphyxiation hazards such as soft sleep surfaces and loose bedding, including pillows, quilts, comforters, and sheepskins. Infants who sleep in adult beds or on sofas with adults are also at increased risk of SIDS.

Evaluation and Management

Typically, the SIDS victim is found by a caregiver after having been asleep for a variable length of time. An ambulance is called, and most SIDS victims receive some prehospital care prior to arriving at the emergency department. The nature of the situation is such that it is often difficult to tell how long the infant has been pulseless and apneic. In the absence of dependent lividity or rigor mortis, resuscitation is indicated and should follow

Table 7-1. Risk Factors Associated With SIDS

Infant Factors	Maternal Factors
Male sex	Age <20 years
Preterm birth	Short interpregnancy interval
Low birth weight	Unmarried
Multiple births	Low socioeconomic status
Low Apgar scores	Low educational level
Treatment in an intensive care unit	Inadequate prenatal care
Congenital defects	Illness during pregnancy
Neonatal respiratory abnormalities	Smoking during pregnancy
	Use of addictive drugs
Recent viral illness	
Previous ALTE	
Sibling who died of SIDS	
Prone sleeping position	
Sleeping on a soft surface	
Bed sharing	
Overheating	

the guidelines set forth in the chapter on pediatric cardiopulmonary resuscitation.

The usual cardiac situation encountered is asystole. However, pulseless electrical activity, bradycardia, or rarely other arrhythmias may be encountered. The prognosis for an infant with asystole on arrival to the emergency department is exceedingly poor. Resuscitative efforts are terminated when there is no response to interventions and further efforts are considered futile. The victim is unlikely to survive if there has been no response to adequate cardiopulmonary resuscitation and at least two doses of epinephrine.

During the resuscitation, it is important that the family be kept informed of the progress of the situation. The decision to allow the parents in the room during the resuscitation should be considered based on local practice and the parents' wishes. As soon as possible, the parents should be interviewed regarding the events leading up to the discovery of the infant. Information solicited should include past medical history, present illnesses, current medications, and any history of trauma. The child is carefully examined for any congenital abnormalities, signs of concurrent illness, or evidence of physical abuse. All of this information is carefully documented in the medical record, along with the medical treatment during the resuscitation.

Disposition

In the event that a perfusing rhythm is restored, the child is stabilized to the degree possible and admitted to a pediatric intensive care unit. Further interventions and diagnostic evaluation depend on the patient's condition and likely etiology of the event. The parents should be made aware that the return of spontaneous circulation may be transient, with death occurring subsequently in the intensive care unit. Alternatively, spontaneous circulation may persist, but the child may be declared brain dead due to severe hypoxic-ischemic insult.

After an unsuccessful resuscitation, the parents should be allowed to see and hold the baby and be given the details of the resuscitation and more information about SIDS. Social work and pastoral support should be begun as soon as possible to assist the family. Parental grief and guilt is universal in this situation. It is important to stress the importance of the autopsy, since it helps to confirm the diagnosis of SIDS or establish another etiology for the infant's death. This often helps give the family closure.

THE APPARENT LIFE-THREATENING EVENT

An ALTE is an episode characterized by a combination of apnea (respiratory pause >15 seconds), decreased mental status, color change (pallor or cyanosis), alteration in muscle tone (rigidity or limpness), or choking. The infant usually requires some degree of stimulation or resuscitation, but occasionally recovers spontaneously and is subsequently brought to medical attention. Any infant with an ALTE who has cardiopulmonary compromise upon arrival to the emergency department should be appropriately resuscitated and stabilized. However, the majority will appear well, and the challenge for the emergency department physician is to differentiate between a true life-threatening event and a non–life-threatening occurrence. Most parents are understandably anxious in such a situation, and it may be difficult to obtain accurate information about the patient's current medical history.

Differential Diagnosis

The differential diagnosis of an ALTE is extensive because apnea is the final common pathway for many disease processes seen in infants (Table 7-2). Common causes of ALTE include laryngospasm secondary to gastroesophageal reflux and apnea secondary to viral upper

Table 7-2. Differential Diagnosis of an Apparent Life-Threatening Event

Central Nervous System
   Seizure
   Meningitis/encephalitis
   Head trauma (e.g., child abuse)
   Increased intracranial pressure (e.g., congenital
      hydrocephalus)
   Apnea of prematurity
   Idiopathic central apnea

Respiratory System
   Upper airway obstruction (e.g., nasal congestion)
   Laryngospasm (e.g., gastroesophageal reflux)
   Bronchiolitis (e.g., respiratory syncytial virus)
   Pneumonia

Cardiovascular System
   Arrhythmia (e.g., prolonged QT syndrome)
   Myocarditis
   Severe anemia
   Hemorrhage (e.g., child abuse)

Systemic/Metabolic/Other
   Sepsis
   Hypoglycemia
   Inborn error of metabolism
   Toxins/drugs
   Factitious (e.g., Munchausen's syndrome by proxy)

respiratory infections, bronchiolitis, or pneumonia. Other important though less common etiologies include seizures, meningitis, sepsis, occult trauma secondary to child abuse, arrhythmias secondary to prolonged QT syndrome, and inborn errors of metabolism. A probable cause of the ALTE can be found after thorough evaluation in approximately 50 percent of patients, leaving the remaining 50 percent with an unexplained ALTE. The risk of SIDS should be carefully evaluated in any infant with an unexplained ALTE. However, the exact relationship between ALTE and SIDS is not clear. Therefore, older terms for ALTE such as "near-miss SIDS" and "aborted SIDS" are misleading and no longer appropriate.

History

The parents should be questioned closely about the details of the ALTE, especially regarding the infant's respiratory effort, skin color, mental status, muscle tone, the duration of the event, and the degree of resuscitation required prior to evaluation in the emergency department.

True apnea must be distinguished from the normal periodicity of breathing that occurs during infancy. The parents are usually unable to accurately estimate the duration of the ALTE due to their own anxiety during the event, therefore the association of apnea or respiratory difficulty with pallor or cyanosis is significant. Normal periodic breathing is not associated with skin color changes. Facial color changes are common in infants with a history of choking or gagging, and it is important to distinguish true cyanosis from the more common facial redness and flushing. The infant's mental status during the event is also important. An infant who remains awake and alert during an event is unlikely to have suffered prolonged hypoxia or an acute neurological event such as a seizure. Likewise, the history of muscle tone can provide important information. Hypotonia associated with apnea or color change implies significant hypoxia or decreased cerebral perfusion, while hypertonicity is characteristic of seizures. A history of apnea that required vigorous physical stimulation or cardiopulmonary resuscitation is ominous and implies a true life-threatening event.

Information is also gathered concerning any recent illness that may have contributed to the ALTE. A history of fever alerts the physician to the possibility of sepsis or meningitis. A preceding respiratory illness implies the possibility of apnea due to upper respiratory obstruction, bronchiolitis, or pneumonia. Vomiting and diarrhea can lead to hypoglycemia or significant electrolyte abnormalities. A history of regurgitation with feedings suggests the possibility of laryngospasm secondary to gastroesophageal reflux. The infant with a preexisting neurological disorder may be at increased risk of seizures. Intentional or unintentional trauma can lead to apnea due to severe head and chest injuries or exsanguination secondary to occult intracranial, intrathoracic, or intraabdominal hemorrhage.

A family history of other infants with sudden death alerts the physician to the possibility of inherited disorders, such as inborn errors of metabolism or the prolonged QT syndrome. A history of a sibling with SIDS is a recognized risk factor for sudden death. In addition, cases of multiple infant deaths due to child abuse within a family have been reported. Finally, the possibility of factitious ALTE due to Munchausen's syndrome by proxy must be considered in the infant who repeatedly presents with an ALTE or other unexplained illnesses. The physician should be alerted to the possibility of child abuse or Munchausen's syndrome by proxy if the history is inconsistent and the parents' reaction to the situation is abnormal.

Evaluation and Management

The initial evaluation of the ill-appearing infant should be directed at identifying and stabilizing immediate life-threatening conditions. Attention is focused on establishing a patent airway and adequate breathing and circulation. Vital signs are obtained, cardiac monitors are placed, and intravenous access established as needed. Pulse oximetry and rapid bedside glucose and hemoglobin determinations will give immediate feedback as to whether the infant is hypoxic, hypoglycemic, or anemic. An arterial blood gas analysis is a sensitive indicator of overall physiologic status and is useful in any infant who appears unstable. After the initial evaluation is completed, a more thorough head-to-toe examination of the infant is performed. This secondary survey is directed at identifying any physical findings that may elucidate the etiology of the ALTE.

The many diagnostic studies to be considered in the evaluation of an ALTE reflect the diverse differential diagnosis. Selection should be guided by the presentation of the infant. For example, if a serious bacterial infection is suspected, a complete blood count, blood culture, urinalysis with urine culture, and lumbar puncture are performed prior to initiation of age-appropriate antibiotics. Nasopharyngeal swabs for viral identification are considered when a viral respiratory infection is suspected, especially respiratory syncytial virus. A chest radiograph is obtained for any infant with respiratory or cardiac abnormalities. In addition, a bedside electrocardiogram is useful to assess for cardiac pathology including prolonged QT syndrome, Wolff-Parkinson-White syndrome, myocarditis, or anomalous left coronary artery with myocardial ischemia. If the history suggests a seizure, serum electrolytes, glucose, blood urea nitrogen, serum creatinine, calcium, magnesium, and phosphorus are obtained. Consideration is given to obtaining a computed axial tomography scan of the head, skeletal survey, and drug screen if child abuse is suspected. When an inborn error of metabolism is suspected, blood for glucose, ammonia, amino acids, and urine for organic acids are obtained. Other studies may be indicated, depending on the clinical scenario.

Disposition

An infant may be discharged from the emergency department if a detailed history does not indicate that a true apneic event has occurred as long as the infant is doing well and has a normal physical examination. Examples of such a situation include periodic breathing mistaken for apnea or a minor coughing or gagging episode. A reasonable period of observation in the emergency department during which the infant is asymptomatic while sleeping and feeding is important, but does not prove that the prior event was insignificant and does not rule out recurrence. After parental education, the infant may be discharged home with specific instructions for follow-up in 24 hours with a primary care provider or return to the emergency department sooner if any problems occur. Any infant with a history of true apnea, pallor, cyanosis, limpness, or unresponsiveness requiring vigorous physical stimulation or cardiopulmonary resuscitation is excluded from outpatient consideration. If there is any question about the nature of the event, the parents' ability to care for the infant at home, or the adequacy of follow-up, it is best to err on the side of caution and admit the infant for observation and monitoring.

Any infant with a true life-threatening event is placed on a cardiopulmonary monitor and admitted to the hospital after emergency department evaluation. Further studies that may be considered include an electroencephalogram to evaluate for the possibility of seizures and a pneumogram to delineate central and obstructive apnea. An esophageal pH probe study and barium swallow are helpful in identifying gastroesophageal reflux. Any infant who is unstable is admitted to the pediatric intensive care unit.

BIBLIOGRAPHY

American Academy of Pediatrics Task Force on Infant Sleep Position and Sudden Infant Death Syndrome: Changing concepts of sudden infant death syndrome: Implications for infant sleeping environment and sleep position. *Pediatrics* 105(3):650–656, 2000.

Emery JL, Howat AJ, Variend S, et al: Investigation of inborn errors of metabolism in unexpected infant deaths. *Lancet* 2:29, 1988.

Gilbert-Barness E, Braness LA: Cause of death: SIDS or something else? *Contemp Pediatr* 9:13, 1992.

Guntheroth WG, Lohmann R, Spiers PS: Risk of sudden infant death syndrome in subsequent siblings. *J Pediatr* 4:520, 1990.

Ramanathan R, Coruin MJ, Hunt CE, et al: Cardiorespiratory events recorded on home moniters. *JAMA* 285:2199-2207, 2001.

Reece RM: Fatal child abuse and sudden infant death syndrome: A critical diagnostic decision. *Pediatrics* 91:423, 1993.

Schwartz PJ, Stramba-Badiale M, Segantini A, et al: Prolongation of the QT interval and the sudden infant death syndrome. *N Engl J Med* 338:1709–1714, 1998.

Willinger M, James LS, Catz C: Defining the sudden infant death syndrome (SIDS): Deliberations of an expert panel convened by the National Institute of Child Health and Human Development. *Pediatr Pathol* 11:677, 1991.

8

Discontinuation of Life Support

Brian A. Bates

HIGH-YIELD FACTS

- In the emergency department, the decision to terminate resuscitation is usually based on the patient's response to advanced life support. Death is defined by the failure to generate a spontaneous perfusing rhythm despite standard resuscitative measures.

- In children, the failure to respond to 2 standard doses of epinephrine is highly correlated with death. This is not an "official" standard, however, and, in the absence of such a standard of care, the physician must decide in an individual situation when she or he feels comfortable in withdrawing advanced cardiac life support (ACLS).

- The risk is that prolonged resuscitative efforts will ultimately succeed in generating a perfusing rhythm in a patient with terminal or extremely severe neurologic impairment, who then languishes in a vegetative state.

- Cold-water drowning is perhaps the most common clinical situation in which very long resuscitations have occasionally produced viable survivors. In any situation in which the patient is hypothermic, resuscitation is generally continued until the patient is adequately warmed.

- Resuscitation is not indicated, either in the emergency department or in the field, for patients with rigor mortis, dependent lividity, or decapitation.

- Terminally ill children may have advance directives in the form of do-not-resuscitate (DNR) orders. Such directives require a written statement from the patient's attending physician and are revocable at any time.

- In the past, medical personnel were commonly taught procedures, particularly intubation, using patients who had expired in the emergency department or who were dead on arrival. Ethically, the practice of postmortem endotracheal intubation has support, since it is a noninvasive procedure that does not mutilate the patient and can provide a practitioner with life-saving skills.

- Patients who suffer brain death but who are candidates for organ donation may be identified in the emergency department, and it may be justifiable to approach family members to discuss the possibility of organ donation.

To withhold or withdraw life support from a child is a very difficult decision for both parents and physicians. It is especially difficult in an emergency department, where the patient's past medical history is likely to be unavailable and there is inadequate information to decide quickly whether to withhold support. Even in patients with obvious terminal disease, there is often no do-not-resuscitate (DNR) order, and the patient's personal physician may be unavailable in a timely fashion. In such a situation, denying the patient advanced life support can precipitate an emotional and medicolegal disaster.

In the emergency department, the decision to terminate resuscitation is usually based on the patient's response to advanced life support. Death is defined by the failure to generate a spontaneous perfusing rhythm despite standard resuscitative measures. However, once cardiopulmonary resuscitation is initiated, there are no absolute guidelines to determine how long the effort is continued until death is declared. In children, the failure to respond to 2 standard doses of epinephrine is highly correlated with death, but this is not an "official" standard, and, in the absence of such a standard of care, the physician must decide in an individual situation when she or he feels comfortable in withdrawing advanced cardiac life support (ACLS). The risk is that prolonged resuscitative efforts will ultimately succeed in generating a perfusing rhythm in a patient with terminal or extremely severe neurologic impairment, who then languishes in a vegetative state.

There are certain medical situations that appear to justify prolonged resuscitations. Cold-water drowning is perhaps the most common clinical situation in which very long resuscitations have occasionally produced viable survivors. In any situation in which the patient is hypothermic, resuscitation is generally continued until the patient is adequately warmed.

Resuscitation is not indicated, either in the emergency department or in the field, for patients with rigor mortis, dependent lividity, or decapitation.

Terminally ill children may have advance directives in the form of DNR orders. Such directives require a written statement from the patient's attending physician and are revocable at any time. When a patient arrives in the emergency department with a DNR order, it is reviewed by the attending physician with the parents or legal guardian. There are often time limits on DNR orders, and other hospital-specific guidelines may exist.

In the past, medical personnel were commonly taught procedures, particularly intubation, using patients who had expired in the emergency department or who were dead on arrival. Ethically, the practice of postmortem endotracheal intubation has support, since it is a noninvasive procedure that does not mutilate the patient and can provide a practitioner with life-saving skills. More invasive procedures are performed only with the consent of the parents or guardian. When the patient is to be referred to the medical examiner, invasive procedures are avoided.

In the event that patients who undergo resuscitation in the emergency department develop a perfusing rhythm, they are transferred to an intensive care unit, where a definitive assessment of the patient's neurologic status is carried out. The ability of technology to sustain cardiopulmonary function despite cessation of neurologic activity has led to the development of criteria for brain death. Brain death is generally considered as the irreversible cessation of all neurologic activity and justifies the withdrawal of medical support. It is extremely unlikely that, in an acute insult, brain death will be declared in the emergency department. In some situations, such as severe head trauma, it may be obvious that a terminal neurologic insult has occurred, and it may be appropriate to advise the parents or guardian of this. Patients who suffer brain death but who are candidates for organ donation may be identified in the emergency department, and it may be justifiable to approach family members to discuss the possibility of organ donation.

BIBLIOGRAPHY

American Heart Association and International Liaison Committee on Resuscitation: Ethical aspects of CPR and ECC and pediatric advanced life support, in *Guidelines 2000 for Cardiopulmonary Resuscitation and Emergency Cardiovascular Care. Circulation* 102(suppl 1):I-12–I-21 and I-291–I-342, 2000.

Chipman C, Adelman R, Sexton G: Criteria for cessation of CPR in the emergency department. *Ann Emerg Med* 10:11, 1981.

DeBard ML: Cardiopulmonary resuscitation: Analysis of six years' experience and review of the literature. *Ann Emerg Med* 10:408, 1981.

Eliastam M: When to stop cardiopulmonary resuscitation. *Topics Emerg Med* 1:109, 1979.

Ludwig S, Kettrick RG, Parker M: Pediatric cardiopulmonary resuscitation: A review of 130 cases. *Clin Pediatr* 23:71, 1984.

9

Death of a Child

William R. Ahrens

HIGH-YIELD FACTS

- In contrast to patients who die in the hospital or in hospice, the majority of patients who are pronounced dead in emergency departments die suddenly and survivors are confronted with the loss of a loved one with no prior psychological preparation.

- The majority of emergency physicians feel that managing the death of a child is far more stressful than managing the death of an adult; some feel it is the most difficult aspect of their job.

- The immediate reaction of family members to the sudden loss of a child is disbelief, even though many say they knew before being told that their child had died. A sense of guilt is probably universal.

- The process of dealing with the patient's death begins with and should be considered an important part of the resuscitation.

- After the patient is pronounced dead, it is the attending physician who is responsible for telling the parents.

- The physician must introduce him- or herself, make eye contact and address the parents by name. The language used must be direct and nonjudgmental and it cannot be overemphasized that the deceased patient should be referred to by his or her name.

- Most, but not all, parents find that spending time with the child is helpful. In certain cases, some family members will want to hold the body, but reluctance to do this is normal for others and is neither a pathological response nor indicative of abuse.

- There are many support groups available for parents who have lost children. For many surviving family members, such support groups are extremely helpful.

- Dealing with the effect of the death of a child on the emergency department staff is also problematic. Some emergency physicians and other staff members utilize grief-counseling services, but this service is by no means universally available.

- It is likely that educating physicians and staff in the best way to communicate the death of a child to parents does help to alleviate some of the anxiety that the situation entails. At the very least, it creates a mutually supportive culture within the department regarding the management of death.

Dealing with death is a fact of life for the emergency physician. In contrast to patients who die in the hospital or in hospice, the majority of patients who are pronounced dead in emergency departments die suddenly and survivors are confronted with the loss of a loved one with no prior psychological preparation. They receive the news from strangers in the potentially chaotic, intimidating environment of a busy emergency department, and are required to make heart-wrenching decisions in a brutally short period of time. It is the challenge of the emergency department staff to create an environment in which bereaved survivors are treated with consideration and empathy, in a way such that informing the loved ones of a child's death is a constructive first step in the long process of healing.

EFFECTS ON PHYSICIANS AND PARENTS

In general, emergency physicians find it emotionally difficult to deal with the death of a patient, and this is particularly true when the patient is an infant or child. The majority of emergency physicians feel that managing the death of a child is far more stressful than managing the death of an adult; many feel it is the most difficult aspect of their job. Physicians often feel guilty and inadequate after a failed pediatric resuscitation, even when they know that the patient had no chance of recovery. Many feel impaired for the remainder of their shift. Few have had any formal training in how to tell parents that their child is dead. This may contribute to the fact that many parents leave the interview with the impression that the physician is cold and uncaring, a phenomenon that has profound long-term effects on the way survivors grieve. Family members who perceive the physician or staff as uncaring often believe that they are being held responsible for their child's death. This is particularly true for babies who die of sudden infant death syndrome (SIDS).

The immediate reaction of family members to the sudden loss of a child is disbelief, even though many say they knew before being told that their child had died. A sense of guilt is probably universal. Parents describe the experience in the emergency department as one that is replayed "like a tape" thousands of times in their minds, often for years after the event. They can often recall very minute details, and can recite verbatim exactly what they were told and by whom. This is the normal reaction to a traumatic event. Long-term effects on families are less clear and more difficult to study. The loss of a child certainly has profound implications for surviving siblings, whose entire relationship with the family suddenly changes, and who in some way may themselves feel responsible for their brother or sister's death. Grandparents too feel profound loss. While some say that divorce is more common in families who lose children, this is bitterly disputed by many bereaved parents.

THE INTERVIEW

Given the reality that the vast majority of pediatric patients who arrive pulseless and apneic will die in the emergency department, the process of dealing with the patient's death begins with and should be considered an important part of the resuscitation. Parents should be placed in a private, quiet room with adequate seating. A member of the resuscitation team is designated to communicate with the family. Ideally, this is a senior member of the team; it is neither desirable nor fair to give this difficult job to a junior member inexperienced in delivering bad news. One of the most common complaints of families whose loved one died in an emergency department is that they were not kept informed of the progress of the resuscitation. There are some families who will want to be present during the resuscitation. There is a growing body of research that indicates that this is helpful for both the family and staff. The decision to allow or invite family members into the resuscitation room depends largely on the comfort level of the team performing the resuscitation. However, family presence is becoming more common in such situations.

After the patient is pronounced dead, it is the attending physician who is responsible for telling the parents.

Every effort should be made to secure the department so sufficient time can be spent talking to the family. If possible, the physician should be seated during the interview. Many parents will already be aware that the child has died. The physician must introduce him- or herself, make eye contact, and address the parents by name. The language used must be direct and nonjudgmental and it cannot be overemphasized that the deceased patient should be referred to by his or her name: "I am very sorry, but Brendon has died," or "I am very sorry to have to tell you that Becky is dead" are both acceptable examples. Many physicians tend to use euphemisms in an attempt to "soften the blow." While this is understandable, it is a grave mistake and such language as "the baby expired" or "the little guy didn't make it" is deeply resented by parents, who universally perceive it as depersonalizing their child. Parents should be told that every reasonable effort was made to save the child. It is neither desirable nor effective to review the details of the resuscitation.

AFTER THE INTERVIEW

Family members are offered an opportunity to spend time with the dead child after the interview. Before this is done, resuscitation equipment is removed, the body is cleaned and preferably wrapped in a clean blanket. Most, but not all, parents find that spending time with the child is helpful. In certain cases some family members will want to hold the body. A reluctance to do this is normal for others, and is neither a pathological response nor indicative of abuse.

Most cases of sudden death require mandatory autopsies. It is important that this process is explained to family members, and that they are told how to follow-up on the results if they so desire. In cases in which the cause of death is unknown in the emergency department, parents should not be told they will feel better once they know the results of the postmortem examination; at least in cases of SIDS, this is not universally true. In many instances, the patient's personal physician may be available to discuss the autopsy, and there are some coroners who are very experienced in discussing postmortem results with bereaved family members.

Because most pediatric patients suffer arrests involving prolonged tissue asphyxia, they are rarely candidates for organ transplant. However, most are eligible to donate heart valves, skin, and corneas. While asking family members about potential tissue donation immediately after the death of their child is extremely difficult, there are at least some people who retrospectively wish they had been approached. In some states all deaths are reported to regional organ banks, where experts in asking families about donating organs or tissue are available to initiate the process.

An integral part of the grieving process involves processing memories. The vast majority of family members who have a child die in an emergency department would like a physical memento of the patient. These include a lock of hair and/or an ink print of a hand or foot, or a plaster mold of a hand or foot. Some would like it at the time of the patient's death, others some time later. The patient's clothes and other personal items should also be returned. Many neonatal intensive care units have "memory boxes" containing mementos of the baby which are given to parents. It is likely that unless one has experienced the loss of a child oneself, it is impossible to fully comprehend the value such items have to grieving parents. Parents who decline them at the time of the child's death can be told they will be saved, and are available if they change their minds.

FOLLOW-UP CARE

There are many support groups available for parents who have lost children. The Sudden Infant Death Syndrome Alliance has chapters in all 50 states. For many surviving family members, such support groups are extremely helpful, and for some people bonds formed in these groups result in a long-term commitment. All family members who have children die in the emergency department should be made aware of the existence of the appropriate support group.

Some family members feel that follow-up contact from the emergency department after their loved one's death is beneficial, though this does not appear to occur frequently. Such follow-up is a chance to reinforce the sympathy of the emergency department staff, and to offer the family the resources of the institution in arranging long-term support.

MANAGEMENT OF GRIEF AMONG EMERGENCY DEPARTMENT STAFF MEMBERS

Dealing with the effects of the death of a child on the emergency department staff is also problematic. At least some emergency physicians and presumably other staff members utilize grief-counseling services when the hospital provides them, but this service is by no means universally available. While critical incident stress debriefing is commonly utilized, there is no data that confirm that it is efficacious. The format of such counseling is not standardized, and though some people may benefit from it, others may not. It is likely that educating physicians and other staff members in the best way to communicate the death of a child to parents does help to alleviate some of the anxiety that the situation entails. At the very least, it creates a mutually supportive culture within the department regarding the management of death. There are several modalities that have been successfully utilized, including role playing, hearing from parents whose children have died in an emergency department, and incorporating "death-telling" into an advanced life-support curriculum. Indeed, it is to be hoped that all advanced life-support courses will in the near future include the management of death, since death is the end result in the vast majority of cases of cardiopulmonary arrest.

Even under optimal circumstances and with sufficient education, managing the death of a child in an emergency department will always be difficult. This is in large part due to the fact that such deaths invariably appear senseless. One of the key aspects of parents' recoveries is their attempt to find meaning in their child's life, however short it may have been. An important component of this involves the parents' perception of what their child meant to the emergency department personnel in general and the attending physician in particular. An impression that the physician perceived the patient as a valued human being, and that he or she is truly sorry for the parents' loss plays an incalculably important role in the process of healing. Inherently, this requires the physician to say that he or she is sorry about the parents' loss. The belief on the part of the parents that the physician feels badly about the child's death is for some inexplicable reason vital to their recovery. Parents should never be denied this simple human comfort for fear that it will be taken as an admission of medical malfeasance. It is a rare parent who holds an emergency physician responsible for their child's death. In time, most people will reconcile their child's death in the context of their individual beliefs. It is hoped that as they relive the events in the emergency department, they recall a caring and compassionate staff who sympathized with their loss, and shared with them a sense of the value of their child's life.

SUMMARY

Some suggestions and comments from parents whose children died in emergency departments follow.

- Just let the parents know you're sorry, that everything possible was done.
- Unless it has happened to you, don't say "I know how you feel," because you don't.

- Just be honest; say everything possible was done to save the child.
- Be direct.
- Look the parents in the eyes. Explain that all attempts at resuscitation were performed.
- Tell them how sorry you are, that life isn't fair, and most importantly that it was not their fault.
- Allow your humanity to show. One physician was very compassionate, and he had tears in his eyes.
- Make sure you express how sorry you are and tell the loved ones how it affects the staff.
- It's okay to show emotion; don't be overly clinical.
- The doctor should say "I'm sorry, we did all we could."
- As you well know, once your child is dead, you can never have enough mementos.
- There is no easy way to deliver the news. No one wants the job.

BIBLIOGRAPHY

Ahrens WA, Hart RG: Emergency physicians' experience with pediatric death. *Am J Emerg Med* 15:642–643, 1997.

Ahrens WA, Hart RG, Maruyama N: Pediatric death: managing the aftermath in the emergency department. *J Emerg Med* 15:60–63, 1997.

Oliver RC, Fallat ME: Traumatic childhood death: how well do parents cope? *J Trauma* 39:303–306, 1995.

Sachetti A: Acceptance of family member presence during pediatric resuscitations in the emergency department: effects of personal experience. *Pediatr Emerg Care* 16:85–87, 2000.

Schmidt TA, Tolle SW: Emergency physicians' responses to families following patient death. *Ann Emerg Med* 19:125–128, 1990.

10

Evaluation and Management of the Multiple Trauma Patient

Michael J. Gerardi

HIGH-YIELD FACTS

- Children have psychological and physiologic responses to trauma that are different from those seen in adults.

- The airway is secured while concomitantly stabilizing the neck. The jaw thrust maneuver is used to open the airway and the oropharynx is cleared of debris and secretions.

- Orotracheal intubation is the most reliable means of securing an airway. An uncuffed tube should be used in children <8 years of age.

- *Hypovolemic shock* occurs most commonly after major trauma and is due to blood loss, which makes up 8 to 9 percent of the body weight of a child. Determination of the extent of volume depletion and shock is difficult in children and multiple parameters must be used.

- Vascular access is a difficult procedure under the best of circumstances and is often a reason for delay in transport of a critically ill child. Vascular access can be attempted en route to avoid prolonged stay at the scene and intraosseous (IO) infusion should be used as a quick access for crystalloid infusion if attempts at intravenous cannulation are unsuccessful after 90 seconds.

- For shock, the initial resuscitative fluid should be crystalloid isotonic solution, such as Ringer's lactate or normal saline. Give an initial infusion of 20 mL/kg as rapidly as possible.

- Insert a Foley catheter and use urinary output as a straightforward, readily available monitor: 1 mL/kg/h for children >1 year of age; 2 mL/kg/h for children <1 year of age. Urinary output may help assess perfusion and intravascular status.

- Unique characteristics of the pediatric cervical spine predispose it to ligamentous disruption and dislocation injuries without radiographic evidence of bone injury.

- Controversies arise in diagnosing and managing blunt abdominal injuries. CT with IV, oral, and colonic contrast may be the most sensitive and useful diagnostic modality, but diagnostic peritoneal lavage provides rapid, objective evaluation of possible intraperitoneal injury, especially involving the liver, spleen, and bowel.

- Ultrasound can diagnose most injuries to the liver, spleen, and kidneys, and can document intraperitoneal fluid. Ultrasound is generally not a substitute for CT unless the examiner is very experienced in the use of ultrasound in traumatized children.

Trauma is the leading cause of death in children >1 year of age in the United States. In developed countries, traumatic injuries are the leading cause of morbidity and mortality in children between the ages of 1 and 14 years, and unintentional injury ranks as the leading cause of death from age 1 through age 34 years. Despite the fact that overall mortality from pediatric trauma occurs at one third of the rate of trauma deaths in adults, case-fatality rates for children are higher when compared with adults who have similar injuries. Mortality data alone do not emphasize the profound impact of trauma. Each year, 20 percent of American children receive medical care for an injury. For children <14 years of age, injuries are the leading cause of visits to hospital emergency departments, numbering 7.9 million, and the second leading cause of hospitalization, accounting for >200,000 admissions. Injuries are the leading cause of medical spending for children ages 5 to 21 years. The costs in terms of dollars and lives are impressive: 22,000 lives lost, 600,000 hospitalized, and 16 million seen in emergency departments each year.

The health care cost is approximately $160 billion per year nationally. Average costs for initial hospitalization and ED visits are $5094 and $171 per patient, respectively. There are additional costs to the emotional and financial status of the patients and their families, attributable to the devastating nature of many traumatic injuries. Even minor injuries may have lasting effects causing functional impairment or subtle cognitive or behavioral deficits years after the acute traumatic event. Therefore, physical, emotional, and psychological needs of the child and family must be considered.

NATURE OF INJURIES AND UNIQUE PEDIATRIC ASPECTS

Motor vehicle occupant injuries are the leading cause of injury death among children aged 0 to 19 years. Other major causes of death are homicide, suicide, drowning, pedestrian/motor vehicle accidents, and burns, with the relative risk for each type of injury varying by age group (Table 10-1). Infants (birth to 12 months), toddlers (1 to 3 years), and preschoolers (3 to 5 years) are at greatest risk from falls. Because they have a proportionately larger head and a higher center of gravity, they sustain a high proportion of isolated closed-head injuries. These patients, especially infants and toddlers, are also at risk of child abuse.

School age children (6 to 12 years of age) are most commonly victims of unintentional trauma, especially motor vehicle–related trauma, as pedestrians, bicyclists, or unrestrained passengers. These patients also sustain a large number of closed-head injuries, often in association with other injuries. Adolescents (13 to 19 years of age) are in a transition from childhood to adulthood and require treatment considerations that combine psychological requirements of a child with the physical needs of an adult. These patients engage in many risk-taking behaviors, and are at high risk of homicide and suicide.

Blunt injuries account for 87 percent of all childhood trauma. Penetrating trauma accounts for 10 percent, with the remaining 3 percent due to drowning. Motor vehicle–related incidents account for 40 percent of blunt trauma and are the leading cause of severe injury in children; falls are the second most common etiology. Boys are involved in injuries twice as frequently as girls. Although blunt trauma is the major etiology of injury to children, the rapid increase in penetrating trauma to children in the inner cities has been dramatic.

Children have psychological and physiologic responses to trauma that are different from those seen in adults. An understanding of these anatomic and physiologic differences is a fundamental tenet in providing appropriate, expert care for children.

Due to a child's smaller mass, kinetic energy is distributed over a smaller area and it, therefore, impacts a greater proportion of the total body volume. Musculoskeletal compliance is greater in children and children have less protective muscle and subcutaneous tissue. The increased flexibility and resilience of the pediatric skeleton and surrounding tissues permits external forces to be transmitted to the deeper internal structures. Therefore, internal injury must always be considered, even in the absence of external signs of trauma.

Since a child's head represents a larger percentage of total body mass than that of an adult, head injuries in

Table 10-1. Leading Causes of Trauma in Children by Age Group

<1 Year of Age	1–4 Years of Age	5–9 Years of Age	10–14 Years of Age
Suffocation	Motor vehicle traffic	Motor vehicle traffic	Motor vehicle traffic
Motor vehicle traffic	Drowning and submersion	Drowning and submersion	Drowning and submersion
Drowning and submersion	Fire and burn	Fire and burn	Fire and burn
Fire and burn	Suffocation	Suffocation	Suffocation

children are common and account for a large percentage of serious morbidity and mortality. The head is also a major source of heat loss in a child. The occiput is more prominent in young children, decreasing in prominence from birth until approximately age 10. This should be taken into account when positioning the head for intubation and airway management. The bony sutures are open at birth; they gradually fuse by 18 to 24 months of age. Palpation of the fontanels can provide useful information regarding intracranial pressure. The child's brain, having a higher percentage of white matter than gray matter, may have greater resilience in withstanding blunt trauma. However, it is more susceptible to axonal shearing forces and cerebral edema.

A child's neck is shorter and supports a relatively heavier weight than an adult's, making it especially subject to forces of trauma and sudden movements. A younger child's short, fat neck also makes the evaluation of neck veins and tracheal position difficult.

The most dramatic and critical differences between children and adults are in the airway (Table 10-2). A child's larynx is located in a more cephalad and anterior position. In addition, the epiglottis is tilted almost 45 degrees in a child and is more floppy, making manipulation and visualization for intubation more difficult. Unlike the adult, where the glottis is the narrowest portion of the upper airway, the cricoid cartilage is the narrowest portion of the child's airway. This fact, plus the abundant loose columnar epithelium, limits the size of the endotracheal tube and is the reason that uncuffed tubes should be used in children under 8 years of age.

The pediatric thorax is more pliable due to more flexible ribs and cartilage and there is less overlying fat and muscle. This allows a greater amount of blunt force to be transmitted to underlying tissues. The diaphragmatic muscle is much more distensible in a child. A child's mediastinum is also very mobile. Therefore, the mediastinum and abdominal organs are subject to sudden, wide excursions that can be dramatically seen in tension pneumothorax.

The diaphragm inserts at a nearly horizontal angle from birth until about 12 years of age, in contrast to the oblique insertion in the adult. This, in effect, causes abdominal organs to be more exposed and less protected by ribs and muscle. Therefore, apparent insignificant forces can cause serious internal injury. Children are also primarily diaphragmatic or "belly" breathers, making them dependent on diaphragmatic excursion for ventilation.

The spleen and the liver are in a more caudal and anterior position. Even though the increased elasticity and compliance of a child's connective tissue and suspensory ligaments should protect these organs, they are actually more subject to injury due to increased motion at impact.

Long bones in children are different primarily due to the presence of growth plates or epiphyses and increased compliance (see Chap. 18). The epiphyseal-metaphyseal junctions are relatively weak and ligaments are stronger than the growth plate. This weakness predisposes a child to disturbances of the growth plate. The Salter Harris classification system was created to assist in the diagnosis and management of growth plate injuries. Increased compliance of bone results in significant absorption of energy without radiographic signs of fracture even though there is bony damage. Therefore, the physical examination is often more sensitive than radiographs for growth plate and long bone fractures. Blood supply to bones can also be easily disrupted, resulting in limb length disparity.

Table 10-2. Comparison of Infant and Adult Airways

	Infant	Adult
Head	Large, prominent occiput, assumes sniffing position when supine	Flat occiput
Tongue	Relatively larger	Relatively smaller
Larynx	Cephalad position, opposite C2–3	Opposite C4–6
Epiglottis	"Ω" or "U" shaped, soft	Flat, flexible
Vocal cords	Short, concave	Horizontal
Smallest diameter	Cricoid ring, below cords	Vocal cords
Cartilage	Soft	Firm
Lower airways	Smaller, less developed	Larger, more cartilage

Source: Used with permission from Strange GR (ed): *APLS: The Pediatric Emergency Medicine Course.* Elk Grove Village, IL and Dallas, TX: American Academy of Pediatrics & American College of Emergency Physicians, 1998.

PEDIATRIC TRAUMA SYSTEMS

The differences in the mechanisms and patterns of injury observed in early childhood, late childhood, and adolescence, together with immature anatomic features and the developing physiologic functions of the pediatric patient, result in unique responses to major trauma, which in turn drive the need for specialized pediatric resources. Therefore, the injured pediatric patient has special needs that may be optimally provided in the environment of a children's hospital with demonstrated expertise in and commitment to both pediatric and trauma care. Pediatric trauma centers will usually be located in large metropolitan areas and will have a lead role in the care of the injured child within their trauma systems. Geographic areas with access to a pediatric trauma center should work to integrate this hospital into the regional trauma system through invited participation, appropriate field triage, and interfacility transport of the most critically injured children. When a pediatric trauma center, whether freestanding or affiliated with an adult trauma center, is not available, this role should be fulfilled by the adult trauma center with the largest volume of pediatric patients.

PREHOSPITAL CARE ISSUES

Considerations in the field care of the traumatized child include endotracheal intubation, IV access, immobilization, and rapid transport. Which procedures should be attempted in the field is controversial. The prehospital success rate for endotracheal intubation varies from 48 to 89 percent. It has been demonstrated that trauma deaths can be reduced by 25 percent when a system provides personnel trained to perform aggressive airway management and develops guidelines for ground versus aeromedical transport. However, one computer model demonstrated that children in respiratory distress in urban centers would have a shorter time to intubation if transported by police rather than EMS units. Rural systems as a whole require more aggressive initial treatment in the field due to transport times that are 3 to 4 times greater than those in urban areas.

In the last few decades, there has been a dramatic evolution in the development of trauma systems. Regionalized trauma care is generally believed to confer benefits to the injured but there is not much evidence to date supporting that which seems intuitively obvious. Regardless, the advent of pediatric emergency medicine and emergency medical services for children (EMSC) has led to the development of coordinated systems of care for critically ill and injured children in many parts of the country.

Vascular access is a difficult procedure under the best of circumstances and is often a reason for delay in transport of a critically ill child. It is reasonable for traumatized children to be transported immediately without vascular access if a short transport time is expected. Vascular access can be attempted en route to avoid prolonged stay at the scene. Intraosseous (IO) infusion should be used as a quick access for crystalloid infusion if attempts at intravenous cannulation are unsuccessful after 90 seconds. IO lines can be placed successfully in the field 80 percent of the time.

INITIAL ASSESSMENT AND MANAGEMENT GUIDELINES FOR THE INJURED CHILD

The highest priorities in caring for an injured child are determining whether there are life-threatening disturbances and providing immediate treatment. The next priority is identifying injuries requiring operative intervention and initiating that process. Finally, the child is examined for non–life-threatening injuries and specific initiating therapy is initiated (Table 10-3).

The *primary survey* and initial *resuscitation,* occurring simultaneously, usually require the first 5 to 10 minutes and focus on diagnosing and treating life-threatening disorders. The *secondary survey* continues the assessment with a more thorough physical examination and diagnostic testing. It is an anatomic survey that evaluates in a timely, directed fashion, each body area from head-to-toe. In this fashion, life-threatening injuries are promptly recognized before proceeding to less urgent problems. Trauma and pediatric resuscitation courses emphasize the importance of completing surveys and resuscitation in an orderly fashion to ensure against missing injuries. Children with serious injuries require continual reassessment. Repeat vital signs should be performed every 5 minutes during the primary survey and every 15 minutes while in the ED awaiting transfer or operative intervention.

Primary Survey

The primary survey includes:

- Airway and cervical spine stabilization
- Breathing and ventilation

Table 10-3. Initial Approach to the Pediatric Trauma Patient

1. **Before Arrival**
   Prepare all equipment
   Mobilize trauma team and call for assistance (respiratory therapy, nurses, radiology technician)
   Have O-negative blood on stand-by
2. **First 5 Minutes**
   Assess respiration, oxygenation; ventilate if necessary
   Check pulse oximetry reading
   Cardiac and blood pressure monitoring
   Consider end-tidal CO_2 monitoring if available
   Maintain C-spine immobilization
   Perform needle or tube thoracostomy if tension pneumothorax suspected
   Intubate or attain surgical airway if indicated
   Treat obvious wounds: apply pressure to external hemorrhage; dressing to sucking chest wound
3. **Second 5 Minutes**
   Reassess airway, ventilation, oxygenation, temperature
   Assess perfusion
       Volume resuscitation: 20 mL/kg with crystalloid and repeat as necessary
       Consider un–cross-matched or O-negative blood
   Assess neurologic status
   Send laboratory specimens: type and cross, CBC, amylase, liver transaminases, BUN, creatinine, glucose,
       electrolytes, ABG, urinalysis
   Needle pericardiocentesis, thoracotomy, and aortic clamping, if indicated
   Nasogastric tube, urinary catheter
4. **Next 10 Minutes/Secondary Survey**
   Reassess airway, ventilation, oxygenation, perfusion, neurologic status and disability
   Assess head, neck, chest, abdomen, pelvis, neurologic examination, extremities
   Tube thoracostomy if indicated
   Reduce vascular-compromising dislocations
   Administer drugs: tetanus toxoid, antibiotics, analgesics, sedatives
   Lateral neck, chest, and pelvis radiographs
   ECG
   Start to make arrangements for transfer, admission, and movement to operating room or ICU
5. **Next 10 Minutes**
   Reassess airway, ventilation, oxygenation, perfusion, neurologic status and disability
   Document resuscitation; talk to family
   Splint fractures; dress wounds
   IVP, DPL, CT as indicated
   Consider more invasive monitoring devices central venous line, arterial line

- Circulation and hemorrhage control
- Disability (neurologic screening examination)
- Exposure and thorough examination

This initial survey is a physiologic survey of the patient's vital systems and, if serious physiologic alterations are encountered in the course of the survey, resuscitative care must be performed. A guide to pediatric vital signs is provided in Table 10-4.

Airway

The airway is secured while concomitantly stabilizing the neck. The jaw thrust maneuver is used to open the airway and the oropharynx is cleared of debris and secretions.

Although bony cervical spine injuries are less common in children, they are at high risk for cervical cord injuries. Cervical spine injury should be assumed until a

Table 10-4. Pediatric Vital Signs

Age	Weight,[a] kg	Respiratory Rate	Heart Rate	Systolic BP[b]
Preterm	2	55–65	120–180	40–60
Term newborn	3	40–60	90–170	52–92
1 month	4	30–50	110–180	60–104
6 month–1 year	8–10	25–35	120–140	65–125
2–4 years	12–16	20–30	100–110	80–95
5–8 years	18–26	4–20	90–100	90–100
8–12 years	26–50	12–20	60–110	100–110
>12 years	>40	12–16	60–105	100–120

[a]Weight estimate: $8 + [2 \times \text{age (years)}] = \text{weight (kg)}$.
[b]Blood pressure minimum $70 + [2 \times \text{age (years)}] = \text{systolic blood pressure}$; $\frac{2}{3} \times \text{systolic pressure} = \text{diastolic pressure}$.
Source: From Fitzmaurice LS. *Pediatric Emergency Medicine, Concepts and Clinical Practice.* St. Louis, MO: Mosby-Yearbook Inc. Modified with permission.

normal examination and an adequate cervical spine series are obtained to rule it out.

Ventilation with a bag-valve-mask device is initiated to treat inadequate ventilation. Cricoid pressure must be applied when ventilating a patient with a bag and mask to prevent gastric insufflation.

Indications for endotracheal intubation in the trauma patient are:

- Inability to ventilate the child by bag-valve-mask methods

- The need for prolonged control of the airway

- Prevention of aspiration in a comatose child

- The need for controlled hyperventilation in patients with serious head injuries

- Flail chest with pulmonary contusion

- Shock unresponsive to fluid volume

Orotracheal intubation is the most reliable means of securing an airway. An uncuffed tube should be used in children <8 years of age. Appropriate tube size is approximated by the diameter of the nostril or the diameter of the child's fifth finger. General guidelines based on age are given in Table 10-5. Emergency intubation should always be accomplished via the oral approach in traumatized children. Nasotracheal intubation, besides being extremely difficult in an acutely injured child, is relatively contraindicated due to the acute angle of the posterior pharynx, the necessity of additional tube manipulation, and the probability of causing or increasing pharyngeal bleeding. Other disadvantages are that it has a high complication rate, is time consuming, and may require multiple attempts.

Preparation should always precede intubation and includes guaranteeing the presence of all equipment and drugs necessary to adequately manage an acute airway. This can be accomplished even before an injured child arrives.

Intubation may be necessary to maintain an adequate airway. However, intubation may be difficult due to poor airway visualization, seizures, agitation, or combativeness. Prolonged intubation procedures can lead to intracranial pressure (ICP) elevation, pain, bradycardia, regurgitation and hypoxemia. Rapid sequence induction (RSI) can greatly facilitate intubation and reduce adverse effects significantly (see Chap. 5).

Emergency physicians must be able to secure an airway when unable to perform orotracheal or nasotracheal intubation. There are several options:

- *Cricothyrotomy* has a role for patients in whom there is extensive central facial or upper airway injury or when there have been unsuccessful attempts at orotracheal intubation. However, it is difficult and hazardous in children. It is not recommended under the age of 10 and complication rates are as high as 10 to 40 percent.

- *Tracheostomy* is time consuming and hazardous in the ED, in addition to requiring surgical skill.

- *Needle cricothyrotomy with transtracheal jet ventilation (TTJV)* currently is the preferred surgical method of choice to secure an emergency airway in children.

Table 10-5. Equipment Sizes for Pediatric Trauma

Age	Mask Size	Oral Airway	Nasal Airway	Laryngoscope Blade	Endotracheal Tube (mm)	Foley Catheter
Newborn	Infant	0		0	3–3.5	5–8
6 mo	Infant/child	1	12	1	3.5	8
1 yr	Child (s)	1–2	12	1	4.0	8
3 yr	Child (s)	2	16	2	4.5	10
5 yr	Child (m)	3	16	2	5.0	10
6 yr	Child (m)	3	16	2–3	5.5	10–12
8 yr	Sm med	4	20	2–3	6.0	12
12 yr	Med lg	4–5	24–28	3	6.5	12–16
16 yr	Med lg	5	28–30	3–4	7.0–8.0	14–18

Age	Orogastric Tube (F)	Suction Catheter	Chest Tube	Vascular Catheter	Intraosseous Needle (G)
Newborn	5 or 8 feeding	8	12–18	20–22	
6 mo	8	8	14–20	20–22	17
1 yr	10	8	14–24	20–22	17
3 yr	10	10	16–28	18–22	15
5 yr	10–12	10	20–32	18–20	15
6 yr	12	10	20–32	18–20	
8 yr	14	12	24–32	16–20	
12 yr	14	12	28–36	16–20	
16 yr	16–18	12–14	28–40	14–18	

Permission granted from W.B. Saunders. Schafermeyer RW: Pediatric Trauma in *Advances in Trauma. Emerg Med Clin North Am.* 11:187–205, 1993.

A percutaneous technique and TTJV has several advantages over a surgical cricothyrotomy in the ED:

- Straightforward technique
- Allows adequate ventilation for at least 45 to 60 minutes, allowing time for definitive airway placement
- Plays a central role in those patients in whom intubation is not possible

However, advantages over traditional surgical methodologies have not been scientifically demonstrated, despite being inherently obvious. Some expertise and/or practice are required and the airway is not protected from aspiration. Complications include subcutaneous emphysema, bleeding, and catheter dislodgment. However, the issue of CO_2 retention, although controversial, is overstated and of relative unimportance when airway access and oxygenation are critical. TTJV undoubtedly provides a life-saving and temporary airway, which should be adequate for 45 minutes 2 hours, until endotracheal intubation is can be achieved.

The procedure for TTJV is as follows:

- A 14-gauge angiocatheter of the TTJV needle is connected to a 5 mL syringe with 3 mL of saline.
- The trachea is stabilized with the non-dominant hand and, after the region is prepped, the cricothyroid membrane is punctured at a 30- to 45-degree angle caudally. Special care is required to avoid puncturing the posterior wall of the trachea.
- Placement is verified with aspiration of air.
- The catheter is slid off the needle and placement reconfirmed with the syringe.
- The catheter must be constantly held or secured in place and the jet ventilation tubing is attached to the O_2 source. This O_2 source *must be a*

high-pressure source directly from the wall and not from a regulator valve.

- The PSI can then be adjusted on the pressure gauge. There are no available well-studied guidelines for PSI settings for TTJV in children. However, parameters recommended by practitioners familiar with this technique are shown in Table 10-6. A low PSI must be used initially in children and the provider should look for adequate chest excursion. The PSI can be adjusted upward until adequate chest rise is observed, which is the best indicator of adequate tidal volume. The inspiration:expiration ventilation ratio is 1:3 or 1:4.

Breathing

Acceptable ventilation occurs only if there is adequate spontaneous air exchange with normal O_2 saturation and CO_2 levels. Pulse oximetry is mandatory and end-tidal CO_2 monitoring is an increasingly more common and available technology that should be used to confirm endotracheal tube placement. Severe hypoxemia may be manifested by any combination of and degree of agitation, altered mental status, cyanosis, poor end-organ function, poor capillary refill, and desaturation on pulse oximetry. Children with respiratory failure to any degree should have positive pressure ventilation (PPV) started immediately.

Signs that a child has inadequate ventilation include tachypnea, nasal flaring, grunting, retractions, stridor, and wheezing. Reasons for compromised ventilatory function include depressed sensorium, airway occlusion, restriction of lung expansion, and direct pulmonary injury. Restriction of lung expansion by gastric distention is more likely to occur in children due to increased importance of the diaphragmatic excursion to ventilation in children. This problem is addressed by early placement of oro- or nasogastric tube.

In an obtunded or comatose child, ventilation using a bag-valve-mask device, endotracheal tube, or transtracheal jet ventilation needle should be via a high-flow O_2 source capable of producing chest rise and adequate O_2 saturation.

At this stage of the resuscitation, immediate attention and treatment of tension or hemo-pneumo-thorax, if present or suspected, is required. The classic presentation for pneumothorax of absent breath sounds, tympany, hypotension, and jugular venous distention due to high intrathoracic pressures, is rare in children. Children are especially sensitive to mediastinal shift or twisting in tension hemopneumothoraces. Therefore, needle decompression thoracostomies should be performed immediately if any of the following are present: decreased breath sounds, refractory hypotension, hypoxia, or radiographically confirmed hemopneumothoraces.

Massive hemothorax may present as absent breath sounds, dullness to percussion on the affected side of the chest, and hypotension. Jugular venous distention is not commonly seen because of the low circulatory volume. Operative thoracotomy should be considered when the initial drainage is greater than 15 mL/kg or the chest tube output exceeds 4 mL/kg/h.

The skin wound of an open pneumothorax should be occluded on three sides with a dressing of petrolatum gauze or plastic sheet, leaving one side of the dressing open to act as a flutter valve to minimize the potential for development of a tension pneumothorax. A tube thoracostomy can wait until completion of the primary survey.

Circulation

During the primary survey, the major goals of circulatory assessment and treatment are to diagnose and control both external and internal hemorrhage and assess pulse and perfusion. Vascular access for fluid infusions and phlebotomy are additional goals. Determination of volume status, blood pressure, and perfusion are estimated by assessment of pulse, skin color, and capillary refill time. A palpable peripheral pulse correlates with a blood pressure above 80 mm Hg, and a palpable central pulse indicates a pressure above 50 to 60 mm Hg. A nor-

Table 10-6. Parameters for Transtracheal Jet Ventilation

	Initial PSI	Estimated Tidal Volume
Adult	30–50	700–1000 cc
8 years to young teens	10–25	340–625
5–8 years	5–10	240–340
<5 years	5	100

movolemic euthermic patient's capillary refilling time, assessed after blanching, will be 2 to 3 seconds. If the extremities are cool distally and warm proximally, changes in volume status and perfusion can be followed during therapy by the change in temperature as perfusion of the distal extremities improves or worsens.

Control external hemorrhage by direct pressure or placing pneumatic splints. Application of extremity tourniquets or hemostats to bleeding vessels should be avoided. Application and inflation of a pneumatic anti-shock garment is controversial but may be useful to help control bleeding in the pelvis or lower extremities. As in adults, Trendelenburg position may be of benefit in low-perfusion states to help maintain central circulation.

Absent pulses or cardiac arrest in a child with traumatic injuries portends a poor outcome. In children with penetrating chest or abdominal trauma, a resuscitative thoracotomy can be life-saving if vital signs were recently lost. In children with traumatic arrest from blunt trauma, the outcome is invariably death. During resuscitation of traumatic arrest, standard advanced cardiac life-support algorithms should be followed and there should be early administration of blood products. If chest trauma is present or there has been a deceleration injury, as with an automobile crash or fall, consider the presence of cardiac tamponade, a rare condition in children. Although echocardiography is diagnostic, look for Beck's triad, which consists of hypotension, muffled heart sounds, and jugular venous distention. Fluid boluses should be administered early and can be temporizing but periocardiocentesis and resuscitative thoracotomy can be lifesaving.

Table 10-7. Pediatric Glasgow Coma Scale

	Eye Opening	
Score	**0–1 Year**	**>1 Year**
4	Spontaneously	Spontaneously
3	To shout	To verbal command
2	To pain	To pain
1	No response	No response

	Best Motor Response	
Score	**0–1 Year**	**>1 Year**
6		Obeys command
5	Localizes pain	Localizes pain
4	Flexion withdrawal	Flexion withdrawal
3	Decorticate	Decorticate
2	Decerebrate	Decerebrate
1	No response	No response

	Best Verbal Response		
Score	**0–2 Years**	**2–5 Years**	**>5 Years**
5	Appropriate cry Smiles, coos	Appropriate words and phrases	Oriented, converses
4	Cries	Inappropriate words	Disoriented, converses
3	Inappropriate cry	Cries/screams	Inappropriate words
2	Grunts	Grunts	Incomprehensible sound
1	No response	No response	No response

Note: A score is given in each category. The individual scores are then added to give a total of 3–15. A score of <8 indicates severe neurologic injury.

Obtain vascular access in a rapid, reliable, safe, and technically simple manner with a capability to infuse the greatest possible volume of fluid. Two lines are placed so that blood and medications or fluids can be given simultaneously. Attaining vascular access is practically difficult in children so one functioning intravenous line is all that may be readily achieved and is usually adequate. Intraosseous line placement should be considered early in a severely injured child, even when a blood pressure or pulse are present, if vascular access is difficult. Any fluids, medications, or blood products can be given through this line, which functions as well as central venous access. If central venous access is desired, the femoral vein is the easiest site because of identifiable landmarks and relative ease of the procedure compared to other central venous lines in children.

Disability

Disability is assessed by performing a rapid neurologic examination to determine level of consciousness as well as pupil size and reaction. The Glasgow Coma Scale is a more quantitative measure of level of consciousness (Table 10-7). Although recently found to be less predictive of overall outcomes in children with trauma, it is an extremely useful tool with which to follow their improvement or deterioration.

However, in the midst of a trauma resuscitation, the AVPU system (Table 10-8) can be quite helpful in grossly following mental status changes.

Exposure

Completely undress the patient in order to perform a thorough assessment. Children have a larger body surface area:weight ratio so maintaining the patient's body heat is a constant concern when he or she is exposed.

Table 10-8. AVPU Method for Assessing Level of Consciousness

A	Alert
V	Vocal stimuli: responds
P	Painful stimuli: responds
U	Unresponsive

RESUSCITATION

This phase occurs simultaneously with the primary survey but it is separated in presentation for clarity and organization.

Ensure adequate oxygenation and ventilation of all trauma victims. Vascular access is the next priority via percutaneous or cutdown cannulation of the upper or lower extremity veins. Two large bore intravenous lines should be established, with size guided by the size of available veins. The highest success rate is obtained at the antecubital fossae or the saphenous veins at the ankle (anterior to the medial maleolus). Veins are often visibly absent, difficult to cannulate with an appropriately sized catheter, or collapsed in the face of hypovolemia. In these situations, femoral vein central line or intraosseous infusion into the tibia marrow space are reasonable life-saving alternatives. A third option would be rapid venous cutdown access performed on an antecubital vein or the saphenous vein at either the ankle or in the groin.

Send blood for type and cross-match, complete blood count, serum electrolytes, liver transaminases, and amylase. Liver transaminase elevation in the acute trauma setting serves as a marker of liver injury that might not be clinically apparent. A blood gas needs to be sent in any patient who might have significant volume loss, respiratory compromise, or concomitant toxic exposure (e.g., carbon monoxide poisoning in a burn patient).

Perform an assessment for shock and determine whether or not adequate organ perfusion exists. Shock after trauma is usually hypovolemic. Cardiogenic and neurogenic shock are less likely but need to be considered. Isolated head trauma, except in infancy, is not a cause of shock in children.

Hypovolemic shock occurs most commonly after major trauma and is due to blood loss (Table 10-9). The blood volume of the child makes up 8 to 9 percent of the total body weight. Determination of the extent of volume depletion and shock is difficult in children, and multiple parameters must be used. Hematocrit can be normal in the face of acute blood loss. And blood pressure alone is an insensitive indicator of shock, especially when determining treatment priorities.

Cardiogenic shock after a major childhood injury is rare but could occur due to cardiac tamponade or direct cardiac contusion. It should be suspected if there are dilated neck veins in a patient with decelerating injury, penetrating chest trauma, or sternal contusion. Neurogenic shock presents with hypotension without tachy-

Table 10-9. Therapeutic Classification of Hemorrhagic Shock in the Pediatric Patient

	Blood Loss Percent of Blood Volume[a]			
	Up to 15	15–30	30–40	≥40
Pulse rate	Normal	Mild tachycardia	Moderate tachycardia	Severe tachycardia
Blood pressure	Normal or increased	Decreased	Decreased	Decreased
Capillary refill	Normal	Positive	Positive	Positive
Respiratory rate	Normal	Mild tachypnea	Moderate tachypnea	Severe tachypnea
Urinary output	1–2 mL/kg/h	0.5–1.0 mL/kg/h	0.25–0.5 mL/kg/h	Negligible
Mental status	Slightly anxious	Mildly anxious	Anxious and confused	Confused and lethargic
Fluid replacement (3:1 rule)	Crystalloid	Crystalloid	Crystalloid + blood	Crystalloid + blood

[a]Assume blood volume to be 8–9% of body weight (80–90 mL/kg).

cardia or vasoconstriction. Isolated head injury does not produce shock unless there is significant intracerebral hemorrhage in an infant. Distributive or septic shock should not be a consideration immediately after trauma, even if there is contamination of the abdominal cavity.

Ringer's lactate (LR) or normal saline is the fluid of choice for initial resuscitation of the pediatric trauma victim. Fluid replacement can be divided into two phases: initial therapy and total replacement (Table 10-10). The initial resuscitative fluid should be crystalloid isotonic solution, such as Ringer's lactate or normal saline. Give an initial infusion of 20 mL/kg as rapidly as possible. This is best accomplished by using a 3-way stopcock and pushing boluses rather than trying to infuse via a pump or gravity, especially if the vein cannulation device is smaller than 18 gauge. After a rapid 20 mL/kg bolus over 10 minutes, the child should be reassessed. The fluid bolus should be repeated up to four times if necessary. If the child continues to be unstable, 10 to 20 mL/kg packed red blood cells or whole blood need to be urgently infused. The outline below delineates anticipated fluid needs for different classes of shock. The 3:1 rule is commonly used in replacing lost blood with crystalloid: 300 mL of crystalloid for each 100 mL of blood loss. If the initial hemoglobin value is <7, blood should be given immediately since this level of hemoglobin overwhelms compensatory mechanisms and increases cellular hypoxia.

Clinically assess volume and perfusion status during resuscitation. Vital signs are checked before and after bolus therapy. If a child is not responding appropriately, suspect continued bleeding and look for other causes of refractory shock, such as tension pneumothorax or hy-poxemia. Insert a Foley catheter and use urinary output as a straightforward, readily available monitor: 1 mL/kg/h for children >1 year of age; 2 mL/kg/h for children <1 year of age. Urinary output may help assess perfusion and intravascular status.

While restoring or immediately after attaining adequate perfusion, urinary and gastric catheters should be placed. Blood at the urethral meatus or in the scrotum, or abnormal placement of prostate on rectal examination prohibit catheterization until retrograde urethrogram (RUG) has proven that the urethra is intact. This can be done by instilling gastrograffin into a partially inserted Foley catheter.

Nasogastric tube insertion should be avoided or performed with the utmost care to avoid passage into the brain via a cribiform plate fracture when a patient has blood coming from the ears, nose, or mouth.

Measure and monitor the patient's body temperature. Hypothermia must be avoided and/or corrected. Attention should be paid to using radiant warmers, warmed IV fluids, and covering exposed body parts.

Obtain radiographs at this time, but limit them to cervical spine, chest, and pelvic films until the patient is initially resuscitated.

It is important to obtain surgical consultation in any significantly injured child as early in the evaluation as possible. If notified by EMS of a severely injured child coming to the facility, contact the surgeon on call for trauma or contact the referral center to prepare for early transfer of the critically injured child. Initiation of a transfer protocol, if warranted, should be activated at this time. See Table 10-14 for criteria to guide the decision of when transfer is needed.

Table 10-10. Guidelines for Fluid Resuscitation in Shock

Mild shock (15–25% of blood volume loss)
    Initial volume:
        20 mL/kg LR or NS
        If no improvement, repeat 20 mL/kg LR or NS
    Total volume:
        If improved, run LR or NS at 5 mL/kg/h for several hours
        If child remains stable, adjust intravenous rate downward toward maintenance levels
    Maintenance after volume is restored:
        10 kg: 100 mL/kg/24 h
        10–20 kg: 1000 mL + 50 mL/kg/24 h
        20 kg: 1500 mL + 20 mL/kg/24 h
Moderate shock (25–40% of blood volume loss)
    Initial volume:
        20 mL/kg/LR or NS; repeat immediately if not improved
    If no improvement, alternative therapy includes:
        20–40 mL/kg LR, or NS again, *or* 10–20 mL/kg packed red blood cells, *or* operative intervention
        10–20 mL/kg packed red blood cells if initial Hgb < 7.0
    Total volume:
        If improved, run LR or NS at 5 mL/kg/h for several hours
        If a child remains stable, adjust intravenous rate toward maintenance levels
        May need transfusion depending on clinical response and hematocrit
Severe shock (>40% of blood volume loss)
    Initial volume:
        Push LR or NS until colloid available
        Push packed red blood cells or whole blood
        Surgery
    Total volume:
        Replace loss with type-specific blood

Equipment tables should be readily available in the resuscitation room as an aid in determining tube and catheter sizes. As an alternative, the Broselow tape system can also be used to ensure the use of properly sized equipment.

SECONDARY SURVEY AND DEFINITIVE CARE

Once life-threatening conditions identified in the primary survey are stabilized, perform a timely, directed evaluation of each body area, proceeding from head to toe. Continuously reassess vital signs and abnormal conditions identified in the primary survey at a minimum of every 15 minutes. The components of the secondary survey are:

- complete examination
- history
- laboratory studies
- radiographic studies
- problem identification

Use an AMPLE history to determine the mechanism of injury, time, status at scene, changes in status, and complaints that the child may have:

- **A** - allergies
- **M** - medications
- **P** - past medical and surgical history
- **L** - time of the child's last meal
- **E** - events preceding the accident

Complete laboratory and radiologic studies that were not done during the resuscitation.

A decision regarding disposition can probably be made by this point during most resuscitations.

Head Examination

Reevaluate pupil size and reactivity. Perform a conjunctival and fundal examination for hemorrhage or penetrating injury. Assess visual acuity by determining if the patient can read, see faces, recognize movement, and distinguish light versus dark.

A thorough palpation of the skull and mandible should be done looking for fracture-dislocations. If airway is secure, maxillofacial trauma is a lower priority and the physician should move on quickly.

Cervical Spine

Injuries of the cervical spine (C-spine) are not common in children but the presence of any of the following comorbid conditions increases the risk:

- Injuries above the clavicles
- Injuries from falling >1 floor
- Motor vehicle–pedestrian crash at >30 mph
- Unrestrained or poorly restrained occupant of a motor vehicle crash
- Sports injuries

Children tend to have injuries of the upper C-spine and cord.

In very low–risk injuries, the C-spine can usually be cleared in the ED with a normal lateral C-spine film and a normal clinical examination. Caveats are that cervical spine film must show all seven cervical spine vertebrae and that the patient should be awake, cooperative, and free of other distracting painful injuries before ruling out a cervical injury. The child under control should be able to actively flex, extend, and rotate the neck with no symptoms or signs of spasm, guarding, pain, or tenderness.

Unique characteristics of the pediatric C-spine predispose it to ligamentous disruption and dislocation injuries without radiographic evidence of bone injury. The incomplete development of the bony spine, the relatively large size of the head, and the weakness of the soft tissue of the neck given the larger head size, predispose to spinal cord injury without radiographic abnormality (SCIWORA). Children with high-risk mechanisms of injury should have three views: anteroposterior (AP), an odontoid, and lateral views. Patients with altered sensorium cannot be cleared despite negative films and the collar should remain in place while further testing and imaging studies are completed.

Special considerations are required in four situations:

- The child who requires immediate intubation due to airway compromise should not have airway management delayed waiting for a lateral C-spine film. The safety of oral intubation with in-line C-spine immobilization has been demonstrated in multiple studies.

- If such a child who is intubated is at high risk for C-spine injury, then a CT scan of the upper cervical vertebrae should be done when a head CT scan is performed.

- If an injured patient arrives with a helmet in place and does not require immediate airway intervention, then lateral C-spine can be done prior to removing the helmet. There should be careful attention to maintaining C-spine immobilization while removing the helmet.

- Penetrating injuries to the neck requiring operative intervention should have entry and exit sites denoted with opaque markers on antero-posterior and lateral films of the C-spine.

Chest

The child should be completely exposed to visually inspect for wounds requiring immediate attention. Sucking chest wounds require a sterile occlusive dressing. A flail chest component could be splinted but the patient most likely would need intubation. Roll the patient keeping in-line spine immobilization looking for posterior thoracic penetrating wounds. Look for pneumothorax, hemothorax, or cardiac tamponade by palpating bony parts and auscultating the thorax. Tension pneumothorax may be manifested by contralateral tracheal shift, distended neck veins, and diminished breath sounds. However, a child's small chest size facilitates the contralateral lung's transmission of breath sounds that makes auscultation an insensitive marker for pneumothorax. Neck vein distention is difficult to appreciate and an insensitive marker when assessing for tension pneumothorax. Therefore, a hemodynamically unstable child should undergo immediate needle decompression thoracentesis if there is reason to suspect blunt or penetrating injury to the thorax. After thoracentesis, tube thoracostomy(ies) should be done. Impaled objects protruding from the chest should be left in place until the child undergoes surgery. If the chest radiograph reveals a widened mediastinum or apical cap, and there is a history of significant deceleration injury, aortography is indicated. Although first or second rib fractures increase the likelihood of a vascular injury, their absence does not preclude an aortic injury.

Air lucencies on chest radiography appearing to be of intestinal origin should be considered evidence of a diaphragmatic injury. Any penetrating injury to abdomen or lower chest carries a risk of diaphragmatic injury.

Abdomen

During the secondary survey, determining the exact etiology of an abdominal injury is secondary to determining whether or not an injury actually exists. It is particularly difficult to find retroperitoneal injuries unless there is a high index of suspicion. Signs suggesting abdominal injury include abdominal wall contusion, distention, abdominal or shoulder pain, and signs of peritoneal irritation and shock. Penetrating wounds to the abdomen usually need immediate operative intervention.

Controversies arise in diagnosing and managing blunt abdominal injuries. CT with IV, oral, and colonic contrast may be the most sensitive and useful diagnostic modality (see below under "Imaging"). Diagnostic peritoneal lavage (DPL) provides rapid, objective evaluation of possible intraperitoneal injury, especially involving the liver, spleen, and bowel. It can be considered more sensitive than a CT in diagnosing hollow-viscous injuries, especially early in the evaluation of a child who is a victim of a deceleration injury while wearing a seatbelt (see Table 14-3). It is much less sensitive than CT in diagnosing injuries to the pancreas, duodenum, genitourinary tract, aorta, vena cava, and diaphragm.

DPL is most valuable in deciding whether or not a patient needs immediate laparotomy. Consider performing DPL in the patient requiring urgent anesthesia and nonabdominal surgery, such as evacuation of an epidural hematoma or treatment of a penetrating upper chest injury. Use DPL to help determine the etiology of unexplained hypovolemia and to assist in the evaluation of selected penetrating injuries to the abdomen and lower thorax.

In children, after emptying the bladder with a Foley catheter, use a midline approach above or below the umbilicus. Instill 10 mL/kg of Ringer's lactate if the initial aspirate is not grossly bloody. An aspirate is considered positive if:

- >100,000 red blood cells/mm^3
- >500 white blood cells (WBCs)/mm^3

- a spun effluent hematocrit >2%
- bile, bacteria, or fecal material are found

False positive tests most commonly occur in the face of a pelvic fracture. A positive DPL >100,000 RBCs may be due to a laceration of the liver or spleen but this would not be an indication for surgery. Greater than 80 percent of these patients will stop bleeding under observation without an operative intervention. In these cases, a CT scan is more valuable for evaluating and assessing damage and determining a treatment plan in the stable patient.

Pelvis

Palpate the bony prominences of the pelvis for tenderness or instability. Examine the perineum for laceration, hematoma, or active bleeding. If not checked earlier when placing a Foley, examine the urethral meatus for blood.

Rectal

Perform a rectal examination to determine sphincter muscle tone, rectal integrity, prostatic position, presence of a pelvic fracture, and the presence of blood in the stool.

Extremity Examination

Look at all extremities looking for deformity, contusions, abrasions, intact sensation, penetrating injuries, pulses, and perfusion. The presence of a pulse does not exclude a proximal vascular injury or a compartment syndrome. Palpate long bones circumferentially assessing for tenderness, crepitation, or abnormal movement. Straighten severe angulations of the extremities if possible and apply splints and traction. Open fractures and wounds should be covered with sterile dressings. Look for pelvic fracture(s) by palpation, especially over the anterior iliac spines and pubis. Inspect soft tissue injuries for foreign bodies, irrigate to minimize contamination, and debride devitalized tissues.

Back Examination

Examine the back, particularly in cases of penetrating trauma, looking for hematomas, exit or entry wounds, or spine tenderness. With the neck immobilized if injury or paralysis have not been ruled out, the patient should be rolled for the examination.

Skin

Examine for evidence of contusions, burns, penetration sites, burns, petechiae, and signs of abuse.

Neurologic Examination

Obtain an additional Glasgow Coma Score and perform a more in-depth evaluation of motor, sensory, and cranial nerves. Check the fundi and look for rhinorrhea. Level of consciousness, pupillary examination, and sensorimotor examination, as quantified in the Glasgow Coma Scale, are invaluable in identifying a change in mental status. Presence of paresis or paralysis suggest a major neurologic injury. Conversely, lack of neurologic findings does not eliminate the possibility of a cervical cord injury, especially when the patient has a distracting injury and/or pain other than in the cervical or vertebral area at any level.

Any injured child is at risk for exposure to heat or cold. Due to their relatively larger body surface area, hypothermia can develop in the prehospital setting and/or in the emergency department. Hypothermia may impair circulatory dynamics and coagulation, worsen metabolic acidosis by increasing metabolic demand, and increase peripheral vascular resistance. The likelihood and risks of hypothermia can be minimized with the use of overhead warmers, warmed intravenous fluids, and warm blankets.

Additional Treatment and Tests

Tetanus prophylaxis (toxoid and possibly tetanus immune globulin) should be given. Additional blood chemistry analyses, such as liver transaminases, creatinine, and amylase should be sent. This is also the time to make arrangements for other diagnostic tests.

Consider the psychosocial aspects of traumatic injuries. Permit parents at the child's bedside as soon as the child's clinical status is stabilized.

Burns

Burns are the second most common cause of accidental death among children <4 years of age and may often be a significant part of the problem in a multiply injured patient. For the principles and procedures of burn management, see Chap. 114.

Imaging

A child with major blunt trauma needs three basic radiographs immediately:

- A lateral cervical spine film should be reviewed before proceeding with other films in a stable cooperative patient. If the patient is uncooperative or unstable, other films need to be shot while maintaining cervical spine immobilization.
- Chest films are much more sensitive than clinical examination in smaller children for detecting hemo-pneumo-thoraces. Check for widening of the mediastinum and fractured ribs.
- Pelvic fractures are important clinical indicators in that 80 percent of children with multiple fractures of the pelvis have concomitant abdominal or genitourinary injuries. During the secondary survey, thoracolumbar and extremity films can be completed as indicated.

Based on clinical findings in the primary and secondary surveys, further imaging studies may be needed.

CT Scan of Head

Indications for CT scanning of the brain are:

- GCS <13
- deteriorating neurologic examination
- post-traumatic seizures
- prolonged lethargy
- prolonged vomiting
- loss of consciousness
- amnesia
- confounding medical problems, such as hemophilia (see Chap. 73)

CT Scan of Abdomen

Indications for abdominal CT scanning are:

- A hemodynamically stable victim of blunt trauma with clinical signs of intraabdominal injury
- Hematuria >20 RBCs per high-powered field
- Even minimal hematuria with a history of deceleration injury
- Worrisome mechanism of trauma in the presence of neurologic compromise

Positive findings on abdominal CT are significantly increased if three of the following are present:

- gross hematuria
- lap belt injury

- assault or abuse as a mechanism of trauma
- abdominal tenderness
- trauma score <12

Other indicators that independently increase the positive predictive value of abdominal CT are:

- positive abdominal findings
- worrisome mechanism of trauma
- significant neurologic compromise (GCS <10)

For trauma patients, double-contrast CT should be performed. Dilute gastrograffin (20 mL/kg) is instilled via a nasogastric tube 20 minutes prior to CT scan and intravenous contrast after the initial survey is performed. During the CT, the Foley catheter should be clamped to evaluate the bladder and the nasogastric tube should be pulled into the esophagus to avoid artifact. Dosing for contrast media is outlined in Table 10-11.

Ultrasonography

Ultrasonography may be an alternative to CT in selected cases when CT is not available. Ultrasound can diagnose most injuries to the liver, spleen, and kidneys and can document intraperitoneal fluid. This modality is not a substitute for CT unless the examiner is very experienced in the use of ultrasound in traumatized children.

Table 10-11. Dose of Contrast Media for Radiographic Studies

Age, Years	Dose
Intravenous: 60% Hypaque	
0 to 9	1 mL/0.45 kg bolus
10 or more	50 mL, followed by infusion of 50 to 100 mL during scan
Oral: 1.5% Hypaque (20 mL to 1 L of Fluid Given PO or NG)	
0–2	100 mL
3–5	150–200 mL
6–9	200–250 mL
>9	300–1000 mL
Adult	1000 mL
Oral: Gastrografin, 20 mL/kg via NG Tube 20 Min Prior to Scan	

If intraperitoneal fluid is found by CT or ultrasound with no apparent injury to the spleen or liver, a DPL should be performed. A limitation of CT scanning is the lack of sensitivity in diagnosing injuries to hollow viscous organs (bladder, intestinal perforations/rupture). Consider other diagnostic modalities for motor vehicle crash occupants who have:

- Clinical evidence of lap belt injuries to the abdomen or spine
- Transverse ecchymoses of the abdominal wall with or without abdominal pain or tenderness
- Symptoms or signs of lumbar spine injury with or without spinal cord injury

CT scans in such patients will miss free intraperitoneal air in 75 percent of cases and lumbar spine injuries in 77 percent of cases. Therefore, if a patient is hemodynamically stable, evaluation should include thoracolumbar spine films (especially a lateral) in the resuscitation area, an abdominal film looking for free air (e.g., left lateral decubitus film once C-spine injury is excluded), a cystogram, and a DPL. If injury to bowel or bladder is confirmed, laparotomy is indicated. If non-CT studies are negative but there is evidence of possible retroperitoneal injury, then double-contrast CT is indicated.

Urologic Studies

If a patient has gross blood at the meatus, or the integrity of the urethra is in doubt due to possible pelvic fracture, then a retrograde urethrogram should be performed. Conversely, there is high correlation between blood at the meatus and pelvic fractures. The study is performed by instilling contrast through a Foley catheter that has been inserted into the distal urethra and partially inflated (0.5 to 1.0 mL of saline in the balloon). If the urethra is found not to be damaged, the catheter can be advanced to perform a cystogram.

A "1-shot" intravenous pyelogram is a very useful and reasonable test to perform in the ED to evaluate renovascular status if the patient is too unstable for CT. A 2 to 4 mL/kg bolus of 50 percent diatrizoate sodium (Hypaque) is injected and a film of the abdomen is taken 5 minutes later. This will determine the absence or presence of blood supply to one or both kidneys and it may also show the function of the upper ureters. Knowledge of the status of the blood supply is very important because a renovascular intimal tear with occlusion or vascular disruption must be identified immediately. The warm ischemic time in which to diagnose, repair, and

Table 10-12. Revised Trauma Score[a]

Revised Trauma Score	Glasgow Coma Score	Systolic Blood Pressure (mmHg)	Respiratory Rate (breaths/minute)
4	13–15	>89	10–20
3	9–12	76–89	>29
2	6–8	50–75	6–9
1	4–5	1–49	1–5
0	3	0	0

[a]A score of 0–4 is given for each variable then added (range, 0–12). A score ≥11 indicates potentially important trauma.

avoid irreparable damage to a devascularized kidney is only 6 hours.

INJURY SEVERITY MEASURES

The Trauma Scores

The Revised Trauma Score (Table 10-12) was originally developed for rapid assessment, triage, measuring progression of injury, predicting outcome, and assisting in quality assessment. It is useful in the overall management of trauma patient but is less sensitive for severe injury to a single organ system. It is straightforward to calculate for all trauma patients. It allows for standardization of triage protocols and for scientific comparisons between groups of patients and institutions.

The Pediatric Trauma Score (Table 10-13) was developed to reflect the unique injury pattern in children. It incorporates age into the score.

- Score >8: associated with 100 percent survival
- Score <8: should go to pediatric trauma center
- Score <0: 100 percent mortality

In a study by Nayduch, the Trauma Score had a better predictive value for overall outcome, whereas the Pediatric Trauma Score was a better predictor for appropriate ED disposition. Unfortunately, no trauma score is totally reliable in predicting extent of either injuries or outcomes. For example, Jaimovich reviewed 305 pediatric trauma patients' functional long-term outcomes and found that the current trauma scoring systems fall short in identifying "nonsalvageable" survivors who make meaningful neurologic recovery. In addition, Lieh-Lai's study demonstrated that a low GCS does not always predict the outcome of severe traumatic brain injury and in the absence of hypoxic insult; children with scores of 3 to 5 can recover independent function. Therefore, the Trauma Score or Pediatric Trauma Score can be used to triage patients and predict outcome but exercise caution if used to predict functional outcome.

DISPOSITION/TRANSFER

Triage and Prehospital Care Issues

Prehospital care should include, when appropriate, endotracheal intubation, IV access, immobilization, and

Table 10-13. Pediatric Trauma Score[a]

Variables	+2	+1	−1
Airway	Normal	Maintainable	Unmaintainable
CNS	Awake	Obtunded/LOC	Coma
Body weight	>20 kg	10–20 kg	<10 kg
Systolic BP	>90 mm Hg	90–50 mm Hg	<50 mm Hg
Open wound	None	Minor	Major
Skeletal injury	None	Closed fracture	Open/multiple fractures

[a]A score of +2, +1, or −1 is given to each variable, then added (range −6 to 12). A score ≥8 indicates potentially important trauma. LOC = Loss of consciousness.

rapid transport. It is unresolved which procedures should be attempted in the field or during transport. For example, the prehospital success rate for endotracheal intubation varies from 48 to 89 percent. It has been demonstrated that trauma deaths could be reduced by 25 percent in a system by providing additional airway skills training, using aggressive airway management, and developing guidelines for ground versus aeromedical transport. One computer model found that children in respiratory distress in urban centers would have a shorter time to intubation if transported by police rather than EMS units. Rural systems as a whole require more aggressive initial treatment in the field due to transport times 3 to 4 times greater than those in urban areas.

Vascular access is a difficult procedure under the best of circumstances and is often a reason for delay in transport of a critically ill child. It is reasonable that traumatized children can be transported immediately without trying to attain vascular access at the scene if a short transport time is expected. Second, intraosseous infusion (IO) should be used as a quick access for crystalloid infusion if attempts at intravenous cannulation are unsuccessful after 90 seconds. IO can be placed successfully in the field 80 percent of the time.

Facilities that receive trauma victims should have the appropriate personnel and patient care resources committed at all times. However, a majority of seriously injured children are not brought to comprehensive trauma

Table 10-14. Reasons for Transfer of Pediatric Trauma Patients for Tertiary Care

I. Mechanism of trauma
  A. Falls
    1. Falls >10 feet involving patients <14 years old
    2. Falls from second floor or higher
  B. Motor vehicle–crash passenger
    1. Evidence of high-impact velocity motor vehicle accident
      a. Shattered windshield
      b. Evidence of intrusion into the passenger compartment
      c. Bent steering wheel
    2. Rollover incident with unrestrained victim
    3. Ejection of the patient from the vehicle
    4. Death of an occupant within the same passenger compartment
    5. Extraction time >20 min
  C. Auto versus pedestrian incident at >20 mph and victim <15 years old
  D. Major burns
  E. Blast injuries
II. Physiology
  A. Total trauma score of ≤12
  B. Pediatric Trauma Score ≤8
  C. Unstable vital signs (age appropriate)
  D. Compromise of airway, breathing, or circulation, or need for protracted ventilation
  E. Severely compromised neurologic status (Glasgow Coma Scale of ≤8)
III. Injuries
  A. Penetrating injuries involving the head, neck, chest, and abdomen or groin
  B. Two or more proximal long bone fractures
  C. Traumatic amputation proximal to either the wrist or the ankle
  D. Evidence of neurologic deficit due to spinal cord injury
  E. Flail chest, major chest wall injury or pulmonary contusion
  F. Penetrating head injury, open head injury, or CSF leak
  G. Suspicion of vascular or cardiac injury
  H. Severe maxillofacial injuries
  I. Depressed skull fracture

centers. Children, therefore, can and should receive appropriate care at all hospitals where EMS policies have established the facility as capable of receiving patients with life-threatening conditions. In a hospital without pediatric anesthesia or pediatric surgical consultants, early transfers to a pediatric trauma center, adult trauma center, or pediatric intensive care unit should be considered. Contingency plans for transfers and referral patterns and prearranged agreements between institutions should be established prospectively. Guidelines for transfer to a pediatric trauma center are given in Table 10-14.

Children who appear to have clinical brain death should be considered for continued resuscitation since they may be candidates for organ procurement. If heart, heart-lung, kidney, pancreas, and liver transplantation are considered, pre-mortem management is key to the viability of the organs. Considerations such as these can be undertaken within a facility that has received legal and ethical guidance and support for such undertakings. Sensitive parental consultation and support are paramount. Organ donation may provide traumatized families some consolation and strength in the face of such tremendous grief.

When dealing with a traumatized child, the physician must communicate openly and clearly with the family. Psychological support is needed through the entire hospital course. Disposition and treatment decisions and progress reports need to be presented frequently, succinctly, and with sensitivity. Parents should be allowed to see the child and/or accompany him or her as soon as is practical.

BIBLIOGRAPHY

APLS Joint Task Force: Trauma in Strange GR (ed): APLS: The Pediatric Emergency Medicine Course. Elk Grove Village, IL and Dallas, TX: American Academy of Pediatrics & American College of Emergency Physicians, 1998, pp 59–78.

ACS Committee on Trauma: Advanced Trauma Life Support Manual. Chicago: American College of Surgeons, 2000.

ACS Committee on Trauma: *Trauma Systems in Resources for Optimal Care of the Injured Patient.* Chicago: American College of Surgeons, 1999.

Fleisher G, Ludwig S: *Textbook of Pediatric Emergency Medicine.* Baltimore: Williams & Wilkins, 3d ed, 1998.

Jaffe D, Weson D: Emergency management of blunt trauma in children. *N Engl J Med* 324:1477–1482, 1991.

Nathans AB, Jukovich GJ, Maier RV, et al: Relationship between trauma center volume and outcomes. *JAMA* 285:1164–1171, 2001.

Schafermeyer R: Advances in trauma: Pediatric trauma. *Emerg Med Clin North Am* 1 1:187–205, 1993.

Sheik AA, Culbertson CB: Emergency department thoracotomy in children: Rationale for selective application. *J Trauma* 34:322, 1993.

Teach SJ, Antosia RE, Lund DP, et al: Prehospital fluid therapy in pediatric trauma patients. *Pediatr Emerg Care* 11:5–8, 1995.

Wright JL, Klein BL: Regionalized pediatric trauma systems. *Clin Pediatr Emerg Med* 2:3–12, 2001.

11

Head Trauma

Kimberly S. Quayle

HIGH-YIELD FACTS

- The most common cause of head injury in children is falls. However, more severe injuries are most likely to be caused by motor vehicle collisions, bicycle collisions, and assaults, including child abuse.
- Children with skull fractures are more likely to have an associated intracranial injury; however, intracranial injury may occur in the absence of skull fracture.
- Children with severe injuries, including those with altered mental status, focal neurologic deficits, or penetrating injuries, should undergo emergent computed tomography of the head and prompt neurosurgical consultation.
- Infants and children younger than 2 years may have subtle presentations despite clinically significant intracranial injury.
- Children with minor head injury and no loss of consciousness or brief loss of consciousness may be observed without computed tomography of the head.
- Prevention of hypoxia, ischemia, and increased intracranial pressure is essential for children with severe head injuries.
- Although children have a greater likelihood of survival and recovery from brain injury than adults, they may be more vulnerable to long-term cognitive and behavioral dysfunction.

Each year approximately 22,000 children aged 1 to 19 years die from trauma in the United States and 600,000 sustain injuries necessitating hospital admission. Brain injury causes more death and disability in children than in any other age group. Eighty percent of children who die from multiple trauma have significant head injury,

compared to 50 percent of adult trauma victims. Pediatric brain injury leads to major morbidity, from physical disability, seizures, and mental retardation. The most common cause of head injury in children is falls; however, severe injuries are more likely to be caused by motor vehicle collisions (with the child as occupant or pedestrian), bicycle collisions, and assaults, including child abuse. Males account for two-thirds of head-injured children in all age grops.

PATHOPHYSIOLOGY

Primary brain injury occurs as a result of direct mechanical damage inflicted during the traumatic event. Secondary injuries occur from metabolic events such as hypoxia, ischemia, or increased intracranial pressure. The prognosis for recovery depends on the severity of the injuries. Anatomic features, specific injuries, and intracranial pressure physiology are important components in the pathophysiology of pediatric brain injury.

ANATOMY

The scalp is the outermost structure of the head and is adjacent on its inner surface to the galea, a tendinous sheath connecting the frontalis and occipitalis muscles (Fig. 11-1). Beneath the galea is the subgaleal compartment, a space that may contain loose connective tissue. Large subgaleal hematomas may form in this space. The pericranium lies just below, tightly adhering to the skull. The outer and inner tables of the skull are separated by the diploic space. The thin, fibrous dura is next, and it contains few blood vessels compared to the underlying leptomeninges, the arachnoid, and pia. Small veins bridge the subdural space from the leptomeninges to drain into the dural sinuses. Dural attachments partially compartmentalize the brain. In the midline, the falx cerebri divides the right and left hemispheres of the brain. The tentorium divides the anterior and middle fossa from the posterior fossa, with an opening for the brain stem. Cerebrospinal fluid surrounds the brain within the subarachnoid space. Approximately 72 percent of the adult intracranial volume of 1200 to 1500 mL is attained by 2 years of age, 90 percent by 8 years, and 96 percent by adolescence.

The outer structures protect the brain during everyday movements and minor trauma; however, these usually protective features can inflict damage when significant force is applied or sudden movement occurs. Movement

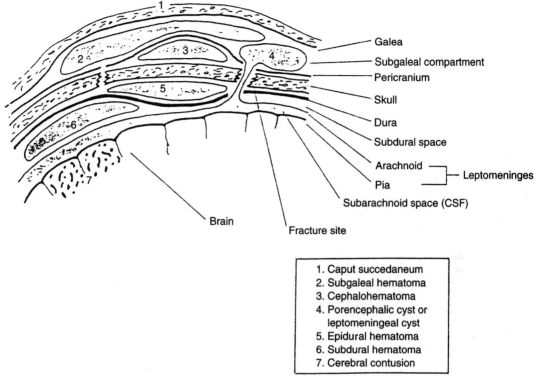

Galea
Subgaleal compartment
Pericranium
Skull
Dura
Subdural space
Arachnoid ──┐
           ├─ Leptomeninges
Pia ──────┘
Subarachnoid space (CSF)

Brain

Fracture site

1. Caput succedaneum
2. Subgaleal hematoma
3. Cephalohematoma
4. Porencephalic cyst or leptomeningeal cyst
5. Epidural hematoma
6. Subdural hematoma
7. Cerebral contusion

Fig. 11-1. Traumatic head injuries. [From Barkin RM, Rosen P (eds): *Emergency Pediatrics: A Guide to Ambulatory Care,* 3d ed. St. Louis: Mosby-Year Book, 1990. Reproduced with permission of Mosby-Year Book, Inc.]

of the brain within the vault along the uneven base of the skull may injure brain tissue. The unyielding, mature skull can contribute to brain injury when brain edema or an expanding hematoma develops. Subsequently, herniation across compartments can cause compression of vital structures, ischemia from vascular occlusion, and infarction.

In infants, the open sutures and thin calvarium produce a more flexible skull capable of absorbing greater impact. Incomplete myelinization contributes to greater plasticity of the brain as well. This flexibility permits more severe distortion between the skull and dura, and the cerebral vessels and brain, increasing susceptibility to hemorrhage. Finally, the disproportionately large size and weight of the head compared to the rest of the body in infants and young children contributes to an increased likelihood of head injury.

SPECIFIC INJURIES

Scalp injuries may bleed profusely since it is richly vascularized. Scalp bleeding can lead to hemodynamically significant blood loss from relatively small lacerations, especially in infants and young children. Open scalp wounds should be carefully explored for skull integrity, depressions, or foreign bodies. The presenting sign of a subgaleal hematoma is an extensive soft tissue swelling that occurs several hours or days after the traumatic event and is commonly associated with a skull fracture. A subgaleal hematoma can persist for several days to weeks.

Linear nondepressed skull fractures occur at the point of impact. The presence of a skull fracture indicates a significant blow to the head, and children with skull fractures are more likely to have an associated intracranial injury. However, the absence of a skull fracture does not exclude the presence of intracranial injury. "Growing fractures" are unique to infants and young children. They may occur after a skull fracture in children under 2 years of age when associated with a dural tear. Rapid brain growth postinjury may be associated with the development of a leptomeningeal cyst, which is an extrusion of cerebrospinal fluid or brain tissue through the dural defect. Thus, children younger than 2 with a skull fracture require follow-up to detect a growing fracture.

Basilar skull fractures typically occur at the petrous portion of the temporal bone, although they may occur anywhere along the base of the skull. Clinical signs suggesting a basilar skull fracture include hemotympanum, cerebrospinal fluid otorrhea, cerebrospinal fluid rhinorrhea, periorbital ecchymosis ("raccoon eyes"), or postauricular ecchymosis (Battle's sign). Radiologic diagnosis often requires detailed computed tomography (CT) imaging of the temporal bone, as plain skull radiographs or routine head CT scans may not be diagnostic.

Epidural hematomas occur as commonly in children as in adults, although they are less likely to be clinically apparent in children. Eighty percent occur in combination with a skull fracture and meningeal artery bleeding; the remainder are venous in origin. While they may be life-threatening, prompt diagnosis leading to surgical intervention makes an excellent outcome possible. Signs and symptoms include headache, vomiting, and altered mental status, which may progress to signs and symptoms of uncal herniation with pupillary changes and hemiparesis.

Acute subdural hematomas occur more commonly in adults than in children. Acute interhemispheric subdural hematomas, which occur more commonly in infants and young children, are often caused by shaking/impact injuries of abuse. Subdural hematomas usually result from tearing of the bridging veins, and typically occur over the cerebral convexities. The mechanism of injury is usually acceleration-deceleration, therefore subdural hematomas are often associated with more diffuse brain injury. Subdural hematomas progress more slowly than epidural bleeds, with symptoms commonly including irritability, vomiting, and lethargy.

Parenchymal contusions are bruises or tears of brain tissue. Bony irregularities of the skull cause these cerebral contusions as the brain moves within the skull. A coup injury occurs at the site of impact, while a contrecoup injury occurs at a site remote from the impact. Intraparenchymal hemorrhages may also occur from shearing injury or penetrating wounds. Signs and symptoms may include decreased level of consciousness, focal neurologic findings, and seizures.

Penetrating injuries result from sharp-object penetration or gunshot wounds. Extensive brain injury is common and severity depends on the path of the object and location and degree of associated hemorrhage.

A concussion is defined as a transient loss of awareness and responsiveness following head trauma. Transient symptoms may include loss of consciousness, vomiting, headache, amnesia, or dizziness.

Diffuse brain swelling occurs three times more often in children than in adults. The swelling usually results from a shearing, acceleration-deceleration injury. Prolonged coma or death may occur.

INTRACRANIAL PRESSURE AND HERNIATION SYNDROMES

The total volume of the intracranial vault is constant. Approximately 70 percent of this volume is brain, 20 percent is cerebrospinal and interstitial fluid, and 10 percent is blood. If one of these three components increases in volume, then the other two compartments must decrease or intracranial pressure rises. The main component of compensation is a displacement of cerebrospinal fluid into the spinal canal. Once this compensatory mechanism is maximized, any additional increases in volume cause elevation of intracranial pressure to abnormal levels (>15 to 20 mmHg). Cerebral perfusion becomes impaired and irreversible ischemic damage to the brain ensues.

An intracranial mass or hematoma will occupy the fixed intracranial space, compress the normal brain tissue, and reduce blood flow. Cytotoxic cerebral edema occurs with fluid accumulation within damaged brain and glial cells. Interstitial cerebral edema results from decreased absorption of fluid following brain trauma. Vasogenic cerebral edema occurs as the endothelial cell barrier is compromised and leakage of fluid into the perivascular brain tissue occurs.

The volume of cerebrospinal fluid may also increase despite the compensatory redistribution of the fluid into the spinal canal. As brain and blood volumes increase, the ventricular spaces become compressed until redistribution is not possible. Additionally, if the cerebrospinal fluid pathways are compressed by edematous tissue, cerebrospinal fluid outflow ceases and ventricular dilation and hydrocephalus occur.

Cerebral blood volume in head-injured children may be increased as a result of brain injury. The mechanisms of autoregulation of cerebral blood flow are complex, however, flow is often increased in head-injured children, possibly due to a loss of normal autoregulatory mechanisms. Hypoxia and hypercapnia from hypoventilation of the injured patient also affect cerebral blood flow. Cerebral hyperemia may contribute to the development of brain swelling in children in the first 24 hours postinjury.

Diffusely or focally increased intracranial pressure may produce herniation. Cingulate herniation occurs as one cerebral hemisphere is displaced underneath the falx cerebri to the opposite side. A transtentorial or uncal herniation is of major clinical significance (Fig. 11-2). A mass lesion or hematoma forces the ipsilateral uncus of the temporal lobe through the space between the cerebral peduncle and the tentorium. This causes ipsilateral compression of the oculomotor nerve and an ipsilateral dilated nonreactive pupil. The cerebral peduncle is compressed causing a contralateral hemiparesis. As the intracranial pressure increases and the brain stem is

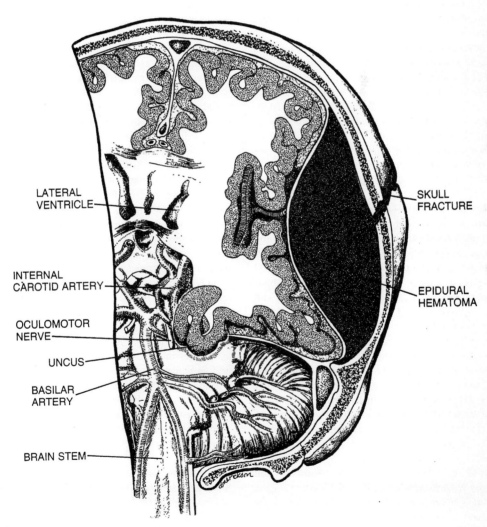

Fig. 11-2. Anterior view of transtentorial uncal herniation caused by a large epidural hematoma. (From American College of Emergency Physicians: *Emergency Medicine: A Comprehensive Study Guide,* 3d ed. New York: McGraw-Hill, 1992. Reproduced with permission of McGraw-Hill.)

compressed, consciousness wanes. If herniation continues, ongoing brain stem deterioration occurs, progressing to apnea and death. Uncal herniation may be bilateral if there are bilateral lesions or diffuse edema. Herniation of the cerebellar tonsils downward through the foramen magnum occurs infrequently in children. Medullary compression from this herniation causes bradycardia, respiratory arrest, and death.

ASSESSMENT

Assessment begins with a detailed history of the traumatic event. The examiner must obtain as many details about the mechanism of injury as possible. Time and location of injury are also important. Symptoms and signs occurring since the injury should be noted, including loss of consciousness, seizures, vomiting, headache, visual changes, altered mental status, weakness, and amnesia. Past medical history should include prior history of seizures, neurologic abnormalities, bleeding disorders, and immunization status. Child abuse should be suspected for a witnessed report of abuse, a history insufficient to explain the injuries present, a changing or inconsistent history, or a developmentally incompatible history.

Physical evaluation begins with the primary assessment. Airway obstruction by the tongue commonly occurs in unconscious children with serious head injury. Blood, vomitus, teeth, foreign bodies, or other debris may obstruct the airway as well. Establish an airway by positioning, suctioning, placing an oral airway, or intubation. Maintain cervical spine control in children with significant head injury until cervical spine injury is excluded. Manually stabilize the cervical spine during laryngoscopy.

Once the airway is established, ventilation is assessed. The examiner should observe chest expansion, auscultate breath sounds, and assess for cyanosis or respiratory distress. Hypoventilation is treated with 100 percent oxygen, bag-valve-mask ventilation, and subsequent intubation of the trachea with consideration of rapid sequence technique.

Compared to awake intubation, the rapid sequence induction (RSI) technique produces an unconscious and paralyzed patient, creating an easier procedure for the physician and providing a better-tolerated procedure for the patient with less discomfort and less intracranial pressure elevation. The RSI technique should also reduce the risk of aspiration in trauma patients, who should be presumed to have full stomachs. The general procedure for RSI is discussed in Chap. 5; however, there are a few points of special note regarding the use of RSI in head trauma patients.

Ketamine is contraindicated in head-injured patients because it increases intracranial pressure. The use of succinylcholine is controversial in head-injured patients due to concerns for increased intracranial pressure associated with its use. Rocuronium, a nondepolarizing muscle relaxant that does not increase intracranial pressure, is an alternative because its onset of action is similar to succinylcholine, but its duration of action is significantly longer. RSI for intubation is contraindicated in patients with major facial or laryngeal trauma or distorted facial and airway anatomy. These conditions may lead to a situation in which intubation or mask ventilation is unsuccessful.

Circulation is assessed by evaluating the heart rate, peripheral pulses, and perfusion. Life-threatening hemorrhage must be controlled and blood pressure maintained, so that adequate cerebral perfusion occurs. Hypovolemic shock is rare after an isolated head injury, although it does rarely occur in infants and young children. Other sources for hypovolemia must be sought.

After the rapid ABC (*a*irway, *b*reathing, *c*irculation) assessment, a primary survey of neurologic disability follows. Level of consciousness should be ascertained and categorized as alert, responsive to verbal stimulus, responsive to painful stimulus, or unresponsive (AVPU). Pupillary response is then evaluated. The remainder of the primary survey is completed prior to returning to a more detailed secondary neurologic examination. The scalp is examined and palpated for depressions. In an infant, the fontanel is evaluated. Signs of basilar skull fracture as discussed earlier should be noted. Extraocular movements, muscle tone, spontaneous movements, and posture are evaluated. An older child should move the extremities in response to the examiner's request. The neck is palpated for tenderness or deformities. Stereotyped posturing should be noted and described. Decorticate posturing signifies damage to the cerebral cortex, white matter, or basal ganglia. Decerebrate posturing suggests damage lower to the midbrain.

In adults and older children, the Glasgow Coma Scale is commonly used to assess and follow the level of consciousness in head-injured patients. The Glasgow Coma Scale evaluates for eye opening, best motor response, and best verbal response (Table 11-1). Use of the Glasgow Coma Scale in infants and young children is limited by this age group's undeveloped verbal skills. Many specialized coma scales for use in children have been developed, however, none have been validated. Evalua-

Table 11-1. Glasgow Coma Scale[a]

Eye opening (E)	Spontaneous	4
	To speech/voice	3
	To pain	2
	No response	1
Motor response (M)	Obeys commands	6
	Localizes pain	5
	Withdraws to pain	4
	Abnormal flexion-decorticate	3
	Abnormal extension-decerebrate	2
	No response	1
Verbal response (V)	Oriented	5
	Confused/disoriented	4
	Inappropriate words	3
	Incomprehensible sounds	2
	No response	1

[a]E + M + V = coma score (range: 3 to 15)

tion of young children and infants following head injury may be difficult, particularly the assessment of mental status and neurologic examination.

The neurologic status of a head-injured child must be regularly reassessed, particularly with regard to level of consciousness and vital signs. The frequency of reassessment is dictated by the condition of the child.

DIAGNOSTIC STUDIES

In children with serious injuries, complete blood count, type and cross-match, electrolytes, and coagulation studies should be done. Arterial blood gases, toxicology screens, and ethanol levels are obtained as indicated. Cervical spine films should be obtained in alert patients with neck pain or neurologic deficits and in all unconscious patients.

Computed tomography (CT) of the head has become the diagnostic method of choice for identification of intracranial pathology in acute head trauma victims. Skull radiographs are not routinely recommended. However, they may be useful in certain clinical situations, such as screening in young infants with scalp hematomas, in cases of suspected nonaccidental trauma, or when CT is not readily available.

Children with severe injuries including those with altered mental status, focal neurologic deficits, or penetrating injuries should undergo emergent head CT and prompt neurosurgical consultation. Children with a

known skull fracture or signs of a basilar or depressed skull fracture should also undergo head CT. Consensus is lacking regarding the management of previously healthy children who are alert with normal, nonfocal neurologic examinations following minor head injury. The American Academy of Pediatrics recently published recommendations for the evaluation of children 2 to 20 years of age with minor head injury, but without multiple trauma, cervical spine injury, preexisting neurologic disorder, bleeding diathesis, suspected intentional head trauma, language barrier, or the presence of drugs or alcohol. This practice parameter recommends observation by a reliable caretaker for neurologically normal children with no loss of consciousness or with brief loss of consciousness. Head CT scans may be obtained for children with brief loss of consciousness if desired by the physician and parents. Children without a history of loss of consciousness, but with a history of seizure, headache, vomiting, or amnesia, may be observed without a head CT if they have an alert mental status and a normal neurologic examination.

Infants and children younger than 2 years may have subtle presentations despite clinically significant intracranial injury. Recently published guidelines provide recommendations for the management of minor head injury in this age group as well. Infants with high-risk findings such as depressed mental status, focal neurologic deficit, signs of depressed or basilar skull fracture, seizure, irritability, acute skull fracture, bulging fontanel, vomiting 5 or more times or for more than 6 hours, or loss of consciousness for 1 minute or longer should undergo prompt CT scanning. A head CT should be considered in infants at intermediate risk with vomiting 3 to 4 times, brief loss of consciousness, or history of resolved lethargy or irritability. Head CT, skull radiographs, or observation may be selected for infants with scalp hematomas, a higher-force mechanism of trauma, a fall onto a hard surface, or unwitnessed trauma. If skull radiographs are chosen based on lack of availability of CT or need for sedation, then the presence of a skull fracture should prompt transport to a facility capable of performing head CT. Infants at low risk who are asymptomatic and have a low-energy mechanism of trauma may be carefully observed by a reliable caretaker.

Patients who do not meet criteria for imaging may be observed at home by a reliable caretaker with careful instructions to return the child to medical attention if symptoms develop, worsen, or persist. Children who have normal head CT scans and normal mental status and neurologic examinations may also be observed at home, as the development of delayed intracranial injuries in these patients is rare. Children with isolated nondepressed skull fractures without intracranial injury may also be observed at home.

TREATMENT

The goal of management of head injury in children is to prevent secondary injury to the brain. Prevention of hypoxia, ischemia, and increased intracranial pressure is essential. Prompt neurosurgical intervention is necessary in the majority of seriously head-injured or multisystem-injured children.

As discussed earlier, endotracheal intubation and controlled ventilation are almost always required for patients with severe head injury. Hypercarbia will increase cerebral blood flow and intracranial pressure, and must be avoided. Hypoxemia may worsen the initial injury or cause secondary brain injury. By following arterial blood gases and adjusting ventilator settings accordingly, it is possible to keep arterial PO_2 and PCO_2 near normal levels, unless the child has underlying pulmonary disease or injury. Moderate hyperventilation (PCO_2 32 to 35 torr) is recommended for management of increased intracranial pressure. In the emergency department setting, modest hyperventilation may be used in unconscious patients, prior to insertion of an intracranial pressure monitor.

Brain perfusion must be preserved by maintaining normal intracranial pressure and normal mean arterial pressure. Cerebral perfusion pressure is equal to mean arterial pressure minus intracranial pressure. An arterial catheter should be inserted for close monitoring of arterial pressure. More invasive cardiovascular monitoring is rarely necessary. Hypotension should be treated with isotonic fluid boluses and inotropic medications as needed to maintain an adequate mean arterial blood pressure and cerebral perfusion pressure.

Mannitol and loop diuretics are often used to maintain optimal intracranial pressure by reducing intravascular volume. Fluid restriction may be used in conjunction; however, cerebral perfusion pressure must be maintained. Syndromes of inappropriate antidiuretic hormone secretion or diabetes insipidus may occur in children with serious head injury; therefore fluid balance and electrolyte status must be followed closely.

Seizures may occur following brain injury. Most children with serious injuries are treated with phenytoin or fosphenytoin either to treat active seizures or for prophylaxis.

Seriously brain-injured children must be monitored in an intensive care setting. Cardiopulmonary monitors, noninvasive blood pressure monitors or indwelling arterial catheters, and urinary catheters are commonly used. Intracranial pressure monitors may be used to detect acute changes in intracranial pressure, to limit indiscriminate therapies to control intracranial pressure, and to reduce intracranial pressure directly by cerebrospinal fluid drainage. The patient should be positioned with a 15° to 30° elevation of the head. Corticosteroids and hypothermia are not routinely used to treat children with serious brain injury. Coordination of the care for these children should involve neurosurgical, pediatric, and critical care physicians, most often in a tertiary care pediatric center.

The care for children with less serious injuries varies. Many children are admitted for observation with serial neurologic examinations. The majority of children who have minor head injuries can be observed safely at home by an adult caretaker with careful, detailed instructions to return if there is a change in condition. If a responsible caretaker cannot be identified, hospital admission for observation for the first 24 hours is warranted.

PROGNOSIS

Although children have a greater likelihood of surviving a severe head injury and are more likely to recover from focal brain injury than adults, they may be more vulnerable than adults to long-term cognitive and behavioral dysfunction after diffuse brain injury. Early identification of neurobehavioral deficits is an important part of follow-up in children with significant head injury.

BIBLIOGRAPHY

Adelson PD, Kochanek PM: Head injury in children. *J Child Neurol* 13:2, 1998.

Committee on Quality Improvement, American Academy of Pediatrics: The management of minor closed head injury in children. *Pediatrics* 104:1407, 1999.

Duhaime AC, Christian CW, Rorke LB, et al: Nonaccidental head injury in infants—the shaken baby syndrome. *N Engl J Med* 338:1822, 1998.

Greenes DS, Schutzman SA: Occult intracranial injury in infants. *Ann Emerg Med* 32:680, 1998.

Klassen TP, Reed MH, Stiell IG, et al: Variation in utilization of computed tomography scanning for the investigation of minor head trauma in children: A Canadian experience. *Acad Emerg Med* 7:739-744, 2000.

Quayle KS: Minor head injury in the pediatric patient. *Pediatr Clin North Am* 46:1189, 1999.

Quayle KS, Jaffe DM, Kuppermann N, et al: Diagnostic testing for acute head injury in children: When are head computed tomography and skull radiographs indicated? *Pediatrics* (Online) 99:11, 1997. http://ww.pediatrics.org/cgi/content/full/99/5/e11.

Sanchez JI, Paidas CN: Childhood trauma: Now and in the new millennium. *Surg Clin North Am* 79:1503, 1999.

Schutzman SA, Barnes P, Duhaime AC, et al: Evaluation and management of children younger than two years with apparently minor head trauma: Proposed guidelines. *Pediatrics,* Accepted for publication.

Zuckerman GB, Conway EE: Accidental head injury. *Pediatr Ann* 26:621, 1997.

12

Evaluation of Children for Cervical Spine Injuries

David M. Jaffe

HIGH-YIELD FACTS

- Upper cervical spine injuries are often fatal and cervical spine injuries should be suspected in blunt trauma victims with cardiopulmonary arrest.

- Due to differences in anatomy and physiology, children sustain proportionally more upper cervical spine and spinal cord injury without radiographic abnormality (SCIWORA) injuries than adults. Many SCIWORA injuries can be detected using MRI technology.

- Standard radiographic screening for children consists of the AP, lateral, and open mouth views; however, in younger or uncooperative children, the open mouth view can be omitted. CT is more sensitive for bony injury and MRI for soft tissue injury.

- Although spine immobilization is indicated when cervical spine injury is suspected and used liberally in American out-of-hospital transport systems, there are documented complications, including restriction of ventilation, pain, improper spine positioning, and interference with other important diagnostic and therapeutic procedures. A recent study has challenged the benefit of out-of-hospital immobilization even among spine-injured patients.

- In-line stabilization, rapid sequence induction and oral endotracheal intubation are the preferred techniques to achieve airway stabilization in children with suspected cervical spine injury.

Few medical disorders are as devastating as the consequences of spinal cord injury. There are approximately 200,000 persons with spinal cord injury in the United States, and between 1 and 10 percent of them are children. The annual direct medical costs of these injuries exceeds $4 billion, and the estimated annual lost earnings totals $3.4 billion. These numbers do not begin to describe the physical and emotional challenges experienced by patients with spinal cord injury.

The emergency physician should maintain a high level of suspicion for possible cervical spine injury to avoid inadvertently causing or worsening cord damage by permitting unnecessary neck motion when an unstable bony or ligamentous injury is present. This legitimate concern raises several questions, the answers to which remain controversial.

- Which children need spinal immobilization, and how is it best achieved?

- If an artificial airway is needed, how should it be provided in children who might have spine injuries?

- How is the cervical spine "cleared"?

EPIDEMIOLOGY

Approximately 1100 children sustain spine injuries annually. In the United States, the incidence of spinal cord injury in children has been estimated at 18 per million, compared to 28 to 50 per million for all age groups.

Motor vehicle-related injuries and falls are the leading causes of spinal cord injuries. Firearms and sports activities are the other major causes. Most sports-related injuries occur among adolescents and young adults. Football, wrestling, gymnastics, ice hockey, pole vaulting, and diving have been associated with fatal or disabling spine injuries.

The case fatality rate was reported as 59 percent in a carefully done epidemiologic study in California. All children in this study who sustained their cord injuries in auto-bicycle or auto-motorcycle crashes died, as did 76 percent of pedestrians struck by an automobile.

Because it is logical to be concerned about spine injuries associated with head injury, it is instructive to compare the epidemiology of spine injury with that of brain injury. Brain injury is associated with 80 percent of traumatic deaths in children. A rough estimate of the incidence of brain injury in children is 1850 per million, approximately 100 times that of spine injury. Two studies in adults found no differences in the rates of cervical spine injury among patients with and without head injury. Another study did show a small increase in spine injury among adults with head injury (4.5 versus 1.1 percent). Since head injury is so common among seriously injured children, the emergency physician will often need to evaluate for spine injury in the presence of head injury. But the absence of head injury does not obviate the need to evaluate for cervical spine injury. Cervical spine injury should also be suspected in the multiply-injured child with absent vital signs.

ANATOMY AND PHYSIOLOGY

The major anatomic components of the cervical spine are the bones, joints, ligaments, and intervertebral disks, as well as the muscles, nerves, and vessels of the neck. The bones consist of the base of the skull and the first 8 vertebrae, C1-C7 and T1. With the exception of the first two, the vertebrae are similar to one another, consisting of a body and an arch that form a ring around the spinal canal, which contains the spinal cord and subarachnoid space (Fig. 12-1). The C1 and C2 vertebrae have unique characteristics (Figs. 12-2 and 12-3). The occiput artic-ulates with articular facets on the lateral arches of C1, which is a ring-like structure. The odontoid process of C2 is articulated with the inner surface of the anterior arch of C1 and serves as a pivot point for rotation of C1 on C2. The atlantoaxial joint is stabilized by a transverse

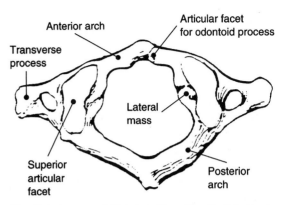

Fig. 12-2. Anatomy of C1 (atlas). (From Bonadio WA: Cervi-cal spine trauma in children: Part I. General concepts, normal anatomy, radiographic evaluation. *Am J Emerg Med* 11:158-165, 1993. Reproduced by permission of W.B. Saunders Company, copyright 1983.)

ligament. Other ligaments that connect the vertebrae are depicted in Fig. 12-4. Intervertebral disks cushion com-pression forces applied to the cervical spine and support the spinal column during bending. Facets and interfacet joints also absorb compression forces and limit flexion. Interfacet joints have synovial membranes and fibrous capsules.

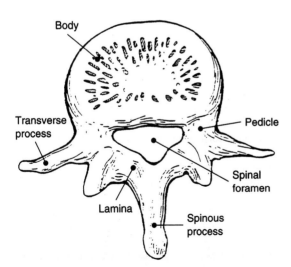

Fig. 12-1. Anatomy of a typical cervical vertebra. (From Bona-dio WA: Cervical spine trauma in children: Part I. General con-cepts, normal anatomy, radiographic evaluation. *Am J Emerg Med* 11:158-165, 1993. Reproduced by permission of W.B. Saunders Company, copyright 1993.)

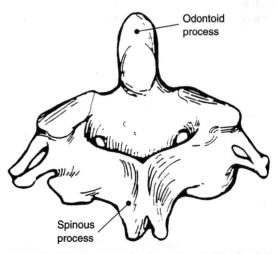

Fig. 12-3. Anatomy of C2 (axis). (From Bonadio WA: Cervical spine trauma in children: Part I. General concepts, normal anatomy, radiographic evaluation. *Am J Emerg Med* 11:158-165, 1993. Reproduced by permission of W.B. Saunders Com-pany, copyright 1983.)

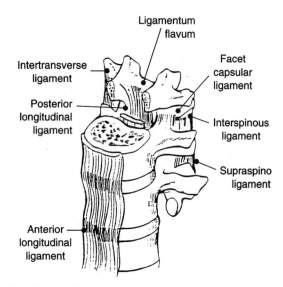

Fig. 12-4. Multilayered section of cervical spine anatomy with anterior and posterior compartments delimited by posterior longitudinal ligament. (From Bonadio WA: Cervical spine trauma in children: Part I. General concepts, normal anatomy, radiographic evaluation. *Am J Emerg Med* 11:158-165, 1993. Reproduced by permission of W.B. Saunders Company, copyright 1983.)

Because the vertebral column undergoes significant developmental changes in childhood, the patterns of injury also differ between children and adults. The biomechanical and anatomic features of the spine attain adult patterns between the ages of 8 and 10 years; however, the adult patterns of injury are not fully manifest until age 15 years. Compared to the adult, the pediatric spine is characterized by greater elasticity of ligaments, joint capsules, and cartilaginous structures; a relatively more horizontal orientation of facet joints and uncinate processes; and wedged anterior surfaces of vertebral bodies (Figs. 12-5 and 12-6). The neck musculature is relatively underdeveloped, and the head is relatively large and heavy. The center of gravity is higher, and the anatomic fulcrum of the spine is at the level of C2 and C3, compared to its location in the lower cervical spine in adults. There is also a greater vulnerability of the vertebral arteries to ischemia, thought to be due to relative instability of the atlantooccipital joint. The major differences in injury patterns between children and adults resulting from these anatomic and biomechanical features are a predisposition for upper cervical spine injuries and for spinal cord injury without radiographic abnormality (SCIWORA) in pediatric patients. Fractures below the

level of C3 account for only about 30 percent of spinal lesions among children less than 8 years of age, whereas they account for 85 percent of those in adults. The reported prevalence of SCIWORA ranges from 1 to 67 percent, but most studies report SCIWORA in 25 to 50 percent of pediatric spinal cord injuries. Flexion-extension views and computed tomography (CT) scans of the spine are normal. Autopsy studies have revealed muscular and ligamentous disruptions, growth plate avulsions, epiphyseal separations, spinal instability, and subdural or epidural spinal hematomas. Some of these injuries can be unstable despite the absence of bony injury. Many of these soft tissue injuries of the spinal cord and ligaments have recently been demonstrated on MRI.

EVALUATION AND MANAGEMENT

Spinal cord injury should be suspected whenever there has been severe multiple trauma; significant trauma to the head, neck, or back; or any trauma associated with high-speed vehicular crashes and falls from heights. A useful diagnostic mnemonic is to evaluate the "six P's":

- Pain
- Position
- Paralysis
- Paresthesia
- Ptosis
- Priapism

Conscious children old enough to talk may complain of pain localized to the vertebra involved. Head injury with diminished level of consciousness, intoxication, or significant injury of another part of the body may make the localization of pain unreliable. The patient's position may indicate a spine injury. A head tilt may be associated with a rotary subluxation of C1 on C2 or a high cervical injury. The prayer position (arms folded across the chest) may signify a fracture in the C4 to C6 area. Paresis or paralysis of the arms or legs should always suggest spine injury. Paresthesia, a "pins and needles" sensation, or numbness or burning may sometimes seem inconsequential, but these symptoms should always be taken as potential indicators of spine injury. Some patients complain of a sensation like an electric shock passing down the vertebral column, especially when attempting to flex the head. Horner's syndrome (ptosis and a miotic pupil) suggests a cervical cord injury. Priapism is present only in about 3 to 5 percent of spine-injured patients, but indicates that the sympathetic nervous sys-

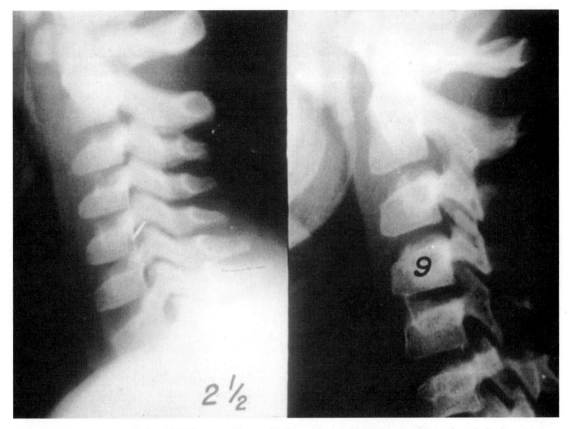

Fig. 12-5. Cross-table lateral view (CTLV) x-ray of 2 year old *(A)* and 9 year old *(B)* for comparison of cervical spine anatomy.

tem is involved. Absence of vital signs has also been associated with otherwise unsuspected spinal cord injury. Absence of the bulbocavernosus reflex in the presence of flaccid paralysis carries a grave prognosis. To elicit the bulbocavernosus reflex, a finger is inserted into the rectum; then the glans of the penis or the head of the clitoris is squeezed. A normal response is a reflex contraction of the anal sphincter.

There are also characteristic cord syndromes (Fig. 12-7):

- Spinal shock
- Brown-Séquard syndrome
- Central cord syndrome
- Anterior cord syndrome

In spinal shock, there is flaccid paralysis below the level of the lesion, absent reflexes, decreased sympathetic

tone, and autonomic dysfunction. Hypotension may occur. Sensation may be preserved, but if it is absent the prognosis for recovery is poor. The central cord syndrome is often associated with extension, which can cause a circumferential pinching of the spinal cord by the ligamentum flavum. The anterior cord syndrome is associated with severe flexion injuries, especially teardrop fractures, in which a fragment of the fractured vertebral body is driven posteriorly into the anterior portion of the spinal cord (Fig. 12-8).

Upper extremity position and function may provide clues not only to the presence of a cervical cord injury, but also to the level of injury. With injuries at C5, patients can flex at the elbows but are unable to extend them; with injuries at C6-C7 they can flex and extend at the elbows; and injuries at the T1 level allow finger and wrist flexion.

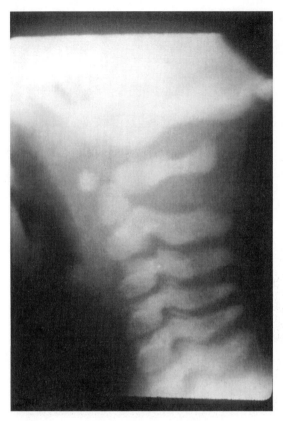

Fig. 12-6. Cross-table lateral view (CTLV) x-ray of neonate.

SPINAL SHOCK

- Flaccid below level of lesion
- Absent reflexes
- Decreased sympathetic tone
- Autonomic dysfunction
  (including hypotension)
- Sensation may be preserved;
  if absent = total cord transection
  (poor prognosis)

CENTRAL CORD

- Diminished or absent upper-
  extremity function
- Preservation of lower-
  extremity function
- Associated with extension
  injuries

BROWN-SÉQUARD

- Hemisection
- Ipsilateral loss of
  - Motor function
  - Proprioception
- Contralateral loss of
  sensation:
  - Pain
  - Temperature

ANTERIOR CORD

- Complete motor paralysis
- Loss of pain and
  temperature sensation
- Preservation of position
  and vibration
- Associated with severe
  flexion injuries

Fig. 12-7. Cord syndromes.

subtle indicators such as stepoffs, subluxations, and malalignments are sought. On the OM view, the alignment of the atlantooccipital and atlantoaxial joints, alignment of the margins of the lateral arches of C1 with C2, and the position of the odontoid between the lateral arches of C1 are evaluated. These bony structures are also examined for fractures.

ANALYSIS OF RADIOGRAPHS

The standard screening series for adults consists of three views:

- Cross-table lateral view (CTLV)
- Anteroposterior view (AP)
- Open-mouth view (OM)

The open-mouth view is used to visualize C1, C2, and the atlantoaxial and atlantooccipital articulations. Because it is difficult to obtain in younger children, the value of requiring the OM view in cervical spine screening has been questioned. The Waters view can be substituted to allow visualization of the odontoid projected through the foramen magnum. The steps in evaluating the CTLV are presented in Fig. 12-9. On the AP view, symmetry of longitudinal alignment of vertebral bodies, facets, pillars, and spinous processes is assessed. Evidence of linear or compression fractures as well as more

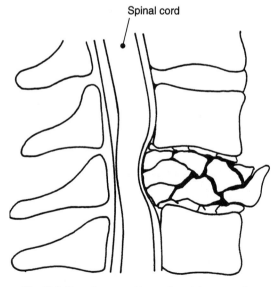

Fig. 12-8. Burst fracture with anterior cord compression.

1. All seven vertebral bodies must be clearly seen, including the C7 to T1 junction.
2. Evaluate proper alignment of the posterior cervical line and the four lordotic curves: anterior longitudinal ligament line, the posterior longitudinal ligament line, the spinolaminal line, and the tips of the spinous processes.
3. Evaluate the predental space (3 mm in adults, 4–5 mm in children).
4. Evaluate each vertebra for fracture and increased or decreased density (e.g., suggestive of a compression fracture, metastatic lesion, osteoporosis).
5. Evaluate the intervertebral and interspinous spaces. (Abrupt angulation of more than 11° at a single interspace is abnormal.)
6. Evaluate if there is fanning of the spinous processes, suggestive of posterior ligament disruption.
7. Evaluate prevertebral soft-tissue distance. (Less than 7 mm at C2 and less than 5 mm at C3–C4 is considered normal.) Note: in children less than 2 years old, the prevertebral space may appear widened if it is not an inspiratory film.
8. Evaluate the antlantooccipital region for possible dislocation.

Fig. 12-9. Criteria for clearing the cervical spine using cross-table lateral view. (From Van Hare RS, Yaron M: The ring of C2 and evaluation of the cross-table lateral view of the cervical spine. *Ann Emerg Med* 21:734, 1992. Reproduced by permission.)

The sensitivity and specificity of the CTLV compared to the gold standard of thin-layer CT in adults have been reported as 82 and 70 percent, respectively. Adding the AP and OM views increased sensitivity to 93 percent and specificity to 71 percent. The predictive value of negative tests was 97 percent for CTLV alone and 99 percent for three views. In a retrospective study of 59 spine-injured children, the AP and CTLV views were sufficient to identify all those who had spine injuries, although other views were necessary to fully delineate the extent of injury.

Other imaging modalities are available when the standard views fail to delineate the cervical anatomy adequately or when clinical suspicion of a cervical spine injury is high despite a negative screening series. These options include the swimmer's view to delineate the lower cervical spine, flexion and extension views, supine oblique views, thin-section tomography, computed tomography, and MRI. Some of these techniques, especially flexion and extension (stress) views, require positioning the head and neck out of neutral position and must be performed under careful medical supervision.

One should not perform stress imaging of the cervical spine in patients who have altered mental status or who are otherwise incapable of clear communication about the effect of such manipulation. MRI is the modality of choice for assessing the supportive soft tissues of the spine and the spinal cord itself. Therefore, MRI can evaluate the extent of injury and offer prognostic information in situations in which cord damage is present, including SCIWORA.

A related and still controversial issue is the appropriate selection of patients for imaging or the concept of "clearing" the cervical spine. The major clinical concern is to avoid missing cervical spine injuries that may be difficult to detect clinically. There is also concern about avoiding a large number of unnecessary radiographs, unnecessary delays in providing other aspects of care while radiographs are being taken and retaken, and unnecessary maintenance of uncomfortable, rigid immobilization. Both clinical practice and recommendations in the literature vary widely. Some recommend that all patients in whom the possibility of cervical spine injury was entertained in the field (i.e., all patients who arrive immobilized in the emergency department) should have radiographic evaluation. Others have suggested more narrow sets of criteria for cervical spine imaging or, alternatively, criteria for those patients who do not need imaging.

In a 1991 study, nine children had a delayed diagnosis of cervical spine injury but all of them had symptoms. Subsequently, a series of adults with cervical spine injury included 11 patients "who had no clinical indication of cervical trauma other than a known mechanism of cervical injury." This series did not specify the mechanism for these patients and depended on the quality of retrospectively collected clinical data.

Two studies of children each suggested a set of criteria for obtaining films. The combination of neck pain or involvement in a motor vehicle crash with head trauma was 100 percent sensitive in identifying 25 cervical spine injuries in a series of 2133 children. Jaffe and colleagues applied the criteria of neck pain or tenderness, limitation of neck mobility, history of trauma to the neck, and abnormal neurologic examination to a series of 206 patients among whom 59 had cervical spine injury. These criteria were 98 percent sensitive. Both of these studies were retrospective as well. Because of the relative infrequency of cervical spine injury among children, the prospective collection of reliable data has been difficult.

As long as there are competing management priorities in the patient with multiple trauma, and as long as there is no perfect diagnostic technique for detecting cervical spine injuries, there will continue to be controversy about how to clear the cervical spine. More than one approach can be defended. The approach of this author is to apply clinical criteria to select a group of children who do not need screening spine films. These include verbal, awake, alert, nonintoxicated children with no significant painful lesions elsewhere and normal neurologic examinations, including normal sensation and mobility in all four extremities. They must also have no spine tenderness, and normal range of motion of the neck (tested last and with care under medical supervision). Even among children who meet these criteria, it is wise to obtain radiographs when the mechanism of injury causes a high transfer of energy to the patient, such as a fall from a height or a motor vehicle collision. The mere presence of a cervical collar, however, is not necessarily an indication for cervical spine radiography. In absence of specific neck-related pathology or neurological deficits to suggest a spine injury, CTLV and AP views to screen for radiologically detectable cervical spine injury are appropriate. However, the presence of any clinical data suggesting spine injury mandates complete imaging of the cervical spine, including CT or MRI imaging when the patient is hemodynamically and neurologically stable. If other emergency procedures need to be done—for example, endotracheal intubation or surgical intervention—these should not be delayed by prolonged attempts to clear the cervical spine in the emergency department. Instead, immobilization can be maintained with the assumption that a spine injury may be present, and the appropriate emergency procedures performed. Later, when the life-threatening problems have been addressed, cervical spine imaging can be completed.

MANAGEMENT

A widely held view regarding the pathogenesis of spinal cord injury is that there are two phases of injury: direct damage that is largely irreversible, and a second phase consisting of ischemia, hypoxemia, and tissue toxicity.

A number of agents, such as free oxygen radicals, are associated with an inflammatory response to injury that may be responsive to medical intervention. Therefore, good trauma management is also good management for spinal cord injuries. The ABC (*a*irway, *b*reathing, *c*irculation) mnemonic popularized by the American College of Surgeons Advanced Trauma Life Support Course has helped providers across the United States establish priorities of care. Careful attention to oxygenation and ventilation is critical. Airway obstruction is common in

trauma victims, and the mandibular block of tissue often obstructs the airway of the supine, unconscious child. Also, the child may be unable to cough or expectorate to clear mucus, vomitus, blood, or other debris. Lifting the mandible with a jaw-thrust maneuver often improves the airway. At the same time, the emergency practitioner must be cognizant of the possibility of a cervical spine injury, which could be worsened by excessive motion of the spine. It is often possible to perform a jaw-thrust maneuver and stabilize the cervical spine at the same time (Fig. 12-10).

Most injured children arrive at the emergency department with good immobilization of the cervical spine. Stiff collars are now made for children as young as 1 year of age. However, the cervical collar alone does not provide adequate immobilization. Cloth tape or straps across the forehead and external orthoses, including a rigid backboard, are usually employed to complete the immobilization (Fig. 12-11). Concern has been raised regarding the immobilization of younger children, who have disproportionately large heads. Use of a flat board may force the head forward, causing the neck to flex. The ideal backboard would be modified with a recess for the young child's occiput. Alternately, the chest may be

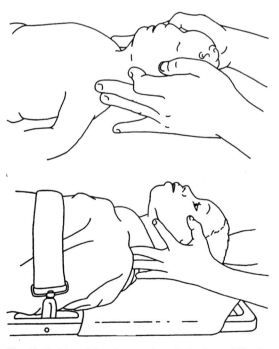

Fig. 12-10. Manual jaw-thrust and cervical spine stabilization in *(A)* an infant and *(B)* a child.

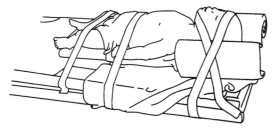

Fig. 12-11. A method for immobilization of an infant.

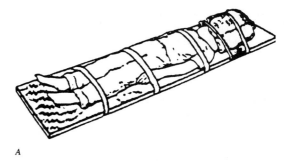

A

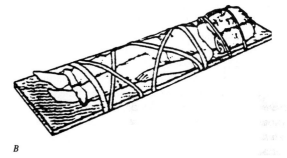

B

Fig. 12-13. Illustrations of *(A)* lateral strap technique and *(B)* cross strap technique. (From Schafermeyer RW, Ribbeck BM, Gaskins J, et al: Respiratory effects of spinal immobilization in children. *Ann Emerg Med* 20:1018, 1991. Reproduced by permission.)

raised by an extra mattress pad or even a support made of sheets or towels (Fig. 12-12). Schafermeyer demonstrated that full supine immobilization reduced the forced vital capacity of healthy children between the ages of 6 to 15 years to 80 percent of unrestricted values (Fig. 12-13). Therefore, it is important for prehospital and emergency care providers to evaluate the effect of immobilization on ventilation, especially when a significant injury or embarrassment of the respiratory system is likely.

Other concerns have been raised about both the methods used to immobilize children and the indications for spine immobilization in out-of-hospital settings. Immobilization has been shown to cause pain in healthy adults

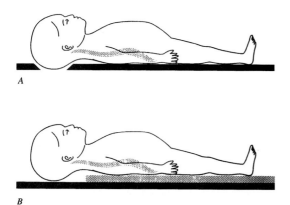

A

B

Fig. 12-12. Backboard modifications for children. *A.* Young child on a modified backboard that has a cutout to recess the occiput, obtaining a safe supine cervical positioning. *B.* Young child on a modified backboard that has a double-mattress pad to raise the chest, obtaining a safe supine cervical positioning. (From Herzenberg JE, Hensinger RN, Dedrick DK, et al: Emergency transport and positioning of young children who have an injury of the cervical spine. The standard backboard may be hazardous. *J Bone Joint Surg* 17:15, 1989. Reproduced by permission.)

that can last as long as 72 hours. A recent intriguing study comparing outcomes in adults with documented spine injuries in New Mexico and Malaysia demonstrated that out-of-hospital immobilization provided no benefit. It is likely that the dogma concerning rigid immobilization of all trauma patients, especially those with low probability of spine injury, may change during the next decade.

The spine-injured patient may have hypoventilation because of diminished diaphragmatic activity or because of intercostal muscle paralysis. Concomitant head or chest injuries and aspiration of gastric contents may further compromise ventilation. Therefore, supplemental humidified oxygen should routinely be provided. Ventilation should be assisted whenever hypoventilation is suspected. If prolonged assisted ventilation is likely, the trachea is intubated to facilitate ventilation, to protect the airway, and to reduce the hazards associated with gastric air accumulation.

Whether or not there is a cord injury, there is often a need to provide assisted ventilation to the multiple trauma victim. Although the bag-mask technique will permit ventilation, its prolonged use increases the likelihood of aspiration of gastric contents. Therefore, the emergency practitioner often faces the need to intubate the trachea prior to completing full evaluation of the cervical spine. There have been a number of studies on cadavers and adult volunteers to suggest that some cervical mobility occurs with laryngoscopy. These studies also suggest that manual in-line stabilization is the best method for minimizing this mobility during laryngoscopy. In children, blind nasotracheal intubation is unreliable because it can be technically difficult. Emergency cricothyrotomy is relatively contraindicated in young children because of the small size of the cricothyroid membrane and the likelihood of causing permanent tracheal damage. When intubation of the trachea is needed, both pediatric surgeons and emergency physicians have adopted the strategy of oral intubation with in-line manual stabilization, which can be provided either from below or above the patient (Fig. 12-14). The rapid sequence induction technique is often indicated, especially when significant brain injury is suspected (see Chap. 5). The emergency physician should never fail to provide an adequate airway for an injured child in order to wait for the cervical spine to be cleared.

Hypotension may be secondary to either hypovolemia or spinal shock. A clue to differentiating these is the pulse. Often the pulse is slow in spinal shock, whereas it is rapid in hypovolemic shock. Adequate fluid (crystalloid, colloid, and blood) is administered to combat hypovolemia. In the case of spinal shock, atropine and vasopressors, such as dopamine, may be needed.

The patient with spinal shock may be more sensitive to temperature variations than other patients and may require warming or cooling if subjected to extreme environmental temperatures either at the scene or during transport. Care should be taken to protect areas of the body that may have lost sensation from hard, protruding objects, as they may cause skin necrosis, especially on long transports.

The results of the second National Acute Spinal Cord Injury Study were reported in May 1990. The investigators reported that high-dose methylprednisolone (30 mg/kg) followed by 5.4 mg/kg/h for 23 hours, if given within 8 hours of acute spinal cord injury, improved the neurologic recovery as compared to placebo or naloxone. Children under the age of 13 years were excluded from the study. The putative mechanism of action is the ability of the steroid at these doses to inhibit oxygen free radical–induced lipid peroxidation. Lipid peroxidation is thought to mediate cell membrane degeneration and to explain other documented tissue-protective effects of

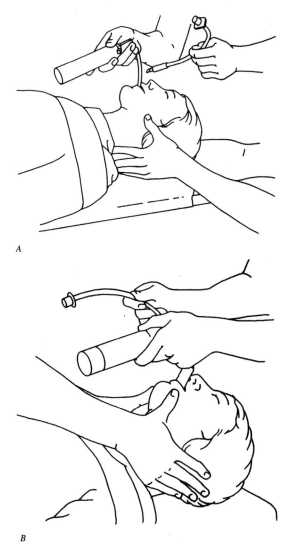

A

B

Fig. 12-14. In-line stabilization for endotracheal intubation: *(A)* above and *(B)* below.

steroids: support of energy metabolism, prevention of posttraumatic ischemia, reversal of intracellular calcium accumulation, prevention of neurofilament degradation, inhibition of vasoactive prostaglandin $F_{2\alpha}$ and thromboxane generation, and retardation of axonal degeneration. Though there have still been no clinical trials confirming the efficacy of this regimen in children, it has become accepted neurosurgical practice to administer glucocorticoids to treat spinal cord injuries.

BIBLIOGRAPHY

Bracken MB, Shepard MJ, Collins WF, et al: A randomized, controlled trial of methylprednisolone or naloxone in the treatment of acute spinal-cord injury. *N Engl J Med* 322:1405, 1990.

Bracken MB, Shepard MJ, Holford TR, et al: Administration of methylprednisolone for 24 or 48 hours or tirilazad mesylate for 48 hours in the treatment of acute spinal cord injury. *JAMA* 277:1597, 1997.

Hauswald M, Ong G, Tandberg D, et al: Out-of-hospital spinal immobilization: Its effect on neurologic injury. *Acad Emerg Med* 5:214, 1998.

Jaffe DM, Binns H, Radkowski MA, et al: Developing a clinical algorithm for early management of cervical spine injury in child trauma victims. *Ann Emerg Med* 16:270, 1987.

Keiper MD, Zimmerman RA, Bilaniuk LT: MRI in the assessment of the supportive soft tissues of the cervical spine in acute trauma in children. *Neuroradiology* 40:359, 1998.

Kewalramani LS, Kraus JF, Sterling HM: Acute spinal cord lesions in the pediatric population. Epidemiological and clinical features. *Paraplegia* 18:206, 1980.

Pang D, Wilberger JE Jr: Spinal cord injury without radiographic abnormalities in children. *J Neurosurg* 57:114, 1982.

Schafermeyer RW, Ribbeck BM, Gaskins J, et al: Respiratory effects of spinal immobilization in children. *Ann Emerg Med* 20:1017, 1991.

13

Thoracic Trauma

Wendy Ann Lucid
Todd Brian Taylor

HIGH-YIELD FACTS

- Serious blunt chest trauma results in rib fractures and pulmonary contusions nearly 50 percent of the time, with pneumothorax (20 percent) and hemothorax (10 percent) occurring less frequently. The overall mortality is about the same for blunt and penetrating trauma.

- Gunshot wounds to the chest are associated with abdominal injuries in 30 to 40 percent of patients.

- Uncertainty as to the side of the tension pneumothorax should not prohibit initiation of empirical treatment if the patient is deteriorating. Decompression of the other side should be done if immediate improvement is not seen with the initial needle or tube thoracostomy.

- Due to the compliance of the ribs and supporting structures, children are particularly susceptible to pulmonary contusion with little external signs of trauma.

- The most common site for aortic disruption in children is at the level of the ligamentum arteriosum and it may be associated with aortic dissection. As in adults, morbidity and mortality is high with injuries to the great vessels.

- Serious thoracic injuries are relatively less common among children and only 15 percent require more than simple chest tube placement. Nevertheless, children surviving to reach an emergency department require rapid evaluation and management. Moreover, proper identification of these injuries allows for early surgical referral and treatment of potentially life-threatening chest injuries.

In an ideal world, all children with thoracic injuries would be treated in trauma centers with pediatric expertise. In reality, a child with thoracic injury can arrive at a nontrauma center and must be managed there until arrangements for transport to an appropriate facility can be made. The decision to discharge, admit, or transfer to a higher level of care must take into account the mechanism of injury, as well as the clinical status of the child. Facility expertise and regional protocols will often dictate these decisions.

MECHANISM OF INJURY

Blunt Thoracic Trauma

Blunt trauma accounts for the vast majority of serious chest injuries in children. The National Pediatric Trauma Registry statistics reveal 83 percent blunt versus 15 percent penetrating trauma injuries. Of the blunt injuries, most are caused by motor vehicle crashes and the remainder are due to falls and bicycle crashes. The mechanism of injury is important due to recognizable patterns of trauma associated with particular injuries. However, *isolated* chest injury is relatively infrequent, due in part to the common mechanisms of blunt trauma in childhood.

While the incidence of thoracic trauma may be low, the associated and concomitant mortality remains high and it is among the most lethal of all childhood injuries. Multisystem trauma mortality is 10 times higher when associated with chest injury. Chest injury therefore serves as a marker of injury severity. Serious blunt chest trauma results in rib fractures and pulmonary contusions nearly 50 percent of the time and pneumothorax (20 percent) and hemothorax (10 percent) less frequently. The overall mortality is about the same for blunt and penetrating trauma. However, children usually die from the primary wound with penetrating injuries and from the associated injuries in blunt chest trauma.

Penetrating Thoracic Trauma

Penetrating trauma accounts for only about 15 percent of thoracic trauma in childhood. The incidence is increasing even among younger children, primarily due to gunshot wounds. These wounds are less often fatal than in adults, probably due to the unintended nature of the injuries and the childhood cardiovascular reserve. Hemorrhagic shock from massive hemothorax accounts for the vast majority of deaths from gunshot wounds, whereas stab wounds more often cause death from tension pneumothorax. Cardiac injury with associated tamponade and major vascular injuries are more often associated with death, and account for the remainder of deaths associated with penetrating thoracic injuries.

Concomitant abdominal injury should be suspected with penetrating trauma at or below the level of the sixth rib anteriorly, below the scapula posteriorly, or when stomach contents, chyme, or saliva are recovered from the chest tube. Gunshot wounds to the chest are associated with abdominal injuries in 30 to 40 percent of patients. Therefore, "isolated" thoracic trauma does not exclude abdominal injury, especially in the presence of abdominal tenderness or developing peritonitis.

PATHOPHYSIOLOGY

Children are somewhat anatomically protected against blunt thoracic trauma, but thoracic trauma remains the second most common cause of traumatic death (15 percent) after head injury. This is due in part to the compliance of the cartilaginous ribs and their ability to dissipate the force of impact, thereby protecting the ribs and underlying structures from injury. However, these same anatomical characteristics can complicate pediatric thoracic trauma. Compliant ribs allow significant trauma to occur to intrathoracic structures (heart, lungs, airways, and vessels) with few or no apparent external signs of trauma. Even bruising, petechiae, and tenderness may be absent. The mobility of the mediastinal structures can lead to rapid ventilatory and circulatory collapse should tension pneumothorax develop.

Several factors lead to decreased respiratory compensation in children sustaining thoracic trauma:

- Proportionally larger oxygen consumption and smaller functional residual capacity of the lungs increase the risk of hypoxia.
- Tachypnea is the chief physiologic response to hypoxia due to limited pulmonary compliance and greater chest wall compliance.
- Younger children are diaphragmatic breathers due to horizontally aligned ribs and immature intercostal musculature. Abdominal trauma often increases early respiratory fatigue, as does multisystem trauma in which air swallowing results in gastric distention that limits diaphragm excursion.

Pulmonary injuries are the most common type of thoracic trauma in children. Blunt trauma tends to cause pulmonary contusion, while penetrating trauma tends to cause lacerations, and either can cause a hematoma. Pulmonary contusions are important because of their association with forceful mechanisms that often result in multisystem injuries. Pulmonary lacerations have a cavitary appearance on chest radiograph, but require surgical repair only when associated with ongoing bleeding or air leakage. Pulmonary hematoma is uncommon and is generally a self-limited injury, rarely progressing to lung abscess.

MANAGEMENT OF THORACIC INJURY

As in all traumatic injuries, priority is initially given to airway, breathing, and circulation before specific injuries are addressed. A variety of conditions can cause airway compromise and all of them can be immediately life threatening. The obvious causes include airway obstruction from foreign body, unconsciousness, and neck trauma. This section assumes that the ABCs (*a*irway, *b*reathing, *c*irculation) of trauma resuscitation have already been initiated.

The physical signs of thoracic injury can be subtle in the pediatric patient, even with severe injury. Respirations may appear shallow rather than labored, and central cyanosis can be absent in hemorrhagic shock due to a relative decrease in unsaturated hemoglobin. Therefore absence of the typical signs for specific injuries does not exclude their existence.

Diagnostic studies and treatment will vary depending on the clinical situation. With thoracic injury, a minimal work-up includes:

- Arterial blood gases
- Hemoglobin/hematocrit
- Chest radiograph
- Pulse oximetry
- Cardiac monitor
- Supplemental oxygen
- Two large-bore intravenous lines

The upright posteroanterior chest radiograph is the mainstay in the evaluation of chest trauma and is most likely to facilitate the diagnosis of small apical pneumothoraces or small hemothoraces. The clinical situation may dictate immediate treatment without a radiograph, or reliance on a more easily obtained supine portable chest radiograph. Use of other diagnostic modalities is dictated by the clinical situation.

Concomitant abdominal and thoracic trauma requires a special approach. Immediate stabilization of the chest wound with a thoracostomy tube is indicated before the patient is placed under general anesthesia. The abdominal injuries are repaired first if the clinical situation allows. After the abdomen is closed, a thoracotomy can be performed if necessary for other injuries and to irrigate the chest if it is contaminated with intestinal contents.

SPECIFIC INJURIES AND MANAGEMENT

Pneumothorax

It is important to appreciate the difference between spontaneous and traumatic pneumothorax. Spontaneous pneumothorax is caused by a ruptured bleb or small distal bronchiole that will easily seal itself and heal quickly. The air is reabsorbed over a few days often without intervention. A small spontaneous pneumothorax can be treated with close observation or simply aspirated and followed with repeated chest radiographs to ensure resolution. At the most, they require a small chest tube that can often be placed anteriorly.

A traumatic pneumothorax is prone to expand and is often associated with significant pulmonary injury. There may be an associated hemothorax and even a small pneumothorax can quickly develop into a more serious tension pneumothorax.

Conservative treatment includes placing a large caliber, lateral, posteriorly directed chest tube for even a small traumatic pneumothorax. A small caliber, lateral or anteriorly placed tube can be used to evacuate a pneumothorax if an underlying hemothorax is not suspected. Even with a very small pneumothorax, a chest tube is mandatory if the patient is to undergo mechanical ventilation (for surgery or respiratory failure) or emergency transport, particularly by air ambulance, because the changes in atmospheric pressure will tend to expand the pneumothorax. Less invasive treatment, for an isolated small traumatic pneumothorax, includes observation for 6 hours with a repeat chest radiograph. If there is no size increase, the patient may be discharged to return in 24 hours for another chest radiograph. This approach may be reasonable in selected cases.

Hemothorax

The mechanism for hemothorax is similar to that for pneumothorax. Injury to the intercostal or internal mammary vessels or lung parenchyma may result in significant bleeding. Bleeding is difficult to quantify on chest radiograph and a chest tube is invariably necessary to evacuate the hematoma and observe for ongoing bleeding. Removal of the hematoma also prevents delayed complications due to fibrosis or empyema.

Massive Hemothorax

Blunt injuries and gunshot wounds typically cause bleeding from lung parenchyma and deep vascular structures, while stab wounds more often bleed from intercostal vessels. Massive hemothorax is rare in children and is usually associated with a powerful force mechanism, such as a high-speed motor vehicle crash, a fall from a great height, or a high-powered or close-range gunshot wound.

Clinical findings include decreased breath sounds and dullness to percussion on the affected side with or without obvious respiratory distress. Pneumothorax may coexist, presenting features of tension pneumothorax and hemothorax. Hypovolemic shock may be an early or late presenting feature. A hemothorax requires a minimum of 10 mL/kg of blood to be visualized on chest radiograph. Any abnormal fluid collection in the traumatic setting is assumed to be blood. Treatment of massive hemothorax requires rapid evaluation and treatment.

Fluid resuscitation should begin with crystalloid in the field. Preparation for transfusion should begin immediately and blood given as the clinical situation warrants. Critical patients may require type-specific or O-negative blood, while more stable patients may be able to wait for cross-matched blood or not need a transfusion at all. Both vital signs and the amount of output from the chest tube should be taken into account when deciding the need for immediate transfusion. Hemoglobin and hematocrit may not be useful initially because rapid blood loss does not allow for equilibration and these tests may not accurately reflect current blood volume.

Thoracostomy tubes should be placed as soon as the diagnosis of massive hemothorax is suspected. A large-caliber (about as wide as the intercostal space) tube should be used and inserted laterally and directed posteriorly to allow for drainage. Consideration should be given to using an autotransfusion chest tube collection system, as this may be the most rapidly available source for blood transfusion. A chest radiograph should be taken soon after chest tube placement to confirm the position and to ensure reexpansion of the lung.

The decision to proceed with a thoracotomy will generally be made by the consulting surgeon. Guidelines include:

- Initial evacuated volume exceeding 10 to 15 mL/kg of blood
- Continued blood loss exceeding 2 to 4 mL/kg/h
- Continued air leakage

In certain circumstances, an emergency thoracotomy may be necessary as a last resort to control bleeding until definitive treatment can be administered. Bleeding may be controlled in this manner by directly clamping the injured area. Various techniques may be necessary depending on the type of injury, and the procedure should only be performed by those trained in these techniques. Aggressive blood resuscitation and continued chest tube suction is a reasonable alternative until a physician with expertise in emergency thoracot-omy is available.

Open Pneumothorax

Open pneumothorax (sucking chest wound) is created when the chest wall is sufficiently injured to create bidirectional flow of air through the wound. The normal expansion of the lung is impossible due to the equalization of pressures between the chest cavity and atmosphere. Inability to generate a negative pressure to expand the lung compromises gas exchange and hypoxia/hypercarbia ensues. The compliant mediastinum in children complicates this condition allowing compression of both lungs with inspiration resulting in paradoxical breathing.

Management of an open pneumothorax depends on the size of the chest wall defect and respiratory status. Breathing patients with small injuries such as knife or gunshot wound can be treated by covering the chest wall defect with a sterile petroleum dressing and placing a thoracostomy tube through a fresh incision. Size and location of the chest tube will depend on the extent of underlying injury. In general, a large caliber tube placed laterally and directed posteriorly should be used, as an underlying hemothorax may be present. Small chest wall defects will seal and heal spontaneously and generally do not require surgical repair.

Prehospital treatment of a sucking chest wound may consist of placing a petroleum dressing with only three sides taped to create a flutter valve to decompress the chest and eliminate the sucking chest wound. This should be converted to a sealed dressing and thoracostomy tube as soon as possible. Chest wall defects too large to adequately seal (such as in a blast injury) or patients not spontaneously breathing will require intubation and ventilatory support. Large wounds will often require urgent thoracotomy to repair the chest wall defect and underlying injuries.

Tension Pneumothorax

Tension pneumothorax occurs when the lung or airway develops a leak through a one-way valve defect allowing air to flow into the pleural cavity without a means of escape. As the amount of air increases, the pressure against the mediastinal structures shifts the mediastinum towards the opposite side and causes vascular compromise of the heart and great vessels. Cardiac decompensation ensues from mechanical impingement of blood flow and hypoxia from respiratory compromise. Immediate action must be taken to relieve the tension to avoid imminent demise.

Causes of tension pneumothorax include barotrauma from severe blunt compression of the chest cavity against a closed glottis and rib fractures that puncture the lung tissue. Penetrating injuries, such as stab wounds, can also cause a tension pneumothorax since the lung is injured without a large enough defect to allow exterior decompression. An open pneumothorax is more common with gunshot wounds.

Many patients with tension pneumothorax present with severe respiratory distress, decreased breath sounds, and hyperresonance on the ipsilateral side. As the tension progresses mediastinal shift leads to contralateral tracheal deviation and distended neck veins due to compromised venous return. Subcutaneous emphysema may dissect superiorly into the neck or inferiorly into the abdomen and scrotal area. Circulatory collapse with hypotension and narrow pulse pressure will result if the tension is not decompressed quickly.

Only completely stable patients should have further treatment delayed for a chest radiograph. In fact, treatment in the field is often required using a needle thoracostomy attached to a flutter valve placed percutaneously via the second intercostal space in the midclavicular line. Care must be taken to avoid the intercostal vessels by placing the needle just over the top of the third rib.

Diagnosis of tension pneumothorax in children is complicated by false transmission of breath sounds. This can confuse the clinical diagnosis; however, uncertainty as to the side of the tension pneumothorax should not prohibit initiation of empirical treatment if the patient is deteriorating. Decompression of the other side should be done if immediate improvement is not seen with the initial needle or tube thoracostomy.

Definitive treatment is accomplished using a large caliber (appropriate for age) thoracostomy tube placed laterally and directed posteriorly to allow drainage of the hemothorax that often accompanies tension pneumothorax in trauma patients.

PULMONARY CONTUSION

Pulmonary contusion can be caused by blunt trauma to the chest wall or by high-speed penetrating trauma, such as a gunshot wound to the chest. Children are particularly susceptible to pulmonary contusion with few external signs of trauma due to the compliance of the ribs and supporting structures.

Injured leaky capillary membranes allow bleeding or oozing of fluid into the interstitial and alveolar spaces and may cause hypoxia and respiratory distress if the injury is large. The analogy of the "bruised lung" carries more significance when the decreased functional residual capacity and higher risk of hypoxia due to the proportionally higher oxygen consumption in children are taken into account.

Initial symptoms range from minimal to severe respiratory distress and the mechanism of injury may be the only early clinical indicator of pulmonary contusion. The initial chest radiograph may not show the classic patchy infiltrate and physical examination may not reveal signs of pulmonary consolidation due to the contracted state of circulation often present in a multisystem injury. Blood gas analysis also may not be diagnostic in the early stages, as the alveolar-arterial gradient may be normal. A high index of suspicion is necessary to identify early pulmonary contusion.

Treatment is directed toward preventing hypoxia and respiratory failure. A search for concomitant injuries is prudent because a force capable of causing a pulmonary contusion often causes other injuries. However, in isolated cases supplemental oxygen and close monitoring are often all that is required. Patients who meet the usual blood gas criteria for intubation will require ventilation with positive end-expiratory pressure (PEEP) of 5 to 10 cmH$_2$O.

Spontaneous resolution of pulmonary contusion is the usual course unless acute respiratory distress syndrome (ARDS) supervenes. Excessive administration of crystalloid and aspiration of gastric contents are two factors that predispose to ARDS and should be avoided.

TRAUMATIC ASPHYXIA

Traumatic asphyxia is not as ominous as its name would suggest and is an injury unique to children due to the increased compliance of the chest wall. It is thought to arise from a severe blow to the chest that results in transmission of pressure through the superior vena cava into the capillaries of the head and neck. This results in a deep violet color of the skin in the head and neck region and is associated with bilateral subconjunctival hemorrhages and facial edema. As the name implies, the patient's appearance can be quite dramatic, but the condition itself is benign. The significance is as a marker for associated head trauma, pulmonary contusions, and intraabdominal injuries. About one-third of these patients will experience a loss of consciousness, but intracranial hemorrhages are rare. Transient and permanent visual disturbances can occur due to retinal hemorrhages and edema.

TRAUMATIC TRACHEAL AND BRONCHIAL DISRUPTION

Traumatic bronchial disruption is rare in children, but is highly lethal. Half of these patients die within the first hour after injury. This condition is due to a shearing force associated with a crush injury to the chest or, more commonly, from severe compression of the chest against a closed glottis. The disruption nearly always occurs adjacent to the carina.

Ipsilateral tension pneumothorax is common and a persistent large air leak or failure of reexpansion of the lung after chest tube placement may be seen. Hemoptysis may also be present. Bronchoscopy is diagnostic and should be considered in patients with these findings.

Small leaks require only a chest tube and observation. Thoracotomy for definitive repair is necessary in more severe cases if bleeding cannot be controlled or tracheal obstruction occurs from tracheal disruption or hematoma. Establishing an airway can be complicated by disruption of the trachea or peritracheal hematoma distorting the airway anatomy. A surgical airway may be necessary and should be placed below the level of the disruption by tracheostomy or cricothyrotomy. Inability to ventilate once an airway has been established requires emergency thoracotomy.

TRAUMATIC ESOPHAGEAL RUPTURE

Traumatic esophageal rupture is virtually unknown in children. It occurs with severe blunt upper abdominal trauma in which stomach contents are forcefully injected into the esophagus against a closed cricopharyngeus muscle causing a rupture of the esophageal wall into the mediastinum. Clinically similar to Boerhaave's syndrome, it progresses rapidly to mediastinitis, sepsis, and death if unrecognized. Death often occurs even with early surgical intervention.

Clinical signs include pain and shock out of proportion to the apparent severity of injury. It may be associated with a pneumothorax that drains stomach contents or bubbles equally and continuously throughout the respiratory cycle. Subcutaneous emphysema may dissect into the neck and be palpable. Although rarely heard in children, Hamman's sign (mediastinal crunch) may be appreciated as a crunching sound with heartbeats. Chest radiograph often reveals mediastinal emphysema and may be the only clue to the diagnosis. Fluoroscopy with water-soluble contrast and\or endoscopy can confirm the diagnosis.

Urgent surgical repair with mediastinal drainage is required. Delayed definitive repair may be necessary with extensive esophageal damage and temporary esophageal diversion may be required.

TRAUMATIC DIAPHRAGMATIC HERNIA

Traumatic diaphragmatic herniation in children is part of the "lap belt" complex, occurring predominantly on the left in the acute setting. It is most often caused by blunt trauma producing a sudden increase in intraabdominal pressure and less commonly by penetrating trauma occurring anywhere between the nipples and umbilicus. Symptoms result not from the hernia itself, but from herniation of abdominal contents into the chest. Right-sided herniation is often delayed and symptoms appear after the abdominal contents have been drawn into the chest. The diagnosis may be obscured until this event occurs, resulting in as many as 90 percent of these injuries being overlooked on the initial evaluation.

Signs may include contusions and abrasions of the upper abdomen and lower chest wall, but herniation can occur without external signs of trauma. Breath sounds may be decreased or bowel sounds heard on the affected side. Chest radiograph findings depend on the status of the abdominal contents and are outlined in Table 13-1.

Acute traumatic diaphragmatic herniation requires surgical repair. However, initial management should concentrate on assuring respiratory status and stabilizing other injuries. A nasogastric tube should be placed to decompress the stomach and intubation with positive pressure ventilation performed if respiratory status deteriorates. With delayed presentations, chest radiograph may demonstrate the pathology. Some cases may require confirmation by fluoroscopy or in rare cases by laparotomy.

RIB FRACTURES

Rib fractures are uncommon in children, but can occur with severe direct blows to the chest. Without a clear history of trauma, and particularly if there are multiple fractures in various stages of healing, child abuse should be suspected. The posterolateral aspect of the ribs is the most susceptible to fracture from all causes. Referred pain from rib fractures can confuse the diagnosis. Upper abdominal tenderness severe enough to mimic peritonitis can result from an intercostal nerve injury associated with a lower rib fracture.

Isolated rib fractures are not identified on the initial chest radiograph as often as 50 percent of the time. Due to the self-limited nature of isolated rib fractures and the importance of other aspects of care, rib radiograph series are of limited value as well as being time consuming, expensive, and difficult to obtain in children. Sternal fractures and costochondral separations are also not easily recognized on chest radiograph or rib series, but should be suspected if there is point tenderness, crepitus, or obvious deformity. All of these fractures are important as markers of injury severity.

Simple rib fractures are well tolerated in children and no specific treatment, other than pain management, is indicated. Atelectasis and respiratory splinting is uncommon. Pain medication and\or intercostal nerve blocks may be necessary depending on the clinical setting.

Table 13-1. Chest Radiograph Findings in Traumatic Diaphragmatic Hernia

---

Chest radiograph with acute herniation of abdominal contents
    Diagnostic with bowel or stomach presenting within the chest cavity
    Presence of the nasogastric tube in the chest
Chest radiograph with diaphragmatic tear but delayed herniation of abdominal contents
    Unexplained elevation of the hemidiaphragm
    Unrelieved acute gastric dilation
    Loculated subpulmonic hemopneumothorax
    Presence of the nasogastric tube in the chest.

Flail Chest

Severe blunt trauma to the chest wall can cause more than two fractures to the same rib. When this occurs in more than two adjacent ribs, the structural integrity of the chest wall is compromised, causing a flail chest. Concomitant pulmonary contusion is common and children tolerate this condition poorly.

Signs and symptoms include varying degrees of respiratory distress and hypoxia along with the classic paradoxical chest wall motion. Tenderness, bruising, and crepitus overlying the flail segments may also be present. Muscle spasm and respiratory splinting may obscure the clinical diagnosis by "stabilizing" and concealing the flail segments on physical examination.

Chest radiograph confirms the diagnosis and often reveals associated pulmonary contusion. Treatment is aimed at preventing hypoxia and respiratory failure and is dependent on the extent of injury and the child's ability to compensate. Supplemental oxygen and close monitoring may be all that is required. The addition of intercostal or epidural nerve block for pain control is preferable to narcotic analgesia due to the potential for respiratory depression. Those meeting the usual blood gas criteria for intubation will require ventilation with PEEP of 5 to 10 cmH$_2$O. External stabilization with Hudson traction and towel clips has been proven to be less effective than the above methods and should no longer be used.

CARDIOVASCULAR INJURIES

Cardiac and great vessel injuries are uncommon in children. The most common cardiovascular injury from blunt trauma is myocardial contusion and from penetrating trauma pericardial tamponade. Rare complications of blunt thoracic trauma include myocardial rupture, myocardial necrosis with subsequent aneurysm, traumatic aortic insufficiency, pericardial laceration, fatal cardiac herniation, coronary artery injury, and cardiac conduction system injury. Traumatic aortic rupture is the most common great vessel injury and is probably underreported since more than 50 percent of victims die before reaching the hospital. Injuries to other vessels are rare except in cases of penetrating trauma involving projectiles.

Cardiac Tamponade

Cardiac tamponade is a life-threatening condition that occurs when fluid (blood or serous fluid) fills the pericardial space to such an extent that venous return is compromised. Stab wounds are the most common traumatic etiology and the overlying wound is a clue to the diagnosis. Gunshot wounds to this area typically cause sudden death and blunt trauma is unlikely to cause this condition acutely. The laceration of the pericardium can be quite small and since the coronary arteries and cardiac chambers are at or near arterial pressure, the pericardial sac fills quickly with blood, causing normovolemic shock and death.

Clinical findings include:

- Presence of a precordial wound
- Tachycardia
- Narrow pulse pressure
- Pulsus paradoxus
- Beck's triad: muffled or distant heart sounds, hypotension, and jugular venous distention (may be absent in the presence of hypovolemia)

Hypotension progressing to pulseless electrical activity (PEA) results unless prompt treatment is initiated.

The chest radiograph typically shows the classic "water bottle" cardiac silhouette. The ECG may show evidence of acute myocardial infarction if a coronary artery has been lacerated or may simply show tachycardia with extremely low voltage.

Bedside echocardiography is diagnostic; however, treatment should not be delayed while waiting for the echocardiogram. Definitive treatment requires thoracotomy, pericardiotomy, and repair of the underlying injury. Although its role has become limited, in certain circumstances pericardiocentesis is both diagnostic and therapeutic. However, there is a high incidence of false negatives, so a negative pericardiocentesis does not necessarily rule out a hemopericardium. With rapid bleeding into the pericardium, blood often clots, making it impossible to relieve the tamponade without a thoracotomy. This technique also carries significant risks, such as myocardial and coronary artery laceration, leading to hemopericardium, pneumothorax, and dysrhythmia. It should not be done unless definitive thoracotomy is not readily available and the patient's condition is rapidly deteriorating. Repeated aspirations may be necessary, so the needle or plastic angiocath is generally left in place until a thoracotomy can be done.

In certain circumstances, an emergency pericardial window may be necessary to open the pericardium and control the bleeding until definitive treatment can be performed. Bleeding may be controlled by directly clamping the injured area. However, the coronary arteries are easily damaged even under the best of circumstances. Therefore this should only be performed by those trained in these procedures. Repeated pericardial aspiration and aggressive blood resuscitation are reasonable alternatives until a physician with expertise in emergency thoracotomy is available.

Myocardial Contusion

The most common cause of myocardial contusion in adults is striking the steering wheel at moderate to high speed. This probably explains why this problem is rare and does not often cause significant morbidity in children. High-speed (gunshot or close-range shotgun) penetrating trauma or blunt trauma applied to the central anterior or in the anteroposterior direction (as opposed to the lateral or oblique direction) can cause myocardial contusion. As in adults, its diagnostic criteria and significance are still unclear.

Diagnosis based solely on clinical criteria is often necessary, and the mechanism of injury is the most significant clue. Typically, there is significant tenderness in the anterior chest or the chest pain is poorly localized. ECG findings are less common in children, and tachycardia is the most common finding. Echocardiograms, while often diagnostic in adults, rarely show abnormalities in children. Myocardial enzymes may be diagnostic, but as in adults, their usefulness and significance are difficult to ascertain. Radionuclide angiography may be useful in selected cases.

Children do not commonly experience ventricular dysrhythmias. However, if the diagnosis of myocardial contusion is suspected, cardiac monitoring should be utilized and significant dysrhythmias treated appropriately. Children injured by a mechanism significant enough to cause a cardiac contusion will usually be observed for other reasons and cardiac monitoring should be instituted in these cases.

Traumatic Rupture of the Great Vessels

Rupture of the great vessels is extremely rare in children, in part due to the higher elastin content of their connective tissue. However, children and adults with Marfan's syndrome are more susceptible due to the intrinsic weakness of their uncrosslinked collagen. Aortic disruption at the level of the ligamentum arteriosum is the most common site in children and may be associated with aortic dissection. As in adults, morbidity and mortality is high with injuries to the great vessels.

Blunt aortic injury is most commonly caused by rapid deceleration, as seen in high-speed automobile crashes and falls from great heights. More than 50 percent of these patients die at the scene. Clinical signs include chest pain that may be localized to the anterior chest, back, or upper abdomen, and a murmur radiating to the back (rarely appreciated). Chest radiograph findings (Table 13-2), although sometimes subtle, can increase suspicion for aortic injury.

Penetrating trauma to the vena cava or pulmonary vessels is more common than penetrating injury to the aorta. Various impaling objects (such as hunting arrows or highway posts) have also been known to cause significant great vessel trauma. A vascular injury should be considered with obvious wounds to the chest associated with hypotension. Hemopneumothorax is invariably associated with these injuries.

With isolated venous or pulmonary vessel injuries, death is usually not immediate and patients often survive to surgery even with severe injuries. Hypovolemic shock is often present initially and may respond to fluid resuscitation only to recur as the slow venous bleeding progresses.

Making the diagnosis can be difficult, especially in children who are not prone to aortic injury. A widened mediastinum is the most common finding, but this alone does not confirm or necessarily warrant an angiogram. CT of the chest may confirm the diagnosis and is less invasive, but can miss small tears and the contrast load may obviate an angiogram if an abnormality is discovered. Early surgical consultation with angiography is the diagnostic modality of choice in the appropriate clinical setting for suspected aortic rupture or dissection.

Definitive treatment requires immediate surgical repair. Initial treatment should be directed toward the ABCs of trauma care and aggressive fluid resuscitation while the surgical team prepares for surgery. Hemopneumothorax should be treated with a thoracostomy tube unless an emergency department thoracotomy is indicated.

Table 13-2. Chest Radiograph Findings in Aortic Injury

Widened mediastinum with obliteration of the aortic knob

Dilation of the ascending aorta

Deviation of the trachea (as evidenced by the endotracheal tube) to the right

Deviation of the esophagus (as evidenced by the nasogastric tube) to the right

Evidence of first and/or second rib fracture

Apical pleural cap (blood at the apex of the lung, seen more commonly on the left)

PROCEDURES

These procedures should only be performed by physicians trained in the techniques and for the appropriate indication.

Thoracostomy Tube Placement for Traumatic Pneumothorax or Hemothorax

The technique is identical for all ages except for size of the tube and depth of insertion. A postinsertion chest radiograph should be obtained to confirm proper placement of the tube and reexpansion of the lung.

Pericardiocentesis

The technique for pericardiocentesis is the same for adults and children. The only essential equipment is a simple 20-mL syringe attached to an 18-gauge $3\frac{1}{2}$-inch spinal needle. Special kits are available that include sterile drapes, large-bore angiocath needle, syringes, three-way stopcock, and an alligator clip with a wire for cardiac monitor guidance. Using cardiac monitor guidance, one will see atypical ventricular depolarization as the needle is advanced toward the myocardium. For the subxiphoid approach, the needle is inserted just left of the xiphoid process aiming for the sternal notch at a 30° to 45° angle. Variations of the technique abound and experience is very helpful.

Emergency Department Thoracotomy

When cardiac arrest occurs following penetrating trauma, immediate thoracotomy may be life-saving. Thoracotomy should only be used for cases in which vital signs have initially been documented and arrest has supervened. Cardiac tamponade is another indication. Survival after emergency thoracotomy in blunt trauma has been universally dismal. External chest compressions, along with attempts to control bleeding and restore blood volume, are a better alternative in these patients. Cross-clamping of the distal thoracic aorta has all but been abandoned, even in adults. Direct finger compression of the proximal abdominal aorta via laparotomy is as effective with less potential for collateral injury.

LAW ENFORCEMENT

Most states require reporting of stab wounds, gunshot wounds, and assaults. Child abuse statutes also require reporting of suspected abuse. As we consider pediatric trauma,

we should also consider our duty to report these injuries to the local authorities and to child protective services.

SUMMARY

As the second leading cause of death in childhood, the skillful management of thoracic injuries cannot be overemphasized. Motor vehicle crashes are the leading mechanism of blunt trauma in childhood, although penetrating trauma is increasing in frequency, especially in older children. Isolated chest trauma is uncommon, so other concomitant injuries must always be addressed in a systematic manner. Because of the pliable rib cage and mediastinal mobility of children, they can suffer significant chest trauma with few external signs. Thus pulmonary contusions and pneumothorax are frequently present without evidence of rib fracture. Most thoracic injuries can be treated nonsurgically with a tube thoracostomy, but the risk of death increases significantly when vital structures are involved.

BIBLIOGRAPHY

Cantor RM, Leaming, JM: Evaluation and management of pediatric major trauma. *Contemp Issues Trauma* 16:229–256, 1998.

Grant WJ, Meyers RL, Jaffe RL, et al: Tracheobronchial injuries after blunt chest trauma in children—hidden pathology. *J Pediatr Surg* 33(11):1707–1711, 1998.

Holmes JF, Brant WE, Bogren G, et al: Prevalence and importance of pneumothoraces visualized on abdominal computed tomographic scan in children with blunt trauma. *J Trauma* 50(3):516–520, 2001.

Karnak I, Senocak ME, Tanyel FC, et al: Diaphragmatic injuries in childhood. *Surg Today* 31(1):5–11, 2001.

Murray JA, Berne J, Asensio JA: Penetrating thoracoabdominal trauma. *Emerg Med Clin North Am* 16:107–128, 1998.

Sanchez JI, Paidas CN: Childhood trauma: Now and in the new millennium. *Surg Clin North Am* 79:1503–1535, 1999.

Tiao GM, Griffith PM, Szmuszkovicz JR, et al: Cardiac and great vessel injuries in children after blunt trauma: An institutional review. *J Pediatr Surg* 35(11):1656–1660, 2000.

APLS Joint Task Force: Trauma, in Strange GR (ed): *Advanced Pediatric Life Support,* 3d ed. Dallas: American Academy of Pediatrics/American College of Emergency Physicians, 1998, pp 59–78.

Schafermeyer RW: Pediatric trauma. *Emerg Med Clin North Am* 11(1):187–205, 1993.

Sivit CJ, Taylor GA, Eichelberger MR: Chest injury in children with blunt abdominal trauma: Evaluation with CT. *Radiology* 171:815, 1989.

14

Abdominal Trauma

Wendy Ann Lucid
Todd Brian Taylor

HIGH-YIELD FACTS

- Blunt abdominal trauma is proportionally more common in children and results in more injuries and deaths than penetrating trauma. However, penetrating trauma is far more lethal as a sole injury.

- Management of pediatric abdominal trauma requires a coordinated effort between the emergency physician, trauma surgeon, and pediatric referral center.

- Care must be taken not to let the head and extremity components of Waddell's triad divert attention from the more subtle findings of intraabdominal injury that may include life-threatening hemorrhage.

- Computed tomography (CT) has eliminated much of the difficulty surrounding the diagnosis of abdominal injuries and is the procedure of choice for stable trauma patients.

- The focused abdominal sonography for trauma (FAST) ultrasound examination evaluates up to six areas of the abdomen with the principal objective of identifying hemoperitoneum.

- Perforations of the duodenum and proximal jejunum are the most common and are usually associated with lap belt or bicycle handlebar injury.

Serious abdominal injuries are relatively common in childhood and account for about 8 percent of admissions to pediatric trauma centers. Only 15 percent of these injuries require surgery and the majority of these are for penetrating wounds. Abdominal trauma is the third leading cause of traumatic death behind head and thoracic injuries, but it is the most common unrecognized cause of fatal injury in children.

Blunt abdominal trauma is proportionately more common in children and results in more injuries and deaths than penetrating trauma. Yet penetrating trauma is far more lethal as the sole injury. Penetrating abdominal trauma accounts for only about 15 percent of the total cases, and of these 6 percent will die primarily from the penetrating wound. Blunt trauma accounts for 85 percent of pediatric abdominal trauma (versus 50 percent in adults), with 9 percent of these patients dying primarily from other associated injuries.

Children are susceptible to different injury patterns than adults. Blunt trauma from automobile accidents causes more than half of the abdominal injuries seen in children and is the most lethal. Penetrating injuries in the pediatric population are increasing. Gunshot and stab wounds are particularly common in young adolescents and 75 percent are inflicted by an assailant as opposed to accidental shootings that occur most commonly from firearms discovered by children in the home. Accidental impalement occurs more often in children <13 years of age and these injuries may involve such diverse items as scissors or picket fences.

Management of pediatric abdominal trauma requires a coordinated effort between the emergency physician, trauma surgeon, and pediatric referral center.

PATTERNS OF INJURY

Motor Vehicle Crashes (Table 14-1)

Multisystem trauma, along with abdominal injury, is common when an automobile strikes a child. Care must be taken not to let the head and extremity components of Waddell's triad divert attention from the more subtle findings of intraabdominal injury that may include life-threatening hemorrhage. The common belief that a unilateral femur fracture can result in hypovolemic shock is questionable, and in this setting further investigation is warranted to evaluate potentially more serious abdominal injuries. In countries in which motorists drive on the right side of the road, the most common injuries are on the left side as children are often struck darting into traffic, and these accidents frequently result in splenic injuries. With unrestrained occupants involved in motor vehicle crashes, head injuries are the most common and lethal injury, but abdominal injuries represent the most common cause of significant blood loss.

The *lap belt complex* (bursting injury of solid or hollow viscera, and rarely disruption of the diaphragm or lumbar spine) is characterized by ecchymosis across the abdomen and flanks (Grey-Turner sign) and occurs in up

Table 14-1. Patterns of Injury by Mechanism

Waddell's Triad	Lap Belt Complex	Fall From a Height
Pedestrian mechanism in child	Restrained occupant in MVC	
Midshaft femur fracture	Blowout diaphragm injury	Head injury
Abdominal injury	Duodenal injury	Multiple long bone fractures
Head injury	Solid organ injury	Chest wall injury

to 10 percent of restrained children. The injury is thought to occur due to an improperly applied restraint that allows the lap belt to ride up and compress the abdomen as the child slides forward under the belt. The overall benefit of avoiding head injuries significantly outweighs any risk associated with seat belts, and proper fitting of restraints should reduce this problem.

Injuries sustained in all-terrain vehicle crashes parallel motor vehicle crashes and have emerged as a frequent cause of abdominal trauma, accounting for a quarter of injuries and 19 percent of deaths.

Bicycle Crashes, Sports Injuries, and Falls

Head trauma remains the predominant injury in bicycle crashes, although abdominal injury can occur if the child is impacted by the handlebars or falls to the ground. Handlebar injuries are particularly obscure, as most children show no serious sign of injury for hours to days after the impact. The mean elapsed time to onset of symptoms is almost 24 hours and as many as one-third are discharged home initially. The seriousness is illustrated by a mean length of stay exceeding 3 weeks for children requiring admission for a handlebar injury. Traumatic pancreatitis is the most common handlebar injury, followed by injuries to the kidneys, spleen, and liver, duodenal hematoma, and bowel perforation. It is prudent to obtain an abdominal CT scan and observe children with a suspicion for this injury.

Sports-related trauma typically produces isolated organ injury due to a direct blow to the abdomen. The spleen, kidney, and gastrointestinal tract are particularly vulnerable. Falls rarely cause isolated serious abdominal injury unless there is a direct blow to the abdomen. Typical injuries seen from falls include trauma to the head and chest wall and multiple long bone fractures.

Child Abuse

Significant abdominal injury occurs in only about 5 percent of child abuse cases, but it represents the second most common cause of death after head injury. The di-

agnosis can be obscured by the inherent delay in seeking treatment, the surreptitious nature of the visit, and the lack of external signs of trauma in up to one-half of these patients.

PATHOPHYSIOLOGY

Certain anatomic features predispose children to multiple rather than single injuries. Proportionally larger solid organs, poorly muscled protuberant abdomen, and flexible thin ribs contribute to the increased incidence of significant abdominal injury and potential for hemorrhage. The diagnosis of a major intraabdominal hemorrhage may be delayed because children have the capacity to maintain normal blood pressure and pulse rate for age, even in the face of significant blood loss. External signs of injury, abdominal tenderness, and absence of bowel sounds seldom give clues to the ultimate need for surgery. Abdominal distention may be due to hemoperitoneum, peritonitis, or most commonly, gastric distention from crying and air swallowing. This can confound the examination by masking or mimicking serious abdominal injury or bleeding. Severe dilation can result in respiratory compromise due to interference with diaphragm motion, gastric aspiration, or vagal dampening of the normal tachycardic response. In children, the primary response to decreased cardiac output is increased heart rate; therefore vagal dampening can lead to precipitous circulatory collapse in the presence of hypovolemia.

MANAGEMENT
General Principles

A team approach in the evaluation and treatment of abdominal injuries, that includes the emergency physician, trauma surgeon, anesthesiologist, and surgical subspecialists, is ideal. In reality, many emergency physicians find themselves as the only physician initially and must approach the injured child in a systematic way, utilizing consultants appropriately and expeditiously. Blunt abdominal injuries rarely require surgical intervention, while penetrating trauma frequently does. Nevertheless, all unstable patients need immediate surgical consultation.

The basic principles of trauma evaluation and resuscitation should be followed in all cases of abdominal trauma. Evaluation of the abdomen is included in both the primary and secondary surveys. The following interventions are particularly important:

- Insertion of a nasogastric tube to decompress the stomach and to check for blood or bile

- A urinary catheter to check for blood and urinary retention, if there is no gross blood at the meatus

- A rectal examination to check for blood, prostate position in males, and rectal tone

- Keep the child NPO due to the possibility of surgery or development of paralytic ileus

- Blood should be obtained for type and cross-match, CBC, serum amylase, and liver transaminases

The mechanism of injury is important and guides the secondary survey and the ordering of specific tests or procedures. With penetrating injury it is important to log roll the patient to inspect the posterior torso for additional wounds. External injuries such as abrasions, lacerations, bruising, and characteristic markings such as tire tracks and seat belt marks should be noted.

Children respond differently to trauma and stress. A traumatized child may be very difficult to examine and may not show the familiar signs of impending demise as seen with adults. History will be limited and the child's reaction to pain may be grossly over- or underexaggerated. A team member should be designated to care for the child's emotional needs and to comfort them through the ordeal of trauma evaluation and treatment.

Penetrating Abdominal Trauma

The diagnosis and treatment of penetrating abdominal injuries in children does not differ greatly from that for adults, and initial management is not dependent on identifying any specific injury. The hollow organs, due to their large volume, are most commonly injured, followed by the liver, kidney, spleen, and major vessels.

In children, the abdomen begins at the nipples, so penetrating wounds between the nipples and the groin potentially involve the peritoneal cavity and should be considered contaminated with a potential for infection. Surgical evaluation, wound debridement, and possible exploration, along with broad-spectrum intravenous antibiotics are necessary in all but the most minor of wounds. Location, size, and possible trajectory of entrance and exit wounds help to identify potential underlying injuries. At a minimum, the following should be performed when there has been significant penetrating abdominal trauma:

- Placement of a nasogastric tube

- Placement of a urinary catheter

- Upright posteroanterior chest radiograph with a lateral, if possible

- Supine, upright, and cross-table abdominal radiographs

- "One shot" intravenous pyelogram for deep penetrating stab wounds and all gunshot wounds

Gunshot wounds to the abdomen require immediate exploration. Most enter the peritoneal cavity and injure organs directly or indirectly through kinetic energy dissipation. The high morbidity and mortality associated with gunshot wounds is due to the destructive force of the missile and its fragments, rapid blood loss, complicated surgical repair, and postoperative complications.

Stab wounds pose the greatest threat to blood vessels. Commonly injured vessels include the aorta, inferior vena cava, the portal vein, and hepatic veins. However, stab wounds enter the peritoneal cavity only one-third of the time and only one-third of these require a visceral repair. Local exploration may be possible to rule out peritoneal penetration in minor stab wounds. Conservative management can be entertained if the patient meets the following criteria:

- No sign of shock or peritonitis with observation for 12 to 24 hours

- No blood in the stomach, rectum, or urine

- No evidence of free abdominal or retroperitoneal air on x-ray

- No history or evidence of bowel or omental evisceration

- Close observation with surgical consultation

Blunt Abdominal Trauma

Both isolated abdominal and multisystem trauma present challenges in the pediatric patient because information is inherently difficult to obtain. Multiple other injuries may overshadow often subtle early abdominal findings and the physical examination may be only 55 to 65 percent accurate. For the emergency physician, the key to management is suspecting the diagnosis and obtaining appropriate studies and consultation. Minor mechanisms, such as falling 2 feet to the ground from a hammock, can result in significant splenic injury with minimal symptoms. Therefore emergency department observation, as well as repeat vital signs and abdominal examinations, may be warranted. Laboratory and radiologic studies may be necessary depending on clinical status, mechanism of injury, and suspicion for injury on physical examination.

Radiographs of the chest (supine or preferably upright posteroanterior plus a lateral) and supine abdomen and pelvis can give important clues to the diagnosis of abdominal injury (Table 14-2). Hemoglobin and hematocrit are seldom useful early in the evaluation, but later may be valuable for comparison to baseline. However, if the initial hematocrit is <30 percent with other signs of impending shock, this suggests significant hemorrhage. An initial hematocrit <24 percent is associated with high mortality, and transfusion should be initiated.

A persistently distended abdomen after nasogastric tube placement, hemodynamic instability not immediately responsive to fluid resuscitation, recurrent hypotension, or signs of peritoneal irritation warrant immediate surgical intervention by a surgeon experienced in pediatric abdominal injuries.

Computed Tomography (CT)

CT has eliminated much of the difficulty surrounding the diagnosis of abdominal injuries and is the procedure of choice for stable trauma patients. Specialized studies should be ordered in consultation with the trauma surgeon to avoid unnecessary delay in definitive treatment. Indications for abdominal and pelvic CT are listed in Table 14-3. CT is useful for evaluation of the liver, kidney, spleen, retroperitoneum, and, to a lesser extent, gastrointestinal injuries. CT identification of pancreatic injury, diaphragm injury, and bowel perforation are much less sensitive and warrant a high index of suspicion with serial abdominal examinations to rule out occult injury.

Use of oral and intravenous contrast media has traditionally been thought to increase the sensitivity of abdominal CT. However, the benefit of oral contrast is being questioned due to the technical difficulty of administration and increased waiting time before scanning, risk of aspiration, and apparent limited value due to frequent lack of bowel opacification.

Diagnostic Peritoneal Lavage (DPL)

Close observation, serial physical examinations, and particularly abdominal CT are utilized to the virtual exclusion of peritoneal lavage in pediatric patients. DPL may still be useful if these other modalities are unavailable or the child must undergo immediate general anesthesia for other injuries. Under these circumstances, DPL can often be performed in the operating suite. However, the usefulness of DPL remains questionable. It is neither organ- nor injury-specific, cannot reliably assess retroperitoneal injury, and the decision to operate for liver or splenic injuries is not based on the amount of intraperitoneal blood in children. In addition, the introduction of air and fluid into the abdomen and the resulting peritoneal irritation make subsequent radiographic and physical examinations more difficult.

The technique for DPL in children is similar to that for adults, although a small supraumbilical incision to avoid the bladder is preferred over the usual infraumbilical approach.

Abdominal Ultrasound

Bedside ultrasound (US) is becoming more readily available and may further reduce the need for DPL. It is particularly useful in the unstable patient as an immediate triage tool and adjunct to the physical examination. As such, it is best used for detecting intraabdominal injuries

Table 14-2. Radiographic Clues in Abdominal Trauma

- A ground-glass appearance of the abdominal cavity may suggest intraperitoneal blood or urine
- Medial displacement of the lateral border of the stomach, as evidenced by the nasogastric tube, suggests splenic laceration or hematoma as the enlarged spleen pushes the stomach aside
- Obliteration of the psoas shadow or renal outline and fracture of the lower ribs suggest renal trauma
- Bleeding from the short gastric vessels gives the fundic mucosa a "sawtooth" appearance
- With nasogastric tube in place, the relative lack of gas in the distal small intestine suggests a duodenal or proximal jejunal hematoma
- Air injected via the nasogastric tube may increase the chance of detecting a pneumoperitoneum indicative of perforated viscus

Table 14-3. Comparison of Techniques for Evaluation of Abdominal Trauma

	Abdominal CT	**Diagnostic Peritoneal Lavage**	**Abdominal Ultrasound**
Indication	Relatively stable patient	Relatively unstable patient	May be used as a triage tool and adjunct to the physical examination
	Multiple trauma or major thoracic, head, or orthopedic (pelvic) injury	Otherwise the same as for CT	Evaluation of pancreatic injury and intraabdominal fluid (presumably blood)
	Physical findings or a mechanism suggesting possible abdominal injury.		May also be used to identify other intraabdominal injuries when CT is not readily available.
	Unexplained hypotension		
	Hematuria (gross or microscopic >20 RBC/hpf), CNS injury, spinal injury, or mental status alteration precluding serial abdominal examination.		
	Declining hematocrit <10 g/dL) or unaccountable fluid and blood requirements		
Advantage	Relatively noninvasive	May be performed on a patient who is relatively unstable or who needs to undergo urgent general anesthesia for other reasons	Available at the bedside and more readily available than CT in some locales
	High sensitivity and specificity		Can be used at the bedside for a FAST examination to evaluate for peritoneal fluid and blood
	Evaluates multiple organ systems simultaneously	Easily and rapidly performed	
Disadvantage	Generally requires intravenous with or without oral contrast	Unless grossly positive, lab results may delay definitive treatment	Not as sensitive as CT
	Time delay	Neither organ- nor injury-specific	
		Cannot assess retroperitoneal injury	
		Decision to operate is not generally based on the amount of peritoneal blood	
		Introduction of air and fluid into the abdomen may alter future diagnostic tests	
		Local peritoneal irritation may alter serial abdominal exams	

that require immediate attention rather than for a definitive diagnosis. It is also useful when CT is not available and its greatest utility is in detecting intraperitoneal hemorrhage and pancreatic injuries.

The use of bedside ultrasound has become part of the core emergency medicine curriculum and is often taught using the "focused abdominal sonography for trauma" (FAST) method. The FAST examination evaluates up to six areas of the abdomen with the principal objective of identifying hemoperitoneum. Children who are hemodynamically unstable with abdominal trauma will require laparotomy regardless of the US and those that are stable are often managed nonsurgically even with abdominal organ injury. Therefore the exact role of US in assessing pediatric abdominal trauma is still being evaluated.

Nuclear Scans

Nuclear scans are not typically used for the evaluation of acute abdominal injury, but can be useful as a follow-up for liver or splenic injuries previously diagnosed by CT.

SPECIFIC INJURIES AND MANAGEMENT

Solid Organs

Spleen

With blunt trauma, the spleen ranks first among the solid abdominal organs susceptible to major hemorrhage and second only to the liver in lethal injury. The typical blunt mechanism of injury is frequently from motor vehicle accidents. A right-sided blow or fall can cause a contrecoup splenic injury. Penetrating injuries of all types can cause splenic injury and, as with liver stab wounds, it is often difficult to determine the extent of underlying injury based on the external signs of trauma. Mononucleosis, common in children, can result in splenic enlargement and predispose to splenic rupture. Patients with this condition should be warned about contact sports or any activity that could cause a blow to the abdomen until the spleen has returned to normal size, a minimum of 4 to 6 weeks.

Although diffuse abdominal pain may be the presenting complaint, typical findings with splenic injury are left upper quadrant abdominal pain, radiating to the left shoulder (Kehr's sign), associated with palpable tenderness on examination. Significant tenderness in the left upper abdomen and/or splenic enlargement should prompt surgical consultation and consideration of a CT

scan. Frank splenic rupture may lead to shock and posttraumatic cardiac arrest. Persistent unexplained leukocytosis or hyperamylasemia also suggests splenic injury.

Abdominal CT is the study of choice to identify splenic injury. Abdominal radiographs may incidentally reveal a medially displaced gastric bubble secondary to the enlarged spleen.

Once a splenic injury has been identified in the stable patient, management is focused on salvaging the spleen. The thick elastic splenic capsule in children and the usual transverse orientation of lacerations parallel to the vessels commonly results in spontaneous cessation of bleeding and allows nonsurgical management in 90 percent of cases.

Conservative management includes initial hospitalization for 7 to 10 days of bed rest, followed by a regimen of limited activity. Although spontaneous healing of splenic lacerations and subcapsular hematomas occurs in the overwhelming majority of cases, delayed spontaneous rupture can occur at any time and is most common on the third to fifth day. The commitment to conservative management includes close observation and frequent examination.

Children who develop hypotension not responsive to volume resuscitation obviously require surgery. When surgery is required for persistent bleeding, all efforts are made to salvage as much spleen as possible. The results of splenorrhaphy or partial splenectomy have been equally as good as nonsurgical management. There is a marked increase in infection and a 65-fold increase in lethal sepsis in children with splenectomy, particularly with encapsulated organisms (*Streptococcus pneumoniae, Haemophilus influenzae, Neisseria meningitidis, Staphylococcus aureus,* and *Escherichia coli*). The pneumococcal and *H. influenzae* (HIB) vaccines should be given to any patient undergoing partial or complete splenectomy, even though antibody response may be inconsistent and temporary.

Liver

The liver ranks second among solid abdominal organs for major hemorrhage and significant injury, but it is the most common source of *lethal* hemorrhage. Mortality from serious liver injuries may be as high as 10 to 20 percent. However, the majority of liver injuries in children are minor and remain undetected unless discovered incidentally by abnormal liver enzymes or imaging studies. CT has revolutionized the diagnosis of liver injury and accounts for the increased recognition of this problem.

Mechanisms of injury are similar to those in splenic trauma. Symptoms depend largely on the extent of injury and range from nonspecific diffuse abdominal pain to posttraumatic cardiac arrest. Significant tenderness in the right upper abdomen and/or liver enlargement should prompt surgical consultation and CT scan evaluation.

Children with liver injuries who are not in shock or who respond to volume resuscitation rarely require surgery to control bleeding. However, nonsurgical management is not without complications. Those requiring late laparotomy have transfusion requirements greater than 50 percent of total blood volume (TBV) during the first 24 hours after injury and bleeding into the biliary tract (hematobilia) are not uncommon. Conservative management includes careful monitoring of vital signs, serial abdominal examinations, and serial hematocrit measurements.

Large stellate liver lacerations and subcapsular hematomas that have eroded through Glisson's capsule rarely stop bleeding without surgery. However, hepatic resection and biliary tree drains are rarely indicated, and direct suturing and drainage can manage most hepatic lacerations. In preparation for surgery, circulating blood volume should be restored since rapid hemorrhage can occur during surgery as blood clots are evacuated during repair.

Pancreas

The pancreas is rarely seriously injured in blunt pediatric trauma due to its deep position in the upper abdomen. However, it is in a fixed position anterior to the vertebral column and vulnerable to a direct blow to the upper central abdomen as seen with bicycle handlebar injury. Pancreatic injuries are notoriously difficult to diagnose.

Traumatic pancreatitis without major pancreatic injury is most common, followed by pancreatic hematomas, and rarely transection of the body or duct. Pancreatic transections often lead to pancreatic pseudocyst formation within 3 to 5 days and result in chronic intermittent attacks of abdominal pain, nausea, vomiting, and weight loss. Acutely, the leakage of pancreatic fluid into the lesser peritoneal sac causes a chemical peritonitis and pancreatic ascites. The classic triad of epigastric pain radiating to the back, a palpable abdominal mass with or without acute peritonitis or ascites, and hyperamylasemia are rarely detected in children.

CT may help identify severe pancreatic injury or evidence of pancreatic edema as an early indication of trauma, but is not as helpful in determining management. Ultrasound may be more useful, but is also unlikely to change the early management. Elevated serum amylase may indicate pancreatic injury, but its absence does not preclude it.

Simple traumatic pancreatitis is treated similarly to other types of pancreatitis with bowel rest, nasogastric suction, intravenous fluids, and pain medication. Severe pancreatic injury will typically require surgical drainage with repair or partial resection of the pancreas. Pancreatic pseudocyst treatment involves 6 to 8 weeks of total parenteral nutrition followed by a surgical drainage procedure.

Abdominal Wall

The muscles of the abdominal wall include the rectus abdominis anteriorly; the internal oblique, external oblique, and transversalis laterally; and posteriorly the erector spinae (sacrospinalis) muscle group, quadratus lumborum, latissimus dorsi, serratus posterior inferior, and the psoas (located deep and posterior). Hematomas of any of these muscles can occur, as well as concomitant injury to the spine and other skeletal structures. The psoas muscle is particularly susceptible to hematoma, even with minor trauma, in patients with a bleeding diathesis such as hemophilia, or those on warfarin.

Tenderness, bruising, swelling, or a mass of the abdominal wall may indicate a hematoma or simply a contusion. However, certain types of ecchymosis are indicative of intraabdominal injury and the onset may occur several hours after the trauma.

- *Grey-Turner sign:* ecchymosis in the abdominal or flank area may represent a retroperitoneal hematoma
- *Cullen's sign:* bluish discoloration around the umbilicus may represent an intraperitoneal hemorrhage

Abdominal wall injuries other than large lacerations are typically self-limited and consideration for other underlying injury is more important, as outlined in the previous sections. Differentiation between abdominal wall and deeper injury can be difficult, so a low threshold for abdominal CT is warranted.

Careful instructions should be given at discharge. Patients and caregivers are instructed to watch for:

- Vomiting
- Increasing pain
- Abdominal distention
- Hematuria
- Fever

Close follow-up should be assured for reexamination within 24 hours for any significant abdominal wall injury.

Hollow Organs

Hollow visceral organs are injured in only 1 to 5 percent of children with blunt abdominal trauma. Of those requiring laparotomy up to 16 percent may have such injuries. Perforations of the duodenum and proximal jejunum are the most common and usually associated with a lap belt or bicycle handlebar injury. Penetrating trauma is more obvious and more likely to show early signs of injury, such as free air.

Without obvious evidence of free air on radiographs, the diagnosis of a perforated viscus in blunt trauma can be difficult. Tenderness may initially be localized and slowly worsen over 6 to 12 hours, accounting for the time necessary for peritonitis or obstruction to occur. Abdominal CT is not particularly sensitive for these injuries, and repeated physical examinations remain the most reliable indicator of enteric disruption. Surgical consultation should be obtained early in the management of these patients. Once the suspected diagnosis of perforated abdominal viscus has been made, treatment is straightforward with laparotomy to repair the injury. Most injuries can be repaired primarily; however, colon perforations often require a diverting colostomy.

Intramural hematomas of the duodenum or jejunum can cause symptoms of intestinal obstruction with pain, bilious vomiting, and gastric distention. The diagnosis can be made with ultrasound or upper GI series, which reveals the "coiled spring" sign. This problem rarely requires surgery. It may cause traumatic pancreatitis with involvement of Vater's ampulla. Treatment is conservative and supportive including nasogastric suction and parenteral nutrition for up to 3 weeks.

When a large abdominal wall defect is present, as with a large stab wound or close-range shotgun wound, evisceration can occur. The bowel should be kept moist with saline-soaked gauze and not allowed to assume a dependent position that would increase edema of the bowel wall.

SUMMARY

Evaluation and treatment of children with suspected abdominal trauma is challenging. Physiologic characteristics of children make vital signs and physical examination less predictive of serious injury than in adults. Therefore other diagnostic clues such as mechanism of injury and maintaining a high suspicion for common injuries are paramount. An awareness of useful diagnostic tests such as abdominal CT and their limitations is also important. When treating the multisystem traumatized child, a systematic approach will lead to identification of less obvious injuries often lurking within the abdomen. Finally, it is wise to identify resources for treatment of pediatric trauma well in advance. The ability to provide definitive care in an efficient manner through trauma teams or expeditious transfer to a trauma center optimizes the chances of survival and limitation of morbidity.

BIBLIOGRAPHY

APLS Joint Task Force: Trauma, in Strange GR (ed): *Advanced Pediatric Life Support,* 3d ed. Dallas: American Academy of Pediatrics/American College of Emergency Physicians, 1997, pp 59–78.

Brown CK, Dunn KA, Wilson K: Diagnostic evaluation of patients with blunt abdominal trauma: A decision analysis. *Acad Emerg Med* 7:385–396, 2000.

Cantor RM, Leaming JM: Evaluation and management of pediatric major trauma. *Contemp Issues Trauma* 16:229–256, 1998.

Melanson SW, Heller M: The emerging role of bedside ultrasonography in trauma care. *Emerg Med Clin North Am* 16:165–189, 1998.

Patel JC, Tepas JJ: The efficacy of focused abdominal sonography for trauma (FAST) as a screening tool in the assessment of injured children. *J Pediatr Surg* 34:44–47, 1999.

Rothrock SG, Green SM, Morgan R: Abdominal trauma in infants and children: Prompt identification and early management of serious and life-threatening injuries. Part I: Injury patterns and initial assessment. *Pediatr Emerg Care* 16:106–115, 2000. Part II: Specific injuries and ED management. *Pediatr Emerg Care* 16:189–195, 2000.

Sanchez JI, Paidas CN: Childhood trauma: Now and in the new millennium. *Surg Clin North Am* 79:1503–1535, 1999.

Schafermeyer RW: Pediatric trauma. *Emerg Med Clin North Am* 11:187–205, 1993.

15

Genitourinary and Rectal Trauma

Wendy Ann Lucid
Todd Brian Taylor

HIGH-YIELD FACTS

- A urinalysis should be performed on all major trauma patients as well as those suspected of having isolated genitourinary (GU) injury.
- Penetrating trauma between the nipples and perineum requires at least a one-shot intravenous pyelogram to rule out GU injuries before surgery.
- Renal trauma can lead to acute tubular necrosis with renal failure, delayed bleeding, infection, or abscess secondary to urinary extravasation. Renin-mediated hypertension can develop weeks to months after the injury.
- Bladder rupture should be considered in children who present with abdominal trauma with gross hematuria, blood at the urethral meatus, inability to void, or little urine upon urinary catheter placement.

The incidence of urinary tract injury in children with multiple trauma is second only to injury of the central nervous system. Although many genitourinary (GU) injuries are of little consequence to the child's overall morbidity and mortality, some may be life threatening if not identified and managed aggressively. Most GU injuries involve the kidneys, but other structures are also important and are often more difficult to evaluate. Most serious GU injuries result from a motor vehicle striking a pedestrian, but penetrating injury continues to increase with the overall increase in violence. Sports-related injuries and child abuse are less frequently recognized mechanisms of injury.

Hematuria heralds the possibility of injury to the kidneys, ureter, bladder, or urethra. As in all major trauma, management of GU injuries begins with the basics of trauma assessment and life support. The kidneys and renal pedicle may be sources for major bleeding and should be considered for patients with hypovolemic shock. A dipstick urine analysis is usually the initial screening test for hematuria in the emergency department. It is highly sensitive for blood but cannot quantify the amount of hematuria or differentiate among myoglobinuria, hemoglobinuria, and true hematuria. Furthermore, in the early postinjury period, not all GU trauma will present with hematuria. The GU system can often be evaluated simultaneously with diagnostic tests being done to evaluate the abdomen. In any event, the GU system should be evaluated before surgery in appropriate cases of penetrating trauma and for patients with significant hematuria.

GENERAL MANAGEMENT PRINCIPLES

Blunt Genitourinary Trauma

More than 90 percent of GU injuries in children follow blunt trauma and more than 10 percent of all children with blunt abdominal injuries will have GU injuries. Children are also more likely than adults to sustain GU injuries from blunt abdominal trauma. After stabilization of the patient's vital functions, specific organ systems are evaluated. The definitive diagnosis of blunt GU injuries may be difficult and demands a systematic approach regardless of whether the patient presents with multiple trauma or isolated injuries to the abdomen, pelvis, or flank. Complications of GU trauma include hemorrhage, urinary extravasation, renal parenchymal damage, infection, delayed hypertension, and renal dysfunction. Injuries to the more vital systems take precedence over the GU system in the initial trauma evaluation and resuscitation, but one must revisit the GU system after these more critical systems are stabilized.

During the physical examination, attention to the abdomen, flank, pelvis, and genitalia will provide clues to possible GU injuries. Unfortunately, in children, the classic findings of flank pain, tenderness, and mass are difficult to elicit, and their absence does not exclude GU injury. As in all trauma patients, the genital and rectal examination should precede the insertion of a urinary catheter. Signs of urethral injury include blood at the meatus or a high-riding prostate.

The usual trauma blood panel, chest radiograph, anteroposterior pelvis film, and abdominal flat plate, often utilized in the evaluation of multiple trauma patients, may provide clues to possible GU injuries. The abdominal radiograph may show loss of the psoas shadow, indicating retroperitoneal blood; scoliosis with concavity to the side of injury; or lower rib or transverse process fractures, all of which are associated with GU trauma. The location of the injury is also a clue to the potential site of injury. Urethral injury may present with blood at the meatus or a high-riding prostate; and a pelvic fracture may herald a bladder injury.

A urinalysis should be performed on all major trauma patients as well as those suspected of having isolated GU injury. If a urine dipstick is positive for blood, a microscopic urinalysis should be performed. Depending on the results of the urinalysis, further diagnostic tests or surgical consultation may be indicated. Although hematuria heralds the possibility of GU trauma, it may also be present without significant injury if there is an underlying renal malformation. Hematuria may be *absent* as much as 50 percent of the time, with renal vascular (pedicle) injury, ureteral injuries, and certain penetrating injuries isolated to the ureters. Therefore, there is no direct correlation between the degree of hematuria and the severity of GU injury. Indications for further GU evaluation include the following:

- gross or microscopic hematuria (>20 RBCs/hpf in children vs. >50 RBCs/hpf in adults)
- abdominal or flank pain
- hematoma
- mass
- flank ecchymosis (Grey Turner sign)
- periumbilical ecchymosis (Cullen sign)
- penetrating trauma that could reasonably expect to injure the GU system (Table 15-1).

Urine output should be monitored to ensure renal perfusion and to exclude bilateral renal artery occlusion or an obstructing process.

Finally, sexual and physical abuse should be considered when evaluating perineal injuries. These injuries may result from the caretakers' ignorance in proper toilet training or from overt abuse. In particular, burns to the perineum, inconsistent mechanism of injury, evidence of previous injury, or the child's own history should prompt further investigation and a report to child protective services and local authorities.

Penetrating Genitourinary Trauma

Penetrating trauma between the nipples and perineum requires at least a preliminary one-shot intravenous pyelogram (IVP) before surgery to rule out GU injuries (Table 15-1). Depending on the location and type of penetrating trauma, other studies may be indicated.

DIAGNOSTIC STUDIES

Computed Tomography

Computed tomography (CT) scan of the abdomen with intravenous contrast is an excellent study for evaluation of the kidneys, with an accuracy of 98 percent. Patients with renal injuries often have concomitant abdominal, retroperitoneal, and pelvic injuries, and CT serves to evaluate many systems at once. Nonionic contrast media should be considered in patients younger than 1 year, those with a history of previous reaction to contrast, unstable patients, and those with underlying renal disease, diabetes, sickle cell anemia, heart or lung disease, dehydration, or other significant medical conditions. Use of

Table 15-1. Indications for Diagnostic Evaluation of the Genitourinary (GU) Tract in Pediatric Trauma

Blunt Trauma
    Multiple trauma
    Gross or microscopic hematuria (>20 RBCs/hpf) or shock
    Palpable flank mass, hematoma, ecchymosis, or tenderness
    Lower rib or thoracic or lumbar spine fractures
    Deceleration injuries (motor vehicle accident or fall from height) with crush injuries to the abdomen or pelvis with
        or without other signs
    Pelvic fracture
Penetrating Trauma
    Any injury that can reasonably be expected to injure the GU tract
    Anticipated surgery for lower chest, abdomen, or pelvics for gunshot or deep stab wound

nonionic media may, however, lead to overestimation of the amount of urinary extravasation, and results of such studies should not be used as absolute criteria for surgery. In addition to identifying specific renal injuries, CT provides information about function and may be more valuable than arteriography when vascular injuries are suspected. Although abdominal CT remains the study of choice for multiply injured children, simple IVP may be more appropriate for isolated renal injuries without shock or significant physical findings (Fig. 15-1, Tables 15-1 and 15-2).

Intravenous Pyelography

A "scout KUB" followed by injection of contrast media (1 to 2 mL/kg, depending on the agent used) and films at 1, 5, and 10 minutes make up the routine emergency IVP. A one-shot IVP at 5 minutes can be substituted in unstable patients in order to document two functioning kidneys. These limited IVPs often do not correlate well with the findings at operation, and a more formal IVP or CT is appropriate for patients who do not require immediate surgery. Prompt bilateral function, with well-defined anatomy, without extravasation, generally excludes major renal injury. Compared with CT, IVP is relatively inexpensive, easy to obtain, and relatively safe and has an accuracy of >90 percent.

Table 15-2. Diagnostic Evaluation of Pediatric Genitourinary (GU) Injury: Patients Meeting Criteria for GU Evaluation

Abdominal CT
Stable patient
Multiple trauma
IVP equivocal or severe injury requiring better definition
IVP
Unstable patient (one - shot IVP)
Isolated GU trauma
Penetrating wounds
Suspected ureteral injury

CT, computed tomography; IVP, intravenous pyelography.

Other Procedures

If CT is unavailable or does not clearly define the injury, other diagnostic procedures may be useful.

Renal ultrasound (US) is less accurate than CT, but it may be useful for following perirenal hematomas or urinomas or to limit radiation exposure in pregnancy. Bedside US and the focused abdominal sonography for trauma (FAST) method, often useful in evaluating abdominal trauma, has limited value for the GU system.

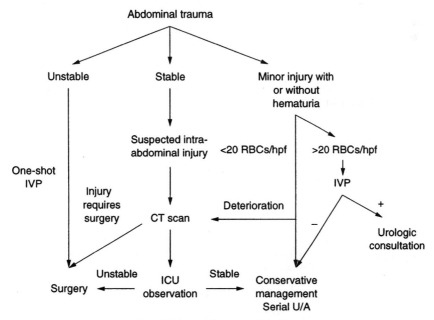

Fig. 15-1. Renal Evaluation After Trauma.

The exact role of US in assessing pediatric trauma remains under investigation.

Retrograde pyelography is useful for delineating ureteropelvic disruption if the IVP is indeterminate. CT cystography is as accurate as a standard cystogram for bladder rupture and can often be done in conjunction with an abdominal CT. Renal angiography has been virtually replaced by CT and digital subtraction angiography, which are less invasive. Radioisotope renal scanning can be used as an alternative for patients allergic to ionic contrast media for evaluation of renovascular injuries.

SPECIFIC INJURIES AND MANAGEMENT

Kidney

Pathophysiology

The kidneys are the second most commonly injured solid organ in blunt pediatric trauma. Although protected by the paraspinous muscles and embedded in fat enclosed in a tough fascial envelope, they are less protected in children. Less perirenal fat, weaker abdominal muscles, more compliant ribs, proportionally larger kidneys, and frequent congenital abnormalities contribute to the high incidence of renal trauma. The substantial force required to cause significant renal injury frequently results in associated abdominal injuries, which may cause hypovolemic shock. Shock due to isolated renal fracture is uncommon since the tight fascial compartment limits the amount of parenchymal bleeding to no more than 25 percent of total blood volume (TBV). Associated injuries, including fractures of the extremities, ribs, skull, pelvis, and spine, head injuries, and spleen and liver lacerations occur in 80 percent of children with renal injuries. Although the management of severe renal injury remains controversial, most renal injuries including contusions and small capsular lacerations are not life threatening and can be managed without surgery.

Mechanism of Injury

Blunt GU injuries occur most commonly with rapid deceleration. The kidneys are crushed against the ribs or vertebral column due to their relatively fixed position within Gerota's fascia, resulting in contusion or parenchymal laceration. For the same reasons, the vascular pedicle can be stretched, resulting in injuries to the renal vein or artery and subsequent thrombosis. Renal pedicle injuries are particularly problematic. They often present with vascular thrombosis, absent hematuria, and

the kidney is nearly always lost despite early surgical intervention.

Penetrating trauma is usually straightforward and is often associated with adjacent visceral injuries. Major penetrating injuries to the kidneys involving extravasation and hemodynamic instability typically require surgery, whereas more minor injuries can be treated conservatively as with most blunt injuries.

Management

Blunt trauma patients without significant concomitant injuries, who present with isolated microscopic hematuria of <20 RBCs/hpf in children (50 RBCs/hpf in adults) require only a follow-up urinalysis in 48 to 72 hours to ensure resolution of the hematuria. If bleeding persists, a formal evaluation should be performed. More significant bleeding and certainly gross hematuria requires urgent investigation. Significant renal injuries or suspicious mechanisms of injury require hospital observation to detect potential progression or associated injuries (Table 15-3 and Fig. 15-1).

Serious GU bleeding occurs in <3 percent of cases and usually requires immediate surgery. This bleeding may be due to direct communication between the renal arterioles and calyx, injury to the renal pedicle, expanding retroperitoneal hematoma, severe kidney laceration causing extensive extravasation, and frank transection of a portion of the main collecting system. Less serious injuries that may require delayed surgical intervention include retroperitoneal extravasation secondary to communication between the renal calyx and the perinephric space and persistent or infected urinoma resulting from a small urinary leak. There is considerable controversy regarding management of grade IV and V injuries (Table 15-3). Ironically, an effort to save the injured kidney with early surgical intervention nearly always results in nephrectomy. Management of moderate and severe renal injuries must be individualized, and early consultation with the appropriate surgeon is important to determine the best course of action. Many urologists prefer conservative management unless there is a definite surgical indication, although associated injuries may require laparotomy in up to 89 percent of cases.

Anomalous kidneys (hydronephrosis, tumor, horseshoe kidney, or polycystic kidney disease) are more easily injured with minor trauma and can present with hematuria of varying degrees. In children, the incidence of anomalous kidneys with renal trauma has been reported to be as high as 15 percent. Due to this high incidence, evaluation by IVP for lower levels of microscopic he-

Table 15-3. Classification of Renal Injury

Grade	Minor Renal Injury	Observation (85%)
I	Contusion	Parenchymal injury without fracture of the parenchyma or capsule as evidenced by delayed or underfilling of the renal calyces on IVP
II	Shallow cortical laceration	Intact capsule with superficial parenchymal laceration without extension into the collecting system; no urinary extravasation on IVP
III	Deep cortical lacerations	Lacerated capsule with superficial parenchymal laceration without extension into the collecting system; no urinary extravasation on IVP
IV	Forniceal laceration	Disruption of the collecting system and parenchymal junction without injury to the parenchyma and capsule
	Major Renal Injury	**Consider Surgery (15%)**
IV	Deep parenchymal laceration	Extension of the laceration into the collecting system with intact or disrupted capsule
V	Shattered kidney	Parenchyma is ruptured in multiple fragments with distortion of the intrarenal collecting structures with intact or disrupted capsule
V	Renal pedicle injury	Laceration or thrombus at the pedicle involving the renal artery or vein as evidenced by lack of contrast in the affected kidney on IVP

IVP, intravenous pyelography.

maturia than adults (20 vs. 50 RBCs/hpf) has been recommended.

Delayed Findings

Renal trauma can lead to acute tubular necrosis with renal failure, delayed bleeding, infection, or abscess secondary to urinary extravasation, and renin-mediated hypertension can develop weeks to months after the injury. Arteriovenous fistula, chronic pyelonephritis, hydronephrosis, chronic calculi, pseudocyst, and hypertension can also occur. Repeat IVP or CT in 3 to 6 months after significant renal injury is prudent to reevaluate the kidneys.

Ureter

Ureteral injuries are uncommon in children, occurring in <5 percent of GU trauma. They occur most frequently as a complication of surgery, but penetrating trauma is the most common external mechanism, accounting for >90 percent of the cases.

About 50 cases of traumatic avulsion of the ureter have been reported. Avulsion occurs most commonly at the right ureteropelvic junction or in the proximal 4 cm of the ureter. It occurs more commonly in children and is invariably due to blunt trauma. This is due, in part, to increased mobility of the childhood spine, allowing the renal pelvis and upper ureter to be compressed against the lower ribs or lumbar transverse processes. The ureter can also be stretched by sudden extreme flexion of the trunk. The diagnosis is difficult to make and often delayed since hematuria can be absent or transient. IVP will usually show extravasation of contrast at the level of the kidney without filling of the ureter. Retrograde pyelography may be necessary to differentiate avulsion from a forniceal tear and to identify the level of the avulsion. Abdominal CT may raise the suspicion for ureteral avulsion, but an IVP or retrograde pyelogram is usually necessary to make the definitive diagnosis. Delayed symptoms include fever, ileus, hematuria, and flank or abdominal pain.

Ureteral transection, irrespective of the cause, is treated with prompt ureteropyelostomy, with or without proximal drainage. The kidney salvage rate is >95 percent. Delay in this diagnosis can cause fistulas, ureteral strictures, and abscesses, and ultimately nephrectomy is frequently necessary.

Bladder

Pathophysiology

Bladder injury represents about one-fourth of all urologic trauma and is due to motor vehicle crash in the vast majority of children. It is often associated with multisystem trauma with a high mortality secondary to associated injuries. Pelvic fracture is associated with injury to the GU system 75 percent of the time, and 10 percent of pelvic fractures result in bladder injury. The bladder has an abdominal position in young children and is more vulnerable to rupture especially when full. Bladder contusions are self-limited and account for about two-thirds of bladder injuries. Penetrating injury to the bladder is much less common.

Iatrogenic bladder injuries may occur during herniorrhaphy (due to the protrusion of the bladder though the inguinal ring), cystoscopy, and umbilical artery cutdown. Umbilical artery cutdown or catheterization may cause urachal-bladder injury due to the closely adherent peritoneum of the urachus and bladder with subsequent intraperitoneal extravasation of urine. It is associated with the triad of oliguria, azotemia, and urinary ascites.

Bladder rupture is associated with a high mortality rate (11 to 44 percent). Mortality increases with delay in diagnosis and may present as persistent hematuria, peritonitis, sepsis, and renal failure following trauma. Bladder rupture is divided into extraperitoneal, intraperitoneal, and combined. With all types, abdominal pain may be absent initially or attributed to pain associated with other abdominal injury or pelvic fracture. Intraperitoneal absorption of urine leads to elevated or rising levels of blood urea nitrogen (BUN) and should raise suspicion for this injury.

Management

In general, bladder rupture should be considered in children with abdominal trauma with gross hematuria, blood at the urethral meatus, inability to void, or little urine upon urinary catheter placement (Table 15-4). Microscopic hematuria suggests potential bladder contusion, but hematuria may be absent even with bladder rupture.

A cystogram is the radiographic study of choice for suspected bladder rupture and has an accuracy of >96 percent (Table 15-5). However, an IVP or abdominal/pelvic CT should be performed before the cystogram to avoid obscuration of the IVP findings by extravasation of dye from the bladder. An IVP alone may diagnose bladder rupture 15 percent of the time but does not exclude rupture. An abdominal/pelvic CT is useful in multiple trauma, but it may not be sensitive enough for bladder injury unless the bladder is fully distended with contrast. With suspected bladder rupture, a retrograde urethrogram should precede attempts to pass a urinary catheter in males due to the high incidence of associated urethral injuries. Cystography should include maximally full, postdrainage, and oblique films to provide the best chance for diagnosis because false-negative cystograms may occur, especially with penetrating bladder injuries.

Due to the broad area of peritonealization of the infant's bladder, extraperitoneal bladder ruptures are more common, and small uncomplicated tears can be managed conservatively with suprapubic or urinary catheter drainage for 7 to 14 days. However, an associated pelvic fracture increases the chances of bladder penetration by a bony spicule and requires surgical exploration and repair.

Intraperitoneal bladder rupture requires surgical exploration, repair, debridement, and bladder drainage. In male infants, a suprapubic catheter is preferred for management in order to avoid complications associated with long-term transurethral catheter drainage.

Table 15-4. Indications for Cystogram in Pediatric Trauma Patients

Penetrating injury to lower abdomen and pelvis
Blunt lower abdominal or perineal trauma with significant microscopic hematuria (>20 RBCs/hpf), gross hematuria,[a] or blood at the meatus[a]
Significant pelvic fracture[a]
Unable to void[a] or little urine with urinary catheterization

[a]A retrograde urethrogram should be considered before attempting urethral catheterization in these instances.

Table 15-5. Findings With Bladder Injury

Cystogram Findings	Radiographic Finding
Bladder contusion	Teardrop shape or elevation of the bladder due to a perivesical hematoma without extravasation of contrast. Lateral deviation and obliteration of the soft tissue planes by pelvic hematoma may also be present.
Extraperitoneal bladder rupture	Postvoid films with significant rupture reveal a tyical "sunburst" pattern as the contrast extravasates outside the peritoneal cavity. However, there may only be small streaks of contrast with minor bladder ruptures.
Intraperitoneal bladder rupture	Extravasation into the peritoneal cavity around the bowel and intraabdominal organs and or in the pericolic gutters, giving a typical hourglass appearance.

Urethra

Pathophysiology

Urethral injuries predominantly occur from blunt trauma (80 percent motor vehicle accidents) and are less common in children due to a more flexible pelvis. Causes include pelvic fracture, straddle injuries, and urethral manipulation. This injury can result in strictures, incontinence, impotence, diverticulae, fistulas, and chordee. The urethra is divided into two sections by the urogenital diaphragm:

- The proximal (posterior) section extends from the neck of the bladder to the urogenital diaphragm.
- The distal (anterior) section extends from the urogenital diaphragm to the meatus.

In males, proximal urethral injuries occur when the bladder is pulled upward, shearing against the relatively fixed portions of the urethra at the urogenital diaphragm, the symphysis pubis, and the bladder neck. Partial or complete vesicourethral avulsion may occur. Female urethral injuries are extremely rare but can occur at the bladder neck and vesicourethrovaginal septum, resulting in urethrovaginal fistula or vaginal stricture. Ninety percent of proximal urethral injuries are associated with pelvic fractures. Symptoms include difficulty voiding; blood at the urethral meatus (90 percent); abdominal pain; instability of the pelvis indicating pelvic fracture; and, in males, a high-riding, floating, or boggy prostate.

Distal urethral injuries are less common and may result in urethral strictures. Direct blows, such as straddle injuries, cause the bulbous urethra to be forced against the symphysis pubis. In males, the injury may go unrecognized until the stricture develops long after the traumatic event is forgotten. In females, labial hematomas may result in urinary retention, which is amenable to catheter drainage. With significant straddle injury, examination under sedation or anesthesia is essential to assess the extent of urethral injury and possible vaginal involvement in females. Symptoms include difficulty voiding and discoloration and edema due to extravasation of blood or urine into the scrotum, perineum, and abdominal wall or along the shaft of the penis.

Management

Early urologic consultation is recommended. Although controversy remains as to the best long-term management, for the emergency physician it is most important to recognize the potential for urethral injury and to avoid iatrogenic complications. Care should be taken to avoid converting partial tears of the urethra into transections by injudicious attempts to pass urethral catheters. Indications for retrograde urethrogram before catheter placement are listed in Table 15-6. Extravasation of contrast media with some contrast also in the bladder indicates partial urethral tear. Extravasation alone indicates a complete transection. In the absence of extravasation, the urinary catheter should be advanced gently into the bladder and a cystogram performed to rule out bladder injury.

CT is not useful in the diagnosis or evaluation of urethral injuries although it is often performed for associated injuries and may occasionally reveal associated bladder or posterior urethral injuries.

Scrotal and Testicular Injuries

Pathophysiology

Injuries to the external male genitalia result from the testis being forced against the pubic ramus. Common

Table 15-6. Indications for Retrograde Urethrogram in Pediatric Trauma Patients

Penetrating injury to lower abdomen and pelvis suspected of involving the lower genitourinary tract
Blunt lower abdominal or perineal trauma with significant microscopic hematuria (>20 RBCs\hpf), gross hematuria, or blood at the meatus
Significant pelvic fracture
Inability to void
High-riding, floating, or boggy prostate in males
Discoloration or edema due to extravasation of blood or urine into the scrotum, perineum, or abdominal wall or along the shaft of the penis
Laceration of the vagina secondary to significant trauma

mechanisms of injury include straddle injury from a bicycle handlebar (particularly from BMX racing), seat, or center bar. Less common injuries include birth trauma, sports injuries, dog bites, and arthropod envenomations. Although genital trauma is relatively common, those requiring surgical intervention in childhood are relatively rare due to the mobility and small size of the testis. However, testicular or appendage torsions, testicular dislocation, epididymitis, hematocele, hematoma, pyocele, hydrocele, and rupture of the testicle all can occur after trauma and make the decision regarding surgical intervention difficult. Salvage of the testis or fertility is dependent on rapidly differenting testicular torsion, rupture, and dislocation from other nonsurgical injuries. Examination of the testis is often complicated by the presence of a hematoma or hematocele. In addition, edema, ecchymosis, and tenderness of the testis may be present with any of the common etiologies.

Management

Significant straddle injuries should be screened with a radiograph of the pelvis to rule out fracture of the pubic ramus. Testicular tissue is fragile and prone to rapid necrosis. Failure to diagnose testicular torsion or rupture can lead to atrophy, loss of spermatogenesis, and hormonal function, as well as psychological consequences. Obvious cases of testicular torsion, rupture, and dislocation require immediate urologic consultation and surgical exploration. Epididymitis, hematocele, hematoma, hydrocele, and testicular appendage torsions may be treated conservatively but may require surgical exploration to differentiate them from a more serious problem. Diagnostic tests, only if immediately available, should be used when the possibility of serious injury or torsion is less likely. A delay of 4 to 6 hours in obtaining diagnostic tests may result in the loss of the testis.

Therefore, urologic consultation should be obtained before ordering diagnostic tests to determine the feasibility and logistics of the evaluation.

Doppler ultrasound is usually readily available and is often used in the evaluation of scrotal or testicular trauma. It easily differentiates hematoceles and abscess from testicular rupture and testicular blood flow, reducing the likelihood of testicular torsion. Equivocal findings may require a ^{99m}technetium radionucleotide scan, but this test is less readily available and may inordinately delay the diagnosis. In choosing the best diagnostic method for scrotal trauma, the entire clinical setting and rapid availability of tests should be considered. Surgical exploration remains the most rapid and definitive method for evaluation of significant scrotal trauma, and other modalities should be reserved for less obvious cases.

Once testicular torsion, rupture, dislocation, and large expanding hematoma have been excluded, the patient may be discharged with urologic follow-up. The use of a scrotal support and cold packs may be beneficial.

Testicular or epididymal rupture results from direct trauma when the testis is forced against the pubic ramus, causing tearing of the inelastic tunica albuginea with extrusion of the seminiferous tissue. Rupture should be suspected when there is a recurrence of pain with delayed onset of scrotal swelling from several hours to 3 days after the injury. Complications include epididymo-orchitis characterized by localized redness, warmth, swelling, and fever. Although somewhat rare in children, testicular rupture is probably underdiagnosed and often confused with hematocele. Such confusion may result in initial nonoperative treatment with subsequent delayed exploration and frequently results in orchiectomy. Early surgical exploration should be performed with suspected testicular rupture.

Testicular dislocation occurs when the testis is forcibly displaced from the scrotum into the inguinal, acetabular, crural, perineal penile, or abdominal region or extruded from the scrotum through a laceration. Mechanisms for this injury are similar to those of other scrotal injuries and, although rare, dislocation should be considered when an empty hemiscrotum is present after trauma. Frequent symptoms include scrotal pain, nausea, and vomiting. Closed relocation of the testis may be possible, and a urologic consultation should be obtained along with diagnostic tests to evaluate the integrity of the testis.

Penile Injuries

Pathophysiology

Penile injuries occur from a variety of mechanisms, although complications of circumcision remain the most common. Other causes include direct blows (from toilet seats, falls, and sports injuries), zipper entrapment of the foreskin, and tourniquet injuries. The vast majority of these injuries are minor and can be treated conservatively. However, major trauma to the perineum may require fluid resuscitation, surgical intervention, and consideration of associated genitourinary trauma. Urinalysis should be performed with any significant penile injury.

Management

Superficial lacerations of the penis can be repaired similarly to any other laceration, but consideration for injury to deeper structures should be given if there is marked swelling, ecchymosis, or blood at the meatus.

Fracture of the penis occurs with rupture of the corpora cavernosa from a tear in the tunica albuginea, often resulting in a large subcutaneous hematoma. It most often occurs when the erect penis is forced against a solid object, such as the pubis, during sexual intercourse. The patient hears a "cracking" sound followed by pain, swelling, and deformity of the penis. Penile fractures can be treated conservatively unless there is severe penile deformity or urethral involvement. Urologic consultation is important to determine the best management in individual cases.

Zipper injuries to the foreskin occur when the zipper entraps the foreskin and retraction of the zipper is either impossible or too painful. Boys 3 to 6 years of age are most susceptible as they quickly zip up their pants after urinating. Treatment involves using bone cutters or a similar device to break the bridge of the sliding piece of the zipper, allowing it to fall apart and release the entrapped foreskin. Local anesthesia and sedation is usually not required.

Tourniquet injuries may be heralded by balanitis, paraphimosis, or cellulitis of the penis in an infant. This may occur when a band of hair surrounds the coronal groove and cuts into the shaft of the penis. The injury is usually localized, but may extend into the urethra and corpora. Removal of the band and treatment of infection is usually all that is required. Follow-up with urology is necessary if deeper injury is suspected.

Vulvar and Vaginal Injuries

Pathophysiology

Perineal trauma, in girls, often results from blunt trauma, such as straddle injuries. Stretching of the perineum from sudden abduction of the legs (doing the splits) can cause tears, and various penetrating injuries occur. Child abuse should be considered when the reported mechanism or history does not match the injuries. Typical injuries include vulvar hematomas; vaginal tears or lacerations; and urethral, rectal, or bladder injuries. Complications of perineal trauma include urinary retention, secondary infection, and urinary tract infection.

Management

Vulvar injuries are usually minor and can be treated with rest and cold packs. Significant straddle injuries should be screened with a pelvis radiograph to rule out fracture of the ramus. Large or expanding vulvar hematomas may require surgical drainage and are susceptible to secondary infection. The hematoma and edema can result in urinary retention and may require a urethrogram or cystoscopy to rule out urethral injury; a suprapubic catheter may be necessary. Minor linear abrasions of the vulva or vagina may result from masturbation and can become secondarily infected, requiring antibiotics.

Vaginal injuries usually result from penetration through the hymenal opening, although severe blunt injury to the pelvis may also cause damage. Most vaginal injuries are minor, but complete vaginal examination is warranted to exclude significant injury. Large lacerations can cause significant bleeding and even shock. Injury to adjacent organs is also possible including the bladder, urethra, ureters, peritoneum, or rectum and retroperitoneal hematoma.

Sexual abuse is estimated to occur in one of five girls during childhood. Abuse should be considered with all perineal injuries and the possibility of sexually transmitted disease recognized. The injuries seen with sexual abuse are usually minimal and the forensic aspect of these injuries is usually more important.

Rectal Trauma

Pathophysiology

Rectal injuries are very uncommon in childhood and are primarily caused by impalement. The injuries are often significant and lead to frequent surgical intervention for either diagnostic evaluation or repair of the injury. Lacerations can occur anywhere from the anal sphincter to well within the rectum. Lesions as far as 10 cm from the anal margin have been reported and may occur with minimal signs of external trauma. Concomitant vaginal injury may be present in females.

Management

Complete evaluation of rectal impalement is necessary, and few children will cooperate with anoscopy without sedation or general anesthesia. Therefore, with a history of impalement with or without significant signs of external trauma, a surgical consultation is warranted. In younger children, the history of impalement may be absent as they present with an acute abdomen or ileus and rectal perforation may only be discovered on laparoscopy.

Retroperitoneal Structures

Pathophysiology

Injuries to other retroperitoneal structures (kidneys, duodenum, pancreas, ureters, and bladder) are covered in separate sections above. The remaining structures consist of blood vessels that are rarely injured in blunt trauma except with rapid deceleration or severe physical abuse. Penetrating trauma is much more likely to cause significant vascular injury with or without other associated organ injury.

Upper retroperitoneal injury typically results in a retroperitoneal hematoma that is confined to the retroperitoneal space. However, the peritoneal membrane can be disrupted, causing massive intraperitoneal hemorrhage. Lower retroperitoneal injury is often associated with pelvic fracture and involves the iliac vessels, with venous injuries being more common than arterial.

Management

Injuries to the upper retroperitoneum are usually associated with multiple severe trauma that often takes precedence over these injuries. However, significant blood loss can result from retroperitoneal injury, resulting in hypotension and shock. The retroperitoneal structures are difficult to evaluate clinically due to their location, and therefore injuries to this area should be considered when hypovolemia cannot be otherwise explained. In the stable patient, CT shows these structures well and can help in determining the extent of the injury. Retroperitoneal injuries are often discovered on laparotomy performed for other more obvious injuries or in the patient requiring immediate intervention. With pelvic fractures, even in the absence of arterial injury, significant bleeding can occur, and attention to volume resuscitation is warranted.

SUMMARY

The approach to childhood GU trauma continues to evolve. Nevertheless, most blunt renal injuries in children are minor, with <10 percent requiring surgery except for high-grade injuries such as pedical or renal pelvis injuries. Since early surgery leads to nephrectomy >90 percent of the time, management that is more conservative is often employed unless there is hypotension with ongoing hemorrhage or urinary extravasation. Diagnostic testing is often useful in identifying GU injuries in children and is often a by-product of tests being done for other reasons in the evaluation of multisystem trauma. Hematuria is the hallmark for GU trauma, and obtaining urine for analysis is key to the evaluation even with minor trauma.

BIBLIOGRAPHY

Ahn JH, Morey AF, McAninch JW: Workup and management of traumatic hematuria. *Emerg Med Clin North Am* 16:145–164, 1962.

Advanced Pediatric Life Support Joint Task Force: Trauma, in Strange G (ed): *Advanced Pediatric Life Support: The Pediatric Emergency Medicine Course,* 3d ed. Dallas: American Academy of Pediatrics/American College of Emergency Physicians, 1998, pp 59–78.

Christopher NCD: Genitourinary tract trauma in the pediatric patient. *Emerg Med Rep* 5:113–120, 2000.

Fleisher G: Prospective evaluation of selective criteria for imaging among children with suspected blunt renal trauma. *Pediatr Emerg Care* 5:8, 1989.

Gausche M: Genitourinary trauma, in Barkin RM (ed): *Pediatric Emergency Medicine: Concepts in Clinical Practice,* 2d ed. St. Louis: Mosby-Yearbook, 1992, pp 355–370.

Rothrock SG, Green SM, Morgan R: Abdominal trauma in infants and children: Prompt identification and early management of serious and life-threatening injuries. Part I: Injury patterns and initial assessment. *Pediatr Emerg Care* 16:106–115, 2000.

Rothrock SG, Green SM, Morgan R: Abdominal trauma in infants and children: Prompt identification and early management of serious and life-threatening injuries. Part II: Specific injuries and ED management. *Pediatr Emerg Care* 16:189–195, 2000.

Schafermeyer RW: Pediatric trauma. *Emerg Med Clin North Am* 11:187, 1993.

16

Maxillofacial Trauma

Alan E. Jones
Stephen A. Colucciello

HIGH-YIELD FACTS

- Maxillofacial trauma in children more often results in soft tissue injury than facial fractures.
- Up to 55 percent of seriously injured children with facial trauma also have intracranial injury, a much higher percentage than occurs with adults.
- The most urgent complication of facial trauma is airway compromise, which is most often associated with mid or lower face injury.
- The CT scan has become the definitive diagnostic test for precise delineation of maxillofacial fractures.
- The mandible is the facial bone most frequently involved in posttraumatic developmental deformities.
- Timely referral of nasal fractures is of significant concern, as these injuries may have a profound effect on subsequent nasal and maxillofacial development.

Accurate bony alignment is important in the growing child, and missed fractures or inappropriate treatment may result in permanent facial deformity. A child with severe maxillofacial injury requires a team approach involving emergency physicians, pediatricians, general surgeons, maxillofacial specialists, and radiologists. Emergency specialists must recognize and prioritize injuries, manage the airway, stabilize the patient, read initial radiographs, and make appropriate consultations.

INCIDENCE

Children have a lower incidence of facial fractures compared with adults. Less than 5 percent of all facial fractures occur in children younger than 12 years , and <1

percent occur in children younger than 6 years. This lower incidence is multifactorial and includes the protected environment of childhood as well as anatomic differences between children and adults. Great structural differences exist between birth and 10 years of age, with marked changes in bone composition and anatomy. Large fat pads in young children cushion impact and lessen forces transmitted to the facial bones. These children have a high ratio of cancellous bone to cortical bone, which provides greater resilience and leads to a higher incidence of incomplete and greenstick fractures. This contrasts with the comminuted fracture pattern seen in adults.

Fracture site distribution tends to shift from the upper aspect of the face in younger children to the lower face in older children. In early childhood, the skull is particularly prominent, whereas the face and mandible are small. This results in a high incidence of skull fractures in the younger age group. Development of paranasal sinuses weakens the anterior facial skeleton. In one study, no LeForte fracture or unclassified maxillary sinus fracture occurred under 5 years of age, prior to pneumatization of paranasal sinuses. For this reason, in children under 5, orbital and frontal skull fractures predominate, whereas in older children, maxillary and mandibular fractures become more prominent. The highest incidence of facial fractures in children occurs between the ages of 8 and 10 years, and the most frequently fractured bones are the nose (45 percent), mandible (32 percent), orbit (17 percent), and zygoma/maxilla (5 percent). The most common facial fractures in injured children requiring hospitalization are mandibular fractures. By the early teen years, the frequency and pattern of maxillofacial injury begins to mirror that found in adults.

ETIOLOGY

Motor vehicle crashes, including auto/pedestrian incidents, are the most frequent cause of facial injury, followed by falls, sporting injuries, and gunshot wounds. Altercations and sports-related injuries are significant causes of facial fractures in older children, accounting for up to 36 percent of injuries. Maxillofacial injuries due to child abuse occur and have a high incidence of associated head and neck bruising. Skull fractures are particularly common in child abuse.

ASSOCIATED INJURIES

Children with serious maxillofacial fractures often have associated injuries, in particular skull fractures and

119

intracranial trauma. Up to 55 percent of seriously injured children with facial trauma may also have intracranial injury, a much higher percentage than occurs with adults. This is due to the high energy necessary to disrupt the pediatric facial skeleton. Temporal bone fractures occur, often in conjunction with mandibular fractures when force is transmitted along the mandible to the temporal bone. These temporal bone fractures are found most frequently in younger children. Periorbital fractures lead to intraocular injury in up to 10 percent of patients, mandating a careful ophthalmologic exam in these situations. Cervical spine fractures are rare in young children, but when present, usually occur in the upper three cervical vertebrae. In severe multiple trauma, the cervical spine should be evaluated with a three- or five-view series, and a careful neurologic examination is paramount.

EMERGENCY MANAGEMENT

The most urgent complication of facial trauma is airway compromise, which is most often associated with mid and lower face injury. Simple maneuvers, such as chin lift-jaw thrust and oropharyngeal suctioning, provide immediate benefit.

Infants under the age of 3 months are obligate nose breathers, and nasal or midface trauma can lead to complete airway obstruction. Mandibular fractures can result in loss of support of the tongue and occlusion of the upper airway. These fractures may also produce hematomas of the floor of the mouth, which can displace tongue and obstruct the airway. In this situation, the physician should open the mouth and pull the tongue forward, either manually or with a large suture or towel clip. In children for whom cervical spine injury is not a consideration or has been ruled out, the child should be allowed to sit up and lean forward. If simple airway maneuvers do not suffice, orotracheal intubation with in-line immobilization is necessary. Nasotracheal intubation should be avoided with midface trauma to prevent passage of the tube into the cranial vault. Nasotracheal intubation is also difficult in the young child, due to the presence of large adenoids. Uncontrolled bleeding into the pharynx may require intubation. If severe oropharyngeal bleeding persists, the pharynx must be packed with absorbent gauze to prevent aspiration when uncuffed endotracheal tubes are utilized.

If the child cannot be intubated, the physician must establish an airway surgically. Avoid emergency cricothyroidotomy in children younger than 12 years of age. In children below this age cricothyroidotomy causes numerous complications, including subglottic stenosis and tracheolaryngeal injury. Emergency tracheostomy results in fewer long-term complications, but is time consuming and requires great expertise. Percutaneous transtracheal jet ventilation is an excellent temporizing measure in these situations. Insert a needle into the cricothyroid membrane, and use oxygen at 50 psi (directly from the wall without a Christmas tree adaptor) with a 1:3 inspiration to expiration ratio.

Severe nasal hemorrhage may lead to aspiration and should be initially controlled by applying pressure to the external nares. If bleeding continues, nasopharyngeal packing should be considered. A Foley catheter is an effective emergency intervention. Insert the catheter along the floor of the nose, inflate the balloon in the nasopharynx, pull it anteriorly, and then place an anterior pack.

HISTORY

Obtain history regarding circumstances of injury from parents and prehospital care providers, as well as from the child, if possible. Determine mechanism and time of injury and assess for loss of consciousness. Question the child about any visual problems, facial anesthesia, or pain with jaw movement.

PHYSICAL EXAMINATION

Inspection of the face may reveal areas of swelling, ecchymosis, or deformity. In addition to face-to-face inspection, a view from the child's head looking down or from the chin looking up may reveal otherwise unappreciated asymmetries. Posttraumatic Bell's palsy provides evidence of a temporal bone fracture. Carefully palpate the entire face starting with the skull. Areas of bony deformity and crepitus will guide x-ray studies.

Eyes

The eyes must be evaluated for the presence of the pupillary light reflex. Hyphema, subconjunctival hemorrhage, and extraocular motions must be assessed. Subconjunctival hemorrhage is an important sign that often occurs in association with orbital, zygomatic, or maxillary fractures. Note the presence of proptosis or enophthalmos. Unequal pupil height may indicate orbital floor fracture. Lids must be retracted for adequate visualization of the globe, and visual acuity must be documented. Complete ocular examination is important in periorbital trauma because of the high incidence of globe injury (see Ch. 17).

Periorbital ecchymosis may occur in a wide variety of settings. Raccoon's eyes secondary to basal skull fracture usually occur 4 to 6 hours after a traumatic event, whereas direct trauma to the periorbital region may result in more immediate bruising. Bilateral periorbital ecchymosis also occurs in conjunction with LeFort II and III fractures.

Carefully palpate the *entire* orbital rim for tenderness or deformity. Many physicians neglect careful palpation of the superior orbital rim, concentrating instead on the inferior rim. Anesthesia above or below the eye may be secondary to supraorbital or infraorbital nerve injury and often occurs in conjunction with fractures.

Telecanthus, an increased width between the medial canthi of the eyelids, with flattening of the medial canthus, is associated with nasal ethmoidal injury. In this situation, the medial canthal ligaments are torn or underlying bone is avulsed from the nasal orbital complex. When telecanthus is present or there is tenderness over the medial orbital rim, a bimanual test for naso-ethmoidal-orbital stability can help detect a fracture. Insert a clamp into the nose, and press the tip intranasally against the medial orbital rim opposite the canthal ligament. Apply counter pressure with a palpating finger against the external surface of the canthal ligament. A fractured medial orbital rim will move between the clamp and index finger. Topical intranasal anesthesia may be necessary to do this maneuver in the awake patient.

Subcutaneous emphysema about the eyes and maxillary area indicates a communication with a sinus or nasal antrum and may erupt when the child blows his or her nose.

Ears

Examine the pinna for presence of subperichondral hematoma. The ear canal must be examined for lacerations and cerebrospinal fluid (CSF) leak. Battle sign, ecchymosis over the mastoid area, appears several hours after injury resulting in basilar skull fracture. The presence of hemotympanum should also raise suspicion for this injury. Tympanic membrane rupture may occur with mandibular condyle fractures.

Midface

Careful simultaneous palpation of the zygomatic arches is used to detect flattening of the arch. Intraoral palpation of the arch is also helpful in detecting minimally

displaced fractures. LeFort III fractures produce elongation of the midface. LeFort fractures may also be identified by manipulation of the central maxillary arch. Grasp the central maxillary arch above the central incisors and attempt to mobilize the midface. LeFort classification is based upon which structures move anteriorly with traction. Specific LeFort fractures are outlined in detail later in the chapter.

Nose

The examining physician must carefully palpate the nose for crepitus and deformity, as edema may obscure bony anatomy. Examine the inside of the nose for septal hematoma, which may be recognized by a bluish, bulging mass on the septum, or by the subjective impression of an abnormally wide septum. Pressure with a cotton swab will detect the presence of a soft, doughy swelling.

With any significant facial trauma, it is important to assess for CSF rhinorrhea. A drop of bloody nasal secretions on a sheet, towel, or tissue paper will form a double ring in the presence of CSF leak. This ring or halo sign, however, is not specific for CSF and may occur in the presence of normal nasal secretions.

Intraoral and Mandibular Examination

Injury of the inferior orbital nerve or inferior alveolar/mental nerve produces anesthesia of the upper or lower lip, respectively. Injury may be secondary to fracture of the bony canal or direct nerve contusion.

The emergency physician must observe movement of the patient's jaw through a full range of motion. Deviation to one side usually indicates ipsilateral subcondylar fracture, since dislocation of the jaw occurs infrequently in children. Difficulty in jaw movement may be secondary to mandibular fractures, injury to the temporomandibular joint, or a depressed zygoma impinging upon the mandible or muscles of mastication. Trismus and malocclusion also occur with such injuries.

It is important to palpate the condyles during jaw motion. This is easily done by placing the examining fingers in the external ear canal, and feeling the motion of the temporomandibular joint (TMJ) while the child opens and closes his or her mouth.

Children, unlike adults, may suffer traumatic diastasis of the hard palate along the midline. To detect this injury, the physician must apply a distracting pressure upon the dental arches. Grasp and manipulate each tooth to assess for laxity and remove teeth that are in danger of falling into the airway. Permanent teeth may be saved in saline moistened gauze. Stress the mandible with lateral and medial pressures on the dental arches, and subsequently apply up and down manual pressure to test for bony disruption. The cooperative child should be asked to bite down upon a tongue blade. Subsequent torque applied to the tongue blade will result in pain and reflex opening of the child's mouth in the presence of a mandibular fracture.

Facial Lacerations

Key to evaluating facial lacerations is an understanding of the relationship between the skin and the underlying vital structures. Injuries to the medial third of the upper or lower eyelids may result in lacrimal apparatus disruption. The course of the facial nerve and parotid duct must be kept in mind during examination. Facial nerve injury will result in paralysis on the ipsilateral side. Suspect laceration of the parotid duct if saliva enters the wound, or if blood is expressed at Stensen's duct. These signs may be elicited by massage of the parotid gland. Parotid duct injury is possible if a deep wound crosses a line drawn from the tragus to the midportion of the upper lip. The buccal branch of the facial nerve also parallels this line. Facial nerve injuries must be surgically repaired if they occur posterior to a vertical line drawn through the lateral canthus. Injuries anterior to such a line are usually not repaired.

RADIOGRAPHY

The choice of radiographic studies depends on the degree of injury and clinical stability of the child. Management of associated intracranial, thoracic, and abdominal injuries always takes precedence over imaging of the face. In the severely injured child, radiographs of the face, including computed tomography (CT) scans, may be deferred for several days, after life-threatening injuries have been addressed and the child's condition is stabilized. Multiple diagnostic modalities may be required.

Utilizing three radiographic views of the face (Waters, posteroanterior [PA], and lateral films) the vast majority of facial bone fractures can be detected. These plain films provide an excellent screening tool for maxillofacial trauma. The Waters view (occipital-mental) is the single most valuable radiologic study for the midface, as it demonstrates the continuity of the orbital rims. It may also demonstrate an air/fluid level in the maxillary sinus, which indicates blood secondary to maxillary fracture.

The PA (or Caldwell) view images the ethmoidal and frontal sinuses, as well as the naso-ethmoidal complex. A cross table or upright lateral view may demonstrate an air/blood level in the sphenoid or ethmoidal sinuses, thus providing a clue to occult fracture. Apart from these three basic views, additional studies may provide valuable information in particular settings.

The panoramic (Panorex) radiograph defines the total anatomy of the mandible, including the teeth, whereas the Towne's view images the condyles and ramus of the mandible. The submental vertex view (jug-handle or zygomatic arch view) demonstrates the zygomatic arches and the base of the skull.

Radiographs of the nose are of limited usefulness. They are difficult to read because of multiple suture lines and the large amount of cartilage in a young child. Nasal radiographs may be inaccurate, with many false-positives and -negatives. Surgical decisions are based more on cosmetic appearance and ability to breathe through the nose than on radiographic findings.

Computed Tomography

The CT scan has become the definitive diagnostic test for precise delineation of maxillofacial fractures. Some authorities recommend routine CT scanning for every case of significant facial trauma. CT further defines injuries seen on plain film, or it may be the initial imaging study of choice for patients with clinically obvious complex fractures. Specialized CT techniques, such as coronal views, thin slice scans (1.5 to 3 mm) and three-dimensional reconstruction assist in surgical planning for these complex injuries. CT is particularly helpful in the presence of orbital fractures and evaluates the status of orbital contents. In children with neurologic findings, a facial scan may be performed after the head scan, obviating the need for plain films of the face. It is a serious error to perform a CT scan of the face in a critically injured, unstable child. Treatment of serious, life-threatening injuries always takes precedence over facial imaging, and critical interventions must never be delayed for CT scans of the face.

To obtain a high-quality scan, children may require sedation and, in some cases, paralysis and intubation. Agents useful in sedation include narcotics, such as fentanyl; benzodiazepines, such as midazolam; barbiturates; sedative hypnotics, such as chloral hydrate; and combination agents. Short-acting, intravenously administered, reversible agents are the safest choice. Avoid ketamine in patients with head trauma, as it may raise intracranial pressure.

SPECIFIC INJURIES

Nasal Fractures

Nasal fractures are the most commonly encountered pediatric facial fracture, accounting for up to 45 percent of the total. Initial control of hemorrhage is obtained with external digital pressure. If nasal packing is used, care must be taken to ensure that packing is not placed intracranially. A particularly severe type of nasal fracture that occurs mostly in children is the "open book" type, where nasal bones separate in the midline along the suture.

Initially, nasal fractures may go undiagnosed secondary to edema and the difficulty in interpreting radiographs. Some physicians elect not to perform radiographs at all in cases of suspected nasal fracture and will make referrals based on physical examination and reports of difficulty breathing through the nose. If radiographs are deferred, the child should be rechecked in 3 to 4 days after swelling has subsided to reassess for deformity or septal deviation. This reexamination may be performed by the emergency specialist or the consultant. For optimal repair of displaced nasal fractures, consultation should take place within 5 to 6 days post injury, after which time fractures begin to unite and manipulation becomes increasingly difficult.

It is critical that emergency physicians recognize and treat septal hematomas. An untreated septal hematoma results in collapse of the septum and a "saddle" deformity of the nose. These hematomas may on rare occasion become infected and lead to septal perforation. Upon diagnosing a septal hematoma, the physician should use a #11 blade to make an L-shaped incision through the mucoperiosteum along the floor of the nose and extend the incision vertically. The hematoma will then be evacuated through the flap. Subsequent packing of the nasal antrum prevents reaccumulation, and the child must be referred to the appropriate specialist. Timely referral of nasal fractures is of significant medical and legal concern, as these injuries may have a profound effect on subsequent nasal and maxillofacial development.

Nasal-Ethmoidal-Orbital Fractures

Nasal-ethmoidal-orbital (NEO) fractures occur when the bony structures of the nose are driven backward into the intraorbital space. Fortunately, these injuries are rare in children. Telecanthus presents secondary to avulsion of one or both medial canthal ligaments. If this injury is suspected, perform the bimanual test for mobility as previously described. Radiographic evaluation should be with a CT scan of the face to include coronal views. Associated injuries include orbital and optic nerve problems, as well as lacrimal system disruption.

Orbital Fractures

The most common orbital fracture is the blowout fracture, which occurs when a blunt object, often a ball or fist, strikes the globe. The intraorbital pressures increase suddenly and contents decompress through the orbit, most commonly the floor. Blowout fractures can also occur through the medial wall, the roof, and even the greater wing of the sphenoid bone. This may lead to entrapment of the inferior ocular muscles, with subsequent diplopia on upward gaze. Evaluation for associated ocular injury such as hyphema, retinal contusion, lens dislocation, and corneal lacerations must be performed and visual acuity documented (see Chap. 17). The Waters view may reveal a soft tissue mass projecting into the sinus cavity, known as the *teardrop sign.* The *open bomb bay door sign* refers to depression of the bony fragments into the sinus. CT scans provide accurate visualization of blowout fractures.

Patients with NEO or orbital fractures should be instructed not to blow their nose. Because patients with subcutaneous emphysema have a fracture into a sinus or the nasal antrum, many practitioners use antibiotics to cover common sinus pathogens. Such prophylaxis, however, has not been conclusively proved to reduce complications. First-generation cephalosporins, trimethoprim/sulfamethoxazole, amoxicillin, or erythromycin are frequently utilized in outpatients. Urgent consultation is required in the presence of exophthalmus or extraocular muscle entrapment. In these situations, orbital contents must be surgically released and the area of blowout covered with implants or bone grafts. Many cases of posttraumatic diplopia associated with blowout fractures may be due to muscle or nerve injury and not true mechanical entrapment. CT evaluation and the forced duction test help distinguish these conditions.

Frontal Sinus and Supraorbital Fractures

Supraorbital fractures involve the superior orbital rim or orbital roof. Exophthalmus and ptosis may be present with impairment of upward gaze. The *superior orbital fissure syndrome* results in paralysis of extraocular muscles, ptosis, and anesthesia in the ophthalmic division of the trigeminal nerve. The *orbital apex syndrome* is a combination of the superior orbital fissure syndrome plus optic nerve damage and results in blindness. These syndromes represent surgical emergencies and require immediate consultation and decompression.

Linear nondisplaced fractures of the anterior wall of the frontal sinus may be treated with observation and antibiotics in either an inpatient or outpatient setting. If the posterior wall is involved, a CT scan will evaluate the possibility of depression and underlying brain injury. Posterior wall fractures should prompt neurosurgical as well as maxillofacial consultation.

Maxillary Fractures

Maxillary fractures are very uncommon in young children, but the incidence increases with age, as the paranasal sinuses develop. Because of the high degree of energy required to fracture the pediatric face, associated injuries, particularly intracranial, must be suspected.

Malar Fractures

The malar complex is often broken in a tripod fashion, with fractures at the infraorbital rim, across the zygomatic-frontal suture and along the zygomatic-temporal junction. Inward displacement of this fragment may result in impingement upon the mandible, giving rise to impaired mouth opening and trismus. The zygomatic arch itself is frequently fractured in isolation.

LeFort Fractures

Fractures to the midface are classified according to the LeFort system, based on the horizontal level of the fracture. LeFort I is a transverse fracture that separates the hard palate from the lower portion of the pterygoid plate and nasal septum. Traction on the upper incisors produces movement of only the hard palate and dental arch. LeFort II or pyramidal fracture separates the central maxilla and palate from the rest of the craniofacial skeleton. Mobilization of the upper incisors will move the central pyramid of the face, including the nose. LeFort III, also known as craniofacial dysjunction, separates the facial skeleton from the rest of the cranium. The entire face, including inferior and lateral portions of the orbital rim, move as a unit. "Pure" LeFort fractures are found more often in textbooks than in clinical practice. Fractures often do not fit the LeFort classification and demonstrate a mixed pattern—perhaps a LeFort II on one side and a LeFort III on the other. LeFort fractures may result in lengthening of the midface, occlusal abnormalities, and orbital ecchymosis and may be associated with

basilar skull fractures. CT scans are essential in their evaluation.

Children with LeFort fractures must be admitted and carefully assessed for associated injury. A maxillofacial specialist should be involved in their care.

Mandible Fractures

Mandible fractures are the second most common facial fracture, following nasal bone injury. Because of its U-shaped structure, fractures of the mandible are often multiple. Blows or falls to the chin result in symphyseal or perisymphyseal injury, whereas lateral blows are more likely to produce body or angle fractures on the injured or contralateral side. The most frequently injured areas are the condyle (70 percent), followed by the body, angle, and symphysis. Younger children suffer isolated condylar fractures and may present with deviation of the jaw to the affected side and trismus. Unlike the situation with adults, dislocation of the TMJ is very unusual in this age group. Physical examination is key in diagnosing these injuries, as radiographs may be nondiagnostic. Greenstick fractures, especially in the area of the condyles, are not well visualized on plain films. Because the Panorex view does not visualize the symphyseal area well, an occlusal view of the mandible is helpful in suspected symphyseal injury. The Towne's and lateral oblique views delineate the body and ramus.

The mandible is the facial bone most frequently involved in posttraumatic developmental deformities. Crush injuries to the condyle prior to the age of 5 years have the greatest potential for developmental arrest, whereas condylar fractures in later childhood may be self-correcting. Arrested development results in severe facial deformity, micrognathia, and ankylosis of the TMJ. Raise the possibility of subsequent growth disturbances with the parents—the younger the child, the more likely the complications.

Treatment of mandibular fractures is based on age, state of dentition, fracture location, bony integrity, and the presence of associated injuries.

Soft Tissue Injuries

Tissues that are clearly devitalized need *conservative* debridement. Emphasis must be placed on irrigation, foreign body removal, and cosmetic approximation of important landmarks such as the vermillion border of the lip and margins of the eyebrows. Eyebrows must not be shaved, as their regrowth is unpredictable. Hematomas of the pinna must be relieved, otherwise a chronic deformity of cauliflower deformity of the ear may result. Drain hematomas of the external ear by either needle aspiration or formal incision, and then apply a pressure dressing to prevent reaccumulation.

Repair of lacerations to the salivary duct or to the lacrymal drainage system must be performed by a specialist. These repairs are achieved over a stent.

Despite the possibility of brisk bleeding, never blindly clamp inside a facial laceration due to the risk of injury to nerves or parotid duct. Direct pressure will control bleeding. Children may require sedation to ensure cooperation in the treatment of either complex or intraoral lacerations. Control of the tongue is necessary in glossal injury, and a large stitch placed in the tip of the tongue will retract it during suturing.

Penetrating wounds to the posterior pharynx occur when a child falls while carrying a pencil or foreign body in his or her mouth. Such wounds endanger carotid artery, jugular vein, and cranial nerves. Sophisticated studies, such as color flow Doppler, angiography, or magnetic resonance imaging may be indicated after specialist consultation.

PAIN MANAGEMENT AND ANESTHESIA

Acute maxillofacial trauma produces injuries that are often extremely painful due to the presence of high numbers of nociceptive neurons in surrounding structures. Repair is frequently difficult in the uncooperative child and often requires the use of local and systemic analgesics, either alone or in combination.

Local anesthesia is the primary method of achieving immediate pain control. Nerve blocks rely on the deposition of anesthetic solutions in areas of nerve trucks and are an especially helpful technique. The most useful maxillofacial nerve blocks in acute injury are mental, inferior alveolar, infraorbital, and supraorbital. These procedures require patient cooperation, and in the uncooperative child local wound infiltration becomes the procedure of choice.

Systemic analgesia, either enteral or parenteral, is often necessary for adequate pain control in the acute setting. Dose-appropriate use of nonsteroidal antiinflammatory agents, opioids, or a combination of the two will be required for pain relief. In cases of lengthy repairs or uncooperative patients, implementation of conscious sedation may be necessary for adequate patient and physician comfort and safety. Both early and adequate analgesia will significantly aid the clinician in the immediate management of the suffering child.

CONCLUSIONS

Maxillofacial trauma in children more often results in soft tissue injury than facial fractures. When fractures do occur, associated injuries, particularly intracranial, may be present. Fractures heal rapidly over 2 to 3 weeks, and repair must be undertaken before bony union occurs. Conservative management is often the rule.

Late reduction of a fracture may result in unsatisfactory cosmesis secondary to arrested growth and distorted dentition. Aggressive airway management, assiduous search for associated injuries, and early consultation are the keys to successful emergency management of pediatric facial trauma.

BIBLIOGRAPHY

Antonyshyn O: Principles in management of facial injuries, in Georgiade GS, Riefkohl R, Levin LS (eds): *Plastic, Maxillofacial, and Reconstructive Surgery.* Baltimore: Williams & Wilkins, 1997.

Chase DC: Maxillofacial injuries, in Buntain WL (ed): *Management of Pediatric Trauma.* Philadelphia: WB Saunders, 1995, pp 200–218.

Dodson TB, Kaban LB: Special considerations for the pediatric emergency patient. *Emerg Med Clin North Am* 18:539–547, 2000.

Druelinger L, Guenther M, Marchand EG: Radiographic evaluation of the facial complex. *Emerg Med Clin North Am* 18:393–410, 2000.

Ellis E, Scott K: Assessment of patients with facial fractures. *Emerg Med Clin North Am* 18:411–448, 2000.

Koltai PJ, Rabkin D: Management of facial trauma in children. *Pediatr Clin North Am* 43:1253–1275, 1996.

LeFort R: Etude experimentale sur les fractures de le machoire superieure. *Rev Chir* 23:208,360,479, 1901.

Rhea JT, Rao PM, Novelline RA: Helical CT and three-dimensional CT of facial and orbital injury. *Radiol Clin North Am* 37:489–513, 1999.

Schultz RC: Facial fractures in children and adolescents, in Cohen M (ed): *Mastery of Plastic and Reconstructive Surgery.* Boston: Little, Brown, 1995, pp 1188–1198.

Yagiela JA: Anesthesia and pain management. *Emerg Med Clin North Am* 18:449–470, 2000.

17

Eye Trauma

D. Mark Courtney
Stephen A. Colucciello

HIGH-YIELD FACTS

- A history of exposure to power tools or metal striking metal should raise the suspicion of an intraocular foreign body.

- Children with sickle cell disease or coagulopathy are more likely to suffer complications associated with a hyphema.

- Visual acuity is the vital sign of the eye and should be documented in every child with an ocular injury or visual complaint.

- Be concerned about the appearance of a corneal abrasion in the absence of known trauma as this may represent herpetic dendrites rather than corneal abrasions.

- Obtain an ophthalmology consultation in the emergency department on all patients with hyphemas.

- A caustic injury to the eye (acid or alkali) is one of the few situations in which treatment must occur prior to examination and visual acuity testing. Copious irrigation with normal saline takes precedence over all but life-saving interventions and should begin at the time and site of exposure.

Ocular trauma is the leading cause of noncongenital blindness in individuals younger than 20 years of age. Every year in the United States over 150,000 children injure an eye. Recreational and sports injuries are more prevalent in the pediatric population than they are in adults. In addition, ocular trauma may occur as a consequence of child abuse.

In preschool children, most injuries are due to falls, motor vehicle collisions, and accidental blows to the eye. Between 5 and 15 years of age ocular trauma occurs twice as often in males. This is also the age group in which sports-related injuries become an important factor, especially baseball, ice hockey, racquet sports, soccer, archery, and fishing injuries. Fireworks and the notorious BB gun remain significant causes of pediatric eye injury.

Children who sustain visual loss prior to age 7 may develop deprivational amblyopia.

HISTORY

Obtain a full history and note any preexisting eye abnormality and whether or not the child normally wears glasses. A history of exposure to power tools or metal striking metal should raise the suspicion of an intraocular foreign body. Inquire as to whether the child is having double vision. If so, determine whether the diplopia is monocular or binocular. Monocular double vision implies a problem with the lens or retina, whereas double vision that occurs only with both eyes open is associated with periorbital fractures or extraocular muscle injury.

Past medical history is also important. Children with sickle cell disease or coagulopathy are more likely to suffer complications associated with a hyphema.

PHYSICAL EXAMINATION

The physical examination of the eye should be performed early in the emergency department (ED) course, after any life-threatening injuries have been excluded or addressed. Progressive lid edema can prevent an adequate examination of the eye.

Visual Acuity

Visual acuity is the vital sign of the eye and should be documented in every child with an ocular injury or visual complaint. In trauma, the best predictor of ultimate visual outcome is initial visual acuity. Assessment should be done *before* intervention—except in the case of major trauma or caustic exposure. Topical anesthetic may be given before testing visual acuity to decrease pain and blepharospasm.

If the child wears glasses, measure acuity with the glasses on. If the glasses have been lost or damaged, correct refractive error by having the child look through a pinhole in a piece of paper. Lack of correction with pinhole testing suggests pathology in the retina or optic nerve.

Evaluate preliterate children with an Allen or "E" chart and move a toy or a light to test the young child's ability to track with each eye. If the child is unable to read an eye chart, ask him or her to finger count at 3 feet; if that fails, due to visual loss, assess for light perception.

Test visual fields in older children in the usual fashion. Younger children will glance toward a toy brought into the field of view. Do not forget to grossly inspect the eyes and assess extraocular movement in a rush for the slit lamp examination.

Adnexae

To avoid missing subtle signs of trauma, begin the examination with the lids and periorbital structures and work centrally in a focused fashion. Examine the lids for swelling or penetrating injury and inspect for ecchymosis. Retract swollen lids with a finger in most cases, but lid retractors or bent paper clips can be used in the case of massive lid edema. Periorbital soft tissue air indicates fracture into a sinus or nasal antrum and is most commonly seen with a blowout fracture. Examine the eye for normal lacrimal drainage. *Epiphora,* tears spilling over the lid margins, may be secondary to injury of the canalicular system.

Conjunctiva and Sclera

Examine the conjunctiva for injection and presence of ciliary flush around the iris (perilimbal injection). Check for chemosis (edema of the conjunctiva), which can be seen in globe rupture. Look at the sclera carefully for any disruption or penetration. The location of any subconjunctival hemorrhage should be documented.

Pupils, Iris, Lens, and Anterior Chamber

Evaluate the pupils for any asymmetry or irregularity. Congenital anisocoria may be detected by obtaining history from the parents. Pupillary dilatation may occur with direct blows to the eye (posttraumatic mydriasis), with anticholinergic medication, or with a third nerve palsy. A blown pupil in a conscious patient is not due to a herniation syndrome. Pilocarpine drops will constrict a pupil that is dilated secondary to a third nerve lesion but will have no effect on pharmacologic mydriasis. The emergency physician should also never overlook the possibility of a glass eye. The ED staff does not soon forget such an oversight.

The lens should be transparent and the margins should not be visible. Examine the anterior chamber for abnormal shallowness or depth. To specifically assess optic nerve function, perform the swinging flashlight test. Swing the flashlight from eye to eye. A pupil that ini-

tially dilates when illuminated by light has a sensory (afferent) defect (Marcus Gunn pupil).

Fundoscopic Exam and Intraocular Pressure

The vitreous should be clear, allowing visualization of the retina. However, visualization of the retina does not completely exclude retinal detachment, as many cases are anterior and thus undetectable with a direct ophthalmoscope. Do not measure intraocular pressure if globe rupture or penetrating injury is apparent, as this may herniate ocular contents. Normal intraocular pressure is between 15 and 20 mm Hg.

EQUIPMENT

The basic equipment for a standard pediatric eye exam includes the following:

- Visual acuity charts (Snellen and Allen "E" chart)
- Pen light
- Ophthalmoscope
- Wood's lamp
- Slit lamp
- Ocular spud
- Fluorescein strips
- Shiotz tonometer or Tono-Pen
- Morgan lens
- Metal eye shields

MEDICATIONS

Topical anesthetics, such as 0.5% tetracaine or proparacaine, have an onset of action within 1 minute and typically last for 15 to 20 minutes. Topical anesthetics should never be prescribed for home use, as prolonged lack of sensation and loss of normal protective reflexes may lead to corneal damage. Cycloplegics such as homatropine (2 to 5 percent) and cyclopentolate hydrochloride (1 to 2 percent) dilate the eye and decrease pain by overcoming ciliary spasm. Always document the use of such medications. Avoid atropine due to its extremely long duration of action.

Steroids are useful in some inflammatory conditions but may lead to glaucoma, cataract formation, and acceleration of fungal and herpetic infections, resulting in visual loss. Never use ocular steroids without first consulting an ophthalmologist. Evaluate the need for tetanus prophylaxis in all patients with ocular injuries. To administer medications to young or uncooperative children, lay them down, secure the head, and place the drop in the medial canthus. Eventually the child will open the eyes and the medication will reach the conjunctiva.

SPECIFIC INJURIES

Lid Lacerations

Minor lacerations, superficial to the tarsal plate, that do not involve the lid margins and that are associated with no suggestion of injury to deeper structures may be repaired by the emergency physician. Other lacerations require specialty repair.

Consider the possibility of globe penetration or injury to deeper structures whenever an eyelid is lacerated. Because eyelids have no subcutaneous fat, the appearance of fat in a wound suggests underlying globe injury. Lacerations involving the medial third of the upper or lower lids are high risk as they may involve the lacrimal system. One way to detect injury of the lacrimal system is to instill fluorescein in the eye and then use a Wood's lamp to check the wound for fluorescence.

Injuries to the lid margins are also problematic as they may result in deformity of the lids and abnormal lid movement if repair is not precise. If the levator palpebrae muscle is injured and not repaired, posttraumatic ptosis will result. Trauma involving the tarsal plate (which only exists in the upper lid as a dense band of fibrous tissue) indicates a complex laceration. Plastic surgery or ophthalmologic consultation should be obtained for repair of any of these lacerations described above.

Subconjunctival Hemorrhage

The most important aspect of the evaluation of subconjunctival hemorrhage is to rule out other, more serious injury. With significant blunt trauma, a subconjunctival hemorrhage may hide a scleral rupture. Clues to such a severe globe injury include decreased visual acuity, severe pain, photophobia, and extension of hemorrhage beyond the limbus. Consider the possibility of a periorbital fracture in patients with traumatic subconjunctival hemorrhage. Lateral hemorrhages in particular are frequently associated with zygomatic fractures (tripod fractures).

In the more common instances of minor trauma or Valsalva maneuvers, with no evidence of severe globe injury, parents should be reassured, told that spontaneous resolution will occur over 2 weeks, and informed of the dramatic color changes that may occur.

Corneal Abrasion

Children with corneal abrasions complain of a foreign body sensation, pain, and photophobia and present with marked blepharospasm and a red eye. Infants may present with only crying. Use tetracaine or proparacaine prior to examination to decrease blepharospasm and pain.

A few drops of fluorescein placed in the conjunctival sac followed by examination under a Wood's lamp or the cobalt blue light of a slit lamp will result in marked fluorescence of corneal abrasions. Make sure that no foreign body is present and that there is no evidence of penetration of the sclera. Multiple vertical striations (ice-rink sign) usually indicate a retained foreign body under the upper lid. Careful examination with lid eversion should reveal the offending agent.

Be concerned about the appearance of a corneal abrasion in the absence of known trauma. This may represent herpetic dendrites rather than corneal abrasions. If this finding is present, test to see whether the corneal reflex is equally brisk in each eye by gently touching the cornea with a wisp of cotton (either before topical anesthesia or after the anesthesia has worn off). Herpetic lesions may decrease the corneal reflex in the involved eye. Patients may have concurrent oral or genital herpes. In the case of herpes keratitis, ophthalmologic consultation is required.

Treat corneal abrasions with ophthalmic antibiotics to prevent secondary infection. The multiple layers of the cornea normally provide a barrier against infection from common organisms such as *Pseudomonas* sp. and *Staphylococcus aureus,* and injury to this barrier may lead to secondary infection. One drop of antibiotic solution applied every 4 to 6 hours for 4 days is sufficient. Ointment in young children and infants can be given at the same frequency by applying a 1-cm length inside the lower eyelid. Several drops of a mydriatic agent such as cyclopentolate 1 percent or homatropine 5 percent applied 2 to 3 times a day for 1 to 2 days will decrease ciliary spasm and provide comfort.

Eye patching is no longer recommended for corneal abrasion. It has not been shown to speed healing or decrease pain, and it may increase infection risk if prophylactic antibiotics are not given due to the patch. The exception to this is corneal abrasion associated with Bell's palsy and incomplete lid closure. Any patch should be rechecked and removed in 24 hours. Some centers suggest that all abrasions should be rechecked in 24 to 48 hours to assess healing. Others tell patients to return if they are still symptomatic after 48 hours. Symptoms and redness should gradually decrease each day. If not, secondary infection, retained foreign body, or corneal erosion should be suspected.

Traumatic Iritis

Patients with posttraumatic iritis usually present 1 to 2 days after blunt trauma to the eye, complaining of photophobia, pain, and tearing. They often have marked blepharospasm and perilimbal injection (ciliary flush). Test for pain on accommodation by having patients first look across the room at a distant object and then quickly focus on the examiner's finger held several inches away. If near gaze causes pain, there is a high probability of iritis. The pupil may be large or small. Posttraumatic miosis develops secondary to spasm of the pupillary sphincter muscle, whereas posttraumatic mydriasis results when sphincter fibers are ruptured. Slit lamp examination will usually reveal cells in the anterior chamber, the hallmark of iritis.

Treat with a long-acting topical cycloplegic, such as 5 percent homatropine, 4 times a day for 1 week, oral antiinflammatory medication, and dark sunglasses to decrease pain. Symptoms may persist for up to 1 week. Although ocular steroids decrease inflammation, prescribe them only after consultation with the ophthalmologist who will see the patient in follow-up.

Hyphema

A hyphema is defined by blood in the anterior chamber. Hyphemas are almost always secondary to blunt trauma. The blood may layer out or may present initially as a diffuse red haze that takes hours to settle. Hyphemas are described by the percentage of the anterior chamber that is filled with blood. A 100 percent hyphema, known as an "eight ball," may cause complete loss of light perception. Hyphemas are easily overlooked in cases of massive lid edema, and for this reason, early lid retraction is necessary for the diagnosis. Older children with hyphemas usually complain of pain, whereas young children may present with somnolence. However, decreased mental status should not be attributed to the hyphema until intracranial injury has been ruled out. Other injuries associated with hyphema include lens dislocation, vitreous hemorrhage, and retinal damage. A large untreated hyphema may result in permanent corneal staining with subsequent loss of visual acuity and deprivational amblyopia. Often it is not the initial hyphema that causes serious morbidity but the rebleed that can occur in several days as the clot breaks down. Rebleeding occurs in up to 16 to 25 percent of patients and may obstruct the aqueous outflow system, causing increased intraocular pressure. Patients with rebleeding have a significantly worse prognosis. Because hemoglobinopathies, particularly sickle cell disease, sickle cell trait, and sickle thalassemia, predispose to rebleeding and other complications, it is critical to determine whether any of these conditions exist in the child with hyphema.

Initial treatment involves bed rest with the head elevated 30 degrees. Shield the involved eye, taking care not to touch or apply pressure to the eye. Obtain an ophthalmology consultation in the ED on all patients with hyphemas.

The subsequent treatment of hyphemas is controversial. Traditionally, all patients have been admitted and placed on strict bed rest. However, older children and reliable adults are now being treated with bed rest at home if they have only a microhyphema (circulation of red blood cells only, with no layering) and daily reexamination for 5 days is possible. Some specialists utilize antifibrinolytics such as aminocaproic acid to reduce rebleeding. The decision as to use of mydriatics, ocular steroids, osmotic agents, or acetazolamide should be left to the ophthalmologist. Acetazolamide or osmotic agents are contraindicated in patients with sickle cell disease due to increased risk of bleeding. Patients should avoid aspirin or other platelet-active medications, as these increase the risk of rebleeding.

Lens Injury

Blunt ocular trauma may result in lens subluxation or dislocation. Subluxation may cause monocular diplopia, whereas dislocation results in profoundly blurred vision. The lens may sublux either posteriorly or anteriorly, resulting in a deep or shallow anterior chamber and a visible lens margin. *Iridodonesis* is a shimmering or shaking of the iris provoked by rapidly changing gaze and is associated with posterior dislocation.

Acute blunt trauma to the eye can cause a cataract if the capsule of the lens is disrupted. The lens subsequently absorbs fluid, taking on a cloudy appearance. Lens injuries should be referred to an ophthalmologist.

Retinal Injury

Retinal trauma often occurs in conjunction with other eye injuries. Older children with retinal injury complain of light flashes or a "curtain" over the visual field. Central vision will be spared if the macula remains unaffected.

Fundoscopy may reveal a variety of hemorrhage patterns. Preretinal hemorrhages are boat shaped, with a horizontal "deck," whereas superficial hemorrhages are flame shaped. Deep hemorrhages are round, with a purple-gray color. The shaken baby syndrome causes linear retinal hemorrhages and associated exudates. Any suspicion of retinal detachment or injury requires ophthalmology consultation.

Retrobulbar Hemorrhage

Bleeding behind the globe may result in deficits in extraocular motion and lead to proptosis or bulging of the eye. Subsequent compromise of the optic nerve produces an afferent pupillary defect (Marcus Gunn pupil). In cases of severe proptosis, progressively worsening vision, and potential optic nerve injury, surgical decompression may be necessary. In rare instances, a lid release procedure (lateral canthotomy) may be required in the ED.

Conjunctival and Scleral Lacerations

Perform a slit lamp examination on all children with conjunctival lacerations to assess for deeper scleral violation. Scleral rupture from blunt trauma often occurs at the insertions of the intraocular muscles or at the limbus. Clues to the presence of scleral disruption include decreased visual acuity, an abnormal anterior chamber, low intraocular pressure (<6), and a positive *Sidle* test. To perform the Sidle test for scleral laceration, place fluorescein on the cornea and observe the suspicious area under the cobalt blue light of the slit lamp. A swirling dilution of fluorescein secondary to leaking aqueous denotes scleral disruption. If a scleral laceration is seen, tonometry is contraindicated. The additional pressure against the eye from the tonometer can extrude the iris.

Treat small conjunctival lacerations with topical antibiotic drops alone. Sutures are not usually necessary. If the patient has deeper injury (i.e., scleral laceration), place an eye shield on the child, administer intravenous antibiotics, provide adequate sedation, and obtain an ophthalmology consultation.

Corneal and Scleral Foreign Bodies

Patients with a superficial foreign body are in pain. Their eye is usually red and tearing, and verbal children will complain of "something in my eye." Corneal abrasions, however, will present in a similar mode.

Perform a thorough examination in all patients by doubly everting the lids after anesthetizing the cornea. This may be done with a cotton swab placed on the middle of the upper lid and folding the lid upward over the swab. Look carefully for a foreign body on the inner surface of the lids. Attempt removal with a cotton applicator soaked in topical anesthetic. In older cooperative children, remove more tenacious foreign bodies under slit lamp guidance using an eye spud or 25-gauge needle on a tuberculin syringe. A foreign body sensation may persist even after removal due to an underlying corneal abrasion. Iron-containing foreign bodies may leave rust rings that may result in photophobia and decreased visual acuity. Some emergency physicians refer these to a specialist, whereas others use an ophthalmic burr to remove superficial rings.

After removing a foreign body, check for additional foreign bodies and abrasions. Instill both a mydriatic agent and a topical antibiotic and recheck the child in 24 hours. Prescribe appropriate analgesia including narcotic agents if appropriate. If a foreign body penetrates the corneal stroma or the sclera, consult an ophthalmologist for evaluation in the ED.

Intraocular Foreign Body

Intraocular foreign bodies are vision-threatening injuries that may be easily overlooked. The key to identification of an intraocular foreign body is to consider it. Ask specific questions about risk factors. Exposure to power tools and metal striking metal, such as a hammer on a nail, predisposes to occult intraocular foreign body.

Certain foreign bodies place the patient at greater risk than others. Iron (siderosis) and copper (chalcosis) are particularly toxic to the eye, whereas glass and plastic are less inflammatory. Organic foreign bodies pose a high risk for intraocular infection.

Children with intraocular foreign bodies may have decreased visual acuity, pupillary distortion, and relatively little pain. A foreign body penetration through the cornea may damage the iris, causing a teardrop-shaped pupil that will "point" to the perforation site.

A number of imaging modalities can detect intraocular foreign bodies. Although larger metallic objects may be seen by routine radiography, a computed tomography scan of the orbit provides greater resolution if the foreign body is small. Ocular ultrasound is highly sensitive for both metallic and nonmetallic penetrations. Magnetic resonance imaging (MRI) accurately detects organic, plastic, and glass particles but may cause further injury if mistakenly used in the case of metal objects. In such cases, the MRI magnet may move the foreign body, causing greater damage.

Cover the involved eye with a metal eye shield and keep the child at rest. Administer broad-spectrum intravenous antibiotics, usually a first-generation cephalosporin and an aminoglycoside.

Topical antibiotics are not indicated with penetrating globe injuries and, in particular, antibiotic ointments should be avoided as they can produce intraocular granulomas and obscure examination.

Should a child with penetrating globe injury require emergency intubation, some authorities suggest a nondepolarizing blocker, such as rocuronium, in place of succinylcholine. Succinylcholine and ketamine may increase intraocular pressure and could theoretically extrude intraocular contents. However, use of succinylcholine has occurred in penetrating eye injury, and association with additional eye damage has not been reported.

Foreign Bodies In Situ

Foreign bodies that protrude from the eye, such as a nail or wire, must be left in place and removed in the operating room. At all costs, resist the urge to "yank it out."

Chemical Injuries to the Eye

A caustic injury to the eye (acid or alkali) is one of the few situations in which treatment must occur prior to examination and visual acuity testing. Copious irrigation with normal saline takes precedence over all but lifesaving interventions and should begin at the time and site of exposure. Extent of caustic injury is dependent on the quantity, the pH, and the duration of the exposure (i.e., time to irrigation). Alkali injuries result in the most serious damage to the eye by causing liquefaction necrosis with saponification of ocular tissues and deep penetration. Acids produce a coagulation necrosis resulting in a protein barrier that blocks further penetration. Complications of caustic injuries include blindness, perforation, corneal neovascularization, secondary glaucoma, cataract formation, and retinal damage.

Begin irrigation in the prehospital setting immediately after injury. Upon arrival at the ED, the child may require sedation with a rapidly acting intramuscular or intravenous agent to allow irrigation of the eye, but topical anesthesia alone may be adequate. If particulate matter remains in the eye, pour liter bottles of irrigant into the eye while retracting the lids to wash the particles out. Perform double lid eversion to expose the fornices and irrigate or swab out any caustic particulate matter. When irrigating the eyes, a Morgan lens (a contact lens connected to intravenous tubing) is useful. An alternative to the Morgan lens is a nasal oxygen cannula placed on the bridge of the nose, which can be connected to intravenous bags of normal saline. This allows bilateral irrigation of the eyes through the nasal prongs.

Never attempt to neutralize acids with alkalis or vice versa, as the resultant heat release will further damage the eye. Lavage the eyes for at least 20 minutes, ideally with 2 L of normal saline. Irrigation may be beneficial for up to 24 hours after alkali exposure. In cases of bad alkali exposure, continuously irrigate the eyes until stopped by the ophthalmologist. Use litmus paper to check the pH in the conjunctival sac after 20 minutes of irrigation, and continue irrigation until the pH is between 7.4 and 7.6. If irrigation is stopped, recheck the pH after 10 minutes to ensure a stable level.

Hydrofluoric acid exposure is a unique situation and may require irrigation with a magnesium oxide solution. Consult a poison center for the latest recommendations.

Ultraviolet Keratitis

Ultraviolet keratitis occurs when children are exposed to prolonged glare from snow or when they stare at an eclipse. Unprotected vision of an eclipse can also cause severe retinal damage and blindness. Older children who watch a welder's torch or use tanning booths without special glasses may also suffer this injury. Photophobia and eye pain usually occur 8 to 12 hours after exposure and, for this reason, patients with ultraviolet keratitis generally present at night. They exhibit both scleral and perilimbal injection accompanied by tearing and blepharospasm. Slit lamp exam using fluorescein shows thousands of punctate, shallow lesions on the cornea (keratitis), which looks as if it had been sandblasted. Treat with cycloplegia and oral analgesia. Ultraviolet keratitis is usually bilateral and generally heals in 24 to 48 hours.

Thermal Burns

Because of reflex blinking, lids are more often damaged from thermal injury than is the globe. Eyelashes and eyebrows are often burned. Evaluate for corneal injury with the slit lamp in the usual fashion with and without fluorescein staining, and apply topical antibiotics to burned lids. Third-degree burns to the eye and periorbital tissues require admission.

CONCLUSIONS

The emergency physician is often the first and many times the only physician to evaluate ocular trauma. Proper identification depends primarily on the consideration of the potential for injury, and on the performance of a thorough, systematic examination. Unfortunate sequelae can often be avoided through timely identification and appropriate specialty consultation. Any eye injury regardless of acuity should be considered an opportunity for physicians to inform parents and patients about protective eyewear and risk reduction behavior.

BIBLIOGRAPHY

Brunette DD, Ghezzi K, Renner GS: Ophthalmologic disorders, in Rosen P, Barkin R (eds): *Emergency Medicine: Concepts and Clinical Practice*. St. Louis: CV Mosby, 1998, pp 2698–2719.

Ferrari LR: The injured eye. *Anesth Clin North Am* 14:125–150, 1996.

Marshall DH, Brownstein S, Addison DJ, et al: Air guns: The main cause of enucleation secondary to trauma in children and young adults in the greater Ottawa area in 1974–93. *Can J Ophthalmol* 30:187–192, 1995.

Napier SM, Baker RS, Sanford DG, et al: Eye injuries in athletics and recreation. *Surv Ophthalmol* 41:229–244, 1996.

Rubin SE, Catalano RA: Ocular trauma and its prevention, in Nelson LB (ed): *Harley's Pediatric Ophthalmology*. Philadelphia, W. B. Saunders; 1998, pp 482–498.

Smith GA, Knapp JF, Barnett TM, et al: The rockets' red glare, the bombs bursting in air: Fireworks-related injuries to children. *Pediatrics* 98:1–9, 1996.

Tingley DH: Consultation with the specialist: Eye trauma: Corneal abrasions. *Pediatr Rev* 20:320–322, 1999.

18

Orthopedic Injuries

Valerie A. Dobiesz
Russell H. Greenfield

HIGH-YIELD FACTS

- Pediatric patients have unique patterns of injuries and fractures due to the immaturity of bone and the dynamic nature of skeletal growth. Fractures account for 10 to 15 percent of all childhood injuries.

- Fractures are more common than ligamentous injuries or sprains in children due to the relative weakness of the physis or growth plate.

- Injuries to the physis may lead to long-term growth abnormalities or growth arrest. Injuries to the physis occur in up to 18 percent of all pediatric fractures.

- Radiographs are more difficult to interpret and findings can be much more subtle in children than adults, as the physis is radiolucent and there are secondary ossification centers. Comparison views of the uninjured extremity can be helpful.

- The majority (75 percent) of physeal fractures are Salter II fractures, and most of these are found after the age of 10 years.

- Up to 50 percent of fractures in children younger than 1 year are the result of nonaccidental trauma.

Trauma to the immature skeleton often results in unique patterns of skeletal injuries. Diagnosis of skeletal injuries in children is difficult because associated physical findings may be subtle, and the confusing nature of pediatric bone x-rays can render interpretation difficult. However, only by making an accurate diagnosis and providing appropriate emergency care can complications be avoided. An understanding of the unique characteristics of growing bone provides the background necessary to anticipate and treat specific childhood orthopedic injuries.

THE PEDIATRIC SKELETON

Growing bone is less dense and more malleable than mature bone due to fewer lamellar components and greater porosity. Children's bones are thus able to absorb more energy and withstand greater force before breaking. When a fracture does occur, propagation of the fracture line is diminished, making comminution less likely. These properties account for injuries that are unique to children, such as incomplete (greenstick) and torus or buckle fractures, as well as plastic deformation or bowing injuries, in which bending of the bone occurs without fracture.

Children's bones are in a dynamic state of growth, and new bone is laid down at fracture sites according to local stresses. This remodeling corrects some longitudinal malalignment and permits the acceptance of greater degrees of angulation with metaphyseal fractures. Remodeling will occur if a fracture is adjacent to a hinged joint, if angulation is <30 degrees in the plane of motion, and if the child has at least 2 more years of bone growth remaining. However, the potential for bony remodeling does not obviate the need for precise anatomic fracture reduction in the presence of rotational deformities, excessive degrees of angulation, or displaced intraarticular fractures.

The periosteum enveloping growing bones is stronger and thicker than mature periosteum and contributes to the lower incidence of open fractures in children. It separates from bone more easily and is thus more resistant to tearing, usually remaining intact on one side of a fracture site. This periosteal sleeve decreases the amount of fracture displacement and can be used to the physician's advantage during fracture reduction. The immature periosteum possesses increased osteogenic capability, and new subperiosteal bone is rapidly laid down. Children's bones heal quickly, and nonunion is rare.

The presence of a physis (epiphyseal plate or growth plate) accounts for the location of some childhood fractures, as well as for specific complications associated with pediatric orthopedic injuries. The growth plate is the weakest structure in the pediatric skeleton and also the place where anatomic alignment of fracture fragments is most critical in order to avoid growth imbalance and deformity. Up to 18 percent of children's fractures involve a growth plate.

Physeal injuries occur more often than ligamentous tears in children because the developing ligaments are more resistant to stress than the adjacent bony structures. Situations in which a sprained ligament would be diagnosed in an adult should prompt the diagnosis of a growth plate injury in a child. Forces capable of producing joint subluxations or dislocations in adults result in a separation at the epiphysis in children because of the relative strength and laxity of children's ligaments.

With certain childhood fractures, especially diaphyseal femur fractures, some degree of overriding of the fracture fragments is actually desirable. Subsequent to the injury there is an increase in blood flow to the growth plate, resulting in accelerated longitudinal bone growth. The overriding and associated shortening of the bone compensate for this rapid longitudinal growth.

Table 18-1. Fracture Terminology

Anatomic location
  Epiphysis: present at the end of each long bone; completely cartilaginous at birth except at distal femur; secondary ossification centers develop that replace cartilage over time
  Apophysis: traction epiphysis; nonarticular site of ligament and tendon attachment (example: distal humeral condyles); not directly involved in longitudinal growth but contribute to bony contour
  Physis (growth plate) or epiphyseal plate: cartilaginous structure between epiphysis and metaphysis responsible for longitudinal bone growth; injury may result in growth disturbance or arrest
  Metaphysis: flared end of diaphysis adjacent to physes representing new bone; structurally weak area; diaphyseal: central shaft of long bone
Diaphyseal: central shaft of long bone
  Articular: involves portion of epiphysis comprising joint surface
  Epicondylar: distal humeral site of muscle attachments
  Supracondylar: part of metaphysis located cephalad to condyles and epicondyles
  Transcondylar: across the condyles of humerus or distal femur
  Intercondylar: intraepiphyseal; fracture disrupts articular surface and separates condyles from one another
  Subcapital: metaphyseal area of proximal femur and radius
Fracture pattern
  Avulsion: bone fragment pulled off by action of tendon or ligament
  Longitudinal: fracture line follows long axis of bone
  Transverse: fracture line at right angle to long axis of bone
  Oblique: fracture line angled at 30–60 degrees from long axis of bone
  Spiral: encircling oblique fracture (has torsional component)
  Impacted: fracture ends compressed together
  Comminuted: any fracture with more than two fracture fragments
  Bowing: (plastic deformation) significant bend in bone without fracture; commonly seen in ulna and fibula in association with fracture of respective paired bone
  Torus: "buckle fracture," metaphyseal compaction of trabecular bone and buckling of cortical bone
  Greenstick: incomplete fracture of cortex on convex (tension, elastic phase) side of bone with only a bend in cortex of concave side (compression, plastic phase); most common fracture pattern in children
  Pathologic: fracture through abnormal, weakened bone (examples: tumors, osteomyelitis, cysts, inherited metabolic disorders)
Fracture fragment positions
  Alignment: refers to longitudinal relationship of one fragment to another
  Displacement: deviation of fracture fragments from anatomic position (displacement of distal fragment described in relation to proximal one; varus displacement: toward midline of body; valgus displacement: away from midline of body)
  Angulation: direction of apex of angle formed by fracture fragments (will be opposite to direction of displacement of distal fragment)
  Distraction: degree to which fracture surfaces are separated
  Bayonet deformity: overlapping fracture surfaces with resultant shortening
  Butterfly fragment: wedge-shaped fragment arising at apex of force applied to shaft of long bone

TERMINOLOGY

In order to communicate meaningfully with consultants and determine the best method of treatment, it is important to grasp the principles of fracture nomenclature and classification systems. The precise anatomic location and morphology of a given fracture should be described using specific terminology. Table 18-1 outlines terms commonly used to describe fractures, and Fig. 18-1 is a diagram demonstrating anatomical terms related to the immature bone.

A break in the skin overlying and communicating with a fracture converts the injury to an open fracture. The major treatment principles concerning open fractures in adults apply to children as well. Operative wound debridement, fracture reduction, and antibiotic administration are mandated in order to promote healing and prevent infectious complications.

PHYSEAL INJURIES

Physeal (epiphyseal plate, growth plate) injuries are more common than generally appreciated, accounting for up to 18 percent of all pediatric fractures. In the early

1960s, Salter and Harris developed the most widely used classification system for fractures involving the growth plate. Modifications were introduced by Ogden some years later. Both systems are based on the radiographic appearance of the fracture and describe the degree of involvement of the growth plate, epiphysis, metaphysis, and joint. These classifications have both prognostic and therapeutic implications (Table 18-2, Fig. 18-2).

Any fracture that involves the growth plate may result in growth disturbance, limb length inequality, and deformity. Parents should be made aware of this fact at the time a physeal injury is diagnosed.

Most fractures classified as Salter-Harris type I or II can be treated with closed reduction. Growth disturbances often complicate type III to V fractures, and these injuries often require operative intervention. Due to severe injury to the growth plate in type V fractures, growth disturbances can occur regardless of the method of treatment.

BIRTH TRAUMA

Fractures of the clavicle, humerus, hip, and femur occur frequently during difficult deliveries. The initial diagnosis

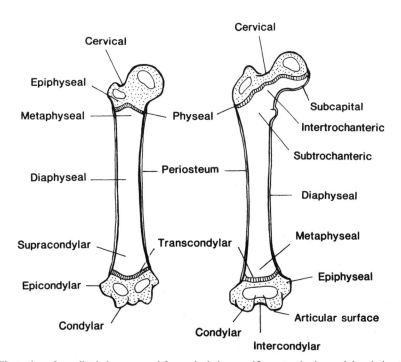

Fig. 18-1. Illustration of a pediatric humerus and femur depicting specific anatomic sites and descriptive terminology.

Table 18-2. Classification of Epiphyseal Injuries

Type	Description
	Salter-Harris System
I	Complete separation of the epiphysis and most of the physis from metaphysis. Prognosis for normal growth is good. Commonly results from shearing force in newborns and young infants. May be seen in victims of abuse. Diagnosis may be difficult; if radiographic studies are normal but patient is tender over the growth plate immobilization and orthopedic referral are recommended.
II	Fracture line propagates along physis and extends into metaphysis; result is displaced metaphyseal fragment, often with epiphyseal displacement. Most common epiphyseal injury; associated with low risk of growth disturbance. Usually occurs in children over 10 years of age.
III	Fracture line extends from physis through epiphysis to articular surface of the joint. Anatomic reduction necessary to restore normal joint mechanics and prevent growth disturbance, bony bridging, and posttraumatic arthritis.
IV	Fracture line begins at articular surface, crosses the epiphysis and growth plate, and extends into the metaphysis, splitting off a metaphyseal fragment (example: humeral lateral condyle fractures). Open reduction and internal fixation usually required to ensure anatomic reduction and avoid angular deformity and loss of joint function. Significant incidence of growth disturbance.
V	Results from longitudinal compression of the growth plate. Rare injury associated with apparently normal x-rays. Diagnosis usually made in retrospect when premature closure of the physis and growth abnormalities develop.
	Additional Types From the Ogden System
VI	Peripheral shear injury to borders of growth plate. Angular deformity may develop due to formation of osseous bridge between metaphysis and epiphysis.
VII	Intraarticular intraepiphyseal injury where ligament pulls off distal portion of epiphysis rather than tearing.
VIII	Fracture through region of metaphysis with temporary disruption of circulation.
IX	Fracture involving significant damage to or loss of periosteum.

is often infection or pseudoparalysis until an x-ray confirms the presence of a fracture (Fig. 18-3).

CHILD ABUSE

A high index of suspicion for nonaccidental trauma must always be maintained when evaluating an injured child. Most child abuse occurs between birth and 2 years of age. Up to 50 percent of fractures in children younger than 1 year of age are the result of nonaccidental trauma.

Clues to the presence of nonaccidental trauma include a significant delay in seeking medical attention and details of the mechanism of injury that are inconsistent with the type of fracture sustained. The developmental level of the patient must also be considered when deciding whether or not the reported mechanism of injury is consistent with physical and radiographic findings.

Determining that a child has been abused involves medical, legal, and moral responsibilities. Historical aspects of the injury, physical and radiographic findings, and an evaluation of the social interactions between family members must all be considered when making the diagnosis of nonaccidental trauma. Certain radiographic findings are suggestive of nonaccidental trauma but not confirmative in and of themselves (Table 18-3). The presence of long bone fractures in a young child should raise the possibility of child abuse. Femur fractures in the nonambulatory child and nonsupracondylar fractures of the humerus are both highly suggestive of abuse. Spiral fractures, however, are common in both accidental and nonaccidental trauma.

Fractures of the metaphyseal-epiphyseal junction are virtually pathognomonic for child abuse. These long bone "corner" fractures are frequently bilateral and result from periosteal avulsion of bone and cartilage secondary to violent twisting forces or downward pull on an

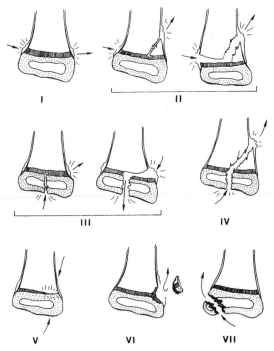

Fig. 18-2. Classification of growth plate injuries described by Salter and Harris (I to V) and Ogden (VI to VII).

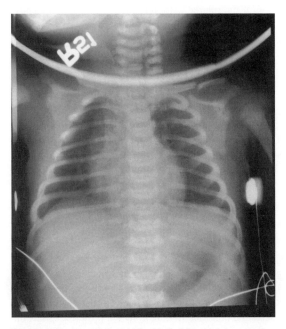

Fig. 18-3. Fracture of the middle third of the clavicle secondary to shoulder dystocia in a newborn.

Table 18-3. Radiographic Findings Suggestive of Child Abuse

High Risk for Abuse

  Metaphyseal lesions
  Posterior rib fractures
  Scapular fractures
  Spinous process fractures
  Sternal fractures

Moderate Risk for Abuse

  Multiple fractures, especially bilateral
  Fractures of different ages
  Epiphyseal separation
  Vertebral body fractures and subluxations
  Digit fractures
  Complex skull fractures

Low Risk for Abuse

  Clavicular fractures
  Long bone shaft fractures
  Linear skull fractures

extremity. A chip of bone or larger "bucket handle" fracture may be present on the radiograph. The injury may not be visible on initial radiographs but will be identifiable 7 to 10 days later as new subperiosteal bone formation (Fig. 18-4).

A skeletal survey should be performed on any child younger than 2 years of age when abuse is suspected. The survey should include anteroposterior (AP) and lateral views of the chest, AP views of the pelvis, AP views of all extremities, including the hands and feet, lateral views of the lumbar and cervical spine, and AP and lateral views of the skull. Oblique views of the thorax increase the yield in detecting rib fractures. A follow-up skeletal survey is recommended 2 weeks after the initial study to increase the diagnostic yield when abuse is strongly suspected.

CLINICAL EVALUATION

Resuscitative efforts and attention to potentially life-threatening injuries take precedence. Once the patient has been stabilized, a complete history and physical examination can be performed.

Pain and fear complicate the evaluation of the injured child. History should be obtained both from the patient, if age appropriate, and from any witnesses to the injury.

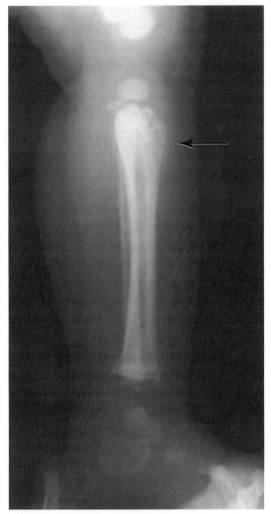

Fig. 18-4. Periosteal reaction with metaphyseal irregularity in a 3-month-old (arrow). This metaphyseal corner fracture is highly suggestive of nonaccidental trauma.

An accurate history should include the time of the event, mechanism of injury, direction and degree of force involved, and history of previous injury. Histories that are vague or inconsistent with the injury suggest the possibility of nonaccidental trauma. Past medical history and developmental milestones should also be addressed.

The injured limb should be observed and palpated to assess for any deformity, swelling, pain, or abnormal motion. Examination of both the joint above and the joint below the site of injury must be included in the evaluation. Careful inspection of the surrounding soft tissues may reveal a break in integrity that signals open communication with the fracture site. A thorough assessment of the neurovascular status of the extremity should be performed prior to and after any attempts at manipulative reduction. Serial assessments during the patient's course will ensure that a developing compartment syndrome is discovered early.

Liberal use of radiographs is advisable because of the difficulty in obtaining an adequate history and performing a physical examination in young children, and due to the relative paucity of physical findings associated with certain childhood fractures. At least two views perpendicular to each other should be obtained, usually an AP and lateral view. The films should include the joints above and below the injury site since dislocations can occur with diaphyseal fractures (e.g., Monteggia fractures). The injured extremity should be splinted *before* the patient goes to the x-ray suite to prevent further injury. Comparison views of the noninjured extremity may be helpful but are not routinely recommended.

THERAPEUTIC CONSIDERATIONS

Pain medication should be provided as needed and local or regional blocks considered after a thorough neurovascular assessment has been performed. Immobilization of the injured extremity, including the joints above and below the fracture, will prevent further injury and may make the patient more comfortable. Open fractures, fractures that are significantly displaced or angulated, fractures associated with neurovascular compromise, and fractures involving a growth plate require immediate orthopedic consultation. Most nondisplaced fractures can be splinted by the primary care physician and referred for definitive care within 3 days.

Casts are not usually applied until 1 to 2 days after the time of injury to allow swelling to diminish. Splints allow visual inspection of the involved area while still maintaining adequate immobilization.

A sling and swathe provides sufficient immobilization for most injuries between the sternoclavicular joint and the elbow, whereas posterior arm splints are useful with elbow, forearm, and wrist injuries. In both cases the elbow should be flexed to 90 degrees and the forearm placed in neutral position. An ulnar gutter splint immobilizes fractures of the fourth and fifth fingers, and a thumb spica splint stabilizes injuries involving the scaphoid bone and thumb. Long leg posterior splints immobilize the knee and stabilize the distal femur as well as the proximal and middle tibia and fibula. Short leg posterior splints provide stable immobilization for ankle and foot injuries.

Prior to discharge, the proper use of ice and elevation should be described and instructions given to return immediately for repeat evaluation should severe pain, swelling, or change in color develop. Children's fractures heal much more quickly than similar injuries in adults, so fracture reduction and orthopedic follow-up must take place as soon as possible after the injury. Young children do not usually require physical therapy as even long-term immobilization rarely results in joint stiffness or loss of function.

BIBLIOGRAPHY

Bachman D, Santora S: Orthopedic trauma, in Fleisher GR, Ludwig S (eds): *Textbook of Pediatric Emergency Medicine.* Baltimore: Williams & Wilkins, 2000, pp 1236–1244.

Bright RW: Physeal injuries, in Rockwood CA, Wilkins KE, King RE (eds): *Fractures in Children.* Philadelphia: JB Lippincott, 1996, pp 87–186.

Canale, ST: Physeal injuries, in Green NE, Swiotkowski MF (eds): *Skeletal Trauma in Children,* vol 3. Philadelphia: WB Saunders, 1998, pp 17–58.

DiScala, C, Sege R, et al: Child abuse and unintentional injuries: A 10-year retrospective. *Arch Pediatr Adolesc Med* 54:16–22, 2000.

Jones E: Skeletal growth and development as related to traums, in Green NE, Swiontkowski MF (eds): *Skeletal Trauma in Children.* Philadelphia: WB Saunders, 1998, pp 1–16.

Leventhal JM, Thomas SA, Rosenfield NS, et al: Fractures in young children: Distinguishing child abuse from unintentional injuries. *Am J Dis Child* 147:87, 1993.

Ogden JA, Ogden DA, Ganey TM: Biological aspects of children's fractures, in Rockwood CA, Wilkins KE, Beaty JH (eds): *Fractures in Children.* Philadelphia: JB Lippincott, 1996, pp 19–52.

Peterson HA: Physeal and apophyseal injuries, in Rockwood CA, Wilkins KE, Beaty JH (eds): *Fractures in Children.* Philadelphia: JB Lippincott, 1996, pp 103–166.

Salter RB, Harris WR: Injuries involving the epiphyseal plate. *J Bone Surg [Am]* 45A:587, 1963.

Section on Radiology: Diagnostic imaging of child abuse. *Pediatrics* 105:1345–1348, 2000.

19

Injuries of the Upper Extremities

Timothy J. Rittenberry
Russell H. Greenfield

HIGH-YIELD FACTS

- Most clavicle fractures heal well without complication, and reduction is rarely necessary.
- Children are more likely to suffer a Salter-Harris type II fracture separation of the proximal humerus than a true shoulder dislocation.
- Fracture at the junction of the middle and distal third of the humerus is associated with radial nerve injury.
- Indirect radiographic evidence of elbow fracture includes the presence of a posterior fat pad, an exaggerated anterior fat pad, and abnormal radiocapitellar or anterior humeral lines. Further evidence may be obtained from normal comparison views.
- Supracondylar fractures of the humerus are associated with acute and delayed neurovascular compromise and require immediate orthopedic consultation.
- The medial epicondyle must be identified in its extraarticular position after reduction of a posterior elbow dislocation.
- Fracture-separation of the distal humeral physis may be the result of physical abuse.
- Fracture of the radius or ulna requires x-ray evaluation of the elbow and wrist to rule out the presence of a Monteggia or Galeazzi fracture.

THE CLAVICLE AND ACROMIOCLAVICULAR JOINT

The clavicle is the most commonly fractured bone during delivery and is the fourth most commonly fractured bone in older children. A direct blow from a fall is the most common cause. The vast majority of injuries involve the area between the middle and distal thirds of the clavicle (>90 percent). Young children sustain incomplete injuries (greenstick or torus fractures), whereas older children and adolescents present more often with displaced fractures.

Fractures of the medial clavicle are rare in children. The medial clavicular epiphysis is the last growth plate in the body to close, allowing physeal injuries to occur up to age 25. In contrast to adults, in whom sternoclavicular joint dislocations occur, children are most likely to experience Salter-Harris type I or II fracture, with or without epiphyseal separation. Accurate diagnosis of medial clavicular fractures is often difficult. Lordotic x-ray views may be helpful.

Shoulder compression during delivery often results in fracture of the clavicle. The injury may be asymptomatic or present as pseudoparalysis (the infant will not move the arm but hand and forearm movement is normal). Exuberant callus formation calls attention to the fracture a few weeks later. Initially the deformity worries parents, but remodeling occurs and results in a normal appearance of the bone in 6 to 12 months. Older patients present with pain and may have an obvious deformity.

A careful search for associated vascular injury is mandatory in the presence of a displaced clavicle fracture. Pulse changes and significant swelling may signal laceration or compression of the subclavian vessels, especially with posterior displacement of the fracture fragments, prompting emergent orthopedic and vascular consultation. Injury to the underlying lung occurs infrequently.

Most clavicle fractures heal well without complication, and reduction is rarely necessary unless significant overriding is present. Injuries due to birth trauma only require careful handling of the infant. Young children are placed in either a sling or a shoulder strap; older patients can be managed with a sling and swathe. Operative intervention is indicated in the presence of an open fracture or vascular complication.

Direct trauma to the distal clavicle produces metaphyseal fractures in young children rather than true acromioclavicular joint separations, as seen in adolescents and adults. Avulsion of bone and periosteum occurs rather than ligamentous tearing. Weighted x-ray views are not routinely recommended. The fracture heals well with the use of a sling and swathe, and surgery is only rarely indicated.

SHOULDER DISLOCATIONS

The same forces that result in shoulder dislocation in adults usually cause displaced Salter-Harris type II fracture separation of the proximal humerus in young children. As with adults, when pediatric shoulder dislocations do occur, anterior dislocations are much more common than posterior or inferior dislocations.

Inspection of the anteriorly dislocated shoulder reveals loss of the normally rounded contour, creating a squared-off appearance. The arm is held in slight abduction and external rotation, and the humeral head may be palpated anterior to the glenoid fossa. Radiographs should include an anteroposterior (AP) view of the shoulder and either a true scapular lateral or transaxillary view. In general, adequate analgesia and relaxation should be provided before attempting reduction with either traction-countertraction, scapular manipulation or external rotation techniques. Posterior shoulder dislocations can occur following seizures or electrical injuries. The arm is held in adduction and internal rotation. The anterior shoulder appears abnormally flat, and the displaced humeral head may be palpable posteriorly. Orthopedic consultation is recommended in all cases of posterior shoulder dislocation.

Axillary nerve damage may accompany shoulder dislocation. Sensation over the deltoid muscle should be assessed before and after reduction. Other complications include greater tuberosity fractures, damage to the glenoid labrum, the Hill-Sachs deformity (a compression fracture of the posterolateral humeral head), rotator cuff injury, and recurrent dislocation.

HUMERUS FRACTURES

Nearly 80 percent of the longitudinal growth of the humerus takes place at the proximal humeral epiphysis. Accordingly, fractures involving the growth plate of the proximal humerus may result in growth disturbances culminating in significant limb length inequality. Fortunately, Salter-Harris fracture types III, IV, and V are rare in this region.

However, Salter-Harris type I and type II fractures of the proximal humerus are frequently encountered. Type I fractures and proximal metaphyseal injuries, including greenstick and torus fractures, occur in youngsters aged 5 to 11 years. Children of age 11 to 15 years suffer the majority of proximal humerus fractures, usually type II injuries. Most proximal humerus fractures are nondisplaced due to the presence of a strong periosteal sleeve.

Routine radiographic evaluation should include at least two views of the humerus at right angles to each other. Films should include the distal clavicle and acromion to rule out associated injury.

Most fractures of the proximal humerus heal well with only a sling and swathe. If the proximal humeral epiphysis is displaced more than 50 percent, angulation is greater than 40°, or significant malrotation is present, reduction with pinning or internal fixation may be required.

Proximal and distal humerus fractures are much more common than diaphyseal injuries. Most humeral shaft fractures are the result of a direct blow to the area. The degree of displacement depends on the location of the fracture and the surrounding muscle attachments, which may pull the fragments out of alignment. A torsional force from a fall or severe twist may result in a spiral diaphyseal fracture. Nonaccidental trauma should be suspected in children under 3 years of age with spiral humerus fractures.

Mid-shaft fractures heal well even with angulation of up to 15 to 20° and as much as 2 cm of overriding, due to bony remodeling and longitudinal overgrowth that occurs in response to the fracture. A sling and swathe should be applied to young children. A sugar tong splint can be used for adolescents.

Fractures involving the junction of the middle and distal thirds of the humerus may be associated with injury to the radial nerve. Motor and sensory functions should be assessed initially and following any manipulation. Acute radial nerve palsy has an excellent long-term prognosis, with reports of 80 to 100 percent recovery of function.

THE ELBOW

With injury in the area of the elbow, radiographic interpretation is complicated by the presence of numerous epiphyses and ossification centers that appear and fuse at different, but characteristic ages. Matters are further complicated by the need for precise anatomic reduction of fracture fragments in order to avoid both early and late complications.

An adequate radiographic evaluation of the elbow consists of an AP view with the joint in extension and a true lateral view with the elbow flexed at a right angle. The anterior fat pad is located within the coronoid fossa and normally appears as a small lucency just anterior to the fossa on a true lateral x-ray of the elbow. The posterior fat pad sits deep down in the olecranon fossa and is not visible under normal circumstances. The presence of a posterior fat pad on a true lateral view of the elbow is always abnormal and suggests blood within the joint capsule. Joint space fluid collections may also cause the

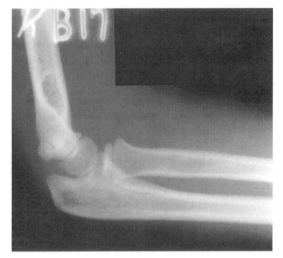

Fig. 19-1. Fracture through the medial epicondyle extending into the olecranon fossa. Note the posterior fat pad sign, signifying the presence of blood within the joint space.

anterior fat pad to be pushed away from the joint and appear as a wind-blown sail—the "sail sign." These abnormal fat pad signs are radiographic evidence of occult fracture of either the distal humerus, proximal ulna, or radius (Fig. 19-1) and can only be detected with the elbow fully flexed at 90°.

There are two reference lines that are useful in assessing elbow radiographs and helping to identify occult injury. The anterior humeral line, drawn along the anterior cortex of the distal humerus on a true lateral view of the elbow, should normally intersect the middle third of the capitellum distally. Posterior displacement of the capitellum may be consistent with an otherwise radiographically inapparent supracondylar fracture. The radiocapitellar line is drawn down the axis of the proximal radius on the true lateral view of the elbow and should bisect the capitellum regardless of the degree of flexion or extension present. Failure to do so suggests the presence of an occult radial neck fracture or radial head dislocation. Any question about the anatomic relationships can be further investigated using comparison views of the uninjured elbow.

SUPRACONDYLAR HUMERUS FRACTURES

A fall onto an outstretched hand causing violent hyperextension of the elbow is the usual mechanism of injury with supracondylar fractures of the distal humeral meta-

physis. The olecranon process is forcibly thrust into the olecranon fossa, resulting in fracture with posterior displacement of the distal fragment (Fig. 19-2). Supracondylar fractures account for 50 to 60 percent of all elbow fractures in children 3 to 10 years of age.

Supracondylar humerus fractures are associated with a high incidence of early neurovascular complications. Although puncture or actual laceration of the brachial artery are rare, the vessel may be compressed or contused or may undergo vasospasm at the fracture site. Signs of significant distal ischemia such as pallor and cyanosis of the fingers, prolonged capillary refill, or absence of the radial pulse indicate the need for prompt reduction of the fracture. If the vascular status is not improved, then surgical exploration is indicated. Patients are at risk of developing a forearm compartment syndrome. Unrecognized, this will lead to Volkmann's ischemic contracture and a nonfunctional hand and wrist. Forearm pain with passive flexion or extension of the fingers or distal parasthesias are ominous early signs of compartment syndrome. Nerve impairment occurs in 10 to 20 percent of children with supracondylar fractures, yet the prognosis for return of function is good. Radial, median, and ulnar nerve injuries, in descending order of frequency, have all been reported. A late complication of supracondylar humerus fractures is cubitus varus, a change in the carrying angle of the elbow.

The potential for significant complications with supracondylar humerus fractures mandates accurate diagnosis and urgent orthopedic consultation. Rotational and angular deformities must be meticulously reduced in order to preserve normal elbow function and prevent vascular compromise. Most children are admitted for 24 to 48

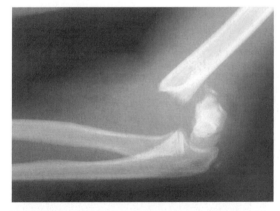

Fig. 19-2. Comminuted supracondylar fracture with large joint effusion. The patient required fasciotomy and skin grafting due to neurovascular compromise.

hours of observation so that the neurovascular status of the extremity can be reassessed frequently. Open reduction and internal fixation may be necessary.

THE MEDIAL AND LATERAL CONDYLES

Fractures involving the articular surface of the lateral condyle (capitellum) comprise 15 percent of all pediatric elbow fractures. The peak in incidence is at 6 years of age. The most likely mechanism of injury involves a fall on the outstretched arm with forearm supination or elbow flexion. Salter-Harris type IV fractures are common. The fracture fragment may become displaced and rotated, and the diagnosis is radiographically obvious if the ossified capitellum is notably displaced from the trochlea or radiocapitellar line. Clinically, swelling and tenderness are most pronounced at the lateral elbow. Although lateral condyle fractures are not usually associated with acute neurovascular injuries, they require aggressive intervention to prevent later complications such as nonunion, loss of elbow mobility, and growth arrest of the lateral condylar physis leading to eventual cubitus valgus and tardy ulnar palsy. Management is usually operative in all but nondisplaced fractures.

Fractures of the articular surface of the medial condyle, or trochlea, occur only rarely, but when present require precise anatomic reduction due to the intraarticular nature of the injury (Fig. 19-3). The most frequent complications associated with medial condylar fractures are nonunion and ulnar nerve neuropraxia.

MEDIAL EPICONDYLAR FRACTURE

The epicondyles are located just proximal to the articulating surface of the distal humerus. The medial epicondyle is a traction apophysis to which the forearm flexors are attached. Fractures of the medial epicondyle are rarely encountered in children younger than 4 years of age, occurring most commonly in children aged 7 to 15 years. These may occur as an avulsion injury due to a fall on the arm with forced hyperextension of the wrist and fingers. The vast majority of medial epicondylar fractures, however, are associated with elbow dislocations, occurring approximately 50 percent of the time (Fig. 19-4). The medial epicondyle may dislocate and then block reduction or become entrapped intraarticularly. The medial epicondyle *must* be identified as extraarticular after any elbow reduction. A more insidious injury to the medial epicondyle may occur with repetitive traction stress by the forearm flexors (Little Leaguer's elbow). Treatment is usually nonoperative, with severe displacement or ulnar nerve dysfunction considered relative indications for operative management.

FRACTURE-SEPARATION OF THE DISTAL HUMERAL PHYSIS

Although uncommon, this injury is important because of its association with nonaccidental trauma, such as with violent arm twisting. When present in children under

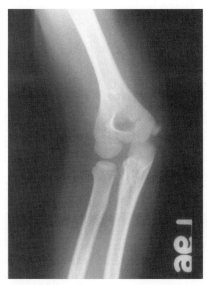

Fig. 19-3. Nondisplaced fracture of the medial condyle in a 5-year-old.

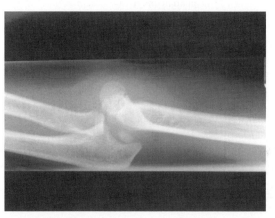

Fig. 19-4. Posterior elbow dislocation with avulsion of the medial epicondyle.

3 years of age, physical abuse should be suspected. The fracture can also occur following birth trauma. This injury is rare past age 3, after which supracondylar fractures predominate. Differentiation from elbow dislocation can be very difficult due to the lack of capitellar ossification. Orthopedic consultation is warranted, and closed reduction usually provides adequate healing.

ELBOW DISLOCATIONS

Pediatric elbow dislocations occur infrequently, since most forces that would result in dislocations in adults usually cause fractures in children. When elbow dislocations do occur, they are usually the result of a fall onto the slightly flexed, outstretched arm in an adolescent. As with adults, most dislocations are posterior.

Associated fractures are the rule and most commonly involve fracture of the medial epicondyle, coronoid process, radial head, or olecranon (Fig. 19-4). Significant damage to the surrounding soft tissues also occurs, with damage to the neighboring nerves more common than brachial artery injury. Recovery of function of the ulnar nerve can be expected, but the prognosis is less optimistic with median nerve injury. Vascular compromise complicates up to 7 percent of pediatric elbow dislocations.

Most dislocations can be reduced after providing adequate analgesia and muscle relaxation. The elbow should be flexed to 60 to 70° and the forearm placed in supination. The proximal humerus is then stabilized by an assistant while longitudinal traction is applied at the wrist. Upon successful reduction the elbow should be gently flexed and immobilized and the neurovascular status of the arm reappraised. A postreduction radiograph should be obtained with attention to verifying the location of the medial epicondyle as extraarticular.

RADIAL HEAD SUBLUXATION

This most common pediatric elbow injury is called "nursemaid's elbow" or "pulled elbow." It occurs when abrupt axial traction is applied to the wrist or hand of the extended, pronated forearm of a child under 5 years of age, causing the annular ligament to slip free of the radial head and become entrapped between the radial head and capitellum. Left-sided injuries occur more commonly due to traction by predominantly right-handed adults walking at the child's side.

A history of the patient being lifted by the arm may be obtained, but the precipitating event is often neither witnessed nor recognized. On presentation the child appears comfortable yet refuses to reach for objects with the affected arm. On examination the forearm is held in pronation with the elbow in slight flexion. There is a remarkable lack of swelling and only mild tenderness over the radial head. The child resists all attempts at passive range of motion. Radiographic evaluation is not necessary in the presence of a clear history of precipitating arm traction.

Whether by supination or pronation, successful reduction of the subluxed radial head usually occurs after one or two attempts. A time-honored method is to place one finger over the radial head while the forearm is supinated and flexed at the elbow. A palpable or audible "pop" usually signals successful reduction. Typically the patient again reaches for objects with the affected arm within 5 to 10 minutes of reduction. No further treatment is necessary. If radiographs are obtained, the child often returns with normal arm movement after active positioning and inadvertent reduction by the technologist.

Several attempts at reduction may be necessary before the patient resumes normal use of the arm. Occasionally, radial traction prior to supination and flexion is necessary. If the subluxation occurred several hours earlier, it may be longer before normal function of the arm is observed. If normal use does not follow reduction attempts, alternative diagnoses should be considered. In such a situation, with the presence of normal radiographs, approximately 60 percent will have nonreduced radial head subluxation, 10 percent will have soft tissue injury, and only 20 percent will have occult fracture. Immobilization with prompt orthopedic follow-up is indicated. Recurrence rates have been reported as high as 30 percent.

FRACTURES OF THE RADIUS AND ULNA

The clavicle is the only bone broken more frequently than the radius and ulna during childhood. Three quarters of all injuries involve the distal third of the forearm. Although an isolated fracture of one of the bones can occur, a high index of suspicion must be maintained for concomitant injury to the paired bone. The force precipitating a readily apparent injury may be transmitted to the paired bone and result in bowing, a greenstick fracture, or dislocation at a location distant from the obvious fracture site. For this reason forearm x-rays should always include the wrist and elbow. Most fractures of the radius and ulna heal without significant complications.

A fall onto an extended, supinated arm with a valgus stress can result in fracture of the radial head or neck. Most proximal radius fractures in young children involve the narrow metaphyseal neck since the head is cartilaginous until ossification begins at age 5 years. Salter-

Harris type I and type II radial neck fractures are most common. Salter-Harris type IV radial head fractures may be encountered in older children. Proximal radius fractures can occur in conjunction with elbow dislocations and are often associated with concomitant injury to the medial epicondyle, olecranon, and coronoid process.

An abnormal fat pad sign or abnormal radiocapitellar line on x-ray points to the presence of an occult radial head or radial neck fracture. Minimally displaced or nondisplaced fractures can be treated in a posterior splint with the elbow flexed at 90°. Complications include restriction of pronation and supination, as well as myositis ossificans.

Olecranon fractures occur commonly in combination with other elbow injuries, such as radial head dislocations, radial neck fractures, and fractures of the medial epicondyle. Isolated olecranon epiphyseal fractures are rare and are usually due to a direct blow to the posterior elbow. Nondisplaced injuries may be treated in a posterior splint. Healing usually takes place without complications, although nonunion and ulnar nerve neuropraxia do occur infrequently.

Most forearm diaphyseal fractures are either greenstick or bowing injuries. Both bones may suffer greenstick or bowing injuries, or one bone may have a greenstick fracture while the paired bone is bowed (Fig. 19-5). The potential for remodeling of a bowing injury, or plastic deformation, is minimal in children older than 4 years. Bowing may restrict pronation and supination as well as result in permanent deformity of the extremity.

Overriding of fracture fragments in the presence of an isolated fracture of one of the forearm bones suggests either a Monteggia or Galeazzi fracture. An isolated fracture of the proximal ulna may be associated with concomitant dislocation of the radial head (Monteggia fracture). This combined injury may be inadvertently

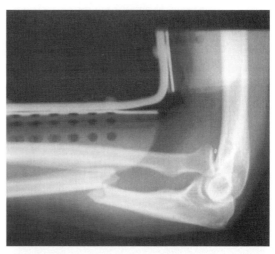

Fig. 19-6. Fracture of the proximal ulna with radial head dislocation (Monteggia fracture). A line bisecting the proximal radius completely misses the capitellum.

overlooked initially because attention is focused on the obvious ulnar fracture. An aberrant radiocapitellar line on plain x-ray is evidence of the accompanying radial head dislocation (Fig. 19-6). Closed reduction is usually successful. A fracture at the junction of the middle and distal thirds of the radius in association with distal radioulnar joint dislocation is called a Galeazzi fracture and is rare in children (Fig. 19-7).

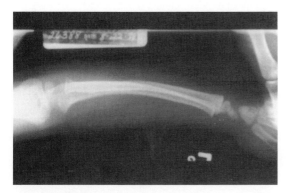

Fig. 19-5. Illustration depicting a greenstick fracture of the radium with associated plastic deformity of the ulna. Radiographic appearance of mid-shaft bowing injury of both the radius and ulna.

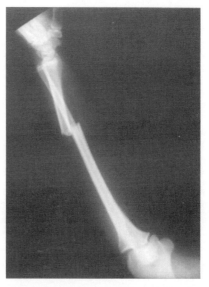

Fig. 19-7. Galeazzi fracture in a 16-year-old.

Fractures of the distal third of the radius and ulna are among the most common orthopedic injuries in children 6 to 12 years of age, often occurring after a fall onto an outstretched hand. Torus fractures of the distal radius and ulna are frequently encountered and can be treated in a long arm splint (Fig. 19-8). The distal radial physis accounts for almost 80 percent of the longitudinal growth of the radius, but significant growth disturbance secondary to injury rarely occurs. Tenderness over the physis of the distal radius with a normal radiograph suggests nondisplaced Salter-Harris type I injury, and splinting with orthopedic follow-up is appropriate.

The capacity for angular remodeling after forearm fracture is great, but rotational remodeling does not oc-cur and rotational abnormalities must be accurately corrected. The strong periosteal sleeve of the bones makes nonunion rare. Complications are uncommon, but vascular compromise or compartment syndrome can develop with any forearm fracture.

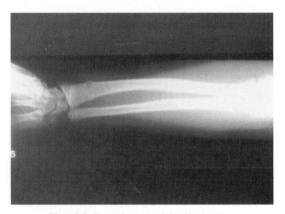

Fig. 19-8. Torus fracture of the distal radius.

BIBLIOGRAPHY

Green NE: Fractures and dislocations about the elbow, in Green NE, Swiontkowski MF, (eds): *Skeletal Trauma in Children.* Vol 3. Philadelphia: WB Saunders, 1998, pp 259–317.

Kennington RT, Dwyer BJ, Phillips WA: Avoiding misdiagnosis with pediatric arm injuries. *Emerg Med Rep* 11:189, 1990.

Ogden JA: Injury to the immature skeleton, in Touloukian RJ (ed): *Pediatric Trauma.* St. Louis: Mosby Yearbook, 1990, pp 411–415, 420–428, 433–434.

Rittenberry TJ, Townes DA: Pediatric orthopedics: The upper extremity, in Hart RG, Rittenberry TJ, Uehara DT (eds): *Handbook of Orthopaedic Emergencies.* Philadelphia: Lippincott-Raven, 1999, pp 420–437.

Schunk JE: Radial head subluxations: Epidemiology and treatment of 87 episodes. *Ann Emerg Med* 19:1019, 1990.

Snyder HS: Radiographic changes with radial head subluxation in children. *J Emerg Med* 8:265, 1990.

Villalba K, Kroger KJ: Upper extremity injuries, in Reisdorff EJ, Roberts MR, Weigenstein JG (eds): *Pediatric Emergency Medicine.* Philadelphia, WB Saunders, 1993, pp 948–960.

Wilkens KE: Fractures and dislocations of the elbow region, in Rockwood CA, Wikins KE, Beaty JH (eds): *Fractures in Children.* Philadelphia: Lippincott-Raven, 1996, Vol 3, pp 420–437.

20

Injuries of the Hand and Wrist

Dennis T. Uehara

HIGH-YIELD FACTS

- The normal cascade of the resting hand shows increasing flexion from the index to little fingers and from the distal interphalangeal (DIP) joints to the metacarpophalangeal (MCP) joints. Deviation from this normal cascade implies a tendon laceration.

- Arterial bleeding from a volar laceration indicates that the digital nerve is also lacerated. In the hand, the digital nerve is superficial to the digital artery, so a volar laceration of the artery must cut the nerve first.

- Firm pressure over the volar aspect of the forearm will cause passive motion of the fingers, demonstrating tendon integrity. This test may be used in frightened or uncooperative children.

- A Salter-Harris type III fracture of the distal phalanx may not be seen on x-ray because the epiphysis in young children may not be ossified. Look for a mallet deformity and inability to extend the DIP joint.

- Carpal fractures are rare in children due to the elasticity imparted by the cartilage surrounding the carpal bones. As in adults, scaphoid fractures are the most commonly encountered carpal fracture.

- A volar dislocation of the proximal interphalangeal (PIP) joint may be irreducible if the proximal phalangeal condyle becomes button-holed between the central tendon and the lateral band. In addition, the central slip is sometimes avulsed, resulting in a delayed boutonnière deformity. These patients should be referred to orthopedics.

- Always test for joint stability by active range of motion performed after reduction of a dislocation. Stability through a full range of motion implies that the joint will respond well to conservative treatment by splinting.

Pediatric hand and wrist injuries are commonly seen in emergency practice. In the younger age group, the injuries are often isolated to the fingers and are the result of a crushing mechanism. Thirty-eight percent of these injuries occur in children younger than 5 years of age and 80 percent from birth to 10 years. Most occur in the middle finger and to the distal phalanx. Approximately 25 percent of such injuries result in fractures. Amputations and tendon injuries are found occasionally. In the older age groups, injuries tend to occur as a result of athletic competition. Hand and wrist injuries occur in 3 to 9 percent of all sports injuries. Sprains are the most common, followed by contusions and fractures. Commonly encountered injuries include radius fractures, scaphoid fractures, ligamentous injuries to the wrist and fingers, dislocations of the DIP and PIP joints, and phalangeal fractures.

Pediatric hand fractures represent 5 to 7 percent of all pediatric fractures. These injuries are sometimes difficult to diagnose and may be associated with long-term morbidity. This makes appropriate initial evaluation and treatment imperative. Fortunately, healing is rapid, tendon and joint complications are rare, and their ability to remodel is remarkable.

PHYSICAL EXAMINATION

Observation

The physical examination of the hand begins with observation. One should look for lacerations, puncture wounds, soft tissue swelling, deformity, and color. The resting hand should demonstrate increasing flexion from the index through little finger and increasing flexion of the joints, from the DIP through MCP joints. Disruption of this normal cascade implies a laceration to an extensor or flexor tendon. A complete flexor tendon laceration results in straightening of the finger due to the unopposed extensors. A complete extensor tendon laceration results in flexion of the finger due to the unopposed flexors.

Malrotation as a result of a phalangeal or metacarpal fracture will occasionally occur. Alignment may appear normal in extension but be grossly abnormal with the fingers flexed. Malrotation may lead to significant cosmetic and functional impairment, so the diagnosis should be made on initial presentation to avoid permanent disability. A useful method to test for malrotation is to have the patient alternately flex the fingers to the palm. Each finger converges to the same place on the palm, the tubercle of the scaphoid. Patients with significant malrotation will violate this pattern with the affected finger. Another method is to compare the planes of the fingernails with the fingers in flexion. The nail plates should be approximately parallel and symmetric to the opposite hand. Any abnormal tilting is evidence of a rotational deformity.

Palpation

Gently performed palpation of the injured hand can give significant information. This must be performed delicately since the pediatric patient is likely to be afraid and unwilling to allow examination freely. The examination should be performed with the patient's hand resting comfortably on a flat surface. One may use a fingertip or an object such as the eraser end of a pencil or the end of a cotton-tipped applicator to find the exact area of maximal tenderness. Maximal tenderness over the radial or ulnar aspect of an interphalangeal joint indicates a collateral ligament tear. Tenderness over the volar aspect of an interphalangeal joint indicates volar plate injury. Tenderness over the ulnar aspect of the thumb MCP joint indicates a gamekeeper's thumb (torn ulnar collateral ligament of the thumb). Pain over the anatomic snuff box is presumptive evidence for a scaphoid fracture. Erythema, warmth, swelling, and tenderness over the distal finger pad confirms the diagnosis of a felon.

Circulation

Circulation is best assessed by observing color and testing for capillary refill and temperature of the skin. A cyanotic edematous hand indicates venous insufficiency. A pale cool hand or a finger with poor capillary filling indicates arterial insufficiency. Doppler ultrasound or an Allen test may determine adequacy or circulation. Brisk arterial bleeding can be managed by pressure. Blindly clamping arterial bleeders may cause further harm by damaging nerves, arteries, tendons, and muscle. Arterial bleeding from a volar laceration implies laceration of the digital nerve since these nerves are located superficial to the artery.

Sensation

Senation in the cooperative patient is best tested by two-point discrimination. Each digital nerve is alternately tested. This may be performed with a bent paper clip gently touching the tip of the finger along the longitudinal axis. The distance between the tips of the paper clip begins at 1 cm and is then made closer until the patient can no longer recognize one from two points. Normal two-point discrimination is 3 to 5 mm. In children too young or too afraid to cooperate, two other methods of sensory testing have been reported: loss of skin wrinkling and loss of sweating. After the hand is soaked in warm water for 30 minutes, the skin wrinkling usually seen is lost after digital nerve injury. Skin sweating is responsible for the "tackiness" of the fingertips and relies on intact sympathetic innervation. Following digital nerve injury, the ability to sweat is lost, and the skin takes on a smooth, silky texture. This may be tested by moving a smooth object, such as the barrel of a pen, over the fingertip. In the injured finger the barrel will move smoothly; in the normal finger there will be resistance. Even under the best of circumstances, such testing will be challenging in the emergency department. As always, a high index of suspicion is required for successful diagnosis.

Motor

The ulnar, median, and radial nerves can be evaluated by three gross motor tests of function. The ulnar nerve is tested by having the patient abduct the index finger against resistance while palpating the first dorsal interosseus muscle. The median nerve is tested by having the patient palmar abduct the thumb against resistance while the examiner palpates the belly of the abductor pollicis brevis muscle, located on the radial aspect of the thenar eminence. The radial nerve is tested by having the patient extend the fingers and wrist against resistance.

Tendon

Examination of the hand for tendon injury is particularly difficult in the pediatric age group. The child's pain, anxiety, and unwillingness to cooperate, as well as partial tendon lacerations, all conspire to thwart the unwary examiner. The flexor digitorum profundus is tested by immobilizing the PIP and MCP joints and allowing the patient to flex the DIP joint against resistance. The flexor pollicis longus is tested by immobilizing the MCP joint of the thumb and allowing the patient to flex the interphalangeal (IP) joint. The flexor digitorum superficialis is tested by immobilizing the MCP joint and allowing the patient to flex the PIP joint against resistance. This test does not work for the index finger since the flexor digitorum profundus cannot be immobilized. To test the index finger, have the patient hyperextend the DIP joint with force against the thumb (thumb index pinch). If the patient is able to do this, the superficialis is intact. Patients with a superficialis laceration will not be able to hyperextend the DIP joint but will accomplish pinch by flexion of the DIP joint. The flexor carpi radialis is tested by flexing and radially deviating the wrist against resistance. The flexor carpi ulnaris is tested by flexing and ulnarly deviating the wrist against resistance.

Since evaluating young patients is difficult, depending on age and willingness to cooperate, other tests may be required to determine tendon function. With the elbow resting on the table, allow the wrist to naturally fall into flexion. It is noted that the fingers fall into extension. When the wrist is relaxed in extension, the fingers fall into the normal cascade of flexion. This normal flexion and extension of the fingers relies on an intact tendon system. Another method to assess the flexor tendons is palpation of the forearm to create passive motion of the fingers. This is performed by pressing or squeezing the forearm at the junction of the middle and distal thirds on the ulnar-volar surface. This will cause flexion of the fingers, especially the ulnar three fingers. A similar test can be performed for the flexor pollicis longus by pressing on the distal forearm on the mid-volar aspect. An intact flexor pollicis longus will result in flexion of the interphalangeal joint of the thumb. The extensor tendons are tested as described in Table 20-1.

FRACTURES OF THE PHALANGES

Distal Phalanx

Pediatric distal phalanx fractures are either crush or hyperextension injuries. Crush injuries are quite common, usually resulting from entrapment in a closing door. In these injuries, the soft tissue damage is more significant than the orthopedic injury. Wound care must be meticulous, the nail bed approximated with absorbable suture, the nail plate replaced in the eponychial fold, and the finger splinted.

Table 20-1. Extensor Tendons of the Hand

Compartment	Tendon	Insertion	Test of Function
First	Abductor pollicis longus	Dorsum of the base of the thumb metacarpal	Extension and abduction of the thumb
	Extensor pollicis brevis	Dorsum of the base of the thumb proximal phalanx	Extension and abduction of the thumb
Second	Extensor carpi radialis longus and extensor carpi radialis brevis	Dorsum of the base of the index metacarpal Dorsum of the base of the long metacarpal	Making fist while extending the wrist
Third	Extensor pollicis longus	Dorsum of the base of the thumb distal phalanx	Lifting the thumb off the surface of the table while the palm is flat on the table
Fourth	Extensor digitorum communis	Dorsum of the bases of the proximal phalanges	Extension of the fingers at the MCP joints
	Extensor indicis proprius	Dorsum of the base of the index finger proximal phalanx	Extension of the index finger at the MCP joint with the hand in a fist
Fifth	Extensor digiti minimi	Dorsum of the extensor hood of the little finger	Extension of the little finger while making a fist
Sixth	Extensor carpi ulnaris	Dorsum of the base of the little finger metacarpal	Extension and ulnar deviation of the wrist

A hyperflexion force applied to the tip of the finger may result in one of two types of pediatric injuries (Fig. 20-1). In the preadolescent, an open Salter-Harris type I or II fracture occurs with a mallet deformity. Treatment consists of wound care, replacement of the nail plate, and splinting of the DIP joint in slight hyperextension with an aluminum splint. In the adolescent hyperflexion injury, an open displaced Salter-Harris type III fracture occurs. These injuries are treated by wound care, closed reduction, and splinting in slight hyperextension. If adequate reduction is not obtained, then open reduction and Kirschner-wire fixation is performed. It is important to recognize the mallet deformity present in both of these injuries and treat and refer appropriately.

Middle and Proximal Phalanx

Middle and proximal phalangeal fractures commonly occur at the physis. These fractures are usually Salter-Harris type II fractures (Fig. 20-2). They are reduced by flexion of the

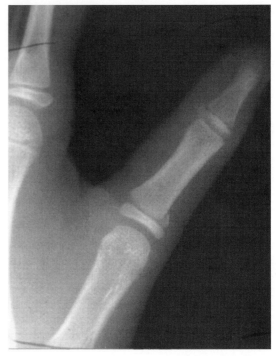

Fig. 20-2. Salter-Harris type II fracture of the proximal phalanx of the thumb.

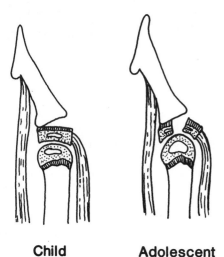

Child   Adolescent

Fig. 20-1. Mallet injuries are caused by avulsion of the extensor tendon from the distal phalanx or from a fracture of the dorsal base of the distal phalanx. An extension lag at the distal interphalangeal (DIP) joint is present, and the patient is unable to actively extend the DIP joint. In children a Salter-Harris type I or II fracture is seen. In the adolescent, a Salter-Harris type III fracture occurs. These fractures may be difficult to detect radiographically since the epiphysis is not fully ossified in children. Inability to actively extend the DIP joint and a mallet deformity reveal the extent of injury. *Source:* Uehara DT: Injuries of the hand and wrist, in Strange, Ahrens, Lelyveld, Schafermeyer (eds): *Pediatric Emergency Medicine: A Comprehensive Guide.*

MCP joint and adduction of the finger. The wrist is placed in an ulnar gutter splint, and the patient is referred to an orthopedist. Salter-Harris type III fractures are ligament or tendon avulsion injuries. Displaced fractures usually require Kirschner-wire fixation. Fractures of the phalangeal shaft are not common in children and when they do occur are often undisplaced or minimally displaced. Splinting and referral is all that is necessary. Displaced fractures of the shaft or neck require splinting and acute referral.

METACARPAL FRACTURES

Metacarpal fractures may occur in the epiphysis, physis, neck, shaft, or base. The neck fracture is the most common and is equivalent to the adult boxer's fracture. These fractures rarely require reduction and can be treated with an ulnar gutter splint with orthopedic referral. A displaced intraarticular fracture of the base of the thumb metacarpal, equivalent to the adult Bennett's fracture, is rare in children. These fractures are unstable Salter-Harris type III fractures and are treated by open reduction and Kirschner-wire fixation. Most other metacarpal fractures are undisplaced or minimally displaced and are treated initially by splint immobilization. Displaced fractures can generally be treated with closed reduction and splinting, but occasionally Kirschner-wire fixation is required.

CARPAL FRACTURES

Fractures of the carpal bones in children are exceedingly rare. The carpus is surrounded by cartilage that acts as a "shock absorber." Fractures are more likely to occur in the distal radius and ulna. Scaphoid fractures are the most commonly encountered of the carpal bone fractures. In the pediatric population, the peak age is in early adolescence, with the mechanism of injury being a fall on the outstretched hand. Physical examination may reveal limitation of range of motion from pain and swelling and tenderness in the "anatomic snuff box." As in the adult, initial x-rays often appear normal. In a child with this presentation, application of a short arm thumb spica splint for 2 weeks with orthopedic referral is appropriate. Nonunion and avascular necrosis are rare in children because most injuries are avulsions or nondisplaced fractures through the distal third of the bone rather than fractures through the waist, as in adults. Other carpal bone fractures are very rare in children and are treated as in adults with splinting and orthopedic referral.

FRACTURES OF THE WRIST

Fractures of the wrist are common in children, with that of the distal radial metaphysis being the most commonly encountered childhood fracture (Fig. 20-3). The mechanism is usually a fall on the outstretched hand. Physical examination may reveal swelling, deformity, and tenderness, indicating a displaced fracture. Commonly, there is no noticeable swelling or deformity. One must search for the point of maximal tenderness that identifies the location of the fracture. One study documented point tenderness and reduction of grip strength of at least 20 percent as predictors of radius fracture. Radiographs should be used liberally to identify these occult fractures. Salter-Harris type I and II fractures are commonly seen. Undisplaced and minimally displaced fractures are splinted and referred. When present, displacement is almost always dorsal and, when significant, requires reduction and immobilization in a long arm cast.

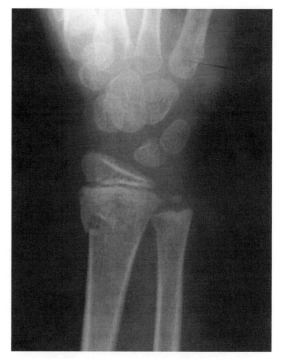

Fig. 20-3. Undisplaced distal radius fracture.

DISLOCATIONS

Distal Interphalangeal Joint

DIP dislocations result from a hyperextension force. This dislocation generally displaces dorsally and is often open, due to the tight adherence of skin to bone in this area. Reduction is usually uncomplicated and consists of traction countertraction followed by flexion. Test active motion to ensure that the extensor and flexor tendons are functioning and that the volar plate is not interposed in the joint.

Proximal Interphalangeal Joint

PIP dislocations can occur in dorsal, volar, radial, or ulnar directions. Dorsal dislocations are the most common. These dislocations occur as a result of an axial load with concomitant hyperextension. Reduction is accomplished through slight hyperextension and longitudinal traction applied to the middle phalanx while correcting the ulnar or radial deformity. The finger is then gently flexed into position. Active range of motion is tested, and stress testing of the collateral ligaments and volar plate is performed. The finger is placed in a splint immobilizing the PIP (20° to 30° of flexion) and MCP joints (60° to 70° of flexion). Orthopedic referral is recommended. Volar dislocations are rare and may be irreducible due to entrapment of the proximal phalangeal condyle between the central tendon and lateral band. These dislocations may result in avulsion of the central slip of the extensor tendon leading to a late boutonnière deformity. Orthopedic referral is required.

Metacarpophalangeal Joint

MCP joint dislocations sometimes occur in the pediatric age group. As in the adult, the thumb MCP dislocation is the most common (Fig. 20-4). It occurs as a result of a hyperextension force, usually from a fall on an outstretched hand. Dislocations may be simple reducible or complex irreducible. In the simple reducible dislocation,

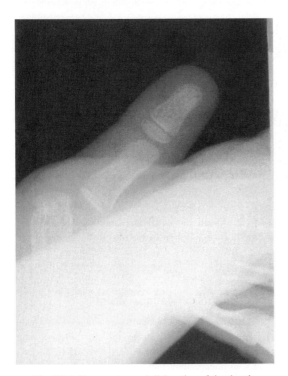

Fig. 20-4. Carpometacarpal dislocation of the thumb.

the proximal phalanx assumes a dorsal point at a 90° angle to the metacarpal. This dislocation can be reduced by gentle traction countertraction. Joint stability is assessed, the finger splinted, and the patient referred. The complex irreducible dislocation has the same mechanism of injury but here, the proximal phalanx assumes a bayonet position parallel to the metacarpal. The volar plate is interposed in the joint, and the metacarpal head may also be trapped in the substance of the intrinsic muscles. Closed reduction is impossible. This dislocation can only be reduced by open reduction. Some authors recommend one attempt at gently performed closed reduction. Vigorous traction is to be avoided since this may convert a simple reducible dislocation to a complex irreducible one.

Carpometacarpal Joint

Carpometacarpal dislocations are rare in the pediatric age group. These injuries are generally a result of violent trauma that result in multiple dislocations or multiple fracture dislocations. These injuries require prompt orthopedic consultation for surgical intervenion.

BIBLIOGRAPHY

Doraiswamy NV: Childhood finger injuries and safeguards. *Injury Prev* 5:298–300, 1999.

Doraiswamy NV, Baig H: Isolated finger injuries in children—incidence and aetiology. *Injury* 31:571–573, 2000.

Huurman WW: Injuries to the hand and wrist. *Adolesc Med* 9:611–625, 1998.

Kocher MS, Waters PM, Micheli LJ: Upper extremity injuries in the paediatric athlete. *Sports Med* 30:117–135, 2000.

MacGregor DM, Hiscox JA: Fingertip trauma in children from doors. *Scot Med J* 44:114–115, 1999.

Mahabir RC, Kazemi AR, Cannon WG, et al: Pediatric hand fractures: A review. *Pediatr Emerg Care* 17:153–156, 2001.

Mastey RD, Weiss AP, Akelman E: Primary care of hand and wrist athletic injuries. *Clin Sports Med* 16:705–724, 1997.

Pershad JM, Monroe K, Kinh W, et al: Pediatric wrist injuries. *Acad Emerg Med* 7:1152–1155, 2000.

Rettig A: Epidemiology of hand and wrist injuries in sports. *Clin Sports Med* 17:1152–1155, 1998.

Rockwood CA, Wilkins KE, King RE: *Fractures in Children,* 3d ed. Philadelphia: JB Lippincott, 1991.

21

Injuries of the Pelvis and Hip

Edward P. Sloan
Russell H. Greenfield

HIGH-YIELD FACTS

- Unstable pelvic fractures are present when there are multiple breaks in the pelvic ring. Suspect visceral injuries due to high-kinetic energy trauma.

- An anteroposterior pelvis radiograph and a pelvic CT scan are the best tests for determining the extent of injury when pelvic fractures are present.

- The most common hip dislocation is posterior.

- Reduction of a hip dislocation should take place prior to 12 hours after the injury. Complications include avascular necrosis of the femoral head, degenerative arthritis, and sciatic nerve injury.

- Hip fractures involve either the epiphysis (transepiphyseal) or the femoral neck and trochanters (cervicotrochanteric).

- Slipped capital femoral epiphysis is a disruption of the capital femoral physis that can occur over time. It is most common in overweight adolescent males and is diagnosed on the anteroposterior or frog-leg view of the pelvis.

- Legg-Calvé-Perthes disease is an idiopathic avascular necrosis of the femoral head that is most common in Caucasian children between 4 and 9 years of age. Radiographs demonstrate a small femoral head and epiphyseal collapse as a result of avascular necrosis.

- Femur fractures are common, with peak incidence at the age of 3 years. The most commonly fractured portion of the femoral shaft is the middle third.

- A spiral femur fracture in a nonambulatory infant or child suggests child abuse.

- Distal femoral epiphyseal fractures in children are significant because they can cause growth disturbances in the lower extremity.

PELVIC FRACTURES

The pelvis in the growing child is more elastic and pliable than in the adult, allowing significant displacement to occur without causing a fracture. There are three ossification sites in the pelvis that meet at the acetabulum and form the triradiate cartilage, which itself can be disrupted with pelvic trauma.

Isolated or single breaks in the pelvic ring are considered stable pelvic fractures. Although common in osteoporotic elderly adults, these injuries are relatively uncommon in children. High-kinetic energy trauma, such as is seen in motor vehicle crashes or pedestrian accidents, can cause multiple disruptions in the pelvic ring to occur, rendering the pelvis unstable. Multiple breaks in the pelvic ring can exist as bilateral pubic rami fractures, which cause a free-floating pubis (Fig. 21-1). An unstable pelvis also is seen with a vertical double break in the pelvic ring, which is termed a Malgaigne fracture. This injury involves both a disruption of the pubis anteriorly and the sacroiliac joint posteriorly. These trauma mechanisms can also cause isolated sacral fractures to occur without a disruption of the sacroiliac joint or the other bones of the pelvis.

Compression injuries to the pelvis can cause acetabular fractures or injury to the triradiate cartilage. These injuries are relatively rare, and are often seen in association with hip dislocations. When this occurs, growth arrest can occur, causing the formation of a shallow, dysplastic acetabulum (Fig. 21-2). Avulsion fractures of the pelvis often occur as a result of muscle traction stress in adolescent athletes. These fractures are usually caused by the strong contraction of the sartorius and hamstring muscles, which results in damage to the anterior superior and inferior iliac spines or ischial tuberosity. These are stable injuries that can be managed conservatively.

The examination of a child with a possible pelvic fracture includes direct observation of the pelvis for areas of ecchymosis and swelling. The pelvis can be stressed by pressing posteriorly on the iliac crests and by applying direct pressure on the symphysis pubis. When pain, crepitus, or movement of the pelvic ring in noted, then a pelvic fracture should be suspected. The pelvis should

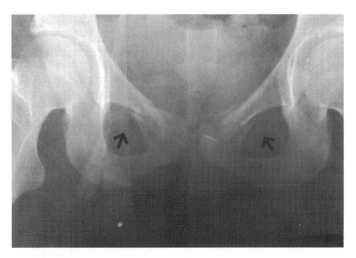

Fig. 21-1. Bilateral superior pubic rami fractures. Associated injury to the bladder and urethra should be suspected.

also be palpated for point tenderness when an avulsion fracture is suspected. In the setting of multiple blunt trauma with a suspected unstable pelvic fracture, not only must the pelvis fracture be addressed, but also the evaluation and diagnosis of blunt injury to the pelvic viscera must be completed. This includes a careful examination of the abdomen, rectum, and vagina. In most cases, an anteroposterior (AP) pelvis radiograph is adequate to diagnose pelvic fractures. The pelvic CT scan will further identify the full extent of the boney injury and the status of the pelvic viscera.

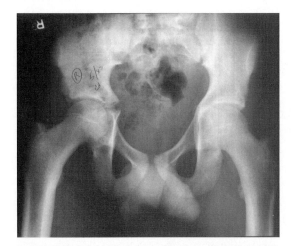

Fig. 21-2. Fracture through the triradiate cartilage of the right acetabulum. Growth arrest is a common complication of this type of injury.

HIP DISLOCATIONS AND FRACTURES

When the pediatric patient presents with hip pain when no apparent trauma has occurred, diagnoses such as transient synovitis and septic arthritis of the hip should be considered, as well as Legg-Calvé-Perthes disease (LCPD) and slipped capital femoral epiphysis (SCFE). In the setting of trauma, hip dislocations and fractures should be considered.

Hip dislocations most often occur in the setting of high-kinetic energy trauma but can occasionally occur as a result of less severe trauma, as is seen with a fall. The hip most commonly dislocates posteriorly, with the leg held flexed and internally rotated at the hip. Anterior hip dislocations are less common, and cause the leg to be flexed and externally rotated. Central hip dislocations cause the femoral head to protrude through the acetabulum into the pelvis such that no rotational deformity is noted on physical examination. In all of these dislocations, there will be significant pain and a marked reduction in the affected hip's range of motion. With all hip dislocations, there is a significant risk that the acetabulum will also be fractured. Because of this risk, a CT scan of the hip and pelvis should be obtained in addition to plain radiographs.

Hip dislocations can cause several complications, including recurrent dislocations, avascular necrosis of the femoral head, degenerative arthritis, and sciatic nerve injury. Hip dislocations and recurrent dislocations can occur because of the pliable nature of the acetabular cartilage and the ligamentous laxity seen in children. Avascular necrosis occurs in up to 10 percent of patients with a traumatic hip dislocation, even when reduction occurs quickly and without acute complication. When closed reduction is delayed greater than 12 hours, the risk of avascular necrosis is increased. When the dislocation causes the acetabulum to be disrupted, joint instability can occur such that operative intervention is required. Surgical intervention is also required if boney fragments are present in the joint post-reduction because these fragments will cause degenerative arthritis. Hip dislocations can also cause the sciatic nerve to be injured. In this case, prompt reduction is required.

Although rare, hip fractures are important because they often can cause avascular necrosis, premature closure of the physis, and resultant shortening and angulation of the lower extremity. Fractures of the hip can involve either the epiphysis (transepiphyseal) or the femoral neck and trochanters (cervicotrochanteric). Transepiphyseal fractures occur often in patients with preexisting SCFE. Cervicotrochanteric fractures can occur in the femoral neck or in the intertrochanteric region of the hip. Depending on the location of the fracture and the amount of displacement of the fracture fragments, open reduction and internal fixation is often required to prevent avascular necrosis and to achieve adequate healing.

SLIPPED CAPITAL FEMORAL EPIPHYSIS

Slipped capital femoral epiphysis (SCFE) is a disruption of the capital femoral physis, similar to the type of injury seen with a transepiphyseal fracture. Unlike the transepiphyseal fracture, which is caused by high-kinetic energy trauma, SCFE is a condition that can occur over time through repeated minor injury and slippage of the femur superiorly and in the anterolateral direction away from the epiphysis.

Although SCFE is more common in adolescent males and in those who are overweight, it can occur in rapidly growing adolescents who are tall and thin. When the symptoms have been present for <3 weeks, the SCFE is considered acute; otherwise, the SCFE is considered chronic. Children may present with a limp and hip pain that radiates to the groin, thigh, or knee. The physical examination may reveal hip tenderness, and possibly will demonstrate limited internal rotation and flexion as well as shortening of the extremity.

Laboratory testing is usually noncontributory to the diagnosis of SCFE. Radiographic studies should include an AP radiograph of the pelvis, lateral hip views, and a frog-leg view of the pelvis. If there is irregular widening of the epiphyseal line or asymmetry between the affected and normal hip, then SCFE should be considered. On the AP or frog-leg view of the pelvis, a line drawn along the superior edge of the femoral neck should transect at least 20 to 25 percent of the epiphysis. When a SCFE is present, this line will no longer pass through the epiphysis as a result of the movement of the femoral neck in the superior and lateral direction relative to the epiphysis (Fig. 21-3). The SCFE is considered to be severe if the amount of slippage is noted to be >50 percent of the metaphyseal width. Because SCFE is bilateral in up to one third of children, a careful examination of the unaffected hip should occur at the time of

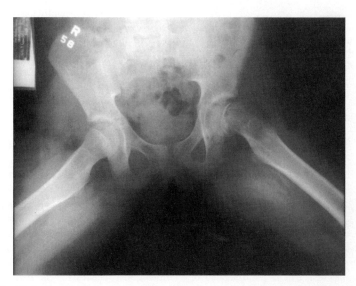

Fig. 21-3. Frog-leg view of the pelvis revealing a slipped left femoral capital epiphysis.

the physical examination and upon review of the radiographs.

When a SCFE is noted, the patient should be discharged with crutches and absolute non–weight-bearing with close orthopedic follow-up. In cases where the slip is acute, the slippage severe, and the pain refractory to therapies, hospital admission may be warranted because operative intervention may be required to optimize patient outcome. SCFE can be complicated by avascular necrosis, early closure of the physis, and degenerative arthritis of the hip.

LEGG-CALVÉ-PERTHES DISEASE

Legg-Calvé-Perthes disease is an idiopathic avascular necrosis of the femoral head. It is more common in boys, with a peak incidence between the ages of 4 and 9 years, with a greater incidence in Caucasian children. It is thought to occur as a result of a thrombotic disorder that causes repeated bone infarction and resorption.

Patients with LCPD may present with a limp, pain in the hip or knee, and limited hip internal rotation and abduction. The pain is often exacerbated by strenuous exercise. As with SCFE, laboratory testing is noncontributory. Radiographic studies, again, should include an AP radiograph of the pelvis, lateral hip views, and a

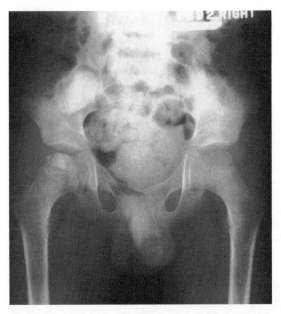

Fig. 21-4. Legg-Calvé-Perthes disease of the left femoral head.

frog-leg view of the pelvis. The radiographs may show a small femoral head, a widened medial joint space, and evidence of epiphyseal collapse as a result of avascular necrosis. If LCPD is suspected and the plain radiographs are normal, a bone scan or MRI should be ordered in follow-up to assist in making the diagnosis (Fig. 21-4). Bilateral hip involvement can occur in up to 15 percent of children.

Treatment should include no weight bearing, crutches, NSAIDs, and close orthopedic follow-up. Parents should be warned that the return to normal activities can be variable, and that some children limp for many years as a result of the LCPD.

FEMUR FRACTURES

Pediatric femur fractures are common, peaking at 3 years of age. Femur fractures can occur as a result of birth trauma, underlying bone pathology, or as a result of child abuse. Abuse should be suspected in the presence of a spiral femur fracture, especially in the nonambulatory child. These spiral fractures often can present without significant swelling, such that the only clue to the injury is the patient's refusal to bear weight on the affected extremity. In older children and adolescents, femur fractures occur more commonly as a result of high-kinetic energy vehicular trauma. Because a significant amount of force is required to fracture the femur, associated injuries should be excluded by a careful physical examination.

The most commonly fractured portion of the femur is the femoral shaft, especially the middle third. Other fractures are considered subtrochanteric, supracondylar, epiphyseal, or shaft fractures involving the proximal or distal thirds of the femur. Although fractures of the femoral shaft cause significant hemorrhage, a unilateral femur fracture most often does not cause marked hypotension. The examination of the affected extremity should exclude an ipsilateral hip dislocation.

Patients with femoral shaft fractures should be admitted for pain control and casting or skeletal traction. In older children, as in adults, when the fracture fragments are displaced and angulated, plates and/or intermedullary rods are sometimes needed to achieve adequate reduction.

Distal femoral epiphyseal fractures are not as common as epiphyseal fractures in other parts of the body, but the incidence of growth disturbance after this injury is high. Premature closure of the epiphysis can have serious consequences for the pediatric patient, since almost 65 percent of the longitudinal growth of the lower extremity can be traced to this growth area. Salter-Harris type II fractures of the distal femoral epiphysis occur most often, usually in older children, and normally heal without complication. Salter-Harris III and IV injuries are uncommon in the distal femoral epiphysis, but when present, require operative intervention to achieve exact anatomic reduction. Salter-Harris V distal femur fractures are usually diagnosed in retrospect when growth disturbances are detected in the injured lower extremity.

Hospital admission is most often required for pain control, to mandate no weight bearing, and to facilitate immediate orthopedic consultation. Complications associated with distal femoral epiphyseal injuries include growth arrest, vascular compromise, peroneal nerve palsy, and recurrent displacement, such that long-term orthopedic follow-up is required for these patients.

BIBLIOGRAPHY

Bachman D, Santora S: Orthopedic trauma, in Fleisher GR, Ludwig S, Henretig FM, et al (eds): *Textbook of Pediatric Emergency Medicine,* 4th ed. Philadelphia: Lippincott Williams & Wilkins, 2000, pp 1435–1478.

Della-Giustina K, Della-Giustina DA: Emergency department evaluation and treatment of pediatric orthopedic injuries. *Emerg Med Clin North Am* 1999;895–922.

Hayes O: Pelvic and lower extremity injuries, in Reisdorff EJ, Roberts MR, Weigenstein JG (eds): *Pediatric Emergency Medicine.* Philadelphia: Saunders, 1992, pp 961–973.

Kehl DK: Slipped capital femoral epiphysis, in Morrisey RT, Weinstein SL (eds): *Lovell and Winter's Pediatric Orthopedics,* 5th ed. Philadelphia: Lippincott Williams & Wilkins, 2001, pp 999–1034.

Loder RT, Aronson DD, Greenfield ML: The epidemiology of bilateral slipped capital femoral epiphysis. *J Bone Joint Surg* 1993;1141–1147.

Offierski CM: Traumatic dislocation of the hip in children. *J Bone Joint Surg* 1981;194–197.

Ogden JA: Injury to the immature skeleton, in Touloukian RJ (ed): *Pediatric Trauma.* St. Louis: Mosby-Yearbook, 1990, pp 415–417.

Quintana EC, Friedman M, Selbst SM: Pitfall in pediatric emergency medicine. *Foresight: Risk Management for Emergency Physicians* 2001;1–3.

Rockwood CA, Wilkins KE, Beaty JH (eds): *Fractures in Children,* 5th ed. Philadelphia: Lippincott Williams & Wilkins, 2001.

Weinstein SL: Legg-Calvé-Perthes syndrome, in Morrisey RT, Weinstein SL (eds): *Lovell and Winter's Pediatric Orthopedics,* 5th ed. Philadelphia: Lippincott Williams & Wilkins, 2001, pp 957–998.

22

Injuries of the Lower Extremities

Edward P. Sloan
Russell H. Greenfield

HIGH-YIELD FACTS

- Ligamentous injuries of the knee are less likely to occur than are epiphyseal injuries. Distal femoral epiphyseal fractures are common, as are avulsion fractures of the tibial spines.

- Osgood-Schlatter disease, also known as traumatic tibial apophysitis, is inflammation and pain due to avulsions at the tibial tuberosity. This painful condition can be managed conservatively in most cases.

- Proximal tibial epiphysis fractures can be significant because they can cause vascular compromise and growth disturbances.

- Spiral tibial shaft fractures are common in children due to twisting injuries and are termed toddler's fracture in those just learning to walk.

- Fibular head fractures can occur as a result of motor vehicle bumper injury in children. In order to exclude a significant peroneal nerve injury, it must be shown that there is no foot drop of the affected extremity (loss of dorsiflexion).

- When examining the child with ankle pain, it is necessary to exclude injuries of the calcaneus, proximal fibula, and base of the fifth metatarsal because these injuries can cause pain similar to that seen with an ankle sprain.

- The most common fracture of the talus is in the neck, which occurs due to forced dorsiflexion. This injury is often complicated by avascular necrosis.

- Bohler's angle may not be as useful in children as in adults in detecting a

calcaneus fracture. When a calcaneus fracture is found, associated injuries, such as lumbar spine, contralateral calcaneus fractures, and renal pedicle disruptions, are less common in children than in adults.

- Midfoot fractures are rare due to the strong fibrous tissues that surround these bones, and are difficult to detect because of the irregularities of these bones. Lisfranc's fracture occurs at the base of the second metatarsal, where the stability of the midfoot is maintained.

- The Jones' fracture is a metatarsal neck fracture distal to the apophysis of the base of the fifth metatarsal. Although the apophysis of the fifth metatarsal runs parallel to the axis of the metatarsal shaft, fractures most often are perpendicular to the axis of the metatarsal shaft.

KNEE AND PATELLAR FRACTURES

Significant knee injuries in children most often result in fractures, as opposed to isolated ligamentous sprains. This is because the knee ligaments have a greater tensile strength than do the epiphyseal growth plates and cartilage. Thus, the same mechanism of injury resulting in a knee ligament disruption in an adult causes an epiphyseal fracture in children whose bones are still growing (generally up to 14 to 16 years of age). Pediatric ligamentous injuries do occur, however, often in conjunction with fractures of the adjacent bones. Avulsion of the intercondylar eminence of the tibia (tibial spine) in children is analogous to anterior cruciate disruption in adults. Also, injury to the knee's medial and lateral collateral ligaments is frequently associated with a fracture of the distal femoral epiphysis. Distal femoral epiphyseal fractures, which are important because of the significant lower extremity growth that occurs in this growth plate, are discussed in Chap. 21.

The presence of a thick cartilage surrounding the osseous center of the patella accounts for the rarity of childhood patellar fractures. Avulsion fractures of the superior or inferior pole of the patella can occur, and may disrupt the extensor mechanism of the knee. Similarly, transverse patellar fractures that require operative intervention occur relatively infrequently. A bipartite patella, which occurs bilaterally in up to 40 percent of children, will demonstrate smooth, contoured boney segments in the superior-lateral portion of the patella.

Knee dislocations are also extremely rare in children, but when they do occur, there are often associated extremity fractures and neurovascular disruption. Floating knee describes the occurrence of both distal femur and proximal tibia-fibular fractures, as is seen when an automobile bumper strikes a child.

When examining the child with a potential knee injury, the emergency physician should consider the possibility of distal femur and femoral epiphyseal fractures, tibial spine and tuberosity avulsions, patellar fracture, fractures of the proximal tibia and tibial epiphysis, and fibular head fracture. The physical examination of the knee should include the following assessments:

- Gross alignment of the knee
- Areas of ecchymosis
- Areas of point tenderness
- Range of motion
- Joint line tenderness
- Traumatic knee effusion
- Ligamentous laxity
- Competence of the extensor mechanism
- Adequacy of distal neurovascular function

OSGOOD-SCHLATTER DISEASE

Osgood-Schlatter disease, also known as traumatic tibial apophysitis, is inflammation and pain due to the avulsion of the chondral portion of the tibial tuberosity. It is thought to be secondary to repeated forceful use of the quadriceps muscle and the knee's extensor mechanism. It is usually seen in physically active teenagers, especially boys between the ages of 14 and 16 years. It occurs bilaterally in up to 25 percent of patients. Patients often complain of pain below the knee exacerbated by physical activity and kneeling. The physical examination reveals tenderness and, possibly, swelling over the tibial tuberosity. The knee radiograph may reveal irregularity or prominence of the tibial tuberosity. Management consists of temporary restriction of activity and relief of pain with nonsteroidal antiinflammatory drugs (NSAIDs), given that this problem is usually self-limited. Rarely, a retained ossicle within the patellar tendon can cause discomfort in adulthood and require surgical excision.

PROXIMAL TIBIA AND TIBIAL SHAFT FRACTURES

The proximal tibial epiphysis is more resistant to injury than the distal femoral epiphysis, making injury to this tibial structure less common when knee trauma occurs. Injuries to this structure and to the proximal tibial metaphysis can occur, however, due to twisting injury in children up to 8 years of age, and due to motor vehicle bumper injuries in older children and adolescents (Fig. 22-1). Because the popliteal neurovascular bundle courses just behind the proximal tibia, posterior displacement of the fracture fragments can cause vascular compromise and/or thrombosis. Significant fracture of the proximal tibia can also cause limb growth disturbances and compartment syndrome, the latter of which occurs due to the interosseous membrane and the other strong fibrous sheaths in the lower extremity.

Tibial diaphysis (shaft) fractures occur commonly in children. Spiral fracture of the tibial shaft in infants and young children due to twisting injury is termed a toddler's

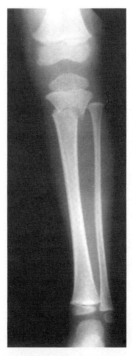

Fig. 22-1. This patient suffered a fracture of the proximal tibial metaphysis after being struck by a car. Complications associated with this injury include damage to the posterior tibial artery and the development of a valgus deformity.

fracture. Motor vehicle bumper trauma more often causes transverse tibial shaft injuries, and may also cause the formation of a butterfly fragment when multiple fractures occur. Stress fractures of the tibial shaft also occur in children, causing pain in the proximal tibial shaft. These children may not recall any acute trauma, but often have recently begun to participate in a new or rigorous activity. Radiographs may reveal a radiolucent line and periosteal reaction of the tibial shaft. Because other diagnoses, such as osteogenic sarcoma and osteomyelitis, must be excluded when this finding is seen, orthopedic consultation is advised when making the diagnosis of a tibial stress fracture.

PROXIMAL FIBULA AND FIBULAR SHAFT FRACTURES

As with the tibia, proximal and fibular shaft fractures occur in younger children due to twisting injuries and, in older children and adolescents, due to motor vehicle trauma. When the fibular head is fractured, injury to the peroneal nerve must be considered. In children with automobile bumper–induced fracture of the proximal fibula, assessment for the presence of foot drop is essential to evaluate for this complication.

Fracture of the fibular shaft can also occur as a result of injury to the ankle. As with the Maisonneuve fracture in adults, a fibular shaft fracture can occur in children as a result of disruption of the distal tibial epiphysis. This occurs when lateral movement of the distal tibial epiphysis causes disruption of the interosseous membrane and an oblique fibular fracture proximal to the ankle mortise. Therefore, children with a significant ankle injury should be examined for proximal fibula tenderness to exclude this type of fibular shaft injury.

ANKLE FRACTURES

Three bones form the ankle joint:

- The weight-bearing distal tibia
- The non–weight-bearing fibula
- The talus, the most proximal tarsal bone

The mechanisms that cause ankle injury in children are similar to those seen in adults. In children, however, the strength of the ankle ligaments makes injury to the distal tibial and fibular epiphysis more likely than a ligamentous disruption. In fact, disruptions of the growth plates of the distal tibia and fibula account for up to 25

percent of all physeal injuries, second only to distal radius physeal injuries.

Medial ankle injuries occur as a result of foot pronation, forced eversion, and external rotation. The distal tibia epiphysis is the weakest structure in the ankle, and Salter-Harris type II fractures of the distal tibia are common (Fig. 22-2). Distal tibial epiphysis disruption, especially Salter-Harris type III and IV fractures, often is complicated by growth arrest. The triplane fracture is a type IV fracture that has multiple tibial epiphysis and metaphysis fragments, requiring operative intervention to assure an optimal outcome.

Supination with forced foot inversion and external rotation cause injury to the lateral ankle structures. Although distal fibular Salter-Harris type I and II fractures can occur, fibular type II and IV fractures generally do not occur. On occasion, the talofibular ligament can cause a fracture of the distal fibular epiphysis, an injury that can be treated as an ankle sprain when seen in isolation.

The physical examination of a child with an ankle injury should also include palpation of the base of the fifth metatarsal, the calcaneus, and the proximal fibula, since

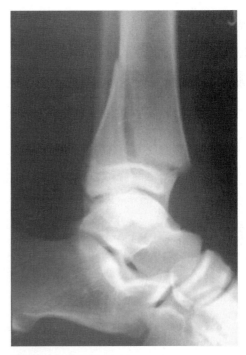

Fig. 22-2. Salter-Harris type II fracture of the distal tibia. An associated greenstick fracture of the fibula commonly occurs with this injury.

all of these structures can be fractured and cause pain suggestive of an ankle injury. The radiographic evaluation of the ankle includes three views:

- Anteroposterior (AP)
- Lateral
- Mortise

The lateral view allows the posterior malleolus, the talus, calcaneus, and the base of the fifth metatarsal to be visualized. On the mortise view, a uniform 3- to 4-mm space between the tibia, talus, and fibula should be visualized as an indication of a stable ankle mortise.

In managing pediatric ankle injuries, it is best to assume a Salter-Harris type I or V injury when the physis is noted to be tender to palpation. Salter-Harris type II to IV injuries, especially those that cause ankle mortise disruption, should be managed aggressively with orthopedic consultation because complications, such as growth arrest, can be seen. In ankle fracture-dislocations in children, unlike in adults, the ankle mortise remains intact and instead, there is displacement of the tibial epiphyseal plate. Forced reduction of the dislocated epiphyseal plate can cause the growth plate germinal layer to be damaged by the fracture fragments. As such, it is only necessary to provide an anatomic reduction with gentle traction if there is vascular compromise or an inability to stabilize the ankle. Otherwise, the reduction can take place after admission for orthopedic repair.

FOOT FRACTURES

Most pediatric foot fractures involve the forefoot and occur due to falls, crush injuries, or lawnmower injuries. The cartilaginous composition of the tarsal bones early in life accounts for their flexibility and the relative paucity of pediatric hindfoot fractures.

The talus is most commonly fractured in its neck due to forced dorsiflexion, which happens in adults with braking in a high-speed motor vehicle crash (Fig. 22-3). Although talus fractures are rare in children, they are important because they are often complicated by avascular necrosis. When talus fractures occur, the ankle should be splinted in plantar flexion, and orthopedic consultation obtained. Transchondral fractures, which occur at the cartilaginous surface of the talar dome, can occur in older children. The clinician must always look at the talar dome on the mortise view to detect irregularities suggestive of a transchondral fracture because chronic pain and arthritis can result from this injury.

Although the calcaneus is the most commonly fractured tarsal, it is injured in children only rarely because

TALAR FRACTURES

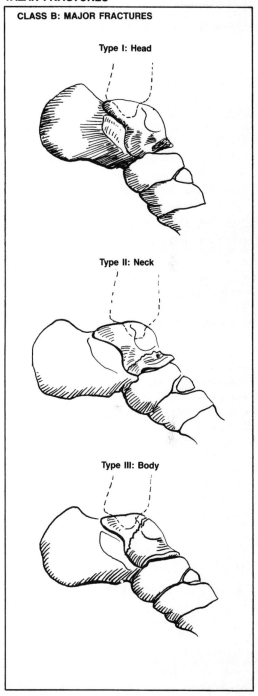

CLASS B: MAJOR FRACTURES

Type I: Head

Type II: Neck

Type III: Body

Fig. 22-3. Talus neck fracture in a child. (Used with permission from King RE, Powell DF: Injury to the talus. In: Jahss MH (ed): *Disorders of the Foot and Ankle,* 2d ed, Philadelphia: Saunders, 1991, p 2308.)

of the elasticity of the tissues that surround it. A fall with a direct load is the most common mechanism (Fig. 22-4). There are three significant differences in pediatric calcaneal injuries as compared with adults. First, Bohler's angle is unreliable in detecting injury in young children because the angle is normally found in nonadolescent children. Second, because comminution occurs less commonly in children, nonoperative therapy is more often successful. Finally, concomitant injury of the lumbar spine, renal pedicle, and contralateral calcaneus are less common in children than in adults.

Fractures of the cuboid, navicular, and cuneiforms usually result from direct trauma to the midfoot. Irregularities of these bones during growth make fracture exclusion difficult, but conservative management usually is effective for such hard to detect injuries. Tarsometatarsal (Lisfranc's joint) fractures can occur as a result of direct trauma, but they usually occur as a result of forced abduction and plantar flexion, as is seen with jumping from the tiptoe position (Fig. 22-5). To exclude this injury, the clinician must make sure that there is no fracture at the base of the second metatarsal, which is firmly anchored by strong interosseous ligaments in a recess next to the first metatarsal. If a fracture is noted in this location, then the other metatarsal bases should be examined for displaced fractures. Orthopedic consultation is indicated for a Lisfranc's fracture because vascular compromise and the need for operative intervention both can complicate this fracture.

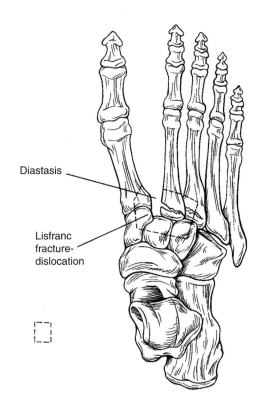

Fig. 22-5. Lisfranc's dislocation of the second metatarsal. (Used with permission from Ogden JA: *Skeletal Injury in the Child,* 2d ed, Philadelphia: Saunders, 1990, p 887.)

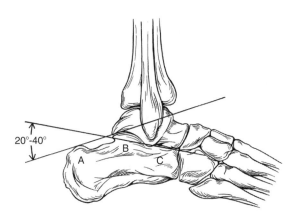

Fig. 22-4. Angles used to assess the calcaneus. *A.* Bohler's angle *B.* Calcaneus pitch. (Used with permission from Shereff MT: Radiographic analysis of the foot and ankle. In: Jahss MH (ed): *Disorders of the Foot and Ankle,* 2d ed, Philadelphia: Saunders, 1991, p 104.)

Metatarsal shaft fractures can occur as a result of direct trauma, twisting force, or axial load on the foot. Metatarsal stress fractures are rare, but can occur in children. Crush injuries that cause multiple metatarsal fractures should be managed conservatively because a compartment syndrome of the foot can occur with multiple fractures and the soft tissue injury. The Jones' fracture is a metatarsal neck fracture that is distal to the apophysis at the base of the fifth metatarsal, which is visible between 8 and 15 years of age. Both the Jones' fracture and avulsion fractures of the metatarsal are transverse in their orientation, whereas the apophysis is oriented parallel to the long axis of the metatarsal (Fig. 22-6).

Phalangeal injuries in children occur due to direct trauma and with the axial loading that can occur with kicking. Once rotational deformity has been excluded, buddy taping the affected toe to the next toe can effectively manage most of these injuries. Phalangeal fractures that occur as a result of the foot being stuck in the spokes of a bicycle wheel are important because of the soft tis-

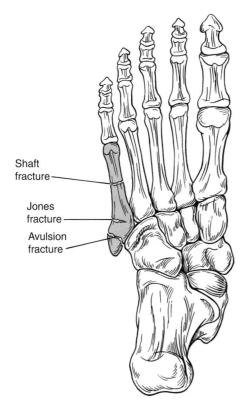

Shaft
fracture

Jones
fracture

Avulsion
fracture

Fig. 22-6. Displaced fracture of the base of the fifth metatarsal in an adolescent. Note that the apophysis is not united. Also, note that the fracture is perpendicular to the metatarsal shaft, and that the apophysis is parallel to the long axis of the metatarsal shaft. (Used with permission from Harris JH, Harris WH, Novelline RA: *The Radiology of Emergency Medicine,* 3d ed, Baltimore: Williams & Wilkins, 1993, p 1032.)

sue trauma that accompanies the fractures, as with a washing machine wringer injury. Neurovascular compromise must be excluded and skin integrity confirmed. Finally, because lawnmower phalangeal injuries in children cause significant morbidity, small children should not ride with parents on a riding mower, nor should teenagers use a walking mower without adequate foot protection.

BIBLIOGRAPHY

Bachman D, Santora S: Orthopedic trauma, in Fleisher GR, Ludwig S, Henretig FM, et al (eds): *Textbook of Pediatric Emergency Medicine,* 4th ed. Philadelphia: Lippincott Williams & Wilkins, 2000, pp 1435–1478.

Della-Giustina K, Della-Giustina DA: Emergency department evaluation and treatment of pediatric orthopedic injuries. *Emerg Med Clin North Am* 1999;17:895–922.

Hayes O: Pelvic and lower extremity injuries, in Reisdorff EJ, Roberts MR, Weigenstein JG (eds): *Pediatric Emergency Medicine.* Philadelphia: Saunders, 1992, pp 961–973.

Mellick LB, Reesor K: Spiral tibial fractures of children: A commonly accidental spiral long bone fracture. *Am J Emerg Med* 1990;8:234–237.

Ogden JA: Injury to the immature skeleton, in Touloukian RJ (ed): *Pediatric Trauma.* St. Louis: Mosby-Yearbook, 1990, pp 415–417.

Rockwood CA, Wilkins KE, Beaty JH (eds): *Fractures in Children,* 5th ed. Philadelphia: Lippincott Williams & Wilkins, 2001.

Sloan EP, Rittenberry TJ: Ankle and foot injuries, in Reisdorff EJ, Roberts MR, Weigenstein JG (eds): *Pediatric Emergency Medicine.* Philadelphia: Saunders, 1993, pp 974–982.

Tenenbein M, Reed MH, Black GB: The toddler's fracture revisited. *Am J Emerg Med* 1990;8:208–211.

23

Soft Tissue Injury and Wound Repair

Jordan D. Lipton

HIGH-YIELD FACTS

- In assessing a child with a minor wound, exclude more serious, sometimes occult, injuries that take precedence in management.

- Always consider nonaccidental trauma, especially when the history and the injury are inconsistent.

- Physical examination of the wound must assess the length and depth of the injury, circulatory status, motor and sensory function, the presence of foreign bodies and contaminants, and the involvement of underlying structures.

- Topical lidocaine-adrenaline-tetracaine (LAT) has been shown to provide effective anesthesia for pediatric facial and scalp lacerations. Use of LAT compares favorably with topical tetracaine-adrenaline-cocaine without the risks and administrative complications of cocaine.

- Irrigation with 5 to 8 psi of normal saline is the method of choice for removing bacteria and debris from most wounds. Low-pressure irrigation with a bulb syringe does not adequately remove bacteria and debris.

- Sharp lacerations of the scalp, trunk, and extremities are rapidly and effectively closed using staples, which induce minimal inflammatory reaction and produce similar cosmetic results to suturing.

- Splint a wound overlying a joint in the position of function for 7 to 10 days.

- Antibiotics are indicated for patients with simple wounds who are prone to infective endocarditis, who have orthopedic prostheses, who have immune-compromising disease, or who present with a wound infection due to inappropriate care at home or with wounds that are more than 12 to 24 hours old. Other indications for antibiotics are for wounds contaminated with feces or saliva, extensive intraoral lacerations, mammalian bites, and any wounds in which there is involvement of cartilage, joint spaces, tendon, or bone.

- Outcome is dependent on wound care after discharge from the ED, so the patient and parents should be given thorough instructions about care of the wound and what to expect. They should be informed that all significant wounds heal with scars, regardless of the quality of care.

Minor trauma and soft tissue injuries are some of the most common reasons for children to present to the emergency department (ED). Despite the frequency of such encounters, they can be terrifying for both the child and parent, and there is great variability in each physician-patient encounter. To maximize cosmetic and functional results, it is important to ensure meticulous wound care and repair, which is simpler when dealing with a calm child. Therefore, overcoming a child's fear and anxiety is a necessary component of wound care.

SKIN AND SOFT TISSUE ANATOMY AND BIOMECHANICS

The skin is composed of the dermis, which provides most of the skin's tensile strength, and the epidermis, which protects the dermis from infection and desiccation. Dermal capillaries are fed by the nutrient vessels of the skin, and the epidermis, which has no blood supply, is fed by diffusion of nutrients from the dermis. The subcutaneous tissue beneath the dermis is composed of loose connective and adipose tissue, large vessels, and nerves.

The appearance and function of a healed wound can be predicted by the magnitude of the tension on the surrounding skin, but there is great intra- and interindividual variability. The most cosmetically pleasing scar results when the long axis of the wound is in the direction of maximal static skin tension, along "Langer's lines" (Fig. 23-1). Examination of the wound in the ED is a reliable method to predict the appearance of the healed wound in the absence of confounding variables, such as

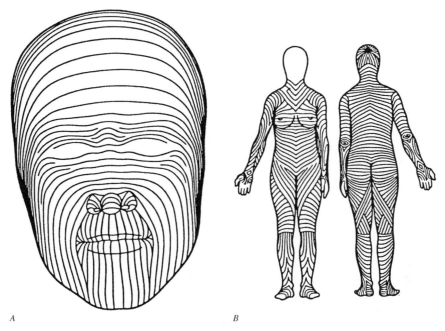

A *B*

Fig. 23-1. Lines of skin tension

the development of wound infection or keloid. Wounds with marked retraction of their edges (≥5 mm) are more likely to heal with wider scars than those with minimal retraction (<5 mm). Dynamic skin tension (caused by joint movements and muscle contraction) also have an impact on the degree of scar formation and postrepair function. A wound intersecting the transverse axis of a joint can result in a significant contracture, since scars do not have the elasticity of uninjured tissue.

Unfortunately, soft tissue wounds often have axes that are perpendicular to the direction of static skin tension or parallel to the dynamic skin tension. Therefore, it is always essential to warn the child and parent of possible adverse cosmetic outcomes, and in some cases referral to a plastic surgeon for follow-up is recommended.

CLASSIFICATION OF MINOR INJURIES

Lacerations

Lacerations are cuts through the skin and, after contusions, are the most common type of soft tissue injury seen in the ED. Lacerations that involve the dermal capillaries bleed and those through the subcutaneous fat produce gaping wounds. The face, scalp, and hands are the most common sites of injury in the pediatric age group. Lacerations generally require more complicated treatment than other minor wounds. Much of this chapter deals with the assessment and treatment of lacerations. All lacerations can be associated with occult injuries and require thorough exploration to detect deeper injuries. The three main classes of lacerations are shear, tension, and compression.

Shear injuries are caused by sharp objects and generally cause little damage to adjacent tissues but can cause nerve, tendon, and vascular damage. Shears usually heal fastest and have the lowest incidence of wound infection.

Tension lacerations occur when stresses cause the skin to tear. There is often associated damage to the surrounding tissues, and these lacerations are irregularly shaped.

Compression lacerations occur during a crush injury and have irregular, often stellate, wound edges. They are often associated with a significant amount of injury to the adjacent skin, they heal most poorly, and they have a higher incidence of wound infection than other types of lacerations.

Abrasions

Abrasions are injuries in which layers of the skin are scraped or sheared away. In superficial abrasions, only the cornified epidermis is removed, there is little or no bleeding, and healing is rapid. Deeper abrasions involving the dermis are prone to bleed and are more susceptible to infection, tattooing, foreign body retention, and other complications.

Contusions and Hematomas

Contusions are the result of crush injuries that produce direct injury to tissues and often injure vessels and nerves. Localized bleeding and edema from increased capillary permeability can cause swelling and pain in the injured area, and on occasion, can result in secondary ischemic injuries. Management of all types of contusions involves elevation of the injured area, application of ice packs intermittently for the first 24 to 48 hours, and careful monitoring of circulation and neurologic function.

Hematomas are localized collections of extravasated blood that are relatively or completely confined within a space or potential space. Hematomas can be associated with most types of minor and major wounds; they must be observed closely for signs of infection and, in some instances, drained.

PREHOSPITAL CARE

Prehospital care of minor wounds, as for all emergencies, includes initial attention to the ABCs (airway, breathing, and circulation). This includes control of bleeding, which can almost always be accomplished by direct manual pressure or use of a pressure dressing. If bleeding is not controlled with these methods, inflation of a sphygmomanometer proximal to the bleeding site on an injured extremity can be safely employed even for prolonged (at least 2 hours) transport times. Always note neurovascular status distal to the injury and assess for associated injuries, prior to nonemergent interventions.

HISTORY AND PHYSICAL EXAMINATION

In assessing a child with a minor wound, first exclude more serious, sometimes occult injuries that will take precedence in management. The history of the injury should include whether the inciting force was blunt or sharp, the time and mechanism of the injury, whether there are other injured areas, and whether there are any possible contaminants or foreign bodies in the wound. Other important information to elicit is the child's tetanus immunization status, whether the child has any medical problems or allergies, any medications that the child takes, and what wound care was received prior to arrival in the ED. Always consider nonaccidental trauma, especially when the history and the injury are inconsistent.

Physical examination of the wound must assess the length and depth of the injury, circulatory status, motor and sensory function, the presence of foreign bodies and contaminants, and the involvement of underlying structures (nerves, tendons, muscles, ligaments, vessels, bones, joints, and ducts). Whereas the sensory-motor examination must precede the administration of anesthesia, the remainder of the examination should rarely be performed without adequate anesthesia. To avoid terror in the child, anxiety in the parents, and frustration for everybody else, use a calm, unhurried, reassuring, and honest approach throughout the evaluation and management.

Test sensation by measurement of two-point discrimination distal to an injury. For children younger than 5 years, use a noxious stimulus, such as a pinprick, to provide a sensory and a partial motor assessment. Since normal autonomic tone produces a degree of normal sweating, denervated fingers do not sweat, which provides a clue to injury. One can use an ophthalmoscope to look for beads of sweat on the involved finger. Evaluate circulation by palpation of peripheral pulses and skin temperature, observation of skin color, and rapidity of capillary refill. Test tendons, muscles, and ligaments distal to an injury, paying special attention to hand and forearm injuries. With cooperative older children, it is possible to test these structures' functions individually; however, with younger, less cooperative children, one must rely on observation of posture, symmetry, and function and exploration of the wound. Use a toy or light pen that requires manipulation by the child to help in evaluating motor function.

MANAGEMENT

Instruments, Sutures, Staples, Tape, and Tissue Adhesives

The selection of the closure technique will depend on the location and nature of the laceration. Sutures, staples, surgical tape, or tissue adhesives may be selected (Table 23-1). Most wound repairs can be accomplished with a few basic instruments and supplies, as follows:

- Needle holder
- Forceps
- Number 15 scalpel (11 for puncture wounds)

- Scissors
- Sutures (Table 23-2), wound adhesive, or staples
- Sterile drape(s)
- Anesthetic agent(s)
- Topical antiseptic
- Normal saline
- Irrigation equipment (large syringe with 18- to 20-gauge needle or plastic catheter)
- Sterile gauze.

A number of needle types are available for use by the emergency physician, and manufacturers generally place a life-size diagram of the needle on each suture package. The most common type of cross-sectional needle configuration used for wound repair is the cutting needle. Cutting needles come in two grades: cuticular and plastic. Plastic needles, which are identified by the letter P next to the needle size, are recommended for ED wound and laceration repair. The other type of curved needle configuration is the tapered needle, which is not commonly used in the ED setting due to difficulty in passing this needle through the epidermis.

Staples have become a frequently used alternative to suturing for selected wounds. Sharp lacerations of the scalp, trunk, and extremities are rapidly and effectively closed using staples, which induce a minimal inflammatory reaction and produce similar cosmetic results to suturing. Do not use staples for repair of hand or face lacerations, and avoid their use in areas of the body that will undergo computed tomography (CT) or magnetic resonance imaging (MRI). They should also not be placed in areas of the scalp that will be subject to prolonged pressure, as they are uncomfortable for the patient.

Steri-strips are an effective alternative for the closure of small linear lacerations that are under minimal tension (Fig. 23-2). Taped wounds are more resistant to infection than sutured wounds and do not require return to

Table 23-1. Advantages and Disadvantages of Common Wound Closure Techniques

Technique	Advantages	Disadvantages
Suture	Time honored Meticulous closure Greatest tensile strength Lowest dehiscence rate	Requires removal Requires anesthesia Greatest tissue reactivity Highest cost Slowest application Highest risk of needle stick
Staples	Rapid application Low tissue reactivity Low cost Low risk of needle stick	Less meticulous closure May interfere with imaging techniques
Tissue adhesive	Rapid application Patient comfort Resistant to bacterial growth No need for removal Low cost Low or no risk of needle stick	Lower tensile strength than sutures Dehiscence over high-tension areas Not useful on hands Cannot bathe or swim
Surgical tape	Least reactive Lowest infection rates Rapid application Patient comfort Low cost No risk of needle stick	Frequently falls off Lower tensile strength than sutures Highest rate of dehiscence Requires use of toxic adjuncts Cannot be used in areas with hair Cannot get wet

Table 23-2. Suture Types and Characteristics

Type and Material	Properties
Nonabsorbable	
Silk	Easy to handle
	Lies flat when tied
	Forms secure knot due to presence of braid
	Induces more tissue reaction and has higher infection potential than other non-absorbables
Cotton	Similar to the properties of silk
Nylon	Synthetic
	Less tissue reactivity and infection potential
	Does not tend to lie flat
	More difficult to handle than silk/cotton
	Decreased knot security due to lack of braid requires more throws per knot
Polypropylene	Similar to the properties of nylon sutures, although slightly easier to handle
Polyester	Infection potential greater than nylon and polypropylene, but less than silk and cotton
	Easier to handle and better knot security than nylon and polypropylene
Metal	Low tissue reactivity and infection potential
	Difficult to handle
	Uncomfortable for patient during healing
Polybutester	Equivalent to nylon and polypropylene in tensile strength and low infection potential
	Stretches easily, thus advantageous for wounds that tend to swell
Absorbable	
Plain gut	Phagocytosed by macrophages
	Maintains tensile strength for ~7 days
	High tissue reactivity and infection potential
Chromic gut	Similar to the properties of plain gut sutures, but maintains tensile strength for ~2–3 weeks
Fast-absorbing	Similar to the properties of plain gut sutures, but breaks down gut within 5–7 days, thus does not require removal with scissors
Polyglycolic acid and polyglactin	Synthetic
	Cause less tissue reactivity and have lower infection potential than gut sutures
	Absorbed by enzymatic hydrolysis
	Braided, thus hold knots well, but have lots of drag through tissues if not coated with materials that reduce friction
	Gradually loses tensile strength over ~4 weeks
Polydioxanone, polyglyconate, and glycoside	Synthetic monofilament (pass more smoothly through tissues)
	Cause less tissue reactivity than gut sutures
	Absorbed by enzymatic hydrolysis
Trimethylene carbonate	Retain ~60% of tensile strength at 28 days

the ED for removal. If applied with an adhesive such as tincture of benzoin, tape should remain in place for several days. Keep benzoin out of the wound, however. Tape can also be used for skin closure of partial-thickness wounds and of wounds that are closed in a layered fashion with well-approximated wound edges. Tape closure is a preferred technique for the repair of multi-ple tangential skin flaps, such as those produced when a child's face hits the windshield in a motor vehicle crash.

Tissue adhesives have been used for many years in Europe and Canada. The recent approval of 2-octylcyanoacrylates (2-OCA; Dermabond) by the Food and Drug Administration (FDA) has offered another option for the repair of pediatric lacerations in the United

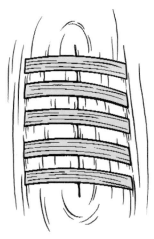

Fig. 23-2. Skin-closure tapes should be applied perpendicular to the wound edges and spaced so that the edges do not gape.

States, thus improving patient care. It is thought that adhesives might replace sutures in one-fourth to one-third of ED laceration repairs, and adhesives are also being used for the closure of many nonemergent surgical incisions.

Analgesia, Local Anesthesia, Nerve Blocks, and Sedation

Analgesia, anesthesia, nerve blocks, and sedation are discussed in more detail in Chapter 24. Most wounds are adequately anesthetized using local infiltration of lidocaine, 1 to 2 percent, with or without epinephrine, and this is still the standard approach. Lidocaine has a rapid onset of action and a duration of action of approximately one-half to 2 hours. Duration of action is prolonged by using epinephrine, but it may increase the risk of infection and should not be used in regions supplied by end-arteries (fingers, nose, lip, ears, genitalia, toes). Consider the use of a longer-acting agent, such as bupivacaine, in order to spare a patient repeated injections if wound repair may be interrupted. Bupivacaine's onset of action is moderate, and duration of action is approximately 2 to 6 hours. For whatever local anesthetic agent is used, take care not to use more than the recommended dose per kilogram of the agent. For plain lidocaine and lidocaine with epinephrine, 4.5 mg/kg and 7 mg/kg are the recommended maximum doses, respectively. Bicarbonate added to lidocaine, in a 1:10 dilution, also reduces pain of injection.

Infiltration is achieved by means of a 25- to 27-gauge needle, injected slowly into the wound margins. Buffer-

ing 9 to 10 mL of 1 percent lidocaine with 1 mL of 8.4 percent sodium bicarbonate has been shown to reduce the pain of injection significantly. When possible, perform infiltration prior to irrigation; however, for grossly contaminated wounds, it is occasionally necessary to irrigate prior to infiltration anesthesia.

Topical lidocaine-adrenaline-tetracaine (LAT), as well as tetracaine-adrenaline-cocaine (TAC), has been shown to provide effective anesthesia for pediatric facial and scalp lacerations. Use of LAT has compared favorably with TAC without the risks and administrative complications of cocaine. Take care to avoid contact of these mixtures with mucous membranes, and do not use them in regions supplied by end-arteries due to the vasoconstrictive effect of the adrenaline. The mixture can be applied to the wound by using saturated sponges, gauze pads, or cotton swabs held in place by a parent or caregiver wearing gloves. Transient anesthesia can also be obtained by applying a solution of 4 percent lidocaine to a wound prior to infiltration anesthesia or to an abrasion that requires mechanical scrubbing.

Use regional nerve blocks for large lacerations and for lacerations in areas where the anatomy will be distorted if local infiltration is performed. They are especially useful for anesthetizing digits. A regional block results in anesthetizing the nerve or nerves that supply a specific anatomic area.

Conscious sedation is usually not required for the management of wounds in children. However, for the child who is too uncooperative to permit adequate wound management, use chemical sedation with agents such as midazolam, fentanyl, nitrous oxide, or ketamine. Both cardiac and respiratory monitoring should be performed during sedation, airway management equipment and reversal agents (naloxone and flumazenil) should be available at the bedside, and the patient should be discharged only when the agents have worn off and the child has returned to his or her presedation level of consciousness.

Some form of physical restraint during wound assessment and management is generally necessary for children younger than 2 years and sometimes is required for children up to 5 or 6 years. Methods used to immobilize a child involve the use of a folded sheet with or without a pillowcase, although commercially available papoose boards may be more convenient. Neither method provides adequate immobilization of the head.

Wound Cleaning and Preparation

Controversy exists as to the proper physician attire during wound care. Some advocate routine donning of goggles, mask, gloves, cap, and gown. Certainly, gloves, mask, and eye protection should always be worn, in keeping with universal precautions.

Hemostasis

Hemostasis is necessary during all stages of wound management and usually is achieved by applying direct pressure with sterile gauze for 10 to 20 minutes. Other methods that can be used for the control of more brisk bleeding include elevation of the wound, application of dilute epinephrine solution (1:100,000) to the wound, infiltration of lidocaine with epinephrine, and packing with absorbable gelatin powder or sponge. Control persistent arterial bleeding in an extremity wound with proximal placement of a blood pressure cuff and inflation to slightly higher than the patient's systolic blood pressure. Alternatively, use tourniquets formed from a Penrose drain, elastic band, or a cut sterile glove for proximal control of bleeding from an injured digit or small extremity. Pay close attention to time limits when using these methods, however (generally limit to 30 to 45 minutes). Electrocauterization of small oozing vessels can also be used for successful hemostasis

Do not suture or clamp vessels blindly because of the risk of injuring adjacent structures. Persistently bleeding small arteries do, however, require ligation. Do not clamp and ligate arteries in the wrists or hands. These require consultation with a hand or vascular surgeon.

Foreign Body Evaluation

After anesthesia, perform wound exploration on all injuries to determine the extent of damage and to remove foreign material. The failure to diagnose foreign bodies in wounds is a frequent cause of litigation against emergency physicians. Inert foreign bodies such as glass or metal should be removed if possible. Radiographs are occasionally required for precise localization of a foreign body, which can be aided by taping a radiopaque marker such as a paper clip to the skin overlying the suspected location. Other studies that can aid in the localization of foreign bodies include xeroradiography, ultrasonography, CT, and MRI. If an inert foreign body is small and cannot easily be removed, it may be left in place and the patient or parent informed of its presence. Organic foreign bodies such as wood unequivocally require removal to prevent inflammatory reactions and infection.

Hair Removal

Since infection rates are significantly greater in wounds that are shaved, remove hair by clipping if it interferes with the procedure. In most wounds, however, even those to the scalp, hair removal is not necessary. Moistening the hair in the area of the laceration with lubricating jelly usually keeps it out of the way. Never shave or clip the eyebrows. They serve as valuable landmarks for alignment during wound repair and, if removed, can take 6 to 12 months to grow back.

Irrigation

Irrigation with between 5 and 8 psi of normal saline is the method of choice for removing bacteria and debris from most wounds. Low-pressure irrigation with a bulb syringe does not adequately remove bacteria and debris from a wound. The pressure delivered by a simple assembly consisting of an 18- to 20-gauge plastic catheter or needle attached to a 30-mL syringe is 6 to 8 psi. Commercial systems to facilitate irrigation are available, including spring-loaded syringes with one-way valves connected to a standard intravenous (normal saline) setup. Regardless of the system used, maintain the tip of the needle somewhere between the wound surface and 5 cm above the intact skin and use 200 to 300 mL of fluid for an average-sized low-risk wound. For increasing size or contamination, use more fluid.

The choice of irrigation fluid is controversial. Normal saline remains the standard fluid, and it is inexpensive, decreases bacterial loads, and reduces wound infection rates. However, it is not bactericidal. Povidone-iodine solution (10 percent) is tissue toxic and has no beneficial clinical effect on wound infection rates. When it is diluted to a 1 percent solution, however, it does not damage tissue but still retains its bactericidal properties. It should be considered as irrigation fluid in moderate- or high-risk wounds.

Antibiotic solutions have been studied for use in irrigation, but they cannot be routinely recommended for uncomplicated wounds. Nonionic surfactant agents (Shur-Clens, Pharma Clens) have been shown to remove bacteria and debris from wounds effectively, but they are much more expensive than normal saline or 1 percent povidone-iodine, do not possess bactericidal activity, and should be reserved for scrubbing rather than irrigating. Hydrogen peroxide has no role in wound irrigation, since it impedes wound healing and has poor bactericidal activity. Benzalkonium chloride, although not as tissue toxic as hydrogen peroxide or 10 percent povidone-iodine, has a limited antimicrobial spectrum and has been associated with stock solution contamination by *Pseudomonas* organisms.

A consequence of, and disincentive to, irrigation is splatter, which can be minimized using one of many techniques. Irrigating through the first web space of the irrigator's hand while cupping the hand above the wound will avoid splatter but will diminish visualization of the wound during irrigation. Attaching a 4 × 4 inch gauze to the irrigation catheter or needle will also provide protection. Commercially available plastic shields (Zerowet) that attach directly to the irrigation syringe provide good protection against splatter while permitting visualization of the wound. An inexpensive version of these plastic shields is formed by puncturing the base of a sterile plastic medication cup with the irrigation needle.

Antisepsis and Scrubbing

Cleanse the skin surrounding the wound prior to wound irrigation and repair. Various antiseptic skin cleansers can be used, including povidone-iodine (Betadine scrub) and chlorhexidene gluconate (Hibiclens). Nonionic surfactants, such as Shur-Clens and Pharma Clens, mechanically lift bacteria from the skin, but possess no bactericidal activity. A gauze sponge folded and placed into the wound will prevent the entry of detergents into the wound itself.

Remove large debris from the wound with forceps and debride devitalized tissue and foreign matter if needed. Avoid mechanical scrubbing of the wound unless there is gross contamination. Although scrubbing can remove debris from the wound, it increases wound inflammation. If it is decided to perform scrubbing, use a fine-pore sponge (e.g., Optipore) to minimize tissue abrasion and a nonionic surfactant to minimize tissue toxicity and inflammation.

Debridement

Debridement is necessary in the management of contaminated wounds or wounds with nonviable tissue. Through removal of contaminants and devitalized tissue from wounds, debridement increases a wound's ability to resist infection, shortens the period of inflammation, and creates a sharp, trimmed wound edge that is easier to repair and more cosmetically acceptable. If the devitalized edge of an irregular wound is debrided, the wound can be undermined to avoid a wide scar.

Primary Wound Closure

Primary closure, using sutures, staples, tape, or tissue adhesive, is performed on lacerations that have been recently sustained (<24 hours on the face and <12 hours on other areas of the body), are relatively clean, and have minimal tissue devitalization.

Prior to beginning closure, identify all the injured layers, such as fascia, subcutaneous tissue, muscle, tendon, and skin. During repair, always match each layer edge to its counterpart and ensure that, when the sutures are placed, they enter and exit the appropriate layer at the same level so that there is no overlapping of layers. A laceration that has been appropriately closed in layers usually does not need large or tight skin sutures to complete the closure. This improves the cosmetic result. However, in hands and feet, placement of deep sutures increases the risk of infection, and they should be avoided in those areas.

The size of suture to be used for wound closure depends on the tensile strength of the tissue in the wound. Use 3-0 suture for tissues with strong tension, such as fascia in an extremity, and 6-0 suture for tissues with light tension, such as the subcutaneous tissue of the face.

Buried Stitch

Deep (buried) sutures serve four key functions and are required for many lacerations to ensure the best cosmetic result:

- They provide 2 to 3 weeks of additional support to the wound after the skin sutures are taken out or the tape is removed. This prevents widening of the scar.
- They help to preserve the normal functioning of the underlying or involved muscles if the muscular fascia is sutured.
- They reduce the likelihood of the development of a hematoma or abscess by minimizing the dead space.
- They avoid the development of pitting in the injured region caused by inadequate healing of the deep tissues.

Unfortunately, deep sutures can result in damage to nerves, arteries, and tendons and, in the extremities, can increase the risk of infection. Since suture material is a foreign body, even in clean or minimally contaminated wounds, use only a few deep sutures. The most common deep suture for laceration repair is the buried knot stitch, where one begins and ends at the base of the wound so as to bury the knot (Fig. 23-3).

The buried horizontal mattress stitch results in passage of suture material at the dermal-epidermal junction, with the knot placed subcuticularly below the dermis. The subcuticular stitch is a running buried suture at the dermal-epidermal junction that is actually used for skin closure (Fig. 23-4). Enter the skin initially approximately 3 mm to 2 cm from one end of the laceration, and allow

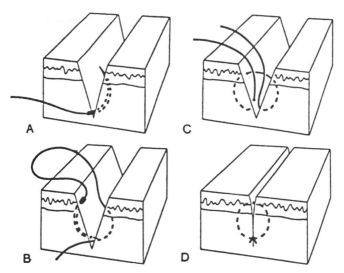

Fig. 23-3. Buried subcutaneous stitch. This is particularly useful when approximating the subcutaneous tissue just beneath the skin edge, because it prevents irritation of the skin edge by the knot.

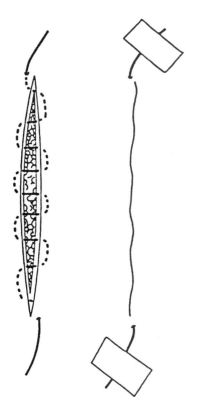

Fig. 23-4. Subcuticular stitch. See text for discussion.

the needle to emerge at the subcuticular plane at the wound apex. Pass the suture through the subcuticular tissue on alternate sides of the laceration. The point of entry of each stitch should be directly across from or slightly behind the exit point of the previous stitch. At the other end of the laceration, burrow the needle again into the dermis to exit the skin 3 mm to 2 cm from the end. Ensure that there is no skin puckering, and then tape the free suture at both ends of the laceration in place. This stitch can be left permanently in place if absorbable suture is used, or can be removed in 2 to 3 weeks if nonabsorbable suture is used. Use of the subcuticular stitch avoids skin suture marks but takes more time than simple interrupted or running sutures.

Skin Closure

Repair the epidermis and superficial layer of the dermis with nonabsorbable synthetic sutures. Place sutures such that the same depth and width is entered on both sides of the incision. A key to cosmetically acceptable closure is edge eversion, which is obtained by entering the skin at a 90-degree angle, and, in some cases, by using a skin hook. For wounds whose edges tend to invert despite proper technique, vertical mattress stitches can be used (see below). The number of sutures used to repair a laceration will vary with each case. For facial lacerations, sutures are generally placed 2 to 4 mm apart and 2 to 3 mm from the wound edge.

Simple Interrupted Stitch

The simple interrupted stitch is used most frequently for skin closure (Fig. 23-5). It involves placing separate loops of suture using proper eversion technique (i.e., entering skin at 90 degrees, including sufficient subcutaneous tissue), followed by tying and cutting each stitch. Although it is time consuming, if one stitch in the closure fails, the remaining stitches will hold the wound together. It is useful for stellate lacerations, wounds with multiple components, and lacerations that change direction. It is also helpful for approximation of landmarks on the skin.

Running Stitch

The running or continuous stitch is well suited for pediatric laceration repair for numerous reasons (Fig. 23-6): first, it is rapid; second, removal is easier; third, the strength of a running stitch is generally greater; fourth, it provides more effective hemostasis; and finally, it distributes tension evenly along its length. The technique cannot be used over joints since, if one point were to break, the entire stitch would unravel.

To begin a simple continuous stitch, place an interrupted stitch at one end of the wound and cut only the free end of the suture. Continue suturing in a coil pattern, ensuring that the needle passes perpendicularly across the laceration with each pass. After each pass, tighten the loop slightly so that tension is equally distributed. To complete the stitch, place the final loop just beyond the end of the laceration and tie the suture with the last loop used as the tail. An interlocking continuous stitch can be used to reduce slippage of loops and for more irregular lacerations (Fig. 23-7). It is performed by pulling the needle through the previous loop each time it exits the skin. It can, however, increase the degree of scarring if the loops are tied too tightly.

Mattress Stitches

The horizontal mattress stitch can be used for single-layer closure of lacerations under tension (Fig. 23-8). It approximates skin edges closely, while providing some eversion, and decreases the time needed to suture because 50 percent of knots are tied. A running horizontal mattress suture can be used in areas of the body where loose skin could overlap or invert easily, such as the upper eyelids (Fig. 23-9).

The half-buried horizontal mattress stitch (corner stitch) is the suture of choice for closure of complex wounds with angulated (V-shaped) flaps (Fig. 23-10). Enter and exit the skin directly across from the flap and course the suture loop within the subcuticular tissue of the flap to maximize blood supply to the tip of the flap.

The vertical mattress stitch is helpful to evert skin edges, but it causes more ischemia and necrosis within its loop than other stitches (Fig. 23-11). It is useful in areas of the body with little subcutaneous tissue. The stitch begins in the same way as a simple interrupted stitch, but after the loop is made, reenter and reexit the skin approximately 1 to 2 mm from the wound edge and tie. A common technique is to alternate vertical mattress stitches with simple interrupted stitches to close a wound.

Knots

The knot used most commonly in the ED repair of lacerations is the surgeon's knot followed by one to four half-knots, usually formed as instrument ties. The single surgeon's knot allows for some give if any tissue edema develops.

Correction of Dog Ears

When wound edges are not precisely aligned, an excess of skin on one or both ends ("dog ears") result. A dog ear can be corrected using the following technique (Fig. 23-12). First, elevate the excess skin with a skin hook and make an oblique incision from the apex of the wound toward the side of the dog ear. Then undermine the flap and lay it flat, excise the excess triangle of skin, and complete the closure.

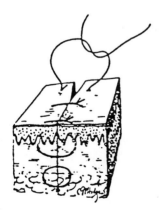

Fig. 23-5. Simple interrupted stitch (with buried subcutaneous stitch). See text for discussion.

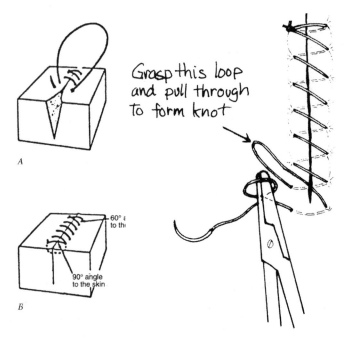

Grasp this loop
and pull through
to form knot

60° a
to th

90° angle
to the skin

Fig. 23-6. The simple continuous stitch. *A/B*. This continuous suture is begun with a single suture that is tied to anchor the rest of the suture. The needle should be passed perpendicular to the skin edge and the suture threads should lie perpendicular to the wound margin, as with the simple interrupted suture. *C*. To finish and tie off this continuous suture, grab the loop formed at the free end after insertion of the needle through the skin at its midpoint with the needle holder and pull on this loop. It will come together as if it were a single thread. Tie the needle end of the suture material and this "looped" free end as a simple interrupted suture would be tied. To complete the simple continuous stitch, a series of square knots is tied, with the loop as one of the ties.

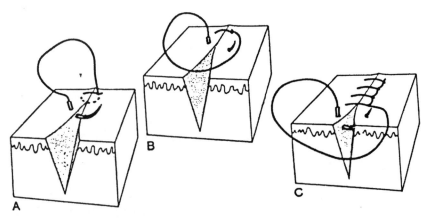

Fig. 23-7. Continuous single lock stitch. See text for discussion.

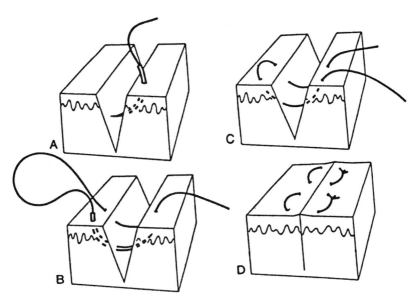

Fig. 23-8. Horizontal mattress stitch. *A.* The needle is passed 0.5–1 cm away from the wound edge deeply into the wound. *B.* The needle is then passed through the opposite side and reenters the wound parallel to the initial suture. *C.* One must enter the skin perpendicularly to provide some eversion of the wound edges and must enter and exit both the wound and skin at the same depth, otherwise "buckling" and irregularities occur in the wound margin. *D.* The suture loop is then tied as shown.

Tissue Adhesives

Tissue adhesives can be rapidly and painlessly applied, often requiring no anesthesia or only painless topical anesthesia with LAT (Fig. 23-13). One must clean and debride the wound in the normal fashion before applying the adhesive. 2-OCA provides enough three-dimensional tensile strength to offer a needleless alternative to sutures for the closure of many facial lacerations and provides comparable cosmetic outcomes. It should be used only topically, with care taken to avoid placing adhesive between wound margins, within the wound, or in the eyes. If lacerations cannot be well approximated manually, or if a significant amount of tension must be used to do so, then the use of an adhesive alone is not appropriate; in these instances, absorbable subcutaneous or subcuticular sutures can be used to relieve tension at the wound edges. At least three or four coats of 2-OCA should be applied to provide adequate strength to the wound. The adhesive usually sloughs off within 7 to 10 days and acts as its own waterproof dressing and antimicrobial barrier. Other advantages of 2-OCA is that it is less expensive to use than sutures and staples and requires no follow-up visit for removal, and patients and parents prefer it.

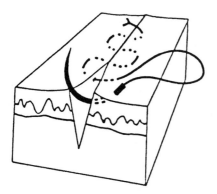

Fig. 23-9. Continuous mattress stitch. See text for discussion.

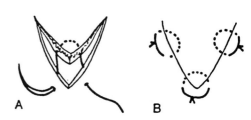

Fig. 23-10. *A,B.* Half-buried horizontal mattress stitch. This minimizes the vascular compromise at a corner flap. See text for discussion.

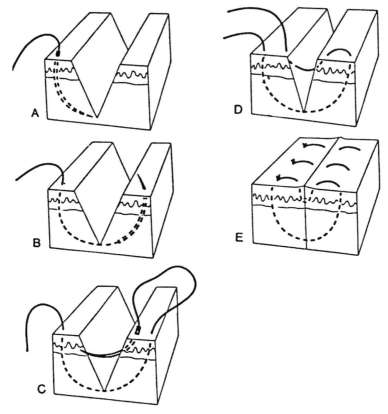

Fig. 23-11. *A–E.* Vertical mattress stitch. See text for discussion.

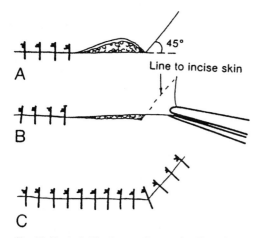

Fig. 23-12. *A–C.* The dog ear. See text for discussion.

Secondary Closure

Secondary closure is a technique that allows wounds to heal by granulation and reepithelialization. It is used to manage ulcerations, drained abscess cavities, deep puncture wounds, older or infected lacerations, and many animal bites. Daily packing is performed with saline-soaked gauze or iodoform gauze strips until granulation tissue closes the potential space.

Delayed Primary (Tertiary) Closure

Delayed primary closure with sutures is performed on wounds 3 to 5 days after they have been initially cleansed, debrided, and packed with saline-soaked gauze. Wounds amenable to this form of closure are those too contaminated for primary closure but not associated with significant tissue loss or devitalization.

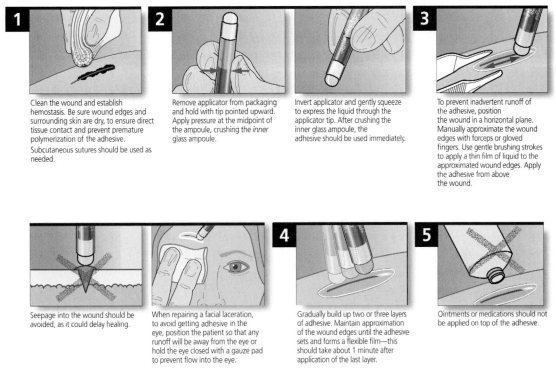

1 Clean the wound and establish hemostasis. Be sure wound edges and surrounding skin are dry, to ensure direct tissue contact and prevent premature polymerization of the adhesive. Subcutaneous sutures should be used as needed.

2 Remove applicator from packaging and hold with tip pointed upward. Apply pressure at the midpoint of the ampoule, crushing the *inner* glass ampoule.

Invert applicator and gently squeeze to express the liquid through the applicator tip. After crushing the inner glass ampoule, the adhesive should be used immediately.

3 To prevent inadvertent runoff of the adhesive, position the wound in a horizontal plane. Manually approximate the wound edges with forceps or gloved fingers. Use gentle brushing strokes to apply a thin film of liquid to the approximated wound edges. Apply the adhesive from above the wound.

Seepage into the wound should be avoided, as it could delay healing.

When repairing a facial laceration, to avoid getting adhesive in the eye, position the patient so that any runoff will be away from the eye or hold the eye closed with a gauze pad to prevent flow into the eye.

4 Gradually build up two or three layers of adhesive. Maintain approximation of the wound edges until the adhesive sets and forms a flexible film—this should take about 1 minute after application of the last layer.

5 Ointments or medications should not be applied on top of the adhesive.

Fig. 23-13. Application of tissue adhesive. (From Ethicon, Inc., a Johnson & Johnson Co.)

Wound Dressing, Drains, and Immobilization

Sutured and stapled lacerations heal best in a moist environment without crust formation between the healing edges. Wounds closed with 2-OCA should not be covered with topical ointments, as they can loosen the tissue adhesive. Thus, after laceration repair with sutures or staples, cleanse the skin of blood and povidone-iodine, and apply a light coat of antibiotic ointment. Since the antibiotic ointment is used for purposes of maintaining a moist environment, and not for protection against infection, a semiporous nonadherent dressing can be applied to the laceration instead (Adaptic, Telpha, Xeroform, or Vaseline gauze). Use a second layer of sterile gauze, or adhesive bandage (Band-Aid) to cover the ointment or nonadherent dressing. Alternatively, use an occlusive or semiocclusive dressing (Op-Site, Tegaderm, DuoDerm, or Biobrane), which reduces the pain associated with dry healing. If there is potential for the formation of a hematoma, apply a pressure dressing, taking care to avoid compression of arterial, venous, and lymphatic circulations.

Drains should not be used in sutured wounds. They act as foreign bodies and promote rather than prevent infection. If a wound is considered a high risk for infection, delayed primary closure should be performed rather than suturing and placing a drain in the wound. Drains should also not be used for hemostasis, which is better achieved by proper laceration repair, electrocauterization, and pressure dressings.

Splint a wound overlying a joint in the position of function for 7 to 10 days. For children, a bulky dressing will act as a splint and minimize motion at the wound, as well as prevent the child from tampering with the wound repair; it is especially helpful for hand and foot wounds.

Prophylactic Antibiotics and Tetanus Prophylaxis

More than 90 to 95 percent of wounds treated in the ED heal without complications if given appropriate wound care. Antibiotics should be considered in a few instances,

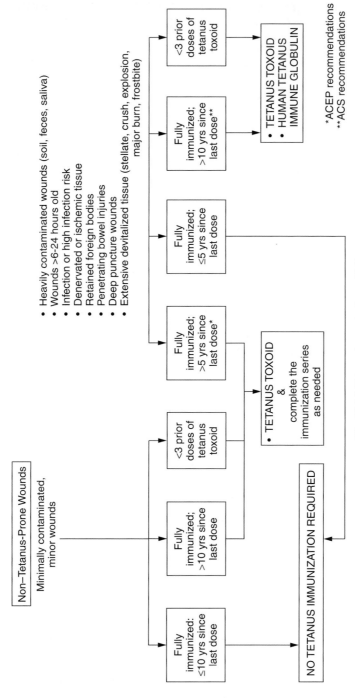

Fig. 23-14. Tetanus immunization guidelines.

however. Antibiotics are indicated for patients with simple wounds who are prone to infective endocarditis or who have orthopedic prostheses. They should also be given to patients who present with a wound infection due to inappropriate care at home, or with wounds that are more than 12 to 24 hours old. Other indications are for wounds heavily contaminated with feces or saliva, which should also be treated with secondary or delayed primary closure. Extensive intraoral lacerations may benefit from a short course of penicillin or erythromycin, and coverage for mammalian bites is discussed below. Consider for antibiotic prophylaxis any wounds in which there is involvement of cartilage, joint spaces, tendon, or bone. Finally, consider prophylactic antibiotics for high-risk wounds (contaminated or devitalized), especially in compromised hosts, such as children with sickle cell disease, diabetes, steroid use, or lymphoma.

When antibiotics are indicated, their effectiveness depends on early administration. The first dose should therefore be given in the ED (preferably within 3 hours of the injury), regardless of the route of administration. The choice of antibiotics depends on the type of wound, although most infections are caused by staphylococci and streptococci that are sensitive to penicillinase-resistant penicillins and first-generation cephalosporins, or erythromycin for penicillin-allergic patients. Wounds contaminated with saliva generally respond to the same agents, and human bites are discussed below. Wounds contaminated with feces require coverage against facultative organisms, coliforms, and obligate anaerobes. Reasonable choices would include second- and third-generation cephalosporins, or the combination of clindamycin and an aminoglycoside. For a fresh-water contaminated wound that requires antibiotic coverage, trimethoprim-sulfamethoxazole and parenteral third-generation cephalosporins are effective in children. Generally, 3 to 5 days of oral antibiotics are prescribed for prophylaxis, but no definitive studies have examined appropriate duration of prophylaxis.

Tetanus prophylaxis begins with appropriate wound care. If the wound is tetanus prone, determine the child's immunization status (Fig. 23-14). If the child has a tetanus-prone wound and was not immunized or only partially immunized, or if his or her immunization status is unknown, treat the child as if he or she has no protection. Give human tetanus immune globulin (HTIG) 250 U IM and complete or initiate primary immunization. If a child has completed primary immunization and has received appropriate boosters, then HTIG is never required.

POSTOPERATIVE WOUND CARE AND SUTURE REMOVAL

Successful outcome of traumatic wounds is partly dependent on wound care after discharge from the ED. Therefore, the patient and parents should be given thorough (preferably written) instructions about care of the wound and what to expect. They should be informed that all wounds of significance heal with scars, regardless of the quality of care. The final appearance of the scar cannot be predicted before 6 to 12 months after the repair. They should be informed about the possibility of infection and that there is always the possibility, despite appropriate management, of a residual foreign body in the wound.

Because lacerations are bridged by epithelial cells within 48 hours, the wound is essentially impermeable to the entry of bacteria after 2 days. Give instructions to keep the dressing in place and the wound clean and dry for 24 to 48 hours. The dressing should be changed only if it becomes soiled or soaked by exudate from the wound. After the initial 1 to 2 days, the dressing may be removed to check for signs of infection, such as erythema, pain, warmth, purulent discharge, excessive edema, or red streaks of lymphangitis. If parental reliability is questionable, the patient should have the wound reexamined in the ED in 2 to 3 days. If there are no signs of infection, instruct the patient or parents to gently wash the wound daily with soap and water to remove dried blood and exudate. Undiluted hydrogen peroxide should not be used, since it may destroy granulation tissue and newly formed epithelium. Generally, the wound should be protected with a dressing during the first week, with daily dressing changes. Once the dressing is removed, patients and parents should be instructed that sunscreen (SPF 15 or greater) should be applied to the scar for at least 6 months when prolonged exposure to the sun is expected, to prevent hyperpigmentation of the scar.

Suture removal should be done at an appropriate time so as to prevent dehiscence of the wound seen with premature removal and to prevent suture track marks and stitch abscesses resulting from late removal (Table 23-3). Children both heal and form suture track marks faster than adults and thus need earlier suture removal. After appropriately timed suture removal, skin tape should be applied, since wound contraction and scar widening will continue to occur for several weeks after an injury.

Table 23-3. Repair of Soft Tissue Injuries by Body Location

Location	Anesthetic	Repair/Material	Type of Closure	Suture Removal (days)
Scalp	Lidocaine 1% with epinephrine	3-0 or 4-0 nylon[a]; ±3-0 polyglycolic acid[b] (galea) Staples if galea intact	Single tight layer with simple interrupted, vertical mattress, or horizontal mattress for hemostasis; galea requires close approximation, but preferably with single-layer closure	7–10 d
Pinna (ear)	Lidocaine 1% (field block)	5-0 polyglycolic acid[b] (perichondrium); 6-0 nylon[a] (skin)	Simple interrupted; stent dressing	4–6 d
Eyebrow	Lidocaine 1% with epinephrine	4-0 or 5-0 polyglycolic acid[b] (and 6-0 nylon)[a]	Layered closure	4–5 d
Eyelid	Lidocaine 1%	6-0 nylon[a] 2-OCA	Horizontal mattress	3–5 d
Lip	Lidocaine 1% with epinephrine or mental node block	4-0 or 5-0 polyglycolic acid[b] or (chromic) gut (mucosa); 5-0 polyglycolic acid[b] (SQ, muscle); 6-0 nylon[a] (skin)	Three layers (mucosa, muscle skin) if through and through, otherwise two layers	3–5 d
Oral cavity	Lidocaine 1% with epinephrine or field block Sedation may be necessary	4-0 or 5-0 polyglycolic acid[b] or (chromic) gut	Simple interrupted or horizontal mattress	7–8 days or allow to dissolve
Face	Lidocaine 1% with epinephrine or field block	4-0 or 5-0 polyglycolic acid[b] (SQ); 6-0 nylon[a] (skin) 2-OCA (skin)	If full-thickness, layered closure	3–5 d
Neck	Lidocaine 1% with epinephrine	4-0 polyglycolic acid[b] (SQ); 5-0 nylon[a] (skin)	Two-layered closure	4–6 d
Trunk	Lidocaine 1% with epinephrine	4-0 polyglycolic acid[b] (SQ fat); 4-0 or 5-0 nylon[a] (skin)	Single or layered closure	7–12 d
Extremity	Lidocaine 1% with epinephrine	3-0 or 4-0 polyglycolic acid[b] (SQ, fat muscle) 4-0 or 5-0 nylon[a] (skin)	Single or layered; splint if over joint	10–14 d (joint) 7–10 (other)
Hands and feet	Lidocaine 1% (lidocaine 2% or bupivacaine 0.25% for field block)	4-0 or 5-0 nylon[a]	Single-layer closure with simple interrupted or horizontal mattress; splint if over joint	10–14 d (joint) 7–10 (other)

(Continues)

Table 23-3. Repair of Soft Tissue Injuries by Body Location (*Continued*)

Location	Anesthetic	Repair/Material	Type of Closure	Suture Removal (days)
Nailbeds	Digital nerve block with lidocaine 2% or bupivacaine 0.25%	5-0 polyglycolic acid[b]		Allow to dissolve

[a]Nylon or polypropylene.
[b]Polyglycolic and (Dexon) or polyglactin (Vicryl).

MANAGEMENT OF SELECTED INJURIES

Abrasions

It is generally sufficient to cleanse abrasions and dress them with a nonadherent dressing or antibiotic ointment and dressing that can be changed daily after cleaning. Deeper abrasions may be treated as skin graft donor sites with cleansing and a fine-mesh gauze dressing. It is important to remove any foreign bodies (e.g., gravel, dirt, or tar) to avoid infection or tattooing ("road rash") of the wound. Anesthesia for the cleansing of abrasions can be difficult, and large abrasions may require general anesthesia or conscious sedation to permit adequate debridement. For smaller areas, topical anesthesia with 2 percent lidocaine or LAT solution, infiltration of local anesthetic, or nerve blocks can be used. Children with large or deep abrasions should have their wounds reexamined in 2 to 3 days for monitoring of healing.

Scalp Lacerations

There are five anatomic layers in the scalp: skin, superficial fascia, galea aponeurotica, subaponeurotic areolar connective tissue, and periosteum. The presence of a rich vascular supply and vessels that tend to remain patent when cut are responsible for the profuse bleeding associated with scalp injuries. Usually, the bleeding is halted by rapid suturing. Other methods to control bleeding include the application of direct pressure, placement of a wide tight rubber band around the scalp, and infiltration of local anesthetics containing epinephrine into the wound. If these techniques are unsuccessful, Raney scalp clips can be used or larger vessels can be ligated.

Before repairing a scalp wound, complete a thorough neck and neurologic examination and palpate the skull for fractures. Palpation will reveal fractures more often than skull radiographs.

The subgaleal layer of connective tissue contains "emissary veins" that drain through vessels of the skull into the venous sinuses within the cranial vault. In scalp wounds that penetrate the galea, bacteria can be carried by these vessels, and a wound infection can result in osteomyelitis, meningitis, or an intracranial abscess. Approximation of galeal lacerations will not only help to control bleeding, but will safeguard against the spread of infection.

Although most lacerations that involve multiple layers of tissue should be closed in layers, scalp wounds are best closed with a single layer of sutures that incorporates the skin, the subcutaneous fascia, and the galea. Some advocate separate closure of the galea with absorbable suture material, which allows its more careful approximation but introduces a foreign body into the wound, thus increasing chances of infection. The ends of the tied sutures should be left longer than usual, and the use of blue nylon may also facilitate removal. Superficial scalp lacerations are also amenable to staple closure, which expedites repair and removal.

Forehead Lacerations

In evaluating a forehead laceration, one must evaluate for central nervous system and neck injuries. Lacerations that are limited to the area above the supraorbital rim can be anesthetized with supraorbital and supratrochlear nerve blocks, thus avoiding tissue distortion associated with local infiltration. As for scalp lacerations, explore for skull fractures and foreign bodies. Close the forehead in layers, beginning with the approximation of the frontalis fascia. Continue the layered closure, taking care to align landmarks such as forehead furrows.

Eyelid Lacerations

The thin, flexible skin of the eyelid is quite simple to suture. However, it is essential that the emergency physician be aware of injuries that require consultation with an ophthalmologist. A thorough eye examination needs to be performed whenever there is a laceration of the eyelid or periorbital region. Also, ensure that the levator palpebrae muscle and its tendinous attachment to the tarsal plate are intact, or ptosis may result. A laceration to the medial aspect of the lower lid often involves the lacrimal duct, which requires repair by an ophthalmologist. If consultation is not required, close lid lacerations in a single layer with 6-0 nonabsorbable suture or fast-absorbing gut, taking care to avoid skin inversion.

Ear Lacerations

Injuries to the ears require expedient cleansing, debridement of devitalized tissue, and coverage of exposed cartilage in order to avoid chondritis. Anesthesia of the external ear is simply accomplished with a field block of the auriculotemporal, greater auricular, and occipital nerves, performed by infiltration at the base of the auricle. Once cleansing and debridement of devitalized tissue is performed, approximate cartilage with 5-0 absorbable suture material placed through the posterior and anterior perichondrium. Keep tension to a minimum to prevent tearing of the cartilage. Next, approximate the posterior skin surface using 5-0 nonabsorbable suture. Finally, approximate the visible surface of the ear using 5-0 or 6-0 nonabsorbable suture, ensuring approximation of landmarks such as folds. No cartilage should be

left exposed. After repair, dress the ear with a mastoid compression dressing, including coverage of the anterior and posterior aspects of the auricle. This prevents accumulation of a perichondral hematoma, which can lead to necrosis of cartilage and subsequent deformity ("cauliflower ear").

Lip Lacerations

Lip lacerations are common in the pediatric age group and require careful attention to ensure a good cosmetic result (Fig. 23-15). Prior to beginning repair, inspect the oral mucosa and teeth for lacerations and trauma. Since local infiltration of anesthetic obscures the lip's landmarks, consider performing a mental nerve block for the repair of lower lip lacerations or an infraorbital nerve block for upper lip lacerations. Otherwise, prior to locally infiltrating the anesthetic, paint a thin line of methy-lene blue along the vermilion border on each side of the laceration, which can be used as a landmark during repair.

After anesthesia, cleanse and irrigate the wound in the usual manner, and then place the first stitch at the vermilion border. If deep sutures are required, leave the initial stitch untied and proceed with deep closure. Through-and-through lip lacerations require three-layer closure. Approximate the orbicularis oris muscle with 4-0 or 5-0 absorbable suture. Close the mucosa with 5-0 absorbable suture to obtain a tight seal. Finally, after irrigation of

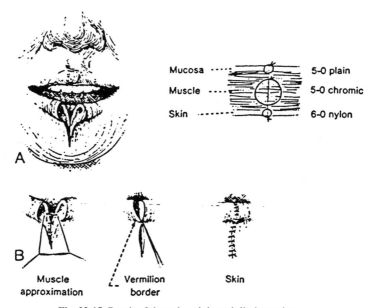

Fig. 23-15. Repair of through-and-through lip laceration.

the outside surface, close the skin with 6-0 nonabsorbable suture material. Four-layer closure, including the subcutaneous layer, can be used to facilitate skin closure. Through-and-through lip lacerations are prone to infection, and prophylaxis with penicillin or erythromycin is recommended.

Fingertip Injuries

Young children often injure fingers in doors and windows. Distal fingertip injuries, even complete amputations, heal remarkably well in children. Therapy of distal fingertip amputations consists first of a digital block or local infiltration, followed by appropriate cleansing and dressing of the wound with antibiotic ointment or nonadherent gauze, and a splint or bulky dressing for protection. Frequent wound checks must then be scheduled with a hand surgeon or the ED to watch for infection.

Prognosis of distal amputations depends on how much of the tip is lost. If the fingernail and nailbed are not involved, prognosis is excellent. If the bone is spared but there is involvement of the nail or nailbed, there may be shortening of the digit. Injuries involving the distal phalanx, especially those at the base of the nail, heal most poorly. More proximal amputations uniformly require consultation with a hand surgeon.

Close nailbed lacerations with 6-0 absorbable sutures. Avoid tying the sutures too tightly and tearing through tissue. Debridement should be kept to a minimum, and the paronychium and eponychium must be prevented from forming adhesions with the nailbed by packing the space with nonadherent gauze or using the nail itself as a stent after repair of the nailbed. If there is an underlying fracture of the distal phalanx, splint the finger and prescribe prophylactic antibiotics (cephalosporin or dicloxacillin).

A paronychium is a cutaneous abscess at the lateral aspect of fingernails or toenails. Since the fingers and toes are vulnerable to trauma during childhood, including nail biting and finger sucking, an acutely painful, swollen, erythematous, and tender paronychia is not an uncommon ED complaint. For fingers, an extensive procedure is rarely required for treatment of a paronychia. Most often, the cuticle (junction between the nail and the skin) can be incised with a number 11 blade, and the abscess can be drained and irrigated with a normal saline-povidone-iodine solution. Systemic antibiotics are needed only when there is an accompanying cellulitis or lymphangitis. Paronychia of the toes are often caused by ingrown toenails; thus removal of the ingrown portion of the nail is required to avoid a recurrence. Since this is a more extensive and painful procedure, a digital nerve block or other anesthesia is mandatory.

A subungual hematoma is a collection of blood under a fingernail or toenail, usually sustained after a direct blow. If the nail is intact, pressure from the hematoma can cause substantial pain. If the hematoma involves less than 25 to 50 percent of the nail bed, trephine the nail using one of a number of techniques. The use of electrocautery has most recently been advocated as the simplest, safest, and least painful method to drain a subungual hematoma. Prior to trephination, cleanse the nail using povidone-iodine, and once blood escapes through the nail, remove the cautery to avoid nail bed damage. Dress the digit with dry sterile gauze and splint for protection. For subungual hematomas involving >50 percent of the nail bed, there is controversy as to what treatment is best. Nail removal used to be advocated, because the risk of nail bed laceration was thought to be much higher. However, this practice has been questioned as long as the nail and surrounding nail fold are intact.

Puncture Wounds to the Foot

Puncture wounds, most often to the foot, have the potential to result in significant morbidity. Cellulitis, plantar space infections, abscesses, retained foreign bodies, and osteomyelitis can result from a benign-appearing wound.

A reasonable approach to puncture wounds of the foot is to obtain a radiograph to exclude bony involvement, air in the joint spaces, and radiopaque foreign bodies. Anesthetize the wound either locally or with a posterior tibial or sural nerve block, and then unroof the puncture site, cleanse and debride the wound, and remove any foreign bodies. If jet irrigation is performed, beware of irrigation fluid that is not returned, which can carry bacteria and debris deeper into the wound, and cause increased swelling of the wound area. The use of prophylactic antibiotics is controversial, but should include *Pseudomonas* coverage, especially if the puncture wound occurs through the sole of a tennis shoe or sneaker. *Pseudomonas aeruginosa* is the most common cause of postpuncture osteomyelitis. Remember that ciprofloxacin and related quinolones cannot be used in children younger than 16 years.

CONSULTATION GUIDELINES

Specialty consultation should be considered for the following:

- Complex or extensive wounds
- Wounds with large tissue defects

- Wounds in which there is tendon, nerve, joint, or critical vessel involvement
- Lacerations involving the parotid or lacrimal ducts
- Lacerations of the eyelid tarsal plates
- Lacerations over fractures
- Facial lacerations in which cosmetic results are a concern
- Wounds about which there is physician uncertainty

BIBLIOGRAPHY

Bruns TB, Robinson BS, Smith RJ, et al: A new tissue adhesive for laceration repair in children. *J Pediatr* 132:1067–1070, 1998.

Christoph RA, Buchanan L, Begalla K, et al: Pain reduction in local anesthetic administration through pH buffering. *Ann Emerg Med* 17:117, 1998.

Hollander JE, Singer AJ: Laceration management. *Ann Emerg Med* 34:356–367, 1999.

Jankauskas S, Cohen IK, Grabb WC: Basic technique of plastic surgery, in Aston SJ, Beasley RW, Thorne CHM (eds): *Grabb and Smith's Plastic Surgery,* 5th ed. Philadelphia: Lippincott-Raven, 1997.

Knapp JF: Updates in wound management for the pediatrician. *Pediatr Clin North Am* 46:1202–1213, 1999

Quinn JV, Wells GA, Sutcliffe T, et al: Tissue adhesive versus suture wound repair at one year: Randomized clinical trial correlating early, three-month, and one year cosmetic outcome. *Ann Emerg Med* 32:645–649, 1998.

Roberts JR, Hedges JR (eds): *Clinical Procedures in Emergency Medicine,* 3d ed. Philadelphia: WB Saunders, 1998.

Schilling CG, Bank DE, Borchert BA, et al: Tetracaine, epinephrine (adrenaline), and cocaine (TAC) versus lidocaine, epinephrine, and tetracaine (LAT) for anesthesia of lacerations in children. *Ann Emerg Med* 25:203–208, 1995.

Trott A: *Wounds and Lacerations: Emergency Care and Closure,* 2d edition. St. Louis: Mosby, 1997.

24

Emergency Department Procedural Sedation and Analgesia

Alfred Sacchetti
Michael J. Gerardi

HIGH-YIELD-FACTS

- The nature of the complaint, the status of the child, the child's response to the problem, and the preferences of the treating clinician determine the analgesic or sedative needs of a patient.

- The degree of monitoring required is determined by the patient, the procedure, and the medications utilized.

- The primary risks of sedation or analgesia for procedures are hypoventilation and hypoxia from respiratory depression, and monitoring should be directed at detection of these problems. For most patients, continuous pulse oximetry will provide both an ongoing assessment of oxygenation as well as a continuous display of heart rate.

- Physicians using these agents must be familiar with their indications, all of their actions, relative contraindications, and potential alternatives.

- One unique side effect of fentanyl is chest wall rigidity, which can occur if the drug is administered too rapidly. This side effect may be reversed with naloxone, although on occasion endotracheal intubation and skeletal muscle paralysis may be required.

- Ketamine produces extremely rapid sedation, analgesia, and amnesia that facilitates painless diagnostic studies as well as painful procedures.

- Caution should be maintained when using combinations of drugs that will not only enhance the desired effects but increase adverse effects, such as respiratory depression. Doses lower than those of either agent alone should be used initially when combining potent agents.

There has been a dramatic transformation over the last decade in the manner in which patients with painful conditions are managed. Previously a footnote in the field of pediatric emergency medicine, procedural sedation and analgesia (PSA) is now recognized as an integral component of the care of any sick or injured child. The ability of emergency medicine practitioners to safely control pain and produce sedation has now been firmly established.

The term *conscious sedation* has been used in an attempt to describe different planes of iatrogenic mental status alteration. Definitions of these planes are based on patient abilities to follow commands and maintain protective airway reflexes. Although applicable in a wide range of patient care settings, such terminology may not be completely applicable in a properly equipped emergency department staffed with a physician competent in pediatric airway management. The term procedural sedation is more appropriate for emergency medicine practice and is defined by the American College of Emergency Physicians as "a technique of administering sedatives or dissociative agents with or without analgesics to induce a state that allows the patient to tolerate unpleasant procedures while maintaining cardiorespiratory function. Procedural sedation and analgesia are intended to result in a depressed level of consciousness but one that allows the patient to maintain airway control independently and continuously."

The degree of sedation needed is determined by the treating physician and the procedure to be performed. Cooperation for a painless diagnostic study, such as magnetic resonance imaging (MRI), will require a different degree of sedation than that necessary for a painful fracture reduction. Patients undergoing rapid sequence intubation or sedation for ventilator management should not be regarded as receiving procedural sedation since the specific intent is to eliminate protective airway reflexes and respiratory drive.

PATIENT ASSESSMENT

The analgesic or sedative needs of any patient are determined by the nature of the patient complaint, the status of the child, the child's response to the problem, and the preferences of the treating clinician.

If the situation permits, children being considered for sedation or analgesia should undergo a focused history pertinent to their chief complaint and relevant past history. Pertinent information for these patients includes:

- past medical problems
- prior sedation or analgesia
- allergies
- upper respiratory infections
- recent meals

Regardless of the response to questions about eating, it is probably prudent to consider every child in the emergency department setting as having a full stomach. Vital signs, including respiratory rate, temperature, and heart rate, should be obtained as well as baseline pulse oximetry.

In addition to a physical examination related to the patient's immediate problem, a brief examination should be conducted of the oral pharnyx, posterior pharnyx, and chest. Because of the relatively larger tongue and more reactive tonsils and adenoids in children, respiratory compromise is more of a concern in children undergoing PSA than adults. In addition, upper respiratory infections (URIs) are common in this population, adding nasal or respiratory tract congestion as another potential source of airway obstruction. None of these are absolute contraindications to administration of sedating agents to a child, but they should be considered by the clinician when determining the manner of a child's procedural sedation.

Any child undergoing PSA in the emergency department (ED) should be assigned an American Society of Anesthesiologists (ASA) score. The ASA scoring system is summarized in Table 24-1. ASA 1 or 2 patients are generally healthy children who are good candidates for PSA in the emergency department; ASA 4 or 5 patients are generally better treated in a formal operating room or procedural unit. ASA 3 patients may be managed in either area depending on the nature of the problem and the capabilities of the treating physician, although consultation with an anesthesiologist may be useful.

A different type of scoring system is also applied for children suffering from isolated painful conditions requiring simple analgesia. Age-specific scoring scales do not classify the risk of the patient for receiving sedatives but rather permit a quantitative comparison of pain relief between assessments and among different examiners. A number of scoring systems have been designed for application to children from infancy through adolescence. Figure 24-1 contains examples of visual analog or ob-

Table 24-1. American Society of Anesthesiologists Physical Status Classification

Class	Characteristics
I	A normal health patient
II	A patient with mild systemic disease
III	A patient with severe systemic disease
IV	A patient with severe systemic disease that is a constant life threat
V	A moribund patient who is not expected to survive without the procedure
E	Emergency procedure

servational scoring systems used in describing painful conditions in patients of various ages.

PATIENT MONITORING

The degree of monitoring required is determined by the patient, the procedure, and the medications utilized.

Patients receiving analgesia for relief of an acute painful condition or simple anxiety alleviation generally do not require any additional monitoring. For example, a child with a clavicle fracture receiving oral acetaminophen with hydrocodone or a patient with abdominal pain receiving a standard dose of morphine generally will not require continuous monitoring beyond repeat vital signs. If unusually high doses of analgesics are required for a patient such as a sickle cell anemia patient still in severe pain after 0.05 mg/kg of hydromorphone, then some form of respiratory or blood pressure monitoring may be warranted. This is generally not a problem since such patients will also require more intensive attention because of the continued severe nature of their pain.

Patients undergoing procedural sedation will usually require some form of additional monitoring. As a general rule electronic monitoring should be in place prior to sedation initiation; however, in difficult circumstances, PSA may begin with bedside monitoring by an appropriately trained nurse or physician while the electronic equipment is being assembled and applied. For any patient undergoing procedural sedation at least one other health care professional should be present to monitor the patient aside from any involved in the performance of the procedure. This clinician should understand monitoring equipment, recognize the signs and symptoms of respiratory depression, and be trained in the management of acute respiratory problems.

Neonatal or Infant Observational Scale

Observation	Score		
	0	1	2
Face	Normal or relaxed	Occasional grimace, frown, withdrawn	Constant frown, grimace, clenched jaw
Cry	No cry	Moans or whimpers	Crying steadily, screams or sobs
Consolability	Content	Reassured by occasional touching, hugging, or talking	Difficult to control or comfort
Legs	Normal relaxed	Uneasy, restless, tense	Kicking or legs drawn up

Visual Pictorial Type Scale

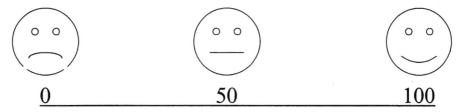

0   50   100

Numeric Visual Analog Scale

0		25		50		75		100

Fig. 24-1. Pediatric pain scales.

The primary risk of PSA is hypoventilation and hypoxia from respiratory depression, and monitoring should be directed at detection of these problems. For most patients, continuous pulse oximetry will provide both an ongoing assessment of oxygenation as well as a continuous display of heart rate. Some newer equipment can provide real time reporting of respiratory rate as well. Cardiac monitoring can be applied depending on department or physician preferences but is generally not needed. Clinicians should recognize that pulse oximetry only reports oxygen status and does not reflect the ventilatory condition of the patient. Children may hypoventilate yet still maintain adequate oxygenation if supplemental oxygen is being provided. For children in whom it is important to maintain normal arterial CO_2 tensions, a continuous end-tidal capnometer may be added to the monitoring equipment. Blood pressure measurements should be obtained prior to sedation in children in whom hypovolemia is a risk based on their clinical presentation or in those in whom hypertension is a historical concern.

The timing and duration of patient monitoring is determined by both the agent used and the procedure performed. At a minimum, any sedated child should have monitoring continued until the clinical effects of their drug therapy have dissipated and the child's respiratory and mental status have approached baseline. This is extremely important in children undergoing acute painful procedures such as fracture reductions. The greatest risk of hypoventilation in these children may occur after the painful stimuli of the procedure have ceased. Conversely, children who initially present extremely agitated and crying vigorously may exhaust themselves and remain sleeping long after the pharmacologic effects of a sedative have passed. As a consequence, the duration of patient monitoring must be determined individually, but it should be maintained long enough to be certain any clinically dangerous effects of administered drugs have resolved.

A flow sheet should be used for all children undergoing PSA. Such forms should include information on:

- ASA class
- relevant past history
- baseline airway, respiratory, and neurologic status
- medications administered and timing
- vital signs
- pulse oximetry
- discharge findings

Discharge of children undergoing PSA should not occur until the child has returned to an appropriate mental and physical baseline. Children should demonstrate the ability to tolerate sips of fluids and to ambulate without assistance unless there is an unavoidable barrier to ambulation, such as lower extremity injury. After-care instructions should reflect the fact that the child has received an agent that may alter mental status and must therefore receive close supervision. Caregivers should be cautioned that normal play activities, such as bike-riding or climbing, should be avoided in the short term and be given specific dietary instructions as well as education in regard to warning signs that may be observed.

Properly staffed and prepared EDs have demonstrated total complication rates <3 percent for all PSA patients with no major problems or deaths found in a national study of children sedated outside the operating room.

ROUTES OF ADMINISTRATION IV, IM, SQ, PO, TM

Most medications given for PSA can be given by a variety of routes. Like every other aspect of procedural sedation, the manner in which a sedative is delivered is a function of the entire clinical scenario and the treating physician's preference.

Intravenous (IV) administration offers the greatest flexibility in terms of titrating medications to a specific patient response. The most significant limitation to this approach is the problem that IV access may present in infants and agitated children. One advantage to the IV route is the potential for initiating patient-controlled analgesia (PCA). PCA permits the patient to control the dose of analgesia and has been shown to be effective in children as young as 5 years of age. IV administration is also the preferred route for a child when multiple doses of medication are anticipated or there is uncertainty regarding the child's response.

Intramuscular (IM) and subcutaneous (SQ) injections provide reliable delivery but should be reserved for drugs with well-established dose-response relationships. Repeated administration of drugs via these routes is painful and places the child in the position of deciding between the pain of their medical condition and the pain of another needle.

Oral (PO) administration should be regarded as similar to IM or SQ delivery routes in that it should be reserved for drugs with predictable actions. The timing of repeat doses can be difficult to determine due to delays in absorption and onset of action. PO administration does have the advantage of being the most comfortable of all routes of administration.

Transmucosal (TM) drug administration is a uniquely pediatric technique. Quicker in onset than PO administrations, TM delivery still is slow enough to make titration of medications difficult. Medications have been successfully delivered transmucosally through the oral, buccal, nasal, and rectal routes. Medications successfully delivered by this route include midazolam, fentanyl, sufentanyl, ketamine, thiopental, methohexital, and diazepam. Transdermal (TD) delivery of analgesic medications has also been described, although this has been reserved primarily for adult patients. In children TD application of topical anesthetics have proved successful in preparation for procedures involving percutaneous punctures.

Inhalation of sedative analgesic agents has been described in children in the ED setting and is a relatively well-tolerated route of delivery. Advantages of this route include ease of delivery and painless administration; the disadvantages stem from the need for specialized equipment and patient cooperation.

SEDATIVE AND ANALGESIC AGENTS

Medications most commonly used for PSA are listed in Table 24-2. Physicians intent on using these agents clinically must be familiar with their indications, all of their actions, relative contraindications, and potential alterna-

Table 24-2. Common Pediatric Procedural Sedation and Analgesic Agents

Medication	Route	Dose (mg/kg)	Typical Maximum (mg/kg)^a	Duration	Comments
Sedative Analgesics					
Meperidine	IV, IM	1.0–2.0	100	3–4 h	Chronic accumulation risk
Morphine	IV, IM, SQ	0.1–0.2	10	2–4 h	
Fentanyl	IV	0.001–0.002	0.05	20 min	Rigidity, apnea, lower dose
	TM	0.005–0.010			<6 mo
Remifentanil	IV	0.001	0.05	4–6 min	Rigidity, apnea
Hydromorphone	IV	0.01–0.02	2		
Hydrocodone	PO	0.2	10	4–6 h	
Codeine	PO	1–1.5	60	4–6 h	
Sedatives					
Diazepam	IV	0.05–0.2	10	2–4 h	
Lorazepam	IV, IM	0.02–0.05	2	6–8 h	
Midazolam	IV, IM	0.01–0.1	2	1–3 h	
Pentobarbital	IV, IM	2.0–5.0	200	2–4 h	
Thiopental	IV	3.0–5.0	500	20 min	Intubation doses
	PR	15–25		1–2 h	
Methohexital	IV	1–1.5	100	20 min	Intubation doses
	PR	18.0–25.0		1–2 h	
Chloral Hydrate	PO	50–75	1,000	10–24 h	Caution post procedure
Propofol	IV	0.25–1.0	75	20 min	Apnea
	Infusion	1–3 mg/kg/h		20 min	
Etomidate	IV	0.1–0.3	30	20 min	
Other Agents					
Ketamine	IV	1.0–1.5	100	30–90 min	
	IM	4.0–5.0		2–4 h	
	PO	5.0–6.0		6 h	
Nitrous Oxide	Inhalation	30–50%		1–2 min	
Diphenhydramine	PO	1.0–1.5	50		
Droperidol	IV, IM	0.01–0.05	5	4–6 h	Possible dystonic reaction
Dexmedetomidine	IV	0.2–0.7 µg/kg/h		5–6 min	Hypotension and bradycardia
Reversal Agents					
Naloxone	IV, IM	0.1	2 mg	20 min	
Flumazenil	IV	0.01	0.2 mg	30 min	

^{a}Typical maximum dose represents dose that is effective in most patients. Since all patients respond differently, it is possible that for some patients a dose in excess of this dose may be required. If such a higher dose is utilized, precautions in monitoring the patient should be taken.

tives. PSA drugs may be divided into four general classes:

- pure analgesics
- sedative analgesics
- pure sedatives
- others

There is no single agent that is ideal for any given scenario, and physician preference and departmental practices play an important role in drug selection. Physicians caring for children should have a working knowledge of multiple agents and be adept at choosing alternate drugs when their drug of choice is inappropriate in a given circumstance.

Pure Analgesic Agents

The medications in this class are

- aspirin
- acetaminophen
- nonsteroidal antiinflamatory drugs (NSAIDs)

These agents are commonly used as antipyretics and for treatment of minor extremity pain. Keterolac, the only parenteral NSAID available in the United States, has proved particularly effective in prostaglandin-mediated conditions, such as biliary or renal colic, although its use in other painful conditions generally requires addition of a supplemental narcotic. Many of the pure analgesics are also combined with narcotic agents for synergistic effects in oral combination therapies.

Sedative Analgesic Agents

Synthetic and naturally occurring narcotic analgesics constitute this class of drugs, and all produce their effect through stimulation of opioid receptor sites in the central nervous system. Differences in the effects of the various clinically used agents result from differential binding preferences for these receptor sites. Narcotic analgesics create dose-dependent pain relief with mild sedative effects. Cardiovascular and respiratory depression may be seen at any dose, although it is generally not clinically significant at standard dosages. More minor adverse effects include nausea and transient itching or urticaria from histamine release. Narcotics may be administered PO, IV, IM, SQ, TM, and even intrathecally. Modifications of narcotic drugs can also produce agents with pure agonist, pure antagonist, and combination effects. Most of the desired actions of the commonly used narcotic agents result from their actions on the mu and kappa receptor sites, and undesired narcotic actions can be reversed through administration of a competitive antagonist such as naloxone or nalmephine.

Morphine may be considered the classic narcotic analgesic and exhibits most of the characteristics of this group. Morphine is generally employed to treat moderate to severe painful conditions, as an adjunct for painful procedures, and occasionally as a sedative hypnotic. It is frequently administered with a phenothiazine or hydroxazine; there is no evidence that addition of these agents either potentiates the analgesic effects of the morphine or decreases the incidence of emesis.

Meperidine is another commonly employed analgesic with clinical characteristics very similar to those of morphine. Unlike morphine, meperidine is metabolized to an active metabolite, normeperidine, which has a longer serum half-life than that of its parent compound. Normeperidine produces a dysmorphic reaction if allowed to accumulate in a child. For this reason meperidine should not be used in children who will require multiple doses of a narcotic over an extended period.

Hydromorphone is a more potent semisynthetic narcotic analgesic similar to morphine and meperidine and is frequently used in pain management protocols for sickle cell anemia patients and in PCA pumps.

Fentanyl citrate is a synthetic short-acting narcotic approximately 100 times more potent than morphine. It has a rapid onset and 20-minute duration of action, making it ideal for brief painful procedures. Unlike other narcotics, fentanyl has little cardiovascular effects, making it attractive in hypovolemic or cardiac patients. One unique side effect of fentanyl is chest wall rigidity, which can occur if the drug is administered too rapidly. This side effect may be reversed with naloxone, although on occasion endotracheal intubation and skeletal muscle paralysis may be required. Fentanyl is also unique in that it is the only narcotic administered through the PO transmucosal route. Provided as a "lollipop," the child is permitted to suck on the fentanyl-containing hard candy vehicle until he or she becomes drowsy. Although effective as a sedative, transmucosal fentanyl produces vomiting in up to 30 percent of children. A cogeniter of fentanyl, sufentanyl has been successfully administered intransally for procedural sedation. Intensive respiratory monitoring is required for children given either of these drugs. Reduced doses should be used in neonates and very young infants, as they are more sensitive to the respiratory depressant effects. Fentanyl has also been incorporated in transdermal patches for use in patients with chronic pain.

Remifentanil is the newest synthetic narcotic analgesic with a 15- to 30-second onset and 4- to 6-minute duration of action. Its potency and cardiovascular effects are similar to those of fentanyl; however, because of its ultrashort duration of action, it is generally delivered as a continuous infusion. Single-bolus injections have been used for PSA. Remifentanil is also used in combination with propofol for nonparalytic rapid sequence intubations, although as yet no specific ED studies involving this technique have been reported. Because of its unique sedative and analgesic characteristics, this drug may be used in short painful procedures. Remifentanil appears to have a wider therapeutic window than fentanyl, and an 80 percent incidence of hypoxia and apnea has been reported with nongeneral anesthesia applications.

Codeine, hydrocodone, and *oxycodone* are less potent narcotic analgesics generally administered orally in combination with a pure analgesic, such as acetaminophen or ibuprofen. Longer-acting preparations of these narcotics have also been formulated for once-a-day oral preparations.

Pure Sedatives

Medications in this group are also referred to as sedative hypnotic agents because of the ability to sedate patients and induce sleep. Most of the agents in this class exert their effect through the gamma-aminobutyric acid (GABA) receptor of central nervous system neurons. GABA receptors are an essential part of the central nervous system's negative feedback loop. Composed of five proteins of three different types, the GABA receptor forms a cell membrane pore. When stimulated, this pore opens, allowing the influx of chloride ions, effectively hyperpolarizing the resting cell membrane. This hyperpolarization makes it more difficult for excitatory neurotransmitters to stimulate that neuron and induce depolarization and nerve conduction. Of the protein types in the GABA receptors, one binds barbiturate class drugs, another binds benzodiazepine class drugs, and one binds GABA.

In addition to decreasing awareness and inducing somnolence, the pure sedatives can also produce cardiovascular and respiratory depression in a dose-related manner.

When sedative hypnotic agents are administered, it is imperative that sufficient medication be administered. Delivery of subtherapeutic doses of any agents in this class will cause disinhibition in the child and may result in agitated, uncontrolled behavior. Treatment of this state is through administration of more of the sedative hypnotic agent to take the child through the plane of disinhibition to one of somnolence.

Barbiturates are the classic pediatric sedative agents. All the medications in this class produce predictable sedation with variability in effects related to their lipid solubility and rate of central nervous system penetration. Drugs used in ED sedation include pentobarbital, thiopental, and methohexital.

Thiopental and methohexital are both extremely rapid-acting anesthesia-induction agents used primarily in the ED setting as part of rapid-sequence intubation protocols. Administered IV, these agents rapidly penetrate the central nervous system and induce profound sedation within 30 seconds. Respiratory depression is a prominent feature of IV administration of these drugs at standard induction doses, and apnea should be anticipated in any child in whom these doses are used. Lower, more slowly administered doses can avoid this problem. Rectal administration of either of these agents has proved effective for sedation of children undergoing diagnostic radiology studies. Absorption via this route may be extremely rapid, and parents holding a child after administration of the drug should be closely supervised, sitting down, and positioned as if the child is already sleeping.

Pentobarbital is a rapid-acting, less-potent sedative hypnotic used primarily in sedation for diagnostic studies. Administered either IV or IM, this agent produces very predictable actions, making it ideal for painless diagnostic studies or procedures. In head-to-head comparisons with benzodiazepines, pentobarbital consistently produces better, more reliable sedation. A modification of the most common protocol for the administration of this drug is as follows:

- Have appropriate vascular access and monitoring.
- Administer 2.5 mg/kg pentobarbital IV over 30 seconds.
- Wait 1 to 2 minutes.
- If the child is not sleeping, administer 1.25 mg/kg pentobarbital IV over 30 seconds.
- Wait 2 to 3 minutes.
- If the child is not sleeping, administer final 1.25 mg/kg over 30 seconds.

Benzodiazepines, like the barbiturates, produce their effect through actions on the GABA receptors. This is why the clinical actions of these two classes of agents are so similar. Unlike the barbiturates, the effects of the benzodiazepines can be reversed with the competitive antagonist flumazenil.

Diazepam and lorazepam are moderate to long-acting anxiolytics with good sedative hypnotic properties. Occasionally used for procedural sedation, these agents are more commonly used for seizure control or agitation management in acute substance abuse or psychosis cases. Both of these drugs can induce skeletal muscle relaxation and have been used to assist reduction of large joint dislocations.

Midazolam is a shorter-acting, more potent benzodiazepine commonly used for procedural sedation in the ED setting. Used alone, this drug can sedate children for diagnostic studies or may be combined with a narcotic analgesic for performance of painful procedures. Midazolam may be given through any number of routes including oral, nasal, rectal, IV, and IM, although the PO and IV routes are most commonly used. A reliable sedative agent, it does have a large and variable therapeutic window in children. Because of this, the potential exists for clinicians to produce a disinhibited state while attempting to sedate a child. Physicians using this drug must feel comfortable administering additional doses of midazolam to reverse this effect in these children. Repeated subtherapeutic doses of midazolam may only lead to a condition in which the child is merely titrated within a state of agitation.

Propofol is an ultra–short-acting sedative hypnotic used for both RSI and PSA. Propofol's mechanism of action is unclear and may relate to both a GABA receptor effect and a direct neuronal membrane action. Propofol is a highly lipid soluble agent that produces clinical effects within one arm brain circulation with a duration of 6 to 8 minutes. For ED procedures such as treatment of large joint dislocations, propofol is generally administered as a 0.5-mg/kg slow bolus and then titrated with repeated 0.1-mg/kg boluses until the desired level of sedation and relaxation is achieved. For prolonged sedation, a propofol bolus is generally followed by a continuous infusion. The pharmacokinetic profile of this drug makes propofol ideal for sedation of patients on ventilators when repeat examinations may be required. Like thiopental and methohexital, propofol will induce apnea and hypotension if pushed rapidly. For induction in preparation for intubation 1 mg/kg is generally administered. Continuous infusions have also been used in sedation for diagnostic studies.

Etomidate is another sedative hypnotic agent that has found application in the ED care of children. Most commonly used as an induction agent for emergency intubations, etomidate has a flat cardiovascular curve and is most useful for hypotensive patients. More recently etomidate has been described as both a sedative and analgesic in short painful emergency department procedures such as fracture reductions.

Chloral hydrate, the traditional oral sedative hypnotic, has an extensive history as a reliable agent for control of pediatric patients for diagnostic procedures. Although effective, chloral hydrate has fallen out of favor because of its long duration of action and the introduction of newer agents. In a direct comparison with oral midazolam, chloral hydrate consistently provided better sedation and control for diagnostic radiographs. Generally given in the range of 50 to 75 mg/kg, chloral hydrate's actions can be seen in 30 minutes, but residual effects may last for up to 36 hours.

Diphenhydramine is an antihistamine with prominent sedative side effects. Marketed as an over-the-counter sleep aid, this medication does have a hypnotic effect that is adequate for children undergoing painless diagnostic studies. Diphenhydramine is particularly effective in a child who is exhausted because of extensive crying.

Dexmedetomidine, related to clonidine, is a central acting α_2-adrenoceptor agonist with potent sedative, analgesic, and anxiolytic actions. This drug is unique in that it does not produce respiratory depression and is utilized predominantly for control of patients undergoing mechanical ventilation. Hypotension and bradycardia are potential side effects with this medication. Clinical trials to date with dexmedetomidine are limited in children, and this drug should be used only for older adolescents.

Other Agents

Ketamine is unique among pediatric PSA agents. As a dissociative agent, it produces a trance-like cataleptic state through disruption of communications between the cortical and limbic systems. Ketamine produces extremely rapid sedation, analgesia, and amnesia that facilitates both painless diagnostic studies and less painful procedures. This agent has mild sympathomimetic effects that can decrease bronchospasm, maintain and even slightly raise systemic blood pressure, and produce tachycardia. Ketamine does increase intracranial pressure and should be avoided in children with head injuries and physical evidence of elevated intracranial pressure. Unlike any of the pure sedatives and sedative hypnotics, ketamine does not produce respiratory depression and in fact may slightly exaggerate coughing and swallowing reflexes. Transient apnea and self-limited laryngospasm have been reported when the drug has been administered by rapid intravenous bolus in extremely young infants. Because ketamine's increase of protective airway reflexes may produce layrngospasm, it should be used with caution in children with excessive airway secretions or brisk oral and posterior pharyngeal bleeding.

Ketamine also produces increased salivation, which can be limited by pretreatment with either atropine or glycopyrrolate. Because of this, care should be taken in the use of this agent in children with active URIs.

Ketamine produces very intense vivid dreams. In children, it is possible to suggest a dream by asking the child what he or she wishes to dream about and reinforcing that idea in conjunction with the administration of the ketamine. The vivid dreams may also result in what are termed emergence reactions, in which the child has what appears to be disturbing hallucinations as the ketamine effect is weaning. These events may appear in up to 50 percent of adults but are relatively rare in children, with mild agitation being reported in about 17 percent of cases and severe agitation in <2 percent. Emergence reactions appear to be related to the child's level of anxiety prior to the procedure, age younger than 5 years, and the existence of underlying medical conditions. Limiting stimuli during recovery may help to lessen these emergence reactions. Emesis occurs in about 17 percent of children older than 5 years of age, but in <4 percent of those under this age. Most of these reactions are self-limited, and acute pharmacologic intervention is not generally required, although administration of a short-acting benzodiazepine in older children or adults may resedate the child during this period. Studies examining prophylactic administration of midazolam in conjunction with the initial ketamine dose have failed to demonstrate any decrease in emergence reactions. Ketamine may be one of the safest of all PSA agents. Patients in whom 10 times the intended dose of the medication was administered demonstrated no significant adverse outcomes.

Droperidol is a butyrophenone whose specific mechanism of action remains unclear. Used commonly for immediate control of agitated patients, this agent may be administered either intramuscularly or intravenously. Its most common ED applications include emesis control and management of acute ethanol intoxication in adolescent or young adult patients. Droperidol has an onset of action of 1 to 5 minutes with a duration of 2 to 6 hours. Although patients are quickly sedated to the point of somnolence, they are easily aroused and maintain protective upper airway reflexes and respiratory drive.

Nitrous oxide is best described as a sedative analgesic that does not function through opioid receptor stimulation. Administered as an oxygen-nitrous oxide mixture, it has an onset of action of 2 to 3 minutes and a similar duration of action. This drug is not metabolized and is excreted only through exhalation by the lungs. The sedation and analgesia produced by this drug is dose dependent and can be intense at higher inhalation concentrations. The minimal concentration with any clinical efficacy is a 30 percent nitrous oxide-70 percent oxygen mixture although true efficacy is probably not achieved under a 50 percent-50 percent mixture. To deliver this drug, patient cooperation is required. Most nitrous oxide systems are designed for self-administration. Modifications have been designed for continuous flow systems applicable to children as young as 4 years of age. The need for specialized equipment and staff training may be a limiting factor in the more widespread use of this modality.

Nitrous oxide is generally used for brief anxiolysis and short painful procedures. In a direct comparison nitrous oxide proved more effective than oral midazolam for laceration repairs.

Because it diffuses freely into any gas-filled cavity, nitrous oxide should not be used for patients with pneumothorax or bowel obstruction.

NONPHARMACOLOGIC SEDATION AND ANALGESIA

Because of their short attention spans and susceptibility to suggestion, children are excellent candidates for nonpharmacologic sedation and analgesia techniques. Distraction either through intensive conversation, story telling, or visual or tactile stimuli are all effective means of diverting a child's attention from a brief painful procedure such as a local infiltration or IV injection. Music via ear phones or videos is another distraction that may be used to occupy a child for performance of a more prolonged procedure.

In newborns, a highly concentrated sugar solution has been shown to decrease observational scores during painful procedures, such as circumcisions. The mechanism of action for this effect appears to be related to induction of central nervous system enkephlins. One to 2 mL of a 50 percent sucrose solution and sucrose-coated nipples have proved effective in decreasing crying in neonates undergoing heel sticks or venipunctures.

Another technique that works well in infants and toddlers is sleep deprivation. For noncritical studies, small children who present in proximity to their normal sleep times may be kept awake beyond this time and then fed and permitted to fall asleep. A mild hypnotic such as diphehydramine may be added to help produce somnolence. This technique is particularly useful in children who are to be discharged for outpatient studies. Depending on the timing of the study, a child can be sleep deprived leading up to the study and then simply allowed to return to physiologic sleep to perform the study. Ideally the caregiver should schedule the test for late morning and awaken the child unusually early the day of the procedure.

SELECTION OF PSA AGENTS

Which PSA agent to employ in any given scenario should be left to the clinician caring for a particular child. Hospital or departmental policies that permit access to a complete choice of medications allow treating physicians to match a child more appropriately to the correct PSA agent. In a study of sedation preferences for posttraumatic head computed tomography (CT) scans, more than 20 different regimens were described. Overly restrictive ED formularies may force performance of a procedure with a less-than-optimal drug and increase the possibilities of an injury or adverse advent.

PSA selection is also dictated by the intended effect on a child. If cooperation for a painless diagnostic procedure is desired, then a sedative hypnotic agent will be the drug of choice. Use of a narcotic analgesic to produce somnolence may require such a large dose that respiratory depression becomes a risk. For the same reasons, use of a pure sedative with no analgesic properties to provide cooperation for a painful procedure is equally inappropriate.

Combinations of different agents may be used to take advantage of the desired properties of each. The most frequent combinations pair short-acting sedatives with short-acting narcotics such as fentanyl/midazolam or fentanyl/propofol. Caution should be maintained with such combinations because not only will the desired effects be enhanced but adverse effects such as respiratory depression may also be increased. Doses lower than those of either agent alone should be used initially when combining potent agents.

Combining a local anesthetic with a sedative can also produce effective patient control. The regional anesthesia permits pain control, and the sedative produces anxiolysis and cooperation for the procedure. Procedures such as lumbar punctures and laceration repairs are examples of where this technique is applied.

Selection of agents is also dependent on the child's age and baseline behavior. One 3-year-old child may hold perfectly still for a 5-minute head CT scan, whereas another may require intravenous access and titrated doses of a sedative hypnotic agent for the same procedure.

Potential agents for different clinical scenarios are listed in Table 24-3.

For very painful acute conditions, some form of a parenteral narcotic is the agent of choice. Less severe pain may be managed with an oral narcotic/acetaminophen or ibuprofen combination. Localized extremity pain from a severe injury such as a femur fracture or crushed finger may best be managed immediately with regional anesthesia such as a femoral or digital nerve block. The options for pain management for acute conditions seem to be age independent, although younger children seem to be at much greater risk of oligoanalgesia than older patients. PCA is an excellent option for any child old enough to use a delivery pump and is particularly useful for constant painful conditions that may take time to resolve, such as sickle cell crisis or pancreatitis.

Sedation options for painless diagnostic studies seems to be more age dependent and much more variable. Adolescents rarely require sedation for radiographic studies, whereas some treatment is frequently needed for infants and small children. Most of the sedative hypnotics will work in these circumstances, and the selection of the agent is as much based on route of delivery as pharmacologic profile. For departments adept at obtaining vascular access, an intravenous route will allow titration of an agent and a shorter clinical duration of action. Infants and small toddlers may be candidates for intramuscular injections or oral or transmucosal drugs.

Multiple comparisons of different sedation options have demonstrated some trends but little conclusive information. Individual studies with the use of oral, nasal, rectal, and parenteral midazolam have demonstrated this to be an effective sedative agent for painless diagnostic studies and as an adjunct for procedures performed with local anesthesia. Midazolam remains the most popular agent recommended for posttraumatic head CTs in children despite head-to-head comparisons demonstrating that ketamine, nitrous oxide, pentobarbital, propofol, and chloral hydrate provide more consistent, more controlled sedation in pediatric patients.

Some outpatient diagnostic studies, such as MRIs, will require pharmacologic interventions to permit completion. The safest means of outpatient sedation for such procedures is to apply the same monitoring criteria used for ED patients. Caregivers should be instructed to return either to the ED or to another area of the hospital with their child at an appropriate time, where proper sedation and monitoring can be initiated. If a free-standing outpatient facility must be used for a procedure, then no sedation should be administered unless that facility has the equipment and staff to perform monitoring to the same extent as that performed in the hospital. If an oral agent must be given, it should not be admin-

Table 24-3. Clinical Scenarios and Possible Sedation Analgesia Options[a]

Scenario	Options		
	1	**2**	**3**
Moderate systemic pain	Morphine	Meperidine	Hydromorphone
Severe systemic pain	Morphine PCA	Fentanyl PCA	Hydromorphone
Fracture care	Regional anesthesia	Ketamine	Fentanyl/midazolam
Urgent diagnostics	Propofol	Pentobarbital	Midazolam
Dislocation	Propofol	Morphine and diazepam	Etomidate
Lumbar puncture[b]	Ketamine	Midazolam	Morphine
Sexual abuse exam	Midazolam	Ketamine and midazolam	Propofol
RSI adjunct	Propofol	Etomidate	Ketamine
Burn care	Nitrous oxide	Ketamine	Morphine
Abscess I&D	Ketamine	Morphine	Remifentanil[c]
Laceration repair	Ketamine	Distraction	Fentanyl/midazolam
Acute agitation control	Droperidol	Lorazepam	Diazepam
Anxiolysis	Lorazepam	Diazepam	Pentobarbital
Nonurgent diagnostics	Sleep deprivation	Diphenhydramine	Midazolam
Scheduled outpatient diagnostic study	Sleep deprivation	Return to ED or sedation unit	Chloral hydrate

[a]This table contains potential sedation or analgesia regimens. Other medications are also applicable for these scenarios, and selection of agents depends on a combination of patient characteristics and individual physician preference. PCA, patient-controlled analgesia; RSI, rapid sequence intubation; I&D, incision & drainage.
[b]Risk of hypoxia with lateral positioning.
[c]Theoretical application at present.

istered until the child is at the facility and under the direct observation of the appropriate staff. Significant morbidity and mortality have occurred during private vehicle transport of children placed in car restraints following administration of procedural sedatives at home. Equally important is the fact that children be maintained under observation until they return to near baseline, prior to the trip home.

CHILDREN WITH SPECIAL HEALTH CARE NEEDS

Children with underlying medical conditions, frequently referred to as children with special health care needs (CSHCN), are becoming more frequent visitors to community as well as academic EDs. These children will require PSA both for problems related to their underlying conditions and for acute problems common to all children. CSHCN are at risk for sedation or analgesic agents being withheld for fear of complications related to preexisting conditions. In reality, these patients are more

appropriate candidates for PSA to avoid undue physiologic or psychological stresses.

The approach to PSA in this population is the same as for any other child, except that selection of the PSA agent must take into account not only the child's acute problem but also preexisting conditions. Whenever possible, coordination of sedation with a child's medication schedule should be attempted. A child on neuropsychiatric or seizure medications who becomes somnolent following routine dosing of the medication may undergo a painless diagnostic study a short time after receipt of their last medication dose. Children with cardiovascular problems should be managed with agents such as fentanyl, which have little blood pressure or heart rate effects. Children with respiratory pathology or anatomic upper airway difficulties may best be served with regional anesthesia or a drug with minimal ventilatory effects such as ketamine. Children with hepatic or renal failure may be more sensitive to drugs and titrated with smaller doses and more prolonged postprocedure observation. Emergency physicians should also not hesitate to involve anesthesiology colleagues to help with CSHCN patients, particularly those who are ASA class 3 or above.

SUMMARY

Safe, effective PSA is an integral part of any child's ED care. Emergency physicians have proved competent and reliable in the delivery of this treatment to ED patients, but they must remain vigilant throughout the administration and recovery from PSA to ensure patient safety and comfort.

BIBLIOGRAPHY

American College of Emergency Physicians: Clinical policy for procedural sedation and analgesia in the emergency department. *Ann Emerg Med* 31:663–677, 1998.

Coté CJ, Notterman DA, Karl HW, et al: Adverse sedation events in pediatrics: A critical incident analysis of contributing factors. *Pediatrics* 105:805–814, 2000.

D'Agostino J, Terndrup TE: Chloral hydrate versus midazolam for sedation of children for neuroimaging: A randomized clinical trial. *Pediatr Emerg Care* 16:1–4, 2000.

Dickinson R, Singer A, Carrion W: Etomidate for pediatric sedation prior to fracture reduction. *Acad Emerg Med* 8: 74–77, 2001.

Green SM, Kupperman N, Rothrock SG, et al: Predictors of adverse events with intramuscular ketamine sedation in children. *Ann Emerg Med* 35:35–42, 2000.

Luhmann JD, Kennedy RM, Porter FL, et al: A randomized clinical trial of continuous flow nitrous oxide and midazolam for sedation of young children during laceration repair. *Ann Emerg Med* 37:1, 2001.

McQuillen KK, Steele DW: Capnography during sedation/analgesia in a pediatric emergency department. *Pediatr Emerg Care* 16:401–404, 2000.

Pomeranz ES, Chudnofsky CR, Deegan TJ, et al: Rectal methohexital sedation for computed tomography imaging of stable pediatric emergency department patients. *Pediatrics* 105: 1110–1114, 2000.

Sacchetti AD, Schafermeyer R, Gerardi M, et al: Pediatric analgesia and sedation. *Ann Emerg Med* 23:237–250, 1994.

Sherwin TS, Green SM, Khan A, et al: Does adjunctive midazolam reduce recovery agitation after ketamine sedation for pediatric procedures? A randomized double-blind placebo controlled trial. *Ann Emerg Med* 35:229–238, 2000.

25

Upper Airway Emergencies

Richard M. Cantor

HIGH-YIELD FACTS

- Acute respiratory emergencies in the pediatric patient are common and may, if improperly treated, result in significant morbidity and mortality.

- The clinician must maintain an awareness of the unique anatomic and physiologic characteristics of the respiratory tract in the growing infant and child.

- Stridor may originate anywhere in the upper airway from the anterior nares to the subglottic region.

- The most common causes of acute upper airway obstruction are croup, epiglottitis, and foreign body obstruction. Additional processes include peritonsillar abscess, bacterial tracheitis, and retropharyngeal abscess.

Acute respiratory emergencies in the pediatric patient are common and may, if improperly treated, result in significant morbidity and mortality. Calm, decisive, and deliberate intervention is mandatory to ensure the most effective outcome. The clinician must maintain an awareness of the unique anatomic and physiologic characteristics of the respiratory tract in the growing infant and child. An expanded knowledge of the most frequent airway problems encountered in children will assist in arriving at the most adequate disposition of these patients. Most importantly, the ability to assess the child in respi-

ratory distress accurately remains the most critical step in patient care.

PATHOPHYSIOLOGY

Upper Airway Considerations

The small caliber of the upper airway in children makes it vulnerable to occlusion secondary to a variety of disease processes and also results in greater baseline airway resistance. Any process that further narrows the airway will cause an exponential rise in airway resistance and a secondary increase in the work of breathing. As the child perceives distress, an increase in respiratory effort will augment turbulence and increase resistance to a greater degree.

Since the young infant is primarily a nasal breather, any degree of obstruction of the nasopharynx may result in significant increase in work of breathing and present clinically as retractions. The large tongue of infants and small children can occlude the oropharynx. Any child who presents with altered mental status will be at risk for the development of upper airway obstruction secondary to a loss of muscle tone affecting the tongue. Occlusion of the oropharynx by this anatomic structure is quite common in this setting. Interventions that can correct this anatomic blockage include either tilting of the head or lifting of the chin.

Older children will frequently present with enlarged tonsillar and adenoidal tissues. Although they rarely cause an upper airway catastrophe, these structures are vulnerable to trauma and bleeding during clinical interventions such as insertion of an oral or nasal airway. The pediatric trachea is easily dispensable due to incomplete closure of semiformed cartilaginous rings. Any maneuver that overextends the neck will contribute to compression of this structure and secondary upper airway obstruction. The cricoid ring represents the narrowest portion of the upper airway and is often the site of occlusion in foreign body aspiration.

Lower Airway Considerations

The lower respiratory tract consists of all structures below the level of the midtrachea including the bronchi, bronchioles, and alveoli. Developmental immaturity of these structures is reflected by a decreased number of these subunits necessary for appropriate oxygenation and ventilation. In addition, the pediatric patient possesses a diminished pulmonary vascular bed. The relatively small caliber of the pediatric lower airway not only predisposes it to occlusion, but even partial obstruction will result in an augmented degree of airway resistance.

Immaturity of the musculoskeletal and central nervous systems can also contribute to the development of respiratory failure. In infancy, the diaphragm remains the primary muscle of respiration. Minor contributions are provided by the intercostal musculature. Any degree of abdominal distention will interfere with diaphragmatic function and cause secondary ventilatory insufficiency. The infant's diaphragm possesses muscle fibers that are more prone to fatigue compared with their adult counterparts. In addition, the chest wall of the pediatric patient is quite compliant, preventing adequate stabilization during periods of increased respiratory distress. Finally, infants are less sensitive to hypoxemia secondary to poor development of central respiratory control, which places this population at risk for insufficient respiratory response to disease states.

SIGNS OF DISTRESS

Regardless of the specific disease process, abnormalities in respiratory function are eventually reflected in physical symptoms and signs ranging from subtle changes to obvious distress. Respiratory distress occurs when there is increased work of breathing or increased respiratory rate in order to maintain respiratory function necessary to meet the body's oxygen and ventilation requirements. Respiratory failure ensues when respiratory efforts cannot maintain adequate respiratory function, either oxygenation or ventilation.

Tachypnea (Table 10-3) represents the most common response of the child to augmented respiratory needs. Central stimulation by the medullary respiratory center is predominantly responsible for this physiologic response. Although most commonly due to hypoxia and hypercarbia, tachypnea may also be a secondary response to metabolic acidosis, pain, or central nervous system insult. Tachycardia represents a protean sign of distress of any etiology in the pediatric patient. This would include the patient with respiratory compromise.

Infants and children readily utilize accessory muscles as a compensatory mechanism necessary to support the increased work of breathing. Intercostal, subcostal, sub- and supersternal, and supraclavicular retractions are commonly seen. In addition, the infant and child, if further compromised, will demonstrate nasal flaring.

Specific attention must be paid to the child who generates a grunting sound at the end of expiration. This physiologic enterprise represents closure of the glottis at the end of expiration, which generates additional positive end-expiratory pressure, which in many disease states is necessary to prevent compromised alveoli from collapse. Grunting represents an ominous sign in the pediatric patient who presents with respiratory distress.

Many infants and children, especially children with upper airway compromise, will assume a "position of comfort," which represents the most adequate anatomic compensation they can generate relative to their disease state. Children with stridor will often assume an upright position, lean forward, and generate their own jaw thrust maneuver to facilitate opening of the upper airway. Patients with upper airway compromise may also prefer to breathe through an open mouth, which suggests dysphagia with inability to swallow secretions, or the general presence of air hunger. Patients with lower airway disease, specifically those with reactive airway components, will assume a "tripod position" consisting of upright posture, leaning forward, and support of the upper thorax by the use of extended arms. This position allows for full use of the thoraco-abdominal axis for the work of breathing.

In situations in which significant excessive negative intrathoracic pressure is generated, venous return will increase to the heart, and left ventricular volume will be compromised. These intracardiac phenomena result in the generation of a pulsus paradoxus of greater than 20 mmHg (normal 0 to 10 mmHg). The presence of an elevated pulsus paradoxus correlates well with severe respiratory distress.

The presence of cyanosis is an ominous sign in the pediatric patient. It represents inadequate oxygenation within the pulmonary bed or inadequate oxygen delivery by the cardiac vasculature. Cyanosis of respiratory origin tends to be central rather than peripheral. A secondary effect of cyanosis may be the development of somnolence. The most common symptoms and signs of hypoxemia include agitation, irritability, and failure to maintain feeding efforts in the young infant. Clinically evident hypoxemia may not appear until pO_2 levels are dangerously low in the anemic child.

By far the most reliable sign of respiratory failure remains the generation of an ineffective respiratory effort by the infant or child and an altered level of consciousness. Auscultation of the chest may reveal decreased air entry, poor breath sounds, and bradypnea as the child progresses toward respiratory failure. Concomitant with hypoxemia in infants is the development of bradycardia. Although bradycardia may also be due to excessive vagal stimulation, hypoxemia should be ruled out in all such cases of respiratory distress.

GENERAL MANAGEMENT PRINCIPLES

Any child with respiratory distress requires supplemental oxygen. Humidified oxygen may be delivered in a variety of ways, including mask with or without rebreather apparatus, nasal prongs, or face tent, or via an oxygen hood. Infants and children who feel threatened by the use of frightening equipment may be placed in the mother's arms and receive oxygen by tubing alone (at maximal flow) or by inserting the end of the tubing in a cup.

Specific diagnostic categories of respiratory distress offer the clinician various therapeutic modalities, which will improve the patient's status (see next section). General evaluative principles that should be applied to the infant or child in distress include the following:

- Standardized approach to the patient in mild to moderate distress:
  - Provide adequate supplemental oxygen.
  - Allow the child to assume a position of comfort.
  - Create a comfortable, nonthreatening environment for both parent and child.
  - Avoid any noxious stimuli in the form of unnecessary procedures.
  - Maintain normothermia and hydration.
  - Assess the degree of respiratory distress, at presentation and at appropriate intervals.
- Arterial blood gases:
  - Measurement of Pa_{CO_2} provides the clinician with an estimate of alveolar ventilatory sufficiency. The absolute value must be interpreted in the face of the amount of respiratory effort the patient must generate to attain that particular Pa_{CO_2}. Therefore, a Pa_{CO_2} of 40, although listed as within normal limits in most references, is less than acceptable when applied to an infant in distress with marked tachypnea. Any degree of fatigue in this patient will promote CO_2 retention and the rapid development of potentially irreversible

respiratory failure. Tachypnea does not guarantee adequate ventilation, since many patients will fail to generate adequate tidal volumes and, in effect, be hypoventilating.

- Pa_{CO_2} provides an estimate of alveolar gas exchange and a measure of the balance between tissue perfusion and metabolic demand. It is important to emphasize that the use of percutaneous oximetry only reflects oxygenation and may, in some circumstances, falsely represent the adequacy of ventilation. The use of oximetry should not replace the use of one's eyes and a stethoscope in evaluating the pediatric patient with respiratory distress.

- The arterial pH represents the balance between metabolic demand and respiratory expenditure. With metabolic acidosis, the respiratory system represents the primary compensatory mechanism for overall balance. In patients with excessive work of breathing, generation of lactate from respiratory musculature may remain uncompensated by hyperventilation, resulting in profound acidemia.

- Recognition of the signs of respiratory failure, including:
  - Decreased level of consciousness (Tables 10-9 and 11-1)
  - Progressive fatigue
  - Increasing work of breathing and respiratory rate
  - Poor color (cyanotic, ashen, or gray)
  - Diaphoresis, retractions, grunting, and flaring
  - Decreased air movement on auscultation
  - Hypoventilation or apnea
  - Acidosis, hypercapnea, or hypoxemia

ASSESSMENT AND MANAGEMENT OF SPECIFIC CLINICAL SCENARIOS

Stridor, the hallmark of upper airway compromise, results from the generation of inspiratory turbulence transmitted against a narrowed lumen. Stridor may originate anywhere in the upper airway from the anterior nares to the subglottic region. In the young infant, stridor is most often the result of a congenital anomaly involving the tongue (macroglossia), larynx (laryngomalacia), and trachea (tracheomalacia). Congenital forms of stridor are often chronic in their presentation.

In the emergency department (ED), the most common causes of acute upper airway obstruction are croup, epiglottitis, and foreign body obstruction. Additional processes include peritonsillar abscess, bacterial tracheitis, and retropharyngeal abscess (Tables 25-1 and 25-2).

Epiglottitis (Supraglottitis)

Epiglottitis represents a true upper airway emergency with life-threatening complications if handled improperly. It may occur at any time of the year and, most importantly, in any age group. Traditionally, it most commonly involves children from 2 to 5 years of age. With the advent of the *Haemophilus influenzae* type b vaccine, the age range has shifted to involve older children. Possible presentations include the following:

- The acute (over several hours) onset of fever, sore throat, and dysphagia with progression to signs of respiratory distress. The child will often assume a position of comfort consisting of voluntary upper airway posturing, i.e., sitting upright, mouth open, with head, neck, and jaw extension. The voice will be muffled, and stridor, if present, may actually be quite minimal in intensity. The clinician will often note that these children appear "toxic." In severe cases, airway and swallowing mechanisms may be compromised to such a degree that profound drooling may ensue.

- Some children will be devoid of any respiratory symptoms. They will, however, complain of a severe sore throat and dysphagia. In the absence of signs of pharyngeal or tonsillar pathology, therefore, epiglottitis must be considered in this subgroup of patients. In addition, the presence of pharyngitis or uvulitis in no way excludes the possibility of epiglottitic involvement.

- Croup-like presentations in patients who fail to respond to traditional therapies should alert the clinician to the possibility of epiglottitis.

- Epiglottitis may occur at any age. Up to 25 percent of pediatric cases will be in infants <2 years of age. Adults will often only complain of a sore throat.

Most cases are caused by *H. influenzae* type b with accompanying bacteremia. Uncommon but reported causative agents include *Streptococcus pneumoniae, Staphylococcus aureus,* and group A beta-hemolytic streptococci. Blood cultures will be positive in 80 to 90 percent of affected individuals.

The most important clinical consideration for patients with epiglottitis remains the fact that, if unrecognized, airway obstruction and respiratory arrest will most certainly occur. Factors contributing to airway and ventilatory deterioration include patient fatigue, aspiration of secretions, and sudden laryngospasm. All maneuvers that agitate the child should therefore be avoided, including separation from parents, alteration of optimal airway posture (lying down), fearful events (rectal temperatures, blood work, radiographs), and gagging (forcible tongue blade examination of the oral cavity, suctioning).

Radiographs should include anteroposterior and lateral views of the soft tissues of the neck. Patients with

Table 25-1. Features of Upper Airway Disorders

Disease Process	Age Group	Mode of Onset of Respiratory Distress
Severe tonsillitis	Late preschool or school age	Gradual
Peritonsillar abscess	Usually >8 yr	Sudden increase in temperature, toxicity and distress, with unilateral throat pain, "hot potato speech"
Retropharyngeal abscess	Infancy–3 yr	Fever, toxicity, and distress after URI or pharyngitis
Epiglottitis	2–7 yr	Acute onset of hyperpyrexia, with distress, dysphagia, and drooling
Croup	3 mo–3 yr	Gradual onset of stridor and barking cough, after mild URI
Foreign body aspiration	Late infancy–4 yr	Choking episode resulting in immediate or delayed respiratory distress

URI, upper respiratory infection.

Table 25-2. Clinical Features of Acute Upper Airway Disorders

	Supraglottic Disorders (Epiglottitis)	**Subglottic Disorders (Croup)**
Stridor	Quiet	Wet and loud
Voice alteration	Muffled	Hoarse
Dysphagia	+	−
Postural preference	+	−
Barky cough	−	+
Fever	++	+
Toxicity	++	−
Trismus	+	−

suspected pneumonia should receive chest views as well. Under no circumstances should the child receive these evaluations if they promote agitation and subsequent worsening of stridor and airway compromise. The clinician must be prepared to emergently intubate and ventilate these patients at all times and in all places within the ED. In most cases, direct visualization and culture of the epiglottis itself will be performed in the operating suite prior to intubation.

The following management guidelines should be followed to avoid undue morbidity and mortality:

- Avoid agitating the child in any way.

- Provide supplemental oxygen in a nonthreatening manner.

- Allow the patient to assume a position of comfort.

- Prepare equipment for bag-valve-mask (BVM) ventilation, endotracheal intubation; needle cricothyrotomy, cricothryrotomy, and tracheostomy.

- Consult an expert in intubation and provision of a surgical airway and alert the operating room.

- Take the child to the operating room for direct visualization of the epiglottis and intubation.

- If the child suffers a respiratory arrest
  - Open the airway.
  - Attempt BVM ventilation (usually effective).
  - If unable to ventilate, intubate! If unable to intubate, perform needle or surgical cricothyroidotomy!

- Provide appropriate intravenous antibiotics (cefotaxime 50 mg/kg every 6 hours).

- Provide adequate sedation and restraint post intubation.

- Transfer the patient to an intensive care unit for further treatment and monitoring.

Croup (Viral Laryngotracheobronchitis)

Laryngotracheitis (croup) is a respiratory infection that diffusely affects the upper respiratory tract. This entity accounts for 90 percent of stridor with fever. The subglottic region is most commonly affected, resulting in edematous, inflamed mucosa with a fibrinous exudate. Agents responsible for croup are multiple, including parainfluenza types 1, 2, and 3, (most common), adenovirus, respiratory syncytial virus (RSV), and influenza. The seasonal predominance (winter) is related to the epidemiology of the most common causative agents.

Children from 1 to 3 years are usually affected. They often present, after several days of nonspecific upper respiratory infection (URI) symptoms, with a characteristic brassy or barking cough that is almost unique to croup. Inspiratory stridor eventually develops, ranging in severity from mild (only when crying or agitated) to severe (present at rest). Temperatures to 102°F are common in the course of the disease; higher temperatures or the presence of a toxic appearance should alert the clinician to carefully consider other diagnoses (atypical epiglottitis or bacterial tracheitis). The usual evolution of symptoms is a worsening of symptoms for 3 to 5 days followed by resolution over a period of days. The vast majority of children tolerate this common disease without significant morbidity; however, a small percentage may develop complete upper airway obstruction.

A variety of croup scores have been developed that quantify and qualify a constellation of physical findings, assisting the clinician in estimating the severity of subglottic obstruction as mild, moderate, or severe (Table 25-3).

Table 25-3. Clinical Croup Score[a]

	Score
Inspiratory Breath Sounds	
Normal	0
Harsh with ronchi	1
Delayed	2
Stridor	
None	0
Inspiratory	1
Inspiratory and expiratory	2
Cough	
None	0
Hoarse cry	1
Bark	2
Retractions and Flaring	
None	0
Flaring, suprasternal retractions	1
As under 1, plus subcostal and intercostal retractions	2
Cyanosis	
None	0
In air	1
In 40% O_2	2

[a]A score of 4 or more indicates moderately severe airway obstruction. A score of 7 or more, particularly when associated with $Paco_2 > 45$ and $Pao_2 < 70$ (in room air), indicates impending respiratory failure.

The most common presentation will be the child with mild croup who may be treated as an outpatient if able to take oral liquids and if well hydrated and if the physician is comfortable with parental reliability. Cool mist therapy may be suggested. The classic technique is to fill the bathroom with steam by running a hot shower. The parents can then sit with the child in this home version of a Turkish bath, for no more than 30 minutes at a time. A car ride in the cool night air with the windows slightly open may also diminish the child's symptoms. Follow-up within 24 hours should always be arranged if the patient is discharged with instructions to return if symptoms worsen.

Patients with a mild to moderate croup score can be discharged if the child improves with cool humidified oxygen therapy, the parents are reliable, and the child is older than 6 months of age.

Patients with a moderate croup score (stridor at rest) are treated as inpatients in most institutions. The purpose of admission is to provide pharmacologic therapy and to observe the child who may be at risk for progression to airway obstruction. The use of oxygen, cool mist, and racemic epinephrine delivered by nebulizer will usually result in symptomatic improvement of the patient for up to 2 hours. The recommended dose for racemic epinephrine is 0.5 mL of a 0.25 percent solution dissolved in 2.5 mL of normal saline. Peak effects have been demonstrated at 10 to 30 minutes, with duration of action lasting up to 2 hours. It is important to remember that a child may experience a return to a pretreatment level of obstruction 1 to 2 hours after therapy. This phenomenon is inaccurately referred to as "rebound." It is not the practice in many pediatric centers to discharge a child after treatment with racemic epinephrine. Recent data, utilized for patients receiving steroids, has advocated the safe discharge of racemic epinephrine recipients after 2 to 3 hours of ED observation. Racemic epinephrine is not believed to shorten the duration of illness.

Although it is unproved, many believe that a child with severe croup may be successfully carried through the episode with racemic epinephrine therapy as often as every 20 minutes (as an inpatient), avoiding the need for intubation.

Corticosteroids in higher doses (dexamethasone, 0.6 mg/kg/dose intramuscularly) seem to be of benefit in preventing the progression of croup to complete obstruction and may shorten the duration of illness. If corticosteroids are being considered (usually for the moderately or severely obstructed patient), they should be administered as soon as feasible.

If a child has severe croup (score ≥10 or a 3 in any category), it is prudent to admit that child to an intensive care setting. Treatment with oxygen, mist, racemic epinephrine, and corticosteroids should be initiated as soon as possible in the ED. Antibiotics may be needed.

Children should be electively intubated for respiratory failure (lethargy, inability to maintain respiratory efforts, Pao_2 <70 on 100 percent oxygen or $Paco_2$ >60), but this decision is best made in the intensive care setting. Children who develop severe upper airway obstruction from this disease do not do so suddenly but rather progress gradually over time. If intubation must be performed in the ED, an endotracheal (ET) tube 1 mm smaller than that calculated for age should be utilized to accommodate the subglottic edema and airway narrowing.

The following regimen is suggested for the patient with croup:

- Avoid agitating the patient, and provide humidified oxygen if indicated.

- Allow the patient to assume a position of comfort (usually in a parent's arms or lap).

- Initially, provide cool, moist air.

- If stridor at rest persists (or fatigue or distress is noted), administer aerosolized racemic epinephrine at a dose of 0.5 mL in 2.5 mL normal saline solution. Patients who receive this intervention are candidates for admission, or, at a minimum, observation within the ED for a period of 2 to 4 hours.

- Administer intramuscular or intravenous dexamethasone, 0.6 mg/kg.

- Intubate if clinically warranted.

- Upright lateral neck radiographs, if desired, should be reserved for patients without suspicion of epiglottitis and close supervision of the patient maintained while the films are obtained.

Bacterial Tracheitis

Bacterial tracheitis, also referred to as membranous tracheitis, is an infection of the subglottic region. There is controversy as to whether this entity exists alone or whether it is a secondary bacterial colonization of a preexistent viral laryngotracheobronchitis. This entity occurs in the same age group as croup; however, these children usually present atypically, with a toxic appearance and high fever. Pus may be produced during spasms of brassy or barking cough. In some cases, the stridor is severe enough to be present during both inspiration and expiration.

Bacterial tracheitis represents a true upper airway emergency since, like supraglottitis, progression to full airway obstruction is possible. It is not prudent to attempt to differentiate this entity from supraglottitis prior to obtaining a definitive airway in the operating room. Upon intubation, a normal epiglottis combined with the presence of pus, inflammation, and in some cases a pseudomembrane in the subglottic region confirms the diagnosis. Cultures most commonly grow *S. aureus,* but *Streptococcus* spp, *H. influenzae,* and *Pneumococcus* are possible. Meticulous endotracheal tube suctioning in a pediatric intensive care unit (PICU) setting will usually maintain airway patency. Broad-spectrum antibiotic coverage that includes coverage for *S. aureus* is required. A third-generation cephalosporin, such as ceftriaxone, is a good initial choice.

Retropharyngeal Abscess

Retropharyngeal abscesses are seen predominantly in children younger than 3 years of age secondary to suppurative cervical lymphadenopathy. Older children may present with this entity, in many instances following penetrating trauma to the posterior oropharynx. Common organisms include group A beta hemolytic *Streptococcus* and *S. aureus.* Symptoms include high fever, muffled voice, difficulty swallowing, drooling, and, less frequently, inspiratory stridor. Dysphagia and drooling are more frequent findings than actual upper airway compromise.

Children with retropharyngeal abscesses can present with a stiff neck and be initially diagnosed with meningitis. The presentation may also mimic supraglottitis when inspiratory stridor is present. Therefore, it is acceptable to make this diagnosis in the operating room on direct visualization.

A high index of suspicion must be maintained to accurately identify the child with a retropharyngeal abscess. Clinically noting a swelling of the wall of the posterior pharynx may make the diagnosis. Given the overlap in presentation with supraglotittis, even if the diagnosis is suspected, it is prudent to first obtain a lateral neck film that will demonstrate swelling of the prevertebral soft tissue at the level of the pharynx and a normal epiglottis and aryepiglottic folds. Attempting to visualize the oral cavity and posterior pharyngeal wall may be made in an older cooperative child as long as agitation does not ensue. In most suspected cases, a computed tomography scan of the neck will identify any soft tissue swelling, and in selected cases, the presence of free air would alert the specialist that surgical drainage may be necessary.

Definitive therapy involves intraoperative drainage of the abscess after securing the airway by endotracheal intubation. Children with cellulitis without a collection of pus should be treated with antibiotics. Airway management for severe or complete upper airway obstruction should include endotracheal intubation under direct visualization (to avoid rupture of the abscess). In children with partial airway obstruction who do not demonstrate signs of respiratory failure, meticulous observation with all equipment and personnel on hand (a PICU setting) is acceptable. Antibiotics must cover the common organisms (*S. aureus, Streptococcus,* and anaerobes). Clindamycin is a good empiric choice.

Peritonsillar Abscess

Peritonsillar abscesses usually affect children over the age of 8 years. They are the most common deep infections of the head and neck, usually representing complications of bacterial tonsillitis, or in some cases, a superinfection of an existent Epstein-Barr infection. Most are polymicrobial in origin, including group A *Streptococcus* (predominant), *Peptostreptococcus, Fusobacterium,* and other mouth flora, including anaerobes.

Historically these patients present with increasing dysphagia and ipsilateral ear pain, with progression to trismus, dysarthria, and toxicity. Drooling is common. Patients will often have a "hot potato" phonation, representing splinting of the palatine muscles during normal speech.

The pharynx will be erythematous, with unilateral tonsillar swelling, which, in some cases, may displace the uvula toward the unaffected side. The soft palate may be displaced medially. Fluctuance may confirm the presence of underlying purulent fluid. Reactive cervical adenopathy is common. Severe, although uncommon, complications have been reported, including sternocleidomastoid spasm and torticollis, fascitis, mediastinitis, and airway obstruction.

The complete blood count will demonstrate an elevated white blood count count. Throat cultures (superficial) should be obtained in all cases. An experienced otolaryngologist should perform direct tonsillar needle aspiration, after adequate sedation/analgesia has been administered. Serologic testing for Epstein-Barr virus infections should be performed as well.

Most patients require admission for drainage, intravenous hydration, and antibiotics (nafcillin or a third-generation cephalosporin). Rarely, selected individuals may be discharged from the ED after careful follow-up is arranged.

FOREIGN BODY OBSTRUCTION

Most foreign body aspirations occur in children younger than 5 years, with 65 percent of deaths affecting infants younger than 1 year. Common offending agents are foods (e.g., peanuts, hard candies, frankfurters) and items commonly found in the home (e.g., disc batteries, coins, marbles). Symptoms range from mild (cough only) to full-blown upper airway obstruction. It is imperative that the clinician maintain a high index of suspicion relative to the possibility of foreign body aspiration, especially in the afebrile child with sudden onset of symptoms. In >50 percent of cases, there is no history of foreign body ingestion or a choking spell.

Most patients will present with symptoms of partial obstruction. Evaluation should include anteroposterior and lateral views of the upper airway extending from the nasopharynx to the carina. More extensive radiographic investigations include inspiratory and expiratory chest radiographs, or bilateral decubital views. Both maneuvers will demonstrate the failure of the affected hemithorax to lose volume because of positioning. These examinations are of great value in diagnosing foreign bodies that are radiolucent. A high index of suspicion must be maintained in all suspected cases. Esophageal foreign bodies, if positioned at the thoracic inlet or carina, can impede the upper airway and cause symptoms and signs of airway obstruction.

Foreign body obstruction should be managed as follows:

- Acute complete obstruction:
  - Children younger than 1 year: give four back blows followed by chest thrusts.
  - Children older than 1 year: employ repetitive abdominal thrusts.

- If unsuccessful, utilize Magill forceps under direct laryngoscopy in an attempt to remove the foreign body.
- If still unsuccessful, attempt vigorous BVM ventilation in preparation for brochoscopy.
- Incomplete obstruction (phonation, coughing present):
  - Provide supplemental oxygen.
  - Allow a position of comfort.
  - Avoid noxious stimuli.
  - Arrange for controlled airway evaluation in the operating room.

SUMMARY

Competency in the management of the pediatric patient with respiratory distress is a necessary skill for the emergency physician. This chapter has provided an outlined overview of the most common upper airway disorders that one will encounter in general practice. Standardized therapeutic interventions will maximize overall clinical outcomes.

BIBLIOGRAPHY

Bernstein T, Brilli R, Jacobs B: Is bacterial tracheitis changing? A 14-month experience in a pediatric intensive care unit. *Clin Infect Dis* 27:458–462, 1998.

Blotter JW, Yin L, Glynn M, et al: Otolaryngology consultation for peritonsillar abscess in the pediatric population. *Laryngoscope* 110:1698–1701, 2000.

Damm M, Eckel HE, Jungehulsing M, Roth B: Management of acute inflammatory childhood stridor. *Otolaryngol Head Neck Surg* 121:633–638, 1999.

Herzon FS, Nicklaus P: Pediatric peritonsillar abscess: Management guidelines. *Curr Probl Pediatr* 26:270–278, 1996.

Hvizdos KM, Jarvis B: Budesonide inhalation suspension: A review of its use in infants, children and adults with inflammatory respiratory disorders. *Drugs* 60:1141–1178, 2000.

Kumar RK, Mashell K: Acute epiglottitis. *J Pediatr Child Health* 34:594, 1998.

Malhotra A, Krilov LR: Viral croup. *Pediatr Rev* 22:5–12, 2001.

Rittichier KK, Ledwith CA: Outpatient treatment of moderate croup with dexamethasone: Intravenous versus oral dosing. *Pediatrics* 106:1344–1348, 2000.

Rosekrans JA: Viral croup: Current diagnosis and treatment. *Mayo Clin Proc* 73:1102–1106, 1998.

White CB, Foshee WS: Upper respiratory tract infections in adolescents. *Adolesc Med* 11:225–249, 2000.

26

Asthma

Kathleen Brown

HIGH-YIELD FACTS

- Inhaled albuterol remains the first-line therapy for acute asthmatic exacerbations.
- The addition of nebulized ipratroprium to the first two to three albuterol doses is associated with a decreased need for hospitalization in pediatric patients with moderate-severe asthma exacerbations.
- Administration of corticosteroids in the ED has been shown to enhance recovery from an acute asthma exacerbation and to decrease rates of hospitalization.
- Methylxanthines have not been shown to offer any benefit over treatment with albuterol in acute asthma exacerbations.
- Magnesium sulfate, heliox, and ketamine have, in some studies, been shown to be of benefit for severe asthma exacerbations, but convincing evidence of their benefit is not available.

Asthma is the most common chronic disease of childhood. It affects at least 5 percent of the population of the United States and accounts for 1 to 5 percent of all emergency department (ED) visits. From 1980 to 1987, the prevalence of asthma and the rate of hospitalization and death due to asthma increased. However, since 1988, the rates of death due to asthma in this country appear to have stabilized. Asthma was the eighth leading cause of death in children aged 5 to 14 years in 1997.

Asthma is traditionally defined as intermittent, reversible obstructive airway disease. It is now known to be a chronic inflammatory disorder of the airways. Clinically it manifests as recurrent episodes of wheezing, dyspnea, chest tightness, and cough. These episodes are associated with variable airflow obstruction that is usually reversible.

ETIOLOGY/PATHOPHYSIOLOGY

The major mechanisms thought to contribute to the pathophysiology of asthma are increased airway responsiveness, inflammation, mucus production, and submucosal edema. Airway responsiveness is defined as the ease with which airways narrow in response to various nonallergic stimuli. These stimuli include inhaled pharmacologic agents, such as histamine and methacholine, and physical stimuli, such as exercise. The level of airway responsiveness is reported to correlate with the severity of asthma symptoms and medication requirements. The critical role of airway inflammation in both the development of obstruction and the degree of hyperresponsiveness has only recently been appreciated. Pathologic specimens from patients demonstrate inflammation of the airways even in the mildest forms of the disease. Increased mucus production and submucosal edema add to the obstruction that occurs secondary to bronchospasm and inflammation.

These three components are synergistic and their relationship can be understood by dividing the mechanisms involved into stages. The early bronchospastic response is a classic antigen antibody reaction. When the patient is exposed to a specific antigen, mast cells are sensitized by reagin or antigen-specific IgE antibody, which attaches to the cell wall. When this sensitized cell is reexposed to the specific antigen, mediators are released, including histamine, leukotrienes, and chemotactic factors that attract inflammatory cells to the area (Fig. 26-1). A predisposition to develop this response may be genetically based. In some patients this initial inflammatory response is secondary to an infection. Whatever the cause of the inflammatory response, it is the convergence of these inflammatory cells that appears to correlate with the late asthmatic response. These inflammatory cells release a number of products that cause damage to the bronchial wall. Eosinophils play a large role in this process. They migrate to the bronchial wall in response to chemotactic substances released by macrophages and are stimulated by mediators such as platelet-activating factor (PAF) to release a number of substances that cause inflammation in the bronchial wall. Histamine is released from mast cells. It causes smooth muscle constriction and bronchospasm and plays a role in mucosal edema and mucus secretion. All inflammatory cells produce products that are the result of the action of phospholipase A2 on their membrane phospholipids. This leads to the formation of PAF and arachidonic acid and its metabolites, including leukotrienes. These products cause smooth muscle contraction and mucosal

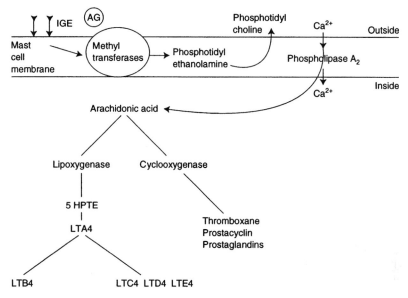

Fig. 26-1. Pathophysiology of asthma.

edema. In addition to mucosal edema, hypersecretion, and bronchoconstriction, these cell products contribute to the sloughing of mucosal cells, which cause a loss of the protective effects of the epithelium and exposure of nerve fibers to irritants. Experimental models show that airway inflammation produces an alteration of the sensory nerve endings that may lead to bronchial hyperreactivity.

Once bronchial hyperactivity is present, nonspecific triggers may produce acute bronchospasm. The most common trigger is an upper respiratory infection. Other common triggers include inhaled allergens, exercise, and cold air. The level of airway responsiveness is not static. It may increase or decrease in response to various factors. Anxiety may potentiate bronchospasm through vagal efferentes. A vicious cycle can develop in which continuous or repeated exposure to allergens in sensitized persons increases airway responsiveness. This is the chronic stage of asthma. Chronic asthma is not always reversible. During the immune response, proliferating fibroblasts deposit extensive networks of collagen that can lead to fibrosis, remodeling of the bronchioles, and irreversible airway disease.

All asthmatics have profound bronchoconstriction in response to cholinergic agonists, such as methacholine chloride, suggesting that the parasympathetic nervous system is involved in the asthmatic response. The bulk of autonomic nerves in human airways are branches of the vagus nerve, whose efferent fibers enter the lung at the hilum and travel along the airways into the lungs. They are found throughout the length of the airways but predominantly along the large and medium-sized airways. Their postganglionic varicosities and terminals supply the smooth muscle and submucosal glands of the airways as well as vascular structures. Release of acetylcholine at these sites results in smooth muscle contraction and release of secretions from the submucosal glands. The level of parasympathetic activity can be augmented by neural reflexes that involve afferent and efferent vagal fibers. Stimuli that result in reflex bronchoconstriction include mechanical stimulation of the airways and inhalation of certain particles, gases, aerosols, and cold and dry air. There is little direct sympathetic innervation of the bronchial tree. However, there are many β2-adrenergic receptors in airway smooth muscle that are responsible for bronchoconstriction. The importance of the sympathetic nervous system is not in maintaining airway tone but in reversing bronchoconstriction.

There are several differences in the anatomy and physiology of a child compared with an adult that make children more prone to obstruction and more vulnerable to respiratory failure. The peripheral airways are smaller and thus offer greater resistance to air flow. Infants do not possess the collateral channels for ventilation that are present in older children and adults. In infancy the diaphragm is the primary muscle of respiration. Any degree of abdominal distention will provide significant interference to diaphragmatic function and secondary ventilatory insufficiency. The infantile diaphragm possesses muscle fibers that are more prone to fatigue. The chest wall of the pediatric patient is more compliant, preventing adequate stabilization during periods of increased respiratory distress.

CLINICAL PRESENTATION

A family history of asthma, atopy, or allergic disease is common. A recent history of an upper respiratory infection or exposure to a specific trigger is usually obtained. The initial history in a child with an acute asthma attack should include the patient's or parents' perception of the severity of the attack, precipitating factors, history of past attacks, medications (last doses, recent changes), and duration of symptoms.

Physical examination should start with a general assessment of the patient's degree of distress. Important clues are alertness, anxiety, fluid status, general health, positioning, ability to speak, and presence of cyanosis. The inability of the patient to lie down is significantly correlated with poor vital signs, abnormal arterial blood gases, and abnormal spirometry. Inability to speak was correlated in one study with hypoxia and a decreased peak flow rate. Vital signs may also have some prognostic value. Fever may point to a more complicated course and significant underlying disease. Increased pulse rate may be a sign of hypoxia. Pulsus paradoxus (a drop in systolic blood pressure of 10 mmHg or more with inspiration) was believed to correlate with a worsening status, but its usefulness has been questioned. Increased respiratory rates are usually seen in asthmatic exacerbations, but respiratory rate may decrease with fatigue in severe asthma. The lung exam may reveal a number of findings including diffuse wheezing. Wheezing results from turbulent airflow and occurs first on expiration alone, progressing to both inspiration and expiration. The wheezing may be localized and may shift in location with time as the relative degree of obstruction may vary with location and time. If airway obstruction is severe, there will be little airflow and the chest may be quiet. Thus wheezing is not a reliable indicator of the degree of obstruction. Lung exam may also reveal diffuse or localized rales, or a persistent cough with a clear lung exam. Air trapping due to occlusion of small airways leads to hyperinflation of the chest, making it a less efficient muscle of inspiration and forcing the use of accessory muscles. The use of accessory muscles is a more reliable indicator of degree of obstruction. The presence of air leak is suggested by asymmetric breath sounds, tracheal deviation, or subcutaneous edema.

LABORATORY AND RADIOGRAPHIC FINDINGS

Typical chest radiograph findings are hyperinflation, peribronchial cuffing, and areas of subsegmental atelectasis. These findings are nonspecific and usually add little to the clinical assessment. Chest radiographs have been shown to change the course of treatment in only 10 percent of asthmatics. Specific indications for a chest radiograph in a known asthmatic include clinical suspicion of consolidation, effusion, pneumothorax, or impending respiratory failure. Children with first-time wheezing should have a chest radiograph to exclude other causes of wheezing (Table 26-1).

Spirometry can be used to assess a patient's degree of respiratory compromise. However, many children are not able to cooperate for spirometry. The simplest spirometry test, peak expiratory flow rate (PEFR), can usually be performed in children older than 5 years. A PEFR of less than 30 to 50 percent of predicted or of the patient's personal best indicates severe airway obstruction.

Oximetry is another tool that may help assess severity. It correlates with ventilation perfusion mismatching and thus degree of obstruction. An initial oxygen saturation of less than 91 percent was correlated with need for admission in one study. A rise in oxygen saturation with treatment was not a determinant of outcome.

Table 26-1. Differential Diagnosis in a Wheezing Infant

Anaphylaxis
Aspiration
Bronchiolitis
Bronchopulmonary dysplasia
Congestive heart failure
Cystic fibrosis
Extrinsic airway compression
Foreign body aspiration
Immotile cilia
Immune deficiency
Mediastinal masses
Pneumonia
Vascular rings

Blood gases may help assess the status of severe asthmatics but are not necessary for management of most acute asthma exacerbations. Hypoxia will be present early because of the ventilation perfusion mismatching. Pco_2 will be decreased early in the disease secondary to compensatory hyperventilation. As the obstruction progresses, the number of alveoli being adequately ventilated and perfused decreases and CO_2 retention occurs. Thus a "normal" or slightly elevated Pco_2 in a patient with an asthma exacerbation may be a sign of muscle fatigue and impending respiratory failure. Eventually the hypoxia and hypercapnia lead to acidosis.

DIFFERENTIAL DIAGNOSIS

The diagnosis of asthma depends on documentation of episodic, reversible airway disease. This is most reliably accomplished by performing pulmonary function tests (PFTS). However, children younger than 6 years are generally unable to perform the tasks needed to get accurate PFTS. Therefore, the diagnosis in small children is usually made on a clinical basis. The diagnosis of asthma should be considered in all children with recurrent wheezing and symptom-free intervals, especially if there is a family history of asthma, atopy, or allergies. A personal history of atopy or allergies is also suggestive of the diagnosis of asthma in a wheezing child. Many children with asthma have their first asthmatic episode prior to 6 months of age. In infants, as in older children, viral infections are the most common trigger for asthma. Both infants who have asthma and those who do not may become infected with respiratory syncytial virus (RSV) or other viruses and develop bronchiolitis as their first or only episode of wheezing. Therefore, in an infant with wheezing, it is often impossible to clinically differentiate between bronchiolitic wheezing and asthma. The most important clue to infantile asthma is a history of recurrent episodes of wheezing or persistent cough.

A list of other possible etiologies for wheezing in an infant or child is provided in Table 26-1. A history of prematurity or ventilatory support will help in identifying the infant with bronchopulmonary dysplasia (BPD). Cardiac examination may reveal other signs of cardiac failure in an infant with wheezing secondary to congenital heart disease. An association of signs and symptoms with feeding may suggest a tracheoesophageal fistula, gastroesophageal reflux, or recurrent aspiration. Clues to identifying the presence of a lower airway foreign body may come from the history (sudden onset, observed aspiration), chest exam (asymmetry), or radiographic studies (localized air trapping). A patient with cystic fibrosis may have clubbing of the digits, poor weight gain, or symptoms of malabsorption. It is often quoted that all that wheezes is not asthma. This is especially true in children, and it is important to remember that even patients who come to the ED with a previous diagnosis of asthma and wheezing may have another etiology for their wheezing. Some patients with chronic cough, recurrent pneumonia, or chronic congestion may have a pathologic process similar to that of an asthmatic and may benefit from the same modes of treatment.

TREATMENT

Every patient with an acute asthma exacerbation needs rapid cardiopulmonary assessment. The choice and intensity of therapy depend on the severity of the exacerbation and the patient's response to initial treatment. Recommended doses are summarized in Table 26-2. Therapies that should be considered in all ED patients with an acute exacerbation of their asthma include oxygen and fluids. Hypoxia can lead to hypoventilation and acidosis, which can cause pulmonary vasoconstriction, pulmonary hypertension, and right heart failure. Asthmatic patients are also often dehydrated due to decreased intake or vomiting and may require intravenous fluids. However, acute asthma is associated with increased secretion of antidiuretic hormone and an increase in capillary permeability and interstitial fluid; thus overhydration may result in pulmonary edema. Antibiotics should be used in asthma only if evidence of concurrent infection exists. Chronic sinusitis, in particular, is thought to cause persistent asthmatic exacerbations.

β-Adrenergic Agonists

Adrenergic bronchodilators remain the first line of emergency treatment of asthma. Bronchodilation is produced by stimulation of β2-adrenoreceptors, which mediate an increase in cyclic AMP via the enzyme adenyl cyclase. Cyclic AMP stimulates binding of calcium ions to the cell membrane, reducing the mycoplasmal calcium concentration, with resultant bronchodilation (smooth muscle relaxation) and stabilization of mast cells (Fig. 26-2). Stabilization of mast cells retards the release of histamine and other inflammatory products. β-agonists also improve mucociliary clearance.

Albuterol is the most commonly used adrenergic agent in this country because it combines a long duration of

Table 26-2. Medications for an Acute Asthma Exacerbation

Medication	Route	Dose
β-adrenergic agents		
Albuterol (5 mg/mL)	Nebulizer	0.15 mg/kg q15–20 min × 3; then q1–4h prn (minimum 2.5 mg, maximum 5 mg)
	Continuous nebulization	0.3–0.5 mg/kg/hr up to 20 mg/hr
90 μg/puff	MDI	4–8 puffs q20min × 3; then q1–4h prn
Epinephrine (1:1,000 solution)	SC	0.01 mg/kg (maximum 0.3 mg)
Tertbutaline (0.1%)	SC	0.01 mg/kg (maximum 0.3 mg)
	IV	Loading dose 10 μg/kg
		Infusion 0.4 μg/kg/min; may titrate up to 6 μg/kg/min
Corticosteroids		
Methylprednisolone	IV	2 mg/kg (maximum 125 mg)
Prednisone/prednisolone	PO	ED dose: 2 mg/kg
		Discharge: 1–2 mg/kg/day × 5 days (maximum 60 mg)
Anticholinergics		
Ipratropium bromide (500 μg/2 mL)	Nebulizer	250–500 μg q20min × 2–3 doses (usually with albuterol); then q2–4h prn
18 μg/puff	MDI	4–8 puffs as needed
Magnesium sulfate	IV	50–75 mg/kg over 20 min (maximum 2.5 g)
Ketamine	IV	Induction: 1–2 mg/kg

action with $β_2$ selectivity. Aerosol therapy is the most commonly used and recommended form of β-adrenergic agents. It has been shown to be as effective as intravenous or subcutaneous therapy and more effective than oral therapy. There are two main methods of delivering aerosolized medications. Numerous studies exist that suggest comparable efficacy of metered dose inhalers (MDIs) and jet nebulization. MDIs are less expensive and more convenient, but they require a cooperative

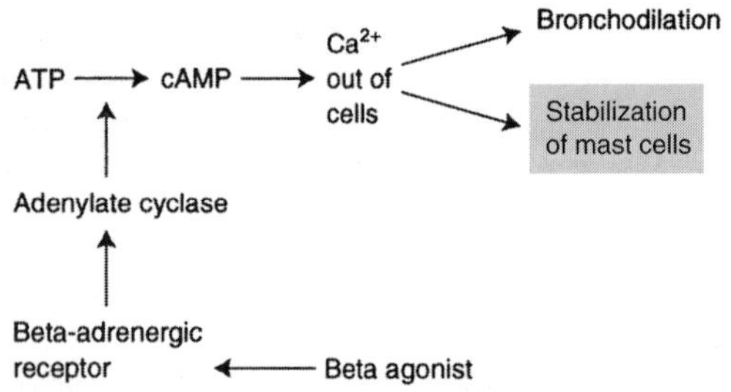

Fig. 26-2. Mechanism of action of β-adrenergic agonists.

(usually older) patient who understands the appropriate technique of administration. One method for enabling younger children to use an MDI more effectively is the use of an aero chamber or spacer, which provides a reservoir of particles for inspiration requiring less coordination of MDI activation with inhalation.

Particles generated by aerosolization vary in size. Only those in the 1- to 5-μm range are useful drug vehicles and are deposited in the lower airways. These represent only 10 percent of the output from an MDI and 1 to 5 percent from jet nebulizer. The rest of the particles escape into the room or are dissolved in mucus membranes and swallowed. Low flow rates and greater breath-holding periods optimize drug deposition in the lower airways. Oxygen flow rates of 6 to 7 L/min are recommended. Doses of up to 0.15 mg/kg every 20 minutes in severe asthmatics, or 0.3 mg/kg every hour in moderate asthmatics, have been demonstrated to be safe and more effective than lower doses. Since so much of the drug escapes into the atmosphere, especially when being delivered to very young children, many physicians will administer "unit doses" (usually 2.5 or 5 mg albuterol/3 mL NS) to all patients regardless of size. Continuous nebulization of albuterol at initial rates of greater than 3 mg/kg/hr has also been shown to be safe and effective. Continuous nebulization is usually started at 10 mg/hr and titrated up or down as needed. The frequency of aerosols or rate of continuous nebulization should be guided by repeat assessments of the patient's clinical status.

Other adrenergic medications are sometimes used in the treatment of acute asthmatic exacerbations. Epinephrine is available as a subcutaneous injection. It is more toxic and no more effective than inhalation of a β_2 selective drug. Parenteral administration (0.01 mL/kg up to 0.3 mL of the 1:1,000 solution subcutaneously) should be reserved for those patients who are unable to generate adequate tidal volume to deliver aerosolized drug to the bronchial tree. Subcutaneous terbutaline (0.01 mg/kg up to 0.25 mg), which is more β_2 specific, may be used as an alternative to subcutaneous epinephrine. It is preferred to subcutaneous epinephrine in the pregnant patient, as subcutaneous epinephrine has been associated with fetal malformations from decreased uterine blood flow.

Intravenous tertbutaline has been shown to be safe and effective in two small studies of pediatric patients with severe asthma exacerbations. Albuterol has also been used as an intravenous medication in other countries. However, intravenous β-agonists have not been shown to have benefit over inhalational therapy. Isoproterenol was used as an intravenous preparation in the past in severe asthmatics. However, it can cause significant cardiac toxicity, especially in hypoxic patients. Therefore isoproterenol is no longer recommended as a treatment for asthma.

Older inhaled β-adrenergic agents (isoetharine, metaproterenol) stimulate β_1 and β_2 receptors, at least theoretically, and have more undesirable side effects than albuterol. Inhaled epinephrine, which is available without a prescription, is much shorter acting than other inhaled β-agonists. Salmeterol is a longer acting β_2-agonist that has a longer duration of action but slower onset than albuterol. It is not intended for frequent repetitive administration. Levalbuterol (Xopenex) is the pure R-isomer of albuterol. It was designed and has been shown in some studies to provide the bronchodilatory effects of albuterol with fewer side effects. However, there are no published trials describing its use in acute asthma exacerbations.

Side effects associated with all β-adrenergic agonists are largely due to sympathomimetic effects and include tremors, anxiety, nausea, headache, vomiting, tachycardia, arrhythmia, hypertension, and hypotension. Non-sympathomimetic side effects include decreased oxygen saturation (secondary to altered V/Q matching), which is common, and paradoxical bronchospasm, which is rare. Metabolic side effects include hypokalemia, hypophosphotemia, hyperglycemia, and lactic acidosis. These side effects are often related to dose and route of administration and rarely require cessation of therapy. However, all patients receiving prolonged β-adrenergic therapy should have their oxygen saturation, heart rate, blood pressure, and serum electrolytes monitored closely.

Corticosteroids

Multiple studies have demonstrated the effectiveness of corticosteroids in the treatment of asthma. Benefits that have been demonstrated include rate of improvement measured by clinical scores and PFTs, increased rate of improvement, decreased duration of symptoms, decreased hospitalization rates, decreased relapse rates, and decreased need for β-agonists. The use of steroids in the treatment of asthma has expanded greatly in the last few years. A clearer understanding of the inflammatory mechanisms involved in the pathogenesis of even mild asthma has led to a greater emphasis on the use of steroids.

Corticosteroids are thought to have two mechanisms of action in improving asthmatic patients. They restore responsiveness to β-adrenergics by increasing receptor numbers and lowering their threshold. Two mechanisms by which they reverse inflammation are inhibition of arachidonic acid metabolites via phospholipase and suppression of the polymorphonuclear (PMN) response to chemotactic stimuli. A number of studies have shown that corticosteroid benefit can occur promptly enough to affect the patient's disposition from the ED. Oral and parenteral corticosteroids are known to be equally efficacious. Following a short course of corticosteroid therapy, adrenal suppression is minimal and clinically insignificant. Toxicity is chiefly related to duration of use and not to dose. Therefore, doses at the top of the dose-response curve should be used and they should be stopped as soon as clinically allowable. In the ED, 2 mg/kg of prednisone or an equivalent dose of another corticosteroid should be given as an initial bolus. This dose can be given orally or intravenously. Recently the use of inhaled steroids in the acutely ill asthmatic patient has been investigated, but a consistent significant benefit has not been reported.

Anticholinergics

Atropine was the first drug used as a bronchodilator. It acts through interruption of parasympathetic transmission to the bronchial tree by decreasing the intracellular cyclic GMP (Fig. 26-3). This decreases the influence of cholinergic nerve endings on bronchial tone and dilates the airways. It fell into disfavor with the discovery of epinephrine in the 1920s mainly because it produces anticholinergic side effects at doses only slightly above those required for bronchodilation. There has been a resurgence of interest in the use of anticholinergic agents in recent years due to our better understanding of the cholinergic mechanisms that control airway caliber, as well as the development of synthetic analogs that are not appreciably absorbed across mucous membranes but retain their anticholinergic properties. Ipratropium bromide (Atrovent) is a quaternary amine that fits into this category. There is evidence that its use in combination with β-agonists in pediatric patients with an acute exacerbation of their asthma is helpful in reducing rates of hospitalization. Side effects include dry mouth and metallic taste.

Methylxanthines

Once a mainstay in the treatment of acute bronchospastic disease, theophylline/aminophylline has been relegated to a second- or third-line role. These methylxanthines are not believed to increase bronchodilation in patients treated maximally with β-agonists. A systematic review of 27 studies in adult asthmatic patients concluded that the use of aminophylline did not result in any additional bronchodilation compared with standard care with β-agonists. Studies in pediatric patients have shown similar results. The frequency of adverse effects was also higher with aminophylline. Aminophylline has a narrow therapeutic-toxic window. Side effects include tachycardia, arrhythmias, nausea, vomiting, headaches, dizziness, and nervousness.

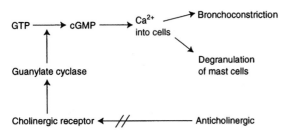

Fig. 26-3. Mechanism of action of anticholinergic agents.

Magnesium

For patients that have not responded to therapy with β-agonists, ipratropium, and corticosteroids, additional therapies may be considered. Magnesium produces bronchodilation via counteraction of calcium-mediated smooth muscle constriction. There has not been a well-designed trial in pediatric patients supporting its efficacy. However, a recent systematic review of the literature on intravenous magnesium for asthmatics of all ages did demonstrate a decrease in admission rate for those with severe acute asthma exacerbations.

Heliox

Inhalation of a blend of helium and oxygen has also been suggested to be helpful for severe asthmatic patients unresponsive to other therapies. Because this mixture is less dense than air, there is less airway resistance and turbulence in the bronchi when it is inhaled. This may lead to decreased work of breathing and delay fatigue and respiratory failure until concurrent bronchodilator and antiinflammatory therapy become effective. Current published literature on this subject is inconclusive as to its benefit, but no significant complications were seen.

Intubation/Mechanical Ventilation

Indications for intubation of an asthmatic patient include:

- Decreased level of consciousness
- Apnea
- Exhaustion
- Rising $Paco_2$ after treatment
- Pao_2 <60 mmHg
- pH <7.2.

An asthmatic may not immediately improve with intubation, since intubation does nothing to change lower airway obstruction. Intubation and mechanical ventilation may also put the patient at risk for serious complications. When intubating an asthmatic patient, the largest diameter tube appropriate for the patient's size is used to avoid increasing resistance even further. Although sedation is normally contraindicated in patients with asthma, sedation and paralysis may be indicated to avoid barotrauma secondary to the child struggling during passage of the endotracheal (ET) tube. A modified rapid sequence induction should be used. The dissociative anesthetic ketamine is known to have bronchodilatory properties and therefore is a good choice for a sedative. Paralysis with succinylcholine may increase secretions but is not contraindicated. Pancuronium is thought to have bronchodilatory properties; however, its long duration of action outweighs this benefit. Vecuronium or rocuronium are recommended by most authors, when muscle paralysis is indicated for prolonged mechanical ventilation as needed in a severe asthmatic exacerbation. Once intubated, patients with asthma will require sedation and paralysis to maintain effective ventilation. They also require a long expiratory time to avoid air trapping due to airway obstruction. The ventilator may be providing a second inspired breath before the first breath has been fully expired (stacking breaths). Intrinsic positive end-expiratory pressure (PEEP) may cause an increase in intrathoracic pressure that leads to decreased venous return to the heart and can cause hypotension. Air trapping also puts the patient at risk for the development of air leaks. Intubated asthmatic patients need to be watched carefully for the development of pneumo-thorax or pneumomediastinum. Sudden changes in the patient's respiratory or hemodynamic status may be due to a tension pneumothorax until proved otherwise. Ventilator settings should be adjusted to provide for adequate oxygenation with as low a peak pressure and PEEP as possible. The use of permissive hypercapnea (P_{CO_2}) levels as high as 70 to 90 mmHg) has been associated with decreased morbidity and mortality rates in intubated asthmatic patients.

DISPOSITION/OUTCOME

The decision to admit or discharge a patient from the ED after treatment for asthma can be difficult. Studies have shown that there is a high relapse rate for patients discharged after treatment, and many patients return to the ED requiring further therapy or hospitalization. Numerous studies have been published attempting to establish objective criteria for admission. Clinical examination and scoring systems perform poorly in identifying patients requiring hospital admission. Various spirometric parameters have also been proposed but have not proved to have adequate sensitivity. To date no objective criteria have been shown to be uniformly helpful in making this decision. The following risk factors have been identified as being associated with mortality:

- Previous intubation (greatest predictor of subsequent death)

- Two or more hospitalizations in the last year
- Three or more ED visits in the last year
- Use of systemic steroids
- Rapid progression of attacks
- Hypoxic seizures
- Severe nighttime wheezing
- Barotrauma
- Self-weaning from medications
- Lack of perception of the severity of the disease
- Poor medical management
- Poor access to medical care
- Smoke exposure

Patients discharged from the ED after an acute asthma exacerbation should be instructed to continue β-agonist use and be placed on a short course of corticosteroids. Steroid bursts for ≤5 days, if done no more than four times a year, do not require tapering. Immune suppression is clinically insignificant in patients with normal baseline immune function. Growth suppression does not occur, and the incidence of adverse psychiatric effects is low. The most commonly used regimen is 1 to 2 mg/kg/day (maximum of 60 mg) prednisone for 5 days. Some suggest a single daily dose given at 7 to 8 AM to coincide with surge in endogenous cortisol production and to minimize adrenal suppression. However, divided doses are usually used to minimize gastrointestinal upset.

Several other drugs are commonly used in the treatment of chronic asthma and should be considered as therapy for the patient being discharged from the ED. Cromolyn sodium prevents mast cell histamine release by stabilizing the mast cell through an unknown mechanism. It is not believed to have any bronchodilating activity and is therefore used only for prophylaxis. It has almost no toxicity. Leukotriene receptor antagonists have recently been introduced as treatment for chronic asthma. Monteleukast has been shown to be safe and effective in children 6 to 4 years of age with asthma. The use of inhaled steroids is encouraged for chronic treatment at home in moderately severe asthmatics. A recent study has shown that the addition of inhaled steroids to oral steroids in patients discharged from the ED can decrease the rate of relapse.

Despite the mortality and morbidity associated with this disease, the prognosis for most children with asthma is good. At least half of all children with asthma will be symptom free by adulthood.

BIBLIOGRAPHY

Afilalo M, Guttman A, Colacone A, et al: Efficacy of inhaled steroids (beclomethasone dipropionate) for treatment of mild to moderately severe asthma in the emergency department: A randomized clinical trial. *Ann Emerg Med* 33:304–309, 1999.

Chiang VW, Burns JP, Rifai N, et al: Cardiac toxicity of intravenous terbutaline for the treatment of severe asthma in children: A prospective assessment. *J Pediatr* 137:73–77, 2000.

Gawchik SM, Saccar CL, Noonan M, et al: The safety and efficacy of nebulized levalbuterol compared with racemic albuterol and placebo in the treatment of asthma in pediatric patients. *J Allergy Clin Immunol* 103:615–621, 1999.

Laviolette M, Malmstrom K, Lu S, et al: Montelukast added to inhaled beclomethasone in treatment of asthma. *Am J Respir Crit Care Med* 160:1862–1868, 1999.

Parameswaran K, Belda J, Rowe BH: Addition of intravenous aminophylline to β-2 agonists in adults with acute asthma. Cochrane Database of Systematic Reviews. Issue 4, 2000.

Qureshi F: Management of children with acute asthma in the emergency department. *Pediatr Emerg Care* 15:206–214, 1999.

Rowe BH, Bota GW, Fabris L, et al: Inhaled budesonide in addition to oral corticosteroids to prevent asthma relapse following discharge from the emergency department: A randomized controlled trial. *JAMA* 281:2119–2126, 1999.

Rowe BH, Travers AH, Holroyd BR, et al: Nebulized ipratropium bromide in acute pediatric asthma: Does it reduce hospital admissions among children presenting to the emergency department? *Ann Emerg Med* 34:75–85, 1999.

Schuh S, Reisman J, Alshehri M, et al. A comparison of inhaled fluticasone and oral prednisone for children with severe acute asthma. *N Engl J Med* 343:689–694, 2000.

Stephanopoulos DE, Monge R, Schell KH, et al: Continuous intravenous terbutaline for pediatric status asthmaticus. *Crit Care Med* 26:1744–1748, 1998.

27
Bronchiolitis

Kathleen Brown

HIGH-YIELD FACTS

- Bronchiolitis is a self-limited, virally mediated, acute inflammatory disease of the lower respiratory tract that results in obstruction of the small airways. Bronchiolitis occurs almost exclusively in infants.

- Bronchiolitis is a clinical diagnosis characterized by rapid respirations, chest retractions, wheezing, and, frequently, hypoxia.

- Respiratory failure may occur secondary to respiratory muscle fatigue or apnea, especially in very young and premature infants.

- Treatment is largely supportive. Routine treatment with bronchodilators or corticosteroids has not been shown to be of benefit.

- Indications for hospital admission are as follows:
  - need for supportive care (oxygen, intravenous fluids)
  - persistent respiratory distress
  - respiratory failure
  - adjusted age < 6 weeks
  - significant underlying disease

Bronchiolitis is a disease of the very young and occurs almost exclusively in children younger than 2 years. An attack rate of 11.4 percent in the first year of life and 6 percent in the second year of life was reported from one center. It is most common between the ages of 2 and 6 months and accounts for approximately 17 percent of all hospitalizations of infants. It is more common in males than females and has a seasonal pattern, being most common in the winter and spring.

Bronchiolitis is an acute inflammatory disease of the lower respiratory tract that results in obstruction of the small airways. The term is used to describe a clinical syndrome that occurs in infancy and is characterized by rapid respirations, chest retractions, wheezing, and, frequently, hypoxia.

ETIOLOGY

The most common etiologic agent in bronchiolitis is respiratory syncytial virus (RSV). RSV is present in up to 75 percent of the infants admitted to the hospital with bronchiolitis and is the primary pathogen during epidemics. Other viruses known to cause bronchiolitis are parainfluenza, influenza, mumps, adenovirus, echovirus, and rhinovirus. *Mycoplasma pneumoniae* and *Chlamydia trachomatis* have also been associated with bronchiolitis. Mycoplasma has been shown to be a cause of bronchiolitis in school age children. Adenovirus is associated with a particularly severe form of bronchiolitis that can lead to a chronic condition known as bronchiolitis obliterans.

PATHOPHYSIOLOGY

Infection produces inflammation of the bronchiolar epithelium, which leads to necrosis, sloughing, and lumenal obstruction. When ciliated epithelium sloughs, it is replaced by cuboidal cells. Increased mucus production and edema contribute further to airway obstruction. The absence of ciliated epithelium prevents adequate mobilization of secretions and debris. Histologic sections of the tracheobronchial tree of patients with bronchiolitis are very similar to those in asthmatics. The bronchioles and small bronchi are obstructed secondary to the submucosal edema, peribronchiolar cellular infiltrate, mucus plugging, and intraluminal debris. The obstruction is not uniform throughout the lungs. This leads to ventilation/perfusion mismatching and resultant hypoxia. The hypoxia leads to compensatory hyperventilation. If the obstruction is severe, hypercapnia may occur. Distal to the obstructed bronchiole, air trapping or atelectasis may occur. The epithelium usually regenerates from the basal layer within 3 to 4 days. However, functional regeneration of the ciliated epithelium usually requires about 2 weeks.

Adenovirus is associated with a particularly severe reaction that is termed bronchiolitis obliterans. In this disease the destruction of the normal ciliated epithelium is extensive. The normal cells are replaced by stratified undifferentiated epithelium with an intense inflammatory response extending to the alveoli. During the reparative phase, extensive fibrosis and scarring lead to obliteration of the small airways.

CLINICAL PRESENTATION

Typically, a child with bronchiolitis will have a prodrome of an upper respiratory tract infection. Parents will describe runny nose, low-grade fever, and decreased appetite for 1 to 2 days prior to the development of tachypnea and evidence of increased work of breathing. However, in some children lower tract symptoms may develop over hours. Often, there will be a family or contact history of upper respiratory tract infection.

Hyperventilation occurs as a compensatory response for hypoxia secondary to ventilation/perfusion mismatching. Respiratory rates $\geq$ 70 to 90/min are not uncommon. Flaring of the nasal alae and use of intercostal muscles may also be present. Respirations are shallow because of persistent distention of the lungs by the trapped air. Wheezing, prolonged expiration, and musical rales are common. The chest is often hyperexpanded and hyperresonant due to the air trapping. The liver and spleen may be displaced downward because of the hyperinflation and flattening of the diaphragm. Thoracoabdominal asynchrony with breathing may be present and correlates with the degree of obstruction. Fever is present in two-thirds of children with bronchiolitis. Despite these findings, the patient often has a nontoxic appearance. Respiratory fatigue may occur since the bronchiolitic infant may increase the work of breathing up to sixfold. Apnea is not uncommon (18 to 20 percent of those hospitalized with RSV bronchiolitis), especially in very young and premature infants. It generally occurs early in the illness, often prior to the onset of other respiratory symptoms.

LABORATORY AND RADIOGRAPHIC FINDINGS

A chest radiograph will reveal hyperinflation in the majority of patients with bronchiolitis. Peribronchial cuffing (thickening of the bronchiole walls) will be seen in about half. There may be areas of subsegmental atelectasis that can be difficult to differentiate from pneumonia. A chest radiograph is useful in ruling out the other disease processes in the differential diagnosis of bronchiolitis. A leukocyte count is usually within the normal range. Viral cultures will usually reveal an etiologic

agent. Rapid tests (complement fixation or indirect immunofluorescent antibody testing) are available for RSV and other viruses in many institutions and may be useful in confirming the diagnosis. Hypoxia is common, and the patient should have oxygen saturations assessed with a pulse oximeter. Hypercarbia will be present in those with more severe obstruction. Respiratory rates > 60 breaths/min correlate well with carbon dioxide retention on blood gases.

DIFFERENTIAL DIAGNOSIS

The differential diagnosis for bronchiolitis is essentially the same as for asthma (Table 26-1). Bronchiolitis may be very difficult to differentiate from infantile asthma. Response to bronchodilators does not exclude bronchiolitis, since some children with bronchiolitis may have some degree of bronchospasm. Since bronchiolitis most commonly occurs in infancy, particular attention should be paid to other processes that may present in infancy. Congenital heart disease, cystic fibrosis, vascular ring, and other congenital anomalies may mimic the findings of bronchiolitis. Infants and toddlers are particularly prone to foreign body aspiration, and this should be considered in a wheezing infant.

TREATMENT

Since most children with bronchiolitis will have some degree of hypoxia, monitoring by oximetry and provision of oxygen is important. Many of these children will have difficulty drinking, secondary to their increased work of breathing. Intravenous hydration should be considered if the patient cannot take adequate oral fluids. However, these patients are also at increased risk for the development of pulmonary edema if they are overhydrated. Avoid fluids in excess of their estimated deficit plus maintenance.

As discussed above, a chest radiograph will often reveal areas of opacity suggestive of pneumonia. Deciding whether to use antibiotics in these patients is often difficult. No significant benefit has been demonstrated from routine antibiotic usage. In the severely ill patient, a broad-spectrum antibiotic, such as cefuroxime, may be warranted to cover for the possibility of a bacterial superinfection until ruled out by appropriate cultures.

The association between bronchiolitis and the development of asthma, a disease in which steroids clearly are of benefit, has led some physicians to advocate steroid use in bronchiolitis. No study has convincingly documented their benefit. In fact, a large controlled multi-institutional study showed corticosteroids to be of no value in the treatment of bronchiolitis. A systematic review of the topic led to the same conclusion. Steroids are not recommended for routine use by most authors. The use of inhaled steroids in children with bronchiolitis has also been studied. No study has shown a benefit of this therapy.

The use of bronchodilators in bronchiolitis is also controversial. Most clinicians believe that bronchodilators produce clinical improvement in some patients with bronchiolitis. However systematic reviews looking at studies of the efficacy of β-agonists in bronchiolitis have not demonstrated a significant benefit of their routine use. The use of nebulized epinephrine has also been recommended by many as therapy for bronchiolitis. It was noted, in some studies, to be superior to salbutamol or albuterol at improving oxygenation and decreasing hospitalization. A systematic review, assessing the use of any bronchodilator therapy in bronchiolitis, demonstrated a modest improvement in clinical scores that was of questionable clinical significance. No difference was found in oxygenation or rates of hospitalization. Most authors in this country recommend that patients with bronchiolitis, especially those with a past history of wheezing, should be given at least a trial of adrenergic bronchodilators. If there is no response to the trial dose, then therapy should be discontinued.

Ribavirin is an antiviral drug that is thought to have some efficacy against RSV. It is a nucleoside analog that interferes with viral protein synthesis. A systematic review of all randomized controlled trials of ribavirin for RSV lower respiratory infection revealed that ribavirin reduces the length of mechanical ventilation, which may lead to a subsequent reduction in total hospital days. Ribavirin has not been shown to significantly reduce mortality or respiratory deterioration, although usage is associated with strong trends toward reduced risks of these outcomes. The current American Academy of Pediatrics recommendations for ribavirin suggest that it should be used based on the particular clinical circumstances and physician's experience.

RSV immunoglobulin has been advocated for treatment of some patients with RSV bronchiolitis. Studies looking at its use in "high-risk" children with bronchiolitis and in previously healthy children with "severe" disease did not show a significant decrease in need for intensive care, mechanical ventilation, or supplemental oxygen. Its use to prevent RSV infection in high-risk neonates has been more successful.

Two to five percent of infants hospitalized for bronchiolitis will develop respiratory failure and require mechanical support. There are no absolute criteria for endotracheal intubation. Suggested indications include $P_{CO_2} > 60$ to 65 mmHg, recurrent apneic spells, decreasing mental status, and hypoxia despite O_2 therapy. Once intubated, these infants have many of the same problems that intubated asthmatics have and are at risk for air trapping and the development of air leaks. There have been reports of the successful use of nasal or endotracheal continuous positive airway pressure in treating patients with bronchiolitis as a means to avoid mechanical ventilation and its complications. There are also reports of successful management of severe bronchiolitis with extracorporeal membrane oxygenation in patients unresponsive to conventional therapy.

DISPOSITION/OUTCOME

Bronchiolitis is a short-lived, self-limited disease that lasts a few days. Most patients do not require admission. The decision as to which child requires admission can sometimes be difficult. One case control study looked at whether oxygen saturation or clinical assessment could be used to predict patients who would return after discharge and require admission and found that they could not. Suggested criteria for admission include the following: age (adjusted for prematurity) < 6 weeks, hypoxemia, persistent respiratory distress, and dehydration. Children with a history of prematurity, congenital heart disease, bronchopulmonary dysplasia, underlying lung disease, or compromised immune function are at the highest risk for morbidity and mortality and should be admitted. Follow-up within 24 hours is recommended for those who are discharged.

The overall mortality rate for infants with RSV bronchiolitis is 1 to 3 percent. The mortality rate for infants within congenital heart disease and RSV bronchiolitis is 37 percent. It has been reported that 15 to 30 percent of infants who are hospitalized with bronchiolitis will require admission to an intensive care unit or ventilatory support. Up to 50 percent of infants with RSV bronchiolitis will go on to have recurrent wheezing. The only factor shown to increase the likelihood of subsequent wheezing is a family history of asthma, or atopy. Whether the initial infection causes changes that predispose to the development of asthma or whether patients with a genetic predisposition to reactive airway disease develop wheezing as a response to infection in infancy is controversial. Patients with bronchiolitis obliterans have a much poorer prognosis. They usually develop debilitating chronic lung disease.

BIBLIOGRAPHY

Cade A, Brownlee KG, Conway SP, et al: Randomized placebo controlled trial of nebulized corticosteroids in acute respiratory syncytial viral bronchiolitis. *Arch Pediatr Adolesc Med* 82:126–130, 2000.

Dobson JV, Stephens-Groff SM, McMahon SR, et al: The use of albuterol in hospitalized infants with bronchiolitis. *Pediatrics* 101:361–368, 1998.

Flores G, Horwitz RI: Efficacy of β-2 agonists in bronchiolitis: A reappraisal and metanalysis. *Pediatrics* 100:233–239, 1997.

Garrison MM, Christakis DA, Harvey E, et al: Systemic corticosteroids in infant bronchiolitis: A meta-analysis. *Pediatrics* 105:44, 2000.

Hall CB: Respiratory syncytial virus a: A continuing culprit and conundrum. *J Pediatr* 135:S2–S7, 1999.

Kellner JD, Ohlsson A, Gadomoski AM, et al: Bronchodilators for bronchiolitis. Cochrane Database of Systematic Reviews. Issue 4, 2000.

Milner AD: The role of corticosteroids in bronchiolitis and croup. *Thorax* 52:595–597, 1997.

Randolph AG, Wang EL: Ribavirin for respiratory syncytial virus infection of the lower respiratory tract. Cochrane Database of Systematic Reviews. Issue 4, 2000.

Richter H, Seddon P: Early nebulized budesonide in the treatment of bronchiolitis and the prevention of postbronchiolitic wheezing. *J Pediatr* 132:849–853, 1998.

Rodriguez WJ: Management strategies for respiratory syncytial virus infections in infants. *J Pediatr* 135:S45–S50, 1999.

28

Pneumonia

Kathleen Brown

HIGH-YIELD FACTS

- The incidence of pneumonia in children varies inversely with age.
- The primary predictor of the etiologic agent for infectious pneumonia is the patient's age.
- Pneumonia is usually part of a sepsis syndrome in the newborn, and in an infant presenting symptoms may be nonspecific.
- The most sensitive finding for diagnosing pneumonia in an infant is tachypnea.
- Most children with pneumonia can be managed as outpatients. Indications for admission include:
  - Hypoxia
  - Respiratory distress
  - Toxic appearance
  - Dehydration
  - Age <3 months
  - Impaired immune function
  - Infections unresponsive to oral therapy
- The presence of underlying disease and the ability of the caregivers to provide care for the child should also be considered.
- Empiric antibiotic therapy should be based on the most likely etiologic organisms based on the child's age and clinical presentation.

Pneumonia is an inflammation of the lung tissue, most commonly caused by an infection and defined by pulmonary infiltrates on a chest radiograph. Pneumonia develops more often in childhood than at any other age. The incidence of pneumonia in children varies inversely with age. The rate drops from 40/1000 in preschool children to 9/1000 in 9- to 15-year-olds. More males than females are affected in all age groups. Seasonal variations occur, especially among viral etiologies. Parainfluenza occurs most commonly in the fall, respiratory syncytial virus (RSV) in the winter, and influenza in the spring. Bacterial pneumonia may occur throughout the year but tends to increase in the colder months when crowding promotes transmission of infectious agents through respiratory droplets. *Mycoplasma pneumoniae* and *Chlamydia trachomatis* disease is endemic, although *M. pneumoniae* may cause epidemic outbreaks, particularly in the fall.

ETIOLOGY

The predominant pathogens that cause pneumonia in infants and children are dependent on:

- Age of the patient
- Vaccination status
- Presence of underlying disease
- Attendance in daycare
- Exposure history

Cases of pneumonia due to a particular agent often occur in clusters, so it is helpful to be aware of recent outbreaks in your locale. Table 28-1 summarizes the most common etiologic agents for pneumonia by age groups in normal healthy children.

Most (60 to 90 percent) of cases of pneumonia are nonbacterial in origin. Viruses responsible for neonatal pneumonia include rubella, cytomegalovirus (CMV), and herpes simplex virus (HSV). RSV, parainfluenza virus, and adenovirus are the most common isolates in those between 1 and 6 months of age; influenza virus and enteroviruses are isolated less frequently in this age group. Children between 6 months and 4 years are most often infected with parainfluenza viruses, adenovirus, and Epstein-Barr virus (EBV). Other viral agents isolated in children with pneumonia include influenza, rhinoviruses, enteroviruses, measles, varicella, rubella, HSV, and EBV.

The immediate newborn period is the only time when bacterial infections are the most common cause of pneumonia. Most infections in this age group are caused by aspiration of the organisms that colonize the mother's genital tract during labor and delivery. The predominant pathogen is group B *Streptococcus,* followed by *E. coli, Klebsiella* spp, and other gram-negative enteric bacilli from the Enterobacteriaceae group. Other less commonly encountered organisms include nontypable *Hemophilus influenzae,* other streptococci (group A and α-hemolytic spp), *Enterococcus, Listeria monocytogenes,* and anaerobic bacteria.

Table 28-1. Common Etiologies of Pneumonia

Age	Viral Agents	Bacterial Agents
Birth–2 weeks	CMV, HSV, Rubella	Group B *Streptococcus* *Escherichia coli* and other coliforms *Listeria monocytogenes*
2 weeks–2 mo	RSV Adenovirus Influenza EBV Parainfluenza	*Staphylococcus aureus* *Haemophilus influenzae* *Streptococcus pneumoniae* *Chlamydia trachomatis*
2 mo–3 yr	RSV Parainfluenza Adenovirus Influenza EBV	*S. pneumoniae* *Mycoplasma pneumoniae* *S. aureus* *H. influenzae*
3–12 yr	Influenza Adenovirus Parainfluenza EBV	*M. pneumoniae* *S. pneumoniae*
13–19 yr	Influenza Adenovirus Parainfluenza EBV	*M. pneumoniae* *S. pneumoniae*

CMV, cytomegalovirus; HSV, herpes simplex virus; RSV, respiratory syncytial virus; EBV, Epstein-Barr virus.

Between 1 and 3 months of life these organisms are still encountered, but much less commonly. Viruses are the most common etiologic agents in this age group. *Streptococcus pneumoniae* is the most common bacterial pathogen. *H. influenzae* type B (HIB), *Streptococcus pyogenes,* and *Staphylococcus aureus* occur less frequently.

Infants in the 3-week to 3-month age group may develop what is referred to as afebrile pneumonia or pneumonitis syndrome. This syndrome is typified by cough, tachypnea, and sometimes respiratory distress in the absence of fever. This syndrome is most commonly caused by viral infections but may also be caused by infections with *C. trachomatis, Mycoplasma hominis,* and *Ureaplasma urealyticum.*

In the preschool age group, viruses still remain the most common etiologic agent of pneumonia, but bacterial pathogens become relatively more common. The most common bacterial pathogen encountered is *S. pneumoniae.* In the past, infections with HIB were almost as common as *S. pneumoniae,* but because of the development of an effective vaccine against HIB, a marked decline in the incidence of infection with this organism has been observed. Other bacteria that are isolated less commonly include *S. aureus,* group A *Streptococcus, Moraxella catarrhalis,* and *Neisseria meningitidis. M. pneumoniae* has been isolated more frequently in this age group in recent studies.

Once children reach school age, *M. pneumoniae* is the most frequent bacterial cause of pneumonia. *S. pneumoniae* remains a common pathogen in this age group. *Chlamydia pneumoniae* is estimated to be the cause of up to 19 percent of adolescent pneumonia.

Gram-negative bacilli, including *Pseudomonas,* should be considered in all patients who have recently been hospitalized. Anaerobic infections should be considered in children with neurologic or anatomic defects that make them prone to aspiration. Unusual causes of bacterial pneumonia in children include *Mycobacterium tuberculosis, Legionella pneumophila, Chlamydia psittaci, Francisella tularensis,* and rickettsial infections. A resurgence of virulent group A *Streptococcus* infection has been associated with sporadic cases of invasive disease including pneumonia and empyema in children. Children with progressive or unresponsive pneumonia should be evaluated for these pathogens. The immunocompromised host is susceptible to all the infectious agents listed above as well as opportunistic organisms such as *Pneumocystis carinii,* CMV, and fungal disease.

PATHOPHYSIOLOGY

Most pneumonias are acquired through aspiration of infective particles. There are a number of mechanisms that normally help protect the lung from infection. Infectious particles are filtered in the nose, or entrapped and cleared by the mucus and ciliated epithelium in the respiratory tract. If a particle makes it to the lung, the agent must contend with alveolar macrophages, and also with systemic, humoral, and cell-mediated immune mechanisms. Infants in the first several months of life also possess passively acquired maternal antibodies that help protect them from pneumococcal and several other infectious agents. Alterations in any of these protective mechanisms may predispose a child to the development of pneumonia. Examples include congenital anatomic abnormalities, congenital or acquired immune deficiencies, neurologic abnormalities that predispose the child to aspiration, and alterations in mucus secretion quality or respiratory epithelium. In a child without any of these predisposing abnormalities, access to the lung is gained by the infectious particles through alterations in the normal anatomic and physiologic defenses. This most commonly occurs secondary to a viral infection of the upper respiratory tract. The virus may spread contiguously to involve the lower respiratory tract and cause a viral pneumonia.

Alternatively, the damage caused by the virus to the normal defense mechanisms may allow pathogenic bacteria to infect the lower respiratory tract. These bacteria may be organisms that normally colonize the child's upper airway, or organisms that are transmitted person to person by airborne droplet spread. Less commonly, bacterial and certain viral pneumonias (e.g., varicella, measles, rubella, CMV, EBV, HSV) may be acquired through hematogenous spread either from a localized source or generalized bacteremia or viremia.

Once in the lung parenchyma, bacteria cause an acute inflammatory response that includes exudation of fluid, deposition of fibrin, and infiltration of alveoli with polymorphonuclear leukocytes followed by macrophages. The exudative fluid in the alveoli creates the characteristic lobar consolidation seen on chest radiograph. Viral agents, *Mycoplasma,* and *Chlamydia* cause inflammation with a predominantly mononuclear infiltrate of submucosal and interstitial structures. This leads to sloughing of the epithelial cells into the airways, as occurs with bronchiolitis.

CLINICAL PRESENTATION

Symptoms and signs of pneumonia vary with the patient's age, the specific pathogen, and the severity of the disease. The typical history in an older child includes fever, pleuritic chest pain, dyspnea, increased sputum production, and tachypnea. However, in very young children, these classic symptoms may be absent. Usually, pneumonia presents as part of a sepsis syndrome in the newborn, whereas in the infant, the symptoms may be nonspecific. These symptoms may include fever without a localizing source, apnea, poor feeding, abdominal pain, vomiting or diarrhea, hypothermia, grunting, bradycardia, lethargy, or shock. In infants younger than 3 months, apnea is a presenting symptom of viral pneumonia.

The history may also give clues as to the etiologic agent. Viral pneumonia is often preceded by upper respiratory symptoms and may be associated with an exanthem. The onset of lower tract symptoms, primarily tachypnea, is usually gradual. Bacterial pneumonia may also be preceded by a viral upper respiratory infection, with a more sudden onset of lower tract symptoms. Fever often accompanied by chills is almost always present. Occasionally pleuritic involvement produces pain with respiratory effort. The parents may report that the child has been lethargic and eating less than usual. Pneumonia due to *S. aureus* is notorious for being particularly rapid in progression of symptoms. A history of chlamydial infection in the mother during pregnancy or conjunctivitis (present in 50 percent of cases) in the infant is suggestive of *C. trachomatis* pneumonia. Pneumonia caused by *M. pneumoniae* is usually seen in adolescents, is usually insidious, and often includes a complaint of a sore throat. Mycoplasma infections generally present with a gradual onset of malaise, fever, and headache. Cough usually begins 3 to 5 days after the onset of illness. Patients with underlying disorders such as sickle cell anemia seem to manifest an increased severity of disease.

The findings on physical examination in patients with pneumonia vary with the patient's age, the microbial etiology, and the severity of the infection. Tachypnea is the most frequent sign of pneumonia in children and may be an otherwise isolated finding in febrile children. A review of studies that looked at clinical findings in children with pneumonia found that the best physical exam finding for ruling out pneumonia in an infant or child is the absence of tachypnea. However, tachypnea is a nonspecific symptom and may occur secondary to fever, anxiety, metabolic disease, cardiac disease, or other respiratory problems. Fever can increase an infant's respiratory rate by 10 breaths per minute for each degree in centigrade elevation. Respiratory rates should be counted over 1 minute. Several studies have shown that rates counted over less time tend to overestimate the rate. Generally accepted standards for what is considered tachypnea in an infant or child are shown in Table 10-4.

Auscultation of the lungs may reveal localized rales, wheezing, and decreased air entry in the affected area. However, auscultatory findings are less reliable in children. When a group of pediatricians were asked to examine 56 children with lower respiratory tract symptoms, there was only fair agreement about most auscultatory findings. In younger children, decreased breath sounds rather than rales are often noted, as the involved areas tend to be ventilated poorly. Grunting respirations are frequently present in infants with pneumonia. Abdominal distention and pain may be present secondary to a paralytic ileus or diaphragmatic irritation in lower lobe pneumonias. More severe pneumonia is associated with deterioration of the patient's mental status, the use of accessory muscles, and the presence of retractions, nasal flaring, splinting, and cyanosis. Infants may demonstrate chest indrawing and paradoxic or seesaw breathing.

Associated physical findings may give clues as to the etiology of the pneumonia. Children with viral pneumonia are more likely to have diffuse findings on chest exam and will often have a component of airway disease producing wheezing, prolonged expiration, and hyperinflation. Bacterial pneumonia tends to produce localized findings on chest exam. Patients with bacterial pneumonia also tend to appear relatively toxic and are almost always febrile. An infant with chlamydial infection is usually afebrile and has a distinct staccato cough (i.e., short, abrupt onset) and diffuse rales on auscultation. Such infants rarely appear systemically ill. Mycoplasmal infection may produce pharyngitis, and rales are present in approximately 75 percent of patients. A variable rash, which may be papular, vesicular, urticarial, or erythema multiforme–like, is present in about 10 percent of patients with *Mycoplasma* pneumoniae.

LABORATORY AND RADIOGRAPHIC FINDINGS

The chest radiograph is considered the customary method for diagnosing pneumonia. Radiographically, viral pneumonias tend to appear as diffuse interstitial infiltrates, frequently with hyperinflation, peribronchial thickening, and areas of atelectasis. Bacterial pneumonias tend to have lobar or segmental consolidation. However, bacterial pneumonias with perihilar interstitial and nodular patterns on radiographs have been reported, and viral

Table 28-2. Empiric Parenteral Antibiotic Therapy for Inpatient Treatment of Pneumonia in Immunocompetent Patients

Age	Therapeutic Agent(s)
0–1 mo	Ampicillin + aminoglycoside or ampicillin + cefotaxime
1–3 mo	Ampicillin + cefotaxime (consider erythromycin or clarithromycin if *Chlamydia* pneumonitis is suspected)
3 mo–5 yr	Cefuroxime, cefotaxime, or ceftriaxone (consider the addition of a macrolide if the patient's course is suspicious for *Mycoplasma pneumoniae*)
>5 yr	Macrolide (consider adding cefuroxime in severely ill patients)
All ages	Add vancomycin, if resistant *Streptococcus pneumoniae* is suspected. If the patient's course is suspicious for *Staphylococcus aureus* infection, consider addition of an antistaphylococcal agent.

pneumonias can cause lobar or segmental consolidations. Several studies have looked at the accuracy of the chest radiograph in differentiating viral from bacterial disease. These studies have demonstrated sensitivities ranging from 42 to 80% and specificities of 42 to 100 percent.

In patients with bacterial pneumonia, as proved by lung puncture, blood cultures are positive 13 percent of the time. In pneumococcal disease, they are positive in about 10 percent of cases. *S. aureus,* HIB, and group A streptococcal pneumonia have a higher incidence (up to 90 percent for HIB) of positive blood cultures. They should be obtained in infants who have high fever, who appear ill, or who require hospitalization. Sputum cultures may also help in identifying the causative organism but are almost impossible to obtain from nontracheostomized children, particularly those younger than 8 years. Cultures of the nasopharynx for viral pathogens and chlamydial, pertussis, and mycoplasma organisms will often reveal the etiologic agent in patients with pneumonias caused by these organisms. These tests may provide useful information for the primary management of the child and should be considered if the test is available and the disease is suspected. Fluorescent antibody tests for *C. trachomatis* and *B. pertussis* are preferable to culture in some settings.

Rapid viral antigen tests exist for a number of organisms but are not widely available in the emergency department (ED), except for RSV identification. Bacterial antigen testing is available in some centers, but it has a poor sensitivity and specificity in diagnosing the etiology of pneumonia. Serologic testing can be done for viruses, mycoplasma, parasites, and fungi, in persistent or puzzling cases. Skin testing for tuberculosis should also be considered in patients not responding to traditional therapy or with apical, cavitary pneumonias. More invasive diagnostic procedures such as endotracheal cultures, percutaneous lung puncture, bronchoalveolar lavage, or open lung biopsy may be necessary in patients with severe disease that is unresponsive to empiric therapy.

The white blood count is usually elevated, with a left shift in bacterial pneumonia, most notably in pneumococcal disease. Typically viral, chlamydial, and pertussis pneumonias will produce lymphocytosis. However, it is not unusual for viral pneumonia to initially provoke a significant polymorphonuclear cell response. An exception to this guideline is in children with sickle cell disease or other hemoglobinopathies, in whom leukemoid reactions (i.e., extreme leukocytosis) may occur. In patients with mycoplasmal pneumonia, the total white blood count and differential count are usually normal,

but the erythrocyte sedimentation rate may be elevated. Chlamydial infections or parasitic infections often produce an eosinophilia. Cold agglutinins have been demonstrated to be positive in 72 to 92 percent of patients with *M. pneumoniae* infection. Cold agglutinins may also be positive in viral infections and are less consistently positive in young children. To perform the bedside test for cold agglutinins, place several drops of blood in a blue-stopper coagulation profile tube and place in ice water for 15 to 30 seconds. The presence of floccular agglutination is considered a positive test, and the agglutination should disappear upon rewarming.

DIFFERENTIAL DIAGNOSIS

Initially, it is important to differentiate pneumonia from noninfectious pulmonary conditions, such as congestive heart failure, atelectasis, primary and metastatic tumors, and congenital abnormalities such as pulmonary hypoplasia or congenital lobar emphysema. The wide variety of conditions that may simulate pneumonia include radiologic imaging problems (i.e., poor inspiration, prominent thymus), recurrent or acute aspiration, atelectasis, tumors, collagen vascular disorders, allergic alveolitis, chronic pulmonary diseases (e.g., cystic fibrosis, asthma), and congenital abnormalities (e.g., pulmonary sequestration). A thorough history and physical exam usually helps to exclude many of these conditions. Differentiating the etiology of pneumonia is more challenging. Clinical and laboratory clues are discussed above.

TREATMENT

All patients should be assessed for hypoxia, and oxygen should be provided if indicated. Additional respiratory support should be provided as dictated by the patient's clinical condition. The patient's fluid status should be assessed and hydration provided if needed. Most children with pneumonia can be managed as outpatients. If a bacterial etiology is suspected, the child should be placed on an appropriate antibiotic. An antibiotic is chosen based on the considerations discussed above regarding the most likely etiologic organisms based on the age and clinical presentation of the patient (Table 28-2).

For outpatient treatment, amoxicillin (40 mg/kg/day) is preferred for children between 3 months and 4 years of age. Alternatively, daily intramuscular ceftriaxone may be used. After 4 years of age and in penicillin-allergic children, a macrolide antibiotic is the preferred initial agent. The patient's primary care provider or the ED should provide follow-up within 1 to 2 days.

Empiric intravenous antibiotic therapy should be provided for patients requiring admission for suspected bacterial pneumonia. Empiric coverage should be guided predominantly by the age of the patient. In the newborn, ampicillin (150 to 300 mg/kg/day every 6 to 8 hours in combination with either an aminoglycoside (gentamycin 2.5-mg/kg/dose every 8 to 12 hours) or third-generation cephalosporin (cefotaxime, 100 to 150 mg/kg/day every 6 to 8 hours) is preferred. The ampicillin provides coverage against *Listeria* and *Enterococcus* species. In children with afebrile pneumonia or "pneumonitis syndrome" (see above), treatment should consist of eryth-romycin or clarithromycin. In children older than 3 months, a cephalosporin alone (cefuroxime, cefotaxime, or ceftriaxone) is sufficient. In children who are unresponsive to this therapy or with a suggestive clinical presentation, *Mycoplasma* and chlamydial infections should be considered. Appropriate coverage is a macrolide antibiotic. If the clinical presentation is suspicious for staphylococcal disease, then appropriate coverage (nafcillin, 150 mg/kg/day every 6 hours) should be added. Ceftazidime or ceftriaxone eradicated noscomial pneumonia in 90 percent of cases, but ceftazidime had improved efficacy against *Pseudomonas aeruginosa,* in a recent report. Children with cystic fibrosis often de-velop acute infectious exacerbations secondary to *S. aureus* and *Pseudomonas,* often with resistance to standard antibiotics.

The duration of therapy varies with the clinical response, predisposing to host factors and suppurative complications. Seven to 10 days of antimicrobial treatment should suffice for most uncomplicated cases. Parenteral therapy, if initiated, should be continued until clinical improvement occurs. Routine follow-up radiographs are not necessary if the patient improves clinically. Whenever the case of pneumonia is complicated or prolonged, roentgenographic follow-up is recommended to ensure complete resolution, which may take 4 to 6 weeks or longer.

If viral pneumonia is suspected, no specific antibiotic therapy is warranted. Patients with viral pneumonia often have a mixture of airway and airspace disease. If the patient has prominent reactive airway disease (bronchiolitis-like) symptoms, bronchodilator therapy should be considered. In RSV pneumonia, ribavirin therapy should be considered utilizing the guidelines discussed for bronchiolitis in Chapter 27. Children with fulminant viral pneumonias, such as varicella in the immunocompromised host, may require treatment with acyclovir. Lymphocytic interstitial pneumonia in HIV-positive children should include a combination of prednisone and zidovudine. Bone marrow and solid organ transplant patients with CMV pneumonia may require ganciclovir and gammaglobulin.

DISPOSITION/OUTCOME

As previously stated, most children with pneumonia can be managed as outpatients. Suggested criteria for admission include the following:

- Hypoxia
- Respiratory distress
- Toxic appearance
- Dehydration
- Age younger than 3 months
- Impaired immune function
- Infections unresponsive to oral therapy.

The presence of underlying disease and the ability of the caregivers to provide care for the child should also be considered. Age younger than 1 year or the finding of a pleural effusion or pneumatocele suggests a pathogen other than *S. pneumoniae* (particularly HIB or *S. aureus*). These infections can be rapidly progressive and are not well tolerated, so strong consideration should be given to hospitalizing these patients. All children discharged with a diagnosis of pneumonia should have clinical follow-up arranged within 24 hours.

Most viral pneumonias will resolve spontaneously without specific therapy. Complications are similar to those for bronchiolitis and include dehydration, bronchiolitis obliterans, and apnea. Apnea is seen commonly in very young infants with RSV or chlamydial or pertussis infections. Pleural effusions can occur with viral pneumonias but are not common. Indications for admitting patients with RSV pneumonia are the same as for RSV bronchiolitis (see Chap. 27).

Uncomplicated bacterial pneumonia usually responds rapidly to antibiotic therapy. Delay in improvement or worsening condition after therapy has begun should prompt an evaluation for possible complications. Complications of bacterial pneumonia include pleural effusions, empyemas, pneumothorax, pneumatoceles, dehydration, and development of additional infectious foci. Pleural effusions will occur in approximately 10 percent of cases of pneumococcal pneumonia. Pneumonia due to HIB will be complicated by pleural effusions in 25 to 75 percent of cases. Other foci of infection are frequently seen with HIB and can include meningitis, septic arthritis, epiglottitis, soft tissue infections, and otitis media. Pneumonias secondary to *S. aureus* have a high rate of complications including empyemas (80 percent) and pneumatoceles (40 percent). Mycoplasmal pneumonia can, on occasion, be complicated by pleural effusions, meningitis, encephalitis, arthritis, and hemolytic anemia.

The mortality rate of childhood pneumonia is <1 percent in industrialized nations, but it accounts for up to 5 million deaths annually in children younger than 5 years of age in developing countries.

BIBLIOGRAPHY

Davies HD, Matlow A, Petric M, et al: Prospective comparative study of viral bacterial and atypical organisms identified in pneumonia and bronchiolitis in hospitalized infants. *Pediatr Infect Dis J* 15:371–376, 1996.

Davies HD, Wang EE, Manso D, et al: Reliability of the chest radiograph in the diagnosis of lower tract respiratory infections in young children. *Pediatr Infect Dis J* 15:600–660, 1996.

DeMuri GP: Afebrile pneumonia in infants. *Prim Care Clin Office Pract* 23:849–860, 1996.

Margolis P, Gadomski A: Does this infant have pneumonia? *JAMA* 279:308–313, 1998.

McCracken GH: Etiology and treatment of pneumonia. *Pediatr Infect Dis J* 19:373–377, 2000.

Nelson JD: Community-acquired pneumonia in children: Guidelines for treatment. *Pediatr Infect Dis J* 19:251–253, 2000.

Schaad UB: Antibiotic therapy of childhood pneumonia. *Pediatr Pulmonol* 18S:146–149, 1999.

Sinanaiotis CA: Community-acquired pneumonia in children: Diagnosis and treatment. *Pediatr Pulmonol* 18S:144–145, 1999.

29

Pertussis

Kathleen Brown

HIGH-YIELD FACTS

- Pertussis occurs most commonly in infants younger than 6 months but can occur in any age group.
- The initial or catarrhal stage is characterized by upper respiratory tract symptoms and lasts 7 to 10 days. This is followed by a paroxysmal phase characterized by episodic bouts of staccato cough lasting 2 to 4 weeks.
- Diagnosis is usually based on history and physical examination. Fluorescent antibody testing is currently the most utilized confirmatory test, but it has a low sensitivity and poor predictive value. The polymerase chain reaction test has a much higher sensitivity.
- The mainstay of treatment is supportive therapy including oxygen for hypoxia and intravenous fluids for dehydration. Erythromycin is effective therapy only if given prior to the paroxysmal stage.
- Prophylactic therapy should be given to close contacts.
- Indications for hospital admission include young age (younger than 1 year), hypoxia, and dehydration.

Pertussis is a respiratory infection most commonly diagnosed in infants younger than 6 months, but it can be seen in any age group. It was a leading cause of morbidity and mortality in children prior to the widespread use of the diphtheria-tetanus-pertussis (DPT) vaccine that became available in the 1950s. Over the next 30 years the number of reported cases fell dramatically to a nadir of about 1000 cases a year in the 1970s. However, in the past decades there has been a fourfold increase in the incidence of pertussis in this country. In 1993 per-

tussis became the most commonly reported vaccine-preventable disease among children younger than 5 years old in the United States.

ETIOLOGY/PATHOPHYSIOLOGY

Pertussis is an infection of the respiratory tract produced by *Bordetella pertussis.* Occasionally, a similar clinical syndrome is produced by *Bordetella parapertussis,* the adenoviruses, or chlamydia. *B. pertussis* is spread by respiratory droplet transmission. Following inhalation, *B. pertussis* organisms attach to the epithelial cells of the respiratory tract. Multiplication of the bacteria leads to infiltration of the mucosa with inflammatory cells. Inflammatory debris in the lumen of the bronchi and peribronchial lymphoid hyperplasia combine to obstruct the smaller airways, causing atelectasis.

Attack rates in susceptible household contacts approach 100%. The incubation period ranges from 7 to 14 days. Clinical infection with pertussis is the only assurance of lifelong immunity. Vaccination gives a high degree of protection for 3 years and then gradually declines in effectiveness for 12 years, after which no protection may be evident. There is no passive immunization in utero, and infants are not considered fully immunized until they have received three vaccine injections. Undervaccination of infants, and an increasing teenage and adult population who have lost immunity, have resulted in an increasing pool for the disease.

CLINICAL PRESENTATION

The disease is characterized by three stages:

- The initial or catarrhal stage is characterized by upper respiratory tract symptoms and lasts for 7 to 10 days.
- This is followed by a paroxysmal phase characterized by episodic bouts of staccato cough lasting 2 to 4 weeks.
- In the convalescent stage the symptoms gradually wane.

Infants in the paroxysmal phase of *B. pertussis* infection will have a history of intermittent coughing spells, often followed by posttussive emesis and sometimes associated with cyanosis. The paroxysms are often provoked by feeding or exertion and can be elicited when using a tongue blade to examine the throat. The cough is staccato in nature, allowing little or no inspiration between coughs. At the termination of a paroxysm, a prolonged slow inspiration occurs. Inspiration through a partially closed glottis produces the characteristic whoop. However, this feature is often absent in infants. Silent paroxysms may occur in infants younger than 6 months. Between bouts of paroxysmal coughing, the physical exam is usually normal. Subconjunctival hemorrhages may be observed secondary to the force of the coughing.

Several studies have confirmed the importance of pertussis as the cause of persistent cough among teenagers and adults. These cases usually go undiagnosed and untreated.

LABORATORY AND RADIOGRAPHIC FINDINGS

Cultures of the nasopharynx may reveal the organism. *B pertussis* grows poorly in blood agar and should be plated on Bordet-Gengou agar. This method of culturing is specific but insensitive and considered too time consuming to be useful for diagnosis. Fluorescent antibody testing is currently the most utilized confirmatory test but has a low sensitivity and poor predictive value. A polymerase chain reaction test has been reported to have a much higher sensitivity. Pertussis generally produces extreme leukocytosis (20 to 50,000), with a predominance of lymphocytes. This may not occur in infants younger than 6 months. Radiographs in patients with *B. pertussis* infection may demonstrate a shaggy right heart border or be normal.

DIAGNOSIS

The diagnosis of pertussis is best made through a careful history and physical examination, coupled with the clinician's awareness of its possible existence. In 1990, the U.S. Council of State and Territorial Epidemiologists adopted uniform case definitions for outbreak-related and sporadic reporting of pertussis infections. In an outbreak of pertussis, a cough lasting for 14 or more days can be considered a case. For a sporadic diagnosis, the patient must meet the cough criterion and also have paroxysms, whoop, or posttussive emesis. It is important to remember that many cases are atypical, especially in infants and children who have been partially immunized and older patients who may present with a chronic cough. In such cases, laboratory testing may be helpful.

TREATMENT

Erythromycin is considered to be the most effective antibiotic. However, unless it is started in the incubation period or early catarrhal stage, it does not modify the course of the disease. Initiation of therapy after the onset of paroxysms (when most patients are diagnosed) is ineffective. The recommended dose is 40 to 50 mg/kg/day in four divided doses for 14 days. Although not clinically proved to be effective as a prophylaxis, erythromycin is recommended for use in close patient contacts. In contacts younger than 7 years of age who have not received the primary vaccination series, a dose should be administered. Hyperimmune globulin is not efficacious as prophylactic therapy.

The mainstay of treatment is supportive therapy. Infants may become hypoxic during paroxysms and benefit from humidified oxygen administration. They may also become dehydrated due to inability to feed and will benefit from intravenous fluids. Apnea spells can occur in infants, especially those younger than 6 months of age.

DISPOSITION/OUTCOME

B. pertussis infections can be complicated by apnea, seizures, encephalopathy, and secondary bacterial pneumonia. The incidence of these complications and death due to pertussis infection is greater in infants younger than 1 year. Such infants must be admitted and placed on a cardiorespiratory/apnea monitor. The mortality rate in children younger than 1 year was 0.6 percent of 10,749 cases reported to the Centers for Disease Control and Prevention between 1980 and 1989.

BIBLIOGRAPHY

Black S: Epidemiology of pertuusis. *Pediatr Infect Dis J* 1(4S):S85–S89, 1997.

Dodhia H, Miller E: Review of the evidence for the use of erythromycin in the management of persons exposed to pertussis. *Epidemiol Infect* 120:143–149, 1998.

Hallander HO: Microbiological and serological diagnosis of pertussis. *Clin Infect Dis* 28S:S99–S106, 1999.

Hampl SD, Olson LC: Pertussis in the young infant. *Semin Respir Infect* 10:58–62, 1995.

Hewlett EL: Pertussis current concepts of pathogenesis and prevention. *Pediatr Infect Dis J* 16S:S78–S84, 1997.

30

Bronchopulmonary Dysplasia

Kathleen Brown

HIGH-YIELD FACTS

- Bronchopulmonary dysplasia (BPD) is a chronic lung disease of infancy that follows neonatal lung disease. Oxygen requirement at 36 weeks corrected post gestational age predicts the development of BPD.

- Infants with BPD, ranging from mild asymptomatic disease to crippling cardiopulmonary dysfunction, may present to the ED with an exacerbation of their chronic lung disease. Exacerbations are most often secondary to viral upper respiratory infections.

- The treatment of an exacerbation in a patient with BPD is mainly supportive. Oxygen, ventilatory support, and fluids are provided if indicated.

- Bronchodilators and corticosteroids are often effective in these patients and are used in a similar fashion to the way they are used for asthma. Diuretics have been shown to improve lung function and survival in some patients.

- Indications for admission include:
  - Respiratory distress
  - Need for ventilatory support
  - New infiltrates
  - Infection with RSV
  - Inability of family to manage exacerbation at home

As the care of neonates with respiratory failure becomes more aggressive and more successful, the incidence of chronic lung disease in infants is increasing. The overall rate of bronchopulmonary dysplasia (BPD) is about 15% for premature infants requiring mechanical ventilation.

The incidence is dependent on birth weight, exceeding 50% in infants less than 750 g at birth, and 40% for infants between 750 and 1000 g. In addition to weight, male sex and white race are risk factors for the development of BPD.

BPD is a chronic lung disease of infancy that follows neonatal lung disease. The original insult may be hyaline membrane disease, apnea, persistent fetal circulation, complex congenital heart disease, or any illness requiring prolonged mechanical ventilation as a neonate. Children with residual lung disease after the neonatal period (28 days of age) are said to have BPD. The lung disease may be characterized by respiratory distress, a supplemental oxygen requirement, and/or significant radiologic and blood gas abnormalities. Previous definitions of BPD were based on the presence of a supplemental oxygen requirement at 4 weeks of age. However, this is not predictive of the development of BPD in infants born at less than 30 weeks' gestation. Oxygen requirement at 36 weeks corrected post gestational age has been shown to be an excellent predictor of the development of BPD in this group of infants.

ETIOLOGY/PATHOPHYSIOLOGY

The pathogenesis of BPD is complex, multifactorial, and not yet fully understood. Mechanical ventilation has been implicated as a causative agent. However, some infants who never receive mechanical ventilation go on to develop the clinical syndrome of BPD. Factors thought to play a role in the development of BPD include host susceptibility, primary or secondary lung injury, and the lungs' response to injury.

An increased incidence of reactive airway disease is found in the families of infants who develop BPD. This suggests that some infants may be genetically predisposed to the development of BPD. The major host susceptibility factor associated with BPD is immature lungs secondary to prematurity. Decreased alveolar and airway number as well as increased dispensability of the airway may predispose premature infants to barotrauma during mechanical ventilation. Immaturity is also associated with a defect in the antioxidant defense system (decreased superoxide dismutase) and a decrease in plasma proteinase inhibitors. The primary lung injury often leads to increased permeability of the lungs and the presence of neutrophils and macrophages. These cells produce proteases and other cytotoxic products including oxygen radicals capable of producing pulmonary membrane damage.

Factors involved in secondary injury include mechanical ventilation, oxygen toxicity, and inflammatory mediators. Mechanical ventilation can cause airway injury, epithelial necrosis, and ciliary dysfunction, all of which are prominent features in infants with BPD. Additional evidence for the role of mechanical ventilation in the development of BPD is the fact that infants ventilated for recurrent apnea without clinically evident primary lung disease sometimes will develop BPD. The use of oxygen in the treatment of infants with lung disease results in the formation of toxic oxygen radicals. Infants (both premature and term) are less able to clear these toxins and may suffer secondary lung injury. The oxygen radicals and inflammatory cells lead to the release of inflammatory mediators such as the products of the arachidonic acid pathway (EG, leukotrienes, platelet activating factor, prostaglandins, thromboxane) and cytokines. These mediators have diverse effects including bronchoconstriction, vasoconstriction, pulmonary hypertension, platelet aggregation, increased vascular permeability, increased oxygen radical and protease production, and increased leukocyte migration and adherence. All of these play a role in the development of secondary lung injury.

The way neonates react to lung injury also plays a role in the development of BPD. The principal histologic finding in the lungs of neonates with BPD is an extensive fibroproliferative response far in excess of the needs to repair the damage that occurred. This may be due to neonates having an increased number of pulmonary neuroendocrine cells (PNEC). These are among the first cells to differentiate in regenerating endothelium and demonstrate a proliferative response to lung injury. Malnutrition, which is frequently seen in sick neonates, may also have profound effects on lung defenses and repair capabilities. The multifactorial nature of the pathogenesis of this disease accounts for the great variability in severity of the clinical presentation of these patients.

CLINICAL PRESENTATION

The clinical spectrum of infants with chronic lung disease ranges from mild asymptomatic disease to crippling cardiopulmonary dysfunction. Patients who are likely to present to the ED are those that have been discharged home from the neonatal intensive care unit, typically at about 3–6 months of age. These children are often on home oxygen, bronchodilators, apnea monitors, and other medications. They will present to the ED with an exacerbation of their chronic lung disease most often secondary to a viral upper respiratory infection. Parents may describe increased respiratory distress, poor feeding, lethargy or irritability, and an increased oxygen requirement.

On physical examination, infants with chronic lung disease will usually be small-for-age and have hyperinflated chests (increased anterior-posterior diameter). They will have tachypnea, rales, wheezes, or areas of decreased breath sounds. They may also have signs of an upper respiratory infection, including fever.

LABORATORY AND RADIOGRAPHIC FINDINGS

A chest radiograph will reveal variable degrees of hyperinflation with areas of "scarring" (cystic or fibrotic areas). Comparison with old films is required to differentiate these areas from acute processes.

Oximetry should be checked on all patients with BPD. The results should be interpreted in light of the baseline level of hypoxia and usual need for oxygen therapy. Blood gas results can be helpful in assessing the more severely symptomatic patient. The results will also need to be compared with previous results, as these children will often have hypercarbia and hypoxia at baseline.

DIFFERENTIAL DIAGNOSIS

In most cases, the diagnosis of BPD will be evident from the history. As many BPD exacerbations are triggered by upper respiratory infections, and often involve reactive airways as part of the pathology, the signs and symptoms of an exacerbation may overlap considerably with that of pneumonia, asthma, or bronchiolitis. Often these problems are coexistent and are the cause of the exacerbation. A chest radiograph can be helpful in identifying pneumonia if the radiograph can be compared to previous films (see above). Testing for RSV will help identify those patients who may need ribavirin therapy.

TREATMENT

The treatment of an exacerbation in a patient with BPD is mainly supportive. Oxygen is provided if indicated. The patient's fluid status is assessed and intravenous fluids provided if indicated. Mechanical ventilation may be necessary for recurrent apnea spells (most commonly with RSV infections), worsening hypercarbia, or refractory hypoxemia.

Bronchodilators are often effective in these patients and should be used as they are for asthma. Systemic corticosteroids are thought to be effective in acute exacerbations, but their chronic use is associated with many side effects. Inhaled steroids have been shown to increase the ability to extubate children who are chronically ventilated but its efficacy in nonventilated patients has not been demonstrated. Parenteral diuretics have been shown to improve lung function and survival in some patients. Studies have looked at the effectiveness of aerosolized furosemide for patients with BPD but no conclusive benefit has been demonstrated.

OUTCOME/DISPOSITION

Some patients who present to the ED with exacerbation due to an upper respiratory infection can be managed at home. However, children with BPD often have a very fragile respiratory status and can become very sick with relatively minor insults. Indications for inpatient management include increased respiratory distress, increasing hypoxia or hypercarbia, or new pulmonary infiltrates. Patients with BPD and RSV infections are at high risk for complications of RSV and are candidates for ribavirin administration and need to be hospitalized. It is important to remember that the home care of these children requires a tremendous amount of work on the part of the parents or other caretakers even when the child is not acutely ill. Parents may have difficulty coping with an exacerbation. This factor should be considered when making a decision to discharge a patient for home care.

BIBLIOGRAPHY

Bancalari E: Corticosteroids and neonatal lung disease. *Eur J Pediatr* 157S1:S31–S37, 1998.

Barrington KJ, Finer NN: Treatment of bronchopulmonary dysplasia. *Clin Perinatol* 25:177–202, 1998.

Brion LP, Primhak RA, Yong W: Aerosolized diuretics for preterm infants with chronic lung disease. Cochrane Database of Systematic Reviews. Issue 4, 2000.

Farrell PA, Fiascone JM: Bronchopulmonary dysplasia in the 1990s: A review for the pediatrician. *Curr Probl Pediatr* 27:129–163, 1997.

Lister P, Iles R, Shaw B, et al: Inhaled steroids for neonatal chronic lung disease. Cochrane Database of Systematic Reviews. Issue 4, 2000.

McColley SA: Bronchopulmonary dysplasia: Impact of surfactant replacement therapy. *Pediatr Clin North Am* 45: 573–586, 1998.

Saugstad OD: Bronchopulmonary dysplasia and oxidative stress: Are we closer to an understanding of the pathogenesis of BPD? *Acta Pediatr* 86:1277–1282, 1997.

31

Cystic Fibrosis

Kathleen Brown

HIGH-YIELD FACTS

- Cystic fibrosis (CF) is a generalized defect in all of the exocrine gland secretions.
- Patients not yet diagnosed with CF may present to the ED with a history of failure to thrive, chronic pulmonary infection, or gastrointestinal problems.
- Patients with known CF most commonly present with pulmonary exacerbation, hemoptysis, or cor pulmonale. Nonpulmonary acute complications include meconium ileus, rectal prolapse, intestinal obstruction, and electrolyte abnormalities.
- First-line therapy for respiratory exacerbations, the primary cause of morbidity and mortality, include bronchodilator therapy and antibiotics.
- Other possible therapies for pulmonary exacerbations include antiinflammatory agents, chest physiotherapy, and mucoactive agents.

Cystic fibrosis (CF) is the most common lethal inherited disease among Caucasians in the United States. It occurs in approximately 1 in 2500 and 1 in 17,000 live births in whites and blacks, respectively. CF is a generalized defect in all of the exocrine gland secretions. Most patients with CF have the classic triad of manifestations:

- Chronic pulmonary disease
- Malabsorption
- Elevated content of sweat electrolytes

There can be considerable individual variation in the severity and the course of the disease.

ETIOLOGY/PATHOPHYSIOLOGY

CF is inherited as an autosomal recessive condition. The CF gene is localized on the long arm of chromosome 7.

The most common mutation that causes CF (DeltaF508), and >600 less-common mutations, have been identified. DNA probes for the normal gene and some mutations are available for detection of patients and carriers. The product of the defective gene in CF is the cystic fibrosis transmembrane conductance regulator (CFTR). This product controls fluid balance across epithelial cells. It acts as a chloride channel activated by cAMP. The decreased chloride transport is accompanied by decreased transport of sodium and water, resulting in dehydrated viscous secretions that are associated with luminal obstruction and destruction and scarring of various exocrine ducts. It is thought that perhaps the high concentration of salt in these secretions inactivates the naturally occurring antibiotic peptide compounds (defensins) that are produced by the airways. This may be why CF patients are chronically colonized with bacterial pathogens. The sweat of patients with CF also contains a high concentration of chloride. This forms the basis for the most important diagnostic test in patients with CF, the qualitative pilocarpine iontophoresis sweat test.

Clinically, the patients are noted to have abnormalities in clearing mucus secretions, a paucity of water in mucus secretions, an elevated salt content of sweat and other serous secretions, and chronic infections of the respiratory tract. The first three are thought to be primary defects and the fourth a secondary event. The chronic mucus plugging and infection leads to hyperinflation, bronchiectasis, and atelectasis. There is a progressive increase in the amount of ventilation/perfusion mismatching and structural changes in the lungs. Eventually most CF patients die of respiratory failure complicated by cor pulmonale.

In patients with CF, the exocrine glands of the pancreas produce viscous, low volume, and bicarbonate- and enzyme-deficient secretions. Pancreatic insufficiency occurs with the obstruction and dilation of pancreatic ducts. Abnormal intestinal mucins and biliary tract secretions have also been implicated in the intestinal malabsorption and obstruction seen in CF.

CLINICAL PRESENTATION

Patients who have not yet been diagnosed with CF may present to the emergency department (ED). Failure to thrive with a history of chronic respiratory and/or gastrointestinal problems is the most typical presentation. However, since the expression of the defect is so variable, many other presentations are possible. The diagnosis should be considered in any case of failure to thrive, atypical asthma (especially with clubbing, bronchiectasis, or purulent sputum), recurrent respiratory infections, or chronic diarrhea. Hypoproteinemia may develop in those with prominent malabsorption. Malabsorption may also lead to symptoms of vitamin deficiencies. A hemorrhagic diatheses secondary to vitamin K deficiency has been described. Patients with clinical findings suggestive of CF should be referred for diagnostic evaluation.

Patients with known CF may present to the ED with a variety of acute complications. The most common of these is a pulmonary exacerbation. Patients will present with a progressive worsening in their chronic lung disease. Often there will be a preceding upper respiratory infection. The patient will have signs of respiratory distress, may be cyanotic, and may progress to frank respiratory failure. Chest examination will reveal diffuse rales, rhonchi, or wheezing. Pneumothoraces are not unusual in patients with CF and should be considered in any patient with an acute deterioration. Many patients with CF will have intermittent blood-streaked sputum that is usually not clinically significant. However, significant hemoptysis (30 to 60 mL) can result from erosion of a bronchial vessel. Less commonly, patients with CF will cough up blood from a bleeding esophageal varices secondary to advanced cirrhosis. Many patients with CF will develop pulmonary hypertension and right ventricular hypertrophy as a result of their chronic lung disease. Congestive heart failure can develop during a respiratory exacerbation. These patients will have signs and symptoms typical of CHF.

Acute nonpulmonary complications of CF include meconium ileus, rectal prolapse, intestinal obstruction, and electrolyte abnormalities. A neonate with meconium ileus will usually have a history of having passed no stool or only a small amount of meconium stool. On physical examination, these patients will have a distended abdomen. They may also have visible peristaltic waves or a palpable abdominal mass. Intestinal obstruction secondary to inability to pass the dry abnormal stool can also occur in older children with CF and is sometimes called meconium ileus equivalent. Like a meconium ileus, these fecal masses can lead to complications including volvulus, intussusception, or intestinal perforation. Rectal prolapse is associated with CF and is most commonly seen in children younger than 3 years old. As patients approach adulthood, they may develop additional complications, such as diabetes mellitus (17 percent of adults), obstructive biliary tract disease (15 to 20 percent of adults), and obstructive azospermia (90 per-

cent of postpubertal males). The elevated sweat electrolyte content gives patients with CF their characteristically salty taste and can lead to acute or chronic electrolyte depletion at any age.

LABORATORY AND RADIOGRAPHIC FINDINGS

A quantitative pilocarpine iontophoresis sweat (sweat chloride) test should be part of the diagnostic evaluation in any patient with suspected CF. This test is time consuming and is usually not available in the ED setting. A referral for an evaluation including this test should be made for any patient in whom the diagnosis is suspected.

In patients with known CF with a pulmonary exacerbation, sputum cultures should be obtained to help guide antibiotic therapy. Past sputum culture results can be helpful in guiding initial therapy. Blood cultures to rule out bacteremia may be indicated in febrile or toxic-appearing patients.

Electrolyte determination will usually reveal low serum sodium and chloride levels. Bicarbonate levels and serum pH are usually elevated. These abnormalities represent renal compensation for the increased salt loss in the sweat. Dehydration and symptomatic electrolyte deficiencies can occur, especially in periods of hot weather. Characteristic electrolytes may provide a diagnostic clue when seen in a patient with other findings suggestive of CF. Patients with significant hemoptysis should have blood sent for a hematocrit, type and cross-match, and prothrombin time. Oximetry should be checked in any patient with increased pulmonary symptoms. Blood gas determinations may be useful in managing a patient with respiratory failure.

Typical radiographic findings of a patient with CF include diffuse peribronchial thickening, hyperinflation, and variable fluffy infiltrates. It is often helpful to compare current films with previous ones in patients with an acute exacerbation. Radiographic studies may be helpful in diagnosing the acute complications of CF. Patients with a sudden change in pulmonary condition should have a chest radiograph to rule out a pneumothorax. Patients with cor pulmonale will have a large heart, as opposed to the narrow heart usually seen in patients with CF, and prominent pulmonary vasculature. Patients with meconium ileus or meconium ileus equivalent will have dilated loops of bowel on an abdominal film. A bubbly granular density in the lower abdomen representing the meconium or fecal mass may also be seen.

DIFFERENTIAL DIAGNOSIS

The expression of the genetic defect in CF is variable, and the disease can present in many different ways. Patients who should be considered for a CF evaluation are discussed above. The pilocarpine electrophoresis test is the most valuable aid in distinguishing patients with CF from those with other diseases.

TREATMENT

Much of the treatment of CF involves issues of chronic care. However, the ED physician may be called upon to manage the acute complications of CF. The most common of these will be pulmonary exacerbations. Therapy is aimed at relieving the mucus plugging and obstruction and treating infection. Oxygen should be administered if indicated by pulse oximetry or blood gas.

The obstructive airway disease in CF is multifactorial and only partially reversible because of the airway inflammation associated with infection and underlying structural damage. Bronchodilators, both β-adrenergic and anticholinergic agents, are often effective, in the short term, in patients with CF. They should be used in patients who respond clinically. Doses are the same as for asthmatic patients. Methylxanthines are sometimes used in the treatment of patients with CF and acute pulmonary exacerbations who are unresponsive to other therapies. If they are used, it is important to remember that patients with CF have increased clearance and therefore require larger or more frequent doses, and drug levels should be monitored.

The patient's recent sputum culture and sensitivity results may be helpful in choosing initial antibiotics. If these results are unavailable, empiric therapy should be aimed at the most common organisms seen in these patients, which are *Staphylococcus aureus,* nontypable *Hemophilus influenzae,* and gram-negative bacilli in infants and young children, and *Pseudomonas aeruginosa,* by the end of the first decade of life. Other pathogens, such as *Burkholderia cepacia, Burkholderia gladioliaspergillus fumigatus,* and nontuberculous mycobacteria are particularly problematic in some patients and are associated with a worse prognosis. Inhaled antibiotics, particularly tobramycin, were found to be safe and effective as maintenance therapy for patients colonized with *Pseudomonas aeruginosa.* This agent is also sometimes used in the setting of an acute exacerbation.

Mucoactive agents, particularly recombinant human deoxyribonuclease (Pulmozyme), has been shown to be safe and effective in patients with stable but severe pulmonary disease. A small study looking at its use in the setting of an acute exacerbation did not show any benefit when it was added to standard therapy. Hypertonic saline has also been proposed as a possible method of clearing secretions in patients with CF. It has been found to increase forced expiratory volume in 1 second in some trials, but there are concerns about its long-term effects on airway infections. Chest physiotherapy and postural drainage techniques are well accepted but not well proved as therapy for clearing secretions in patients with CF.

Antiinflammatory medications are thought to be helpful in the long-term management of patients with CF. Chronic oral steroids at a dose of 1 to 2 mg/kg on alternate days have been shown to be effective in slowing the progression of lung disease in CF but have also been associated with the development of cataracts and growth retardation. Chronic high-dose ibuprofen and inhaled corticosteroids are commonly used. However, reviews of their effectiveness have not demonstrated sufficient evidence to recommend their routine use. Patients with an acute exacerbation who are on chronic steroids should have these medications continued and, due to the potential of adrenal suppression, higher doses should be considered.

Patients with pneumothoraces should be managed in standard fashion. A pneumothorax, which is >10 percent of the area of the hemithorax, should be treated with tube thoracostomy. Tension pneumothoraces should be treated with needle aspiration followed by tube thoracostomy.

Significant hemoptysis (>30 to 60 mL) is an indication for inpatient observation. Vitamin K is indicated if the prothrombin time is prolonged. If bleeding persists, guidelines for replacement are the same as for bleeding from other sources. Massive hemoptysis (>300 mL) may compromise the airway, and ligation or embolization of the bleeding vessel should be attempted with the help of a bronchoscopist and/or thoracic surgeon.

Cor pulmonale may require treatment with oxygen and diuretics, in addition to treatment for the underlying pulmonary disease. Patients with CF and respiratory failure are very difficult to manage. They do not respond as well to mechanical ventilation and have even more complications than patients with other forms of chronic obstructive pulmonary disease. Factors that should be considered include the patient's baseline pulmonary function, the course of the patient's disease, and the expectations of the patient and their parents. In general, patients in whom respiratory failure is precipitated by an acute insult such as a viral pneumonia or episode of status asthmaticus and whose baseline pulmonary function was good should be considered for mechanical ventilation. In patients who have experienced a steady progressive decline in their pulmonary function despite adequate medical therapy, mechanical ventilation is often not warranted. This can be a very difficult decision and should be made in conjunction with the patient's chronic care provider and/or the patient and the patient's parents. Recently a number of patients with CF have undergone heart-lung transplants, with 3-year survival rates reported at >50 percent.

In patients with uncomplicated meconium ileus or meconium ileus equivalent, saline or gastrografin enemas may relieve the obstruction. Laparotomy is indicated if there are signs of perforation, volvulus, or intussusception, or if the medical management is unsuccessful. Patients presenting with dehydration and electrolyte abnormalities should be rehydrated with isotonic saline. Frequent check of serum electrolytes should guide fluid therapy.

OUTCOME

Many more CF patients are now surviving to adulthood. Factors contributing to this improvement in survival include more effective antibiotics, earlier diagnosis, and the prompt recognition and treatment of the serious, acute complications of CF.

BIBLIOGRAPHY

Cheng K, Ashby D, Smythg R: Oral steroids for cystic fibrosis. Cochrane Database of Systematic Reviews. Issue 4, 2000.

Dezateux C, Crighton A: Oral non-steroidal anti-inflammatory drug therapy for cystic fibrosis. Cochrane Database of Systematic Reviews. Issue 4, 2000.

Dezateux C, Walters S, Balfour-Lynn I: Inhaled corticosteroids for cystic fibrosis. Cochrane Database of Systematic Reviews. Issue 4, 2000.

Konstan MW: Therapies aimed at airway inflammation in cystic fibrosis. *Clin Chest Med* 19:101–113, 1998.

Marshall BC, Samuelson WM. Basic therapies in cystic fibrosis. Does standard therapy work? *Clin Chest Med* 19:487–504, 1998.

Ramsey BW: Drug therapy: Management of pulmonary disease in patients with cystic fibrosis. *N Engl J Med* 335:179–188, 1996.

Rosensstein BJ, Zeitlin PL: Cystic fibrosis. *Lancet* 351: 227–282, 1998.

Wark PA, McDonald V: Nebulized hypertonic saline for cystic fibrosis. Cochrane Database of Systematic Reviews. Issue 4, 2000.

32

Congenital Heart Disease

Kelly D. Young

HIGH-YIELD FACTS

- Ductal-dependent lesions typically present with sudden onset cardiogenic shock at 1 to 2 weeks of life and require immediate prostaglandin E_1 infusion.

- Congestive heart failure typically presents in the first 6 months of infancy in children with left-to-right shunting lesions and requires immediate stabilization and medical management.

- Aortic coarctation may present with hypertension and the complications of hypertension. The median age of presentation is 5 years. Blood pressure will be higher in the upper extremities compared with the lower extremities.

- The number of survivors of cardiac surgery for congenital heart lesions is rapidly increasing, and emergency physicians should be aware of common complications, such as arrhythmias, residual or recurrent lesions, and endocarditis.

- Children commonly have benign cardiac murmurs, which are usually softer, lower pitched, and early- to midsystolic compared with pathologic murmurs.

The term "congenital heart disease" encompasses a wide variety of lesions. The emergency physician must be able to not only recognize and manage previously undiagnosed congenital heart disease, but also anticipate complications in a rapidly growing population of sur-

vivors of surgery for congenital heart lesions. This chapter reviews the common presentations and management of cyanotic and acyanotic congenital heart lesions and also discusses complications seen in postoperative congenital cardiac patients.

EPIDEMIOLOGY

Congenital heart lesions occur in approximately 8 in 1000 live births in the United States. This figure includes lesions ranging from severe to mild but does not include common lesions such as bicuspid aortic valve (1 to 2 percent of the population) or mitral valve prolapse. Overall, neither gender is predominant, but individual lesions may be found more commonly in either males or females. About 10 percent of cases can be attributed to genetic causes, with the other 90 percent multifactorial in origin. Many genetic syndromes (e.g., trisomy 21, or Down's syndrome) and teratogens (e.g., congenital rubella infection) are associated with a higher risk of specific congenital heart lesions. Most patients present during infancy (Table 32-1).

PHYSIOLOGY

Fetal Circulation

Oxygenated blood from the placenta enters the fetus through the single umbilical vein. About half of this blood bypasses the liver via the *ductus venosus,* flowing directly into the inferior vena cava (IVC). The majority is then directed from the IVC across the *foramen ovale* into the left atrium, bypassing the right heart and pulmonary circulation. This highly oxygenated blood in the left atrium mixes with pulmonary venous return, enters the left ventricle and the ascending aorta, and perfuses the cerebral circulation. Deoxygenated blood returns from the cerebral circulation by way of the superior vena cava, entering the right atrium, right ventricle, and pulmonary artery. Because pulmonary vascular resistance is high in the fetus, most of this blood bypasses the pulmonary circulation by way of the *ductus arteriosus* and enters the descending aorta. Two-thirds of this descending aorta outflow returns

Table 32-1. Common Presentations by Age

Age	Presentation
0–2 weeks	Ductal-dependent circulatory failure
	Hypoplastic left heart syndrome
	Aortic coarctation, severe
	Aortic stenosis, severe
	Cyanosis
	Tetralogy of Fallot
	Transposition of the great arteries
	Total anomalous pulmonary venous return
	Truncus arteriosus
	Tricuspid atresia and other tricuspid anomalies
2–6 weeks	Congestive heart failure
	Ventricular septal defect, large
	Patent ductus arteriosus
	Atrioventricular canal defect
	Cyanosis
	Truncus arteriosus
	Tetralogy of Fallot
	Tricuspid atresia
6 weeks–6 months	Congestive heart failure
	Ventricular septal defect
	Atrial septal defect
	Atrioventricular canal defect
	Cyanosis
	Tetralogy of Fallot
Childhood–adulthood	
	Murmur
	Ventricular septal defect
	Atrial septal defect
	Patent ductus arteriosus
	Aortic stenosis
	Pulmonic stenosis
	Hypertension
	Aortic coarctation
	Syncope/exercise intolerance
	Aortic stenosis
	Pulmonic stenosis
	Eisenmenger's syndrome
	Arrhythmias
	Atrial septal defect
	Cyanosis
	Eisenmenger's syndrome

to the placenta via the umbilical arteries, and one-third perfuses the lower part of the fetus.

Neonatal Circulation

In the first hours of life, the newborn's pulmonary arterioles dilate, and pulmonary vascular resistance begins to fall, resulting in increased pulmonary blood flow. Separation from the low-resistance placental circuit results in increased systemic blood pressure, which also reduces blood flowing through the ductus arteriosus. The smooth muscle of the ductus constricts in response to increased blood PO_2, and the ductus is functionally closed by 15 hours of life. In the normal infant, it becomes the ligamentum arteriosum by 2 to 3 weeks of age. The foramen ovale closes by 3 months of age.

The neonatal myocardium is less efficient. It requires more oxygen and is less able to increase its contractility. When increased cardiac output is needed, the neonate responds by increasing heart rate. Thus, the physiology of neonates and young infants is one of rate-dependent cardiac output, increased oxygen consumption, and lower systolic reserve, resulting in higher propensity for congestive heart failure. Also, the neonate and young infant differ from the older infant and child, since shunting may still occur via the foramen ovale or a patent ductus arteriosus. Pulmonary vascular resistance is still higher and is responsive to oxygen (decreases resistance), and the right ventricle is still prominent (manifested as right axis deviation on the electrocardiogram).

EVALUATION

History

General health, including growth, development, and susceptibility to respiratory illnesses, should be assessed. Pregnancy, birth, and family history may provide valuable clues to specific genetic or teratogenic etiologies. Symptoms of congestive heart failure should be sought: poor feeding, longer feeding times than the average infant, poor growth or failure to thrive, sweating with feeding, irritability or lethargy, weak cry, increased respiratory effort, dyspnea, tachypnea, and coughing. Ask about cyanosis or cyanotic episodes. Cyanosis is often more noticeable during crying or exercise.

Physical Examination

Check vital signs, including four-extremity blood pressures and pulse quality, in the upper and lower extremi-

ties in the sick infant. Color and general appearance may be a significant clue for classifying the lesion into one of three categories:

- Pink: congestive heart failure, L → R shunt
- Blue: cyanotic heart disease, R → L shunt
- Gray: outflow obstruction, hypoperfusion, and shock.

For cyanosis to be clinically apparent, 3 to 5 g of deoxygenated hemoglobin must be present (correlating to an oxygen saturation of 80 to 85 percent). Therefore, if the child is anemic, cyanosis may be less easily recognized. Peripheral cyanosis, or acrocyanosis, and mottling may be seen in normal newborns. Nailbeds (look also for clubbing) and mucous membranes are the best locations to assess for central cyanosis. Auscultate for murmurs, S1 and S2, and extra sounds. If the child is quiet and comfortable when you first enter the room, take advantage of the situation to auscultate then, before upsetting the child with other elements of the physical examination. Murmurs are commonly heard in normal children (Table 32-2). Generally speaking, normal murmurs are never diastolic, late systolic, or pansystolic. Examine the abdomen for hepatomegaly. Start low in the pelvis, working upward; a normal infant's liver is palpable 1 to 3 cm below the right subcostal margin. Examine the child generally for dysmorphic features suggestive of a genetic or teratogenic syndrome.

Ancillary Tests

Chronically cyanotic children usually compensate with polycythemia. A cyanotic child's oxygen-carrying capacity will be further compromised by anemia, and a "normal" *hematocrit* by usual standards may be inadequate for the cyanotic child. If it is unclear whether the child's oxygenation is decreased due to a heart lesion or severe respiratory illness, the *hyperoxia* test may be used. Apply 100 percent oxygen for several minutes. The child with pure respiratory disease will generally respond with some improvement in PO_2 level or oxygen saturation, whereas the child with intracardiac right-to-left shunting due to congenital heart lesion will not. A *chest radiograph* (CXR) should be obtained to evaluate cardiomegaly, individual chamber enlargement, and pulmonary vascularity. An *electrocardiogram* (ECG) should be evaluated for conduction and rhythm disturbances, chamber forces, and rare ischemic changes. A pediatric handbook must be consulted, as ECG normals vary greatly by age, especially among infants and young

Table 32-2. Normal Benign Cardiac Murmurs

Murmur	Age	Character	Positioning	Etiology	Differential Diagnosis
Still's vibratory	Most common benign in children 2–6 yr old, can occur infant to adolescent	I–III/VI early systolic ejection murmur, left lower sternal border to apex, twanging musical quality	Louder when patient supine	Postulated to be from ventricular false tendons	VSD murmur is harsher
Pulmonary flow murmur	Child to young adult	II–III/VI crescendo-decrescendo, early to midsystolic, left upper sternal border, 2nd intercostal space	Louder when patient supine, increased on full expiration	Flow in the pulmonary outflow tract	ASD has fixed split S2; pulmonic stenosis has higher pitched, longer murmur, ejection click
Peripheral pulmonic stenosis	Newborn to 1 yr old	I–II/VI low pitched, early to midsystolic ejection murmur in the pulmonic area and radiating to axillae and back	Increased with viral respiratory infections, lower heart rate, decreased with tachycardia	Turbulence at the peripheral pulmonary artery branches due to narrow angles in infants	Significant branch pulmonary artery stenosis in Williams syndrome; congenital rubella has higher pitched murmur, extends beyond S2; older child
Supraclavicular or brachiocephalic	Child to young adult	Crescendo-decrescendo, systolic, low-pitched, above the clavicles, radiating to neck, abrupt onset and brief	Decreases with rapid hyperextension of the shoulders	Flow through the major brachiocephalic vessels arising from the aorta	Idiopathic hypertrophic subaortic stenosis: louder with Valsalva and softer with rapid squatting. Aortic stenosis: higher pitched, ejection click
Venous hum	Child	Faint to grade VI, continuous, humming, low ant. neck to lateral sternocleidomastoid muscle to ant. chest infraclavicular	Louder when sitting, looking away from murmur; softer when lying, with compressed jugular vein or head turned toward murmur	Turbulence from the internal jugular and subclavian veins entering the superior vena cava	Patent ductus arteriosus has machinery murmur, not compressible, bounding pulses
Mammary souffle	Pregnant, lactating, rarely adolescent	High-pitched, systole into diastole, ant. chest over breast, varies day to day		Plethora of vessels over chest wall	Patent ductus arteriosus has machinery murmur, doesn't vary day to day

Table 32-3. Duration of ECG Intervals (Values in Seconds)

Age	P-R Limits	QRS Limits	QTc Limits
0–7 d	0.08–0.12	0.04–0.10	0.34–0.54
7–30 d	0.08–0.12	0.04–0.07	0.30–0.50
1–3 mo	0.08–0.16	0.05–0.08	0.32–0.47
3–6 mo	0.08–0.12	0.05–0.08	0.35–0.46
6–12 mo	0.08–0.14	0.04–0.08	0.31–0.49
1–3 yr	0.08–0.16	0.04–0.08	0.34–0.43

Source: Modified from Dittmer DS, Grebe RM: *Handbook of Circulation.* Philadelphia: WB Saunders, 1959, p 141.

children. Age and chamber differences may seem intimidating to the clinician, but a few basic principles may provide a guide (see also Tables 32-3 and 32-4):

- The ECG is most often used to evaluate chamber size and conduction disturbances. Ischemic changes are rare.
- Sinus bradycardia must be recognized in the sick infant.
- Intervals are analyzed for drug effects and for long Q-T syndrome.
- Neonatal right-sided forces such as right axis deviation and right ventricular hypertrophy will take on adult form by age 3 to 4 years.
- Abnormal axis or chamber hypertrophy may suggest subclinical congenital defect.
- Right bundle branch block is common, and left bundle branch block is rare.
- Ischemic changes are rare and differ from those in

Table 32-4. Age-Specific QRS Axis

Age	Range	Mean
1–7 d	80–160	125
1–4 weeks	60–160	110
1–3 mo	40–120	80
3–6 mo	20–80	65
6–12 mo	0–100	65
1–3 yr	20–100	55

Source: From Hakim SN, Toepper WC: Cardiac disease in children, in Rosen P, Barkin RM (eds): *Emergency Medicine: Concepts and Clinical Practice II.* St. Louis, MO: Mosby-Year Book, 1992, p 546.

adults. Q waves greater than 35 msec, ST elevation greater than 2 mm, or ventricular arrhythmia in the setting of a worrisome clinical setting may indicate ischemia. T-wave changes are common in children and are rarely ischemic.

CLASSIFICATION

Lesions are usually classified as cyanotic or acyanotic and subclassified according to whether pulmonary blood flow (PBF) is increased, normal, or decreased. Cyanotic lesions can be remembered by the "5 T's":

- Tetrology of Fallot (TOF)
- Tricuspid anomalies including tricuspid atresia and Ebstein's anomaly
- Truncus arteriosus
- Total anomalous pulmonary venous return (TAPVR)
- Transposition of the great arteries (TGA)

Tetralogy of Fallot and the tricuspid anomalies result in decreased PBF, whereas truncus arteriosus, TAPVR, and TGA result in increased PBF.

Hypoplastic left heart syndrome (HLHS) also causes cyanosis and increased PBF. Acyanotic lesions causing increased PBF often present with congestive heart failure (CHF); such lesions are ventricular septal defect (VSD), atrial septal defect (ASD), patent ductus arteriosus (PDA), and atrioventricular septal defect or AV canal defect. Acyanotic lesions with normal or decreased PBF include pulmonary stenosis (PS), aortic stenosis (AS), and aortic coarctation.

BRIEF SURVEY OF INDIVIDUAL LESIONS

Tetralogy of Fallot is the most common cyanotic congenital heart disease seen in children older than 4 years. It consists of right ventricular (RV) outflow obstruction with resultant right ventricular hypertrophy (RVH), a large VSD, and an overriding aorta. Patients have a loud, harsh, pansystolic murmur in the left sternal border, and often a single S2. CXR shows a boot-shaped heart (couer en sabot), decreased PBF, and in 25 percent, a right-sided aortic arch. ECG shows right axis deviation (RAD) and RVH. Severity ranges widely, and depends on the degree of RV outflow obstruction.

Tricuspid atresia must be accompanied by an intra-atrial right-to-left shunt (ASD or patent foramen ovale). Tricuspid atresia is rare, and findings depend on the presence or absence of a VSD, and resulting RV presence or hypoplasia. *Ebstein's anomaly* is a displacement of the tricuspid valve into the RV. Severity varies widely depending on the degree of displacement.

Truncus arteriosus involves a single arterial trunk supplying both the pulmonary and systemic circulation. A VSD is usually present. Initially there may be no or mild cyanosis. A murmur is detected in the first few days, pulses are bounding, and there is a single S2. The patient may have symptoms of CHF and recurrent pulmonary infections. CXR shows cardiomegaly and increased PBF. ECG shows left ventricular hypertrophy (LVH), RVH, or both.

Total anomalous pulmonary venous return has many variations depending on whether it is total or partial (from one to four veins connecting anomalously to a location other than the left atrium, usually the right atrium) and where the veins connect. Cyanosis is mild to moderate, depending on the degree of mixing of the right and left circulations. There is often little murmur, but the S2 is widely split. CXR may show a "snowman" appearance, and ECG may show RVH, RAD, and right atrial enlargement (RAE).

Transposition of the great arteries is the most common cyanotic lesion to present in the first week of life. The right ventricle feeds the aorta, whereas the left ventricle feeds the pulmonary artery. Mixing via an ASD or patent foramen ovale, VSD, or PDA must occur to sustain life, as the pulmonary and systemic circulations are in parallel. Symptoms include cyanosis and tachypnea in the first days of life; there is often no murmur. CXR may be normal or may have an "egg on a string" appearance. ECG shows RAD and RVH but may be normal in the first days of life. If the mixing lesion is small, the patient presents early with cyanosis. If there is a large VSD, the infant may present with CHF and cyanosis at 2 to 6 weeks of age.

Hypoplastic left heart syndrome is a rare anomaly in which the right ventricle perfuses both circulations via the pulmonary artery. The systemic circulation is perfused through the PDA. Management includes the entire range of no treatment, palliative surgery, and cardiac transplantation, depending on the parents' choice and resources available.

Ventricular septal defect is the most common congenital heart lesion, accounting for 20 percent. Small VSDs have a high rate of spontaneous closure. A harsh pansystolic murmur is heard in the left lower sternal border. If the defect is large, respiratory symptoms and congestive heart failure develop in the first 3 months of life. (As pulmonary vascular resistance decreases, left-to-right shunting via the VSD increases.) CXR may be normal or show signs of CHF. ECG may show LVH, RVH, and left atrial enlargement (LAE) if the defect is large.

Atrial septal defect accounts for 12 percent of congenital heart lesions. Many patients are asymptomatic and undiagnosed until childhood or even adulthood. A soft systolic ejection murmur of increased pulmonic flow is heard in the left upper sternal border, and S2 is widely split and fixed (does not close with respiration). CXR shows right-sided chamber enlargement and increased PBF, and ECG shows an RSR' in lead V1, often right bundle branch block (RBBB), and an increased PR interval.

Patent ductus arteriosus occurs in 8:1000 premature infants and 2:1000 full-term infants. A continuous machinery-like murmur is heard in the left second intercostal space, first appearing at 2 to 5 days of age. (Before that, the pulmonary vascular resistance is high enough that there is not significant left-to-right shunting through the ductus.) Because of the diastolic runoff into the PDA, pulses are bounding. Infants may develop CHF, or may compensate with myocardial hypertrophy and present later with exercise intolerance. CXR shows increased PBF and possible cardiomegaly. ECG is normal or shows LVH. Premature infants often respond to indomethacin with closure of the PDA.

Atrioventricular septal defect or AV canal is associated with Down's syndrome. Symptoms include those of CHF, poor growth, and frequent respiratory infections. CXR shows increased PBF and cardiomegaly. ECG shows an increased PR interval, RAE and/or LAE, and RVH. The axis is often superior (extreme left axis deviation).

Pulmonary stenosis often produces no symptoms and may be recognized when a murmur is noted during routine physical examination. Once it is moderate to severe, there may be cyanosis on exertion, syncope, RV failure, and even sudden death. An ejection click is typically heard before the systolic ejection murmur in the left second to third intercostal space. CXR shows a prominent main pulmonary artery and normal to decreased PBF. ECG may be normal or show RVH.

Aortic stenosis is often associated with a bicuspid aortic valve and may be asymptomatic, although severe aortic stenosis can present as shock in an infant. Once symptomatic, patients complain of dyspnea on exertion, fatigue, abdominal pain, increased sweating, and exertional syncope (indicative of critical aortic stenosis). An ejection click is heard before the systolic ejection murmur in the right upper sternal border, radiating into the neck. There may be a left ventricular thrill or heave. CXR shows normal PBF. ECG shows LVH.

Aortic coarctation accounts for 10 percent of congenital heart lesions. The narrowing most commonly occurs just distal to the left subclavian artery branch. Symptoms range from CHF in infancy to hypertension in childhood or adulthood. (The median age at referral is 5 to 8 years old.) Blood pressure is elevated in the upper compared with the lower extremities, and femoral pulses are weak or absent. Children may complain of pain in the legs after exercise. A systolic ejection murmur at the apex radiates to the interscapular back. There may be a diastolic murmur of aortic regurgitation as well. In some patients a thrill is felt in the suprasternal notch. CXR is normal initially, but may show notching of ribs 3 through 8 posteriorly as collateral circulation develops. ECG shows LVH in the severely affected infant. Children may present with complications of hypertension, including intracranial hemorrhage.

COMMON PRESENTATIONS

Rather than memorizing a slew of individual lesions, the emergency physician should concentrate on a few scenarios of presentation common to groups of lesions. These scenarios require rapid emergency care and management to prevent further decompensation and cardiac arrest. Knowledge of the exact lesion is not necessary to provide the critical management needed in these cases.

Ductal-Dependent Lesions and Cardiogenic Shock

Lesions completely dependent on a patent ductus arteriosus for systemic or pulmonary blood flow present with acute onset circulatory failure and shock when the ductus closes, typically within the first week of life. Such lesions include HLHS, severe aortic coarctation, interrupted aortic arch, and lesions such as pulmonary atresia or TGA without another mixing lesion such as a VSD. No symptoms or signs of congenital heart disease may have been noted prior to presentation, in the newborn nursery or at home. Ductal-dependent cardiac failure should be suspected in any infant in the first week of life with sudden-onset circulatory collapse leading to hypoperfusion, hypotension, severe acidosis, and cyanosis. Infants may present in the second week of life, but rarely present beyond 2 weeks old.

The mainstay of therapy for suspected ductal-dependent cardiac shock is prostaglandin E_1 (PGE_1) infusion. PGE_1 maintains the patency of the ductus. It is bolused initially at 0.1 μg/kg and then infused at 0.1 μg/kg/min. Adverse effects include hyperthermia, apnea, hypotension, rash, tremors, focal seizures, and bradycardia. Nevertheless, PGE_1 is critical for infants in ductal-dependent cardiac shock and should be begun in the emergency department. One should be prepared to manage the infant's airway and breathing in the case of apnea and add inotropic medications as needed for circulatory support. Other etiologies for shock must be entertained and treated as well, such as sepsis. A pediatric cardiologist must be consulted immediately and the patient admitted to the pediatric or neonatal intensive care unit.

Congestive Heart Failure

A common scenario is that of an infant 2 to 6 months old with a left-to-right shunting lesion (VSD, PDA, AV canal defect, or, less commonly, an ASD alone) resulting in volume overload and CHF. Excessive pressure load from left-sided obstruction (e.g., aortic coarctation, aortic stenosis) may also result in CHF. Causes other than congenital heart lesions include myocardial dysfunction (e.g., cardiomyopathies) and dysrhythmias.

Symptoms are gradual in onset and include the following:

- Poor feeding (increased time to feed)
- Poor growth
- Sweating
- Irritability or lethargy
- Weak cry
- Increased respiratory effort
- Dyspnea
- Tachypnea
- Chronic cough or wheeze
- Increased frequency of respiratory infections

Physical examination may reveal the following:

- Tachypnea
- Retractions
- Nasal flaring
- Wheezing
- Rales (although less commonly than in adults)
- Tachycardia
- Gallop rhythm
- Hyperactive precordium

- Murmur
- Poor peripheral pulses with delayed capillary refill
- Hepatomegaly (a cardinal sign of CHF in infants)

Jugular venous distension and peripheral edema, often seen in adults with CHF, are rarely seen in young children. If present, edema is best appreciated in the eyelids, sacrum, and legs. CXR shows cardiomegaly (cardiothoracic ratio >0.55 in infants, >0.50 for children over 1 year old) and increased pulmonary vascularity. When evaluating for cardiomegaly, remember that infants often have a prominent thymus overlying the heart shadow; the thymus gives an appearance of an enlarged mediastinum and will be apparent as anterior to the heart on the lateral film. ECG findings depend on the specific lesion.

Treatment includes oxygen to keep saturations about 95 percent. Overoxygenating the patient may lead to pulmonary vascular dilation and worsened failure. The infant should be kept in a semireclining position (such as when in an infant car seat) if possible. Fluid and sodium restriction are necessary, and Lasix should be given at 1 mg/kg intravenously. In consultation with a pediatric cardiologist, the patient should be started on digoxin. A pediatric handbook may be consulted for digitalization doses. Patients may require sedation, but careful attention must be paid to maintaining airway and breathing. Preparations should be made for endotracheal intubation and ventilatory support in the event that they are needed. If a patient's respiratory status is borderline for artificial ventilation, a trial of continuous positive airway pressure (CPAP) may be applied nasally in an attempt to avoid the need for intubation. If the patient is in shock, fluids must be used judiciously (boluses of only 5 mL/kg, if at all), and inotropic support with dopamine or dobutamine may be more appropriate. Complete blood count, chemistry panel, calcium level, rapid bedside glucose test, and arterial blood gas should be assessed. Vital signs including blood pressure, cardiac rhythm, and oxygen saturation should be monitored continuously.

Hypoxemic "Tet" Spells

Sudden-onset spells of increased cyanosis may occur in young children with tetralogy of Fallot and, less commonly, in other complex lesions with decreased PBF, such as tricuspid atresia. Various theories exist regarding the initiation of a spell. The classic explanation of sudden "clamping down" of the pulmonary infundibulum right ventricular outflow tract, leading to increased right-to-left shunting, although not a complete explanation, provides a useful model. The increased right-to-left

shunting leads to hypoxemia, cyanosis, and acidosis. Attempts at compensation occur via hyperventilation and decreased systemic vascular resistance (SVR) to increase cardiac output. Decreased SVR and increased venous return result in further shunting, rounding out a vicious cycle of ongoing shunting and hypoxemia.

Symptoms include a sudden increase in cyanosis, restlessness, irritability or lethargy, and occasional syncope. Hyperpnea is a cardinal symptom of hypoxemic spells. Previously appreciated murmurs of left-to-right shunting may disappear during a spell. Spells are most common in children younger than 2 years and often occur when SVR is naturally decreased: in the morning after awakening, after a feed, after defecation, and after a bout of crying. The "tet spell" may occur in a previously acyanotic patient and may be the first presentation of a child with previously unrecognized congenital heart disease. Spells must be differentiated from seizures, CHF, respiratory disease, and diabetic ketoacidosis. Differentiating factors include history of congenital heart disease, profound cyanosis unresponsive to oxygen, and typical clinical presentation.

The child should be kept as calm as possible, in a position of comfort with a parent present. Avoid unnecessary painful or stressful procedures. Oxygen should be given, although it will have little effect in shunt-induced hypoxemia. The child should be placed in a knee-chest position (to simulate squatting) to increase SVR. Older children may even have a history of squatting on their own to abort spells. Morphine, 0.1 to 0.2 mg/kg, intravenously or subcutaneously, is the traditional first-line medical therapy, although the exact mechanism by which it "breaks" the spell is unknown. A fluid bolus of 10 mL/kg normal saline intravenously should be given, to counteract the vasodilating effects of morphine and to ensure adequate preload, on which pulmonary flow is dependent. Successful therapy will be evidenced by improved pulse oximetry, decreased cyanosis, decreased hyperpnea, and a calmer child. If the above therapies are unsuccessful, propranolol 0.1 to 0.2 mg/kg by a slow intravenous route (mechanism of action unclear) or phenylephrine 0.1 mg/kg intravenously followed by an infusion of 2 to 10 μg/kg/minute (α-agonist resulting in increased SVR) may be used, usually in consultation with a cardiologist. If all else fails, general anesthesia may be necessary.

Presentations in Older Children and Adults

Clinically inapparent lesions are frequently discovered by recognition of a murmur during routine physical examination. Common lesions include ASD, small VSD, PDA, PS, AS, and aortic coarctation. Patients with an

ASD will also be noted to have a fixed, split S2. Adult patients with unrepaired ASD may present with atrial arrythmias, often in the fourth decade of life. Patients with PDA and AS may present with dyspnea on exertion and fatigue. Patients with critical AS may present with syncope. Patients with critical PS may present with cyanosis on exertion, right-sided heart failure, or syncope. Patients with aortic coarctation are often diagnosed during evaluation for hypertension. They may present with symptoms resulting from the hypertension such as headache, intracranial hemorrhage, dizziness, palpitations, or epistaxis. Occasionally, they may complain of claudication due to decreased perfusion of the lower extremities.

Eisenmenger's Syndrome

Patients with a large left-to-right shunt left unrepaired, either by choice or because the lesion was never recognized, gradually develop pulmonary vascular disease due to the increased volume overload. When pulmonary hypertension becomes severe enough, the direction of shunting will reverse to right to left, and cyanosis ensues. This typically occurs in adolescence to early adulthood. Patients may complain of decreased exercise tolerance, dyspnea on exertion, hemoptysis, palpitations due to atrial arrhythmias, and symptoms of hyperviscosity due to chronic polycythemia (vision disturbances, fatigue, headache, dizziness, paresthesias, and even cerebrovascular accident). Brain abscesses can occur with right-to-left passage of an infected embolus. On exam, the murmur may have disappeared with the disappearance of left-to-right shunting, and S2 is loud due to the pulmonary hypertension. CXR shows decreased vasculature (pruned pattern), and ECG shows RVH. Although no definitive therapy exists other than heart-lung transplant, patients should avoid dehydration, heavy exertion, altitude, vasodilators, and pregnancy, which is associated with a high mortality rate. Symptoms of hyperviscosity may be treated with phlebotomy and isovolemic replacement. Patients should be medically managed by a cardiologist to optimize cardiac function as long as possible.

CARE OF THE POSTCARDIAC SURGERY CONGENITAL HEART PATIENT

Categories of Repair

Patients with true complete repairs generally lead a normal life after repair. True complete repairs are typically performed successfully for ASD, VSD, PDA, aortic coarctation, and TGA (switch procedure). Repairs of TOF, AV canal, and valve obstructions typically result in anatomic repairs with residual lesions, and late complications may occur. Repairs requiring prosthetic materials such as pulmonary atresia, truncus arteriosus, and prosthetic valve replacements will require replacement of the prosthetic material due to growth of the child or degeneration of the material. Physiologic repairs improve the patient's blood flow physiology but do not result in normal cardiac anatomy. These palliative repairs, which include the Fontan operation for lesions resulting in a functionally single ventricle, and the Senning and Mustard operations for TGA (now less common than the switch procedure) invariably produce late complications.

Postoperative Complications

Arrythmias are the most common problem and may present with symptoms of palpitations, decreased appetite, emesis, and decreased exercise tolerance. Arrhythmias may be a result of the surgical repair, the underlying lesion (e.g., Ebstein's anomaly), or medical therapy (e.g., digoxin toxicity). Supraventricular tachycardia (SVT) is the most common clinically significant arrhythmia and is seen in lesions repaired with atriotomy (Senning, Mustard, Fontan, ASD repair, TAPVR repair). Bradycardia due to sinoatrial nodal disease is seen in 20 percent of patients status post Fontan repair, and first-degree block may occur after AV canal repair. Ventricular arrhythmias occur uncommonly after VSD or TOF repair and are decreasing further due to increased use of transatrial approaches to repair. RBBB is common after VSD, TOF, and AV canal repairs. Premature ventricular contractions are benign if isolated and unifocal (order a 24-hour Holter monitor test); a cardiologist should be consulted if they are frequent, coupled, or multifocal. Isolated, infrequent premature atrial contractions are common in normal and postcardiac surgery patients.

Residual or recurrent lesions occur as a complication of repair, due to incomplete success of the repair, outgrowing prosthetic materials, or from conduit stenosis. Coarctations recur in 10 percent of repaired patients. Recurrent stenosis after PS or AS repair is common, as is aortic insufficiency after AS repair. Recurrent stenosis may be recognized by a new murmur or a change in exercise tolerance. A residual small VSD around the borders of the patch is present in 15 to 25 percent of patients after VSD or TOF repair; most close spontaneously within 6 to 12 months.

Endocarditis is a significant complication seen in congenital heart patients before and after surgical repair. The rate in patients with uncorrected congenital heart disease is 0.1 to 0.2 percent per patient-year; this decreases to 0.02 percent after correction for many lesions. Unrepaired complex congenital heart disease carries the highest risk, at 1.5 percent per patient-year. ASDs of the ostium secundum type are the lowest risk lesions and do not require prophylaxis for procedures, even if unrepaired. Patients with repaired ASD, VSD, PDA, aortic coarctation, and PS (no mechanical valve) without resid- ual lesions, and patients status post heart transplantation or pacemaker insertion also carry a low risk and do not require prophylaxis. Patients status post AS or TOF repair and those with prosthetic valves remain at high risk. Antibiotic prophylaxis should be given to patients at high risk prior to invasive procedures likely to produce bacteremia. See Table 32-5 for procedures requiring prophylaxis and antibiotic regimens used.

Table 32-5. Endocarditis Prophylaxis

Procedures For Which Prophylaxis Is Recommended

Dental and periodontal procedures
Replacement of avulsed teeth
Tonsillectomy and/or adenoidectomy
Surgery involving respiratory mucosa
Rigid bronchoscopy
Sclerotherapy for esophageal varices
Esophageal stricture dilation
Endoscopic retrograde cholangiography
Biliary tract surgery
Surgery involving intestinal mucosa
Prostatic surgery
Cystoscopy
Urethral dilation

Prophylactic Regimens

Amoxicillin 50 mg/kg (maximum 2 g) orally 1 hr before procedure
   If unable to take oral medication:
      Ampicillin 50 mg/kg (maximum 2 g) IM or IV 30 min before procedure
   If allergic to penicillin:
      Clindamycin 20 mg/kg (maximum 600 mg) orally 1 hr before procedure
      Cephalexin or cefadroxil 50 mg/kg (maximum 2 g) orally 1 hr before procedure
      Azithromycin or clarithromycin 15 mg/kg (maximum 500 mg) orally 1 hr before procedure
   If unable to take oral medication and allergic to penicillin:
      Clindamycin 20 mg/kg (maximum 600 mg) IV 30 min before procedure
      Cefazolin 25 mg/kg (maximum 1 g) IM or IV 30 min before procedure
   For genitourinary and gastrointestinal (excluding esophageal) procedures, high-risk patient
      Ampicillin 50 mg/kg (maximum 2 g) *and* gentamicin 1.5 mg/kg (maximum 120 mg) IM or IV within 30 min
         of procedure. Six hours later, ampicillin 25 mg/kg (maximum 1 g) IM or IV *or* amoxicillin 25 mg/kg
         (maximum 1 g) orally
   For genitourinary and gastrointestinal (excluding esophageal) procedures, high-risk patient allergic to penicillin
      Vancomycin 20 mg/kg (maximum 1 g) IV over 1–2 hr *and* gentamicin 1.5 mg/kg (maximum 120 mg) IM or
         IV; complete within 30 min of procedure
   For genitourinary and gastrointestinal (excluding esophageal) procedures, moderate-risk patient
      Amoxicillin or ampicillin as above
   *For genitourinary and gastrointestinal (excluding esophageal) procedures, moderate-risk patient allergic to
      penicillin:*
      Vancomycin as above (without gentamicin)

Other complications common in patients with congenital heart disease include poor growth, electrolyte disturbances due to medications, cerebral embolus in patients with right-to-left shunts (healthcare workers should be particularly careful to avoid air embolus during intravenous line placement), and increased susceptibility to respiratory illnesses. Cardiac patients may have a particularly difficult time with respiratory syncytial virus infections.

SUMMARY

Emergency physicians should concentrate on recognition and management of a few common presentations seen in congenital heart disease patients, especially ductal-dependent circulatory failure and congestive heart failure. Physicians are unlikely to be able to determine the specific lesion in the emergency department without an echocardiogram, and knowledge of the exact lesion is often unnecessary for appropriate therapy. The number of adolescent and adult survivors of congenital heart disease repair is rapidly increasing, and these patients are subject to certain complications that emergency physicians must be prepared to recognize and manage.

BIBLIOGRAPHY

Brickner ME, Hillis LD, Lange RA: Medical progress: Congenital heart disease in adults (part 1). *N Engl J Med* 342:256, 2000.

Brickner ME, Hillis LD, Lange RA: Medical progress: Congenital heart disease in adults (part 2). *N Engl J Med* 342:334, 2000.

Clyman RI: Ibuprofen and patent ductus arteriosus. *N Engl J Med* 343:728–730, 2000.

Gewitz MH, Vetter VL: Cardiac emergencies, in Fleischer GR, Ludwig S (eds): *Textbook of Pediatric Emergency Medicine,* 4th ed. Philadelphia: Lipincott Williams & Wilkins, 2000, pp 659–700.

Li MM, Klassen TP, Waters LK: Cardiovascular disorders, in Barkin RM (ed): *Pediatric Emergency Medicine: Concepts and Clinical Practice,* 2d ed. St. Louis: Mosby-Year Book, 1997, pp 634–669.

O-Laughlin MP: Congestive heart failure in children. *Pediatr Clin North Am* 46:263, 1999.

Overmeire BV, Smets K, Lecoutere D, et al: A comparison of ibuprofen and indomethacin for closure of patent ductus arteriosus. *N Engl J Med* 343:674–681, 2000.

Pelech AN: Evaluation of the pediatric patient with a cardiac murmur. *Pediatr Clin North Am* 46:167, 1999.

Rosenkranz ER: Pediatric surgery for the primary care pediatrician, part I: Caring for the former pediatric cardiac surgery patient. *Pediatr Clin North Am* 45:907, 1998.

Toepper WC, Hakim SN: Cardiac disorders, in Rosen P, Barkin R (eds): *Emergency Medicine: Concepts and Clinical Practice,* 4th ed. St. Louis: Mosby-Year Book, 1998, pp 1159–1168.

33

Congestive and Inflammatory Heart Diseases

William C. Toepper
Joilo Barbosa

HIGH-YIELD FACTS

- Congestive heart failure (CHF) is multifactorial. Management is directed at the cause.

- Tachypnea, failure to thrive, or diaphoresis with feeding, accompanied by an abnormal lung exam, hyperactive precordium, gallop, and hepatomagaly suggest CHF. Oxygen, sedation, diuresis, and inotropic support are the mainstays of therapy.

- Myocarditis should be suspected in the wheezing, febrile child who does not respond to bronchodilators. Grunting, CHF, and cardiomegaly on chest radiography suggest the diagnosis.

- The older child with pericarditis presents with pleuritic or positional chest pain, fever, tachycardia, friction rub, and electrocardiographic changes. Natural history is usually benign.

- The at-risk patient with endocarditis presents with unexplained fever, myalgia, new murmur, and elevated acute-phase reactants.

- The diagnosis of acute rheumatic fever should be based on the Jones criteria. Incidence of valve involvement is reduced with early aggressive management.

CONGESTIVE HEART FAILURE

Congestive heart failure (CHF), the physiologic state in which cardiac output is unable to meet tissue metabolic demands, has many etiologies (Table 33-1). Cardiac output is determined by four factors:

- *Preload,* or filling volume, is increased in left-to-right shunts.

- *Afterload,* or the resistance the ventricles face upon ejection of blood, is important in outlet obstruction or systemic hypertension.

- *Contractility* is altered in cardiomyopathy.

- *Rate* can either be too slow, resulting in inadequate output, or too fast, decreasing diastolic filling (Table 10-3).

In CHF, end-organ hypoperfusion explains most clinical features (Table 33-2). Decreased flow to the kidney results in renin/angiotensin-based salt and water retention and an increased circulating volume. In addition, angiotensin-2, a potent vasoconstrictor, increases vascular resistance, resulting in a rise in blood pressure. Sympathetic discharge, due to decreased oxygen delivery, results in improved contractility. Redistribution of blood from skin and skeletal muscle to heart, brain, and kidney improves vital function. As the disease process worsens, physiologic mechanisms are unable to keep up. Overcompensation results in symptoms. Salt and water retention produces edema. Increased adrenergic response and tachycardia cause inadequate diastolic filling. Diaphoresis during feeding is secondary to catecholamine release. Decreased skin perfusion results in mottling and pallor. Increased systemic vascular resistance increases myocardial demand, causing hypertrophy or dilation. Valve insufficiency or myocardial ischemia can cause further decrease in cardiac output.

Clinically, infants in CHF are irritable, feed poorly, and have poor weight gain. An acute weight gain may be due to edema. Diaphoresis during feeding is especially suggestive of CHF. Volume overload may present insidiously with respiratory symptoms such as cough or chest congestion. The lack of fever and rhinorrhea helps differentiate CHF from infection. A respiratory infection such as respiratory syncytial virus (RSV) can cause decompensation in the child with pulmonary outflow obstruction. Symptoms may overlap. Abnormal vital signs such as unexplained tachycardia or tachypnea with normal temperature may suggest cardiac disease. Early, blood pressure may be elevated due to increased adrenergic activity. Low blood pressure and delayed capillary refill develop later as cardiogenic shock ensues. High blood pressure may also suggest coarctation of the aorta or primary hypertension with a subsequent decrease in cardiac output due to ventricular dysfunction. Signs of CHF include adventitial lung sounds and a hyperactive precordium.

Table 33-1. Etiologic Basis of Congestive
Heart Failure

Preload (Volume Overload)
  Left-to-right shunt: VSD, PDA, AV fistula
  Anemia: iron deficiency, sickle cell, thalassemia
  Iatrogenic
Afterload (Increased SVR)
  Congenital: coarctation of the aorta, aortic stenosis
  Systemic hypertension
Contractility
  Inflammatory: infectious (myocarditis)
  Rheumatic: rheumatic fever, early Kawasaki, SLE
  Toxin: digoxin, Ca^{2+} channel/β-blocker, cocaine
  Traumatic: cardiac tamponade, myocardial contusion
  Metabolic: electrolyte abnormality, hypothyroidism

VSD, ventricular septal defect; PDA, patent ductus arteriosus;
AV, arteriovenous; SLE, systemic lupus erythematosus.

An abnormal precordial examination is highly suggestive of chamber abnormality. Routine palpation in normal infants provides a baseline for comparison. Displaced PMI, right ventricular lift, or palpable murmur is strongly suggestive of CHF. A pathologic murmur or gallop rhythm is characteristic. The abdomen is palpated for hepatomegaly, a common finding in pediatric CHF. Facial edema and anasarca are late signs. Pedal edema and neck vein distention are rare.

The chest radiograph is a reliable tool for measuring volume overload. It is difficult to distinguish right- from left-sided chamber enlargement in children, and the electrocardiogram (ECG) may be helpful. Other radiographic signs include increased pulmonary vascular markings, interstitial fluid, or pulmonary edema. The ECG, in addition to assessing chamber enlargement or hypertrophy, is useful in picking up dysrhythmia or ST/T-wave changes. The echocardiogram may be diagnostic. Ultimately the child in severe or refractory congestive heart failure may require pulmonary arterial catheterization to determine whether preload, afterload, contractility, or rate is responsible.

Therapy is directed toward the cause. Examples include interventional techniques for obstructive lesions, exchange transfusion for profound anemia, or pericardiocentesis for cardiac tamponade. When the cause is unknown, empiric therapy is initiated. This includes positioning, sedation (morphine sulfate), supplemental oxygen, and intravenous fluids to relieve the work of feeding.

Pharmacologic therapy is also directed at the specific cause. Fluid overload is treated with furosemide 1 mg/kg/dose intravenously or intramuscularly. Digoxin improves contractility by both blocking the sodium-potassium pump and increasing intracellular calcium, making actin-myosin bridging more forceful. Digoxin also slows heart rate and relieves diaphoresis through adrenergic withdrawal. It is useful in the stable well-known patient but is contraindicated in CHF associated with acute myocarditis because of its arrhythmogenic

Table 33-2. Symptom-Based Assessment of Congestive Heart Failure

Signs/Symptoms	Mechanism	Treatment
Pulmonary Venous Congestion		
Tachypnea	L → R shunt	Diuresis
Wheezing	Pulmonary edema	Oxygen
Rales	Poor oxygenation	Sedation
Poor feeding		
Irritability		
Systemic Venous Congestion		
Hepatomegaly	Increased right-sided filling pressure	Diuresis (spironolactone)
Peripheral edema		
Impaired Cardiac Output		
Decreased pulses	Decreased contractility and perfusion	Digoxin
Delayed capillary refill		Pressors
		Afterload reduction

Table 33-3. Oral Dosing Guidelines for Digoxin[a]

Age and Weight	Acute Digitalization (μg/kg)[b]	Maintenance
Premature infant	20	5 μg/kg/day
Full-term infant	30	4–5 μg/kg q12h
2–24 mo	40–50	5–10 μg/kg q12h
>24 mo	30–40	4–5 μg/kg q12h

[a]IV dose is 75% of PO dose.
[b]Daily dose = 1/2 given initially, then 1/4 given at 8 hr and 1/4 given at 16 hr.

effects on the irritable myocardium. Dosing is outlined in Table 33-3. Amrinone is also a positive inotrope with the additional benefit of decreasing pulmonary vascular resistance. It may be beneficial in digoxin-refractory patients. Its potent vasodilatory effects may cause hypotension. β-Blockers may also have a role in chronic CHF. They "upregulate" cell wall receptors, increasing contractility. The decision to begin digoxin, amrinone, or β-blockers is best made in consultation with a pediatric cardiologist or intensivist. An algorithmic approach to CHF is presented in Fig. 33-1.

The child in moderate to severe CHF will require the intensive care unit or transfer to a tertiary care facility. Intubation may be necessary to improve oxygenation and provide positive end-expiratory pressure (PEEP), useful in pulmonary edema. Inotropic support includes dopamine to increase contractility and blood pressure, dobutamine for its more pronounced effect on contractility, and epinephrine to improve blood pressure (Table 33-4).

In the setting of low output with increased systemic resistance, such as in hypertensive cardiomyopathy, afterload reduction with angiotensin-converting enzyme (ACE) inhibitors may be helpful. Contraindications include patients with renal insufficiency and those with right-to-left shunts. In right to left shunt, the systemic circulation may improve at the expense of the pulmonary circulation.

```
              Identify the cause

     Easily                 Not easily correctable
  correctable?                 or ill defined?


        Example                 Supportive care
  cardiac tamponade        IV-NPO-Na⁺ restriction
         SVT                 Oxygen-oximetry
                             Upright position
Treat cause                  Cardiac monitor
Pericardiocentesis           Sedation
valsalva, adenosine, etc.    (morphine, 0.05mg/kg IM)


             Continued assessment

      Empiric therapy based on clinical suspicion


Preload          Afterload         Rate          Contractility

diuresis        Load altering    Alter rate        Digoxin
(furosemide,       agents                          Pressors
1 mg/kg IV)     (Table 33-5)    (Chapter 34)    (Tables 33-3 &
                                                     33-4)


                     SEVERE?

             Intensive Care Unit

                 Consider:
              Intubation-PEEP
        Pulmonary artery catheter
          Pressors/vasodilators
        Other (ECMO, balloon pump)
```

Fig. 33-1. Management of acute congestive heart failure in children.

Table 33-4. Inotropic Agents: Dosage and Pharmacologic Effects

Drug	Dose (μg/kg/min)	Increased HR	Increased Contractility	Increased Afterload	Vasodilation
Dopamine	1–5	1+	1+	0	renal
	6–20	2–3+	3+	1–3+	0
Dobutamine	2–10	1+	3+	0	1+
Epinephrine	0.05–1	3+	3+	0–3+	0–2+
					(dose dependent)
Norepinephrine	0.05–0.5	2+	3+	4+	0
Isoproterenol	0.1	3+	2+	2+	0
					(bronchial smooth muscle)

In severe cases, such as myocarditis with cardiogenic shock, the weakened myocardium ineffectively pumps against increased afterload. Vasodilators such as sodium nitroprusside may be helpful. It has venodilator and arteriolar dilator effects and is easily titratable (Table 33-5).

MYOCARDITIS/PERICARDITIS

Inflammatory diseases of the myocardium and pericardium can be confused with other infectious or pulmonary diseases. Myocarditis and pericarditis can be subtle in their early presentation and be misdiagnosed. Complaints include cough, wheeze, congestion, fever, or tachypnea. Subtle clues and a high index of suspicion may suggest a cardiac diagnosis. Bronchospasm responding poorly to conventional therapy may suggest early myocarditis. Wheezing in the febrile child or in a child without a history of asthma should include a chest x-ray looking for cardiomegaly or pulmonary congestion. Other signs and symptoms include poor feeding, cyanosis, and grunting. Myocarditis should be considered in any child who deteriorates despite aggressive treatment for bronchospasm or reactive airway disease. Murmur, gallop rhythm, rales, or organomegaly, coupled with ECG changes or cardiomegaly, may confirm suspicion.

The etiologies of myocarditis and pericarditis overlap. Viruses (enterovirus, varicella, mumps), bacteria (*Haemophilus influenzae*, *C. diphtheria*, *M. tuberculosis*), rickettsia, fungus, and parasites are known causes. Most cases are idiopathic. Inflammatory etiologies include acute rheumatic fever, Lyme disease, and collagen vascular disease. Certain toxins such as cocaine may cause myocarditis. Anomalous origin of the coronary arteries may cause myocarditis in the infant. HIV-associated myocarditis not due to opportunistic infection is often discovered at autopsy.

Myocarditis carries a grave prognosis, with 35 percent mortality. The hallmark presentation, CHF, includes gallop rhythm, hyperactive precordium, and hepatomegaly. Pulmonary findings such as wheezing or tachypnea are often confused with bronchospasm. Fever with muscle or joint tenderness help support the diagnosis. Presentation is often fulminant, with cardiogenic shock, acidosis, or syncope secondary to dysrhythmia. Chest radiography may demonstrate cardiomegaly. Pulmonary vascular congestion is a poor prognostic sign. Other prognostic indicators include the acuity of onset of CHF, a cardiac index <3 L/min, and a northwest axis. ECG findings include diffuse ST-T-wave changes, low voltage, interval prolongation, and ectopy.

Ventricular ectopy signals diffuse myocardial involvement with risk of sudden death. Arterial blood gas, acute viral serologies, and cardiac enzymes may help in management. Emergent echocardiogram should be considered. The definitive diagnostic procedure, right-sided endocardial biopsy, may be indicated in the most severe cases.

Initial management includes the treatment of CHF. Bed rest, oxygen, fluid restriction, diuresis, and inotropic support may be necessary. Invasive monitoring should be considered. Digoxin is contraindicated because of its potential to cause dysrhythmia. An aggressive approach to dysrhythmia may prevent sudden death. Meticulous supportive care of acid-base derangements, metabolic abnormalities, and fluid status may be life-saving. Corticosteroids and other immunosuppressants are rarely used.

Ultimately transplantation may be required for end-stage cardiomyopathy due to myocarditis. Rejection and infection may complicate the initial posttransplant period. Rejection, or lymphocytic infiltration with myocyte destruction, is suspected in the setting of lethargy, poor feeding, fever, CHF, and dysrhythmia. Echocardiogram or biopsy may be necessary. Infection, a more common complication, should be approached individually. Transplant patients handle most infections well. Exceptions include the steroid-dependent or asplenic child. Cytomegalovirus and *Pneumocystis carinii* infections are most common early after transplantation, when immunosuppression is highest.

Unlike myocarditis, pericarditis usually follows a benign clinical course. Presenting symptoms include pleuritic or positional chest pain, abdominal pain, dyspnea, and fever. Signs include a pericardial friction rub and tachycardia. The ECG can be diagnostic, with diffuse ST-segment elevation and PR depression. Low voltage and electrical alternans signal significant effusion.

Treatment for uncomplicated pericarditis is supportive and directed toward treating the organism, toxin, or metabolic derangement. Inflammation and pain can be treated with nonsteroidal antiinflammatory agents. Hospitalization and cardiology input are suggested. Occasionally, admission to an intensive care setting is necessary in an ill-appearing child or one with large effusion. However, most cases of pericarditis are self-limited and will follow a benign clinical course.

In the setting of significant effusion with an ill-appearing child, constrictive pericarditis should be considered. Constrictive pericarditis is usually bacterial (*Staphylococcus aureus, H. influenzae, Streptococcus pneumoniae*). Treatment consists of antibiotics, emergent pericardiocentesis, and operative pericardial window. In some cases effusion is minimal, but a thickened stiff pericardium results in cardiac tamponade. Tamponade is rare in viral or idiopathic pericarditis but should be considered when heart sounds are distant, or in the presence of pulsus paradoxus or jugular venous distention.

ENDOCARDITIS

Bacterial endocarditis occurs in children with congenital heart disease or central venous catheters or in adolescents who use intravenous drugs. Seeding can occur via dental caries, skin infections, and manipulation of the airway, gastrointestinal tract, or genitourinary tract. Staphylococcal and streptococcal species predominate, with HACEK organisms (*Hemophilus, Actinobacillus, Cardiobacterium, Eikenella, Kingella*) and *Candida* as occasional offenders. Diagnosis is suspected in the at-risk patient in the presence of unexplained fever, weakness, myalgia, and arthralgia. A new murmur is present in fewer than 50 percent of cases. Other findings may include congestive heart failure secondary to valvular insufficiency, petechiae, or new neurologic findings. Adult cutaneous hallmarks such as Janeway lesions or Osler nodes are rare. Blood culture will identify the organism in 90 percent of cases. Other supportive data include elevated acute-phase reactants such as white blood cell count or erythrocyte sedimentation rate, anemia, hematuria, or embolic infiltrates. The echocardiogram has a 70 to 80 percent detection rate, with failure occurring in children who have complex congenital heart disease.

Antibiotic therapy can be more specifically directed if started after the specific organism is identified. However, in the sickest patients, appropriate broad-spectrum coverage can be started in consultation with a consultant. Bacteremia will persist in some patients despite antibiotics. Removal of vegetation or valve replacement may be indicated. Other sequelae for which surgery may be required include threatened or recurrent embolization, severe valve failure, recalcitrant arrhythmia secondary to vegetation, or myocardial abscess. Pulmonary or neurologic emboli are dependent on the location of the vegetations and presence of intracardiac shunting. Overall endocarditis carries a mortality rate of 6 to 14 percent and should be strongly considered in the high-risk patient.

Because of the high mortality rate, prevention of endocarditis is key. The emergency physician plays an important role in endocarditis prophylaxis. Indications are dynamic. American Heart Association guidelines for at-risk patients and procedures are summarized in Tables 32-5 and 33-6.

Table 33-5. Load-Altering Agents

Drug	Dose	Comments
Nitroprusside	1–10 μg/kg/min IV	Cyanide toxicity
Captopril	Infants: 0.1–2.0 mg/kg PO q8–12h	Neutropenia, cough, proteinuria
Nitroglycerin	2–10 μg/kg/min IV	Use not well established in children
Amrinone	0.5–2 mg/kg, then 5–10 μm/kg/min IV	Hypotension

Table 33-6. Endocarditis Prophylaxis in Cardiac Conditions[a]

Endocarditis Prophylaxis Recommended

High risk
  Prosthetic valves
  Previous bacterial endocarditis
  Complex cyanotic malformations
  Surgical systemopulmonary shunts
Moderate risk
  Rheumatic or acquired valvular dysfunction
  Hypertrophic cardiomyopathy
  MVP with regurgitation or thickened leaflets
  Most other complex cardiac malformations

Endocarditis Prophylaxis Not Recommended

Isolated secundum ASD
Repaired secundum ASD, VSD, PDA, without residua after 6 mo
Innocent murmurs
Previous Kawasaki syndrome without valvular dysfunction
Previous rheumatic fever without valvular dysfunction
Cardiac pacemakers and implanted defibrillators

ASO, atrial septal defect; VSD, ventriculoseptal defect; PDA, patent ductus arteriosus; MVP, mitral valve prolapse.
[a]This table lists selected conditions but is not meant to be all inclusive.
Source: Adapted from Dajani AS, Taubert KA, Gerber MA, et al: Prevention of bacterial endocarditis: Recommendations by the American Heart Association. *JAMA* 277:1794, 1997.

ACUTE RHEUMATIC FEVER

Valve involvement characterizes the carditis of acute rheumatic fever. The acute phase begins 2 to 3 weeks after a group A streptococcal illness. Jones criteria are outlined in Table 33-7. Typically, carditis follows arthritis and can involve the three layers of the heart. A benign acute phase can be followed years later with valvular insufficiency. Mitral insufficiency is most common and is characterized by a holosystolic, high-pitched, blowing apical murmur radiating to the axilla. Regurgitant aortic murmurs are middiastolic, high-pitched, and blowing, located at the base, radiating into the neck. Other cardiac findings include tachycardia, gallop rhythm, pericardial rub, or congestive heart failure. The ECG may demonstrate PR prolongation, conduction delays, left ventricular hypertrophy (LVH), or dysrhythmia. Echocardiography is helpful in the follow-up of patients with rheumatic heart disease and may have a role in the evaluation of patients without murmur or with subclinical heart involvement.

Treatment during the acute phase includes hospitalization and bed rest. Cardiac rehabilitation follows. High-dose aspirin is begun upon confirmation of the diagnosis. Penicillin or erythromycin is given to eradicate residual streptococci. Corticosteroids are controversial and may have a role in the treatment of carditis or chorea. Long-term follow-up of patients with rheumatic fever includes surveillance for recurrence, endocarditis prophylaxis, and treatment of chronic failure. Patients without early cardiac involvement are unlikely to develop delayed valvular disease.

CHEST PAIN IN CHILDREN AND ADOLESCENTS

Considerable anxiety is associated with chest pain, and the child is no different in this respect. Parents are often concerned about a cardiac etiology. It is a common complaint but rarely as serious as in adults. The cause of chest pain in the pediatric population is usually benign. In the rare case of cardiac pain, disease processes are generally less serious than those in adults.

Table 33-7. Guidelines for the Diagnosis of Initial Attack of Rheumatic Fever (Jones Criteria, 1992 Update)

Major Manifestations

Carditis
Polyarthritis
Chorea
Erythema marginatum
Subcutaneous nodules

Minor Manifestations

Clinical findings
   Arthralgia
   Fever
Laboratory findings
   Elevated acute phase reactants
      Erythrocyte sedimentation rate
      C-reactive protein
   Prolonged PR interval

Supporting Evidence of Antecedent Group A Streptococcal Infection

Positive throat culture or rapid streptococcal antigen test
Elevated or rising streptococcal antibody titer

If supported by evidence of a preceding group A streptococcal infection, the presence of two major manifestations or of one major and two minor manifestations indicates a high probability of acute rheumatic fever.

Most children with chest pain look well. Causes include musculoskeletal, pulmonic (pneumonitic, pleuritic, or asthmatic), traumatic, or gastrointestinal pain. Approximately one-third of cases will have no obvious underlying pathology.

The cases of most concern are those involving children with known cardiac disease, chest pain during exercise, or syncope. Unexplained abnormal vital signs or dysrhythmia also suggest serious disease. Cardiac pain due to myocarditis is accompanied by cough, shortness of breath, malaise, and fatigue. Pericarditis pain is a sharp, substernal pain that worsens with inspiration. Sitting forward can often relieve the pain. Chest pain and a new murmur suggest aortic stenosis or hypertrophic cardiomyopathy. Fixed cardiac output results in exertional pain, dyspnea, ischemia, or syncope. Patients with suspected hypertrophic cardiomyopathy or aortic stenosis should be screened for LVH. Those with LV strain or S-T/T-wave abnormalities are at higher risk for ischemia or sudden death.

Rarely, patients will present with myocardial ischemia. Teens and younger adults at risk for premature atherosclerosis or ischemia include those with a history of Kawasaki disease, cocaine use, familial hyperlipidemia or hypercholesterolemia, collagen vascular disease (particularly systemic lupus erythematosus), glue sniffing, and chronic steroid use. The index of suspicion is the most reliable tool in the at-risk patient.

Evaluation includes a thorough history and physical examination. Time and attention both aid in the diagnosis of chest pain and convey a sense of security that is reassuring to the family. Risk factors are different in children and adolescents, especially those with congenital or structural heart disease. Ancillary tests, such as chest radiography and ECG, may be helpful in suspected LV outlet obstruction or when pulmonary disease requires confirmation. Occasionally, an ECG or chest x-ray is required for parental reassurance, a mandatory condition for discharge. Most children with chest pain look well and can be safely discharged. A logical explanation for the pain and plans for follow-up should be provided. Symptom control may be as important as making the diagnosis. Nonsteroidal antiinflammatory agents or acetaminophen should be prescribed. Activity level and back-to-school expectations should be explained. Overall, a calm, thorough clinical evaluation done by a confident team of emergency personnel is essential in diffusing the fear of a frightened child and nervous family.

BIBLIOGRAPHY

Chinnock R, Sherwin T, Robie S, et al: Emergency department presentation and management of pediatric heart transplant recipients. *Pediatr Emerg Care* 11:355–369, 1995.

Committee on Rheumatic Fever, Endocarditis, and Kawasaki disease, American Heart Association: Guidelines for the diagnosis of rheumatic fever. *JAMA* 268:2069, 1992.

Dajani AS, Taubert KA, Gerber MA, et al: Prevention of bacterial endocarditis: Recommendations by the American Heart Association. *JAMA* 277:1794, 1997.

Feldman AM, McNamara D: Medical progress: Myocarditis. *N Engl J Med* 343:1388–1398, 2000.

O'Laughlin MP: Congestive heart failure in children. *Pediatr Clin North Am* 46:263–273, 1999.

Shannon KM: Arrhythmias in congenital heart disease. *Curr Treat Options Cardiovascular Med* 1:373–379, 1999.

Zavaras-Angelidou KA, Weinhouse E, Nelson DB: Review of 180 episodes of chest pain in 134 children. *Pediatr Emerg Care* 8:189–193, 1992.

34

Dysrhythmias in Children

William C. Toepper

HIGH-YIELD FACTS

- Dysrhythmias in children are classified according to rate, QRS width, and clinical stability.
- Sinus bradycardia in the neonate always requires aggressive investigation and prompt resuscitation.
- Infants with paroxysmal supraventricular tachycardia (PSVT) present in a low output state with irritability, poor feeding, tachypnea, and diaphoresis.
- Vagal maneuvers and adenosine convert most episodes of PSVT. Verapamil is contraindicated in children <2 years of age.
- Accessory pathway is the most common mechanism for PSVT in the child, but is difficult to appreciate during PSVT. Digoxin may precipitate ventricular tachycardia (VT) and is only used under the supervision of a pediatric cardiologist.
- Atrial fibrillation or flutter associated with accessory pathway disease or hypertrophic cardiomyopathy puts a child at high risk for 1:1 conduction, ventricular tachycardia, and sudden death.
- The electrocardiogram (ECG) is important in the evaluation of the syncopal patient, looking for wide complex tachycardia, long QT syndrome (QTc >0.46 s), or hypertrophic myocardopathy (LVH).

Disorders of rate and rhythm in the pediatric population are rare. Worrisome dysrhythmias, such as ventricular tachycardia, can be asymptomatic in children and have a benign natural history. Others, such as supraventricular tachycardia, have predictable etiologies based on age and little possibility for coronary artery-related decom-

pensation. Rhythm disturbances, such as sinus bradycardia, can be life-threatening in the neonate.

Atrial fibrillation is rare in children and must be approached differently from atrial fibrillation in the adult because many interventions used in adults can cause 1:1 conduction, followed by ventricular dysrhythmia, and possible death. The physician should be cautious in applying the usual adult practice to children suffering from similar rhythm disturbances. Mechanisms differ, treatment varies, and complications due to atherosclerosis are negligible.

Dysrhythmias in children are usually the result of cardiac lesions. In contrast, dysrhythmia in the adult is often sequela of chronic hypertension, lung disease, or coronary artery disease. Noncardiac causes, such as hypoxia, electrolyte imbalance, toxins, and inflammatory disease, must be considered in the child, as should cardioactive drugs, such as digoxin or over-the-counter cold remedies. Initial evaluation of the child with idiopathic or unexplained dysrhythmia includes an echocardiogram. Dysrhythmia associated with structural or congenital heart disease has a poorer prognosis than that with structurally normal heart.

Age is an important consideration in the child with dysrhythmia. Some ventricular dysrhythmias disappear with age. Other conditions associated with an escape pacemaker, worsen with age. The ventricular rate in third degree heart block may be adequate for the 2-month-old child but will not provide an adequate cardiac output for the child at age 12. Age is also a factor in the clinical presentation of the dysrhythmia. The infant, unable to verbalize, may present with poor feeding, tachypnea, irritability, or signs of a low output state. The older child presents with specific symptoms, such as syncope from decreased cerebral blood flow, chest pain from decreased coronary blood flow, or palpitations. Adolescents involved in competitive athletics with syncope, palpitations, or worrisome chest pain, should be investigated promptly.

The initial emergency management of dysrhythmias is dependent on three factors:

- rate
- QRS width
- clinical stability

Normal heart rate and blood pressure (see Table 10-4) help establish stability. In addition, decisions should be based on 12-lead ECG interpretation. Single-lead monitor strips can be misleading. Rapid rates can appear supraventricular in origin in the child with sinus tachycardia. Children tolerate most rhythm disturbances well, providing ample time for precise interpretation. A brief review of the natural history and management of pediatric rhythm disturbances follows.

SLOW RATES

Sinus Bradycardia

Sinus bradycardia can be a manifestation of serious underlying disease or a normal physiologic variant. Each child must be approached individually. The athletic heart is approached differently from neonatal bradycardia requiring resuscitation. Serious causes include hypoxia, hypothyroidism, or increased intracranial pressure. Sinus bradycardia can be a manifestation of calcium channel blocker, beta-blocker, or digoxin toxicity. Treating the underlying condition corrects the rate. If the cause is unclear and oxygenation and ventilation are adequate, an unstable patient is given epinephrine 1:10,000, 0.01 mg/kg IV/IO, and atropine, 0.02 mg/kg.

Atrioventricular Blocks

Complete atrioventricular (AV) block may be congenital or acquired. Congenital block associated with structural disease, such as A-V canal, has a poor prognosis. Congenital block associated with maternal collagen vascular disease has a better prognosis. Maternal antibodies cause fibrosis and destruction of the conduction system. Rates of 50 to 80 bpm are typical in complete AV block. Symptoms are rate dependent, with rates >50 rarely symptomatic. An alternative explanation for instability must be pursued in heart rates approaching 80. Complete AV block is suspected in utero in the setting of sustained fetal bradycardia, polyhydramnios, and congestive heart failure (CHF). Treatment of neonatal symptomatic bradycardia due to AV block includes control of CHF, atropine or isoproterenol, and temporary transcutaneous, transthoracic, or umbilical transvenous pacing.

Acquired third degree block is associated with myocarditis, endocarditis, rheumatic fever, cardiomyopathy, Lyme disease, or tumor. Postoperative blocks are less common today because of advances in intra-operative mapping. Postop blocks may last for years or occur years after surgery. Unlike congenital third degree block, QRS complexes are usually wide. Treatment is similar, except patients with syncope must be paced immediately.

Pacemakers in Children

The indications for pediatric pacemakers differ from indications in adults. The most common is symptomatic brady-

cardia. Occasionally, an asymptomatic child with an extremely low heart rate needs pacing. Postop or acquired AV blocks require permanent pacing beyond 10 to 14 days. Other indications include the long Q-T syndrome and cardioinhibitory syncope lasting >10 seconds.

Advances in adult pacemakers have improved the management of children with dysrhythmia. Most permanent pediatric pacemakers are transvenous. Epicardial units are reserved for premature infants and those with right-to-left shunts. Choice of mode depends on disease. For example, children with sinus disease require atrial pacing. Ventricular pacing is unnecessary because AV conduction is normal. Children with congenital or acquired AV block require dual chamber pacing. Isolated ventricular pacing is employed in the very young. Most units can be programmed to sense, demand, or inhibit at the atrial or ventricular level, depending on the needs of the child. Also, they may be programmed to sense motion or breathing.

Syncope or palpitations in a child with a pacemaker suggests malfunction. Chest radiography may reveal wire fracture or lead displacement. Most malfunctions are not mechanical and require external reprogramming. Uncaptured paced beats outside the refractory period require investigation. If the problem is not easily resolved, the patient should be admitted.

Temporary transvenous pacemakers are rarely necessary in children. Transthoracic pacing via pericardiocentesis catheter should be considered in the very unstable infant. Most temporary pacing is transcutaneous. If transcutaneous pacing is ineffective, a 3 to 6 F transvenous pacemaker can be placed via a femoral sheath. The balloon-tipped pacing catheter is advanced until ectopy is noted. Atrial placement is preferred over ventricular leads to avoid perforation or valve incompetence, but must be guided by clinical need. Fluoroscopic guidance is desirable but may be impractical in the unstable patient. After proper positioning, the catheter is connected to the pacemaker and maximum current is chosen. Upon successful capture, current is then decreased until capture is lost. This is the threshold current. The current is then set at 200 percent threshold. Sensitivity can be adjusted to allow for asynchronous pacing (low sensitivity) or overriding by native sinus pacemaker (high sensitivity).

FAST RATES

Paroxysmal Supraventricular Tachycardia

The most common dysrhythmia in the child is paroxysmal supraventricular tachycardia (PSVT). PSVT is differentiated from sinus tachycardia by its abrupt onset, rates >230 bpm, the absence of normal P waves, or by little rate variation during stressful activities, such as phlebotomy. Symptoms of PSVT in infants include poor feeding, tachypnea, and irritability. They may appear ill or septic. Infants tolerate PSVT well but usually present within 24 hours of onset. Occasionally, it is associated with fever, infection, drug exposure, or congenital heart disease, but it is usually caused by one of two mechanisms. Younger children are more likely to have accessory pathway tachycardia, which is very important in choosing treatment.

AV reciprocating tachycardia or accessory pathway tachycardia is most common in children. Conduction during PSVT is usually orthodromic, with antegrade AV conduction and retrograde accessory pathway conduction (Fig. 34-1). Conduction during sinus rhythm can be via the accessory pathway, resulting in a short PR interval and appearance of a delta wave. This characterizes the Wolff-Parkinson-White (WPW) syndrome. Some accessory pathways only conduct retrograde during bouts of PSVT and are termed "concealed" because they are not apparent on surface ECG.

The other mechanism, AV nodal reentry, is more common in adults, but may be responsible for one third of cases of PSVT in adolescents. Within the AV node, fast pathways with long refractory periods are blocked during a PAC, allowing for anterograde conduction down

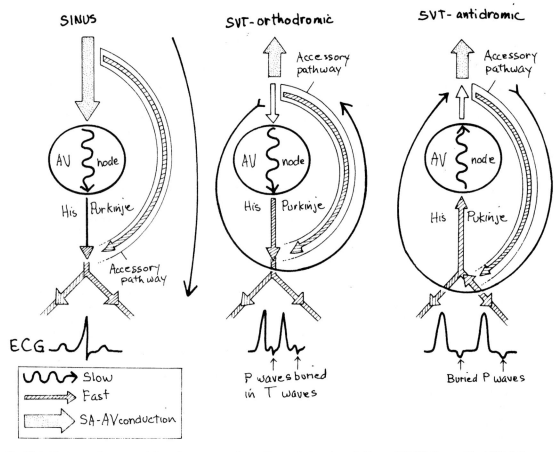

Fig. 34-1. Diagrammatic representation of accessory pathway disease during sinus rhythm and PSVT. Sinus—Short PR, delta wave, characteristic of WPW; Orthodromic-fast retrograde conduction through accessory pathway leads to reentry. His-Purkinje conduction is normal, complexes are narrow. Retrograde P waves are abnormally directed and buried in T wave; Antidromic (rare)—fast antegrade conduction through accessory pathway leads to abnormal His-Purkinje conduction and wide complexes. Retrograde P waves are abnormally directed and buried in T waves.

the slow tract. The impulse then propagates up the fast tract, initiating reentry. Distinguishing nodal from accessory pathway PSVT is difficult during episodes of PSVT. Negative P waves in II, III, and avF, may indicate retrograde conduction through the accessory pathway but they are usually buried in the QRS complex. Pointed or peaked t waves suggest retrograde P waves. P waves are almost never seen in AV nodal reentry. Lack of delta wave during sinus rhythm does not rule out concealed accessory tracts. Information from parents may be helpful, but first episodes of PSVT or unstudied children make diagnosis in the ED difficult.

Unstable PSVT is treated with synchronized cardioversion, 0.5 J/kg, increasing to 2 J/kg as needed. If unsuccessful, esophageal overdrive pacing may be necessary. Vagal maneuvers may convert stable patients. A bag containing ice and some water is placed over the nose and forehead for intervals of 15 to 20 seconds. Ocular pressure or nasogastric stimulation is discouraged. If ice water fails, adenosine, 0.1 mg/kg followed by 0.3 mg/kg, is recommended. Adenosine terminates nodal and accessory pathway tachycardia by blocking adenosine receptors in the AV node and slowing conduction. Transient side effects include headache, flushing, and chest pain. Rhythm disturbances, such as atrial fibrillation, accelerated ventricular rhythm, and wide-complex tachycardia, may require resuscitation. Other side effects include bronchospasm, apnea, and asystole. Adenosine can be used in hypotension but should be avoided in the patient on theophylline. Immediate recurrence rate approaches 50 percent.

Digitalis is commonly used to prolong AV nodal conduction and refractoriness of fast and slow tracts (see Table 33-3). It can promote accessory pathway conduction and ventricular tachycardia; therefore, it is best used in the well-known stable patient with AV nodal reentry. A pediatric cardiologist should be consulted prior to administration. It may take hours to work and if cardioversion is necessary, there is a risk of ventricular fibrillation.

Verapamil is reserved for children >2 to 3 years of age. Hypotension, cardiovascular collapse, and death have occurred in infants. Older children with stable but recalcitrant PSVT may respond to IV verapamil, 0.1 mg/kg slowly. Calcium chloride, 10 mg/kg, and IV saline should be available to treat hypotension.

If the above measures fail or PSVT resumes, procainamide or propranolol may be useful. Procainamide is preferred in narrow complex tachycardia thought to be ventricular. A 5- to 15-mg/kg bolus is given over 20 to 30 minutes, watching for hypotension. Propranolol, 0.1 mg/kg IV, is useful in WPW or other accessory pathway diseases.

Any infant with new onset PSVT should be hospitalized. Structural heart disease must be ruled out. Infants are likely to have accessory pathway disease and require further therapy. A child with immediate recurrence is at higher risk for repeat episodes or recalcitrant PSVT. EPS to determine mechanism and efficacy of treatment may be necessary. Surgical ablation may be required.

Atrial Flutter and Fibrillation

Atrial flutter and fibrillation in children are rare. Children with congenital heart disease, rheumatic fever, or dilated cardiomyopathy are at highest risk. Patients with atrial flutter or fibrillation, in combination with an accessory pathway or hypertrophic cardiomyopathy, are at high risk for sudden death. Unstable patients are cardioverted with 0.5 J/kg. Overdrive pacing 10 to 20 beats per minute faster than the flutter rate may also be effective. The long-term prognosis of children with congenital heart disease and atrial fibrillation or flutter may depend on the elimination of all flutter activity. Cardioversion may be the only option. Patients with long-standing atrial disease associated with a diseased sinus node are at risk for bradycardia or asystole on termination. Pacing must be available.

Premature Ventricular Contractions

Premature ventricular contractions (PVCs) in the infant and young child are rare. Unifocal PVCs begin appearing in healthy children during adolescence. The patient is usually asymptomatic and has a normal physical examination, chest x-ray, and ECG. Unusual morphology, such as multifocal PVCs, coupling, or the "R on T" phenomenon, are rarely cause for emergency intervention in the asymptomatic child with normal Q-T interval. Continuous ECG monitor may define and quantify the PVCs. PVCs that diminish during exercise or stress are benign and require no therapy. Patients with myocarditis, cardiomyopathy, congenital heart disease, or who are postoperative from cardiac surgery, are at greater risk and may require treatment. Syncope or exercise-induced PVCs may also require therapy. Lidocaine, procainamide, propranolol, or amiodarone may be useful using guidelines similar for ventricular tachycardia (see "Ventricular Tachycardia").

Accelerated Idioventricular Rhythm

Accelerated idioventricular rhythm (AIVR) is a benign pediatric dysrhythmia that has the appearance of ventricular tachycardia. Rates are rarely faster than 150 bpm. AIVR begins gradually with fusion beats and is a monomorphic, wide-complex rhythm that originates from an accelerated ventricular focus. Diagnosis can be difficult in the new patient. Patients with AIVR are stable. Unstable wide-complex tachycardia is not AIVR and should be converted immediately. AIVR rarely responds to medication but can be a warning of a residual hemodynamic abnormality associated with corrected congenital heart disease.

Ventricular Tachycardia

Ventricular tachycardia (VT) is rare in children and can be confused with other forms of tachycardia. Ventricular tachycardia is distinguished from PSVT by wide QRS complexes, >0.08 to 0.09 seconds, depending on age. Complexes as narrow as 0.06 seconds have been noted in infantile VT. Wide complexes can be seen in PSVT but this is rare. Antegrade accessory pathway conduction can result in wide and bizarre-looking QRS complexes that simulate VT. Rates averaging 250 bpm are rarely helpful in differentiating PSVT from VT but may be helpful in distinguishing VT from AIVR, with average rates of 150. AV dissociation with P wave and QRS independence can also help distinguish VT from PSVT.

Idiopathic ventricular tachycardia is occasionally encountered in a child who is completely asymptomatic and has a normal heart. It is usually not treated. Serious causes, such as electrolyte disturbance, toxins, or myocarditis, should be considered. Structural heart disease, tumor, cardiomyopathy, or long QT syndrome may be the cause. VT in the setting of a diseased heart or congenital lesion is much more ominous than with normal anatomy. It usually requires aggressive evaluation and treatment. Recurrent exercise-induced syncope is often due to VT. The initial work-up may be negative. A search for a small myocardial tumor, early cardiomyopathy, or occult myocarditis may be necessary. EPS or biopsy may be necessary to guide treatment.

Regardless of etiology, unstable wide-complex tachycardia should be synchronously cardioverted with 2 to 4 J/kg. Any patient in cardiorespiratory arrest should be defibrillated. Upon conversion, lidocaine is begun, 1 to 2 mg/kg bolus, followed by 15 to 50 μg/kg/min infusion. It is also the initial drug of choice for stable VT that requires treatment. Amiodarone, 5 mg/kg over 1 hour, may also be useful. Procainamide may be useful for wide-complex tachycardia of uncertain origin because of its effect both above and below the AV node. An initial dose of 10 to 15 mg/kg over 30 to 45 minutes

is followed by 20 to 80 μg/kg/min drip. Adenosine is safe and may be useful in the rare case of PSVT with aberrancy. It should be used only in stable situations when other traditional therapies have failed.

Ventricular Fibrillation

Ventricular fibrillation is treated with defibrillation, initially at 2 J/kg and subsequently at 4 J/kg. Correction of precipitating factors, such as acidosis, hypoxia, or metabolic derangements, aids in conversion. Ventricular fibrillation may be under appreciated in children with drowning, toxin, and neurologic or trauma-related arrests. Early defibrillation could improve outcome.

OTHER CARDIAC CONDITIONS ASSOCIATED WITH DYSRHYTHMIAS

Long Q-T Syndrome

Jervell and Lange-Nielsen first described the association of syncope, sudden death, deafness, and long Q-T interval in 1957. In 1963, Romano described the syndrome in normal-hearing patients. Congenital long Q-T syndrome (LQTS) is an inherited syndrome characterized by paroxysmal ventricular tachycardia and torsades de pointes. It can be emotionally induced or stress related and can progress to ventricular fibrillation and sudden death. Acquired Q-T prolongation associated with type IA antiarrhythmics, drugs, anorexia nervosa, bulimia, and electrolyte derangements can also predispose to dysrhythmia. The congenital form is the most common form affecting the child.

Diagnosis is suspected in the syncope patient with a family history of syncope or sudden death, unusual seizures, drop attacks, or congenital deafness. A QTc >0.44 seconds is a sign of delayed repolarization; >0.5 seconds is highly associated with sudden death. T wave alternans is also seen.

The cause of congenital LQTS is unclear. Some researchers hypothesize that an imbalance between the right- and left-sided sympathetic cardiac innervation leads to sudden rushes of left-sided sympathetic activity, resulting in torsades de pointes, ventricular tachycardia, ventricular fibrillation, and death. New data suggest that abnormalities in genetically programmed cation channels are responsible for intrinsic cardiac vulnerability. This is further supported by the genetic basis of the syndrome and its similarity to acquired long Q-T abnormalities. Both theories help explain treatment modalities. Beta blockers help control sympathetic rushes and decrease the incidence of syncope. Some patients remain symptomatic and require sympathetic ganglionectomy or pacing. Research into the channel-based theory may lead to therapy directed specifically at the ion defect. The channel theory may help explain the effectiveness of magnesium in treating torsades de pointes. Mortality from untreated congenital LQTS approaches 50 percent. Recognition in the primary care setting is vital.

Hypertrophic Cardiomyopathy

Hypertrophic cardiomyopathy (HC) is characterized by a hypertrophied, nondilated left ventricle. Symptoms include chest pain, dyspnea, syncope, or sudden death. Clinical presentation varies. Some patients are asymptomatic. The majority of symptomatic adults suffer from CHF secondary to insufficient diastolic filling. Dysrhythmias include atrial fibrillation and ventricular tachyarrhythmia, the leading causes of sudden death. Outflow obstruction is rare. Mortality rates of 3 percent are probably overestimated due to sampling bias and may lead to an overly aggressive approach to therapy. This is especially true of the asymptomatic individual. However, pediatric HC tends to be more serious, with mortality rates in infants approaching 6 percent. Other risk factors include advanced symptoms at diagnosis, LV dysfunction, and a family history of sudden death. Atrial fibrillation is especially dangerous in the HC patient.

Signs of HC include late systolic murmur and paradoxical splitting of S_2. LV or septal hypertrophy on ECG is a poor prognostic sign. Echocardiogram is diagnostic. Therapy depends on the clinical manifestation. Beta

blockers are the mainstay of therapy for CHF, effective in relieving dyspnea and chest pain. Beta blockers have no effect on rates of sudden death. Atrial fibrillation should be controlled because of its association with rapid ventricular rate and decreased outflow. Amiodarone may be effective but has also been associated with sudden death in some symptomatic patients. Implantable defibrillators may be preferred. Dual chamber pacing and surgical myectomy may be necessary for significant outflow obstruction.

BIBLIOGRAPHY

Ganz LI, Friedman PL: Supraventricular tachycardia. *N Engl J Med* 332:162–173, 1995.

Gillette PC, Case CL, Oslizlok PC, et al: Pediatric cardiac pacing. *Cardiol Clin* 10:749–754, 1992.

Kugler Jd, Danford DA: Management of infants, children and adolescents with paroxysmal supraventricular tachycardia. *J Pediatr* 129:324–338, 1996.

MacLellan-Tobert SG, Porter CJ: Accelerated idioventricular rhythm: A benign arrhythmia in childhood. *Pediatrics* 96:122–125, 1995.

Meldon SW, Brady WJ, Berger S, Mannenbach M: Pediatric ventricular tachycardia: A review with 3 illustrative cases. *Pediatr Emerg Care* 10:294–300, 1994.

Roden DM, George AL: The cardiac ion channel: Relation to management of arrhythmias. *Annu Rev Med* 47:135–148, 1996.

Sacchetti A, Moyer V, Baricella R: Primary cardiac arrhythmias in children. *Pediatr Emerg Care* 15:95–98, 1999.

Spirito P, Seidman CE, McKenna WL, Maron BJ: The management of hypertrophic cardiomyopathy. *N Engl J Med* 336:775–785, 1997.

35

Peripheral Vascular Disease

William C. Toepper
Joilo Barbosa

HIGH-YIELD FACTS

- Children with high-normal blood pressure require close follow-up and nonpharmacologic management; those with blood pressure >95th percentile (severe hypertension) require evaluation, consultation, and pharmacologic management.

- A hypertensive emergency is any elevation of blood pressure resulting in potential end-organ damage. Blood pressure reduction must begin immediately and should proceed cautiously.

- Hypertensive urgency is defined as a minimally symptomatic elevation of blood pressure with potential for end-organ damage. The goal is improvement over 24 to 48 hours.

- The single greatest risk factor for thromboembolic disease in children is an indwelling central venous catheter.

- Disease patterns for pulmonary embolism in children and adolescents are similar to those in adults, yet diagnosis and management is often delayed or inappropriate.

HYPERTENSION

Hypertension in children is rare, but new data suggest that adult essential hypertension has its roots in childhood. Blood pressure in children is age, sex, and height dependent. The National High Blood Pressure Education Program has updated the norms for children. Table 35-1 provides a concise guideline. Children with systolic or diastolic blood pressures consistently above the 95th percentile have *severe* hypertension. Evaluation, therapy,

and consultation are essential. Blood pressure between the 90th and 95th percentile is high-normal and is referred to as *significant* hypertension. Significant hypertension requires observation, follow-up, and nonpharmacologic therapy. Prompt evaluation for high-normal blood pressure is necessary in the very young child.

Hypertension in children is usually due to an underlying illness or treatable condition. Neonatal hypertension is commonly due to renovascular disease, coarctation of the aorta, or kidney malformation. Children younger than 6 years of age probably suffer from renal parenchymal disease, coarctation, or renovascular disease. Essential hypertension emerges between the ages of 6 and 10 years and is the leading cause of hypertension in the adolescent.

Blood pressure is measured in a comfortable seated position. The infant should be lying down and quiet. Feeding and upright positioning can falsely elevate blood pressure. If severe hypertension is suspected, blood pressure should be determined in both arms and one leg with an appropriate cuff. The bladder should encircle the arm without overlapping by more than 2 cm, and the bladder width should be at least 40% arm circumference. The manufacturers' suggested markings are reliable in the busy emergency department. Small cuffs falsely elevate blood pressure, and large cuffs falsely underestimate blood pressure. Systolic pressure is determined at the onset of the first sound. The fifth Korotkoff sound or the disappearance of sound determines diastolic pressure. If auscultation is difficult, Doppler or oscillometric methods can be used. Automated devices are reliable in infants and young children. In the older child manual blood pressure should be taken several times over several weeks to months before chronic hypertension is diagnosed.

Neonatal Hypertension

A detailed list of causes of hypertension in the child is presented in Table 35-2. Neonatal hypertension deserves additional comment. Unlike children and adults, hypertensive neonates are rarely asymptomatic. Irritability, poor feeding with failure to thrive, and respiratory distress may suggest congestive heart failure. Seizure may be the first manifestation of severe hypertension in the infant. Blood pressure should be checked in any infant with first presentation of seizure. Infants younger than 1 month with systolic readings >100 mmHg may be hypertensive; those with readings >110 mmHg require aggressive evaluation and treatment. Hypertension in neonates and infants is usually due to renal or vascular disease. Renal artery thrombosis from an umbilical

Table 35-1. Classification of Severe Hypertension

Age (yr)		Male @ 50th Percentile Height[a] (95th Percentile BP)	Female @ 50th% Height[a] (95th Percentile BP)
1			
	Systolic BP	>102	>104
3			
	Systolic BP	>109	>107
	Diastolic BP	>65	>66
6			
	Systolic BP	>114	>111
	Diastolic BP	>74	>73
10			
	Systolic BP	>117	>119
	Diastolic BP	>80	>78
15			
	Systolic BP	>131	>128
	Diastolic BP	>83	>83

[a]Normal blood pressures (BPs) in very tall children will be higher than the values presented. Normal BPs in short children will be lower. All-inclusive tables are referenced in the above Task Force report.

Source: Adapted from National Heart, Lung and Blood Institute: Report of the Task Force on Blood Pressure Control in Children—1987. *Pediatrics* 79:1–25, 1987.

catheter is not uncommon. Congenital heart disease should be considered.

Essential Hypertension

Essential hypertension has no specific underlying pathology, yet many factors contribute to its development. Obesity, poor physical fitness, and family history are risk factors. Sodium intake has not been shown to correlate with blood pressure in children or adolescents, but moderate reductions are recommended for early hypertension. It is unlikely that essential hypertension poses any immediate risk to the child, but evidence suggests that ventricular dysfunction and hemodynamic changes in adulthood begin before the age of 20 years. The adolescent with essential hypertension should be counseled about drugs that may elevate blood pressure or the use of birth control pills.

Clinical Manifestations

Most hypertensive children are asymptomatic. Signs and symptoms may suggest the etiology in newly discovered hypertension. Glomerulonephritis may present with hematuria or weakness due to azotemia and anemia. Re-

cent pharyngitis suggests poststreptococcal disease and warrants antibody testing. Coarctation of the aorta is suspected with diminished femoral pulses, collateral circulation, and hyperactive precordium. Examination of the abdomen may reveal tumor or trauma. Renovascular anomalies are associated with bruits, blunt abdominal trauma, or café-au-lait spots. Acute or severe elevations of blood pressure may lead to hypertensive emergencies. A hypertensive emergency is any elevation of blood pressure resulting in potential end-organ damage. Blood pressure reduction must begin immediately and should proceed cautiously. Hypertensive emergencies include encephalopathy, congestive heart failure, nephropathy, eye ground changes, and seizures. Symptoms include headache, dizziness, visual changes, nausea, emesis, or altered level of consciousness.

Assessment

The initial evaluation of the hypertensive child depends on the age and clinical picture. The likelihood of identifying a cause is directly related to the blood pressure and indirectly related to the age of the child. Young children with significant hypertension should have a complete blood count, electrolytes, renal functions, uric acid, urinalysis,

Table 35-2. Causes of Hypertension in Children

Drugs and Poisons	**Central Nervous System**
Cocaine	Increased intracranial pressure
Sympathomimetic agents	Encephalitis
Amphetamines	**Cardiac**
Phencyclidine	Coarctation of the aorta
Corticosteroids	Aortic insufficiency
Cyclosporine	**Metabolic**
Lead	Hypercalcemia
Antihypertensive medication withdrawal	Hypernatremia
Renal	**Miscellaneous**
Glomerulonephritis	Essential hypertension
Henoch-Schönlein purpura	Anxiety and pain
Hemolytic-uremic syndrome	Preeclampsia
Congenital malformation	Porphyria
Polycystic kidneys	Systemic lupus erythematosus
Renovascular	Bronchopulmonary dysplasia
Renal artery stenosis	
Renal vein thrombosis	
Endocrine	
Pheochromocytoma	
Congenital adrenal hyperplasia	
Oral contraceptives	

and renal ultrasound, looking for renal disease. Chest radiograph, electrocardiogram, and echocardiogram are indicated if cardiac involvement is suspected.

Older children with mildly elevated blood pressure should have urinalysis and measurement of renal functions. A lipid profile may be helpful. Intervention is rare and may only require reassurance and repeat blood pressure in a quiet outpatient setting. Older symptomatic children with significantly elevated blood pressure may require further evaluation. Hospitalization is indicated for hypertensive emergencies and for acute hypertension due to serious diseases such as hyperthyroidism. Hospitalization may be necessary for asymptomatic significant hypertension when the social situation is unreliable.

Management

The management of mild hypertension in children begins with lifestyle changes. Weight loss and exercise play a key role. A low-sodium diet is a good idea but may be impractical. Other efforts include a limitation of

alcohol and tobacco use in the home and a low-fat, low-cholesterol diet for all members of the family. The prevention of cardiovascular disease in adults begins in childhood within the family.

A hypertensive emergency with acutely elevated blood pressure and end-organ injury requires prompt but controlled reduction (Table 35-3). The goal of treatment with parenteral therapy is a gradual reduction in blood pressure, 20% initially, with complete control by 2 to 3 days. Hypertensive emergencies rarely occur in previously normotensive children. Drug ingestion, glomerulonephritis, or pheochromocytoma must be considered. Acutely elevated blood pressure due to high intracranial pressure may not require immediate reduction.

Hypertensive urgency is defined as a minimally symptomatic elevation of blood pressure with potential for end-organ damage. The goal is improvement over 24 to 48 hours. Slow reduction with oral agents prevents hypotension or rebound tachycardia. Overly aggressive reduction may result in end-organ hypoperfusion or loss of cerebral autoregulation. Helpful agents are listed in Table

Table 35-3. Therapy for Hypertension in Children

Indications for Nonpharmacologic Intervention Strategies

Systolic or diastolic blood pressure (BP) >90th percentile (high-normal)

Indications for Initiation of Antihypertensive Drugs

Significant diastolic hypertension
Evidence of target organ injury
Symptoms or signs related to elevated BP

Use of Parenteral Therapy

Indicated in acute severe hypertension, such as with acute glomerulonephritis, hemolytic-uremic syndrome, head
  injuries, or any risk of target organ damage

Therapeutic Goals

Diastolic BP <90th percentile
Minimal side effects
Use of the least amount of drug necessary to effectively reduce BP
High degree of patient compliance

Source: Adapted from the National Heart, Lung and Blood Institute: Report of the Task Force on Blood Pressure Control in Children—1987. *Pediatrics* 79:1–25, 1987.

35-4. The most commonly used antihypertensives are listed in Table 35-5. A brief discussion follows, with the agents most useful in hypertensive emergencies given in italics.

ACE Inhibitors

Angiotensin-converting enzyme (ACE) inhibitors interfere with the formation of angiotensin II, a potent vasoconstrictor. Decreased angiotensin II results in decreased aldosterone and norepinephrine. ACE inhibitors also reduce renal vascular resistance, increasing renal blood flow and benefiting cardiac function. Captopril is effective in young children. Enalapril with once-daily dosing is a popular alternative. Side effects include dry cough, rash, angioedema, neutropenia, proteinuria, hyperkalemia, and elevation of creatinine. ACE inhibitors are contraindicated in bilateral renal artery stenosis and pregnancy.

Calcium Channel Blockers

Calcium channel blockers reduce blood pressure by inhibiting calcium influx into the cytosol and decreasing smooth muscle contraction force. Significant side effects include tachycardia and negative inotropy, normalizing within weeks. Other side effects include constipation, somnolence, peripheral edema, and headache. *Nifedipine* is most commonly used in children. Sublingual routes may be used for hypertensive emergency when intravenous access is impossible. Significant

Table 35-4. Drugs Useful in Pediatric Hypertensive Crises

Drug	Dose
Nitroprusside	0.5–1 mcg/kg/min up to 8 mcg/kg/min
Labetalol	0.2–2 mg/kg IV
Nifedipine	0.25–0.5 mg/kg po
Esmolol	0.5 mg/kg IV over 1–2 min, then 0.2 mg/kg/min
Diazoxide	1–5 mg/kg/dose IV up to 150 mg
Hydralazine	0.2–0.4 mg/kg IV; repeat twice prn

Table 35-5. Pharmacologic Management of Hypertension in Children

	Initial Dose (mg/kg/dose)	Maximum/day (mg/kg)	Frequency
ACE Inhibitors			
Captopril	1.5	6	tid
Enalapril	0.15	1	bid
Calcium Channel Blockers			
Nifedipine	0.25	3	tid-qid
Diuretics			
Hydrochlorothiazide	1	2–3	bid
Furosemide	1	12	bid-qid
Spironolactone	1	3	bid-qid
α-Adrenergic Agents			
Prazosin	0.05–0.1	0.5	tid-bid
Clonidine	0.05–0.1	0.5–0.6	qid
β-Blockers			
Propranolol	1	8	bid
Atenolol	1	8	bid-qd
Vasodilators			
Minoxidil	0.1–0.2	1	bid

hypotension can result. Oral administration yields a more predictable response. Long-lasting preparations are recommended for chronic therapy but may be limited by tablet strength.

Diuretics

Diuretics decrease intra- and extravascular volumes. Homeostatic mechanisms neutralize this effect, quickly leading to resistance. The most commonly used agents are loop diuretics, thiazides, and potassium-sparing diuretics for aldosterone-dependent hypertension. All of these are among the safest medications to use initially. Side effects of loop diuretics include hypercalcemia, hyperlipidemia, and hypokalemia. Thiazides cause calciuria, hyperlipidemia, and hypokalemia.

α-Adrenergic Blocking Agents

Peripheral α-antagonists such as prazosin result in smooth muscle relaxation with minimal reflex tachycardia. Central α-agonists such as clonidine act by decreasing sympathetic activity. Their peripheral effects on the presynaptic α_2-receptors cause a decrease in norepinephrine release. Side effects include dry mouth and sedation. Clonidine should be tapered to prevent the development of severe rebound hypertension.

β-Adrenergic Blocking Agents

β-Blockers bind cardiovascular, renin/angiotensin, and central nervous system receptors. Immediate decrease in heart rate and cardiac output result. A mild increase in the blood pressure due to unopposed α-effect is short-lived. Propranolol traverses the blood-brain barrier and has central effects. β-Blockers are well absorbed orally but have considerable first-pass effect. Side effects, less common in children, include bradycardia, bronchospasm, and sleep disturbances. They can also adversely affect glucose metabolism and cause elevation of triglyceride levels.

α- and β-Adrenergic Blocking Agents

Labetalol has both α- and β-blocking effects. The β-effects predominate. It is well absorbed orally but has a high first-pass drug metabolism. It is indicated mainly for intravenous use in hypertensive crises.

Vasodilating Agents

The two most common direct vasodilator agents are *minoxidil* and *hydralazine.* Minoxidil is highly effective but is limited by side effects. Diuretics and β-blockers control fluid retention and compensatory tachycardia. Hypertrichosis is the most prominent side effect.

Nitroprusside is a powerful vasodilator that is very useful in the treatment of hypertensive emergencies. It has a prompt onset of action and short duration. A drop in the blood pressure is dose related; pressure returns to baseline within 5 minutes of cessation. Cyanide toxicity can result from prolonged use or in the very young infant. Thiocyanate levels should be monitored and, if the levels are increasing, another blood pressure agent should be used. There are many other safe administration issues that should be reviewed before giving this agent. *Diazoxide,* a potent arterial smooth muscle dilator, can cause hypotension, coma, or renal failure. A safe, controlled reduction is achieved by using 1- to 2-mg/kg boluses every 10 minutes.

THROMBOEMBOLIC DISEASE IN CHILDREN

Virchow's triad (increased viscosity, decreased flow, and disruption of endothelial integrity) is not limited to adults. This classic description of the physiologic state that allows for pathologic clotting can apply to children and adolescents. The phenomenon is rare, yet thromboembolic (TE) disease may go undetected in children. Children and adolescents tolerate incidents that might be devastating to the adult. The use of indwelling catheters and other technologic advances that predispose to TE events will increase in the future.

Risk Factors

Most data are limited to small clinical series and autopsy studies. Risk factors for thrombophlebitis, deep vein thrombosis (DVT), and pulmonary embolism overlap (Table 35-6). Adult risk factors pertinent to the child or adolescent include prolonged immobilization and oral contraceptive pills. The TE rate is lower in children because of less vulnerability during postoperative states and lower incidence of neoplasia and heart disease. However, most children with TE complications have serious underlying disease such as liver disease or nephrotic syndrome. The single greatest risk factor is an indwelling central venous catheter. Another risk is congenital hypercoagulable predisposition, which may play a factor in approximately 25% cases of significant TE complications.

Hypercoagulability is most often caused by activated protein C resistance, but it may be due to deficiency of protein S or C or antithrombin. These conditions are usually clinically silent in the child but may be unmasked by oral contraceptive pills or minor trauma. The homozygote will present in the first few hours with purpura fulminans, a devastating and often fatal disease. Purpura fulminans is characterized by rapidly progressive hemorrhagic dermal necrosis. It is treated with fresh frozen plasma.

Table 35-6. Major Risk Factors for Thromboembolic Disease

Adolescents	Children	Adults
Oral contraceptives	Hydrocephalus	Oral contraceptives
Trauma	Trauma	Trauma
Elective abortion	Congenital heart disease	Pregnancy
Surgery	Infection	Surgery
Prolonged immobilization	Neoplasia	Neoplasia
Collagen vascular disease	Prolonged immobilization	Heart disease
Intravenous drug abuse	Surgery	Collagen vascular disease
Rheumatic heart disease	Dehydration	Protein S deficiency
Dehydration	Protein S deficiency	
Obesity		
Renal transplantation		
Protein S deficiency		

The heterozygote may go unrecognized until challenged by one of many risk factors. Early recognition of a congenital deficiency is detected by a thorough family history for clotting disorders. Diagnosis of a congenital hypercoagulable state during a TE event is difficult because large thromboses cause temporary deficiencies of clotting factors. When congenital hypercoagulability is suspected, certain drugs (OCPs) must be avoided.

Deep Vein Thrombosis

DVT in children is most often related to indwelling catheters. Clinical exam may be unreliable. Many central line clots are asymptomatic. These should not be considered benign. Swelling is the most reliable clinical sign. The limb may also be tender, warm, and red. Symptoms of upper extremity central line thrombus include headache, facial swelling, and difficulty with infusion.

DVTs not related to central lines most commonly affect the iliofemoral vein and can extend into the vena cava. There is limited diagnostic experience in children. Venogram is considered the study of choice. Noninvasive studies in adults, particularly Doppler ultrasound flow studies, are approaching the sensitivity of venogram and may be utilized in children, especially when venogram is contraindicated or unavailable. Central line dye infusions are unreliable for determining the extent of a catheter-related thrombus.

Right Atrial Thrombosis

Right atrial thrombus is usually related to a central line, but it may occur in congenital heart disease. Patients are young and often asymptomatic. Diagnosis is made on echocardiogram. Symptoms include central line malfunction, fever, or congestive heart failure. Treatment may include surgery, especially for larger thrombus or if medical management is unsatisfactory.

Pulmonary Embolism

Pulmonary embolism (PE) is also underrecognized in children and adolescents. Acute PE in adults may represent the third most frequent cause of death in the United States and is especially significant in the acutely hospitalized patient. The incidence of PEs in pediatric autopsies appears to be around 4 percent, or 1/1000 hospital admissions. Approximately one-third of those PEs may have contributed to mortality. The rarity of the disease and the lack of familiarity on the part of pediatricians

may explain why diagnosis and treatment require a good index of suspicion.

PEs in children are almost always associated with a disruption of endothelial integrity. The disruption is usually proximal and includes central venous catheters or congenital heart disease with endocarditis. In contrast to a 90 to 99 percent rate in adults, only 42 percent of PEs in children are associated with DVT. Emboli need not be massive to cause problems in children. Catheter-associated pulmonary hypertension from chronic seeding is also devastating.

Disease patterns in adolescents are similar to those in adults, yet diagnosis and management are often delayed or inappropriate. Presenting symptoms include pleuritic chest pain (84 percent), dyspnea (58 percent), cough (47 percent), and hemoptysis (32 percent). Objective findings include hypoxia (pO_2 < 80 percent), abnormal chest x-ray (50 percent), tachypnea (42 percent), or fever (32 percent). A classic presentation is rare in children, and no clinical marker is completely predictive. Clinical suspicion is based on a combination of risk factors and clinical findings.

The ventilation/perfusion scan is safe in children. Interpretation of low or medium probability scans can be difficult. Pulmonary angiography is considered safer than unwarranted heparin, a drug known for iatrogenic mishaps.

Treatment of Thromboembolic Disease

Initial treatment of TE disease is anticoagulation. Heparin, 75 U/kg intravenous bolus, is followed by an infusion of 20 U/kg/h. Heparin is adjusted to maintain the APTT at 60 to 85 seconds. Therapy continues for 5 to 10 days. Protamine can reverse the effects of heparin and is dosed based on most recent heparin administration. Protamine, 1 mg/100 U heparin, is appropriate if given within 30 minutes of most recent heparin administration. Low molecular weight heparin is also being used. It is more predictable, may be more effective, and has fewer bleeding complications. Subcutaneous administration is also easier than maintaining an intravenous drip. The overall cost is comparable to heparin. Dose is age adjusted, with newborns requiring the greatest dose per weight.

The oral agent warfarin is begun as early as day 1. The dose, 0.2 mg/kg, is modified to attain an international normalized ratio (INR) of 2 to 3. Maintenance for the first TE lasts 3 to 6 months. Local recurrence and postphlebitic syndrome (persistent pain, swelling, pigmentation, induration, and ulceration) may occur. Investigation into congenital hypercoagulable state is required after resolution.

Thrombolytic therapy is used to restore catheter patency. Urokinase is preferred to streptokinase to avoid allergic phenomena with repeated dosing. The dose of urokinase is 0.3 mL (15,000 U) over 2 to 4 hours. Thrombolytic therapy for massive PE or DVT is occasionally indicated, but safety and efficacy have not been determined.

Management also includes prophylaxis of high-risk patients. Children with previous thromboembolic events, strong family histories of hypercoagulability, dilated cardiomyopathy, or indwelling catheters should be considered for prophylaxis. There is no evidence that perioperative prophylaxis is beneficial in children. Catheter prophylaxis is via heparin flushes. Inpatient DVT prophylaxis for adolescents is low-dose heparin, 5000 U/dose.

BIBLIOGRAPHY

Andrew M, Michelson AD, Bovill E, et al: Guidelines for antithrombotic therapy in pediatric patients. *J Pediatr* 132: 575–588, 1998.

David M, Andrew M. Venous thromboembolic complications in children. *J Pediatr,* 123:337–346, 1993.

Evans DA, Wilmott RW: Pulmonary embolism in children. *Pediatr Clin North Am* 41:569–584, 1994.

Flynn JT, Pasco DA: Calcium channel blockers: Pharmacology and place in therapy of pediatric hypertension. *Pediatr Nephrol* 15:302–316, 2000.

National Heart, Lung and Blood Institute: Report of the task force on blood pressure control in children—1987. *Pediatrics* 79:1–25, 1987.

National High Blood Pressure Education Program Working Group on Hypertension Control in Children and Adolescents: Update on the 1987 Task Force Report on High Blood Pressure in Children and Adolescents: A working group report from the National High Blood Pressure Education Program. *Pediatrics* 98:649–658, 1996.

Sinaiko AR: Hypertension in children. *N Engl J Med* 335: 1968–1973, 1996.

Temple ME, Nahata MC: Treatment of pediatric hypertension. *Pharmacotherapy* 20:140–150, 2000.

36

Age-Specific Neurologic Examination

Susan Fuchs

HIGH-YIELD FACTS

- The neurologic examination of the pediatric patient changes with age.
- Most of the pediatric neurologic examination can be obtained by observation alone.
- The persistence of primitive reflexes in the infant is indicative of central nervous system pathology.

Performing a neurologic examination on an infant or child is more difficult than examining an adult; it is therefore imperative that the evaluation be goal-oriented. The actual presence of a neurologic disorder, its location, and the appropriate evaluation and management all need to be determined in a short period. The issue is further complicated by the fact that the neurologic system in the infant is an evolving organ and the evaluation changes with age.

HISTORY

An accurate history obtained from the parents and child provides important information. Even children younger than 5 years can provide details if the questions are phrased appropriately. The history of the presenting complaint focuses on the major symptom, its duration, factors that exacerbate the problem, and associated complaints. The history includes the length of pregnancy, intercurrent infections, maternal drug history, method of delivery, and perinatal events, such as the need for re-suscitation or prolonged hospitalization. The developmental history includes the age when the child reached certain milestones, such as rolling over, sitting without support, standing, climbing, and running. A brief history regarding language development may be helpful. It may be useful to compare the patient's development with that of other siblings, which is often information that the parent can easily recall. If the child attends school, then poor grades, poor attention span, or other school problems will also provide important information. Review of the family history is important, as several neurodegenerative disorders are transmitted as recessive genes, whereas other disorders such as seizures and migraine headaches are often found in family members.

GENERAL PHYSICAL EXAMINATION

The physical examination includes height, weight, and head circumference, all of which are plotted on growth curves and compared with norms or prior measurements. Heart rate, respiratory rate, and blood pressure are evaluated. The general appearance of the child is important to note, as are obvious dysmorphic features. Cutaneous lesions such as café au lait spots, depigmentation, or angiomas are clues to phakomatoses. The presence of an unusual body odor may be a clue to a metabolic disorder. A thorough examination of the head, ears, neck, heart, lungs, and abdomen is performed.

NEUROLOGIC EXAMINATION

Toys, penlights, bubbles, and even the reflex hammer can be useful adjuncts to an examination, since a wealth of information is obtained by observing the child's behavior during play. Uncomfortable procedures such as fundoscopy and evaluation of pain sensation are left until the end of the examination.

A quick mental status examination is performed by asking the child to give his/her name, age, and birthday. Names of brothers, sisters, pets, or stuffed animals can be substituted. For older children and adolescents, questions about the date, month, and place are also appropriate.

If the child has an altered mental status, a quick assessment is performed using the APVU system (see Table 10-9). A more formal infant Glasgow Coma Scale (GCS) has been developed to assess younger patients (see Table 10-8).

After the child's mental status has been assessed, the neurologic evaluation continues with examination of the skull, looking for macrocephaly, microcephaly, or craniosynostosis. Palpation of the fontanelles for size as well as for pulsations can reveal increased intracranial pressure. Auscultation of the skull with the child standing, listening over both globes, the mastoid region, and temporal fossa, may reveal abnormal intracranial bruits that are heard with angiomas, hydrocephalus, and some tumors. Although many normal children have bruits, those that are especially loud or accompanied by a thrill indicate pathology. Transillumination over the frontal and occipital regions is done in a darkened room and may provide evidence of hydrocephalus, hydrancephaly, or Dandy-Walker cysts.

The evaluation of specific neurologic functions begins with the cranial nerves. The function of cranial nerve I is smell. Although this is not usually tested during the emergency department neurologic examination, it can be done by inhalation of an irritant such as ammonia or a comparison between two smells. The olfactory nerve is not functional in the newborn, in whom its role is performed by the fifth nerve. Cranial nerve II is tested by using visual acuity charts, or, in an infant, by offering objects to grab. While doing this, one can also check visual fields by bringing the objects slowly into the field of vision and noting when the infant's head or eyes turn to the object or by asking a young child to say "yes" or "now" when they first see the object. Pupillary response to light is an indication of an intact second nerve, as this requires reception by the second nerve and outflow from the third nerve. A fundoscopic exam is performed, noting the disc, retina, and macula. Of note, the blink reflex does not appear until 3 to 4 months of age.

The function of cranial nerves III, IV, and VI is evaluated by observing the size of the pupils, the eye position at rest, and the integrity of the extraocular muscles. A penlight or a toy can be moved across six positions of gaze, with the mother holding the child's head still, covering each eye in turn if necessary. Abnormalities that may be detected include lateral and downward deviation of an affected eye with third nerve paralysis, medial deviation with sixth nerve involvement, strabismus secondary to muscular imbalance, and nystagmus.

Cranial nerve V is assessed by asking the patient to open and close the mouth, which involves the use of the temporalis and masseter muscles. Trigeminal nerve lesions will result in deviation of the jaw to the affected side. Although the corneal reflex is another way to test this nerve, it is rarely needed except in comatose individuals. Cranial nerve VII is assessed by asking the child to smile or show the teeth and to close the eyes tightly against resistance. Upper motor neuron disorders affecting cranial nerve VII spare the upper part of the face, which receives innervation from both sides of the brain, whereas lower motor neuron disorders produce both upper and lower facial weakness. The sense of taste to the anterior two-thirds of the tongue is via cranial nerve VII and can be assessed by placing a cotton swab dipped in sugar or salt on the tongue. Cranial nerve VIII is roughly evaluated by ringing a bell or clinking a set of keys and observing whether the infant or child turns to the sound. The use of a tuning fork is usually not required. However, with an abnormal Weber test, there is lateralization of sound to one side when a tuning fork is placed in the midline. The sound is lateralized to the side of a conduction defect and away from a sensory deficit. In a search for nystagmus, vestibular function can be roughly evaluated by having a child "spin like a top" in both directions. Evaluation of phonation and the gag reflex tests cranial nerves IX and X, and watching the position of the tongue at rest and when extended tests cranial nerve XII. With a lesion of cranial nerve XII, the tongue deviates to the affected side. Cranial nerve XI supplies the sternocleidomastoid and trapezius muscles, which can be tested by evaluating the patient's ability to rotate the head and shrug the shoulders.

After testing mental status and cranial nerves, the child is evaluated for the presence of motor weakness. Observing the infant crawl, or the child walk or run, provides clues regarding which muscle groups require formal testing. Pronator drift is performed by having the child raise his or her arms above the head with the hands facing each other or outward with the palms up and the eyes closed. A positive drift is hyperpronation of the hand or movement of the weak side downward. To test weakness of the lower extremities, ask the child to lie on the stomach and maintain the knees in a bent position. For children, upper extremity and shoulder strength can be tested by holding them by their legs and asking them to walk on their hands (like a wheelbarrow). For infants older than 8 months, this can be modified by watching for the parachute response. The infant is held in the prone position (near the abdomen) over a soft surface and then moved quickly toward the surface (as if falling). The infant should extend the arms and wrists and be able to support the body weight on the arms.

Testing coordination involves assessment of cerebellar function, which may be difficult in young children. Although some may be able to perform finger-to-nose testing, it may only be possible to have the patient reach for an object and then watch for a tremor or overreaching. Rapid pronation-supination of the hand, repeated tapping of the examiner's hand ("high fives"), or tapping the foot can also help define pyramidal or extrapyramidal lesions. The tandem gait (heel to toe) walk is often difficult for the child to comprehend and can be difficult to interpret.

Sensory evaluation can be performed on an older child who understands the difference between sharp and dull or who can compare sensation between two areas, but such evaluation is not reliable in most young children and is almost impossible to perform in infants. One quick way to test sensation is to place a tuning fork over a bony prominence and watch for a look of surprise from the infant.

The Romberg test is commonly used to evaluate cerebellar function, but it is also useful for sensation. Ask the child to stand with the feet together, arms crossed in front of the body. If this is impossible, there is a cerebellar problem. If it is successful, ask the child to close the eyes. If he or she has trouble with balance or with feeling the feet on the floor, then a posterior column lesion or peripheral neuropathy is likely. A true cerebellar positive Romberg sign is when the child almost falls down as opposed to wavering a little.

Many primitive reflexes are present at birth that disappear as the child grows. In certain neurologic diseases, these reflexes persist and serve as markers of pathology (Table 36-1). The Moro reflex is elicited by placing the infant in the supine position, elevating the head to 30 degrees, and allowing it to fall back into the examiner's hand. The appropriate response is extension and abduction of the shoulders, followed by adduction of the arms. An abnormality signifies a diffuse process affecting the central nervous system. The tonic neck reflex is provoked by turning the head to the side while the child is supine. The arm and leg on the side to which the neck is turned assume an extensor posture and the opposite arm and leg flex. The normal child will attempt to break the reflex position. Persistence of this reflex beyond 6 to 9 months can indicate a central nervous system lesion. In the palmar grasp reflex, an object placed in the infant's hand will produce flexion and the object will be grasped. Persistence of involuntary grasp can indicate infantile hemiplegia. In the root reflex, stroking the infant's cheek causes the mouth to be turned to the direction of the stimulus.

Standard deep tendon reflexes are relatively easy to evaluate, provided that the child is cooperative or can be distracted. These include the jaw jerk, which is elicited by placing one finger below the lower lip of a slightly open jaw and tapping the reflexes downward: the biceps, triceps, radial, patellar, and ankle reflexes. During their evaluation, one side is compared with another. Clonus is an exaggerated movement that indicates increased reflex excitability. Sustained ankle clonus is abnormal, but several beats may be normal in some children. The Babinski reflex involves stimulation of the plantar surface of the foot from the heel along the lateral border of the sole, crossing over the distal end of the metatarsals to the big toe. A positive response is dorsiflexion of the big toe with separation (fanning) of the other toes; it indicates pyramidal tract pathology. However, a positive Babinski reflex can be seen in most normal 1-year-olds and may exist until 2½ years of age.

Table 36-1. Normal Reflexes

Reflex	Appearance	Disappearance (mo)
Moro	Birth	5–6 mo
Palmar grasp	Birth	6 mo
Plantar grasp	Birth	8–15 mo
Root response	Birth	3–4 mo
Tonic neck	Birth	5–6 mo

BIBLIOGRAPHY

Menkes JH: *Textbook of Child Neurology,* 5th ed. Baltimore, Williams & Wilkins, 1995.

Mickel HS: The neurologic exam in the emergency setting, in Tintinalli JE, Krome RL, Ruiz E (eds): *Emergency Medicine: A Comprehensive Study Guide,* 5th ed. New York: McGraw-Hill, 2000, pp 1415–1422.

Swaiman KF: Neurologic examination after the newborn period until 2 years of age, in Swaiman KF, Ashwal A (eds): *Pediatric Neurology: Principles & Practice,* 3d ed. St Louis: Mosby, 1999, pp 31–38.

37

Altered Mental Status and Coma

Susan Fuchs

HIGH-YIELD FACTS

- For coma to occur, there must be an insult to both cerebral hemispheres or to the reticular activating system.
- Decorticate posturing signifies dysfunction of the cerebral hemispheres with an intact brainstem.
- Decerebrate posturing signifies a lesion of the midbrain.
- Intussuception can have a "neurologic" presentation ranging from lethargy to obtundation.

The term *altered mental status* refers to an abberation in a patient's level of consciousness. It always implies serious pathology and mandates an aggressive search for the underlying disorder. More precise terminology describes the degree of altered mental status and has important implications for differential diagnosis and management, as follows:

- *Lethargy* is a state of reduced wakefulness in which the patient displays disinterest in the environment and is easily distracted but is easily arouseable and can communicate.
- *Delirium* is characterized by disorientation, delusions, hallucinations, fearful responses, irritability, and sensory misperception.
- *Obtundation* is severe blunting of alertness with a decreased response to stimuli.
- *Stupor* exists when the patient can only be aroused by extremely vigorous and repeated stimulation.
- *Coma* occurs when a profound reduction in neuronal function results in unresponsiveness to sensory stimuli. It constitutes the most severe

manifestation of altered mental status. Coma is further categorized depending on the area of the brain affected.

Several scoring systems exist that permit standardized, objective, and reproducible assessment of the degree of altered mental status and allow effective communication among health care providers. The most widely used is the Glasgow Coma Scale (GCS), which scores three responses:

- Eye opening
- Best verbal response
- Best motor response

The GCS has been modified so that it can be applied to infants and children (see Table 10-8).

PATHOPHYSIOLOGY

In general, patients with altered mental status have suffered a diffuse insult to the brain. For patients with no history of trauma, metabolic abnormalities, toxic ingestions, and infectious etiologies such as meningitis and encephalitis are the common causes. The more severe the insult, the greater the alteration in mental status.

For coma to occur, the underlying abnormality must involve damage to either both cerebral hemispheres or to the ascending reticular activating system, which transverses the brainstem through the upper pons, midbrain, and diencephalon and plays a fundamental role in arousal. Coma does not result from isolated injury to one cerebral hemisphere but can result from damage to the reticular activating system, despite a normally functioning cerebral cortex.

Coma can result from structural damage to tissue, infectious processes, metabolic derangements, toxic ingestions, and inadequate cerebral perfusion. Metabolic, infectious, and toxic etiologies tend to produce diffuse but symmetric deficits, such as confusion, that precede other abnormalities, such as motor deficits. Structural lesions result in focal deficits that progress in a predictable pattern. Supratentorial lesions produce focal findings that progress in a rostral-caudal fashion, whereas subtentorial lesions result in brainstem dysfunction followed by a sudden onset of coma, cranial nerve palsies, and respiratory disturbances. The causes of coma are listed in Table 37-1; many of these are included in the mnemonic "tips from the vowels."

Table 37-1. Etiology of Altered Mental Status Based on the Mnemonic
"Tips From the Vowels"

Mnemonic Device	Category	Cause
A	Abuse	Head trauma
		Shock
E	Epilepsy (and other causes of seizures)	Hypernatremia
		Hypocalcemia
		Hypoglycemia
		Hyponatremia
		Postictal state
		Status epilepticus
	Endocrine	Addison's disease
		Hyperthyroidism
		Hypothyroidism
		Inborn errors of metabolism
	Electrolyte disorders	Hypercalcemia
		Hypernatremia
		Hyponatremia
I	Infection	Brain abscess
		Encephalitis
		Meningitis
		Sepsis
		Subdural empyema
	Intussusception	Neurologic presentation
O	Overdose	Alcohol
		Carbon monoxide
		Lead
		Opiates
		Salicylates
		Sedatives
U	Uremia (and other metabolic causes)	Hemolytic uremic syndrome
		Hepatic encephalopathy
		Hypoxia
		Renal failure
		Reye's syndrome
T	Trauma	Child abuse
		Head trauma
		Hemorrhage
	Tumor	
I	Insulin-related problems	Diabetic ketoacidosis
		Hyperglycemia
		Hypoglycemia
		Ketotic hypoglycemia
		Nonketotic hypoglycemia
P	Psychogenic	Diagnosis of exclusion
S	Shock	Anaphylactic
		Cardiogenic
		Hemorrhagic
		Hypovolemic
		Neurogenic
		Septic
	Stroke (and other CNS lesions)	Arteriovenous malformations
		Hemorrhage
	Shunt-related problems	Hydrocephalus
		Shunt dysfunction

HISTORY

The history of a patient with altered mental status focuses on identifying the underlying abnormality. Events prior to the onset of mental status changes are elicited, including prior headache, febrile illness, trauma, and drug ingestion. Associated symptoms such as vomiting, diarrhea, or respiratory difficulties are important clues. Past medical history, including diabetes, seizure disorder, or underlying heart or kidney disease, is elicited. A prior history of similar episodes may imply an underlying metabolic abnormality, such as an inborn error of metabolism.

PHYSICAL EXAMINATION

The physical examination focuses on assessing the degree of neurologic impairment and localizing the lesion responsible for the patient's altered mental status. Particular attention is paid to the vital signs, including temperature. Many systemic illnesses that result in central nervous system dysfunction are associated with profound abnormalities in basic physiologic parameters. Conversely, primary central nervous system pathology often affects cardiovascular and respiratory status. Airway, breathing, and circulation must be evaluated and managed prior to the remainder of the examination.

Examination of the head includes palpation for hematoma or fracture, evaluation of the position of the eyes, reactivity of the pupils, and a funduscopic examination looking for papilledema or retinal hemorrhages. The ears and nose are examined for evidence of bleeding, and the neck is examined for evidence of tenderness or rigidity. Auscultation of the head and neck for bruits is performed. In an infant, palpation of the anterior fontanelle for fullness, depression, or pulsations can provide quick information about intracranial pressure.

Even the odor of the breath may provide clues as to the etiology of altered mental status. For example, diabetic ketoacidosis may be characterized by a fruity smell, hepatic coma by a musty odor, and uremic encephalopathy by a urine-like smell.

The skin is examined for jaundice, petechiae, or purpura. The chest is auscultated for signs of respiratory pathology, and the abdomen is palpated for the presence of hepatosplenomegaly or masses. The abdominal examination is especially important in infants, in whom intussusception is a potential cause of altered mental status. The general neurologic evaluation focuses on an exact description of the patient's mental status, which provides a baseline for comparison during the course of

illness. The cranial nerves and motor function are assessed for potentially localizing findings, which may indicate a mass lesion. For patients with severely depressed mental status, it is especially important to evaluate the response of the extremities to a painful stimulus. The biceps, triceps, patellar, and Achilles reflexes are tested for strength and symmetry, and the patient is evaluated for the presence of a Babinski response, which indicates an upper motor neuron lesion.

For patients in coma, the area of the brain involved can be localized by examination of body position, pupil size and reactivity, respiratory pattern, and spontaneous and induced eye movements.

The patient's posture is the most obvious physical manifestation of illness. In decorticate posturing the arms are flexed and the legs extended. This position implies dysfunction of the cerebral hemispheres with preservation of the brainstem. Decerebrate posturing is characterized by extension of both upper and lower extremities with internal rotation, which may occur during examination as a response to pain. It implies a lesion at the level of the midbrain. In the event of uncal herniation, decerebrate posturing can be unilateral (although ipsilateral pupillary dilation is likely to occur first). Flaccid paralysis implies a diffuse lesion involving both hemispheres and brainstem.

The patient's respiratory pattern is another obvious clue to the nature of coma. Consistent hyperventilation can occur as compensation for a metabolic acidosis, such as occurs in diabetic ketoacidosis or severe salicylate toxicity. It can also occur in lesions of the midbrain and lower pons. Cheyne-Stokes respiration is characterized by periods of tachypnea followed by apnea. It signifies a bilateral hemispheric abnormality with an intact brainstem. In some cases it implies impending temporal lobe herniation. Ataxic breathing is characterized by an irregular rate and depth and can occur with lesions at the level of the pons and medulla.

Examination of the pupils is a fundamental part of the neurologic examination of the comatose patient. Small, reactive pupils imply metabolic lesions affecting the cerebral hemispheres, or a lesion in the medulla. Pinpoint, nonreactive pupils can result from a metabolic derangement or a lesion in the lower pons. Midposition and fixed pupils imply a lesion in the midbrain or upper pons. In the presence of coma, a unilateral dilated pupil can imply third nerve compression from uncal herniation. In the late phase of herniation, the pupil is nonreactive. Bilateral fixed pupils can imply tectal herniation and can be seen in severe hypothermia. In some cases they imply severe permanent brain damage.

Reflex eye movements help to delineate a brainstem lesion. Tests include the oculocephalic (doll's eye) reflex and the oculovestibular (caloric) response. To test the oculocephalic reflex, the head is passively moved from side to side. When brainstem function is intact, the eyes move together toward the side opposite that which the head is turned. With a lesion of the cerebral hemispheres, the horizontal doll's eye reflex is intact, whereas in lesions of the midbrain and upper pons it is impaired. In lesions of the lower pons and medulla it is absent. It can also be abnormal secondary to medications used for sedation. The doll's eye maneuver is easily performed in the emergency department. It is contraindicated if neck trauma is suspected.

The oculovestibular response is evaluated by elevating the patient's head to 30 degrees and irrigating one or both ear canals with cold water. In normal patients, irrigation produces lateral nystagmus with the quick phase away from the irrigated ear. An aysmmetric response can be seen with brainstem lesions, and bilateral loss can be seen with metabolic or structural brainstem lesions. In the unconscious patient, only the slow deviation to the irrigated ear is seen. If warm water is used instead, the quick phase is toward the irrigated ear (COWS = cold opposite, warm same).

LABORATORY TESTING

All patients with altered mental status should have a bedside glucose determination, and the serum glucose should be checked. Other helpful studies include complete blood count with differential and platelets, electrolytes, calcium, renal functions, and urinalysis. In some cases, arterial blood gas and serum ammonia are indicated. Patients who may have ingested a toxin require a toxicology screen. Infants suspected of suffering from inborn errors of metabolism require testing for urine and serum amino acids, liver function, thyroid function, plasma free fatty acids, and serum carnitine. If infection is suspected, cultures are obtained from the blood, urine, and cerebrospinal fluid. Lumbar puncture is withheld until increased intracranial pressure is excluded.

Radiographic examination of the cervical spine is performed if there is any suspicion of trauma. If physical examination findings suggest a structural lesion, suspected herniation, or increased intracranial pressure, a computed tomography scan should be performed. An electroencephalogram is useful to diagnose seizures and some metabolic and infectious disorders but is not an emergency department procedure, unless needed to diagnose status epilepticus.

THERAPY

The first priority in the emergency department management of a patient with altered mental status is stabilization of the airway, breathing, and circulation. Intubation is required for patients with altered mental status who have lost protective airway reflexes and who are at risk for aspiration. Intubation is also indicated for patients with evidence of critically increased intracranial pressure (ICP).

All patients receive oxygen, naloxone, and, if hypoglycemia is suspected, 0.5 to 1.0 g/kg of glucose. Patients who are hypotensive are resuscitated with crystalloids. Fluids are titrated carefully for patients who may have increased intracranial pressure, in whom overaggressive hydration can precipitate herniation. Hypotension is avoided, since it can result in cerebral hypoperfusion and ischemia.

Hyperventilation produces vasoconstriction of the cerebral arteries and has been used as the treatment for impending herniation due to elevated ICP. However, the P_{CO_2} is best not reduced below 30 to 35 torr because severe vasoconstriction and cerebral ischemia can result. Mannitol or furosemide may be useful adjuncts for patients with severely increased ICP, but careful fluid balance must be maintained to avoid hypotension.

Additional therapy is directed at maintaining normal body temperature, controlling seizures, and correcting any acid-base or electrolyte abnormalities. Further management in the emergency department may include the administration of antibiotics, or antidote therapy in the case of toxins.

DISPOSITION

Patients with significant alteration in mental status are best managed in an intensive care unit. For patients with milder disease, the decision to admit to the hospital or discharge from the emergency department largely depends on the etiology of the problem.

SPECIAL CONSIDERATIONS

Several causes of altered mental status and coma are characteristic of the pediatric population and deserve special mention. None are common, but all represent serious problems that confront the emergency physician.

Lead Encephalopathy

Although lead toxicity severe enough to cause encephalopathy is now uncommon, it is a consideration in the differential diagnosis of any child with profoundly altered mental status or coma. Lead encephalopathy can be associated with increased ICP and seizures. Patients with lead encephalopathy often have a history of pica, and parents may have noted abdominal pain, constipation, and vomiting prior to the development of encephalopathy. The evaluation and management of lead encephalopathy is discussed in Chapter 97.

Intussusception

Intussusception is a fairly common gastrointestinal emergency in children younger than 3 years. Although this entity commonly presents with episodes of intermittent abdominal pain and vomiting, there is a "neurologic presentation" in which the child manifests a depressed level of consciousness that can range from lethargy to obtundation. The overall appearance of the patient can mimic shock, with fulminant sepsis a consideration. In some cases the abdominal exam may reveal a mass, and rectal examination shows hemepositive or "currant jelly" stools. Intussusception is discussed in detail in the section on gastrointestinal surgical emergencies.

Reye's Syndrome

Reye's syndrome is a disorder characterized by the acute onset of encephalopathy, often developing about 2 weeks following a viral infection. The diagnosis is based on the presence of encephalopathy, elevated liver enzymes, and the presence of microvesicular fatty changes in the liver. The exact pathophysiology is unknown, but it may involve the interaction of salicylates and certain viruses, especially influenza and varicella. Many feel that the decreased use of aspirin in the treatment of these illnesses may have contributed to the decline of Reye's syndrome. Others suggest that the decline is due to advances in diagnosis of inborn errors of metabolism (especially medium-chain acyl-CoA dehydrogenase [MCAD] deficiency).

The syndrome begins with unremitting vomiting and can progress from lethargy to disorientation, combativeness, and, in severe cases, coma. The encephalopathy is characterized by increased ICP, which at high levels can lead to cardiovascular and respiratory instability and often death. The increased ICP appears to be the predominant factor in influencing outcome. The mechanism resulting in encephalopathy is unknown.

Reye's syndrome in the United States occurred mainly in children younger than 12 to 13 years, but, especially in the United Kingdom, it has been described in patients younger than 1 year. In infants, vomiting may be less prominent, and, unlike older patients, seizures are common.

The encephalopathy is associated with elevated liver function tests, and serum ammonia is generally three times normal. Characteristically, serum bilirubin is only slightly elevated and jaundice is absent. Hypoglycemia is common in infants and in patients with severe encephalopathy. Fatty microvesicular metamorphosis of the liver can be confirmed by biopsy. At an ultrastructural level, mitochondrial abnormalities may be present and may reflect a fundamental lesion in the syndrome.

A system has been developed that categorizes Reye's syndrome into five stages of severity according to the degree of encephalopathy:

- Stage 1: lethargy, with an otherwise normal neurologic examination
- Stage 2: stupor or combatativeness, with inappropriate verbal response
- Stages 3 to 5: increasing degrees of coma.

In a clinical situation, it can be difficult to distinguish stage 2 from stage 3. A distinguishing characteristic is that, in stage 2, the patient's response to pain is generally purposeful, whereas in stage 3 the response to pain is decorticate.

If the diagnosis of Reye's syndrome is entertained, aggressive management is indicated. To avoid overhydration and worsening of cerebral edema, intravenous fluids are administered at or slightly below maintenance requirements. Hypoglycemic patients may require D10 or D15. Patients who are not arousable to voice or light pain are candidates for elective intubation and ventilation. In practice, this occurs at stage 2. Mannitol or furosemide may be required for control of ICP. Some centers institute intracranial pressure monitoring to guide therapy. In some cases, barbiturate coma and decompressive craniotomy have been utilized, but their efficacy is unknown. The need for a liver biopsy to confirm the diagnosis is controversial.

Early intervention can potentially avert the progression of encephalopathy and avoid serious morbidity and mortality. Patients with stage 1 disease usually recover completely. Surviving patients with more severe encephalopathy can suffer permanent neuropsychiatric impairment.

Inborn Errors of Metabolism

Numerous inborn errors of metabolism can present early in life with vomiting, seizures, and altered mental status. Some, including disorders of branched chain amino acids and ketogenesis (such as MCAD and carnitine deficiency) can result in metabolic acidosis. Others, including disorders of ureagenisis such as like arginosuccinic aciduria, citrullinemia, and ornithine transcarbamylase (OTC) deficiency are not associated with metabolic acidosis. Laboratory diagnosis involves examination of urine and plasma for amino acids, organic acids, and carnitine. Appropriate consultation is required to outline and obtain the specific therapies that exist for some of these disorders.

Hypoglycemia

In any patient with altered mental status, hypoglycemia is a consideration. Although it is usually caused by fasting or the administration of exogenous insulin in known diabetics, it is associated with many serious disease states, including sepsis. In the pediatric population, there are also some special diagnostic considerations. Hypoglycemia is discussed more fully in the section on endocrinologic emergencies.

Ketotic Hypoglycemia

Ketotic hypoglycemia occurs in young children, generally between 18 months and 5 years of age. There is often a history of low birth weight. It accounts for up to 50 percent of cases of recurrent hypoglycemia in children.

Attacks are often associated with intercurrent illness or fasting and often occur in the morning. Ketone formation is provoked by hypoglycemia and ketonuria is generally present. Patients respond to the administration of glucose but do not respond to glucagon. The exact pathogenesis is unknown. Children tend to "outgrow" the syndrome.

Nonketotic Hypoglycemia

When a physiologically normal child is hypoglycemic, ketones are formed from the breakdown of fat. The absence of ketones can imply an enzyme defect in fatty acid oxidation such as MCAD. Other causes include hyperinsulism, which occurs with endogenous sources of insulin that can be secondary to a lesion such as nesidioblastosis or islet cell adenoma. In children with recurrent hypoglycemia who do not have ketonuria, evaluation includes urine for organic acids and insulin levels. Referral to an endocrinologist is indicated.

Congenital Adrenal Hyperplasia

In a child with congenital adrenal hyperplasia, hypoglycemia may result from the absence of cortisol. A constellation of symptoms such as lethargy, vomiting, dehydration, and altered mental status should suggest this disorder. Virilization may be present or absent. Emergency treatment includes intravenous fluid therapy with saline and glucocorticoid administration.

BIBLIOGRAPHY

Jennet B, Teasdale G: Aspects of coma after severe head injury. *Lancet* 1:878, 1977.

Orlowski JP: Whatever happened to Reye's syndrome? Did it ever really exist? *Crit Care Med* 27:1582–1587, 1999.

Plum F, Posner JB: *The Diagnosis of Stupor and Coma,* 3d ed. Philadelphia: FA Davis, 1980.

Sarnaik AP: Reye's syndrome: Hold the obituary. *Crit Care Med* 27:1674–1676, 1999.

Taylor DA, Ashwal S: Impairment of consciousness and coma, in Swaiman KF, Ashwal S (eds): *Pediatric Neurology: Principles and Practice.* St Louis: Mosby, 1999, pp 861–872.

Vannucci RC, Wasiewski WW: Diagnosis and management of coma in children, in Pellock JM, Myer EC (eds): *Neurologic Emergencies in Infancy and Childhood,* 2d ed. Boston: Butterworth-Heinemann, 1993, pp 103–122.

38

Seizures
Susan Fuchs

HIGH-YIELD FACTS

- For febrile patients, the etiology of the fever should be investigated if it has not been determined on physical examination. A lumbar puncture is performed in any patient suspected of having a central nervous system infection.

- For most patients with a generalized seizure, no focal findings on physical examination, and no history of trauma, there is little use for a computed tomography (CT) scan. Neuroimaging should be reserved for those with focal seizure, abnormal neurologic examination, suspected intracranial mass lesion, or infection.

- A magnetic resonance image is generally preferable over a CT scan as small tumors, hamartomas, or temporal lobe lesions are seen better. If trauma is suspected, CT scan is preferred for detection of acute hemorrhage.

- Any child who experiences a first focal seizure or who has an abnormal neurologic examination should be considered for hospital admission, with neurologic consultation. If the child has a first focal seizure, a nonfocal neurologic examination, a negative emergency department workup, and is stable, further workup, can be performed on an outpatient basis, in consultation with the child's primary physician, neurologist, and the parents or caretakers.

- For patients with a history of an isolated seizure, the decision to initiate therapy should be made in conjunction with a pediatric neurologist.

- Neonatal seizures are commonly related to perinatal asphyxia, metabolic abnormalities, especially hypoglycemia and hypocalcemia, central nervous system infections, and perinatal hemorrhage, but central nervous system infections in neonates can also present with seizures. Less commonly, seizures are related to inherited metatabolic abnormalities, including urea cycle defects and abnormalities in amino acid metabolism.

- For patients in whom an inherited metabolic defect is considered, serum ammonia is measured, as are serum and urine amino acids. Some defects are associated with metabolic acidosis; therefore an arterial blood gas and serum lactate are indicated.

- Phenobarbital (10 to 20 mg/kg intravenously) is the drug of choice for neonatal seizures, with phenytoin (10 to 15 mg/kg) the second choice. In refractory seizures, pyridoxine (50 to 100 mg intravenously) is indicated, to treat the potential for pyridoxine-dependent seizures.

- For the first simple febrile seizure, there are no required laboratory studies other than a bedside glucose determination.

- Benzodiazepines are usually effective treatment of actively seizing patients but are not useful for long-term seizure control. The administration of a long-acting antiseizure medication, such as phenytoin or phenobarbital, is indicated after seizures are controlled with benzodiazepines.

A seizure results from a paroxysmal electrical discharge of neurons within the brain. These discharges occur in various locations and may spread in different directions and at different speeds, resulting in several types of seizures, each with its own clinical manifestation. Epilepsy is defined as two or more unprovoked seizures. The incidence of childhood epilepsy is 40 per 100,000 children per year, with an incidence of 120 in 100,000 in the first year of life.

CLASSIFICATION

Seizures are fundamentally classified as partial or general. Partial seizures were formerly known as focal seizures. Partial seizures are subdivided as follows:

- Partial simple seizures, in which there is no impairment in consciousness
- Complex partial seizures, in which consciousness is impaired
- Partial seizures that evolve into secondary generalized seizures.

Generalized seizures are categorized by type of clinical seizure (EG, absence, myoclonic, tonic).

Simple partial seizures can have motor manifestations that remain focal or that spread (march) to other motor groups. They can also occur without motor involvement but with complex somatosensory symptoms and autonomic or behavioral manifestations. In general, simple partial seizures involve one cerebral hemisphere.

In addition to differing from simple partial seizures by alteration in consciousness, a predominant aspect of complex partial seizures is the presence of psychomotor automatisms, which are activities that occur during the seizure and for which the patient is amnestic. They can include such activities as chewing or swallowing, gestures such as clapping, or repetitive verbalizations. Postictal disorientation is a feature of psychomotor automatisms. Complex partial seizures can be simple at their onset, with alteration in consciousness developing as the seizure progresses, or they can begin with alteration of consciousness. Abnormalities in complex partial seizures can be unilateral or bilateral and can include both frontal and temporal regions of the cerebral hemispheres.

Partial seizures are further categorized into simple, complex, and those that evolve to secondary generalized seizures.

Generalized seizures involve both hemispheres of the brain and are classified by the type of clinical seizure, which can be divided into two broad groups. Absence (petit mal) seizures, are nonconvulsive and are characterized by an abrupt and brief loss of awareness (<15 seconds), which may include staring or eye blinking, without postictal confusion. It is often possible to induce these seizures by hyperventilation.

There are multiple manifestations of generalized seizures characterized by convulsions. Myoclonic (minor motor) seizures consist of unilateral or bilateral muscle contractions. The old classification of grand mal seizures now encompasses three distinct types of seizures: clonic seizures are characterized by rhythmic jerking and flexor spasms of muscles, tonic seizures by sustained muscle contraction resulting in rigidity, and tonic-clonic seizures by a combination of both. Atonic seizures involve a loss of muscle tone, which causes the child to fall to the floor.

Several distinct types of epilepsy occur only in children. Benign childhood epilepsy, also known as Rolandic epilepsy, has an onset between 3 and 13 years of age, often occurs upon awakening, and consists of facial movements, grimacing, and vocalizations. Diagnosis is based on finding midtemporal or centrotemporal spikes on an electroencephalogram (EEG).

West syndrome involves infantile spasms, characterized by sudden tonic contractions of the extremities, head, and trunk. The classic EEG finding is hypsarrhythmia. Lennox-Gastaut syndrome has its onset at 1 to 8 years of age and consists of multiple seizure types. These children often have seizures every day, and there is an associated deterioration in intelligence, as well as behavior disorders. It is diagnosed by the EEG finding of diffuse spikes and slow waves. The etiology can be primary (idiopathic) or secondary to infections, hypoxia, ischemia, intracranial hemorrhage, and degenerative disorders.

Neonatal seizures, febrile seizures, and status epilepticus are special syndromes and are discussed in detail in the following sections.

THE FIRST SEIZURE AND RECURRENT SEIZURES

The majority of children who present to the emergency department (ED) with seizures have suffered from a febrile convulsion or an exacerbation of a known seizure disorder. However, on occasion a patient may have experienced a first nonfebrile seizure, or may be experiencing recurrent manifestations of an atypical, undiagnosed seizure disorder. Aside from fever, the most common causes of seizures in children include infections, trauma, toxic exposures, and failure to take prescribed anticonvulsants. In addition, childhood seizures are often idiopathic. A more thorough list is included in Table 38-1.

History

In a patient with a suspected seizure, it is necessary to elicit detailed information regarding the episode itself, as well as preceding events. A clear description of the patient's level of consciousness during the episode, memory of the event, and any postictal phenomena are important in categorizing the seizure. Abnormal motor movements are noted and characterized as localized or general. Information regarding abnormal eye movements, facial grimacing, lip movements, and urinary or

Table 38-1. Etiology of Childhood Seizures

Infections	**Inborn Errors of Metabolism**
Meningitis	**Vascular**
Meningoencephalitis	Intracranial hematoma
Brain abscess	Embolism
Trauma	Infarction
Hemorrhage: epidural, subdural	Hypertensive encephalopathy
Posttraumatic	**Tumor**
Intoxication	**Psychological**
Lead	Hyperventilation
Cocaine	Breath-holding spells
PCP	**Congenital**
Amphetamine	Malformations
Aspirin	Birth asphyxia
Carbon monoxide	Neurocutaneous syndromes
Theophylline	**Other**
Drug Withdrawal (Anticonvulsants)	S/P DPT immunization
Metabolic	**Seizure Disorder**
Hypoglycemia	Noncompliance
Hyponatremia	Inadequate drug level
Hypernatermia	
Hypocalcemia	
Hypomagnesemia	

fecal incontinence is elicited. It is important to document the duration of the episode. Patients are questioned regarding the presence of any associated aura or somatosensory manifestations, such as visual or auditory hallucinations. If there have been recurrent episodes, a pattern may be evident, such as a predilection for the event to occur upon wakening, or when the patient is fatigued. A history of fever, trauma, prior seizures, drug use or withdrawal, underlying medical disorders, perinatal problems, developmental milestones, and a family history of seizures will help direct further evaluation.

Physical Examination

If the child is actively seizing, stabilzation and treatment are priorities. However, most children will have stopped seizing by the time of evaluation, and a thorough physical examination is required. Complete vital signs including temperature, heart rate, respiratory rate, and blood pressure are obtained. Determining the child's level of consciousness is important, as in the postictal period he or she may be sleepy or confused; if the level of consciousness does not return to normal within 1 hour after the seizure, additional studies may be needed. The head circumference is measured in a young infant to detect micro- or macrocephaly, and the head is palpated in any child with trauma to detect hematomas or skull fractures. Examination of the eyes includes an assessment of pupillary reactivity, establishing whether gaze is conjugate or disconjugate, and a funduscopic exam to detect papilledema or retinal hemorrhages. The presence or absence of meningismus and photophobia should be documented.

A thorough neurologic examination is performed. In some patients, examination may reveal Todd's paresis, a transient paralysis that can follow a seizure. It is usually unilateral and may involve both the face and extremities. The skin should be examined for petechiae, café au lait spots, and adenoma sebaceum.

Laboratory Evaluation

A bedside glucose check is performed on all patients to detect hypoglycemia. Other laboratory studies are based on the type of seizure and likely etiologies but will usually include a complete blood count, electrolytes, and glucose. Calcium, magnesium, phosphorus, and toxicology screens are obtained if they are clinically indicated, as are more complicated studies such as lead level and urine amino acids. If the child has been on antiseizure medication, a drug level is obtained.

For febrile patients, etiology of the fever should be investigated if not determined on physical examination. A lumbar puncture is performed in any patient suspected of having a central nervous system infection. However, if there are focal findings on physical examination or suspicion of a mass lesion, the lumbar puncture is delayed pending computed tomography (CT) of the brain.

Radiologic Evaluation

For most patients with a generalized seizure, no focal findings on physical examination, and no history of trauma, there is little use for a CT scan. Neuroimaging should be reserved for those with a focal seizure, an abnormal neurologic examination, a suspected intracranial mass lesion, or infection. Magnetic resonance imaging (MRI) is preferable to a CT scan as small tumors, hamartomas, or temporal lobe lesions are seen better. If trauma is suspected, a CT scan is preferred as an acute hemorrhage can be detected, but MRI is preferred for brain damage and old hemorrhage detection.

Electroencephalogram (EEG)

An EEG is the study of choice in the evaluation of childhood seizures. The most beneficial one is during a seizure (ictal EEG), but this is rarely possible. An EEG performed right after a seizure will probably show diffuse slowing, so it should be performed a few days to weeks after the seizure. Any focal finding warrants further studies, whereas a specific pattern can confirm the diagnosis of some types of seizures. An abnormal EEG (diffuse or focal) is also the most important predictor of seizure recurrence. Unfortunately, a normal EEG does not rule out a seizure disorder.

Disposition

Any child who experiences a first focal seizure or who has an abnormal neurologic examination should be considered for hospital admission, with neurologic consultation. If the child has a first focal seizure, a nonfocal neurologic exam, a negative ED workup, and is stable, further workup can be performed on an outpatient basis, in consultation with the child's primary physician, neurologist, and the parents/caretakers. A child with a first general-ized seizure does not necessarily need to be admitted and, depending on the type of seizure and etiology, may not require treatment until an EEG is performed.

Many parents will be uncomfortable taking their child home due to fear of another seizure. It is important to stress to parents that there is no evidence that a single seizure damages the brain. There is no way to absolutely predict seizure recurrence. However, it is increased when there is an underlying neurologic problem or an abnormal EEG. Other risk factors include partial seizures, a family history of seizures, prior febrile seizures, and the presence of Todd's paresis after a seizure. The duration of seizure, status epilepticus, age at first seizure (except focal motor seizures in infants younger than 2 years), and even treatment after a first seizure have no bearing on recurrence.

Many anticonvulsants are available, some of which have efficacy for certain types of seizures. Especially for patients with a history of an isolated seizure, the decision to initiate therapy should be made in conjunction with a pediatric neurologist (Table 38-2).

NEONATAL SEIZURES

These are seizures that occur during the first 28 days of life, although most occur shortly after birth. Because the cerebral cortex is immature, seizures in neonates can be extremely subtle, consisting only of lip smacking, eye deviation, or apnea. Motor activity can appear normal.

Neonatal seizures are commonly related to perinatal asphyxia, metabolic abnormalities, especially hypoglycemia and hypocalcemia, central nervous system infections, and perinatal hemorrhage. Central nervous system infections in neonates can also present with seizures. Less commonly, seizures are related to inherited metabolic abnormalities, including urea cycle defects and abnormalities in amino acid metabolism. These defects often become apparent after the infant begins feeding and usually cause lethargy, vomiting, and poor feeding as well as seizures. A rare cause of refractory seizures in neonates is inherited pyridoxine deficiency, which is inherited as an autosomal recessive trait (Table 38-3).

History

Information obtained in neonates with seizures should include the following:

- Gestational age of the patient
- Maternal infections

Table 38-2. Anticonvulsant Choice—Daily Oral Medications

Seizure Type	Drug of Choice (in order of preference)
Absence	Ethosuximide (Zarontin) 15–40 mg/kg/d bid
	Valproic acid (Depakene) or divalproex (Depakote) 10–45 mg/kg/d bid or qid
	Clonazepam (Klonopin) 0.05–0.3 mg/kg/d tid
	Lamotrigine (Lamictal) 5–15 mg/kg qd or bid if given alone; 1–5 mg/kg qd or bid when given with valproic acid
Atonic	Valproic acid, clonazepam, ethosuximide
Myoclonic	Valproic acid, clonazepam, lamotrigine
Partial	Carbamazepine (Tegretol/Carbatrol) 10–30 mg/kg/d bid or qid
	Phenytoin/fosphenytoin 4–8 mg/kg/d bid
	Valproic acid
	Phenobarbital 2–8 mg/kg/d qd/bid
	Primidone (Mysoline) 12–25 mg/kg/d bid/qid
	Gabapentin (Neurontin)[a] 30–45 mg/kg/d tid
	Oxcarazepin (Trileptal)[a] 20–40 mg/kg/d bid
	Tiagabine (Gabatril)[a] 1–2 mg/kg/d bid/qid
Generalized, tonic-clonic	Carbamazepine, phenytoin, phenobarbital, primidone, valproic acid, lamotrigine, topiramate (Topamax)[a] (5–10 mg/kg/d bid)
Infantile spasms	ACTH, prednisone

[a]Drug not FDA approved for children.

- Maternal drug use during pregnancy
- Maternal fever during labor
- Premature rupture of membranes
- Duration of labor
- Method of delivery
- Complications during delivery
- Need for the newborn to be aggressively resuscitated, which may indicate perinatal asphyxia
- Feeding pattern and the type of formula (important for a child who has a seizure after 3 days of age, when inherited metabolic defects become more likely)

Laboratory Evaluation

Bedside glucose determination, serum glucose, and electrolytes, calcium, and magnesium are obtained. In most instances, a lumbar puncture for bacterial and viral cultures, cell count, protein, glucose, and Gram's stain is performed as soon as possible. For patients in whom an inherited metabolic defect is considered, serum ammonia is measured, as are serum and urine amino acids. Some defects are associated with a metabolic acidosis; therefore arterial blood gas and, if possible, serum lac-

tate are indicated. Cranial ultrasound or CT can be useful to diagnose hemorrhage.

Treatment

The initial treatment is aimed at securing an adequate airway and ensuring oxygenation. If hypoglycemia (<40 mg/dL) is found, 5 to 10 mL/kg of $D_{10}W$ is administered intravenously, followed by an infusion of $D_{10}W$. Phenobarbital (10 to 20 mg/kg intravenously) is the drug of choice for neonatal seizures, with phenytoin (10 to 15 mg/kg) the second choice. In refractory seizures, pyridoxine (50 to 100 mg intravenously) is indicated, to treat the potential for pyridoxine-dependent seizures. Other metabolic abnormalities such as hypocalcemia (<7 mg/dL) and hypomagnesemia are corrected. Hypomagnesemia may be made worse by giving calcium.

FEBRILE SEIZURES

A febrile seizure is a seizure accompanied by a fever without evidence of intracranial infection, intracranial abnormality, toxins, or an endotoxin, such as *Shigella* neurotoxin. Febrile seizures usually occur between 6

Table 38-3. Causes of Neonatal Seizures

Hypoxia/Anoxia (Intrauterine or Perinatal)

Cerebral Ischemia (Secondary to Hypoxia/Anoxia)

Hemorrhage

Subarachnoid (birth trauma)
Subdural (birth trauma)
Intraventricular/intracerebral (prematurity)

Infection

Meningitis: group B streptococci, *Escherichia coli*
Meningoencephalitis: herpes, cytomegalovirus,
    toxoplasmosis

Metabolic

Hypoglycemia (especially first day of life)
Hypocalcemia (days 3–14)
Pyridoxine (vitamin B_6) deficiency

Drug Withdrawal

Narcotics

Inborn Errors of Metabolism (Days 4–7)

Aminoacidurias
    Maple syrup urine disease
    Phenylketonuria
Urea cycle defects: citrullinemia
Organic acidurias: proprionic acidemia

Structural Anomalies

Lissencephaly

Hereditary Disorders

Tuberous sclerosis

---

months and 5 years of age. Most febrile seizures are self-limited, generalized, and last for <15 minutes, in which case they are classified as simple. A complex or atypical febrile seizure lasts more than 15 minutes, occurs more than once in a 24-hour period, or has a focal component. Following a febrile seizure, children will usually have a postictal period during which they are lethargic, irritable, or confused.

Approximately 2 to 5 percent of all children will have a febrile seizure. They occur most commonly in children younger than 2 years. Twenty-five to 30 percent of children who have one febrile seizure will have a recurrence. The rate of recurrence is increased if the first seizure occurs before 1 year of age, is most likely in the first 6 to 12 months after the first seizure, and is not affected by the height of the fever or duration of the original seizure. Risk factors that correlate with an increased risk of subsequent epilepsy include a prolonged or unilateral seizure, a prior neurologic deficit, and a family history of epilepsy.

Any illness that causes fever can provoke a febrile seizure. The seizure usually occurs during the early phase of the infectious illness. Commonly implicated etiologies include upper respiratory tract infections, pharyngitis, otitis, pneumonia, gastroenteritis, urinary tract infections, and roseola. Febrile seizures can also occur after immunizations.

The history should focus on the presence of a preceding febrile illness. A description of the seizure and its duration is obtained from a witness. Preexisting neurologic abnormalities, developmental delay, and a family history of seizures are obtained to provide information regarding the risk of recurrence.

In most cases, the seizure will have terminated upon arrival in the ED, but the child may still be postictal. If the child continues to seize, anticonvulsant therapy as described in the section on status epilepticus is indicated. A complete physical examination focuses on determining the etiology of the fever, with particular attention to excluding central nervous system infection. In a febrile seizure the neurologic examination is normal. If a neurologic deficit exists, consider another etiology for the fever.

Laboratory Evaluation

A bedside glucose determination is done on all patients. For the first simple febrile seizure, there are no required laboratory studies. Complete blood count may be helpful for children with complex febrile seizures or if history or physical examination warrants it. It should be understood that the complete blood count may not be reliable, since the seizure may result in an elevated white blood cell count. If no source of fever has been determined by physical examination, a blood culture, urinalysis, and urine culture may be helpful. Electrolytes, calcium, and glucose are usually normal but may be useful if the history is compatible with an electrolyte imbalance. For example, a child with gastroenteritis in whom hyponatremia is a possibility will require electrolyte determination. The greatest controversy surrounds the need to perform a lumbar puncture in a child who has had a febrile convulsion. A child over 18 months who is nontoxic, with a normal mental status, and who has no evidence of neck pain or stiffness does not require a lumbar puncture. In a child who is still postictal or non-communicative (younger than 12 months) or who has received prior antibiotics, detecting meningismus may be difficult. In this situation, a lumbar puncture should be strongly considered.

Other studies such as skull radiographs, CT scan and even EEG are rarely helpful and not warranted after the first simple febrile seizure, unless history or physical findings suggests some underlying pathology.

Therapy

The initial management of the patient with a febrile seizure includes stabilizing the airway and ensuring adequate oxygenation. If the seizure persists for more than 10 minutes, anticonvulsant therapy is indicated.

Acetaminophen 15 mg/kg po or pr or ibuprofen 10 mg/kg po is administered to reduce the fever.

The benign nature of these seizures and the low risk of recurrence outweigh the benefits of the medications used, given their side effects. The ultimate decision should be made jointly between the parents and primary care physician. The medication commonly used is phenobarbital, which has been associated with undesirable side effects on behavior and mood. Valproic acid is an alternative; however, it can cause gastrointestinal upset and liver dysfunction. The use of oral or rectal diazepam prophylaxis at the time of fever has been studied and was found to be effective in reducing the risk of recurrence, but it also results in side effects including ataxia, lethargy, and irritability. Unfortunately, the use of antipyretic agents without concurrent anticonvulsants is not useful to prevent recurrent febrile seizures.

Disposition

Patients with febrile seizures may be discharged with follow-up by their primary care provider unless an underlying infection precludes discharge. If a bacterial infection is the etiology of the fever, it is treated with appropriate antibiotics. Parental reassurance and education regarding the benign nature of febrile seizures, the low risk of recurrence, and the low incidence of subsequent epilepsy are part of the discharge instructions.

STATUS EPILEPTICUS

Status epilepticus is a seizure lasting >30 minutes or two or more seizures without recovery of consciousness in between. Status can present in several forms, including generalized (convulsive and nonconvulsive) and partial seizures (convulsive and nonconvulsive). More than 50 percent of cases of status occur in children younger than 3 years of age, with the most in the first year of life. Approximately one-third of cases of status epilepticus are the initial presentation of epilepsy, one-third occur in patients with known epilepsy, and one-third occur due to an isolated brain injury/insult.

Etiologies for status epilepticus overlap those for a first seizure and include central nervous system infection, medication change or noncompliance in children on anticonvulsant therapy, head trauma, hypoxia, metabolic disorders, toxic ingestions, tumor, vascular lesions, and progressive neurologic disorders. Therefore, laboratory and diagnostic studies are similar to those for a first, or recurrent seizure, depending on the presumed etiology.

Initial therapy consists of meticulous attention to maintaining patency of the airway and adequacy of oxygenation and ventilation. Venous access is secured as soon as possible.

Head positioning, using the chin lift and jaw thrust, may open the airway, and an oral or nasal airway can be inserted. Oral suctioning may be required, so this should be available. High-flow oxygen is administered to all patients via mask or bag-valve-mask ventilation, and cardiac status and pulse oximetry are monitored continuously. Intubation may be necessary to oxygenate and ventilate the patient adequately. In addition, when administering anticonvulsants, especially benzodiazepines, intubation may be necessary because of respiratory depression.

After intravenous access is obtained, a bedside glucose determination is performed, and blood is drawn for complete blood count, electrolytes, BUN, glucose, calcium, and magnesium. For patients on anticonvulsant therapy, drug levels are obtained, and in some patients a toxicology screen may be indicated. If the glucose is <60 mg/dL, 0.5 to 1.0 g/kg of dextrose is given as $D_{25}W$, 2 to 4 mL/kg or $D_{50}W$ 1 to 2 mL/kg. If vascular access cannot be obtained, intraosseous access is an acceptable alternative in children younger than 6 years. In adolescents and adults, thiamine 100 mg intravenously is also given.

Drug therapy requires a clear plan, prompt administration of anticonvulsants in adequate doses, and with attention to side effects, such as hypoventilation or apnea. Benzodiazepines are effective for treatment of an actively seizing patient. Lorazepam (Ativan) has an onset of action of 2 to 3 minutes and a relatively long half-life of 12 to 24 hours. Side effects, although less frequent and of shorter duration than those of diazepam, include respiratory depression and sedation. The dose is 0.05 to 0.10 mg/kg, up to a maximum of 8 mg. Diazepam (Valium) is useful for control of seizures. It has an onset of action of 1 to 3 minutes, but its half-life of 15 to 20 minutes means that repeated doses are often required. The dose is 0.1 to 0.3 mg/kg, administered slowly by intravenous push. Side effects include respiratory depression, hypotension, sedation, and bradycardia. Diazepam can also be given rectally, using the intravenous formulation in a dose of 0.5 mg/kg for the first dose and 0.25 mg/kg for any subsequent dose, to a maximum of 20 mg. With rectal administration the onset of action is usually within 5 to 10 minutes. There is also a rectal gel form of diazepam (Diastat) available, with the dose via this formulation of 0.5 mg/kg for 2–5 yrs, 0.3 mg/kg for 6–11 yrs, and 0.2 mg/kg for $\geq$12 yrs. (It is available in several premeasured sizes: 2.5, 5.0, and 10 mg.) Midazolam (Versed) is a benzodiazepine that is rapidly absorbed after intramuscular injection and is an alternative to other benzodiazapines when it is impossible to obtain intravenous or intraosseous access. The dose is 0.1 mg/kg, with an onset of action in approximately 15 minutes.

Because benzodiazepines are not useful for long-term seizure control, the administration of a long-acting anti-seizure medication is indicated after seizures are controlled with benzodiazepenes. Phenytoin, when given intravenously, has rapid brain deposition but takes longer to control the seizure than a benzodiazepine (10 to 30 minutes). The loading dose is 20 mg/kg, which must be given slowly, 50 mg/min in adults or 1 mg/kg/min in children <50 kg. Side effects include hypotension and cardiac conduction disturbances (widened QT interval and arrhythmias), which if they occur should prompt a slower infusion or stopping the medication. Phenytoin will precipitate in glucose solutions, so it should be given directly into the vein, or in saline. Long-term seizure control can be accomplished by repeating half of the initial dose in 2 to 3 hours (intravenously or po) and then continuing the medication on a bid schedule (4 to 8 mg/kg), following serum levels.

Fosphenytoin is a new water-soluble prodrug of phenytoin. The conversion is 1.5 mg fosphenytoin = 1 mg phenytoin = 1 mg phenytoin equivalents (PE). (Therefore, 150 mg fosphenytoin = 100 mg phenytoin =100 mg PE, and all doses listed below are in phenytoin equivalents.) The intravenous loading dose is 20 mg PE/kg, which can be given at a rate of 3 mg PE/kg/min up to 150 mg PE/min. The only side effects are pruritus and paresthesias (groin). Because it is in a neutral solution and does not contain propylene glycol, it can also

be given intramuscularly (same dose as intravenously); however, peak levels are reached in 3 hours.

Phenobarbital is still a useful drug for treating status epilepticus, and it remains the drug of choice for neonatal seizures. Peak brain levels are reached in 10 to 20 minutes, and its duration of action is >48 hours. The loading dose is 20 mg/kg IV given slowly at 100 mg/min. Side effects include respiratory depression (additive with benzodiazepines), sedation, and occasionally hypotension. If seizures stop before the entire loading dose is given, the remainder can be given intravenously or even orally within 1 to 2 hours. Long-term therapy can be initiated in 24 hours using 2 to 8 mg/kg/day given twice a day, monitoring drug levels to avoid oversedation.

If status persists after giving one dose of a benzodiazepine followed by phenytoin or phenobarbital, an additional dose of benzodiazepine can be given. If the seizure persists after phenytoin was given, phenobarbital can be administered (or vice versa). In such cases, the risk of apnea is high, so assisted ventilation and possibly intubation may be required.

For refractory status, pentobarbital, diazepam, or midazolam may be given as continuous infusions. Pentobarbital is given as a loading dose of 5 to 20 mg/kg intravenously followed by an infusion of 0.5 to 3 mg/kg/h, to keep the level between 20 to 50 µg/mL and to produce burst suppression on the EEG, or cessation of epileptic activity. Vasopressors are often needed with pentobarbital coma, and the patient should be weaned off of the infusion to determine whether status has stopped. Diazepam is infused at a rate or 2 mg/kg/h, or midazolam is given initially as a loading dose of 0.15 mg/kg, then 0.5 to 1 µg/kg/min, and titrated upward (up to 4 µg/kg/min) over 60 minutes until there is cessation of seizures or burst suppression on the EEG. Other options include the use of intravenous propofol (3 to 6 mg/kg/h) or inhalation anesthetics such as isoflurane.

Therapy of nonconvulsive status epilepticus is similar to that of convulsive status, using a benzodiazepine, phenytoin, or fosphenytoin. For absence status a benzodiazepine can be followed by oral or nasogastric ethosuximide, valproic acid (oral, ng, pr, or intravenously), or clonazepam. (Do not give both valproic acid and clonazepam.) The dose for rectal valproic acid is 20 mg/kg of the liquid formulation, 30 to 60 mg/kg via ng, or 5 mg/kg intravenously.

Disposition

Any child who has received lorazepam or a long-acting anticonvulsant medication should be admitted to the hospital. Since diazepam is short acting, if no other drugs have been given, admission decisions can be individualized. Intensive care admission is obviously needed for any child still in status, requiring assisted or mechanical ventilation, or in whom the evaluation has revealed an etiology requiring close monitoring.

BIBLIOGRAPHY

American Academy of Pediatrics, Committee on Quality Improvement, Subcommittee on Febrile Seizures: Practice parameter: Long-term treatment of the child with simple febrile seizures. *Pediatrics* 103:1307–1309, 1999.

American Academy of Pediatrics: Provisional Committee on Quality Improvement, Subcommittee on Febrile Seizures: Practice parameter: The neurodiagnostic evaluation of the child with a first simple febrile seizure. *Pediatrics* 97:769–775, 1996.

Baumann RJ, Duffner PK: Treatment of children with simple febrile seizures: The AAP practice parameter. *Pediatr Neurol* 23:11–17, 2000.

Camfield PR, Camfield CS: Pediatric epilepsy: An overview, in Swaiman KF, Ashwal S (eds): *Pediatric Neurology: Principles and Practice,* 3d ed. St. Louis: Mosby, 1999, pp 629–633.

Dreifuss FE: Partial seizures (focal and multifocal), in Swaiman KF, Ashwal S (eds): *Pediatric Neurology: Principles and Practice,* 3d ed. St. Louis: Mosby, 1999, pp 646–660.

Haafiz A, Kissoon N: Status epilepticus: Current concepts. *Pediatr Emerg Care* 15:119–129, 1999.

Holmes GL, Riviello JJ: Midazolam and pentobarbital for refractory status epilepticus. *Pediatr Neurol* 20:259–264, 1999.

Kriel RL, Birnbaum AK, Cloyd JC: Antiepileptic drug therapy in children, in Swaiman KF, Ashwal S (eds): *Pediatric Neurology: Principles and Practice,* 3d ed. St. Louis: Mosby, 1999, pp 682–718.

Meek PD, Davis SN, Collins DM, et al: Guidelines for non-emergency use of parenteral phenytoin products: Proceedings of an expert panel consensus process. *Arch Intern Med* 159:2639–2644, 1999.

Pellock JM: Status epilepticus, in Swaiman KF, Ashwal S (eds): *Pediatric Neurology: Principles and Practice,* 3d ed. St. Louis: Mosby, 1999, pp 683–691.

Sabo-Graham T, Seay AR: Management of status epilepticus in children. *Pediatr Rev* 19:306–309, 1998.

Stafstrom CE: The pathophysiology of epileptic seizures: A primer for pediatricians. *Pediatr Rev* 19:342–351, 1998.

Tasker RC: Emergency treatment of acute seizures and status epilepticus. *Arch Dis Child* 79:78–83, 1998.

39

Syncope

Susan Fuchs

HIGH-YIELD FACTS

- Most syncope in children is neurocardiogenic.
- Situational events that cause a Valsalva-like maneuver can cause syncope.
- Prolonged Q-T syndrome is an uncommon but important cause of syncope in children.
- A "tilt-table" test may help to diagnose neurocardiogenic syncope.

Syncope refers to a sudden and transient loss of consciousness and postural tone. Although in the pediatric age group it accounts for less than 1 percent of emergency department visits, 15 to 50 percent of children will have experienced a syncopal episode by age 18. Syncope can be a manifestation of serious underlying pathology and always warrants careful evaluation. Unlike the adult population, in which syncope often results from malignant cardiac arrhythmias, in the pediatric population it is more often secondary to neurally mediated causes and is therefore discussed in the section on neurologic emergencies.

PATHOPHYSIOLOGY

The pathophysiology of syncope varies with etiology (Table 39-1), but it always results from momentarily inadequate delivery of oxygen and glucose to the brain. Syncope can result from inadequate cardiac output, which can be secondary to obstruction of blood flow, or to an arrhythmia. It can also result from inappropriate autonomic compensation for the normal fall in blood pressure that occurs on rising from a sitting or supine position. Respiratory disturbances, especially hyperventilation that results in hypocapnia and cerebral vasoconstriction, can also cause syncope.

HISTORY

The first component in the evaluation of a patient with syncope is to determine that momentary loss of consciousness actually occurred. It is common for patients to confuse acute dizziness or vertigo with loss of consciousness. For patients who did indeed lose consciousness, the events antecedent to the syncopal episode are elicited. A sudden change in posture, emotional excitement, respiratory difficulty, palpitations, and any history of trauma are essential information. Past history of syncope is sought, as is any history of medication or drug ingestion that would explain a precipitous fall in blood pressure. Patients are queried carefully about any history of heart disease.

An important consideration in any patient with a history of loss of consciousness is the possibility that the patient may have suffered a seizure. In contrast to syncope, seizures are usually accompanied by some form of muscle twitching or convulsions, and are usually followed by a postictal phase, during which the patient has mental status changes. Convulsions are unusual during syncopal episodes except during very severe events, and patients generally have normal mental status upon recovery from the episode.

PHYSICAL EXAMINATION

The physical examination focuses upon establishing the hemodynamic stability of the patient. Particular attention is paid to vital signs, especially to pulse and orthostatic blood pressure. A positive "tilt test" is a decrease in systolic blood pressure by 20 mmHg accompanied by an initial elevation in heart rate (20 beats per minute), which can be followed rapidly by bradycardia and syncope. The patient's mental status is carefully evaluated, and a full neurologic examination is performed.

For all patients, a careful cardiac examination is indicated. The regularity of the pulse is noted, as is the quality of the peripheral pulses. The heart is auscultated carefully to detect the presence of a murmur that may indicate congenital heart disease, especially aortic stenosis. The presence of gallops, rubs, thrills, or carotid bruits is noted. The quality and presence of all peripheral pulses are evaluated. Diminished pulses should prompt blood pressure measurements in all extremities to check for coarctation of the aorta.

Table 39-1. Causes of Syncope

Neurocardiogenic (Vasodepressor)

Orthostatic hypotension
Environmental triggers
Excess vagal tone
Situational syncope
Reflex syncope (pallid breath-holding spells)

Cardiac

Arrhythmias
  Supraventricular tachycardias
  Atrial flutter
  Wolfe-Parkinson-White syndrome
  Ventricular tachycardia
  Ventricular fibrillation
  Conduction disturbances
    Atrioventricular block
    Prolonged QTc
    Sick sinus syndrome
Obstructive lesions
  Aortic stenosis
  Pulmonic stenosis
  Idiopathic hypertrophic subaortic stenosis
  Mitral stenosis
  Coarctation of the aorta
  Tetralogy of Fallot
  Anomalous origin of the left coronary artery
  Tumors
Other
  Myocarditis
  Pericarditis
  Cardiac tamponade
  Cardiomyopathy
  Pulmonary hypertension

Noncardiac

Metabolic
  Hypoglycemia
  Hypocalcemia
  Hypomagnesemia
Toxic
Seizures
Psychogenic
  Hyperventilation
  Hysteria

LABORATORY STUDIES

The selection of laboratory studies of use in the evaluation of the syncope patient is largely guided by the history and physical examination. For a patient with a history of fasting or diabetes, blood glucose is indicated. In the presence of pallor or a history of blood loss, hemoglobin measurement is obtained. Electrolyte abnormalities are uncommon, but if an arrhythmia is suspected, then serum potassium, calcium, and magnesium are measured. Other studies including arterial blood gas, toxicology screening, and pregnancy testing may be indicated in certain clinical scenarios.

For all patients with a history of syncope, a 12-lead electrocardiogram is indicated. This provides information concerning potential conduction defects or arrhythmias. Special attention is paid to determination of the corrected QT interval (QTc), since prolonged QT syndrome is a cause of syncope in children. If abnormalities are seen, or if a cardiac abnormality is strongly suspected, further evaluation will include a 24-hour ambulatory (Holter) monitor and cardiology consultation.

SPECIFIC ETIOLOGIES OF SYNCOPE

Neurocardiogenic (Autonomic, Vasodepressor, Vasovagal) Syncope

The most common syncope in children is neurocardiogenic (vasodepressor or vasovagal) syncope. There is a sudden, brief loss of consciousness due to vasodilatation and decreased peripheral resistance, resulting in decreased arterial pressure, hypotension, bradycardia, and then decreased cerebral blood flow (Bezold-Jarisch reflex). Current theories suggest that the systemic vasodilation and the changes in heart rate and blood pressure are caused by sympathetic withdrawal, rather than increased parasympathetic (vagal) activity. Orthostatic hypotension may be a result of volume depletion, anemia, or drugs, but it can also be due to a paradoxic response to the vasodepressor reaction. A tilt-table test can be performed by a cardiologist to diagnose true neurocardiogenic syncope. A positive tilt-table test response, consisting of an initial increase in heart rate followed by bradycardia and syncope, may warrant drug therapy if frequent episodes occur.

Environmental factors, such as prolonged standing, heat, fatigue, crowding, or hunger, can trigger syncope. Emotional stress or a recent illness can also play a role. Patients may have symptoms beforehand such as blurred vision, dizziness, nausea, or pallor. This is what is commonly referred to as a "simple faint." Placing the person in a supine position with the head down usually results in improvement, although the patient may still complain of dizziness.

Another autonomic cause of syncope is excess vagal tone, which can imitate cardiac causes of syncope, as the children will have a low resting heart rate, junctional rhythms, and depressed sinoatrial node function. Exercise can increase this vagal tone and lead to syncope. Therefore, a history of syncope during exercise should prompt a full evaluation to rule out cardiac etiologies.

The term situational syncope can be used for those patients that have syncope triggered by specific events. The common denominator is that these actions are accompanied by a Valsalva-like maneuver. This includes coughing, micturition, hair-grooming, diving, weight-lifting, and sneezing. Another form is carotid sinus syncope, which occurs with head rotation or pressure on the carotid sinus. This can occur with shaving or tight collars.

Breath-holding spells are another example of reflex syncope. The age of onset of breath-holding spells is 6 to 18 months. There are actually two types of breath-holding spells:

- The pallid breath-holding spell is a form of reflex syncope. Pallid breath-holding spells are usually provoked by some mild antecedent trauma (usually to the head). The child may gasp and cry, then become quiet, lose postural tone and consciousness, and become pale. The child may have clonic movements in more severe episodes. They regain consciousness in less than 1 minute, but may be tired after the episode.

- A cyanotic breath-holding spell is often precipitated by anger or frustration. The child cries, becomes quiet and holds the breath in expiration. This apnea is associated with cyanosis and there may be a loss of consciousness, limpness, or opisthotonic posturing, with recovery usually within 1 minute.

Cardiac Syncope

Cardiac syncope is important to exclude, as this is the type that is truly life threatening. The differential in this subgroup includes arrhythmia, obstruction, and cyanosis. Arrhythmias that result in a heart rate that is too fast or too slow can cause a decrease in cardiac output and lead to decreased cerebral perfusion. Included in this group are supraventricular tachycardia (SVT), atrial tachycardia, Wolff-Parkinson-White syndrome, atrial flutter, ventricular tachycardia, and ventricular fibrillation. Conduction abnormalities such as AV block, sick sinus syndrome (may occur after cardiac surgery), and long QT syndrome (QTc > 440 msec) may be present. All these problems should be excluded by evaluation of a 12-lead electrocardiogram (ECG) and rhythm strip. If the problem is intermittent, 24-hour Holter monitoring and referral to a cardiologist should be included in the evaluation. Obstructive lesions can impair cardiac output and cerebral blood flow, leading to syncope. These include congenital lesions such as aortic stenosis, pulmonic stenosis, idiopathic hypertrophic subaortic stenosis (IHSS), mitral stenosis, coarctation of the aorta, tetralogy of Fallot, and anomalous origin of the left coronary artery. Acquired lesions include cardiac tumors and conditions secondary to myocarditis, pericarditis, cardiac tamponade, and cardiomyopathy. Evaluation includes a 12-lead ECG, chest radiograph, and prompt cardiology referral. The presence of chest pain and syncope with exercise, as well as a murmur on physical examination, can suggest left ventricular outflow obstruction due to IHSS or aortic stenosis. Cyanosis with or without syncope can result from increased resistance to pulmonary blood flow, causing an increase in the right-to-left shunting of blood. These spells can occur in children with tetralogy of Fallot, tricuspid atresia, and Eisenmenger's syndrome. Primary pulmonary hypertension can cause dyspnea on exertion but can also cause syncope from inadequate cardiac output.

Noncardiac Syncope

Noncardiac causes of syncope include neurologic, metabolic, psychological, and toxicologic problems. Seizures should be considered whenever there is a loss of consciousness, especially if accompanied by increased muscle tone or tonic-clonic movements. If syncope occurs while the child is in a recumbent position, a seizure is a likely diagnosis. The diagnostic workup should proceed based on the most likely etiology and type of seizure.

Hypoglycemia is the main metabolic disorder that can cause syncope. Prior to a loss of consciousness there is often a period of confusion and weakness. Hypocalcemia and hypomagnesemia can also cause syncope, but this is secondary to the arrhythymias generated by these disorders.

Psychological causes of syncope include hyperventilation and hysteria. Hyperventilation results in hypocapnia, which causes cerebral vasoconstriction and decreased cerebral blood flow. The patient may complain of shortness of breath and numb fingers before syncope ensues. Hysterical syncope occurs when the patient mimics a loss of consciousness and falls to the ground without injury. No abnormalities of heart rate, blood pressure, or skin color are detected, and clues regarding surrounding events may point to the correct diagnosis.

Drug-induced syncope can be caused by prescription

drugs, over-the-counter medications, or drugs of abuse. Drugs of abuse such as cocaine are well known to result in syncope as well as more serious cardiac arrhythmias. Marijuana, alcohol, and opiates can all cause a loss of consciousness. Inhalant use can result in ventricular tachycardia and death. Antihypertensive agents, phenothiazines, calcium channel blockers, nitrates, and barbiturates can block the increased blood pressure response, and β-blockers and digitalis will block the tachycardia needed to respond to decreased systemic vascular resistance prior to syncope. Some of the newer antihistamines can cause prolonged QT and even torsades de points, if given with macrolides or ketoconazole.

TREATMENT

Although most children will not require specific therapy, treatment should be based on the etiology and frequency of syncopal episodes. A child with hypoglycemia requires glucose, and one with anemia or hypotension may benefit from intravenous fluids while a workup for the etiology is ongoing. If a cardiac etiology is suspected, depending on the urgency of the situation, further studies could be performed on an inpatient or outpatient basis, but activity restrictions may be needed while awaiting evaluation. Treatment of a child with orthostatic syncope with β-blockers or mineralocorticoids should await formal tilt-table testing. If a neurologic etiology is suspected, treatment with anticonvulsive medications should be based on neurologic consultation. If the emergency department evaluation and workup is negative, with the likely etiology being a simple faint, reassurance

may be all that is needed. Avoidance of specific triggers or environmental factors can prevent most attacks. Those with a prodromal phase can be taught to sit or lie down before the loss of tone and consciousness occurs.

DISPOSITION

Most patients with syncope can be discharged from the emergency department with appropriate follow-up. Those who require admission have conditions with a cardiac origin that require urgent evaluation: arrhythmias (SVT, atrial flutter, ventricular tachycardia or fibrillation), conduction abnormalities (third-degree AV block, sick sinus syndrome), or newly diagnosed or worsening of obstructive lesions (aortic stenosis, pulmonic stenosis, IHSS). In addition, patients with arrhythmias precipitated by drugs require inpatient monitoring, for at least the half-life of the offending agent.

BIBLIOGRAPHY

Chaves-Carbello E: Syncope and paroxysmal disorders other than epilepsy, in Swaiman KF, Ashwal S (eds): *Pediatric Neurology.* St. Louis: Mosby, 1999, pp 763–772.

Kapoor WN: Syncope. *N Engl J Med* 343:1856, 2000.

Lewis DA, Dhala A: Syncope in the pediatric patients: A cardiologist's perspective. *Pediatr Clin North Am* 46:205, 1999.

Prodinger RJ, Reisdorff EJ: Syncope in children. *Emerg Med Clin North Am* 16:617, 1998.

Roddy SM: Breath-holding spells and reflex anoxic seizures, in Swaiman KF, Ashwal S (eds): *Pediatric Neurology.* St. Louis: Mosby, 1999, pp 759–762.

40

Ataxia

Susan Fuchs

HIGH-YIELD FACTS

- Ataxia can result from a variety of lesions, including damage to the peripheral nerves, spinal cord, cerebellum, and cerebral hemispheres. One of the most common etiologies is drug intoxication, especially with alcohol or phenytoin.

- Findings of cerebellar dysfunction include nystagmus, staggering, wide-based gait, and titubation. In addition, a sensory examination for light touch and pinprick, position, and vibration sense should be performed because lower extremity sensory impairment can cause ataxia.

- In a patient with acute ataxia, the history and physical examination focus on excluding acute infectious etiologies, such as meningitis or encephalitis, lesions that result in increased intracranial pressure, such as hemorrhage and tumors, and toxic ingestions.

- A common cause of ataxia in children younger than 5 years is acute cerebellar ataxia, a postinfectious phenomenon that often occurs about 2 weeks after a viral illness. The onset of ataxia is insidious and predominantly affects the gait, although dysmetria, nystagmus, and dysarthria can occur.

- In children, the most common cause of intermittent ataxia is a migraine headache that involves the basilar artery. Besides ataxia, associated symptoms include blurred vision, visual field deficits, vertigo, and headache.

- Chronic progressive ataxia has an insidious onset and progresses slowly over weeks to months. The differential diagnosis consists of brain tumors, hydrocephalus, and neurodegenerative disorders.

- The combination of ataxia, headache, irritability, and vomiting in a child younger than 6 years is characteristic of a medulloblastoma.

- Hereditary causes of ataxia include spinocerebellar ataxias, of which Freidrich's ataxia is the most common. This autosomal recessive ataxia, which usually manifests before 10 years of age, is characterized by ataxia, nystagmus, kyphoscoliosis, cardiomyopathy, and distal muscle wasting.

- Patients with progressive ataxia require an aggressive evaluation in the emergency department. All patients are examined for signs of increased intracranial pressure, which in some cases can be severe enough to result in the threat of uncal herniation.

- The emergency department evaluation of chronic nonprogressive ataxia consists of ensuring, by a careful history and physical examination, that the problem is indeed stable.

Ataxia is a disorder of intentional movement, characterized by impaired balance and coordination. It can variably affect the trunk or extremities. Severe truncal ataxia is sometimes referred to as titubation. Ataxia of the extremities can result in a wide-based gait or can cause dysmetria, which is the tendency of the limbs to overshoot a target, with subsequent movements attempting to correct the overshoot.

PATHOPHYSIOLOGY

Ataxia can result from a variety of lesions, including damage to the peripheral nerves, spinal cord, cerebellum, and cerebral hemispheres. Lesions of the cerebellum can be further categorized as affecting the hemispheres, which results in limb ataxia, or the midline vermis, which causes truncal ataxia. The anatomy of the cerebellum is such that lesions in a single hemisphere cause ipsilateral limb manifestations. Damage to the spinal cord can cause ataxia when the patient stands with the eyes closed, which is referred to as a Romberg's sign.

Metabolic and systemic disorders can also cause ataxia. One of the most common etiologies is drug intoxication, especially with alcohol or phenytoin.

EVALUATION

True ataxia must be distinguished from problems with similar neurologic manifestations. Vestibular disorders can cause vertigo, a sensation of abnormal movement or spinning that can cause a severe gait disturbance, nausea, and vomiting. Vertigo is often accompanied by nystagmus. Myopathies can be confused with nystagmus, as can peripheral neuropathies. On physical examination, myopathies are characterized by muscle weakness, whereas peripheral neuropathies are accompanied by decreased reflexes. Chorea is a disorder characterized by involuntary movements and incoordination. It is distinguished from ataxia in that it occurs at rest, whereas ataxia is manifested during intentional movement.

Physical Examination

Vital signs and a thorough physical examination should be performed. Findings of cerebellar dysfunction include nystagmus, staggering, wide-based gait, and titubation. Specific neurologic tests include the following:

- Finger to nose with eyes closed (to look for intention tremor)
- Finger to nose to (examiner's) finger (tests cerebellar integrity when limb strength and sensation is intact)
- Heel-to-shin maneuvers (test cerebellar integrity when limb strength and sensation are intact)
- Rapid alternating hand movements (tests cerebellar function)
- Heel and toe walking (with hemispheric lesions there is a tendency to veer in one direction)
- Tandem gait (with hemispheric lesions there is a tendency to veer in one direction)
- Walking in a circle (with hemispheric lesions there is a tendency to veer in one direction).

In addition, a sensory examination for light touch and pinprick, position, and vibration sense should be performed because lower extremity sensory impairment can cause ataxia.

For diagnostic purposes, it is useful to categorize ataxia as acute, intermittent, or chronic. Chronic ataxia is further categorized as progressive or nonprogressive (Table 40-1).

Table 40-1. Causes of Ataxia

Acute
Postinfectious
Acute cerebellar
Polymyoclonus/opisthotonos
Posttraumatic
Hematoma
Mass
Infection
Meningitis
Encephalitis
Polyneuritis
Posterior fossa tumors
Intoxications
Alcohol
Anticonvulsants
Cyclic antidepressants
Sedative-hypnotics
Chronic
Progressive
Tumor
Abscess
Hydrocephalus
Degenerative
Intermittent
Migraine
Seizures
Metabolic
Multiple sclerosis
Nonprogressive
Cerebral palsy
Sequelae of
Head trauma
Lead poisoning
Cerebellar malformations
Dandy-Walker cysts
Agenesis
Hypoplasia

ACUTE ATAXIA

Acute ataxia generally has an onset of <24 hours. Drug toxicity and infections are the most common etiologies. Acute metabolic processes, such as hypoglycemia, are also implicated, although they are usually accompanied by multiple systemic manifestations.

In a patient with acute ataxia, the history and physical examination focus on excluding acute infectious etiologies, such as meningitis or encephalitis, lesions that result in increased intracranial pressure, such as hemorrhage and tumors, and toxic ingestions. Central nervous system infections are usually characterized by fever and headache, and often by mental status changes. The physical examination may reveal neck stiffness. Lesions that cause increased intracranial pressure are associated with headache and vomiting, and the physical examination may reveal papilledema. In the case of a cerebellar hemorrhage, the onset of ataxia is extremely sudden, whereas with posterior fossa tumors, the history will usually reveal a more protracted process. Toxic ingestions are likely in patients on anticonvulsants and are especially common in toddlers. Acute ataxia can also occur after head trauma, in which it can result from a cerebellar hemorrhage or basilar skull fracture.

Any ataxic patient in whom an acute infectious process is considered requires a lumbar puncture. It is imperative that, prior to lumbar puncture, increased intracranial pressure be excluded by computed tomography (CT) scan of the brain. In any case in which ingestion of a toxic substance is suspected, a toxicology screen is indicated. Specific toxins to assess include anticonvulsants, tricyclic antidepressants, sedative/hypnotics, and alcohol.

Certain causes of acute ataxia are almost unique to the pediatric population and deserve special mention. Guillian-Barre syndrome can also present with ataxia, although the associated findings of areflexia and, in the Miller-Fisher variant, ophthalmoplegia, distinguish it from acute cerebellar ataxia.

Acute Cerebellar Ataxia

A common cause of ataxia in children younger than 5 years is acute cerebellar ataxia. The onset of ataxia is insidious and predominantly affects the gait, although dysmetria, nystagmus, and dysarthria can occur. Acute cerebellar ataxia is thought to be a postinfectious phenomenon and often occurs 2 weeks after a viral illness. Ataxia has been reported after infection with varicella, influenza, mumps, echovirus 6, coxsackie B virus, and other viruses. It is a self-limiting illness with an excellent prognosis. Acute cerebellar ataxia is a diagnosis of exclusion.

Myoclonic Encephalopathy of Infancy

Myoclonic encephalopathy of infancy (polymyoclonus-opsoclonus) is another cause of acute ataxia. This syndrome occurs in association with occult neuroblastoma, viral disease, aseptic meningitis (especially mumps), and unknown or miscellaneous causes. It is differentiated from acute cerebellar ataxia by its association with opsoclonus (rapid, chaotic conjugate eye movements), which occur in association with polymyoclonia (severe myoclonic jerks of the limbs and trunk or head). Diagnostic tests that should be initiated in the emergency department (ED) include chest and abdominal CT, urine vanillylmandelic acid (VMA), and lumbar puncture to exclude aseptic meningitis. Treatment for the parainfectious form includes ACTH and oral glucocorticoids. Unfortunately, for those without an underlying cause, intellectual impairment is often associated with this movement disorder.

Chronic Intermittent Ataxia

Chronic intermittent or recurrent ataxia occurs as acute episodes that are similar in nature. In children, the most common cause of intermittent ataxia is a migraine headache that involves the basilar artery. Besides ataxia, associated symptoms include blurred vision, visual field deficits, vertigo, and headache. In a child experiencing the first basilar migraine, it is essential to exclude an acute infectious process, toxic ingestion, or mass lesion.

Partial complex seizures can also cause intermittent ataxia but are often associated with alteration of consciousness and possibly characteristic motor manifestations.

Rarely, inborn errors of metabolism result in intermittent ataxia. These include maple syrup urine disease, Hartnup's disease, urea cycle defects, multiple carboxylase deficiencies (biotinidase deficiency), and ataxia with vitamin E deficiency.

Patients with intermittent ataxia may not require radiographic or laboratory evaluation in the ED if they present with a known diagnosis. Patients suspected of having seizures are referred for an electroencephalograph. The rare patient suspected of having an undiagnosed inborn error of metabolism is referred to a pediatric endocrinologist.

CHRONIC PROGRESSIVE ATAXIA

Chronic progressive ataxia has an insidious onset and progresses slowly over weeks to months. The differential diagnosis consists of brain tumors, hydrocephalus, and neurodegenerative disorders.

The combination of ataxia, headache, irritability, and vomiting in a child younger than 6 years is characteristic of a medulloblastoma. Cerebellar astrocytomas are located in the cerebellar hemispheres and cause ipsilateral limb ataxia, headache, and double vision. They occur most commonly in school-aged children. Brainstem gliomas present with ataxia and are often accompanied by cranial nerve palsies or spasticity. In some cases posterior fossa tumors have a relatively acute presentation.

Hydrocephalus, whether congenital or acquired, can cause ataxia due to stretching of frontopontocerebellar fibers. It is often accompanied by headache and vomiting and, when the patient presents late in the course of illness, can be associated with critically increased intracranial pressure.

Neurodegenerative diseases are a group of inherited disorders that can cause spinocerebellar degeneration and progressive ataxia. These include Refsum's disease and Bassen-Kornzweig syndrome (abetalipoproteinemia), which are treatable by diet (dietary restriction of phytanic acid and the addition of vitamin E, respectively).

Other hereditary causes of ataxia include spinocerebellar ataxias, of which Freidrich's ataxia is the most common. This autosomal recessive ataxia, which usually manifests before 10 years of age, is characterized by ataxia, nystagmus, kyphoscoliosis, cardiomyopathy, and distal muscle wasting.

Patients with progressive ataxia require an aggressive evaluation in the ED. All patients are examined for signs of increased intracranial pressure, which in some cases can be severe enough to result in the threat of uncal herniation. A CT of the brain is indicated in any patient with signs of a mass lesion or hydrocephalus. Many of these patients are candidates for an emergency placement of a ventricular shunt. For patients with signs of increased intracranial pressure, fluid therapy is restricted to two-thirds of maintenance requirements to reduce the risk of herniation. Patients with suspected neurodegenerative diseases are referred to a pediatric neurologist for further evaluation and specific diagnosis.

NONPROGRESSIVE ATAXIA

Chronic nonprogressive ataxia may be a sequela of head trauma, meningitis, or lead poisoning. It can also result from congenital malformations, such as cerebellar agenesis or hypoplasia or the Chiari type I malformation (herniation of the cerebellar tonsils into the foramen magnum).

The ED evaluation of chronic nonprogressive ataxia consists of ensuring, by a careful history and physical examination, that the problem is indeed stable. Patients with an unknown diagnosis may benefit from CT or magnetic resonance imaging of the brain.

BIBLIOGRAPHY

Swaiman KF: Muscle tone and gait disturbances, in Swaiman KF, Ashwal S (eds): *Pediatric Neurology: Principles and Practice,* 3d ed. St. Louis: Mosby, 1999, pp 54–62.

Swaiman KF: Movement disorders and disorders of the basal ganglia, in Swaiman KF, Ashwal S (eds): *Pediatric Neurology: Principles and Practice,* 3d ed. St. Louis: Mosby, 1999, pp 801–831.

Swaiman KF: Cerebellar dysfunction and ataxia in childhood, in Swaiman KF, Ashwal S (eds): *Pediatric Neurology: Principles and Practice,* 3d ed. St. Louis: Mosby, 1999, pp 787–800.

41

Weakness

Susan Fuchs

HIGH-YIELD FACTS

- Upper motor neuron diseases usually present with asymmetrical weakness contralateral to the lesion and are associated with hyperreflexia, increased muscle tone, and the absence of atrophy or fasciculations. Lower motor neuron diseases present with symmetrical weakness that can be isolated to specific muscle groups and are associated with findings of decreased muscle tone and depressed reflexes.

- Involvement of bulbar muscles is manifested by cranial nerve findings, facial muscle weakness, and chewing or swallowing difficulties. Bulbar involvement can occur in both upper and lower motor neuron disorders.

- Neuropathies are disorders of nerves and tend to produce more prominent distal muscle weakness, hypesthesias or paresthesias, and decreased reflexes, especially early in the disease.

- Myopathies are disorders of muscle and can be inflammatory or congenital. Inflammatory myopathies usually involve proximal muscles and are often associated with muscle pain or tenderness.

- For patients old enough to cooperate, motor strength in the extremities is evaluated and rated on a scale of 1 to 5:
  - 0, total lack of contraction
  - 1, trace contraction
  - 2, active contraction without gravity
  - 3, movement against gravity
  - 4, movement against resistance
  - 5, normal motor strength

- Guillain-Barré syndrome often starts with nonspecific muscular pain, most often in the thighs. The pain is followed by weakness, which is most often symmetrical and distal, progresses upward, and, in some cases, results in total paralysis within 24 hours.

- Transverse myelitis is a syndrome characterized by acute dysfunction at a level of the spinal cord that can occur as an isolated phenomenon or as part of another illness. For a patient with signs of a rapidly advancing spinal cord lesion, it is imperative to exclude a treatable mass lesion that could be compressing the cord, by promptly obtaining a magnetic resonance image or contrast myelography.

- Tick paralysis is caused by a neurotoxin from the Rocky Mountain wood tick or the Eastern dog tick. Several days after the tick attaches, the patient begins to experience ataxia and difficulty walking; if the tick is not removed, flaccid paralysis and death can result.

- Food-borne botulism results from ingestion of toxins contained in improperly canned foods. Diarrhea and vomiting are followed by neurologic symptoms, such as blurred vision, dysarthria, and diploplia, followed by weakness of the extremities.

- Infant botulism is caused by colonization of the intestinal tract by spores of *Clostridium botulinum* and has been related to the ingestion of contaminated honey. A prominent manifestation is constipation; when the condition is severe, the infant can develop difficulty sucking and swallowing and can become hypotonic.

The differential diagnosis of weakness is vast, and the child who presents with this complaint requires a thorough evaluation. The term "weakness" can refer to a general phenomenon that affects all or most of the body or may refer to a specific area, such as an extremity. The specific complaint can include generalized fatigue, refusal to walk, limp, increased clumsiness or falling, pain, loss of bowel or bladder function, or focal motor weakness. In infants, weakness can imply lethargy, poor feeding, or poor head control. Slowly progressive forms of weakness may be due to congenital disorders. The child may present at a time when the weakness is mild, yet progressive. Others may have paralysis at the time of presentation. The primary focus in this chapter is on weakness arising from neuromuscular disorders.

PATHOPHYSIOLOGY

The pathophysiology of weakness varies with the etiology and the specific area affected. Terms that are applied to neuromuscular disorders include the following:

- Paresis, which implies a complete or partial weakness
- Paralysis, which is a loss of function
- Paraplegia, paralysis of the lower half of the body
- Quadraplegia, involving all limbs; both paraplegia and quadriplegia usually result from a spinal cord lesion.
- Hemiplegia, involving one side of the body, generally results from a lesion in the brain.

Abnormalities of the neuromuscular system are further classified as arising from an upper or lower motor neuron unit. The upper motor neuron unit arises in the cerebral cortex, traverses the brainstem, and travels down the spinal cord. Upper motor neuron diseases usually present with asymmetrical weakness that is contralateral to the lesion and are associated with hyperreflexia, increased muscle tone, and the absence of atrophy or fasciculations. The lower motor neuron unit includes the anterior horn cells, peripheral nerve, neuromuscular junction, and muscle fibers. Lower motor neuron diseases present with symmetrical weakness that can be isolated to specific muscle groups and are associated with findings of decreased muscle tone and depressed reflexes. Depending on whether the disorder is acute or chronic, atrophy and fasciculations may be present.

Involvement of bulbar muscles is manifested by cranial nerve findings, facial muscle weakness, and chewing or swallowing difficulties. Bulbar involvement can occur in both upper and lower motor neuron disorders.

Another distinction that should be made in the patient presenting with weakness is between a myopathy and neuropathy. Neuropathies are disorders of nerves and tend to produce more prominent distal muscle weakness, hypesthesias or paresthesias, and decreased reflexes, especially early in the disease. Myopathies are disorders of muscle and can be inflammatory or congenital. Inflammatory myopathies usually involve proximal muscles and are often associated with muscle pain or tenderness. Reflexes become decreased late in the disease. Congenital myopathies tend to involve specific muscle groups and can present at birth with hypotonia and weakness, or in older children with a more insidious progression.

DIAGNOSIS

History

It is vital to distinguish between acute and chronic disorders, since this information will direct the remainder of the workup. The location of the initial weakness is elicited, and weakness is established as focal or general. Focal weakness is further characterized as predominantly proximal or distal. The rate of progression of symptoms is characterized as acute, which implies minutes to hours, subacute, meaning hours to days, and slowly progressive, which involves a prolonged period. Acute onset or rapid progression implies spinal cord compression or a vascular event involving the spinal cord or brain. Subacute progression can be due to infection, inflammation, or tumor. Slowly progressive symptoms imply a chronic or congenital disorder. Defining the progression of symptoms is facilitated by asking the parents questions regarding progressive difficulty in walking, recent difficulty climbing up or down stairs, or inability to go from a sitting to standing position unaided. The loss of developmental milestones implies a degenerative disorder.

The patient and parents are questioned regarding symptoms preceding the onset of weakness, such as recent illness, fever, headache, neck or back pain, and loss of bowel or bladder function. A history of recent trauma to the head or neck and the presence of underlying medical problems, such as sickle cell disease or hemophilia, is sought. Prior episodes of weakness may point to an intermittent metabolic problem, such as dyskalemic paralysis. A family history of weakness suggests a congenital disorder, such as muscular dystrophy, myotonic disorders, metabolic muscle disease, or myasthenia gravis. A history of exposure to drugs or heavy metals suggests poisoning. A pertinent travel history is indicated, since weakness can be a manifestation of entities such as tick paralysis or black widow spider bites. A careful antenatal history is indicated to rule out a perinatal insult, as is an immunization history to evaluate the possibility of a vaccine-related complication.

Physical Examination

The physical examination begins as the child is placed in the room, with observation of mental status, posture, gait, the ability to get on the examining table, or to sit unaided. The vital signs are assessed, with particular attention to respiratory rate and effort. Many neuromuscular disorders, such as Guillan-Barré syndrome, botulism, myasthenic crisis, and tick paralysis, are associated with a risk of respiratory failure and warrant repeated evaluation of the patient's respiratory status. Blood pressure and pulse are carefully monitored, since some neuromuscular disorders, such as Guillan-Barré syndrome, are associated with autonomic instability.

The patient's general appearance is noted, with attention given to general muscular development and the presence of kyphosis, scoliosis, or lordosis with a protuberant abdomen, which can all suggest a congenital disorder, such as Duchenne muscular dystrophy. The patient's facial expression is noted. Lack of facial expression, snarl, or slack jaw suggest myasthenia gravis. Ptosis can be due to myasthenia or myotonic dystrophy. The inability to close one eye with a concomitant facial droop suggests Bell's palsy. Gross inspection of the muscles is performed, noting the presence of wasting, fasciculations, or hypertrophy.

The neurologic examination includes an evaluation of pupillary size and reactivity and the remainder of the cranial nerves. If possible, the fundus is examined and the visual fields are assessed. For patients old enough to cooperate, motor strength in the extremities is evaluated and rated on a scale of 1 to 5, as follows:

- 0, total lack of contraction
- 1, trace contraction
- 2, active contraction without gravity
- 3, movement against gravity
- 4, movement against resistance
- 5, normal motor strength

For infants who cannot cooperate with the examination, it is possible to perform a general assessment of muscle tone and integrity by holding the baby under the arms and placing the feet on the bed. Infants with normal tone will not slide through an examiner's hands and will actively kick both legs against the resistance of the bed. Older children can be asked to walk on their toes and heels to detect weak ankle flexors and dorsiflexors, respectively. The ability to walk on the heels but not the toes suggests intraspinal pathology.

Deep tendon reflexes at the knees, ankles, elbows, and wrists are elicited. Hyperreflexia or sustained clonus indicates an upper motor neuron lesion, whereas absent or decreased reflexes imply a problem in a lower motor distribution. Other reflexes to be noted include the anal wink and abdominal and cremasteric responses.

Sensory evaluation includes touch, pain, position, vibration, and temperature. Touch and pain are evaluated by assessing soft versus sharp stimulation and two-point discrimination. Position sense is assessed by asking the child to indicate the direction in which an examiner moves a finger or toe. Temperature sensation can be assessed by the use of a cold stethoscope or by touching the child with cold or warm water.

The sensations of touch and position-vibration do not cross in the spinal cord on their way to the brain, whereas those of pain and temperature do. An abnormality of touch and position on one side and pain and temperature on the other suggests a cord lesion. The unilateral loss of all sensations suggests a brain lesion. A stocking and glove distribution of sensory loss suggests a peripheral neuropathy.

Laboratory Evaluation

The laboratory evaluation is based on the provisional diagnosis. Generally, a complete blood count, serum electrolytes, and magnesium are indicated. Elevated serum creatinine kinase is nonspecific but is found in children with active inflammatory myopathies and may be elevated in chronic myopathies. Urine is assessed for the presence of myoglobin and, in selected cases, is used for toxicology screening.

For patients with a suspected spinal cord lesion, radiographs are indicated. Even if they are negative, any patient suspected of having a developing lesion of the spinal cord requires evaluation by magnetic resonance imaging (MRI) or contrast myelography. If neither is available, computed tomography (CT) of the spine may be helpful.

For patients with suspected central nervous system lesions, a CT of the brain is indicated. Some patients may require a lumbar puncture. Poliomyelitis is associated with monocytosis and elevated cerebral spinal fluid protein. Guillan-Barré syndrome is associated with a characteristic albumino-cytologic dissociation.

Electromyography and nerve conduction studies are indicated if lower motor neuron disease is suspected, but they are not emergency department (ED) procedures.

SPECIFIC CAUSES OF WEAKNESS

Weakness due to certain causes is common enough in the pediatric ED population to justify specific discussion.

Guillain-Barré Syndrome

Also known as acute inflammatory demyelinating polyradiculoneuropathy, Guillain-Barré syndrome occurs in both children and adults. It is more common in the adult patient population. The pathogenesis is unknown, but it is thought to result from an immune response to an antecedent viral infection that triggers demyelination of nerve roots and peripheral nerves. The syndrome often starts with nonspecific muscular pain, most often in the thighs. The pain is followed by weakness, which is most often symmetric and distal. Weakness progresses upward and, in some cases, results in total paralysis within 24 hours. Cranial nerve involvement is common. Deep tendon reflexes are usually absent, but plantar responses remain downgoing. Autonomic involvement can produce labile changes in blood pressure and bowel and bladder incontinence. The degree of weakness and the rate of progression of disease vary considerably. Laboratory findings are generally not helpful, although spinal fluid analysis may reveal a high protein.

The basic treatment for Guillain-Barré syndrome is supportive care. In some cases, mechanical ventilation is necessary, and this requirement is associated with a poorer prognosis. Attention is given to fluid and electrolyte balance, heart rate, and blood pressure. Steroids and other immunosuppressive agents are of questionable value. Plasmapheresis may shorten the course of disease, as may therapy with intravenous gammaglobulin.

Transverse Myelitis

Transverse myelitis is a syndrome characterized by acute dysfunction at a level of the spinal cord. It can occur as an isolated phenomenon or as part of another illness and, as such, it represents a syndrome rather than a distinct entity. The onset can be insidious but is usually over 24 to 48 hours. Patients may initially complain of paresthesias and weakness of the lower extremities. Progressive weakness usually results and a sensory level is established, most commonly in the thoracic area. Flaccid paralysis and decreased reflexes are characteristic early in the process but are later followed by increased muscle tone.

For a patient with signs of a rapidly advancing spinal cord lesion, it is imperative to exclude a treatable mass lesion that could be compressing the cord, such as an epidural abscess or hemorrhage. This is usually done by MRI or contrast myelography.

Most patients with transverse myelitis recover some function. Corticosteroids may benefit some patients.

Tick Paralysis

Tick paralysis is caused by a neurotoxin from the Rocky Mountain wood tick *(Dermacentor andersoni)* or the Eastern dog tick *(Dermacentor variabilis)*. The tick produces a neurotoxin that prevents liberation of acetylcholine at neuromuscular junctions. Small children are likely victims. Several days after the tick attaches, the patient begins to experience ataxia and difficulty walking. If the tick is not removed, flaccid paralysis and death can result. Removal of the tick is generally curative.

Botulism

Infection with *Clostridium botulinum* can produce three neurologic diseases. Ultimately, symptoms result from a toxin generated from spores of the bacteria that inhibits release of acetylcholine at the prejunction of terminal nerve fibers.

Food-borne botulism results from ingestion of toxin contained in improperly canned foods. Diarrhea and vomiting are followed by neurologic symptoms, often secondary to cranial nerve dysfunction. Blurred vision, dysarthria, and diplopia can occur and can be followed by weakness of the extremities. Mucous membranes of the mouth and pharynx may be dry. Deep tendon reflexes may be weak or absent. Antitoxin may be effective in food-borne botulism.

Wound botulism results from infection of a contaminated wound. Clinically, it is usually indistinguishable from food-borne botulism. Treatment includes wound debridement and antibiotic therapy. Antitoxin may also be useful.

Infant botulism is caused by colonization of the intestinal tract by spores of *Clostridium botulinum,* which release toxin that is systemically absorbed. It has been related to the ingestion of contaminated honey. A prominent manifestation is constipation. When the disease is severe, the infant can develop difficulty sucking and swallowing and can become hypotonic. Symmetrical paralysis can develop, with involvement of cranial nerves.

Diagnosis is by isolating the toxin in the infant's stool. Electromyography is also useful. The management of infant botulism is supportive and may require mechanical ventilation. Treatment with antitoxin and antibiotics does not seem to be of benefit.

Myasthenia Gravis

The term myasthenia gravis comprises a group of diseases characterized by easy fatigability. Most commonly, associated anti-acetylcholine receptor antibodies destroy the postsynaptic membrane of the myoneural junction, resulting in decreased transmission of nerve impulses. It is the most common disorder of the myoneural junction in children. In children, the striated muscles innervated by the cranial nerves are particularly affected. The diagnosis is usually established by demonstrating improvement in muscle strength after administration of the anticholinesterase edrophonium (Tensilon). The three basic categories of myasthenia gravis in the pediatric population are as follows:

* Transient neonatal variety
* Persistent neonatal form
* Juvenile myasthenia gravis

Neonatal transient myasthenia gravis occurs in infants born to mothers with the disease and is caused by maternal anti-acetylcholine receptor antibodies that cross the placenta. It affects 10 to 15 percent of infants whose mothers have myasthenia gravis. In its severe form, it can cause problems with sucking and swallowing and ventilatory insufficiency. Treatment is with neostigmine or pyridostigmine. The disease usually improves in 4 to 6 weeks.

Persistent neonatal myasthenia gravis may be autoimmune in nature or of a hereditary variety. Symptoms usually appear on the first day of life and, in more severe cases, include ptosis, swallowing difficulties, and respiratory insufficiency. In less severe cases, the onset can be insidious and clinical manifestations of muscle weakness more subtle. Symptoms may be severe enough to require nasogastric feeding and ventilatory support. Pharmacologic therapy is with anticholinesterase agents.

Juvenile myasthenia gravis is similar to that seen in adults. It commonly has its onset at around 10 years of age. Ptosis, ophthalmoplegia, and weakness of other facial muscles are commonly present. Symmetrical limb weakness is usually present, although focal weakness of the ocular muscles can occur. The disease tends to become worse throughout the day. Both remissions and exacerbations are common, and up to 50 percent of affected children may develop seizures. The primary treatment is with anticholinesterase agents. In refractory or severe cases, immunosuppressive agents, plasmapheresis, or thymectomy may be necessary. Erythromycin therapy can exacerbate symptoms and is avoided.

Myasthenic Crisis

Occasionally, exacerbations of symptoms can occur that result in profound weakness, difficulty swallowing secretions, and respiratory insufficiency. This can be associated with antibiotic therapy, central nervous system depressants, antiarrythmics, and hypokalemia. Patients with myasthenic crisis will usually respond to a challenge with edrophonium. If a myasthenic crisis is suspected, the patient is admitted to a unit where respiratory status can be monitored.

Cholinergic Crisis

Patients with myasthenia gravis can also suffer from overdose of anticholinesterase medications, which can provoke a cholinergic crisis. Unfortunately, the symptoms of cholinergic excess are similar to those of a myasthenic crisis. In both, increasing weakness is the predominant finding. Patients suffering a cholinergic crisis may also have associated vomiting, diarrhea, and hypersalivation. In patients with obvious severe cholinergic excess, atropine may be useful in drying airway secretions. However, in most cases, it will be difficult to distinguish between a cholinergic crisis and an exacerbation of myasthenia, and hospital admission and close observation are indicated.

Bell's Palsy

Bell's palsy is a condition that results in unilateral facial weakness. In severe cases, there can be total paralysis of the facial muscles. It is thought to result from swelling and edema of cranial nerve VII, the facial nerve, as it traverses the facial canal within the temporal bone. As such, it is a peripheral neuropathy, and the distribution of the weakness reflects the territory innervated by the facial nerve. The nerve has motor, sensory, and autonomic functions and, in addition to supplying the muscles of the face, innervates the lacrimal and salivary glands as well as the anterior two-thirds of the tongue. In most cases, Bell's palsy is idiopathic. Certain conditions are associated with unilateral facial weakness, including viral infections, otitis media, Lyme disease, and temporal bone trauma.

Symptoms may begin with ear pain, which is followed by the development of facial weakness, characterized by a drooping mouth and inability to close the eye on the affected side. In some cases, lacrimation and taste are impaired. Inability to close the mouth can make eating and drinking difficult.

The lesion is defined as a peripheral neuropathy, as opposed to a lesion of the central nervous system, by the fact that Bell's palsy affects the muscles of the forehead on the side of the lesion. In a lesion of the central nervous system, the forehead is spared, because it receives innervation from both sides of the brain. A lesion in one cerebral hemisphere will cause weakness confined to the lower part of the face. Laboratory studies are usually normal.

The prognosis of Bell's palsy is generally good, with recovery usually beginning in 2 to 4 weeks. Steroid therapy may be beneficial if started early in the course of illness. Treatment includes lubricating solutions for the eye on the affected side to maintain moisture of the cornea. Patients with inability to close the eye may require patching. In young children, ophthalmologic consultation may be advisable.

Myopathies

Myopathies are diseases that affect skeletal muscle. They are relatively uncommon in children, and, in most cases, a child affected with a myopathy will present to the ED with a known diagnosis. Many myopathies are congenital, although some result from spontaneous mutations.

Muscular Dystrophies

Muscular dystrophies are disorders associated with progressive degeneration of muscle, resulting in relentlessly increasing weakness. The many different varieties of muscular dystrophy vary in their mode of inheritance, age of onset, muscles involved, progression of disease, and ultimate outcome. The most common is Duchenne muscular dystrophy, usually an X-linked recessive disorder. Clinical manifestations usually become apparent at about age 3, when patients begin to develop weakness of the hip girdle and shoulder muscles. Patients may have difficulty standing and characteristically rise from all fours by placing their hands on the thighs and pushing up (Gower's sign). The disease is characterized by a progressive loss of muscle strength.

In the later stages, cardiomyopathy is common and scoliosis can result in pulmonary insufficiency. Survival beyond early adulthood is rare.

Periodic Paralysis

Periodic paralysis is an example of a metabolic myopathy that results in muscle weakness without involvement of the central or peripheral nervous system. The disease is primarily autosomal dominant. There are three varieties, characterized by associated hypokalemia, hyperkalemia, and normokalemia.

Episodes of hypokalemic periodic paralysis have their onset during the first or second decade of life. They are often precipitated by excitement or ingestion of carbohydrate meals. Paralysis usually begins proximally and spreads distally. The patient may be areflexic. The episode can last for many hours. Attacks tend to decrease with age. Serum potassium during an attack is usually decreased compared with a baseline value. Treatment with potassium during an attack may be helpful. Long-term therapy with acetazolamide may reduce the number of attacks. Severely affected patients can develop permanent muscle weakness.

Hyperkalemic periodic paralysis is also an autosomal dominant condition associated with intermittent attacks beginning in the first or second decade of life. Attacks can be provoked by periods of rest following heavy exertion. Weakness can develop rapidly and last for hours. The respiratory muscles are usually spared. Some patients develop myotonia during attacks. The serum potassium is elevated above baseline values, although the degree of hyperkalemia varies. In severe cases, standard therapy for malignant hyperkalemia is indicated. As in patients with hypokalemic periodic paralysis, chronic weakness can develop. Treatment with acetazolamide may also be beneficial.

Normokalemic periodic paralysis can be provoked by exposure to cold, activity, and alcohol. The serum potassium does not change during an attack. Treatment with sodium during an attack may improve weakness.

DISPOSITION

The disposition of a patient with weakness depends on the degree of disability and the nature of the underlying problem. In any patient in whom the development of respiratory compromise is a possibility, hospital admission and close observation is recommended.

BIBLIOGRAPHY

Barkin RM: Paralysis and hemiplegia, in Barkin RM, Rosen P (eds): *Emergency Pediatrics*. St. Louis: Mosby, 1984, pp 210–213.

Freeman JM: Diagnosis and evaluation of acute paraplegia. *Pediatr Rev* 4:327, 1983.

Leshner RT, Teasley JE: Pediatric neuromuscular emergencies, in Pellock JM, Myer EC (eds): *Neurologic Emergencies in Infancy and Childhood,* 2d ed. Boston: Butterworth-Heinemann, 1993, pp 242–261.

Miller G: Myopathies of infancy and childhood. *Pediatr Ann* 18:439, 1989.

Patterson MC, Gomez MR: Muscle disease in children: A practical approach. *Pediatr Rev* 12:73, 1990.

Rodenberg H, Gratton M, Bennett J, et al: Left upper extremity weakness in an 18-year old man. *Ann Emerg Med* 20:672, 1991.

Swaiman KF (ed): *Pediatric Neurology: Principles and Practice,* 2d ed. St. Louis: Mosby, 1994, pp 1385–1520.

42

Headache

Susan Fuchs

HIGH-YIELD FACTS

- Most headaches in children are benign.
- A headache worsened by coughing, sneezing, or lying down may be due to increased intracranial pressure.
- Pseudotumor cerebri causes headache in the absence of a mass lesion.
- Complicated migraines are associated with transient neurologic disturbances.
- Psychogenic headaches tend to be chronic and nonprogressive.

Headaches are common in childhood. As many as 75 percent of children experience a headache by the age of 15 years. Although they usually do not result from serious disease, headaches are sometimes the manifestation of life-threatening illness. It is incumbent on the emergency physician to distinguish those headaches that result from benign self-limited processes from those that can result in serious morbidity or mortality. Headaches can be classified as organic, vascular, functional, or psychological. In addition, headache may be related to structures other than the calvarium or its contents. The brain itself is not sensitive to pain, but there are pain-sensitive structures in the skin, the muscles, the vascular sinuses, the intracranial blood vessels, and the meninges at the base of the brain. Inflammation, dilation, irritation, and displacement of the pain-sensitive areas can result in a headache.

ORGANIC HEADACHES

Organic headaches usually result from a process that causes increased intracranial pressure or from an inflammatory process that is usually infectious in nature.

An organic disorder is likely in the following circumstances:

- Acute headache with a neurologic deficit
- Headache accompanied by a fever and neck stiffness
- A chronically progressive headache
- Headache that wakes a patient from sleep
- Headache that increases with straining or coughing

Processes associated with increased intracranial pressure include brain tumors, hydrocephalus, hypertensive encephalopathy, pseudotumor cerebri, and acute hemorrhage, both spontaneous and traumatic. Infectious etiologies include meningitis, encephalitis, and brain abscesses. In essence, all causes of organic headaches are potentially life threatening.

Brain Tumors and Hydrocephalus

The presence of a headache that is made worse by lying down, or that comes on with coughing, sneezing, or straining at stool and then disappears, suggests increased intracranial pressure. Headaches associated with disorders related to increased intracranial pressure are of a progressive nature. Papilledema is often found on funduscopic examination. A complete neurologic examination may disclose other abnormalities, such as ataxia with a cerebellar tumor, or cranial nerve findings with hydrocephalus. Differentiation of these disorders is by computed tomography (CT) scan or magnetic resonance imaging (MRI), with appropriate consultation if hydrocephalus or a tumor is found.

Pseudotumor Cerebri

Pseudotumor cerebri is a condition associated with increased intracranial pressure in the absence of a mass lesion or other obvious etiology. It results from impaired reabsorption of cerebrospinal fluid (CSF). It is associated with high doses of vitamin A and steroid therapy and is especially common in obese adolescent girls. Patients may have papilledema on examination. The CT scan in such patients often reveals small ventricles and an enlarged cisterna magna. Lumbar puncture will reveal an opening pressure >20 cmH$_2$O, with normal protein, glucose, and cell count. Therapy includes serial lumbar punctures to relieve acute symptoms and acetazolamide to reduce the formation of CSF.

Hypertensive Encephalopathy

Severe elevation in blood pressure can cause headache and if untreated can result in the development of encephalopathy and seizures. This should be suspected in a patient with a severe headache whose diastolic blood pressure is greater than the 95th percentile for age. In young children, the development of hypertension is often secondary to an acute illness, such as fulminant glomerulonephritis. It can also be secondary to acute exacerbations for patients with known hypertension. In severe cases, hypertension can result in cardiac as well as neurologic dysfunction. Since other causes of increased intracranial pressure can also occasionally result in hypertension, it is essential that they be excluded.

The blood pressure is checked in all extremities to evaluate for coarctation of the aorta. The laboratory evaluation includes a complete urinalysis, to look for blood, protein or casts, serum electrolytes, and renal functions.

Acute therapy in the emergency department (ED) is individualized, based on complete physical examination findings, degree of hypertension, and past history of hypertension. Patients with encephalopathy and seizures require rapid reduction of blood pressure with an agent such as nitroprusside. The patient is admitted for blood pressure control and complete evaluation.

Acute Hemorrhage

The child presenting with a severe headache of sudden onset, with or without neck or back pain, may have suffered an intracranial hemorrhage. The patient's mental status can range from normal to coma. Focal findings may or may not be present. Spontaneous intracranial hemorrhage usually results from either a ruptured aneurysm or arteriovenous malformation. It can also occur in association with coagulopathies. The diagnosis and management are further discussed in the section on cerebrovascular accidents.

Meningitis/Encephalitis/Brain Abscess

The association of headache with a fever and stiff neck implies an infectious etiology, such as meningitis, encephalitis, or brain abscess. If there are no focal findings or signs of increased intracranial pressure on physical examination, a lumbar puncture is performed and will provide the diagnosis. CSF is sent for culture, cell count, protein, and glucose, with viral cultures and bacterial antigen detection as available and as directed by cell count. If there are focal neurologic abnormalities or signs of increased intracranial pressure, a brain abscess is possible and a CT scan or MRI of the brain with and without contrast is performed prior to a lumbar puncture to avoid the potential for herniation. Hospital admission

is required for children with these problems, and neurologic examination, electrolytes, and fluid status need to be monitored closely.

VASCULAR HEADACHES

Migraine headaches are an example of recurrent headaches. Several theories exist as to their etiology. The vascular hypothesis is that vasoconstriction results in focal neurologic signs or an aura, followed by vasodilation and pain. The neurogenic theory is that afferent inputs to the brainstem result in a slowly spreading neuronal depression followed by dilation and inflammation of the vasculature innervated by the trigeminal nerve. These theories have actually been combined into the trigeminal vascular hypothesis. This theory considers migraine an inherited sensitivity of the trigeminal nerve vascular system. The trigeminal nerve, when stimulated, releases substance P, which in turn causes degranulation of mast cells, histamine release, and release of serotonin from platelets. This results in vasodilation and exudation of plasma into tissues. Ultimately this causes distension of cranial arteries and headache. Serotonin (5-HT) appears to be a key mediator, but there are at least five serotonin receptor subtypes, each with a different role.

Migraines tend to be recurrent, with symptom-free intervals of varying lengths in between episodes. The headache tends to be unilateral, throbbing or pulsating, is often associated with nausea and vomiting, and is relieved with sleep. There is a genetic predisposition to migraines, with a positive family history in 70 to 90 percent of cases. Boys are more commonly affected until puberty, when girls become more predisposed. There are several potential triggers of migraines including emotional stress, missing a meal, lack of sleep, environmental factors (bright lights, loud noises), certain foods (such as chocolate, hot dogs, smoked meats, Chinese food, caffeine-containing beverages, cheese, and aspartame), and certain drugs (such as oral contraceptives, antihypertensive medications, cimetidine, and H_2 blockers).

Although there is an International Headache Society classification for migraines with and without aura, one problem encountered in children is that these criteria lack sensitivity. A pediatric revision modifies the migraine without aura (common migraine) criteria, because in children, the headache may be unilateral or bilateral and may last only an hour (or up to 48 hours), rather than 2 to 48 hours, as in adults.

Migraine with aura (previously called a classic migraine) occurs less frequently in children than in adults.

It is usually preceded by an aura that can be visual or somatosensory in nature. Visual symptoms include scotomas, blurring, and abnormalities in the perception of lights. Somatosensory disturbances may consist of abnormal smells, distorted perception of images, or even focal motor weakness. The aura can be very brief or last for up to an hour. The headache then follows, which is unilateral or bilateral, especially in the frontal or temporal area. It is often associated with nausea or vomiting and is relieved by sleep.

Migraine without aura (common migraine) is the most common type of migraine in children. It is differentiated from the classic migraine by the lack of a definable aura. However, the child will often complain of malaise, nausea, or irritability prior to the onset of the headache. When the headache occurs, it is severe and throbbing, unilateral or bifrontal or bitemporal in location. The headache may be aggravated by routine physical activity and is accompanied by nausea and/or vomiting, photophobia, or phonophobia.

A complicated migraine is associated with transient neurologic disturbances, which include ophthalmoplegia and hemiparesis. The deficits are thought to result from cerebral vasoconstriction resulting in ischemia and edema, and they resolve spontaneously.

A variant of vascular headache fairly common in childhood is the basilar artery migraine, which results in ataxia and vertigo, at times accompanied by visual disturbances. The headache is usually occipital in location. Confusional migraine can result in confusion, agitation, and an altered level of consciousness. This may occur after minor head trauma. The Alice in Wonderland syndrome is a migraine variant that results in distortion of spatial relationships. Ophthalmoplegic migraine results in orbital pain and a third nerve palsy. The headache can occur during, after, or before the nerve dysfunction. Hemiplegic migraine is the existence of a headache and recurrent hemiparesis. Visual field defects and aphasia can also occur. The headache is usually contralateral to the hemiparesis.

Benign paroxysmal vertigo can also be considered a migraine variant. This occurs in children 2 to 6 years old and consists of sudden, brief episodes when the child cannot stand upright without support. There is no loss of consciousness, but nystagmus is often seen. The episode lasts for several minutes, and then the child recovers completely.

ED treatment of migraines consists of providing analgesia and treating associated symptoms such as nausea during the acute attack. Analgesics such as acetaminophen (initial dose of 20 mg/kg, then 10 to 15 mg/kg q4h) or ibuprofen (1 to 12 years of age: 10 mg/kg q4–6h; >12 years of age: 200 to 400 mg q4h) may be effective. It should be noted that once a migraine is ongoing, gastric motility and absorption of medications are reduced, so parenteral medications may be more effective. Sumatriptan is a selective 5-HT agonist that is given as 6 mg subcutaneously. Dihydroergotamine mesylate (DHE) 0.5 to 1.0 mg over 3 minutes intravenously for children older than 10 years may also be beneficial, especially if given with metoclopramide. For nausea, antiemetics such as promethazine (0.25 to 1 mg/kg PO, IM, IV, or rectal q6h), metoclopramide (1 to 2 mg/kg IV—may need to use with diphenhydramine to avoid extrapyramidal symptoms) or chlorpromazine (0.5 to 1.0 mg/kg q4–6h PO, 0.5 to 1.0 mg/kg q6–8h IV or IM) have been used.

Long-term management of migraines depends somewhat on whether the child has an aura. Older children and adolescents who have an aura can take ergotamine compounds (orally, take one to two 1-mg tablets at the onset of attack, and another tablet 20 minutes later if no improvement). Isomethetene mucate, dichloralphenazone, and acetaminophen (Midrin) has also been used (two tablets at onset, then another tablet 1 hour later if no improvement).

Prophylaxis involves avoidance of known triggers, as well as techniques such as relaxation therapy and biofeedback. Those children who have frequent headaches and those with headaches that are unresponsive to abortive measures should be placed on prophylactic medications after consultation with a neurologist. Medications such as propranolol, amitriptyline, carbamazepine, valproic acid, cyproheptadine, and naproxen sodium have all been used.

FUNCTIONAL HEADACHES

Tension-Type Headaches

Tension-type headaches (muscle contraction or stress headache) tend to be chronic and nonprogressive in nature, with the pain described as band-like, bilateral, or generalized. There is no accompanying aura, and nausea is rare. The headache can last for 30 minutes to days and can be accompanied by photophobia or phonophobia but is not aggravated by physical activity. The pathophysiology is thought to result from prolonged muscle contraction, resulting in muscle ischemia.

Tension-type headaches are generally managed with mild analgesics, such as acetaminophen and ibuprofen. Reassuring the family that the problem is not organic and advising the patient to avoid precipitating factors, such as stress, is an important part of therapy. In some cases, treatment with amitriptyline is of benefit.

Cluster Headaches

There are two distinct patterns for these headaches. In the episodic form there are frequent headaches for a period of 1 to 3 months, followed by remission. In the chronic form (20 percent of patients), there is no period of remission. They usually occur at the same time, with extreme pain, described as throbbing deep and around one eye. The attacks often occur during sleep and awaken the patient. The eye often becomes teary and swollen, and the same eye is always affected. The headache may spread to the forehead and cheek, and there is often ipsilateral nasal congestion. The cheek may become flushed and warm. These headaches usually last 10 minutes to 3 hours (average <1 hour). Patients are unable to lie down or rest because of the pain. Treatment often consists of oxygen, but sumatriptan has been used.

Psychogenic Headaches

Psychogenic headaches tend to be chronic and nonprogressive and are characterized by vague complaints and nonspecific symptoms. They may result from stress, adjustment reactions, conversion reactions, depression, and malingering.

OTHER HEADACHES

Included in this group are problems that originate outside the calvarium but that can result in headache, either directly or through referred pain. They include sinusitis, dental caries or abscess, pharyngitis, temporomandibular joint abnormalities, head trauma (postconcussion or posttraumatic syndrome), and ophthalmologic problems, such as refractive errors or astigmatism. Toxic exposures, especially to carbon monoxide, can also cause headache.

BIBLIOGRAPHY

Annequin D, Tourniare B, Massiou H: Migraine and headaches in childhood and adolescence. *Pediatr Clin North Am* 47:617–631, 2000.

Forsyth R, Farrell K: Headache in childhood. *Pediatr Rev* 20:39–45, 1999.

Rothner AD: Headaches, in Swaiman KF, Ashwal S (eds): *Pediatric Neurology: Principles & Practice,* 3d ed. St, Louis: MO: Mosby, 1999, pp 747–758.

Winner PK: Headaches in children. *Postgrad Med* 101:81–90, 1997.

43

Hydrocephalus

Susan Fuchs

HIGH-YIELD FACTS

- Hydrocephalus refers to the excess accumulation of cerebrospinal fluid (CSF). Most cases result from congenital or acquired obstructions to the flow of CSF from the brain to the spinal canal.

- Infants with hydrocephalus are often diagnosed on routine examination by finding head circumference disproportionately large for age or splitting of the cranial sutures.

- Older children with hydrocephalus will usually complain of headache, which is often progressive in nature, worse in the morning, awakens the patient from sleep, and is exacerbated by lying down or straining.

- It is imperative to begin treatment in the unstable patient before herniation occurs. Patients who are lethargic on presentation, those with a Glasgow Coma Scale <8, or those who deteriorate in the emergency department are intubated following rapid sequence induction procedures and ventilated to maintain Pco_2 between 30 and 35 torr.

- Patients who do not respond with an improved mental status after intubation and controlled ventilation may benefit from diuretic therapy with mannitol or furosemide.

- After the patient is stabilized, a computed tomography scan or magnetic resonance image of the brain is performed to define the lesion and plan definitive treatment.

Hydrocephalus refers to the excess accumulation of cerebrospinal fluid (CSF). This can occur due to obstruction of CSF flow, reduced absorption, or excess production. Most CSF is produced by the choroid plexus and absorbed by the arachnoid villi and granulations. Flow di-

rection is from the lateral to third to fourth ventricles to the basal cisterns. It then divides between the spinal subarachnoid space and the subarachnoid cisterns via the interhemispheric and sylvian fissures. Although there are several ways to categorize hydrocephalus based on the site of excess fluid collection, the primary concern in the emergency department is determining the etiology of the problem and instituting appropriate treatment.

Most cases of hydrocephalus result from congenital or acquired obstructions to the flow of CSF from the brain to the spinal canal. Congenital malformations include the Arnold-Chiari malformation, which is elongation and downward displacement of the medulla into the fourth ventricle, and the Dandy-Walker syndrome, which causes obstruction at the outlet of the fourth ventricle. Beyond the neonatal period, the most common causes of acquired hydrocephalus are mass lesions, which include tumors, cysts, and abscesses. Other acquired causes of hydrocephalus are meningitis, encephalitis, posthemorrhagic adhesions, and vascular malformations.

CLINICAL PRESENTATION

The clinical presentation of hydrocephalus depends on the age of the patient and the rate at which it develops.

Infants with hydrocephalus are often diagnosed on routine examination by finding head circumference disproportionately large for age or splitting of the cranial sutures. The unfused sutures of the infant allow the calvarium to expand and function as a pressure relief phenomenon. When the limitations of suture expansion are reached, intracranial pressure begins to rise precipitously, and the infant may experience irritability, poor feeding, or other behavioral changes. When intracranial pressure becomes severely elevated, the infant develops vomiting and lethargy, which can signal impending herniation. In addition to split sutures, the physical examination may reveal a bulging anterior fontanel and engorged scalp veins. Dysfunction of cranial nerve III may result in loss of upward gaze, or the "sundown or setting-sun" sign. Bobble-head doll movements may also occur, especially with aqueductal stenosis or a third ventricle cyst.

Older children with hydrocephalus will usually complain of headache, which is often progressive in nature, worse in the morning, awakens the patient from sleep, and is exacerbated by lying down or straining. The child may suffer visual symptoms that are difficult to specify, but may result in the patient being perceived as unusually clumsy. Gait disturbances can occur, especially ataxia, which is characteristic of children with posterior fossa tumors. As with infants, older children develop vomiting as intracranial pressure begins to become severely elevated. Papilledema is a late finding in children and is rarely found in infants, but it implies a severe increase in intracranial pressure.

MANAGEMENT

In the emergency department, the primary goal of management of the child with hydrocephalus is the assessment and control of elevated intracranial pressure. Patients may be quite stable or in imminent danger of herniation. Specific signs of herniation depend on the part of the brain involved. In uncal herniation, there is compression of the third cranial nerve with dilation of the ipsilateral pupil and contralateral hemiparesis. Herniation of the cerebellar tonsils through the foramen magnum is preceded by headache and stiff neck and characterized by fixed, dilated pupils. The loss of leg function on one side suggests herniation under the falx. Central herniation occurs when both cerebral hemispheres compress the midbrain and results in decreased level of consciousness, constricted pupils, and Cheyne-Stokes respirations.

It is imperative to begin treatment in the unstable patient before herniation occurs. Patients who are lethargic on presentation, those with a Glasgow Coma Scale <8, or those who deteriorate in the emergency department are intubated following rapid sequence induction procedures. Prior to intubation, ventilation with a bag-valve-mask device to attain a Pco_2 between 30 and 35 torr may provide sufficient cerebral vasoconstriction to reduce intracranial pressure enough to avert herniation. Ventilation is continued after intubation, keeping oxygenation and blood pressure within normal values. Patients who do not respond with an improved mental status to intubation and ventilation may benefit from diuretic therapy with mannitol (0.25 to 1 g/kg) or furosemide (1 mg/kg). It is appropriate to elevate the head of the bed 15 to 30 degrees.

After the patient is stabilized, a computed tomography scan or magnetic resonance image of the brain is performed to define the lesion and plan definitive treatment. Therapy usually includes placement of an intracranial pressure monitoring device by a neurosurgeon. In dire circumstances, a percutaneous ventricular tap may be performed.

BIBLIOGRAPHY

Ashwal S: Congenital structural defects, in Swaiman KF, Ashwal S (eds): *Pediatric Neurology: Principles and Practice,* 3d ed. St Louis: Mosby, 1999, pp 234–273.

Kotagal S: Increased intracranial pressure, in Swaiman KF, Ashwal S (eds): *Pediatric Neurology: Principles and Practice,* 3d ed. St Louis: Mosby, 1999, pp 945–953.

44

Cerebral Palsy

Susan Fuchs

HIGH-YIELD FACTS

> - Cerebral palsy is a common condition associated with "special needs" children who require care in emergency departments.
> - The major abnormality in all forms of cerebral palsy is abnormal muscle tone.
> - Breakthrough seizures are common.
> - Respiratory problems, often resulting from chronic aspiration, commonly result in emergency department visits in cerebral palsy victims.
> - Severely impaired patients may require a multidisciplinary approach in the emergency department.

Cerebral palsy (CP) is a nonprogressive motor disorder reported to occur in 1.2 to 2.5 in 1000 children. It is usually evident within the first 2 to 3 years of life. The brain injury that results in cerebral palsy can occur during the antepartum, peripartum, or postnatal period. The actual cerebral injury is a hypoxic-ischemic event that results in specific lesions. Although the disorder is not in itself an emergency department diagnosis, children with cerebral palsy have associated problems that often result in emergency department visits. The emergency department physician must realize that each child with cerebral palsy has different abilities and problems and that each family has different parent-child relationships and coping mechanisms.

CLINICAL PRESENTATION

There are several forms of CP, with the classification systems based on the extremities involved, tone, and the ability to perform normal activity. The major disorder is of muscle tone, but there can also be neurologic disorders such as seizures, vision disturbances, and impaired intelligence.

Spastic CP includes several variants: spastic quadriparesis, spastic diplegia, and spastic hemiplegia. Spastic CP is the most common variant, with 70 to 80 percent of children with CP in one of these groups.

Spastic quadriparesis is characterized by a generalized increase in muscle tone, deep tendon reflexes, and rigidity of the limbs on both flexion and extension. Although the lower extremities are generally more severely affected, in severe forms the child is stiff and assumes a posture of decerebrate rigidity. Many children have pseudobulbar involvement, resulting in swallowing difficulties and recurrent aspiration. Intellectual impairment is severe, and half have a tonic-clonic seizure disorder.

Spastic diplegia is characterized by bilateral spasticity, with greater involvement of the lower extremities than the upper. It is the most common form of CP diagnosed in preterm infants. Early in life, when rigidity predominates, the legs are held in extension and in a scissored pattern due to adductor spasm. As spasticity progresses, flexion of the hips and knees develops, ultimately leading to contractures. In those less severely affected, dorsiflexion of the feet with increased ankle tone results in toe-walking. Other manifestations include convergent strabismus, delayed speech development, and seizure disorders. Intellectual impairment parallels the motor deficit.

Spastic hemiparesis is a unilateral paresis that usually affects the upper extremity more than the lower. Some degree of spasticity and flexion contracture usually results. One of the initial symptoms is fisting, which is an exaggerated palmar grasp reflex. The gait may be circumductive, with swinging of the affected leg like an arc. The extent of functional impairment varies, with fine movements of the hand affected most. Sensory impairment, growth disturbance, and involuntary movements of the affected limbs can occur. In addition, facial weakness, visual disturbances, and seizures can occur.

Another classification of CP is extrapyramidal or dyskinetic, which accounts for 10 to 15 percent of cases. Dyskinesia is difficulty performing voluntary movements. The variants are based on the types of movement and defects in posture more than the tone, with all four extremities involved to varying degrees. Athetoid CP involves slow, continuous writhing motions and usually involves the distal limbs. Ballismus is characterized by violent, jerky motions of the arms and legs. Choreic CP movements result from disorganized tone and can involve the limbs, face, or trunk. Those with tremulous CP have involuntary, rhythmic contractions of opposing muscles.

The remaining forms of CP are less common and include rigid (5 percent), atonic (hypotonic), and ataxic (1 percent). Ataxic CP presents with a wide-based gait and truncal ataxia. There are many children (10 to 15 percent) who have a mixed form of CP, with two or more types of the above-mentioned forms. This group can be difficult to diagnose, as the expression of CP may change during their early years.

COMPLICATIONS

Many complications can occur in the patient with CP, with the type depending on the degree of the patient's impairment. The most common problem in CP patients presenting to the emergency department is breakthrough seizures. The management of seizures is discussed in Chapter 38.

Respiratory difficulties also commonly present to the emergency department. Chronic aspiration can result in reactive airway disease and, for some patients, chronic hypoxia and hypercarbia. Acute pneumonia is common after aspiration and is often difficult to diagnose in patients whose baseline chest radiographs are abnormal. Poor coughing mechanisms contribute to pulmonary pathology. In CP patients with evidence of pneumonia, aggressive antibiotic therapy is indicated. Admission to the hospital may be necessary if the child is unable to take oral antibiotics or needs chest physiotherapy or supplemental oxygen. In many cases, functional lung impairment mandates a low threshold for hospital admission. The management of patients with bronchospasm includes aggressive therapy with bronchodilators.

Many children with cerebral palsy have significant feeding difficulties that require placement of a gastrostomy tube or button, with or without a fundoplication. In some patients a gastrojejunal feeding tube is inserted. Malfunction of either tube can result in vomiting, especially for patients without a fundoplication. Feeding tube malfunction can also result in the inability to deliver feedings and medications, which predisposes to dehydration and subtherapeutic levels of anticonvulsants. When the tube needs to be replaced, correct positioning is confirmed by an abdominal radiograph, accompanied by the injection of radiopaque contrast.

Many patients with CP who are significantly impaired are not toilet trained and are vulnerable to urinary tract infections and perineal skin breakdown that can result in infection. In addition to a chest radiograph to rule out pneumonia, all febrile CP patients require a urinalysis and urine culture.

Although there is no cure for CP, an important goal of emergency department management is ensuring that the child is receiving adequate overall therapy through a multidisciplinary approach and that the family is comfortable with the child's management.

BIBLIOGRAPHY

Davis DW: Review of cerebral palsy, part I: Description, incidence and etiology. *Neonatal Network* 16:7–11, 1997.

Perlman JM: Intrapartum hypoxic-ischemic cerebral injury and subsequent cerebral palsy: Medicolegal issues. *Pediatrics* 99:851–859, 1997.

Swaiman KF, Rusman BS: Cerebral palsy, in Swaiman KF, Ashwal S (eds): *Pediatric Neurology: Principles & Practice*, 3d ed. St. Louis, MO: Mosby, 1999, pp 312–324.

45

Cerebrovascular Syndromes

Susan Fuchs

HIGH-YIELD FACTS

- In children, hemorrhagic strokes are as common as ischemic strokes, with a hemorrhagic incidence of 1.9/100,000/yr versus 1.2/100,000/yr for ischemic strokes.

- Ischemic strokes are caused by vascular occlusion of an artery, usually due to thromboembolism (arterial ischemic stroke) or occlusion of venous sinuses or cerebral veins (sinovenous thrombosis). The ratio of arterial ischemic stroke (AIS) to sinovenous thrombosis (SV) is 3:1, with a neonatal and male predominance.

- A history of cardiac disorders, especially complex congenital heart disease or a prosthetic heart valve, should raise suspicion of an embolic phenomenon. A history of sickle cell disease is also extremely important to determine, as 25 percent of patients will develop cerebrovascular problems.

- Although magnetic resonance imaging (MRI) is more sensitive in detecting infarcts, especially smaller ones and infarcts of the brainstem and cerebellum, a computed tomography (CT) scan is superior to the MRI in detecting hemorrhage acutely (<12 hours). The CT scan with contrast may also miss small hemorrhages, arteriovenous malformations, or aneurysms and may even be normal within the first 12 hours after an ischemic stroke.

- If available, magnetic resonance angiography can be done at the time of the MRI to visualize the flow through the cerebral arteries. MRI can also be used with MRV to diagnose sinovenous thrombosis.

- For patients in whom a hemorrhagic stroke is suspected and in whom the CT scan is negative and there are no signs of increased intracranial pressure, a lumbar puncture is indicated. Particularly with a small subarachnoid hemorrhage, the CT scan may not reveal blood.

- The key function of the emergency department is stabilization of the patient's respiratory and cardiovascular status, especially the blood pressure. In the event of an ischemic infarct, a precipitous decline in blood pressure is avoided, since it can worsen cerebral ischemia, but if hypotension is present, careful fluid resuscitation and inotropic support may be needed.

- Serum glucose should be monitored closely as hypoglycemia can worsen the effect of the stroke, and hyperglycemia can increase infarct size.

- Specific therapy is directed at the etiology of the stroke, such as correction of clotting abnormalities, antibiotics for infections, antiepileptic medication for seizures, and surgery for evacuation of a hematoma. For patients with sickle cell disease, exchange transfusion is indicated for ischemic stroke.

Although they are uncommon in children compared with adults, both ischemic and hemorrhagic strokes do occur. Ischemic strokes can be divided into arterial ischemic strokes and sinovenous thrombosis. Arterial ischemic strokes are characterized by the rapid onset of focal neurologic abnormalities, including hemiplegia, sensory abnormalities, and an altered level of consciousness. Children younger than 4 years of age may have a seizure just prior to or after the stroke, a syndrome known as HHE (hemiconvulsions, hemiplegia, and epilepsy). Sinovenous thrombosis may present with diffuse neurologic signs and seizures, whereas hemorrhagic strokes usually present with severe headache, decreased level of consciousness, seizures, and focal signs.

In children, hemorrhagic strokes are as common as ischemic strokes, with a hemorrhagic incidence of 1.9/100,000/yr versus 1.2/100,000/yr for ischemic strokes.

Ischemic strokes are caused by vascular occlusion of an artery, usually due to thromboembolism (arterial ischemic stroke) or occlusion of venous sinuses or cerebral veins (sinovenous thrombosis). The ratio of arterial ischemic stroke (AIS) to sinovenous thrombosis (SV) is 3:1, with a neonatal age and male predominance.

The arterial circulation to the brain is via the anterior (carotids) and posterior (vertebral and basilar) arteries, which link via communicating arteries to form the circle of Willis. Cerebral arteries can thrombose due to damage to the arterial wall or emboli. Infarction occurs when there is damage to cerebral tissue, resulting in ischemia, hypoxia, and depletion of energy and carbohydrate stores. The extent of neuronal damage depends on the length of time (e.g., in transient ischemic attacks the deficit is usually <1 hour), the availability of collateral

Table 45-1. Predisposing Conditions for Ischemic Stroke

Cardiac

Congenital heart disease
Rheumatic heart disease
Bacterial endocarditis
Arrhythmias
Cardiomyopathy
Prosthetic heart valves
VSD/ASD
Patent foramen ovale

Infection

Meningitis
Encephalitis (especially varicella)

Vasculopathy

Moyamoya disease
Postradiation vasculopathy

Systemic Disorders

Systemic lupus erythematosus
Polyarteritis nodosa
Leukemia
Nephrotic syndrome
Inflammatory bowel disease
Takayasu's arteritis
Dermatomyositis
Rheumatoid arthritis
Diabetes mellitus

Hematologic Disorders

Sickle cell disease
Protein S and C deficiencies
Antithrombin III deficiency
Polycythemia
Hemolytic uremic syndrome
Thrombotic thrombocytopenic purpura
Idiopathic thrombocytopenic purpura

Acquired Prothrombotic States

Lupus anticoagulant/anticardiolipin antibodies
Plasminogen deficiency

Trauma

Head injury
Neck injury
Intraoral trauma
Child abuse

Drugs

Cocaine
Oral contraceptives
Antineoplastic agents (EG, L-asparaginase)
Steroids
LSD
Amphetamines
Alcohol

Metabolic Disorders

Homocystinuria
Hypoglycemia
Mitochondrial encephalomyopathy (MELAS)
Hyperlipidemia

Neurocutaneous Syndromes

Neurofibromatosis
Sturge-Weber syndrome
Tuberous sclerosis

Hereditary Disorders

Ehlers-Danlos syndrome
Fabry's disease

Vasospastic Disorders

Migraine

VSD, Ventriculoseptal defect; ASD, atrial septal defect.

Table 45-2. Conditions Predisposing to Hemorrhagic Stroke

Vascular Malformations	**Drug**
Aneurysms	Amphetamines
Arteriovenous malformations	Phenylpropanolamine
Cavernous malformation	Cocaine
Coagulation Defects	**Head Trauma**
Hemophilia	Child abuse
Disseminated intravascular coagulation	**Brain Tumors**
Idiopathic thrombocytopenia purpura	**Infection**
Vitamin K deficiency	Herpes simplex
Anticoagulation treatment	Varicella
Leukemia	
Aplastic anemia	**Congenital Syndromes**
Factor deficiencies	Ehlers-Danlos Syndrome
Systemic Disorders	Neurofibromatosis
Hypertension	Tuberous sclerosis
Hepatic failure	
Sickle cell disease	

circulation, and the metabolic needs of the brain (e.g., seizures increase the metabolic demand).

In children, risk factors associated with AIS include cardiac disease, coagulation disorders, dehydration, infection, vasculitis, cancer, metabolic disorders, moyamoya, sickle cell anemia, and perinatal complications. In some cases, no risk factor is defined, whereas in others there may actually be multiple risk factors. This is in stark contrast to adults, in whom arteriosclerosis is the leading risk factor.

Sinovenous thrombosis can occur due to thrombophlebitis, hemoconcentration, or coagulation abnormalities. Occlusion of the sinuses or other cerebral vessels results in increased venous pressure, which, if sudden and severe, leads to increased intracranial pressure and decreased cerebral perfusion. In some cases (more than in AIS), the vessels leak and the infarcts become hemorrhagic. In addition, there is a risk of developing communicating hydrocephalus after sinovenous thrombosis.

Risk factors associated with SV are prothrombotic disorders, dehydration, systemic infection, head and neck infections (otitis, mastoiditis, sinusitis), hematologic disorders, drugs, cardiac disease, cancer, and perinatal complications. The underlying diseases that cause AIS and SV are listed in Table 45-1.

Hemorrhagic strokes involve the rupture of cerebral blood vessels with leakage of blood into the brain parenchyma, subarachnoid space, or ventricular system. The location of the hemorrhage defines the two major types of stroke (intracerebral [intraparenchymal] and subarachnoid) and separates the pathophysiology, risk factors, and clinical findings.

Intracerebral hemorrhage occurs when arteries or veins rupture into intracerebral areas or brain parenchyma. Damage occurs to the blood-brain barrier, resulting in cerebral edema; when large, the hematoma can cause a mass effect. The greatest risk factor is head trauma, followed by aneurysms and vascular malformations.

Subarachnoid hemorrhage results from rupture of an aneurysm (usually proximal arteries at the circle of Willis) or an arteriovenous malformation (AVM). Secondary effects include ischemic infarction due to blood in the subarachnoid space, causing vasospasm in the cerebral arteries, and hydrocephalus. Risk factors include disorders associated with vascular malformations, aneurysms, and hypoxia in neonates. However, hemorrhagic strokes are occasionally associated with systemic diseases and coagulopathies. These conditions are summarized in Table 45-2.

DIAGNOSIS

History

The presenting signs and symptoms of a stroke depend somewhat on the type of stroke. Arterial ischemic strokes usually have a rapid onset, so there may be little in the history to warn of the impending event. Patients often suffer sudden collapse, seizures, or loss of focal neurologic function (especially hemiplegia). A history of recurrent headaches, transient ischemic attacks, or focal seizures may be obtained, but these do not provide a specific diagnosis. An older child with a sinovenous thrombosis may present with slowly progressive signs, such as fever, vomiting, or headache. A young infant may have dilated scalp veins, eyelid swelling, and a large anterior fontanelle.

An older child with a hemorrhagic stroke may have a history of severe headache, or neck pain (subarachnoid hemorrhage), or subtle focal neurologic signs (cranial nerve palsies), but in most cases, the presentation is acute.

A history of cardiac disorders, especially complex congenital heart disease or a prosthetic heart valve, should raise suspicion of an embolic phenomenon. The presence of fever and headache should raise concern about meningitis. However, systemic infections such as mycoplasma, Rocky Mountain spotted fever, and others, have been associated with cerebral infarction. A recent infection with varicella is of concern, as postvaricella angiopathy can include basal ganglia infarction and stenosis of large arteries. Inherited coagulation disorders such as deficiency of protein C, protein S, antithrombin III, and plasminogen, or the presence of factor V Leiden, anticardiolipin antibody, or lupus anticoagulant can all lead to thromboembolism.

A history of sickle cell disease is extremely important to determine, as 25 percent of patients will develop cerebrovascular problems. The presence of systemic lupus erythematosus and other forms of vasculitis such as polyarteritis nodosa, mixed connective tissue disease, or Takayasu's arteritis have all been associated with arterial ischemic and sinovenous thrombosis.

Metabolic disorders, such as homozygous homocystinuria (hyperhomocysteinemia), which have a thrombotic effect, can cause arterial and venous thrombosis. Fabry's disease can lead to lacunar infarcts, and hyperlipidemia has also been associated with childhood strokes. The MELAS syndrome (mitochondrial myopathy, encephalopathy, lactic acidosis, and stroke-like episodes) is characterized by nausea, vomiting, headaches, seizures, hemiparesis, and cortical blindness. Neurocutaneous disorders such as neurofibromatosis, Sturge-Weber syndrome, and tuberous sclerosis are all associated with both ischemic and hemorrhagic strokes.

Any history of trauma is significant and suggests a hemorrhagic lesion. However, intraoral trauma can cause dissection of the carotid artery, and injury to the vertebral arteries can occur after neck trauma.

Children who have had radiation for optic gliomas or pituitary or suprasellar tumors can develop postradiation vasculitis.

Adolescents in particular are questioned regarding illicit drug ingestion, particularly cocaine. Additional questions are directed toward detecting one of the underlying etiologies noted in Tables 45-1 and 45-2.

Physical Examination

Stabilizing the patient is the first priority, since seizures may occur in younger children at the time of or shortly after the stroke. Complete vital signs include temperature and blood pressure. If trauma is suspected, the head and neck are immobilized. A thorough examination includes auscultation over the head, eyes, and carotid arteries listening for bruits, as well as a careful auscultation of the heart for murmurs, clicks suggestive of valvular disease, arrhythmias, or indications of prior cardiac surgery. The eyes are examined for extraocular movements, pupillary responses, and visual field testing if possible. The eyes will look toward the lesion if the cerebral hemisphere is involved, but away with brainstem involvement. The skin is examined for petechiae, café au lait spots, neurofibromas, or telangiectasias.

Neurologic assessment includes determination of degree of weakness, cranial nerve dysfunction, and the side and extent to which the extremities are involved. If the facial muscles and tongue are involved, there is dysarthria, but involvement of the basal ganglia, thalamus, or cerebral hemispheres can result in aphasia. It may be difficult to detect sensory impairment due to aphasia.

Some disorders that can be confused with a stroke include complicated migraines, partial seizures, Todd's paralysis, brain tumors, brain abscesses, and subdural hematoma. Most will be diagnosed during the workup of the suspected stroke.

Diagnostic Evaluation

Baseline lab studies include a complete blood count with differential and platelet count and coagulation times. If sickle cell disease is a possibility, sickle prep and hemoglobin electrophoresis is performed. Further coagulation studies are indicated if hemophilia or other coagulopathies, such as protein S or C or antithrombin III deficiencies, are suspected. Other studies should include electrolytes, BUN, creatinine, glucose, and sedimentation rate, as well as a urinalysis looking for red cells or protein. Additional studies such as antinuclear antibodies, drug screens, lipid profile, blood culture, urine for culture, and amino acids are ordered as warranted. An electrocardogram (ECG) and an echocardiogram should be performed on all children in whom underlying heart disease is suspected.

Imaging studies provide information that will help differentiate an ischemic from a hemorrhagic stroke and will help direct treatment. Although magnetic resonance imaging (MRI) is more sensitive in detecting infarcts, especially smaller ones and infarcts of the brain stem and cerebellum, a computed tomography (CT) scan is superior to the MRI in detecting hemorrhage acutely (<12 hours). The CT scan with contrast may also miss small hemorrhage, AVMs, or aneurysms and may even be normal within the first 12 hours after an ischemic stroke. The test of choice for the ED depends on the availability of CT scan versus MRI. If available, magnetic resonance angiography (MRA) can be done at the time of the MRI to visualize the flow through the cerebral arteries and does correlate well with angiography. MRI can also be used with MRV to diagnose sinovenous thrombosis. The visualization of a thrombus and the absence of a flow-related signal provide the diagnosis.

The gold standard to visualize intracranial and extracranial vessels is cerebral angiography. Other modalities that may prove useful include single-photon emission CT (SPECT), Doppler imaging of the carotid arteries, transcranial Doppler, and transcranial ultrasound.

For patients in whom a hemorrhagic stroke is suspected and in whom the CT scan is negative, with no signs of increased intracranial pressure, a lumbar puncture is indicated. Particularly in a small subarachnoid hemorrhage, the CT scan may not reveal blood. The cerebrospinal fluid (CSF) is evaluated for the presence of red blood cells, which, in the absence of a traumatic lumbar puncture, indicates hemorrhage, especially if the blood does not clear during CSF collection. In some cases the CSF may appear xanthrochromic, which is also consistent with hemorrhage.

TREATMENT

The key function of the ED is stabilization of the patient's respiratory and cardiovascular status, especially the blood pressure. In the event of an ischemic infarct, a precipitous decline in blood pressure is avoided, since it can worsen cerebral ischemia. If hypotension is present, careful fluid resuscitation and inotropic support may be needed. If there are signs of impending herniation, mannitol (0.25 to 1 g/kg intravenously over 20 minutes) and controlled ventilation may be required. Serum glucose should be monitored closely as hypoglycemia can worsen the effect of the stroke, and hyperglycemia can increase the infarct size. Maintenance of normal body temperature is also important, as hyperthermia can worsen ischemic brain damage. Specific therapy is directed at the etiology of the stroke, such as correction of clotting abnormalities, antibiotics for infections, antiepileptic medication for seizures, and surgery for evacuation of a hematoma. In patients with sickle cell disease, exchange transfusion is indicated for ischemic stroke (see Chap. 2). Although antithrombotic agents are used commonly in adult ischemic stroke patients, there still exists the risk of extension of an infarction or conversion to a hemorrhagic stroke. Depending on the etiology of the stroke in children, there may be a use for some of these agents, but dosing and efficacy still need to be determined for some therapies. The use of steroids is indicated only if there is proven vasculitis with progression of stenosis, but they are rarely indicated in the ED.

DISPOSITION

Children who have suffered strokes are admitted to an intensive care setting for close monitoring of blood pressure, fluid status, temperature, and neurologic function.

BIBLIOGRAPHY

DeVeber G: Cerebrovascular disease in children, in Swaiman KF, Ashwal S (eds): *Pediatric Neurology: Principles and Practice.* St. Louis: Mosby, 1999, pp 1099–1124.

Scott PA, Barsan WG: Stroke, transient ischemic attack and other central focal conditions, in Tintinalli JE, Kelen GD, Stapczynski JS (eds): *Emergency Medicine: A Comprehensive Study Guide,* 5th ed. New York: McGraw-Hill, 2000, pp 1430–1440.

Solomon GE: Acute therapy of childhood stroke, in Pellock JM, Myer EC (eds): *Neurologic Emergencies in Infancy and Childhood,* 2d ed. Boston, Butterworth-Heinemann, 1993, pp 179–207.

46

The Febrile Child

Nattasorn Plipat
Suchinta Hakim
William R. Ahrens

HIGH-YIELD FACTS

- The approach to fever in the pediatric patient is age dependent, reflecting the implications of bacterial infection in the context of an evolving immune system.

- Neonates younger than 28 days old are susceptible to organisms from maternal flora, especially group B *streptococcus, Escherichia coli,* and *Listeria monocytogenes.* Because they are presumed to localize bacterial infections poorly, virtually any bacterial infection in these patients is considered to be capable of disseminating and causing serious bacterial infection.

- Environmentally acquired encapsulated organisms become the chief pathogens starting between the ages of 28 days and 2 to 3 months and remain so throughout the rest of childhood.

- For patients between 3 and 36 months of age, the immune system has presumably matured to the extent that disseminated infection from a bacterial focus is much less likely. However, up to 2 percent of patients in this age group, with temperatures >39°C, who appear well and have no focus of infection on physical examination, will have positive blood cultures—a situation referred to as occult bacteremia.

- Widespread use of the new conjugate pneumococcal vaccine will markedly reduce invasive infections with *Streptococcus pneumoniae* and make the use of white blood cell counts, blood cultures, and empiric antibiotics in febrile children 3 to 36 months of age without a source of infection unnecessary.

- Observation of the infant or toddler while taking the history provides a wealth of information regarding the child's general appearance that is useful in categorizing the patients as "sick" or "not sick."

- Especially in infants, overwhelming infection can cause apnea. It is important to realize that apnea can be intermittent and that the patient may appear stable between episodes.

- Children who are inconsolable or appear worse when held or rocked by their parents are demonstrating true irritability, which may indicate central nervous system infection.

- Petechiae or purpura are ominous findings that suggest fulminant meningococcemia.

Body temperature is normally maintained within a very narrow range, despite exposure to widely varying environmental temperatures. Body temperature is controlled by a complex system that regulates the balance between heat production and heat loss. Heat production depends on metabolic and physical activity. Heat loss occurs through radiation, evaporation, convection and conduction. Most heat loss occurs through radiation, and evaporative loss accounts for much of the remainder. The thermoregulatory center is located in the preoptic region of the anterior hypothalamus.

Fever is a centrally mediated increase in body temperature that results when some stimulus causes an upward adjustment in the "set point" of the

The authors would like to thank Dr. Stanford Shulman for his gracious review of this chapter.

thermoregulatory center. It is compensated for by mechanisms that increase heat loss. Fever is produced by pyrogens, released from leukocytes and other phagocytic cells, which act on the thermoregulatory center. Fever is distinct from the rise in body temperature that occurs in heat illness, when environmental factors exceed the body's ability to dissipate heat.

Although the exact definition is somewhat arbitrary, fever is usually considered to be present with a rectal temperature $\geq$ 38.0°C (100.4°F). Children tend to have higher temperature than adults. Body temperature also exhibits circadian rhythm and is highest in the afternoon.

There are a variety of ways to measure body temperature. Oral and skin temperatures are lower than rectal temperatures by approximately 0.6°C (1°F) and 1°C (2 to 2.5°F), respectively. Oral temperatures are not recommended in young children, and skin temperatures obtained from the axilla or forehead are unreliable. Tympanic temperatures are lower than rectal temperatures.

Fever most commonly occurs as a response to infection, but it may be due to immune-mediated or collagen vascular disease and is associated with many malignancies. During infection, moderate fever is probably beneficial because it enhances host defense reactions. Rapidly rising temperature, however, may be associated with febrile convulsions. Hyperpyrexia, defined as a core temperature > 41.1°C (106°F), can result in complications such as central nervous system damage and rhabdomyolysis.

About 20 percent of pediatric patients presenting to the emergency department (ED) have fever as a sign or symptom. The vast majority of these patients have benign illnesses that are caused by viruses and are therefore self-limited, or result from bacterial infections that are amenable to outpatient therapy. A very small percentage of patients suffer from life-threatening infections. It is the emergency physician's challenge to identify these patients.

The approach to fever in the pediatric patient is age dependent, reflecting the implications of bacterial infection in the context of an evolving immune system. In essence, neonates and young infants are considered to be deficient in the ability to localize and neutralize bacterial infections. It must be realized that the exact age groups are somewhat arbitrary and are not precisely based on scientific understanding of the immune response. Rather, the management of the febrile child is based on cumulative clinical experience and a growing body of research that is challenging traditional treatment. The exact age at which the developing immune system reaches adequate maturity is unknown. For example, how is a 3-week-old different from an 8-week-old in its ability to handle bacteremia?

It is also important to realize that, although predictable organisms tend to affect different age groups, there is significant crossover. For example, pneumococcal infection is usually associated with infants older than 2 to 3 months but can occur at younger ages. Conversely, group B *Streptococcus,* usually a pathogen in neonates, has been reported in a 5-month-old infant.

THE AGE GROUPS

Neonates younger than 28 days old are susceptible to organisms from maternal flora, especially group B Streptococcus, *Escherichia coli,* and *Listeria monocytogenes.* Since neonates mount febrile responses poorly, the height of the fever does not necessarily correlate with the severity of the illness. Septic neonates may be hypothermic. Because they are presumed to localize bacterial infections poorly, virtually any bacterial infection in these patients is considered to be capable of disseminating and causing serious bacterial infection (SBI).

Infants between 28 days and 2 to 3 months of age constitute the next major category. Environmentally-acquired encapsulated organisms become the chief pathogens from this period throughout the rest of childhood. The traditional approach to febrile infants in this age group has usually included an aggressive workup to search for bacterial illness, followed by hospitalization and empiric antibiotic therapy until cultures of blood, cerebrospinal fluid (CSF), and urine were negative. In many centers, management now includes an effort to define a subgroup of these patients as being at particularly low risk for a serious bacterial infection and therefore candidates for outpatient management. An important concept in this approach is that in this age group virtually any bacterial infection, probably with the exception of acute otitis media, is still considered to be potentially capable of disseminating and causing serious infection.

Patients between 3 and 36 months of age constitute the next traditional age group and present a challenge in emergency management. The immune system has presumably matured to the extent that disseminated infection from a bacterial focus is much less likely. However, up to 2 percent of patients in this age group, with temperatures >39°C, who appear well and have no focus of infection on physical examination, will have positive blood cultures—a situation referred to as occult bacteremia. The management of this subsegment of patients is the subject of intense controversy and ongoing investigation.

After 36 months of age, the management of the non-immunocompromised febrile pediatric patient is similar to that of the healthy adolescent and adult.

PRESENTATION

The history of the present illness is obtained from the person most familiar with the patient. Observation of the infant or toddler while taking the history provides a wealth of information regarding the child's general appearance that is useful in categorizing the patients as "sick" or "not sick."

Information solicited includes the time of onset of the fever and the method used to determine that the patient was febrile. A temperature measured by a caretaker familiar with a thermometer is much more accurate than a history noting that the patient "felt warm." Attempts to treat the fever prior to arrival in the ED are solicited, since antipyretic therapy may result in a normal temperature in triage in a patient with a potentially serious febrile illness. Inappropriate treatment, such as bundling a febrile infant or sponging with alcohol, may also be noted, and the caretaker can then be educated on proper management of fever.

The caretaker is questioned regarding his or her perception of the severity of the patient's illness. Helpful information in neonates and infants includes the patient's general level of activity, feeding, and interaction with the environment. In older patients, a history of play activity is helpful. It is important to attempt to elicit a sense of the child's mental status, but it must be remembered that asking about the presence of "irritability" or "lethargy" introduces terminology into the history that may have a different meaning to the caretaker than to the physician.

The history of the patient's general behavior is followed by questions regarding associated symptoms. A large percentage of infectious illnesses in the pediatric population involve the respiratory tract. The combination of rhinorrhea, cough, and sore throat suggests upper respiratory infection. Acute otitis media is often associated with these symptoms. Infection involving the lower respiratory tract is often characterized by a history of coughing, wheezing, or noisy breathing. In neonates and infants, difficulty in bottle-feeding is the equivalent of dyspnea on exertion and implies significant respiratory distress. Especially in infants, overwhelming infection can cause apnea, which parents may perceive as difficulty breathing. It is important to realize that apnea can be intermittent and that the patient may appear stable between episodes.

Gastrointestinal symptoms are also common in the febrile pediatric patient. Vomiting or diarrhea usually indicate an infectious process involving the gastrointestinal tract, such as viral or bacterial gastroenteritis. However, vomiting and diarrhea can also occur as nonspecific findings in other infections, including otitis media and pyelonephritis, and may occur in association with life-threatening infections such as meningitis and overwhelming sepsis. Information sought regarding vomiting includes frequency, character (projectile or nonprojectile), and whether it contains blood or bile. For patients with diarrhea, the frequency and character of the stool is ascertained. Stool that contains blood is associated with bacterial enteritis, which in neonates and young infants is a potentially serious infection.

The caretaker may also be aware of skin or musculoskeletal manifestations of illness. Many infections and inflammatory diseases are associated with rashes, some of which are transient and whose presence may be established only by a careful history. Musculoskeletal manifestations of infectious and inflammatory illnesses associated with fever include arthritis, arthralgia, and, in some cases, a history of refusal to walk or use a limb.

A history of exposure to an individual with a similar illness is an important clue that may be obtained in the history. Many infectious illnesses are highly contagious and affect multiple members of a household. They range in severity from the benign common cold to serious diseases such as tuberculosis.

It is also important to document the patient's immunization history. Although immunizations provide significant protection from many deadly diseases, their complications can prompt an ED visit. These include febrile reactions that often occur following diptheria-pertussis-tetanus (DPT) vaccine. However, DPT has now been replaced by diphtheria-tetanus-acellular pertussis (DTaP) vaccine, which is significantly less likely to provoke a fever. Mild measles-like illness can occur 6 to 12 days after immunization with measles-mumps-rubella (MMR) vaccine.

It is also essential to elicit a history of medications used during both the current and any recent febrile illness. In addition to antipyretics, patients may be taking antibiotics prescribed by a physician for the current illness in either the patient or siblings. Inappropriate treatment with outpatient oral antibiotics may mask symptoms of serious disease, as in the case of partially treated meningitis. Knowledge of prior therapy is also necessary in deciding current treatment in such cases as recurrent or resistant otitis media.

PHYSICAL EXAMINATION

The physical examination of the febrile pediatric patient is roughly divided into general assessment and detailed evaluation that focuses on identifying a specific site of infection.

It is impossible to overemphasize the importance of the general assessment in guiding the evaluation and management of the pediatric patient. It is largely the general assessment that determines whether the patient is "sick" or "not sick." The general assessment is essentially a gestalt and results from a combination of observation, experience, and the intangible factor of "clinical judgment." However, on analysis, the general assessment is compiled from fairly objective information. It is a fundamental principle that, in neonates and very young infants, the limited development of the patient makes clinical assessment more difficult, even for the experienced clinician. Attempts to apply reproducible scales of observation to this age group in order to predict the presence of SBI have met with mixed results. Although it is certain that an "ill appearing" infant has a relatively high probability of having an SBI, a well appearance does not rule out potentially serious illness.

The most important factor to assess is the patient's mental status, which is evaluated by observing the patient's interaction with the environment, especially with the parents. Older infants and children should recognize their parents and demonstrate curiosity about their surroundings. After 5 to 6 months of age, "stranger anxiety" is appropriate and is not to be construed as irritability. In younger infants, the presence of a social smile is an important finding that implies well-being. A social smile is generally expected to be present by 6 to 8 weeks of age. In neonates too young to have developed a social smile, the baby's state of alertness and desire to breast- or bottle-feed are noted. Virtually all pediatric patients should be consolable. Patients who are inconsolable or appear worse when held or rocked by their parents are demonstrating true irritability, which may indicate central nervous system infection.

Anxiousness and lethargy are also signs of serious illness. In the patient with fever, these findings suggest overwhelming infection. In neonates and infants, noting the quality of the cry can also provide adjunctive information regarding the patient's mental status. A strong, lusty cry is normal, whereas a weak or high-pitched cry indicates distress.

Concomitant with the assessment of mental status, the patient's hydration and perfusion are assessed. For patients who appear dehydrated, the history will usually indicate fluid losses secondary to vomiting or diarrhea. In a febrile patient in whom peripheral perfusion is diminished but who has no history compatible with fluid loss, septic shock is possible. In practice, most patients with significantly decreased perfusion also have depressed mental status.

It is also important to realize that in neonates and infants depressed mental status and signs of impaired perfusion can occasionally be intermittent. This presumably occurs because of the young cardiovascular system's inability to compensate until late in the course of an overwhelming infection. A parent may give a history of finding an infant ashen, mottled, and lethargic or even apneic at home. Nevertheless, the patient may have responded to stimulation alone and may appear relatively well on arrival in the ED. Conversely, a patient who appears well on arrival in the ED may suddenly decompensate, only to respond to stimulation or fluid resuscitation to such a degree that the presence of serious illness is doubted. Any febrile pediatric patient with a history of even a momentary decrease in mental status or perfusion is presumed to have an overwhelming infection until proved otherwise.

In the stable febrile patient, the general assessment is followed by a complete physical examination in an attempt to determine the cause of the fever. The skin is evaluated for the presence of an exanthem, many of which are associated with specific infectious diseases. Localized erythema indicates cellulitis. The presence of petechiae always calls to mind the possibility of meningococcemia, especially in an ill-appearing patient.

The examination of the head focuses on the anterior fontanel, which should be flat and soft. A tense or bulging fontanel suggests increased intracranial pressure that may be caused by meningitis. The fontanel closes at about 18 months of age. The eyes are evaluated for conjunctival injection or discharge. Periorbital redness or swelling suggest cellulitis. All pediatric patients require careful examination of the ears, since otitis media is the most common bacterial infection identified in this age group. The criteria for diagnosis are discussed in Chapter 67. The nose is examined for the presence of clear discharge, which accompanies many upper respiratory infections, or purulent drainage, which may indicate sinusitis. The oral cavity is evaluated for the presence of an exanthem, pharyngeal erythema, tonsillar enlargement, or exudate. Specific infectious lesions are discussed in Chapter 67.

The neck is evaluated for the presence of adenopathy or other localized swelling. Localized neck swelling can occur in adenitis and with infection of congenital anomalies, such as brachial cleft or thyroglossal duct cysts. Although it is important to attempt to determine whether the neck is supple and easily flexed and extended, this is not a reliable way to exclude meningitis in infants younger than 1 year of age.

The chest is evaluated for the presence for retractions, which signify increased work of breathing and, in the absence of stridor, indicate lower respiratory track pathology. Auscultation may reveal wheezing, which may indicate reactive airway disease or acute bronchiolitis. Rales are infrequently heard in pediatric patients, especially infants, even in the presence of well-documented bacterial pneumonia. Percussion of the chest while listening with the stethoscope is more sensitive for determining an area of pneumonic consolidation.

The heart is evaluated for the character of the valve sounds. Muffled heart sounds in a febrile patient may indicate a pericardial effusion, whereas a new or unexplained murmur may indicate infective endocarditis or an inflammatory process such as acute rheumatic fever.

The abdomen is evaluated for the presence of tenderness, guarding. or rebound, which may indicate a surgical problem, such as appendicitis. The size of the liver and spleen is evaluated. Many infectious illnesses, especially those of viral etiology, are associated with hepatosplenomegaly.

The extremities are evaluated for the presence of erythema or swelling, especially of the joints. In infants, range of motion is assessed. In older children, the gait can easily be observed for the presence of a limp. Both osteomyelitis and septic arthritis are more common in children than in adults, and although neither is a very frequent cause of fever, early diagnosis is imperative to avoid morbidity.

MANAGEMENT

The Septic-Appearing or Toxic Child

Sepsis is a clinical condition in which an infectious illness results in systemic toxicity and can ultimately result in irreversible shock. In healthy infants and children, it is virtually always caused by a blood-borne bacterial illness. Neonates and immunocompromised children are also vulnerable to sepsis caused by herpesvirus. Bacterial sepsis is far more common in neonates and young infants than in healthy older children or adults. It is a major challenge for the emergency physician to recognize bacterial sepsis in its early stages.

The clinical manifestations of sepsis are somewhat age dependent. Neonates may present with a history of poor feeding, decreased activity, somnolence, respiratory difficulty, or apnea, or parents may merely complain that the baby "is not acting right." Older infants may have similar symptoms, but the baby's neurologic development may be such that the caretaker can give more specific details of the behavioral abnormalities.

Failure to recognize the parents is an ominous sign that signifies impaired perfusion of the central nervous system.

In most patients, either the history or the physical examination reveals fever. In a small percentage of patients, however, the temperature is normal and, especially in very ill neonates, hypothermia can be present. The physical examination may reveal evidence of decreased peripheral perfusion, including capillary refill delay of >2 seconds, cool, pale extremities, or diminished peripheral pulses. In the pediatric patient, blood pressure is an unreliable indicator of sepsis. In the initial stages, the blood pressure can be normal, the extremities warm, and the pulse bounding. As shock progresses, perfusion deteriorates. Only in the final stages does blood pressure fall. There may be tachypnea and tachycardia out of proportion to the degree of fever. Petechiae or purpura are ominous findings that suggest fulminant meningococcemia.

The successful treatment of sepsis depends on early recognition. Any potentially septic patient requires careful monitoring and strict attention to the maintenance of airway, breathing, and circulation. In relatively stable patients, supplemental oxygen and maintenance of hydration may suffice. In unstable patients, intubation, mechanical ventilation, and aggressive circulatory support, including massive volume resuscitation, invasive monitoring, and the use of pressors, may be necessary. Antibiotic therapy is tailored to the specific situation and is based on the most likely pathogen for the age group (Table 46-1).

Febrile Infants Younger Than 28 Days Old

There is little controversy regarding the treatment of neonates with fever. The management of the febrile patient younger than 28 days old is based on the assumption that the patient's immune system is inherently unable to localize and contain a bacterial infection. Therefore, any bacterial infection is considered serious and life threatening, and any febrile neonate may be suffering from a bacterial illness. Another fundamental assumption is that in this age group even the most experienced clinician is unable to distinguish the patient in the early stages of sepsis from the patient with a benign febrile illness.

Febrile neonates are examined for a focus of fever. Most patients with a definable cause of fever have otitis media, soft tissue infection or evidence of bacterial enteritis, in which case Salmonella is a possible etiology. Blood-borne pathogens include group B Streptococcus,

Table 46-1. Most Common Pathogens in Childhood Bacterial Sepsis

Age Group	Pathogens (Pending Cultures)	Antimicrobial	Initial Dose (mg/kg)
0–1 mo	Group B *Streptococcus,* Enterobacteriaceae, *Staphylococcus aureus, Listeria monocytogenes, Staphylococcus epidermidis*	Ampicillin	50–100
		+	
		gentamicin	2.5
		or	
		ampicillin	50–100
		+	
		cefotaxime	50
1–3 mo	Group B *Streptococcus, S. aureus, Streptococcus pneumoniae, Hemophilus influenzae*	Ampicillin	50–100
		+	
		cefotaxime	50
		or	
		ampicillin	50–100
		+	
		ceftriaxone	50–100
		or	
		ampicillin	50–100
		+	
		chloramphenicol[a]	25
3–24 mo	*S. pneumoniae, Neisseria meningitidis, H. influenzae, S. aureus*	Cefotaxime	50
		or	
		ceftriaxone	50–100
		or	
		ampicillin	50–100
		+	
		chloramphenicol[a]	25
>24 mo	*S. pneumoniae, H. influenzae, S. aureus, N. meningitidis*	Cefotaxime	50
		or	
		ceftriaxone	50–100
		or	
		ampicillin	50–100
		+	
		chloramphenicol[a]	25
Immunocompromised	*S. aureus, Proteus, Pseudomonas,* Enterobacteriaceae	Vancomycin	15
		+	
		ceftazidime	50
		+	
		ticarcillin	75
		or	
		tobramycin	2.5
		or	
		gentamicin	2.5

[a]Primarily used in parts of the world in which cephalosporins are unavailable.

E. coli, and *L. monocytogenes.* It is assumed that even patients with a focus of bacterial infection may be bacteremic and have potentially seeded their CSF.

The laboratory evaluation of the febrile neonate includes a complete blood count and cultures of blood, CSF, and urine. It is imperative that the urine culture be obtained by catheterization or by suprapubic tap, since a bag specimen is unreliable and can obscure the diagnosis. In the neonatal period, the urinalysis may be unremarkable in up to 50 percent of children with a documented positive urine culture. Patients with diarrhea or a history of bloody or mucoid stool require a stool culture. Stool microscopy is considered significant if there are >5 red blood cells (RBCs) or white blood cells (WBCs) per high-power field.

Treatment of the febrile patient younger than 28 days of age includes hospitalization and, in many centers, empiric therapy with ampicillin and either an aminoglycoside or a cephalosporin, such as cefotaxime or ceftriaxone, until all cultures are negative. Any evolution in the management of this group of patients awaits further understanding of the developing immune system, the pathogenesis of specific bacterial infections, and the outcome of outpatient treatment in selected patients.

Febrile Infants 28 Days to 3 Months Old

The management of febrile infants 28 days to 3 months of age is a matter of some controversy. Essentially the same principles apply to this age group as for neonates, and until recently, most centers managed the two groups the same way, although in many centers, the upper age cutoff for a "full septic workup" and admission for empiric antibiotic therapy has been 2 rather than 3 months. This reflects the paucity of data regarding the ability of the developing immune system to contain a bacterial infection. Clinical experience has shown that:

- Most well-appearing febrile infants from 28 days to 2 to 3 months of age do not have documentable bacterial infections.

- Those who have appropriately treated bacterial infections do well.

- Many patients admitted under a "rule-out sepsis" protocol suffer iatrogenic complications.

These observations have resulted in efforts to identify patients with an exceedingly low probability of having a SBI who would be candidates for outpatient management. These efforts were accompanied by the development of ceftriaxone, a cephalosporin that provides an ad-

equate drug level for 24 hours and that has the ability to penetrate the CSF. The availability of ceftriaxone made it possible to provide essentially the same antibiotic therapy to an outpatient that would be provided for a hospitalized patient.

Current data support the following approach to the well-appearing febrile patient between 28 days and 3 months of age. First, the child is evaluated for a focus of infection. Virtually any bacterial infection except otitis media is considered to be an SBI. Infants with evidence of infection of the soft tissue, joint, or bone are pancultured and admitted for appropriate antibiotic therapy. If no source of infection is found, laboratory data are obtained in an effort to classify the infant as low or high risk for bacterial infection. Low-risk criteria are somewhat debatable but in general include a WBC count between 5,000 and 15,000/mm^3, a band count below 1,500/mm^3, a normal urinalysis, a normal CSF and, in patients with diarrhea, stool microscopy with <5 WBCs per high power field. WBCs in the stool reflect the potential for *Salmonella* enteritis.

Infants who are classified as low risk appear to have a low probability of having an SBI (<1 percent). There is currently support for discharging these patients from the ED provided that there is close follow-up. Some favor empiric therapy with ceftriaxone, which can be administered intramuscularly at a dose of 50 mg/kg. This provides parenteral coverage for most bacterial pathogens that result in bacteremia in this age group. Patients receiving ceftriaxone should return to the ED or see their pediatrician in 24 hours for a second dose. Infants who develop positive blood cultures are treated on an individual basis.

Given the extremely low risk of an SBI in this group, another management option is discharging the patient without antibiotic treatment, with a presumed diagnosis of viral infection. In this scenario, extremely close follow-up is necessary. In this management strategy, a lumbar puncture may not be necessary, because the risk of partially treating occult meningitis by the empiric administration of antibiotics is not a consideration.

Outpatient management of febrile patients in this age group is not universally accepted. Especially if there is any question regarding the reliability of follow-up, inpatient treatment should be strongly considered.

Infants 3 to 36 Months of Age

Fever with a Focus of Infection

Infants who are older than 3 months presumably have acquired sufficient immunologic integrity that the risk of dissemination of a bacterial infection is low. However, it must be realized that this age group spans a wide range and that in clinical practice a 90-day-old infant is managed far more conservatively than a healthy 36-month-old. The management of these patients is based on the nature of the infection.

Certain focal bacterial infections are associated with a high likelihood of bacteremia. This is especially true in infections caused by *Hemophilus influenzae* type B, including epiglottitis, buccal and periorbital cellulitis, and some cases of septic arthritis. The potential for bacteremia with this highly invasive organism always mandates an aggressive workup. Blood cultures are indicated, and a lumbar puncture should be strongly considered. As discussed below, incidence of *H. influenzae* B infection has dramatically decreased since the introduction of HIB vaccine. Other infections often associated with bacteremia are soft tissue infections secondary to *Staphylococcus aureus* and *Salmonella* enteritis, which can be especially problematic in younger infants.

Fever without a Focus of Infection

This category of patient presents a significant challenge, largely because of the high volume of such patients in the ED. The major concern in this group in the phenomenon of occult bacteremia, the clinical situation in which a relatively well-appearing febrile infant with no focus of bacterial infection has a positive blood culture. Much research has been done in an attempt to identify patients who are bacteremic, to determine the outcome of patients with bacteremia and to define treatment strategies in potentially bacteremic patients.

Seeding of the bloodstream with bacteria is presumably a result of colonization of the nasopharynx with offending organisms. Bacteremia often provokes a fever but may be clinically silent and the patient may appear well.

Occult bacteremia occurs primarily in patients with a temperature of ≥39°C. At lower temperatures, the risk of bacteremia is much lower. Beyond 39°C, there is a direct correlation between the height of fever and the probability of bacteremia. Prior to the use of HIB vaccine, the prevalence of occult bacteremia ranged from 2.8 to 11.6 percent. The most common cause was *Streptococcus pneumoniae,* which accounted for 60 to 85 percent of cases. The second most common was *H. influenzae* type B, which accounted for 5 to 20 percent. Since the first HIB vaccine was licensed in 1987, the incidence of invasive *H. influenzae* infections in children younger than 5 years has decreased by more than 96 percent. In

most recent studies in the post-HIB vaccine era, the current rate of occult bacteremia is 1.6 to 1.9 percent. The most common pathogen remains *S. pneumoniae* (85 to 92 percent of cases). Other agents are Salmonella, *Neisseria meningitidis,* group A Streptococcus, and group B Streptococcus. No *H. influenzae* type B was isolated in recent studies.

There is no laboratory test for definitely diagnosing or excluding bacteremia in the ED. However, the WBC count is of some value as a screening test, because the likelihood of bacteremia is directly correlated with the degree of elevation of the WBC count. The combination of a temperature >40°C and a WBC > 15,000 mm^3 increases the probability of bacteremia from about 2.6 to 11 percent. Attempts to correlate the erythrocyte sedimentation rate and C-reactive protein with bacteremia have had limited success, and these add little to the complete blood count. Urinary tract infections account for up to 7 percent of male patients younger than 6 months of age and 8 percent of female infants younger than 1 year of age who have fever without focus. It is imperative that urine for culture be obtained from catheterization or suprapubic aspiration in order to avoid a contaminated culture. This is especially important, since up to 20 percent of pediatric patients with urinary tract infections have an unremarkable urinalysis.

A lumbar puncture is indicated in any patient who appears toxic or has clinical findings consistent with meningitis. It is important to remember that in young infants, early meningitis can be extremely subtle, and a liberal approach toward lumbar puncture is indicated. This is especially true in the event that outpatient management with empiric antibiotic therapy is anticipated.

Chest x-rays are unlikely to be helpful in febrile pediatric patients without pulmonary findings, such as cough and tachypnea. Stool cultures are likely to be useful only for patients who have bloody diarrhea or >5 WBCs per high-power field.

The management of the patient between 3 and 36 months of age who has fever without focus is highly controversial. To a large extent, therapeutic options depend on knowing the outcome of untreated bacteremia. This is difficult to determine, especially in light of the decrease in *H. influenzae* type B infections. Untreated bacteremia with *S. pneumoniae* appears to uncommonly result in morbidity, with perhaps a 6 percent risk for subsequent development of meningitis. For the nonimmunized patient, *H. influenzae,* however, is a much more invasive organism, and the risk of meningitis is up to 26 percent. Other potential secondary infections due to *H. influenzae* include septic arthritis, epiglottitis, and facial cellulitis. Although *N. meningitidis* is an infrequent cause of occult bacteremia, up to half of the affected patients develop meningitis or sepsis.

The fact that at least some patients with occult bacteremia develop serious sequelae raises the issue of whether empiric therapy with antibiotics can avert the potential complications in a safe, cost-effective manner. Management algorithms have been devised using a combination of clinical trials, meta-analyses, and hypothetical models. Evidence suggests that treatment with parenteral antibiotics is beneficial in preventing meningitis for patients with occult bacteremia, when compared with no treatment at all or treatment with oral antibiotics, which are effective against *S. pneumoniae* but not *H. influenzae*. Ceftriaxone has the advantage of providing coverage against *H. influenzae*, which is 40 percent penicillin and amoxicillin resistant. Ceftriaxone also provides antibiotic effect for 24 hours and penetrates the CSF.

One management strategy in the well-appearing infant who is 3 to 36 months of age with a temperature above 39°C is to obtain a screening complete blood count. Those patients with a WBC count $> 15,000/mm^3$ are at increased risk for occult bacteremia and should have a blood culture sent. Male infants younger than 6 months of age and females younger than 2 years of age undergo a urinalysis and urine culture. Any patient who appears toxic has a lumbar puncture performed. Empiric therapy with ceftriaxone 50 mg/kg intramuscularly is then administered. An alternative management strategy is to obtain a blood culture on all patients with a temperature $> 39°C$ and initiate empiric therapy with ceftriaxone. This would result in a large number of patients at low risk of bacteremia receiving treatment, because of the lack of a screening WBC.

Patients who have blood cultures positive for *N. meningitidis* or *H. influenzae* should be recalled to the ED and hospitalized for treatment. If a lumbar puncture was not performed on the initial visit, it should be done on the patient's arrival. Children with a blood culture positive for *S. pneumoniae* who are afebrile and look well receive a second dose of ceftriaxone and a follow-up course of oral penicillin. Patients with pneumococcemia who have persistent fever or are ill-appearing require a repeat septic workup and admission for parenteral antibiotics.

In February 2000, a seven-valent pneumococcal conjugate vaccine was licensed for use among infants and young children. The potential direct and indirect effects of the vaccine are very promising. This vaccine covers almost 90 percent of pneumococcal serotypes responsible for invasive diseases in the United States. Vaccina-

tion of healthy infants would annually prevent up to 12,000 cases of meningitis and bacteremia, 53,000 cases of pneumonia, 1 million episodes of otitis media, and 116 deaths due to pneumococcal infection. In addition, at least 80 percent of antibiotic-resistant serotypes are included in the seven-valent vaccine formulation. The approach to the fully immunized, nontoxic-appearing febrile children will most likely change dramatically as use of the vaccine becomes widespread. The expected reduction of drug-resistant strains should allow physicians to reduce use of empirical broad-spectrum antibiotics. The result would be fewer infections caused by drug-resistant strains and reduced antibiotic pressure that leads to additional resistance. Although the vaccine does not have efficacy against serotypes not included in the vaccine, to date there are no data indicating an increase in disease with non-vaccine serotypes in vaccinated children. Another potential benefit of this vaccine is providing herd immunity, a benefit that is thought to have contributed to the success of the HIB vaccination program.

The management of the febrile patient between 3 and 36 months of age will remain controversial until such time as bacteremia can be excluded. Some authorities believe that neither laboratory evaluation nor empiric antibiotic therapy is indicated in well-appearing febrile children with no focus of infection. All authorities agree that regardless of the ED treatment, close follow-up is the most important factor in ensuring a good outcome.

The Febrile Child Older Than 36 Months of Age

Beyond 36 months of age, the immune system of the healthy child has developed to the point where disseminated bacterial infection is much less common. Even bacteremic patients very uncommonly seed their meninges or develop full-blown sepsis. An exception to this is meningococcemia, which remains a serious disease at all ages.

The older febrile child is evaluated for a focus of bacterial infection. Ancillary studies depend on the clinical scenario. Examples include throat cultures for patients with pharyngitis and chest x-rays for patients with cough or objective pulmonary findings. Urinary tract infections are fairly common in young girls and can at times have somewhat atypical presentations, such as vomiting and diarrhea. Thus a urinalysis is occasionally indicated. Blood counts and cultures are usually not indicated, except in ill-appearing children. Most older febrile patients have viral illness and require no workup.

The Treatment of Fever

Despite the great frequency of the problem, whether to treat fever with antipyretics remains controversial. Although there is no doubt that extremely elevated temperatures (>41°C) can be deleterious, the vast majority of patients with fever do well, and lowering the body temperature may obviate some of the potentially beneficial effects of fever.

Patients who definitely require aggressive treatment are those with a history of febrile seizure and those who are physiologically unstable; in these patients the increased basal metabolic rate can further compromise cardiopulmonary function.

Pharmacologic therapy of fever predominantly consists of treatment with acetaminophen and nonsteroidal antiinflammatory drugs (NSAIDs). Both normalize the temperature set point, probably by inhibiting prostaglandin synthesis.

Acetaminophen is an effective antipyretic and is relatively free of side effects. The dose is 10 to 15 mg/kg every 4 hours. An advantage of acetaminophen is that children are fairly tolerant of overdose.

Aspirin is also an effective antipyretic, but, because of a likely link with Reyes' syndrome, the American Academy of Pediatrics does not recommend aspirin use in febrile children, particularly when fever is suspected to be caused by influenza or varicella.

Ibuprofen has been increasingly used as an antipyretic in pediatric patients. It appears to be as effective as acetaminophen, with a slightly longer duration of action. Its use has not been linked to Reyes' syndrome. The dose is 10 mg/kg every 6 hours.

Body temperature can also be reduced by external cooling, which in small children is easily achieved by bathing. Water temperature should be tepid and not cold enough to induce shivering. Parents should be informed that sponging with alcohol is dangerous. Bathing or sponging should be combined with pharmacologic therapy.

BIBLIOGRAPHY

Alpern ER, Alessandrini EA, Bell LM, et al: Occult bacteremia from a pediatric emergency department: current prevalence, time to detection, and outcome. *Pediatrics* 106:505, 2000.

Baraff LJ: Management of fever without source in infants and children. *Ann Emerg Med* 36:602–614, 2000.

Baraff LJ, Bass JW, Fleisher GR, et al: Practice guideline for the management of infants and children 0-36 months of age with fever without source. *Ann Emerg Med* 22:1198, 1993.

CDC: Preventing pneumococcal disease among infants and young children: recommendations of the Advisory Committee on Immunization Practices (ACIP). *MMWR* 49:1, 2000.

Fleisher GR, Rosenberg N, Vinci R, et al: Intramuscular versus oral antibiotic therapy in young, febrile children. *J Pediatr* 124:504, 1994.

Hausdorff WP, Bryant J, Paradiso PR, et al: Which pneumococcal serogroups cause the most invasive disease: implications for conjugate vaccine formulation and use, Part I. *CID* 30:100, 2000.

Hausdorff WP, Bryant J, Kloek C, et al: The contribution of specific pneumococcal serogroups to different disease manifestations: implications for conjugate vaccine formulation and use, Part II. *CID* 30:122, 2000.

Jaffe DM, Tanz RR, Klein JO, et al: Antibiotic administration to treat possible occult bacteremia in children. *N Engl J Med* 317:1175, 1987.

Lee GM, Harper MB: Risk of bacteremia for febrile young children in the post-*Haemophilus influenzae* type B era. *Arch Pediatr Adolesc Med* 152:624, 1998.

Lieu TA, Ray GT, Black SB, et al: Projected cost-effectiveness of pneumococcal conjugate vaccination of healthy infants and young children. *JAMA* 283:1460, 2000.

McCarthy CA, Powell KR, Jaskiewics JA, et al: Outpatient management of selected infants younger than 2 months of age evaluated for possible sepsis. *Pediatr Infect Dis J* 9:385, 1990.

47

Meningitis

Gary R. Strange
John Marcinak
Steven Lelyveld

HIGH-YIELD FACTS

- Early meningitis is not easy to diagnose. Especially in young infants, signs and symptoms are notoriously nonspecific.

- Organisms enter the cerebrospinal fluid by hematogenous spread or by direct extension from the nasopharynx or other adjacent structures. Many of the pathologic changes are not primarily due to infection but result from the response of the human immune system to the infection.

- Over half of all cases of meningitis are aseptic, and most of these cases have a benign outcome.

- For children younger than 1 month, the predominant organisms are group B *Streptococcus, Escherichia coli,* and *Listeria monocytogenes.*

- The incidence of *Haemophilus influenzae* type b, which was the most common etiologic agent of childhood bacterial meningitis, has dropped dramatically since the introduction of the conjugate vaccine against this organism. *Streptococcus pneumoniae* is now the major cause of infant bacterial meningitis in the United States, and *Neisseria meningitidis* is the most common cause in the 2- to 18-year age group.

- Neonatal cerebrospinal fluid contains more cells and protein and less glucose than that of older children.

- Newborns are generally treated with an initial dose of ampicillin, 100 mg/kg, and an aminoglycoside, such as gentamicin, 2.5 mg/kg. Based on local sensitivities, a cephalosporin active against Gram-negative

bacilli, such as cefotaxime, 50 mg/kg, may be substituted for the aminoglycoside.

- Vancomycin is the only antibiotic to which all strains of pneumococci are susceptible and it is therefore added to a broad-spectrum cephalosporin for comprehensive therapy (vancomycin, 15 mg/kg/dose bid, and cefotaxime, 50 mg/kg/dose tid) for infants and small children.

- In the unstable child, lumbar puncture should be withheld until after stabilization and antibiotic administration.

- Steroids may be beneficial in reducing the sequelae of bacterial meningitis. Major sequelae include hearing loss, seizures, and decreased mental ability.

Over the past 20 years, there has been a significant change in the epidemiology of bacterial meningitis, which is now predominantly a disease of adults. The most important contributor to this change has been the decrease in frequency of *Haemophilus influenzae* type b (which was the most common etiologic agent of childhood bacterial meningitis) since the introduction of the conjugate vaccine against this organism. *Streptococcus pneumoniae* is now the major cause of bacterial meningitis in infants 1 month to 2 years of age in the United States. A heptavalent pneumococcal conjugate vaccine was introduced in 2000 that covers about 80 percent of invasive serotypes and is expected to prevent >12,000 cases of meningitis and bacteremia annually. For children younger than 1 month, the predominant organisms are group B *Streptococcus, Escherichia coli,* and *Listeria monocytogenes. Neisseria meningitidis* is the most common cause in the 2- to 18-year age group.

Over half of all cases of meningitis are aseptic, and most of these cases have a benign outcome. Of the viral causes of meningitis, over 80 percent are seasonal enteroviruses, predominantly echovirus and coxsackievirus. Mumps, herpes simplex, varicella, measles, and arboviruses have all been described as central nervous system pathogens.

PATHOPHYSIOLOGY

Most pathogens enter the subarachnoid space by hematogenous spread. In addition, they may enter through a mechanical disruption, as in a fracture of the base of the skull, or by direct extension from an infection in the ear, mastoid air cells, sinuses, orbit, or other adjacent structure. Under normal circumstances, the blood-brain barrier provides an adequate defense against invasive disease. However, once it is breached, natural defense mechanisms are unable to stop the multiplication of organisms. An alteration in the cerebral capillary endothelial cells ensues, with weakening of the blood-brain barrier.

Many of the pathologic changes of meningitis are not primarily due to infection but result from the response of the human immune system to the infection. A complicated series of interactions among immune, vascular, and central nervous system cells, cytokines and chemokines, matrix metalloproteinases, and free radical molecules is ultimately responsible for many of the changes that occur in bacterial meningitis, including neuronal death. Cytotoxic and vasogenic cerebral edema cause an increase in intracranial pressure that in turn leads to decreased cerebral perfusion pressure, decreased blood flow, regional hypoxia, and focal ischemia of the brain.

PRESENTATION

The "classic" signs and symptoms of meningitis include headache, photophobia, stiff neck, change in mental status, bulging fontanelle, nausea, and vomiting (Table 47-1). The Brudzinski sign occurs when the irritated

Table 47-1. Signs and Symptoms of Meningitis at Presentation

Manifestation	% of Cases
Fever	>95
Lethargy	87–95
Vomiting	54–71
Upper respiratory infection symptoms	46–55
Seizures	22–23
Temperature >38.3°C	59–77
Altered mental status	53–78
ENT infection	22–42
Nuchal rigidity	54–59
Brudzinski sign	10–13
Kernig sign	9–11
Focal neurologic defect	5–6

Source: Adapted from Rothrock SG, Green SM, Wren J, et al: Pediatric bacterial meningitis. *Ann Emerg Med* 21:146–152, 1992.

meninges are stretched, with neck flexion causing the hips and knees to flex involuntarily. The Kernig sign of nerve root irritation is present when the hip is flexed to 90 degrees and the examiner is unable to passively extend the leg fully. Children with meningeal irritation often resist walking or being carried, preferring to remain recumbent, often in a fetal position. These signs and symptoms, related to meningeal irritation, are reasonably reliable in older infants and children, but their absence does not rule out intracranial infection.

The younger the child, the less obvious the signs and symptoms until late in the course of the disease. Neonates and young infants are likely to present with poor feeding, irritability, inconsolability, or listlessness. Nuchal rigidity, the resistance to flexion of the neck in the anteroposterior plane only, has been considered one of the most specific signs of meningitis. However, nuchal rigidity is seen in <15 percent of children with meningitis younger than 18 months and, in one study, was found to be present in 21 percent of children being evaluated for meningitis who were subsequently found to have normal cerebrospinal fluid (CSF).

Meningitis may take either an insidious (90 percent) or fulminant (10 percent) course. If the course is insidious, the patient has a high likelihood of presenting to a physician days before diagnosis with a nonspecific illness. This is especially true when the pathogen is pneumococcus. The duration of illness before diagnosis can be up to 2 weeks, with a median of 36 to 72 hours. Many of these children will have been treated with oral antibiotics before the diagnosis of meningitis is considered. Partial treatment may complicate the diagnostic process, but antibiotic treatment prior to diagnosis of central nervous system infection may also be associated with reduction in disease-related sequelae.

The more fulminant the course, the worse the prognosis. Typically, meningococcal disease presents with a more fulminant course. Concomitant meningococcal bacteremia rapidly progresses to petechiae, purpura fulminans, and cardiovascular collapse. As other causes of pediatric meningitis have been contained, meningococcal disease has become a leading infectious cause of death. A new protein-conjugated group C vaccine is available and has shown efficacy in adolescents, children, and toddlers but is of limited efficacy in infants. No vaccine is yet available for bacteria of serogroup B.

The management of any of the bacterial meningitides may be complicated by hemorrhage into the adrenal cortex, the Friderichsen-Waterhouse syndrome.

DIFFERENTIAL DIAGNOSIS

In the early phases, meningitis may be confused with gastroenteritis, upper respiratory infection, pneumonia, otitis media, or minor viral syndromes. As the alteration of mental status becomes more severe, the diagnoses of encephalitis, subarachnoid or subdural hemorrhage with or without direct trauma or abuse, cerebral abscess, and Reye's syndrome must be considered. Toxic ingestions, seizure disorders, diabetic ketoacidosis, hypothyroidism, and other altered metabolic states may be initially confused with meningitis but do not have the same prodrome or fever. The young child with intussusception may present with vomiting, altered mental status, and cardiovascular collapse. Many of these children are evaluated for meningitis before their diagnosis is clear.

MANAGEMENT

Unstable Patients

Whenever meningitis is suspected, the diagnostic test of choice is the lumbar puncture. However, it is imperative not to neglect the ABCs while performing diagnostic procedures. Care must be taken to ensure proper oxygenation and cardiovascular stabilization. In the unstable child, lumbar puncture should be withheld until after stabilization and antibiotic administration. Although the early administration of antibiotics may prevent recovery of the organism on culture of CSF, early appropriate antibiotic therapy should be the goal. However, studies have not shown a correlation between early treatment and clinical outcome. Drawing of specimens for blood cultures prior to administration of antibiotics provides another avenue for identification of specific pathogens and usually can be accomplished without delaying antibiotic administration.

The unstable patient with meningitis may have respiratory compromise, shock, increased intracranial pressure, seizures, or hypoglycemia. The first priority is to ensure an open airway and adequate ventilation. Supplemental oxygen is always administered. Inadequate ventilation or oxygenation, based on clinical assessment or blood gas results, requires assistance with the bag-valve-mask technique, followed by endotracheal intubation (see Chap. 5).

Patients with evidence of shock are treated with rapid intravenous or intraosseous infusion of crystalloid solution in 20-mL/kg aliquots. However, careful assessment of the need for continuing fluid resuscitation should be used, since fluid overload can lead to worsening of cerebral edema. Fluid restriction is not routinely indicated, so once the patient is stabilized, fluid should be given at the usual maintenance rate.

If signs of increased intracranial pressure (worsening mental status, papilledema, full fontanelle, widening of sutures) develop, elevate the head at 30 degrees and initiate controlled ventilation to keep the $Paco_2$ between 30 and 35 mmHg. Patients who do not respond to controlled ventilation may benefit from the use of diuretic therapy with mannitol (0.25 to 1 g/kg) or furosemide (1 mg/kg).

Seizures are controlled with rapid-acting benzodiazepines followed by phenytoin (see Chap. 38).

The blood glucose level should be rapidly assessed with the use of a glucose oxidase reagent strip. If the blood glucose is <40 mg/dL, administer an infusion of glucose, 250 to 500 mg/kg, as 10 percent dextrose for neonates, 25 percent dextrose for infants younger than 2 years, and 50 percent dextrose for older infants and children.

Stable Patients

In stable patients with manifestations suggestive of meningitis, phlebotomy for diagnostic studies is followed promptly by lumbar puncture. The threshold for clinical suspicion of meningitis should be particularly low for certain patients, as follows:

- Neonates
- Immunocompromised children
- Children who have been in close contact with cases of meningitis
- Children with documented bacteremia

The initial workup includes a complete blood count (CBC), electrolytes, glucose, renal functions, and blood culture. Specific tests may be performed to detect bacterial capsular antigens but are not often helpful in the acute situation.

Once it is safe to do so, a lumbar puncture is performed. The expected laboratory parameters for CSF analysis are age-related (Table 47-2). A low white blood cell count, with a predominantly mononuclear cell type, and normal glucose and protein point to a viral etiology. High protein, low sugar, and elevated polymorphonuclear leukocytes (PMNs) point to a bacterial etiology.

Antibiotic Treatment

Antibiotic treatment is directed by the specific organisms, if known, or by the predominant organisms based on age of the patient, if the specific agent is not known.

Table 47-2. Normal Cerebrospinal Fluid (CSF) Values

Parameter	Preterm Infant	Term Infant	Child
Cell count WBC/mm^3	9 (0–25) WBC/mm^3	8 (0–22) WBC/mm^3	0–7
	57% PMNs	61% PMNs	0% PMNs
Glucose	24–63 mg/dL (mean 52)	34–119 mg/dL (mean 52)	40–80 mg/dL
CSF/blood glucose Ratio	55–105%	44–128%	50%
Protein	65–150 mg/dL (mean 115)	20–170 mg/dL (mean 90)	5–40 mg/dL

Newborns are generally treated with an initial dose of ampicillin, 100 mg/kg, and an aminoglycoside, such as gentamicin, 2.5 mg/kg. Based on local sensitivities, a cephalosporin active against Gram-negative bacilli, such as cefotaxime, 50 mg/kg, may be substituted for the aminoglycoside.

Infants and children are generally treated with a cephalosporin (ceftriaxone 100 mg/kg/dose qd or cefotaxime 50 mg/kg/dose tid). In areas where cephalosporins are of limited availability, the combination of ampicillin, 100 mg/kg/dose qid, and chloramphenicol, 25 mg/kg/dose bid, is an option. If the organism is known to be *S. pneumoniae* or if Gram-positive cocci are seen on Gram's stain of the CSF, penicillin and cephalosporin resistance is possible. Vancomycin is the only antibiotic to which all strains of pneumococci are susceptible, and it is therefore added to a broad-spectrum cephalosporin for comprehensive therapy (vancomycin, 15 mg/kg/dose bid, and cefotaxime, 50 mg/kg/dose tid).

Corticosteroid Treatment

The role of steroids in the management of meningitis is controversial. When given prior to the antibiotic, the antiinflammatory effect of dexamethasone (0.15 mg/kg intravenously) decreases intracranial pressure, cerebral edema, and CSF lactate concentrations. Dexamethasone significantly decreases hearing loss and other neurologic sequelae in meningitis caused by *Haemophilus influenzae* type b. Clinical trials and metaanalyses suggest that dexamethasone therapy improves the outcome for patients with bacterial meningitis due to other agents, but the evidence is not yet conclusive. For *S. pneumoniae,* dexamethasone should be considered, after weighing the potential benefits and risks. In addition, some authorities argue that steroids may strengthen the blood-brain barrier and limit the penetration of intravenously administered antibiotics into the CSF. However, this does not appear to be a significant consideration with commonly used antibiotics such as vancomycin, ceftriaxone, and cefotaxime. Currently, there is no clear consensus on the empiric use of steroids for meningitis when the bacterial agent is unknown.

SEQUELAE

The vast majority of children with aseptic meningitis have a self-limited illness without subsequent problems. In spite of modern antibiotic treatment, the mortality of *H. influenzae* type b meningitis is 5 to 10 percent, and for *S. pneumoniae* meningitis, it is 20 to 40 percent. Up to 20 percent of survivors will have some long-term sequelae. These include mild learning defects, sensorineural hearing loss, afebrile seizures, and multiple neurologic defects, including retardation and blindness. Other neurologic defects, such as hemiparesis, ataxia, cranial nerve palsy, and abnormal extensor reflexes, may be present initially but may resolve in a few months.

BIBLIOGRAPHY

Aronin SI: Bacterial meningitis: Principles and practical aspects of therapy. *Curr Infect Dis Rep* 2:337–344, 2000.

Bonsu B, Harper M: Fever interval before diagnosis, prior antibiotic treatment and clinical outcome for young children with bacterial meningitis. *Clin Infect Dis* 32:566–572, 2001.

Nathan BR, Scheld WM: New advances in the pathogenesis and pathophysiology of bacterial meningitis. *Curr Infect Dis Rep* 2:332–336, 2000.

Quagliarello VJ, Scheld WM: Treatment of bacterial meningitis. *N Engl J Med* 336:708–716, 1997.

Ramsay ME, Andrews N, Daczmarski EB, Miller E: Efficacy of meningococcal serogroup C conjugate vaccine in teenagers and toddlers in England. *Lancet* 357:195–196, 2001.

Rosenstein NE, Perkins BA, Stephens DS, et al: Medical progress: Meningococcal disease. *N Engl J Med* 344:1378–1388, 2001.

Schuchat A, Ropbinson K, Wenger JD, et al: Bacterial meningitis in the United States in 1995. *N Engl J Med* 337:970–976, 1997.

Short WR, Tunkel AR: Changing epidemiology of bacterial meningitis in the United States. *Curr Infect Dis Rep* 2:327–331, 2000.

Wang VJ, Malley R, Flwisher GR, et al: Antibiotic treatment of children with unsuspected meningococcal disease. *Arch Pediatr Adolesc Med* 154:556–560, 2000.

Willoughby RE, Polack FS: Meningitis: What's new in diagnosis and management. *Contemp Pediatr* 15:49–70, 1998.

48

Toxic Shock Syndrome

Shabnam Jain

HIGH-YIELD FACTS

- The Centers for Disease Control and Prevention have formulated a case definition. In the absence of a definitive laboratory marker, the strict application of the case definition undoubtedly excludes many subclinical cases.

- Most cases of toxic shock syndrome (TSS) have been directly associated with *Staphylococcus aureus,* of which 67 percent are phage type 1. A disease that is clinically indistinguishable from TSS can be caused by group A *Streptococcus, Streptococcus pneumoniae,* or *Pseudomonas aeruginosa.*

- The Centers for Disease Control and Prevention have reported a decrease in the annual incidence of TSS, presumably from the increased awareness of risk associated with tampon use.

- Nonmenstrual cases occur in a variety of clinical settings, chiefly associated with postpartum or cutaneous/subcutaneous *Staphylococcus aureus* infections. Predisposing factors include burns, abrasions, abscesses, and nasal packing.

- TSS can mimic many common diseases and should be considered in any patient who has unexplained fever, rash, and a toxic condition out of proportion to local findings.

- In TSS, there is sudden onset of high fever associated with chills, vomiting, diarrhea, myalgia, dizziness, hypotension, and rash. The skin findings may be dramatic and present as a severe erythroderma and erythema of mucus membranes, which fades within 3 days of its appearance and is followed by full thickness desquamation.

- Abnormal laboratory values reflect the multisystem involvement in TSS.

- Management depends on prompt recognition, as well as on the identification of the infectious focus. The focus must be drained and foreign material, such as nasal packing or retained tampon, promptly removed.

- A β-lactamase–resistant antistaphylococcal antibiotic, such as oxacillin or nafcillin, has been the recommended treatment, but clindamycin has recently been recommended as having greater efficacy in TSS.

- The most important initial therapy is aggressive volume replacement. Crystalloids or fresh frozen plasma may be used for the management of hypotension, with pressors added if fluids alone are not sufficient.

Toxic shock syndrome (TSS) is a rare acute febrile disease characterized by high fever, diffuse desquamating erythroderma, vomiting, abdominal pain, diarrhea, myalgia, and nonspecific neurologic abnormalities. It can progress rapidly to hypotension, multisystem dysfunction, and death.

TSS was first described in 1978 in 7 children with *Staphylococcus aureus* infections. In 1980, TSS was noted in menstruating women. An epidemic developed associated with continuous tampon use by women who had vaginal colonization with toxin-producing strains of *Staphylococcus aureus.* With the withdrawal of superabsorbent tampons from the market, menstrual TSS is now rare; however, it continues to occur in children and adults, most commonly associated with cutaneous infections.

The Centers for Disease Control and Prevention have formulated a case definition (Table 48-1). In the absence of a definitive laboratory marker, the strict application of the case definition undoubtedly excludes many subclinical cases.

ETIOLOGY AND PATHOGENESIS

Most cases of TSS have been directly associated with *Staphylococcus aureus,* of which 67 percent are phage type 1. A disease that is clinically indistinguishable from TSS can be caused by group A *Streptococcus, Streptococcus pneumoniae,* or *Pseudomonas aeruginosa.*

The pathogenesis is thought to be related to production of a toxin, currently referred to as toxic shock syn-

Table 48-1. Toxic Shock Syndrome: Criteria for Diagnosis

Fever:	Temperature ≥38.9°C
Rash:	Diffuse macular erythroderma, with subsequent desquamation, particularly of palms and soles
Hypotension:	Systolic blood pressure ≤90 mm Hg for adults and for children, systolic blood pressure <5th percentile for age
	Syncope

Involvement of ≥3 of the following organ systems clinically or by abnormal laboratory tests:

Gastrointestinal:	Vomiting or diarrhea at onset of illness
Muscular:	Severe myalgia or CPK > twice normal
Mucous membranes:	Vaginal, conjunctival, or oropharyngeal hyperemia
Renal:	BUN or serum creatinine > twice normal or pyuria in the absence of a urinary tract infection
Hematologic:	Platelet count <100,000/mm^3
Hepatic:	Evidence of hepatitis (total bilirubin, SGOT or SGPT > twice normal)
Central nervous system:	Disorientation without focal neurologic signs when fever and hypotension are absent

Negative results on the following tests, if obtained:
        Blood, throat, or CSF culture
        Serologic tests for rocky mountain spotted fever, leptospirosis, or measles

drome toxin-1 (TSST-1). It is likely that more than one toxin may be involved, and in some cases, the organism does not produce toxin. The majority of cases are caused by coagulase-positive *Staphylococcus aureus,* although recently, coagulase-negative strains have been isolated.

The most impressive aspect of the pathophysiology of TSS is the massive vasodilatation and rapid movement of serum proteins and fluid from the intravascular to the extravascular space. This results in oliguria, hypotension, edema, and low central venous pressure. Large amounts of fluid are required to restore and maintain blood pressure. The multisystem collapse seen in TSS may be either a reflection of the rapid onset of shock, or may be from direct effects of toxin(s) on the parenchymal cells of the involved organs.

EPIDEMIOLOGY

The Centers for Disease Control and Prevention have reported a decrease in the annual incidence of TSS, presumably from the increased awareness of risk associated with tampon use. Although TSS is most often seen in menstruating women, cases are reported in nonmenstruating women, children, and men. With this decrease in reported cases from menstruating women, the incidence in others has become more significant. Nonmenstrual cases occur in a variety of clinical settings, chiefly as-

sociated with postpartum or cutaneous/subcutaneous *Staphylococcus aureus* infections. Predisposing factors include burns, abrasions, abscesses, and nasal packing.

Although children have a higher incidence of minor *Staphylococcus aureus* infection than adults, the incidence of TSS in children is lower. The location of infection probably plays a great role in the elaboration of toxin. The immunologic status of the individual may also play a role. Studies have shown that patients with TSS do not develop a significant antibody response to TSST-1. Therefore, there is a significant recurrence rate for TSS (30 percent). Secondary cases are milder and occur within 3 months of the original episode; the overall mortality rate is 3 percent in menstrual cases.

CLINICAL MANIFESTATIONS

The diagnosis of TSS is based on clinical manifestations (see Table 48-1). TSS can mimic many common diseases and should be considered in any patient who has unexplained fever, rash, and a toxic condition out of proportion to local findings. Patients with menstrual TSS usually present between the third and fifth day of menses. The symptoms, signs, and laboratory abnormalities reflect multiple organ involvement. There is sudden onset of high fever associated with chills, vomiting, myalgia, dizziness, hypotension, and rash. Additional symptoms include headache, arthralgia, sore throat, abdominal pain, diarrhea, and stiff neck. There may be orthostatic dizziness or syncope. Diarrhea is profuse and watery, and there is protracted vomiting. The skin findings may be dramatic and present as a severe erythroderma and erythema of mucus membranes. The skin rash is diffuse and blanching. It fades within 3 days of its appearance and is followed by full thickness desquamation.

Victims of TSS appear acutely ill. Physical examination may reveal hypotension or orthostatic decrease in systolic blood pressure by 15 mm Hg. In the acute stage, which lasts 24 to 48 hours, the patient may be agitated, disoriented, or obtunded. Hyperemia of the conjunctiva and vagina is seen. Tender edematous external genitalia, diffuse vaginal erythema, scant purulent cervical discharge, and bilateral adnexal tenderness are seen in menstruation-related TSS.

Between the fifth and tenth hospital day, a generalized pruritic maculopapular rash develops in about 25 percent of patients. In all cases, a fine generalized desquamation of the skin, with peeling over the soles, fingers, toes, and palms occurs.

Abnormal laboratory values reflect the multisystem involvement in TSS. No specific laboratory test can make the diagnosis, but there are several frequently found abnormalities. Leucocytosis, with an increase in immature forms, is frequently seen. Platelet count may be low. Azotemia and abnormal urinary sediment are seen with the development of acute renal failure. Liver function tests frequently show some elevation of liver enzymes and bilirubin. Electrolyte abnormalities are variable. With severe hypotension, the patient may be acidotic. Clotting studies are normal or mildly elevated, but few patients show clinical evidence of coagulopathy. Cultures of blood, throat, and cerebrospinal fluid may be useful. Vaginal culture should be done, as well as culture from any identifiable focus of infection. *Staphylococcus* will be cultured from the cervix or vagina of more than 85 percent of patients with menstrual TSS. The majority of the above tests return to normal by 7 to 10 days after onset of illness.

Mild episodes of TSS are more difficult to diagnose. The presence of any combination of fever, headache, sore throat, diarrhea, vomiting, orthostatic dizziness, syncope, or myalgias in a menstruating woman should raise the possibility of TSS. There is no diagnostic laboratory test; the presence of *Staphylococcus aureus* on culture is not diagnostic because non-TSST-1–producing *Staphylococcus aureus* may be cultured from the cervix or vagina of up to 10 percent of well women. However, the presence of desquamation during a febrile illness

should prompt the clinician to obtain cultures for *S. aureus*. Other laboratory data do not reflect multisystem involvement in mild cases. Thus, strong support for the fact that the signs and symptoms did represent mild TSS will depend on the development of the typical desquamation of palms, soles, toes, and fingers.

DIFFERENTIAL DIAGNOSIS

Several other systemic illnesses with fever, rash, diarrhea, myalgias, and multisystem involvement resemble TSS. Kawasaki disease is characterized by fever, conjunctival hyperemia, and erythema of mucus membranes with desquamation. Although it is clinically similar, it lacks many of the features of TSS, including diffuse myalgia, vomiting, abdominal pain, diarrhea, azotemia, thrombocytopenia, and shock. Kawasaki disease occurs typically in children under 5 years of age.

The clinical picture of staphylococcal scarlet fever is also very similar to TSS. They are both illnesses caused by toxin-producing staphylococcus. Pathology specimens or serologic evidence of the exfoliation toxin differentiates the two entities.

Streptococcal scarlet fever is rare after the age of 10 years. The "sandpaper" rash of scarlet fever is distinct from the macular rash of TSS.

Septic shock must always be considered in the differential diagnosis of TSS. The appearance of a rash and the laboratory abnormalities associated with TSS will aid in distinguishing these two entities.

MANAGEMENT

Management depends on prompt recognition, as well as on the identification of the infectious focus. The focus must be drained and foreign material, such as nasal packing or retained tampon, promptly removed. Cultures should be obtained. Antibiotic therapy is essential for recovery from the acute episode, but is also important for eradication of the organism to reduce the recurrence rate. A β-lactamase–resistant antistaphylococcal antibiotic, such as oxacillin or nafcillin, has been the recommended treatment, but clindamycin has recently been recommended as having greater efficacy in TSS. Alternative antibiotics for patients allergic to penicillin include clindamycin, erythromycin, rifampin, and trimethoprim-sulfamethoxazole.

The remainder of therapy depends on the severity and extent of symptoms. The most important initial therapy is aggressive volume replacement. Crystalloids or fresh frozen plasma may be used for the management of hypotension, with pressors added if fluids alone are not sufficient.

Continuous monitoring of heart rate, blood pressure, respiratory rate, urinary output, central venous pressure, and pulmonary wedge pressure is required. As volume resuscitation progresses, chest radiographs, blood gases, and electrolytes need to be followed. Thrombocytopenia may require platelet transfusions. If ARDS occurs, mechanical ventilation will become necessary.

Corticosteroids are recommended, but have not been shown conclusively to affect outcome. There is some evidence that methylprednisone, 30 mg/kg, may reduce the severity of the illness if administered early. The majority of patients become afebrile and normotensive within 48 hours of hospitalization. The erythema disappears within a few days and the muscle pain and weakness resolve in 7 to 10 days.

RECURRENCES

More than half of the patients not treated with a β-lactamase–resistant antibiotic have recurrences. Most recurrent episodes occur by the second month following the initial episode, on the same day of menses as the prior attack. In the majority of patients, the initial episode is the most severe. The prevention of the first episode of TSS involves minimizing the use of high absorbency tampons or the continuous use of tampons and identifying the factors associated with nonmenstrual episodes.

BIBLIOGRAPHY

Andrews MM, Parent EM, Barry M, Parsonnet J: Recurrent nonmenstrual toxic shock syndrome: Clinical manifestations, diagnosis, and treatment. *Clin Infect Dis* 32:1470–1479, 2001.

Baracco GJ, Bisno AL: Therapeutic approaches to streptococcal toxic shock syndrome. *Curr Infect Dis Rep* 1999; 1:230–237.

Centers for Disease Control: Defining the group A streptococcal toxic shock syndrome. *JAMA* 269:390–391, 1993.

Herzer CM: Toxic shock syndrome: Broadening the differential diagnosis. *J Am Board Fam Pract* 14:131–136, 2001.

Kniffin W, Smith R, Stashwick C: Toxic shock syndrome in three adolescent males. *J Adolesc Health Care* 10:166–169, 1990.

Meadows M: Tampon safety: TSS now rare, but women still should take care. *FDA Consum* 2000;34:20–24.

Reiss MA: Toxic shock syndrome. *Prim Care Update Ob-Gyn* 7:85–90, 2000.

Russell NE, Pachorek RE: Clindamycin in the treatment of streptococcal and staphylococcal toxic shock syndromes. *Ann Pharmacother* 34:936–939, 2000.

Stevens DL: Streptococcal toxic shock syndrome associated with necrotizing fasciitis. *Annu Rev Med* 51:271–288, 2000.

Vincent JM, Demers DM, Bass JW: Infectious exanthems and unusual infections. *Adolesc Med* 11:327–358, 2000.

49

Kawasaki Syndrome

Gary R. Strange
Shabnam Jain

HIGH-YIELD FACTS

- The principal pathologic feature of this syndrome is an acute, nonspecific vasculitis that affects the microvessels (arterioles, venules, and capillaries).

- Since there are no pathognomonic laboratory findings, the diagnosis is established clinically by the presence of fever and at least four of five other clinical features.

- Thrombocytosis is a constant feature of the subacute phase, with platelet counts in the range of 500,000 to 3,000,000/mm³. Thrombocytosis is rare in the first week of the illness, appears in the second week, peaks in the third week, and returns gradually to normal about a month after onset in uncomplicated illness.

- Patients with Kawasaki syndrome have a 20 to 25 percent risk of developing coronary aneurysms in the absence of treatment. Those younger than 1 year of age at the onset of disease are at greater risk.

- All patients diagnosed with Kawasaki syndrome should be hospitalized immediately for administration of intravenous gamma globulin (IVGG), aspirin therapy, and cardiac evaluation.

- Corticosteroids have been considered to be contraindicated in Kawasaki disease due to unfavorable results in early studies. However, there is growing evidence of their beneficial effect in immunoglobulin-resistant disease and at least one study showing a decreased incidence of coronary artery aneurysms when corticosteroids were added to conventional therapy.

- The overall mortality rate of Kawasaki syndrome in American children is <1

percent, but it is higher in infants younger than 1 year. The prognosis for patients receiving treatment within the first 8 to 10 days of the illness is excellent.

Kawasaki syndrome (KS), or mucocutaneous lymph node syndrome, is an acute, self-limited, multisystem vasculitis of unclear etiology. KS is the leading cause of acquired heart disease in children in the United States and Japan. The diagnosis is based entirely on fulfilling a defined set of clinical criteria; there are no pathognomonic laboratory findings.

The disease may occur sporadically or in miniepidemics. In the United States, cases occur throughout the year with no definite seasonal occurrence. The peak incidence is in children 18 to 24 months of age, with 80-85 percent of cases occurring under the age of 5 years. It is more common in males, who also have a significantly higher mortality rate from this disease.

ETIOLOGY AND PATHOGENESIS

The etiology is unclear. Clinically and epidemiologically, it appears to be caused by either an infectious agent or the immune response to an infectious agent. Inherent immaturity of the immune system resulting in T-cell unresponsiveness has recently been hypothesized. A number of environmental factors have also been proposed, but no consistent associations have been established.

The principal pathologic feature of this syndrome is an acute, nonspecific vasculitis that affects the microvessels (arterioles, venules, and capillaries). Nearly every organ system is involved. In the heart, the vasculitis results in aneurysm formation in 20 to 25 percent of untreated patients. Inflammatory changes may also be found in vessels in the lung, pancreas, kidneys, spleen, mesentery, and gastrointestinal tract.

CLINICAL FINDINGS

Since there are no pathognomonic laboratory findings, the diagnosis is established clinically. Fever and at least four of five other clinical features (Table 49-1) are required to establish the diagnosis. However, all symptoms need not be present simultaneously, and they may vary in severity, time of onset, and duration. In addition, cases of atypical or incomplete Kawasaki syndrome are in-

Table 49-1. Diagnostic Criteria for Kawasaki Syndrome

Fever persisting for ≥5 days
> *and*

At least four of the following findings:

Bilateral, painless bulbar conjunctival injection without exudate

Mucous membrane changes of the upper respiratory tract, including injected, dry, fissured lips, oral mucosal and pharyngeal injection, and "strawberry tongue"

Peripheral extremity changes, including erythema and edema of hands and feet in the acute phase and periungual and generalized desquamation in the convalescent phase

Polymorphous truncal exanthem

Acute, nonpurulent cervical lymphadenopathy

Findings cannot be explained by some other known disease process

---

creasingly being reported, particularly in infants younger than 6 months. Such infants are more likely to be diagnosed with incomplete clinical criteria, to be treated later, and to be more likely to develop coronary artery aneurysms. It appears that the complete set of diagnostic criteria may be an insenstive indicator for the major complications of the disease. The course of the illness has been divided into three phases.

Acute or Febrile Phase

This phase lasts 7 to 15 days and is the period when most diagnostic clinical features occur. Fever is universal, often high, and usually sustained. It lasts for 7 to 15 days (mean 12 days). It is associated with extreme irritability. The fever is unresponsive to antibiotics or antipyretics.

Cervical adenopathy is another early feature. It is typically not very prominent. Involvement of the anterior cervical chain is most common and may be unilateral. The lymphadenopathy is nonsuppurative and may disappear rapidly.

Bulbar conjunctivitis is bilateral, nonexudative, and usually quite prominent. It may persist for several weeks.

Mucocutaneous changes include bright red erythema of the lips with cracking and peeling, a strawberry tongue (similar to that seen in scarlet fever), and hyperemia of the oral mucous membranes.

Cutaneous changes include rash and changes in peripheral extremities. These changes represent small blood vessel vasculitis and perivasculitis of the dermis and subcutaneous tissues. The rash is polymorphous and develops in most children. It may be morbilliform, maculopapular, or scarlatiniform, but vesiculation does not occur. The rash may actually vary in character from

place to place in a single child. It is mostly seen on the trunk and may be prominent in the diaper area. It accompanies the fever throughout the entire acute phase of the disease and then gradually disappears.

Changes in the peripheral extremities occur within a few days after onset. There may be edema of the hands, fingers, feet, and toes, with induration of the dorsum of hands and feet and erythema on the palms and soles.

There are many other ancillary features and alternate presentations of Kawasaki disease. In fact, involvement of almost any system can occur. Relatively common at presentation and during the initial course are pneumonitis, tympanitis, diarrhea, meatitis and sterile pyuria, hepatitis, abdominal pain, arthritis, and arthralgias. Central nervous system involvement often presents as extreme irritability or, occasionally, as aseptic meningitis. These other clinical findings, although not diagnostic criteria, are helpful in supporting the diagnosis.

Subacute Phase

The subacute phase lasts for approximately 2 to 4 weeks and begins with resolution of fever and elevation of platelet count. It ends with the return of platelet counts to near normal levels.

This phase is dominated by desquamation that may have already begun before the disappearance of fever. Desquamation is a constant feature of Kawasaki disease. It is noted first in the periungual region, with peeling underneath the finger and toenails. It may also be prominent in the diaper area.

Thrombocytosis is another constant feature of the subacute phase, with platelet counts in the range of 500,000 to 3,000,000/mm^3. Thrombocytosis is rare in the first week of the illness, appears in the second week, peaks in the third week, and returns gradually to normal about a month after onset in uncomplicated illness.

It is during the subacute phase that complications such as coronary artery aneurysms and hydrops of the gall bladder develop.

Recovery or Convalescent Phase

This phase may last months to years. It is during this phase that coronary artery disease may first be recognized.

ANCILLARY DATA

Laboratory findings are nonspecific in Kawasaki syndrome. The complete blood count often shows an elevated white blood cell count with a left shift. A mild hemolytic anemia may be present. Elevated platelet counts occur in the subacute phase but are usually normal in the acute phase. Acute-phase reactants (CRP, ESR) are markedly elevated. Urinalysis demonstrates moderate pyuria from urethritis. Bilirubinuria may occur as an early sign of hydrops of the gall bladder.

Chest radiographs may show evidence of pulmonary infiltrates or cardiomegaly. The electrocardiogram may show dysrhythmias, prolonged PR or QT intervals, and nonspecific ST-T wave changes. Two-dimensional echocardiography may demonstrate coronary artery dilation or aneurysms, pericardial effusion, or decreased contractility.

DIFFERENTIAL DIAGNOSIS

The differential diagnosis is extensive because of the nonspecific nature of the clinical features (Table 49-2). Most viral exanthems can be eliminated based on the clinical course, by absence of sufficient diagnostic features, by epidemiologic considerations, and by immunization status. Group A β-hemolytic streptococcal or staphylococcal infection can usually be excluded by isolation of the specific organisms. Toxic shock syndrome occurs in older children and adolescents who present with thrombocytopenia rather than thrombocytosis.

COMPLICATIONS

Cardiovascular

The most serious manisfestation of Kawasaki disease is cardiac involvement. Cardiac involvement may result in coronary aneurysms, valvular insufficiency, congestive

Table 49-2. Differential Diagnosis for Kawasaki Syndrome

Viral Illnesses
Rubeola
Rubella
Epstein-Barr virus infection
Adenovirus infection
Enterovirus infection
Bacterial Infections
Toxic shock syndrome
Scarlet fever
Rickettsial Diseases
Rocky Mountain spotted fever
Rheumatologic Disease
Juvenile rheumatoid arthritis
Systemic lupus erythematosus
Acute rheumatic fever

heart failure, myocardial infarction, dysrhythmias, rupture of aneurysms, and pericardial effusion. It usually occurs in the second week of the illness. Almost all the early deaths and most of the long-term disabilities are related to involvement of the heart. Patients with Kawasaki syndrome have a 20 to 25 percent risk of developing coronary aneurysms in the absence of treatment. Those younger than 1 year at the onset of disease are at greater risk.

It is assumed that during the acute febrile phase of the disease, a pancarditis occurs, with a variable number of children developing coronary vasculitis with necrosis of blood vessel wall, aneurysm formation, or thrombosis. Aneurysm of the coronary arteries may be present at onset or begin as early as the second week of the illness. During the subacute phase, these aneurysms reach their peak development and are usually multiple.

Auscultation of the heart reveals gallop rhythms and distant heart sounds in 80 percent of patients. Rarely, a murmur of mitral regurgitation is heard. Cardiomegaly on chest roentgenography is seen in >30 percent of patients. Electrocardiographic changes are common and include low voltage and ST depression in the first week of illness, as well as PR prolongation, QTc prolongation, and ST elevation in the second and third weeks. Arrhythmias are rare and temporary.

Echocardiography is the most sensitive technique for delineating proximal coronary aneurysms, with a diagnostic sensitivity of 80 to 90 percent. Angiography in selected cases may demonstrate lesions of the peripheral cardiac vessels, including narrowing and infarction. The left coronary artery is more commonly involved, and the proximal parts of the coronary arteries are involved more frequently. Aneurysms may be found in arteries other than the coronaries, including the subclavian, brachial, and axillary. Patients at higher risk for development of coronary artery involvement can be determined based on clinical symptoms and signs (Table 49-3).

Dilation of the coronary arteries due to vasculitis is recognized in about 50 percent of patients, beginning on day 7 to 8 of the illness. These dilations and aneurysms remain even after the acute phase in 10 to 20 percent of untreated patients. In children with risk factors, these aneurysms are increased in frequency to ≥ 50 percent. Following treatment the risk for aneurysm is reduced to 4 to 5 percent.

The most common cause of early death in Kawasaki syndrome is myocardial infarction occurring in the subacute phase, which has been described in approximately 25 percent of reported cases. The child may die from infarction, coronary thromboses, or rupture of an aneurysm. Late death may occur from coronary occlusive disease, rupture of an aneurysm several years after onset, or small blood vessel disease in the heart.

Hydrops of the Gall Bladder

This is an acalculous cholecystitis that has been noted in the second phase of the illness. Hydrops is a self-limiting condition that occurs in 3 percent of patients and is a functional, rather than obstructive distension. These children present with abdominal pain, a soft palpable mass in the right upper quadrant, and abdominal distension. Bilirubinemia may be an early sign of hydrops. Diagnosis can be made by ultrasonography.

Other Complications

These include iridocyclitis or anterior uveitis (in about 80 percent of patients), mastoiditis, necrotic pharyngitis,

Table 49-3. Risk Factors for the Development of Cardiac Sequelae in Kawasaki Syndrome

---

Male sex
Age <1 yr
Prolonged fever (>16 days)
Peripheral white blood cell count $>30,000/\mu L$
Erythrocyte sedimentation rate >101 mm/hr
Electrocardiogram abnormality

---

renal infarcts, gangrene of the fingers and toes, encephalopathy, and subarachnoid hemorrhage.

MANAGEMENT

All patients diagnosed with Kawasaki syndrome should be hospitalized immediately for administration of intravenous gamma globulin (IVGG), aspirin therapy, and cardiac evaluation. Routine testing includes complete blood count with platelets, urinalysis, electrolytes, liver profile, chest radiograph, electrocardiogram, and echocardiogram.

Bed rest, coupled with close cardiac monitoring, is essential. Only by detecting the initial signs of cardiac complications can appropriate critical measures be taken to save the life of a severely affected child.

Early in the course of the illness, IVGG may help decrease the inflammatory response and decrease the incidence of coronary artery aneurysm. The dose of IVGG is 2 g/kg infused over 8 to 12 hours as a single dose. The odds ratio for cardiac sequelae is decreased when IVCC is given before the eighth day of the illness and when the administration period is ≥ 2 days.

Aspirin appears to be another particularly important therapeutic modality. Although it does not have an immediate antipyretic effect, aspirin can reduce the height and duration of fever and may serve as an important antithrombotic factor. It is given in a sequential dosage regimen: high dose (100 mg/kg/day divided into 4 doses) until the 14th day of the illness, followed by low dose (3 to 5 mg/kg/day as a single-day dose). Aspirin is continued until the platelet count has normalized. Salicylate levels should be monitored during therapy.

Corticosteroids have been considered to be contraindicated in Kawasaki disease due to unfavorable results in early studies. However, there is growing evidence of their beneficial effect in immunoglobulin-resistant disease and at least one study showing a decreased incidence of coronary artery aneurysms when corticosteroids were added to conventional therapy.

PROGNOSIS

The overall mortality rate of Kawasaki syndrome in American children is <1 percent. It is higher in infants younger than 1 year. The prognosis for patients receiving treatment within the first 8 to 10 days of the illness is excellent. Most aneurysms resolve within the first year with no apparent sequelae; however, it is doubtful that the coronary arteries return completely to normal.

Reports are just beginning to appear of children who recovered uneventfully from Kawasaki disease, only to develop angina and myocardial infarction between 1 month and 13 years after the acute attack. A careful history of possible Kawasaki disease now appears to be mandatory in all older children or young adolescents presenting for preschool physical examinations. All individuals with a history of Kawasaki disease should be followed and examined at intervals, including those who have no apparent cardiovascular abnormalities.

BIBLIOGRAPHY

American Heart Association Committee on Rheumatic Fever, Endocarditis and Kawasaki Disease: Diagnostic guidelines for Kawasaki disease. *Am J Dis Child* 144:1220–1222, 1990.

Dale RC, Saleem MA, Daw S, et al: Treatment of severe complicated Kawasaki disease with oral prednisolone and aspirin. *J Pediatr* 137:723–726, 2000.

Gersony W: Diagnosis and management of Kawasaki disease. *JAMA* 265:2699–2703, 1991.

Kuijpers TW, Wiegman A, Van Lier RA, et al: Kawasaki disease: A maturational defect in immune responsiveness. *J Infect Dis* 180:1869–1877, 1999.

Levy M, Karen G: Atypical Kawasaki disease: Analysis of clinical presentation and diagnostic clues. *Pediatr Infect Dis* 9:122–126, 1990.

Rowley AH, Shulman ST: Kawasaki syndrome. *Pediatr Clin North Am* 46:313–329, 1999.

Shingadia D, Shulman ST: New perspectives in the drug treatment of Kawasaki disease. *Paediatr Drugs* 1:291–297, 1999.

Shinohara M, Sone K, Tomomasa T, et al: Corticosteroids in the treatment of the acute phase of Kawasaki disease. *J Pediatr* 135:465–469, 1999.

Witt MT, Minich LL, Bohnsack JF, et al: Kawasaki disease: More patients are being diagnosed who do not meet American Heart Association criteria. *Pediatrics* 104:10, 1999.

Yanagawa H, Tuohong Z, Oki I, et al: Effects of gammaglobulin on the cardiac sequelae of Kawasaki disease. *Pediatr Cardiol* 20:248–251, 1999.

50

Common Parasitic Infestations

Steven Lelyveld
Gary R. Strange

HIGH-YIELD FACTS

- Three major groups of parasites cause human disease:
  - Protozoa
  - Helminths
    - Nematodes (roundworms)
    - Cestodes (flatworms)
    - Trematodes (flukes)
  - Arthropods
- Virtually all organ systems are at risk for parasitic infestation, with symptoms depending on the system(s) involved. Arthropods are predominantly surface-dwellers and cause pruritus and rash. Nematodes and cestodes infest the gut, producing diarrhea, abdominal pain, and nutritional derangement, but, along with trematodes, they may migrate to the lungs and solid organs.
- *Ascaris lumbricoides* is the largest and most prevalent human nematode, with an estimated 1 billion cases worldwide. Albendazole (400 mg orally as a single dose) or pyrantel pamoate (11 mg/kg orally as a single dose; maximum 1 g) is curative.
- *Enterobius vermicularis* (pinworm) is present in all parts of the United States and affects individuals of all ages and socioeconomic levels, with the most common presentation being that of a toddler or small child with anal itch. Scotch tape, placed sticky side to perianal skin when the child first awakens and then viewed under low power, is usually diagnostic, but repeated examination may be necessary to find the eggs.

- *Trichuris trichiura* (whipworm) lives predominantly in the cecum and can cause malabsorptive symptoms, pain, bloody diarrhea, and fever but is usually asymptomatic. A heavy worm burden may cause a colitis-like picture and rectal prolapse and can be associated with anemia and developmental and cognitive deficits.
- The hookworms, *Necator americanus* and *Ancylostoma duodenale,* are found between 36° north and 30° south latitude and are one of the most prevalent infectious diseases of humans, with an estimated 1 billion individuals affected. Although a broad spectrum of symptoms is possible, the hallmark of hookworm infestation is the microcytic, hypochromic anemia of iron deficiency.
- Symptoms of shistosome infestation appear only in those with heavy infestation and are commonly frequency, dysuria, and hematuria with *Shistosoma haematobium;* and colicky abdominal pain and bloody diarrhea with the other agents. None of these flukes are endemic in the United States.
- The avian schistosome *Trichobilharzia ocellata* is spread by migratory birds to the freshwater lakes of the northern United States. The cercariae cause dermatitis, known as swimmer's itch.
- Most patients with amoebic infestation carry amebas asymptomatically in the cecum and large intestine. Heavy infestations of *Entamoeba histolytica* produce a colitis-like picture ("gay bowel syndrome") with nausea, vomiting, bloating, pain, bloody diarrhea, and leukocytosis without eosinophilia.
- Resistence of head lice to permethrin is now common, with reported insecticidal activity down to 28 percent in one study. The combination of 1 percent permethrin with trimethoprim/sulfamethoxazole has recently been reported to be 95 percent effective, compared with 80 percent for permethrin alone.

Parasitic diseases are ubiquitous. In spite of advances in sanitation throughout the world, new medications, and the heightened awareness of health care providers, between one-fourth and one-half of the world's population has a parasitic infestation at any given time. An increasingly mobile society has made disease containment nearly impossible. Travel (for business and pleasure), immigration, and the importation of vectors as a consequence of international trade have all led to an increase in disease. The increased number of immunocompromised hosts has also led to an increased expression of these infestations. This chapter reviews the major parasitic infestations causing human disease found in the United States. The reader is encouraged to become familiar with more comprehensive texts on parasitology.

The oral exploratory behavior of the child, coupled with a poor capacity to avoid arthropods, place him or her at particular risk for acquiring parasites. Important factors in the history include the following:

- Camping trips
- Travel to regions with questionable sanitation and water purification practices or a warm climate
- Method of food acquisition and preparation
- Exposure to pets and other animals, both domestic and wild
- Participation in day care
- Living in confined situations
- Mental retardation
- Adolescent drug abuse
- Homosexual contacts
- Sexual abuse
- Blood transfusions

Three major groups of parasites cause human disease, as follows:

- Protozoa
- Helminths
  - Nematodes (roundworms)
  - Cestodes (flatworms)
  - Trematodes (flukes)
- Arthropods

Virtually all organ systems are at risk for infestation, with symptoms depending on the system(s) involved. Arthropods are predominantly surface-dwellers. They cause pruritus and rash. Nematodes and cestodes infest the gut, producing diarrhea, abdominal pain, and nutritional derangement. Along with trematodes, the other helminths may migrate to the lungs and solid organs and are associated with malnutrition and inhibited growth and development. Protozoa may live in the gut for gen-

erations, shedding cysts in the stool. Like helminths, they can also, under proper circumstances, travel throughout the body. Some parasites only begin to produce symptoms months to years after the first exposure. In addition, the symptoms produced depend on the stage of the parasitic life cycle.

The varied and nonspecific symptoms produced place parasitic infestation on the expanded differential diagnosis of most patients presenting to the emergency department. The challenge to the pediatric emergency physician is, therefore, to be aware of the patterns of worldwide distribution of these organisms and the symptoms they produce. It is important not to overlook the possibility of parasitic infestation when treating large numbers of patients with common complaints. A list of common emergency department complaints and the major human parasites that produce them is given in Table 50-1.

NEMATODES (ROUNDWORMS)

Ascariasis

Ascaris lumbricoides is the largest and most prevalent human nematode, with an estimated 1 billion cases worldwide. Although it is most commonly found in tropical and subtropical climates, it is present throughout the United States. Ascariasis is most common in preschool and early school age children.

From an egg measuring 65 by 45 μm, this nematode can grow to a length of 30 cm. After being deposited in the stool, the egg matures over 3 weeks. Upon ingestion, the egg hatches in the small intestine. The larvae burrow through the gut mucosa, enter the bloodstream, and migrate to the lungs. They cause shortness of breath, hemoptysis, eosinophilia, fever, and Loffler's pneumonia as they break through the alveoli, migrate up the bronchial tree, and are swallowed. Maturing to the adult form, *A. lumbricoides* can live freely in the small intestine for up to a year, shedding eggs in the stool. At this stage, it usually remains asymptomatic but can cause gastrointestinal symptoms, including pain, protein malabsorption, biliary duct or bowel obstruction, and appendicitis.

Although stool testing for ova is diagnostic, serologic hemagglutination and flocculation tests are available.

Albendazole (400 mg orally as a single dose) or pyrantel pamoate (11 mg/kg orally as a single dose; maximum 1 g) is curative. Piperazine salts (50 to 75 mg/kg for 2 days) are recommended for ascariasis complicated by intestinal or biliary obstruction, since they cause rela-

Table 50-1. Symptoms of Parasitic Disease

Symptom	Possible Cause
Abdominal pain	*Ascaris, Clonorchis, Diphyllobothrium, Entamoeba, Fasciola, Giardia*. hookworm, *Hymenolepsis, Schistosoma, Taenia, Trichuris*
Anemia	*Babesia, Diphyllobothrium*, hookworm, *Leishmania donovani, Plasmodium* species, *Trichuris*
Asthma	*Ascaris, Strongyloides, Toxocara*
Conjunctivitis and keratitis	Filariae (*Onchocerca volvulus*), *Taenia, Trichinella, Trypanosoma*
Diarrhea	*Dientamoeba, Entamoeba, Fasciola, Fasciolopsis, Giardia*, hookworm, *Hymenolepsis, L. donovani, Palantidium, Schistosoma, Strongyloides, Taenia, Trichinella, Trichuris*
Edema	*Fasciolopsis*, Filariae (*Wuchereria bancrofti*), *Trichinella, Trypanosoma*
Eosinophilia	*Ascaris, Dracunculus, Fasciola*, Filariae (*W. bancrofti, Brugia malayi*) fluke (*Paragonimus westermani, Chlonorchis sinensis, Fasciolopsis leuski*), *Hymnenolepsis*, hookworm, *Schistosoma, Strongyloides, Taenia, Toxocara, Trichinella, Trichuris*
Fever	*Ascaris, Babesia, Entamoeba, Fasciola*, Filariae (*W. bancrofti*), fluke (*C. sinensis*), *Giardia, L. donovani, Plasmodium* species, *Toxocara*, Trichi, *Trichuris, Trypanosoma*
Hemoptysis	*Ascaris, Echinococcus, Paragonimus*
Hepatomegaly	Fluke (*C. sinensis, Opisthorchis viverrini, Fasciola*), *L. donovani, Plasmodium* species, tapeworm (*Echinococcus*), *Schistosoma, Toxocara, Trypanosoma*
Intestinal obstruction	*Ascaris, Diphyllobothrium*, fluke (*Fasciolopsis buski*), *Strongyloides, Taenia*
Jaundice	Fluke (*C. sinensis, O. viverrini*), *Plasmodium* species
Meningitis	*Acanthamoeba*, malaria (*Plasmodium falciparum*), *Naegleria*, primary amebic meningoencephalitis, *Toxocara, Trichinella, Trypanosoma*
Myocardial disease	*Taenia, Trichinella, Trypanosoma* (*T. cruzi*)
Nausea and vomiting	*Ascaris, Entamoeba, Giardia, Leishmania, Taenia, Trichinella, Trichuris*
Pneumonia	*Ascaris*, Filariae (*W. bancrofti, B. malayi*), fluke (*P. westermani*), *Strongyloides, Trichinella*
Pruritus	*Dientamoeba, Enterobius*, Filariae (*O. volvulus*), *Trichuris*
Seizures	*Hymenolepsis, Trichinella, Paragonimus*, tapeworm (*Echinococcus, Cysticercus*)
Skin ulcers	*Dracunculus*, hookworm, *L. donovani, Trypanosoma*
Splenomegaly	*Babesia, Toxoplasma, Plasmodium*
Urticaria	*Ascaris, Dracunculus, Fasciola, Strongyloides, Trichinella*

tively rapid expulsion of the worms. If multiple infestations are present, it is recommended that *Ascaris* be treated first, as treatment of other parasites may stimulate a large worm burden to migrate simultaneously, causing obstruction.

There is controversy in regard to the clinical significance of *Ascaris* infestation. However, about 20,000 deaths annually are attributed to *Ascaris,* mostly due to intestinal obstruction. Preventive therapy in endemic regions may be considered.

Enterobiasis

Enterobius vermicularis (pinworm) is present in all parts of the United States and affects individuals of all ages and socioeconomic levels. The most common presenta-

tion is that of a toddler or small child with anal itch. The egg is oval, approximately 50 by 25 μm in size. It is inhaled or ingested and hatches between the ileum and ascending colon, growing to an adult length of 3 to 10 mm. The adult may live and copulate in the colon for 1 to 2 months. The gravid female migrates to the anus, where it deposits embryonated eggs, usually during early morning hours. When the host stirs, the adult will migrate back into the body, causing symptoms of pruritus ani, dysuria, enuresis, and vaginitis. Scratching and hand-mouth behavior reinoculates the host, and the cycle repeats. Granulomas of the pelvic peritoneum and female genital tract may occur.

Scotch tape, placed sticky side to perianal skin when the child first awakens and then viewed under low power, is usually diagnostic, but repeated examination may be

necessary to find the eggs. Treatment is with albendazole, 400 mg orally. Pyrantel pamoate (11 mg/kg) or
mebendazole (100 mg) may also be used. Each drug is
given as a single dose, with a repeat given 2 weeks later
to remove secondary hatchings.

Trichuris trichiura

Trichuris trichiura (whipworm) is found in southern Appalachia, southwest Louisiana, and other warm rural areas. The life cycle mimics that of *E. vermicularis.* The
eggs are of similar size and configuration, with the addition of a rounded cap at each pole. The adult resembles *E. vermicularis,* with a long whip-like projection at
one end. It lives predominantly in the cecum and can
cause malabsorptive symptoms, pain, bloody diarrhea,
and fever but is usually asymptomatic. A heavy worm
burden may cause a colitis-like picture and rectal prolapse and can be associated with anemia and developmental and cognitive deficits. Albendazole (400 mg) as
a one-time dose may be sufficient, but in heavy infestations, the course of treatment should be extended to 3
days. Mebendazole (100 mg bid for 3 days) may also be
used. Community control should be considered in heavily endemic areas.

Trichinosis

Trichinella spiralis is found throughout the United States,
with increasing prevalence in the Northeast and Mid-
Atlantic states. Although <100 cases of clinical disease
are reported annually, cysts are found at autopsy in the
diaphragms of 4 percent of patients. Current control
efforts include laws governing the feeding of swine des-
tined for sale to the public, specifically the heat treatment of garbage used as feed and recommendations for
the preparation of meat in the home.

Digestive enzymes liberate the encysted larvae, which
lodge in the duodenum and jejunum, grow, and, within
2 days, mature and copulate. The females give birth to
living larvae that bore through the mucosa, become
blood-borne, and migrate to striated muscle, heart, lung,
and brain. Host defenses produce inflammation at each
site. Although a classic triad of fever, myalgia, and periorbital edema has been described, symptoms of gastroenteritis, pneumonia, myocarditis, meningitis, and
seizures can occur.

Although most cases are mild and self-limited, the
history and physical examination, along with elevation
of muscle enzymes and eosinophilia, may suggest the
need for further investigation. Serologic tests are available from the Centers for Disease Control and Prevention. Muscle biopsy is confirmative.

Treatment, with aspirin and steroids, is initially aimed
at reducing the inflammatory symptoms. Mebendazole
(200 to 400 mg tid for 3 days and then 400 mg tid for
10 days) is indicated for severe disease but may not be
effective after encystment.

Hookworms

The hookworms, *Necator americanus* and *Ancylostoma
duodenale,* are found between 36° north and 30° south
latitude and are one of the most prevalent infectious diseases of humans, with an estimated 1 billion individuals
affected. The eggs hatch in the soil, releasing rhabditi-
form larvae 275 μm long that feed on bacteria and organic debris. They double in length, molt, and may survive as filariform larvae for several weeks. Upon contact,
they burrow through the skin, causing pruritus (ground
itch), enter the blood, travel to the lung, and are ingested, like *A. lumbricoides.* Although a broad spectrum
of symptoms is possible, the hallmark of hookworm infestation is the microcytic, hypochromic anemia of iron
deficiency. Each adult hookworm may ingest up to 0.05
mL of blood a day. Children with chronic hookworm
disease may develop a characteristic yellow-green pallor
called chlorosis. Although more commonly seen with
the dog and cat hookworms *(Ancylostoma braziliense),*
these hookworms can also cause the serpentine track of
cutaneous larva migrans. Finding the ova in stool is diagnostic. Albendazole (400 mg qd for 2 to 3 days),
mebendazole (100 mg bid for 3 days), or pyrantel
pamoate (11 mg/kg qd for 3 days) is recommended. Cutaneous larva migrans is usually self-limited, but topical
application of 10 percent thiabendzole, ivermectin (150
to 200 μg orally), or albendazole (400 mg qd for 3 days)
may hasten resolution.

Strongiloidiasis

Strongyloides stercoralis (threadworm) is found in southern Appalachia, Kentucky, and Tennessee. Like the hookworms, it penetrates the skin, producing pruritus and cutaneous larva migrans. Pulmonary and gastrointestinal
symptoms occur as the larvae migrate. The human is a
definitive host. Ongoing autoinfection is slowed by the
host's immune response, but immunocompromised patients and the elderly may suffer fatal infestation. The
rise in the acquired immunodeficiency syndrome (AIDS)
has been mirrored by a rise in reported cases of *Strongyloides* infestation. Infestation is extremely common in in-

stitutionalized mentally disabled children. A definitive diagnosis is made by recovering *Strongyloides* in stool, sputum, or duodenal aspirate. Thiabendazole (50 mg/kg/day divided bid, maximum 3 g/day) for 2 days is recommended. An alternative drug is ivermectin, 200 μg qd for 1 to 2 days. In disseminated strongyloidiasis, treatment may need to continue for up to 2 weeks.

Filarial Nematodes

The filarial nematodes *Wuchereria bancrofti* (elephantiasis), *Onchocerca volvulus* and *Loa loa* (river blindness), and *Dracunculus medinensis* (Guinea worms) cause significant world-wide morbidity. They are rarely encountered in the United States; when they are, it is usually in immigrants from parts of the world where they are endemic.

TREMATODES (FLUKES)

Flukes are oval, flat worms with a ventral sucker for nutrition and attachment. Eggs are shed in the stool of definitive hosts, hatch into miracidia, and enter an intermediate host such as a snail or other crustacean, fish, or bird. They develop into cercariae, which leave the intermediate host to become free living prior to infesting the definitive host on contact with contaminated water. The intermediate host may also be ingested, releasing this infective form of the parasite. Symptoms are produced as the fluke reaches its destination. *Fasciolopsis buski* infests the gut; *Fasciola hepatica, Opisthorchis* (formerly *Clonorchis) sinensis,* and *Schistosoma mansoni* the liver; *Schistosoma haematobium* the bladder; and *Paragonimus westermani* the lung. Acute shistosomiasis is an immune complex, febrile disease associated with early infection. Symptoms appear only in those with heavy infestation and are commonly frequency, dysuria, and hematuria with *S. haematobium* and colicky abdominal pain and bloody diarrhea with the other agents. None of these flukes are endemic in the United States. Praziquantel (40 mg/kg/day divided into 2 doses for 1 or 2 days) is recommended for *S. haematobium, S. mansoni,* and *S. intercalatum.* A higher dose, 60 mg/kg/day divided into 3 doses for 1 day, is recommended for *S. japonica* and *S. mekongi.*

Of particular interest to the pediatric emergency physician is the avian schistosome, *Trichobilharzia ocellata.* Spread by migratory birds to the freshwater lakes of the northern United States, the cercariae cause dermatitis, known as swimmer's itch. The intense reaction produced by host defenses is treated with heat and antipruritics. Severe cases are treated with thiabendazole cream.

CESTODES (FLATWORMS AND TAPEWORMS)

Cestodes attach to the gut of the definitive host with hooks or suckers at the head (scolex), from which grow segmented proglottids. Each proglottid is equipped to produce large volumes of eggs. These eggs, along with terminal proglottids, pass in the stool and are ingested by the intermediate host. The eggs hatch into a larval stage, either cysticercus, cysticercoid, coenurus, or hydatid cysts, depending on the species. Symptoms are produced as these larvae act as space-occupying lesions or cause inflammation. When the intermediate host is ingested by the definitive host, the larvae attach to the intestine and the cycle repeats.

Four cestodes produce most clinical disease seen in the United States:

- *Taenia solium*
- *Taenia saginatum*
- *Diphyllobothrium latum*
- *Echinococcus granulosus*

Taenia solium (pork tapeworm) and *Taenia saginatum* (beef tapeworm) infestations are generally asymptomatic and are diagnosed when a parent brings a proglottid to the emergency department for identification. A history of raw meat consumption may be elicited. Patients occasionally will have gastrointestinal complaints. When *T. solium* enters the cysticercus phase, it may migrate to the heart, brain, breast, eye, skin, or other solid organ. Subcutaneous nodules, visual field defects, focal neurologic findings, acute psychosis, and obstructive hydrocephalus may develop years after infestation. Calcified cysts may be found on plain radiographs, and cysts may be seen as a ring of calcification on computed tomography.

Diphyllobothrium latum (fish tapeworm) is becoming more prevalent with the increased popularity of raw fish. Because *D. latum* absorbs >50 times more vitamin B_{12} than *Taenia,* it causes pernicious anemia.

Echinococcus granulosus (sheep tapeworm) is found in agricultural countries. Most reported cases are from the southeastern United States. Symptomatology is secondary to hydatid cyst formation with mass effect.

Most tapeworms are treated with praziquantel (5 to 25 mg/kg once). *Echinococcus* infection and cysticercosis respond best to albendazole (15 mg/kg/day divided tid for 28 days).

PROTOZOA

Entamoeba histolytica

Entamoeba histolytica is a water-borne single-cell organism. It is found in epidemic proportion after heavy rain in areas of suboptimal sanitation and among closely confined populations. In addition to ingestion of contaminated water, it may be spread by direct human contact, both sexually and in breast milk. Most patients carry amebas asymptomatically in the cecum and large intestine. Heavy infestations of *E. histolytica* produce a colitis-like picture ("gay bowel"). These patients may present with nausea, vomiting, bloating, pain, bloody diarrhea, and leukocytosis without eosinophilia. The amebas live at the base of large flask-shaped ulcers. When the infection is severe, direct inspection will reveal pseudopolyps of normal tissue on a base of ulcerative disease. *E. histolytica* has the capacity to invade the blood, causing abscess formation in the liver, lung, brain, and breast. Diagnosis is confirmed with stool specimen or colonoscopic aspiration. Metronidazole (35 to 50 mg/kg/day divided tid for 10 days) followed by iodoquinol (40 mg/kg/day divided tid for 20 days) is recommended to eradicate this infestation.

Dientamoeba fragilis

Dientamoeba fragilis is a flagellate that lives in the cecum and proximal large bowel and has worldwide distribution. It is generally not invasive, does not form cysts, and closely resembles *Trichomonas,* except for the lack of a flagellum. It may be found in children in day care, causing the local mucosal irritative symptoms of abdominal pain, decreased appetite, diarrhea, and eosinophilia. It is diagnosed when trophozoites are found in the stool, after the use of permanent stains. The treatment is iodoquinol (40 mg/kg/day divided tid for 20 days).

Giardia lamblia

This flagellate thrives in the relatively alkaline pH of the duodenum and proximal small bowel. Infestation occurs after ingestion of contaminated water or other fecal-oral behavior. It is commonly found in day care centers; among travelers, immunocompromised children, and patients with cystic fibrosis; and in association with hepatic or pancreatic disease. Flatulence, nonbloody diarrhea or constipation, abdominal distention, and pain are common symptoms. Fever, weight loss, and fat, carbohydrate, and vitamin malabsorption can occur. Although cysts may appear in the stool, it is often necessary to perform duodenal aspiration to confirm the diagnosis. Metronidazole (15 mg/kg/day divided tid for 5 days) is recommended.

Trypanosomes

The vectors that transmit *Trypanosoma gambiense, Trypanosoma rhodesiense* (African sleeping sickness), and *Trypanosoma cruzi* (Chagas' disease) are not endemic to the United States. However, they may be passed on through blood transfusions and breast feeding from infected adults. Although infestation initially mimics a viral illness, patients will later develop alterations in mental status, myocarditis, megacolon, and megaesophagus. If a history of travel to an endemic area by the parent or child is elicited, serologic tests and biopsy of affected organs are indicated. When the diagnosis has been confirmed, treatment is with nifurtimox, suramin, or melarsoprol.

Malaria

In 1993, 1411 cases of malaria were reported to the Centers for Disease Control and Prevention. Over the past 10 years, the number of cases has remained stable at approximately 1000 a year, one-fourth of which occur in children. Ninety percent of these cases are equally divided between *Plasmodium falciparum* and *Plasmodium vivax.* The remainder are caused by *Plasmodium ovale* and *Plasmodium malariae.* Two-thirds were imported from sub-Saharan Africa. In 1993, three cases of falciparum malaria that could not be traced to immigration or travel were reported in New York City. It is felt that these cases might be the first sign of a resurgence of indigenous malaria. Transmission of all forms of malaria is by direct blood inoculum, usually by the *Anopheles* mosquito. It may also be passed transplacentally to the fetus. Following a 1- to 3-week incubation in the liver, *Plasmodium* enters an asexual erythrocytic cycle. *P. falciparum, P. vivax,* and *P. ovale* have a 48-hour cycle and a preference for reticulocytes, whereas *P. malariae* has a 72-hour cycle and is found in older red blood cells. These cycles produce the classic periodicity of fever and shaking chills. Headache, diarrhea, cough, altered consciousness, jaundice, and disseminated intravascular coagulation leading to cardiovascular collapse can ensue. The mortality rate exceeds 4 percent.

With a high index of suspicion, one looks for the parasite on thick and thin blood smears. *P. falciparum* is characterized by a predominance of ring forms within the red blood cells, banana-shaped gametocytes, and the absence of mature trophozoites and schizonts. *P. malariae, P. vivax,* and *P. ovale* have round gametocytes with mature trophozoites and schizonts on smear.

To prevent infestation in travelers, prophylaxis is recommended beginning 1 week before departure and continuing for 4 to 6 weeks after return. Resistance of *P. falciparum* and *P. vivax* to chloroquine is now spreading. If a person is traveling to a sensitive area, chloroquine (5 mg/kg of base, maximum 300 mg) given once a week is recommended. For resistant areas, mefloquine is the drug of choice. Once someone is infected, chloroquine (10 mg/kg of base, maximum 600 mg, followed by 5 mg/kg of base, maximum 300 mg at 6, 24, and 48 hours) or quinine sulfate (25 mg/kg/day divided tid for 3 to 7 days) and pyrimethamine-sulfadoxine (number of tablets based on age) given on the last day of quinine are recommended. As *P. vivax* and *P. ovale* infestations tend to recur, they should, when identified, also be treated with primaquine phosphate (0.3 mg/kg/day for 14 days).

Babesiosis

Babesia microti has an erythrocytic phase similar to that of malaria. It is transmitted by the deer tick *Ixodes dammini* from a rodent reservoir and is therefore found in the same geographic distribution as Lyme disease (northeastern states, Wisconsin, and Minnesota). When symptomatic, patients present with fever, malaise, hemolytic anemia, jaundice, and renal failure. Upon blood smear inspection, it may be difficult to distinguish *B. microti* from the ring form of *P. falciparum*. Treatment is with clindamycin (20 to 40 mg/kg/day divided tid) and quinine (25 mg/kg/day divided tid) for 7 days. Alternatively, a 7-day regimen of atovaquone (750 mg q12h) and azithromycin (500 mg on day 1 and 250 mg thereafter) has been shown to be effective and to have fewer adverse reactions.

Pneumocystis carinii

Pneumocystis carinii has a low virulence and is found in the latent phase in a large percentage of the American population. When the host is immunocompromised, trophozoites replicate in alveolar spaces and spread through the vascular and lymphatic beds. The patient experiences respiratory distress, fever, and nonproductive cough with limited auscultatory findings. The radiograph may be normal or symmetric interstitial ground-glass infiltrates in the middle and lower lung fields may be seen.

Pneumocystis reactivation occurs in debilitated patients and those with suppressed immune responses. It is found in more than 60 percent of patients with HIV infection. The overall mortality rate in children is 40 percent, rising to 100 percent once radiographic changes occur in untreated non-AIDS patients.

Given the high incidence of asymptomatic carriers, the diagnostic method of choice is silver nitrate-methenamine stain of a lung biopsy specimen in the proper clinical setting. Treatment is with trimethoprim (15 to 20 mg/kg/day) and sulfamethoxazole (75 to 100 mg/kg/day) in 3 or 4 divided doses orally or pentamidine (3 to 4 mg/kg/day) intravenously for 2 to 3 weeks.

Coccidia

Cryptosporidium, Isospora belli, and *Toxoplasma gondii* belong to the protozoan subclass *Coccidia,* which also includes *Plasmodium.* Modes of transmission include direct human contact and ingestion of fecally contaminated food and water. *Toxoplasma* is also transmitted transplacentally, with blood transfusion and organ transplantation. Intermediate hosts include farm animals *(Cryptosporidium),* cats *(Toxoplasma),* and other mammals.

Although some children harbor *Cryptosporidium* and *Isospora* asymptomatically, both organisms can cause a secretory, cholera-like diarrhea after a 2-week incubation. Large volumes of watery, nonbloody, leukocyte-free stool may produce significant dehydration. Fever, headache, and anorexia are followed by malabsorption of lactose and fat. These symptoms are self-limited and last for up to 3 weeks. The oocysts may be shed for an additional month. Immunocompromised children may manifest infective symptoms of the liver, gallbladder, appendix, and lung as well as a reactive arthritis. No toxins have been demonstrated, and the pathogenic mechanism of this spectrum of symptoms is not known. Direct examination of stool with a modified Ziehl-Neelsen stain is the diagnostic method of choice. There is no proven antiparasitic cure. Octreotide (300 to 500 μg tid subcutaneously) may control the diarrhea of patients with HIV.

The trophozoites of *Toxoplasma gondii* have a predilection for the brain, heart, and bone, although they can invade any nucleated cell. Approximately 2500 infants are born annually in the United States with congenital disease, 10 percent of whom have the *Toxoplasma* triad of hydrocephalus, chorioretinitis, and intracranial calcification. The long-term prognosis for these children is poor.

Acquired toxoplasmosis in the immune-competent host is asymptomatic but may produce a subclinical reaction in the reticuloendothelial system. For patients with AIDS and other types of immunocompromise, reactivation produces severe central nervous system involvement and dissemination to the heart and lungs. Between 30 and 40 percent of AIDS patients will develop *Toxoplasma* encephalitis or mass lesions of the brain and cranial nerves. The diagnosis is made by antigen detection or by seeing a ring formation on computed tomography with contrast.

Prompt treatment with pryimethamine (2 mg/kg/day for 3 days and then 1 mg/kg/day for 4 weeks) and sulfadiazine (100 to 200 mg/kg/day for 4 weeks) is recommended. However, there is a high fatality rate once *Toxoplasma* becomes reactivated.

ARTHROPODS

Pediculosis

The parasites *Pediculus humanus capitis* (head louse), *Pediculus humanus corporis* (body louse), and *Phthirus pubis* (pubic or crab louse) are 1 to 2 mm long. They attach 0.8-mm–long eggs (nits) firmly to hair shafts, close to the skin. Lice are transmitted by direct human contact or the sharing of clothing or other personal articles. They are not transmitted to or from domestic animals and are found on children with proper hygiene. They require a hair-bearing surface, with the adult viable for only 2 days and the nit for 10 days off the host. The most common complaint is itching. Phthirus pubis may produce blue-colored macules (maculae ceruleae).

A 10-minute rinse with 1 percent permethrin (Nix®) has been reported to kill adult lice and 90 percent of nits. It may, however, exacerbate the pruritus and erythema. It is too toxic to use near the eyes, where petrolatum is recommended to suffocate the lice. Eyelid lice in prepubescent children should alert the physician to the possibility of sexual abuse. Care must be taken to delouse other family members and the child's environment. A spray of permethrin and piperonyl butoxide should be employed on furniture and bedding used in the previous 2 days. Alternatively, objects can be sealed in plastic bags for 2 weeks until all adults and nits are no longer viable. Dead nits can be removed from hair shafts with a fine-toothed comb.

Resistence to permethrin is now common, with reported insecticidal activity down to 28 percent in one study. The combination of 1 percent permethrin with trimethoprim/sulfamethoxazole has recently been reported to be 95 percent effective, compared with 80 percent for permethrin alone.

Scabies

Sarcoptes scabiei (scabies) are transmitted by direct close and prolonged human contact. Scabies will not flourish on other animals. Following a 3- to 6-week incubation, the 200- to 400-μm-long scabies mite burrows between the fingers and toes as well as in the groin, external genitalia, and axillae, depositing eggs in the tunnel as she goes. The itch is worse at night, with infants sleeping poorly and rubbing their hands and feet together. Small red, raised, papules are formed, which may progress to vesicles and pustules. Secondary excoriations are also present. The diagnosis is made clinically. However, one may scrape burrows or papules overlaid with mineral oil and inspect the scrapings for adults, eggs, and excreta for confirmation. A single application of 5 percent permethrin cream is curative for children older than 2 months. Younger children may be treated with sulfur precipitated in petrolatum. The long incubation period makes treating the entire family advisable. As the parasite lives less than 24 hours off the host, environmental decontamination may not be necessary.

Myiasis

Myiasis occurs when fly larvae invade the human body. Under normal circumstances, these larvae live off decaying organic matter. In very unusual circumstances, particularly with debilitated and malnourished children, maggots may be found in the nasal mucosa, eye, diaper area, or skin. Surgical excision is required and is curative.

BIBLIOGRAPHY

Beigel Y, Greenburg Z, Ostfeld I: Clinical problem-solving: Letting the patient off the hook. *N Engl J Med* 342: 1658–1661, 2000.

Georgiev VS: Chemotherapy of enterobiasis (oxyuriasis). *Expert Opin Pharmacother* 2:267–275, 2001.

Georgiev VS: Necatoriasis: Treatment and developmental therapeutics. *Expert Opin Pharmacother* 9:1065–1078, 2000.

Georgiev VS: Pharmacotherapy of ascarisis. *Expert Opin Pharmacother* 2:223–239, 2001.

Hipolito RB, Mallorca FG, Zuniga-Macaraig ZO, et al: Head lice infestation: Single drug versus combination therapy with one percent permethrin and trimethoprim/sulfamethoxazole. *Pediatrics* 107:E30, 2001.

Krause PJ, Lepore T, Sikand VK, et al: Atovaquone and azithromycin for the treatment of babesiosis. *N Engl J Med* 343:1454–1458, 2000.

Nair D: Screening for *Strongyloides* infection among the institutionalized mentally disabled. *J Am Board Fam Pract* 14:51–53, 2001.

Stanley SL: Pathophysiology of amoebiasis. *Trends Parasitol* 17:280–285, 2001.

Stephenson LS, Holland CV, Cooper ES: The public health significance of *Trichuris trichiura*. *Parasitiology* 121(suppl): S72–S95, 2000.

Windsor JJ, Johnson EH: *Dientamoeba fragilis:* The unflagellated human flagellate. *Br J Biomed Sci* 56:293–306, 1999.

51

Gastroenteritis

Elizabeth C. Powell
Sally L. Reynolds

HIGH-YIELD FACTS

- Acute gastroenteritis is a common pediatric illness; an estimated 80 percent of cases can be attributed to viruses.

- In the United States, most deaths occur in infants.

- Most diarrheal pathogens are transmitted person-to-person through the fecal-oral route or by ingestion of contaminated food or water.

- As most episodes are self-limited, laboratory studies to identify diarrheal pathogens are usually not needed.

- Fluid and electrolyte therapy is helpful for all children. Many can be managed with oral rehydration.

- After rehydration, early feeding with milk or food is recommended.

- A minority of children will benefit from antimicrobial therapy.

Acute gastroenteritis is a common pediatric illness often treated in emergency departments and outpatient clinics. In the United States, most children <5 years old have gastroenteritis 2 or 3 times per year, while children attending day care have approximately 5 illnesses per year. Worldwide, diarrheal diseases are the leading cause of childhood death. In the United States they result in around 500 deaths per year. Most reported deaths in the United States occur in children younger than 1 year of age. Although bacteria and parasites are sometimes isolated, viruses cause 80 percent of gastroenteritis in children.

ETIOLOGY

Viruses

Most cases of gastroenteritis are caused by rotavirus, enteric adenovirus, Norwalk virus, calcivirus, or astrovirus. Rotavirus, the single most commonly identified cause of severe diarrhea in young children, accounts for 30 to 50 percent of cases. Infection with rotavirus results in approximately 70,000 hospital admissions per year. The peak age of incidence is between 3 and 15 months. Illness usually begins with fever and vomiting, followed by watery, nonbloody diarrhea. Symptoms last 5 to 7 days. Rotavirus is spread by the fecal-oral route and typically occurs during winter months. Because many older children have acquired immunity to rotavirus, their symptoms are mild. Enteric adenovirus (serotypes 31, 40, and 41), the second most frequently identified cause of viral diarrhea in children, is responsible for 5 to 10 percent of gastroenteritis cases requiring hospital admission. Ill children have fever and watery diarrhea; respiratory symptoms are rare. The diarrhea lasts 5 to 12 days. Viral transmission is through the fecal-oral route. The Norwalk virus causes epidemic gastroenteritis in older children during winter months. Illness is short, usually lasting <3 days. Fever and myalgia often accompany the gastrointestinal symptoms. Norwalk virus is transmitted person to person, by contaminated food or by airborne droplets. Astroviruses and calciviruses are less frequent causes of gastroenteritis in young children. Symptoms from illness with these viruses are similar to those of rotavirus.

Bacteria

Campylobacter jejuni, Salmonella spp., *Shigella* spp., *Yersinia enterocolitica, Clostridium difficile,* and *Aeromonas* are the usual organisms that cause bacterial gastroenteritis in U.S. children. *Escherichia coli* (enterotoxigenic, enteropathogenic, enteroinvasive), the pathogen responsible for most bacterial diarrhea worldwide, is an uncommon cause of diarrhea in the United States. Although some bacteria can be transmitted person to person, most are spread by contaminated food or water. Infected children usually have fever and blood-streaked or bloody diarrhea. In young children, *Salmonella* and *Shigella* infections are associated with specific complications. Salmonella gastroenteritis is associated with a 5 to 10 percent incidence of bacteremia in infants <1 year of age. Young infants and children who are immunocompromised or who have sickle cell disease are at risk for fecal complications from *Salmonella* infection, which include pneumonia, meningitis, and osteomyelitis. *Shigella* gastroenteritis is associated with seizures in some affected children. Seizure activity may precede the diarrhea. *Yersinia* gastroenteritis can cause mesenteric adenitis or terminal ileitis, with symptoms that mimic appendicitis.

Parasites

Giardia lamblia and *Cryptosporidium* also cause diarrhea in U.S. children. Although less common than rotavirus, *Giardia* is an identified pathogen in children attending day care. It is responsible for both acute and chronic diarrhea. It has a high rate of asymptomatic infection, and in untreated children cysts can be shed for months. *Giardia* has a low minimum infective dose of 10 to 100 cysts, and the cysts can survive on inert surfaces for long periods. These factors increase its transmission. *Cryptosporidium* is spread from person to person. Transmission is aided by asymptomatic carriers and the organism's resistance to chlorine.

PATHOPHYSIOLOGY

The symptoms and stool characteristics of viral, bacterial, and parasitic diarrhea are similar. Host defenses, which include gastric acid production, intestinal motility, active immunity, and normal anaerobic flora, all help to prevent infection. Information about host characteristics and local epidemiology is also useful in patient management.

Viral diarrhea is non-inflammatory. Infection causes lytic damage to small bowel enterocytes that results in shortening of the intestinal villi, loss of absorptive surface, and increased bowel motility. There is loss of brush border enzymes, and carbohydrate malabsorption produces an osmotic diarrhea. Bacterial infection is either noninflammatory, inflammatory, or penetrating (Table 51-1). In the United States, bacterial diarrhea is usually inflammatory. Bacteria infect the bowel wall, usually the

Table 51-1. Pathophysiology and Etiology of Diarrhea

Noninflammatory (Watery)	Inflammatory	Penetrating
Vibrio cholera	*Shigella*	*Salmonella*
Escherichia coli	*Salmonella*	*typhi*
(enterotoxigenic)	*Campylobacter*	*Yersinia*
Staphylococcal	*jejuni*	*Campylobacter*
food poisoning	*Clostridium*	*fetus*
Clostridium	*difficile*	
perfringens	*E. coli*	
food poisoning	(invasive)	
Rotavirus		
Enteric adenovirus		
Norwalk-like virus		
Giardia		
Cryptosporidium		

colon. Some organisms produce cytotoxins, which promote local invasion and may cause systemic effects. Noninflammatory bacterial diarrhea involves the small bowel. Stools are watery because infection alters fluid absorption at the villus tip (enteropathogenic *E. coli*) or because of endotoxin production (enterotoxigenic *E. coli*). Parasitic diarrhea is noninflammatory.

HISTORY AND PHYSICAL EXAMINATION

The history is focused on the child's state of hydration and gastrointestinal symptoms. The parent's report of intake and output of both stool and urine is useful in estimating fluid balance. Diaper weight is helpful in gauging urine output. However, as watery diarrhea looks like urine, parents may overestimate urine production. Although most children with gastroenteritis have 6 to 8 semisolid-to-watery stools per day, in some cases children can have up to 15 to 20 stools per day. Vomiting and crampy abdominal pain usually accompanies the diarrhea. Useful past history includes prior gastrointestinal surgery or inflammatory bowel disease, and other chronic illness or immunodeficiency. Information about current antibiotic use, as well as day care or school exposure, foreign travel, and diet, is helpful.

The physical examination is useful in assessing hydration and in distinguishing gastroenteritis from other enteric illnesses. Weight loss, tachycardia, tachypnea (reflecting acidosis), a flat or sunken fontanel, dry mucous membranes and lack of tears, and decreased skin turgor are all evidence of dehydration (Table 51-2). In gastroenteritis, the abdomen is usually soft and nondis-

Table 51-2. Clinical Assessment of Severity of Dehydration

Signs and Symptoms	Mild Dehydration	Moderate Dehydration	Severe Dehydration
General appearance and condition:			
Infants and young children	Thirsty, alert, restless	Thirsty, restless, lethargic, but irritable or drowsy	Drowsy, limp, cold, sweaty, cyanotic extremities, may be comatose
Older children and adults	Thirsty, alert, restless	Thirsty, alert, postural hypotension	Cold, sweaty, muscle cramps, cyanotic extremities, conscious
Radial pulse	Normal rate and strength	Rapid and weak	Rapid, sometimes impalpable
Respiration	Normal	Deep, ± rapid	Deep and rapid
Anterior fontanel	Normal	Sunken	Very sunken
Systolic BP	Normal	Normal or low	<90 mmHg; may be unrecordable
Skin elasticity	Pinch retracts immediately	Pinch retracts slowly	Pinch retracts slowly (>2 s)
Eyes	Normal	Sunken	Sunken
Tears	Present	Absent	Absent
Mucous membranes	Moist	Dry	Very dry
Urine flow	Normal	Reduced amount, dark	None for several hours
Body weight loss (%)	3–5	6–9	10 or more
Estimated fluid deficit (mL/kg)	30–50	60–90	100 or more

tended and bowel sounds are decreased. However, the abdomen can be tender, and children with severe gastroenteritis may have abdominal distension or an ileus. Stool should be inspected for gross blood and tested for occult blood. Approximately 10 percent of children with gastroenteritis have blood in their stools.

DIFFERENTIAL DIAGNOSIS

Most children with gastroenteritis have mild, self-limited illness. The differential diagnosis includes nonenteric infections, such as otitis media or urinary tract infection, anatomic defects, malabsorption and overfeeding, or other diet problems. Also in the differential are appendicitis and uncommon but serious causes of diarrhea, including intussusception, hemolytic uremic syndrome, and pseudomembranous colitis.

Children with appendicitis have fever, abdominal pain, and vomiting. Up to 15 percent of children have diarrhea, most often when the appendix points toward the pelvis or has perforated. Unlike gastroenteritis, appendicitis causes focal peritoneal signs, which usually become apparent to the examiner over time. Ultrasound or computed tomography may be useful in evaluating children, in whom the diagnosis of appendicitis is particularly difficult to make.

Intussusception and hemolytic uremic syndrome cause bloody diarrhea in afebrile children. Intussusception, most common in children younger than 1 year, is associated with a classic "triad" of colicky abdominal pain, vomiting, and currant jelly stools. A palpable abdominal mass is pathognomonic of this disease. The colicky abdominal pain frequently causes children to draw up their legs. In children without typical symptoms it is difficult to distinguish intussusception from gastroenteritis. Children with hemolytic uremic syndrome are usually younger than 3 years old and have vomiting, abdominal pain, and diarrhea. Hemolytic uremic syndrome is characterized by hemolytic anemia, thrombocytopenia, and nephropathy; physical findings include pallor, petechiae, or purpura.

Children with pseudomembranous colitis are usually febrile and have bloody diarrhea. Pseudomembranous colitis is differentiated from the more common viral or bacterial enteritis by a history of prior or concurrent antibiotic use and toxic appearance, abdominal distension, and grossly bloody stool.

DIAGNOSTIC EVALUATION

Most children with uncomplicated gastroenteritis need no laboratory studies. Stool cultures are useful in febrile children with blood in their stools, during community outbreaks, and for those children who are immunosuppressed. Routine stool cultures in most hospital laboratories include *Campylobacter jejuni, Salmonella,* and *Shigella.* The rotazyme assay, used to detect rotavirus, is helpful to cohort and avoid cross-contamination among inpatients. It is rarely indicated in managing outpatients. Even with a selective approach, many stool cultures will be negative for bacteria, as viral diarrhea is much more common and may be bloody.

In children with clinical evidence of moderate to severe dehydration, electrolytes and blood, urea, nitrogen (BUN) may be helpful. The electrolytes in children with diarrhea and dehydration frequently show abnormal bicarbonate levels (10 to 18 mEq/L). Less commonly, serum sodium is abnormal and the BUN may be elevated. In specific situations, a leukocyte count is helpful. Infants <3 months old with *Salmonella* enteritis are more likely to have bacteremia when the leukocyte count is >15,000/mm^3. *Shigella* is associated with normal total leukocyte count, but an increased number of band forms. *Campylobacter* and *Yersinia* also have leukocyte counts in the normal range.

TREATMENT

Most children with gastroenteritis are successfully managed with oral solutions as outpatients. Children who are dehydrated or appear toxic require hospital admission for IV therapy. Very young children, children with chronic diseases, and children with chronic malnutrition should be evaluated carefully and managed conservatively.

Oral Therapy

Children estimated to be <5 percent dehydrated can usually be managed with oral solutions. For those without dehydration, 10 mL/kg of an oral solution should be given for each stool. Those with mild dehydration (3 to 5 per-

cent) should be given 50 mL/kg of an oral solution followed by ongoing replacement for each stool (10 mL/kg). Emesis volume should be estimated and replaced. The volume goal is around 150 mL/kg per 24 hours. Oral rehydration therapy, particularly in infants, should be done with a solution that contains an appropriate carbohydrate:sodium ratio. Fruit juices and decarbonated soda beverages often contain high carbohydrate and low sodium concentrations. Apple and white grape juice also contain sorbitol, which when ingested in large quantities can exacerbate diarrhea. Commercially available oral solutions have sodium concentrations of 45 to 50 mmol/L. Although products with this sodium concentration are best suited to maintenance use, they can be used to rehydrate otherwise healthy children. Oral solutions are also available commercially in flavored and frozen forms (popsicles); their use may improve compliance in toddlers. Breastfed infants should be nursed through the course of their illness, as breast milk is very well tolerated.

Children who are not dehydrated should be fed an age-appropriate diet through their illness; those who are dehydrated should be fed as soon as they have been rehydrated. This helps to prevent weight loss and speeds recovery. However, food will increase the fecal volume and the diarrhea may transiently appear worse. Foods best tolerated are those that are easily digested and include bananas, applesauce, and other fruits and vegetables; yogurt; lean meats; and complex carbohydrates, such as cereal, rice, noodles, potatoes, or bread. Infants may be given formula after dehydration is corrected. Although some clinicians recommend initial refeeding with lactose-free formula, current data do not show these formulas to be superior to milk-based formulas.

IV Therapy

Children with mL (kg) is given over 20 to 30 min to replace intravascular volume. Following the initial fluid bolus, heart rate, perfusion, and mental status are reassessed for improvement. In otherwise healthy children, a second 20 mL/kg bolus of normal saline is indicated if there is a response to the first bolus, but the heart rate remains elevated or perfusion decreased. In cases of severe dehydration, a *Foley* catheter is placed so that urine output can be measured accurately. Electrolytes and BUN, obtained at the time of intravenous line insertion, are useful to identify acidosis and sodium abnormalities.

Dehydrated children awaiting admission require ongoing management in the emergency department. The fluid deficit is calculated using the estimated percentage of dehydration. For example:

- A 10-kg child estimated to be 10 percent dehydrated has a deficit of 1000 mL.
- The deficit is added to the daily maintenance water requirement, calculated in kilograms:
    - first 10 kg: 100 mL/kg
    - next 10 kg: 50 mL/kg
    - beyond 20 kg: 20 mL/kg
- Ongoing losses from fever, vomiting, and diarrhea are also added. They are estimated at 5 to 10 mL/kg per 24 hours.
- Half of the total amount is given in the first 8 hours and the remaining half over the next 16 hours.
- The estimated 24 hour-fluid requirement for this 10-kg child is:

$$\begin{array}{r} 1000 \text{ mL (maintenance)} \\ + \ 1000 \text{ mL (deficit)} \\ + \ \underline{\ \ 50 \text{ mL (ongoing losses)}} \\ = 2050 \text{ mL} \end{array}$$

- The 20 mL/kg ($\times$ 2) of normal saline (NS) used for rapid rehydration is subtracted from the total, giving 1650 mL.
- Half of this, or 825 mL, is administered over the first 8 hours.
- An appropriate solution is $D_5 0.2$ NS with 20 mEq/KCl/L.

The preceding calculation assumes a normal value for serum sodium. The management of dehydration in cases of serum electrolyte abnormalities is discussed in the section on fluid and electrolyte abnormalities.

Toddlers and older children with mild to moderate dehydration, mild acidosis, and normal sodium values may be discharged from the emergency department after IV rehydration and oral intake.

Antidiarrheal agents and antiemetics are not recommended in the treatment of infectious gastroenteritis. Data suggest that bismuth subsalicylate (Pepto-Bismol) may be of modest benefit in reducing the duration of diarrhea. Because of its cost and need for frequent administration, further confirmation of its practical efficacy is warranted. Although phenothiazines reduce emesis, extrapyramidal reactions limit their usefulness in children.

Most cases of acute gastroenteritis are caused by viruses, and antibiotics are not indicated. Antibiotics are needed to treat specific bacterial infections. *Salmonella* gastroenteritis is treated with antibiotics in infants younger than 3 months, in children with malignancy or who are recipients of immunosuppressive therapy, and in children with sickle cell disease. They are also indicated for severe colitis, fecal infection (osteomyelitis, pneumonia) and bacteremia (Table 51-3). Recommended antibiotics are ampicillin and chloramphenicol. Trimethoprim-sulfmethoxazole is an alternate therapy.

Uncomplicated *Salmonella* gastroenteritis in children and in healthy infants >3 months of age does not require antibiotics, as they do not shorten the duration of illness

Table 51-3. Antibiotics for Diarrhea

Organism	Antibiotic	Recommendations
Salmonella	Ampicillin	Treatment of specific, high-risk patients
	Amoxicillin	Focal infections
	Trimethoprim-sulfamethoxazole	Prolonged carrier state
	Cefotaxime	
	Ceftriaxone	
	Chloramphenicol	
	Fluoroquinolones	
Shigella	Trimethoprim-sulfamethoxazole	Treatment recommended for all cases
	Ampicillin	
	Ceftriaxone—for resistant strains	
Campylobacter	Erythromycin	Treatment shortens illness and prevents relapse
	Azithromycin	
Giardia	Metronidazole	Treatment recommended for symptomatic infections
	Furazolidone or albendazole—when suspension needed	

and may prolong the carrier state during which organisms are excreted.

In *Shigella* gastroenteritis, antibiotics do shorten the course of illness and eliminate the organism from the stool, thus preventing spread, and are therefore recommended. For susceptible strains, ampicillin or trimethoprim-sulfamethoxazole is effective. Amoxicillin is less effective. If the susceptibility pattern is not known or if a resistant strain is isolated, parenteral ceftriaxone or a fluoroquinolone should be given.

Most *Campylobacter* enteritis will resolve spontaneously without antibiotics. However, when given early during the infection, erythromycin and azithromycin shorten the duration of illness and prevent relapse. In some areas, erythromycin is not effective because of resistant organisms. Treatment is then based on sensitivity testing.

Symptomatic infection with *Giardia* should be treated with metronidazole. In children who cannot swallow pills, furazolidone, which is available in a liquid suspension of 50 mg/15 mL, is an acceptable alternative. Albendazole is also an effective treatment of *Giardia* in children; it can be formulated into a suspension and given to children ≥2 years old. The dose is 400 mg by mouth each day for 5 days.

Escherichia coli O157:H7 causes sporadic and epidemic gastrointestinal infections. In an estimated 15 percent of infected U.S. children, the hemolytic-uremic syndrome develops after the diarrhea. Data suggest that antibiotic treatment of children with *E. coli* O157:H7 in-fection increases the risk of the hemolytic-uremic syndrome.

BIBLIOGRAPHY

American Academy of Pediatrics, Subcommittee on Acute Gastroenteritis: Practice parameter: The management of acute gastroenteritis in young children. *Pediatrics* 97:424, 1996.

Cicirello HG, Glass RI: Current concepts of the epidemiology of diarrheal diseases. *Semin Pediatr Infect Dis* 5:163, 1994.

Duggan C, Nurko S: "Feeding the gut": The scientific basis for continued enteral nutrition during acute diarrhea. *J Pediatr* 131:801, 1997.

Figueroa-Quintanilla D, Salazar-Lindo E, Eyzaguirre-Maccan E, et al: A watery diarrheal disease. *N Engl J Med* 328:1653, 1993.

Garcia Pena BM, Mandl KD, Kraus SJ, et al: Ultrasonography and limited computed tomography in the diagnosis and management of appendicitis in children. *JAMA* 282:1041, 1999.

Guerrant RL, Bobak DA: Bacterial and protozoal gastroenteritis. *N Engl J Med* 325:327, 1991.

Kapikian AZ: Viral gastroenteritis. *JAMA* 269:627, 1993.

Pickering LK (ed): *American Academy of Pediatrics Report of the Committee on Infectious Diseases,* 25th ed. 2000, pp 198, 253, 502–503, 511.

Torrey S, Fleisher G, Jaffe D: Incidence of *Salmonella* bacteremia in infants with *Salmonella* gastroenteritis. *J Pediatr* 108:718, 1986.

Wong CS, Jelacic S, Tarr PI, et al: The risk of the hemolytic uremic syndrome after antibiotic treatment of *Escherichia coli* O157:H7 infections. *N Engl J Med* 342:1930, 2000.

52

Nonsurgical Gastrointestinal Problems

Tulika Singh
William R. Ahrens

HIGH-YIELD FACTS

- For children with abdominal pain, the physical examination is usually the most useful tool in determining the cause and the need for surgical intervention. Playful children are unlikely to suffer from surgical lesions: Those with peritoneal inflammation tend to lie still and those with obstructions are usually restless and uncomfortable.

- For children with vomiting or diarrhea, the history and physical examination findings will direct the need for diagnostic testing. In cases where a self-limited infectious process is likely and the patient is not clinically dehydrated, no laboratory studies are necessary.

- Stool cultures are indicated in the evaluation of febrile infants and children who have bloody stools and neonates who have white blood cells in the stool, where it is important to rule out *Salmonella*.

- The mainstay of treatment of constipation consists of dietary manipulation to increase fiber and bulk, decrease fat content, and increase total fluid intake. In neonates and young infants, additional feedings of water in between formula or breast feedings may be all that is needed.

- The most common causes of upper gastrointestinal bleeding in children are gastritis, esophagitis, ulcers, and esophageal varices. In newborns, vitamin K deficiency has been a common cause, but the use of prophylactic vitamin K has markedly reduced the incidence.

- In children, lower gastrointestinal bleeding is rarely life threatening. In the newborn,

swallowed maternal blood may be the cause, but vitamin K deficiency should also be ruled out. In premature infants, necrotizing enterocolitis may cause bleeding. In infants, anal fissures are the most common cause.

- *Colic* is an imprecise term used to describe multiple symptoms (including crying, fussing, and irritability) that occur episodically in infants between 1 and 4 months of age. Intolerance to milk protein is suspected to play a role in causing this syndrome.

- Gastroesophageal reflux (GER) is common in infants, and it too is suspected to be associated with cow's milk allergy. Use of more frequent feedings and thickening the formula with cereal are useful initial interventions.

- In the immediate neonatal period, unconjugated hyperbilirubinemia is of great concern due to the association with kernicterus, an irreversible neurologic disorder that occurs when unbound bilirubin is deposited in the brain.

As many as 10 percent of all pediatric visits to the emergency department result from complaints involving the gastrointestinal system. Traditionally, gastrointestinal problems have been considered to be either medical or surgical. This section will discuss gastrointestinal complaints in terms of presenting signs and symptoms and then focus on specific diseases. Because it is so common, a separate section is devoted to gastroenteritis.

ABDOMINAL PAIN

Approximately 20 percent of individuals will seek attention for abdominal pain sometime before adulthood. The majority of these patients will suffer from medical rather than surgical problems.

The evaluation of abdominal pain can be difficult in any patient and in children may be complicated by the patient's inability to describe the symptoms and adequately localize the complaint. The situation is further complicated by the inherently complex nature of abdominal pain.

Abdominal pain is classified as either visceral or somatic. Visceral pain is transmitted via unmyelinated nerve fibers of the sympathetic chain. It can result from distension of a hollow viscus or from an ischemic process. It can be severe and of sudden onset, with a colicky nature, and is often poorly localized. Somatic pain arises from myelinated nerve fibers arising from the parietal peritoneum. It is often of gradual onset, and more sharply localized than visceral pain. Abdominal pain can also be referred to areas of the body that share innervation through the same afferent neural segments. For example, pain resulting from a splenic rupture is commonly referred to the left shoulder, and diaphragmatic irritation from a lobar pneumonia often results in right-sided abdominal pain. Conversely, many systemic illnesses have prominent gastrointestinal manifestations. Diabetic ketoacidosis can cause abdominal pain and vomiting, while lead poisoning can cause vomiting and constipation (Table 52-1).

History

The evaluation of pediatric patients with abdominal pain begins with an attempt to elicit information that will categorize the etiology of the problem as surgical or medical. Patients and parents are questioned regarding the duration of the pain, its location, severity, and the character of the discomfort. Persistent, nonremitting pain of less than several hours' duration indicates a high likelihood of a surgical etiology, as does pain that is localized to a specific area. Pain that wakes patients from sleep almost always indicates organic pathology, which can be surgical or medical. Crampy or colicky pain usually results from the distension of a viscus. It is most commonly due to gastroenteritis, but can also be seen in surgical emergencies such as a bowel obstruction or intussusception. Sharp, localized pain often indicates peritoneal inflammation, as in appendicitis.

Associated symptoms are solicited in order to narrow the differential diagnosis. Patients are questioned about vomiting, with emphasis on gastric contents and the relation of vomiting to abdominal pain. Patients with diarrhea are asked about the frequency and character of stools, especially the presence of blood or mucus. All patients are asked if there is a history of fever. In older patients a history of dysuria is elicited; in younger children the caretaker is asked if the patient appears to be in pain when urinating. In older females a gynecologic history is taken, with emphasis on the date of the last menstrual period, sexual activity, and the presence of vaginal discharge or bleeding.

Patients with recurrent or chronic abdominal pain are particularly problematic. They are questioned regarding

Table 52-1. Nonsurgical Causes of Abdominal Pain

Age Under 2
   Gastroenteritis
   Colic
   Constipation
   Lead poisoning

Ages 2 to 12
   Psychosocial
   Enterocolitis
   Otitis media
   Constipation
   Child abuse
   Sickle cell disease
   Irritable bowel disease
   Chronic recurrent abdominal pain
   Urinary tract infection
   Henoch-Schönlein purpura
   Diabetic ketoacidosis
   Mesenteric adenitis
   Lead intoxication
   Streptococcal pharyngitis

Age Over 12
   Idiopathic
   Constipation
   Chronic recurrent abdominal pain
   Pregnancy
   Urinary tract infection
   Diabetic ketoacidosis
   Pelvic inflammatory disease
   Sickle cell disease
   Streptococcal pharyngitis
   Mesenteric adenitis
   Psychosocial

associated weight loss, fatigue, arthralgias, melena, or hemochezia, all of which indicate an inflammatory process. For patients in whom no organic etiology of abdominal pain appears likely, the possibility of a psychosomatic disorder exists. This has a wide range of underlying causes, including sexual abuse.

Physical Findings

In children, the physical examination is often the most useful tool in determining the cause of abdominal pain or at least in eliminating a surgical lesion. The examination begins with an assessment of the child's general appearance. Patients with peritoneal inflammation tend to lie still, whereas children with obstruction may be restless or writhe in pain. Playful children are unlikely to suffer from surgical conditions. The examination of the abdomen includes assessment of bowel sounds, tenderness, guarding, rebound, and distension. The size of the liver and spleen are also noted. Especially in toddlers, the examination can be difficult, but is often facilitated by having parents hold children on their laps. While this is less than optimal, it allows for a basic assessment that can at least help exclude an acute surgical emergency.

If there is a history of gastrointestinal bleeding or a surgical emergency is suspected, a rectal examination is indicated and the stool is checked for occult blood. In addition, all pediatric patients with abdominal pain require a genital examination to rule out an incarcerated inguinal hernia as the etiology of the pain.

Diagnostic Testing

Ancillary laboratory tests are generally most helpful in supporting the clinical impression derived from the history and physical examination. In many cases no studies are indicated. In younger children, however, in whom the history and physical examination are less reliable, laboratory studies can help determine the etiology of the problem. An elevated leukocyte count indicates an inflammatory or infectious process. A urinalysis is helpful in excluding a urinary tract infection; it is important that whenever possible a catheterized specimen be obtained. If hepatitis or pancreatitis is suspected, liver function tests and pancreatic enzymes may be helpful. Obtaining electrolytes, serum blood urea nitrogen (BUN), and creatinine is indicated for patients with suspected dehydration. For patients with diarrhea accompanying abdominal pain, a microscopic stool examination revealing red or white blood cells indicates an inflammatory process usually secondary to infectious enteritis.

Abdominal radiographs can be helpful in cases of suspected bowel obstruction. Other diagnostic modalities are discussed as they apply to specific diseases.

VOMITING

Vomiting can be caused by a number of problems in diverse organ systems. Although it most commonly results from a self-limited infectious illness, it may be secondary to serious systemic, metabolic, or central nervous system disorders. In general, the most important aspect of caring for patients with vomiting is to exclude a surgical emergency.

History

The history begins with distinguishing true vomiting from gastric regurgitation, which is common in neonates and infants. In true vomiting, patients expel most of the stomach contents. The circumstances under which the vomiting occurs and its character are important. Postprandial emesis is common for patients with acute gastroenteritis, but can also indicate a bowel obstruction. Posttussive emesis is common in conditions such as asthma and pertussis. The presence of bile in the emesis is never "normal" and always suggests the possibility of an obstructive lesion, especially in infants, where it may signify a malrotation. The appearance of blood in the emesis can indicate a gastrointestinal hemorrhage, although true blood must always be distinguished from substances with which it is easily confused. Patients and parents are questioned regarding associated gastrointestinal symptoms such as nausea, diarrhea, or constipation. Associated abdominal pain is especially worrisome if it is present in between episodes of vomiting. Other constitutional symptoms to solicit include fever, dysuria, flank pain, and, in females, gynecologic complaints. The association of headache with vomiting always raises the index of suspicion for intracranial pathology.

Physical Findings

The physical examination of patients with vomiting is similar to that of patients with abdominal pain. Nongastrointestinal causes of vomiting are excluded, with particular attention paid to the central nervous system. Lethargy, papilledema, and, in infants, splitting of the sutures or a full anterior fontanel indicate increased intracranial pressure. The abdomen is assessed for the presence of distension, the character of the bowel sounds is evaluated, and the presence of tenderness, guarding, or rebound is noted. For patients in whom a surgical problem is not considered likely and in whom there is no evidence of gastrointestinal hemorrhage, a rectal exam is probably not helpful. If, however, a surgical abdomen is considered, a rectal examination is indicated.

Diagnostic Testing

The history and physical examination direct the laboratory evaluation of individual patients. In cases where a self-limited infectious process is likely and patients do not appear dehydrated, no laboratory studies are necessary. For patients in whom a surgical process is possible, a complete blood cell count is indicated. A urinalysis is used to evaluate the possibility of a urinary tract infection, a common cause of vomiting that is notoriously difficult to diagnose clinically. The urine-specific gravity is useful as an indication of the status of the patient's hydration. For patients who appear dehydrated, serum electrolytes, creatinine, and BUN are indicated. For patients with suspected liver disease, a hepatic profile is helpful. Abdominal radiographs are only indicated in cases where bowel obstruction is suspected. Other diagnostic modalities are discussed with specific disease entities.

Management

The treatment of patients with vomiting is also discussed in the sections dealing with specific diseases.

DIARRHEA

As an acute episode, diarrhea with or without vomiting occurs more than 1 billion times per year throughout the world. It is a significant problem for many children presenting to an emergency department, accounting for up to 20 percent of all pediatric outpatient visits, and up to 8 percent of all pediatric hospital admissions. The vast majority of patients with diarrhea are suffering from mild, self-limited infectious illness. However, diarrheal diseases remain a major cause of morbidity and mortality throughout the world.

History

Diarrhea is characterized by an increase in the frequency and a decrease in the consistency of patients' stools. This can range from a slight increase in the number of stools per day to a fulminant loss of water and electrolytes through the gastrointestinal tract. It is important to distinguish between previously normal patients with acute diarrhea and patients with gastrointestinal illness that can result in chronic constipation and overflow diarrhea, such as Hirschsprung's disease or cystic fibrosis (Chap. 53).

For patients with diarrhea, further information is obtained regarding the stool's consistency and color and whether the stool contains blood. The presence of blood usually indicates an infectious etiology, which in children is often due to bacterial enteritis. However, life-threatening events can also cause bloody diarrhea. These include intussusception and the hemolytic uremic syndrome. For patients previously treated with antibiotics, pseudomembranous colitis is a consideration. Severe inflammatory bowel disease can also cause bloody diarrhea and can result in life-threatening toxic megacolon. In young infants, salmonella gastroenteritis can cause bloody diarrhea and is considered a serious infection (Chap. 51).

Patients are questioned regarding associated vomiting, abdominal pain, dysuria, and fever. In young infants, a careful feeding history is obtained. Overfeeding can cause diarrhea, as can formula intolerance. True formula allergy can cause bloody diarrhea, but is not life threatening.

Physical Findings

The physical examination of patients with diarrhea focuses on determining the etiology of the problem and assessing the hydration status of patients. The presence of fever implies an infectious etiology. The tympanic membranes are evaluated for the presence of otitis media, which can be associated with diarrhea. The chest is examined to exclude pneumonia. The abdominal examination focuses on excluding a surgical emergency. The character of the bowel sounds, as well as the presence of tenderness, guarding, rebound, or organomegaly, is noted. In the presence of bloody diarrhea, an abdominal mass indicates a high probability of an intussusception. If there is any history of bloody diarrhea, patients appear ill, or patients are <2 to 3 months old with fever and diarrhea, a rectal examination is indicated and the stool is examined for the presence of red and white blood cells.

Diagnostic Testing

For patients with mild, nonbloody diarrhea who do not appear dehydrated, no laboratory work-up is indicated. A urinalysis or urine culture may reveal an underlying urinary tract infection, which can have diarrhea as its sole manifestation. In febrile patients with bloody diarrhea, a stool specimen is sent for bacterial culture and evaluation for ova and parasites. Neonates with stools positive for white blood cells also have stool cultures performed to rule out *Salmonella.* For patients with bloody diarrhea who are not febrile, a life-threatening process such as intussusception or hemolytic uremic syndrome is excluded. For patients who have been treated with antibiotics, stool is sent for assay for *Clostridium difficile* toxin.

CONSTIPATION

Constipation is a decrease in the frequency of stooling, often associated with a change in the character of the stool. It is a frequent presenting complaint in the pediatric population, especially in neonates with inexperienced parents. There are few life-threatening diagnostic possibilities in pediatric patients with constipation. However, the frequency of the complaint and its association with a few serious diseases mandates that the emergency physician become familiar with its assessment and management.

History

A detailed history is important to differentiate true from perceived constipation. Subjective associated symptoms, such as grunting, straining, or turning red during defecation, are normal, though often considered indicative of constipation. Crying during defecation is disturbing to parents, but also does not mean that babies are constipated. Infants may have a small anal fissure causing pain, but normal consistency of the stool. Rather, it is a deviation from established bowel habits in which stool frequency decreases or consistency changes that indicates constipation. Especially in neonates, it is important to establish the pattern of stooling from birth, since delayed passage of meconium in the first 24 to 48 hours is associated with organic pathology, especially Hirschsprung's disease. In infants, a feeding history is important, since a formula change may be associated with a change in bowel habits. It is also important to establish normal growth and development in infants with constipation, since organic causes of constipation can be associated with failure to thrive. In toddlers and older children, a history of toilet training is elicited, since difficulties in making the transition from diapers can result in psychogenic constipation. Soliciting a history of fecal incontinence, or encopresis, is also important. Associated symptoms to elicit include lethargy, poor feeding, fever, and vomiting. It is axiomatic that these do not result from functional constipation.

Physical Findings

The physical examination of constipated patients focuses on differentiating systemic etiology from an obstruction of the gastrointestinal tract. The general appearance of patients is noted in terms of neurologic status and growth and development. Infants are evaluated for the stigmata of hypothyroidism or the cranial nerve palsies of infantile botulism, both of which can cause constipation. The abdomen is evaluated for the presence of bowel sounds and distension. True constipation may cause mild abdominal fullness, but significant distension

is abnormal. The abdomen is palpated in an attempt to elicit tenderness, which is occasionally present in the left lower quadrant. Constipation should never cause peritoneal findings. A digital rectal examination is performed, along with an occult blood test. Presence of impacted stool in the rectal vault suggests true constipation. Absence of stool in the rectal vault suggests proximal pathology, especially Hirschsprung's disease.

Diagnostic Testing

If there is any abnormality noted on the physical examination or the history is suggestive of a surgical emergency, an abdominal radiograph is indicated to rule out a bowel obstruction or severe colonic dilatation.

Management

The mainstay of treatment of constipation consists of dietary manipulation to increase fiber and bulk, decrease fat content, and increase total fluid intake. In neonates and young infants, additional feedings of water in between formula or breast-feeding may be all that is necessary to break the cycle. A temporary change to a formula low in iron or without iron can result in improvement. Parents are encouraged to provide beans, celery, bran, and other high fiber items to children old enough to have solid foods. Juices made naturally from fruits and vegetables are probably helpful. In some cases, cow's milk may be a contributing factor and a trial of lactose-free milk can be beneficial.

Stool softeners, such as docusate and senna, are generally considered safe for children and may be useful until bowel habits have been reregulated. However, their use does not supersede dietary manipulation. Although not considered a routine treatment, a one-time insertion of a glycerin suppository may be belpful in stimulating a bowel movement in acutely constipated patients.

In severely impacted patients, disimpaction is necessary before initiation of maintenance therapy. It may be accomplished with either oral or rectal medication. Disimpaction with oral medication has been shown to be highly effective when high doses of mineral oil, polyethylene glycol electrolyte solutions, or both are used. Laxatives such as high-dose magnesium citrate, lactulose, sorbitol, senna, or bisacodyl can also be used. Rectal disimpaction may be performed with phosphate soda enemas, saline enemas, or mineral oil enemas followed by a phosphate enema. The use of soap suds, tap water, and magnesium enemas are not recommended because of their potential toxicity. Rectal disimpaction has also been effectively performed with glycerin suppositories in infants and bisacodyl suppositories in older children. Phosphate enemas are not indicated in children <2 years of age or for patients with conditions predisposing them to alteration in absorption and excretion of phosphate, including Hirschsprung's disease, imperforate anus, chronic renal failure, or renal dysplasia. Recurrent use of these products is not recommended.

The management of patients with chronic or recurrent constipation is a problem that is beyond the scope of the emergency physician. These patients are referred to a pediatric gastroenterologist or pediatrician for definitive long-term care.

GASTROINTESTINAL BLEEDING

When compared to the adult population, life-threatening gastrointestinal bleeding in children is uncommon, reflecting the relative infrequency of cirrhosis of the liver and gastrointestinal malignancies in the pediatric age group. However, gastrointestinal bleeding does occur in infants and children. On occasion, it is a manifestation of a life-threatening process.

For the purposes of evaluation and management, gastrointestinal hemorrhage is divided into the categories of upper and lower. Upper gastrointestinal hemorrhages occur proximal to the ligament of Treitz. Lower gastrointestinal hemorrhages occur distal to the ligament of Treitz, most commonly in the colon.

Presentation

Gastrointestinal bleeding can present dramatically, as acute hemorrhage that threatens patients with hemodynamic instability, or as a subtle, chronic process that results in the symptoms of chronic anemia. Hematemesis, or the vomiting of blood, is almost always a manifestation of an upper gastrointestinal hemorrhage. The blood may be bright red or, if digested by gastric acid, have a coffee-ground appearance. The color of the blood is not indicative of the severity of the hemorrhage, and it is important to note that 20 to 40 percent of patients with upper gastrointestinal bleeding do not have hematemesis. Melena refers to the passage of dark, sticky, sweet-smelling stools. While it is difficult to quantitate the rate of blood loss for patients with melena, this condition is usually associated with a loss of at least 2 percent of blood volume. Melena usually results from an upper gastrointestinal hemorrhage. Hemochezia is the passage of bright red blood from the rectum. This usually in-

volves a hemorrhagic process in the lower gastrointestinal tract, especially the colon, but can occur in cases of massive upper gastrointestinal bleeding. In cases of severe hemorrhage hemochezia may appear as pure blood, which can occur in an ulcerated Meckel's diverticulum or avulsed juvenile colonic polyp. More commonly, blood is either mixed with the stool, which usually indicates an infectious or inflammatory process, or is noted as streaks on the outside of the stool, which is commonly seen in lesions of the anus, such as traumatic fissures.

Upper Gastrointestinal Hemorrhage

Etiology

The most common causes of upper gastrointestinal bleeding in the pediatric patient population are gastritis, esophagitis, duodenal ulcers, and esophageal varices. In newborns, vitamin K deficiency is a common cause of upper gastrointestinal bleeding.

Gastritis

Gastritis in pediatric patients is often associated with severe physiologic stress, such as trauma, burns, and sepsis. These situations are associated with alteration of the normal buffering capacity of the gastric mucosa, leading to erosion and bleeding. The use of aspirin can also cause gastritis. Abdominal pain is a common presenting complaint, and vomiting can occur. In severe cases, hematemesis or melena can develop, though life-threatening hemorrhage is uncommon. The primary treatment consists of antacids and H_2 blockers.

Ulcer Disease

Peptic ulcer disease in children has somewhat similar manifestations to that in adults. Up to 70 percent of children with ulcers have a family history of the disease. While infection with *Helicobacter pylori* is rare in children in the United States, it is often associated with gastritis and duodenal ulcers in affected pediatric patients. Noninvasive tests such as *H. pylori* antigen immunoassay in the stool and the C-urea breath test (UBT) are becoming more widely available. Serologic methods are unreliable in young children and have been disappointing with respect to the diagnosis of acute infection and control of therapy success after treatment. The immunologic antibody reaction remains positive for months after successful eradication therapy or spontaneous elimination of the germ. Treatment includes 7 to 14 days of a twice-daily triple-drug regimen with omeprazole, clarithromycin, and amoxicillin.

Older children are likely to have abdominal pain, with or without associated vomiting, and nighttime wakening. Preschool children often suffer gastrointestinal bleeding, obstruction, or perforation. Of these, bleeding is the most common symptom. Patients can suffer from chronic low-grade bleeding, which results in iron deficiency anemia, or they can develop life-threatening hemorrhage, which presents as hemochezia or melena. Stress ulcers are common in pediatric patients with serious illness, such as sepsis, or after major trauma or extensive burns.

Patients with known chronic ulcer disease are managed with antacids and H_2 blocking agents, such as cimetidine and ranitidine. If endoscopy shows an acutely bleeding ulcer, aggressive treatment with antacids to keep the stomach pH >4.5 is indicated. Sucralfate is a topical agent used to coat ulcers and may be useful.

Esophageal and Gastric Varices

Esophageal and gastric varices are associated with intrahepatic and extrahepatic portal venous obstruction, which leads to portal vein hypertension. Extrahepatic portal vein obstruction is usually secondary to catheterization of the umbilical vein or inflammatory omphalitis in the neonatal period. Intrahepatic obstruction is most commonly due to cirrhosis secondary to biliary atresia, which is the most common cause of variceal bleeding in children. Other causes of cirrhosis are neonatal hepatitis, congenital hepatic fibrosis, and cystic fibrosis. Two-thirds of pediatric patients with portal hypertension hemorrhage before 5 years of age. In rare cases, bleeding varices are the presenting manifestation of underlying portal hypertension. They are the most common cause of life-threatening upper gastrointestinal hemorrhage in children. The management of variceal-related bleeding is discussed later.

Newborns

In newborns, vitamin K deficiency can result in gastrointestinal hemorrhage. However, this problem has been largely eliminated by the use of prophylactic vitamin K. In some cases, gastrointestinal hemorrhage occurs for which no cause is found and which usually ceases within 24 hours. Maternal blood may be swallowed and confused with gastrointestinal bleeding in newborns. The origin of the blood can be determined by adding sodium hydroxide to the specimen (the Apt test).

Newborns' blood will remain pink, since fetal hemoglobin resists alkalinization, while maternal blood with adult hemoglobin will turn brown.

Management

In all patients with upper gastrointestinal hemorrhage, it is essential that the hemodynamic status of patients is aggressively assessed and managed. The evaluation and management of hypovolemic shock is covered elsewhere. Briefly, all patients with signs of hemodynamic instability manifested by unstable vital signs, pallor, poor capillary refill, altered mental status, or ongoing blood loss require adequate intravenous access and resuscitation with crystalloid solution. Fluid is administered until hemodynamic stability is restored. Blood is sent for an urgent type and cross-match for packed red blood cells and, if liver disease is present, fresh frozen plasma.

Stable patients with a history of hematemesis are evaluated for the possibility of a nongastrointestinal source of bleeding. Common sites are the nose and gums. Occasionally, a severe pharyngitis can produce blood-tinged sputum that is mistaken for hematemesis. Swallowed blood from epistaxis is also a common cause of hematemesis. All patients are evaluated for the stigmata of chronic liver disease, especially jaundice and hepatosplenomegaly. The skin is examined for signs of bleeding diathesis, such as petechiae or purpura.

Laboratory studies include a complete blood cell count, electrolyte levels, and renal functions. A coagulation profile is indicated in all cases of significant hematemesis. Liver function tests are indicated if hepatic insufficiency is suspected.

Placement of a nasogastric tube is indicated in all patients with a history of hematemesis or an examination that reveals melena. Gastric contents are evaluated for bright red blood or coffee-ground material, the presence of which confirms an upper gastrointestinal hemorrhage. A negative nasogastric aspirate does not conclusively rule out hemorrhage, since up to 16 percent of patients with clear drainage have active bleeding. Thus, patients' overall status is important, especially if there is objective evidence of blood loss or obvious melena. The known or suspected presence of varices is not a contraindication to the insertion of a nasogastric tube.

If the nasogastric aspirate reveals active bleeding, gastric lavage is indicated. The most effective composition of the lavage fluid is controversial. At present, free water appears to be as safe as normal saline, and fears about inducing water intoxication exaggerated. The temperature of the water does not appear to influence the outcome. In addition to confirming the presence of an upper gastrointestinal hemorrhage and bleeding stoppage, nasogastric lavage also clears the stomach of blood, which, in the presence of liver failure, can lead to hyperammonemia and possibly aggravated hepatic encephalopathy. It may also facilitate endoscopy.

In the vast majority of cases of upper gastrointestinal hemorrhage due to gastritis, esophagitis, and ulcer disease, lavage will result in cessation or significant slowing of the bleeding. In hemorrhage that results from bleeding varices, bleeding can be brisk and refractory to lavage. In persistent hemorrhage due to esophageal varices, vasopressin in a dose of 0.1 to 0.4 U/min may control the bleeding. Vasopressin is a hormone that causes systemic vasoconstriction, reduces splenic blood flow, and reduces portal pressure. Possible side effects include ischemia of the extremities or viscera. Somostatin is a hypothalamic extract that decreases splenic flow and may be more effective than vasopressin in controlling variceal hemorrhage. Experience in children is limited.

Variceal bleeding refractory to gastric lavage and vasopressin can be controlled by the insertion of a Sengstaken-Blakemore tube into the stomach and esophagus. This instrument has balloons that can be inflated in the proximal stomach and distal esophagus and can tamponade the bleeding. Depending on the site of hemorrhage, the esophageal component, gastric component, or both may need to be inflated. Accurate placement of the tube is confirmed radiographically. Inflation is usually maintained for >12 hours.

If a gastroenterologist is available, injection of a sclerosing agent into the varices is useful for stopping an acute hemorrhage and preventing rebleeding. If this procedure is available, it may be preferable to inserting a Sengstaken-Blakemore tube.

It is vital for all patients with upper gastrointestinal bleeding to be referred for endoscopy. Even for patients with known varices, a significant number of patients will be bleeding from concomitant gastritis or ulcers. When performed within 24 hours of the onset of bleeding, endoscopy can identify the lesion 90 percent of the time and is therefore superior to barium studies.

Lower Gastrointestinal Bleeding

Lower gastrointestinal bleeding in infants and children differs considerably from that in adults. Malignancies of the colon and diverticulitis are virtually nonexistent in children, which fundamentally alters the approach to both the long-term outlook and acute management. In children, lower gastrointestinal bleeding is rarely life threatening, although on occasion it signifies a serious disease process. Currently, it is possible to identify the etiology in 90 percent of children with lower gastrointestinal hemorrhage.

Etiology

A wide range of entities can result in the passage of blood in the stool. It is useful to approach the problem from an age-group–related perspective. A primary focus of forming the differential diagnosis is excluding surgical causes of gastrointestinal hemorrhage, which are uncommon but are always life threatening. They are discussed in the section on surgical emergencies.

Newborns

Rectal bleeding in the newborn is uncommon. In the immediate neonatal period, it is possible for swallowed maternal blood to be confused with that of the baby's. If a bright red specimen is obtained the two can be distinguished by the addition of sodium hydroxide, which alters the color of the maternal blood, but not that of the newborn's.

Necrotizing Enterocolitis

Necrotizing enterocolitis is an inflammatory condition of the bowel usually associated with significant prematurity. However, up to 10 percent of cases occur in fullterm infants, usually within the first 10 days of life. It is a condition associated with significant morbidity and mortality. Early symptoms include lethargy, poor feeding, temperature instability, and apnea. Abdominal distension can develop and, as the disease progresses, either heme-positive or grossly bloody stools are seen. Physical examination usually reveals an ill-appearing infant with or without abdominal tenderness. The work-up includes a complete blood cell count, serum electrolyte levels, and cultures of the blood, urine, and spinal fluid. Abdominal radiographs may reveal air in the bowel wall (pneumatosis intestinalis). Patients have nothing by mouth, and broad-spectrum antibiotic coverage is initiated. Surgical consultation is indicated. It is discussed further in the section on surgical emergencies.

Coagulopathy

Coagulopathy in newborns is almost always due to vitamin K deficiency, although thrombocytopenia may occasionally occur. In either case, infants may have manifestations of coagulopathy other than bleeding, such as ecchymosis or petechia. Vitamin K–induced coagulopathy has become less common since the advent of prophylactic administration at birth. However, any newborns with significant gastrointestinal bleeding should receive supplemental Vitamin K.

Surgical causes of lower gastrointestinal bleeding in newborns include Hirschsprung's disease and malrotation with volvulus. Both are discussed in Chapter 53.

Infants (1 Month to 2 Years of Age)

Anal Fissures

Anal fissures are the most common cause of rectal bleeding in infancy. Up to 17 percent of rectal bleeding in children is caused by rectal fissures, most often in patients <1 year of age. Patients usually have blood-streaked stools. Infants may also appear to have pain with bowel movements. Occasionally, a rectal fissure can cause pain on defecation severe enough to result in constipation. The fissure is often visible on inspection of the anus. In some cases, an internal fissure can be diagnosed by inserting a small test tube into the anus, which facilitates visualization of the internal anal ring. A severe fissure or rectal tear always raises the question of sexual abuse. The treatment is usually with stool softeners and sitz baths.

Formula Intolerance or Allergy

Formula intolerance can result from a true allergy to cow's milk protein that results in a systemic response to an enterically administered antigen. Up to 8 percent of babies are susceptible. The presentation varies from chronic diarrhea and failure to thrive to grossly bloody stools indicative of severe colitis. Vomiting can also occur and can at times be bloody. Nongastrointestinal symptoms such as eczematous skin reaction or wheezing can occur. Up to 20 to 30 percent of patients intolerant to cow's milk are also intolerant to soy-based formulas.

There is no diagnostic laboratory test, though colonoscopy may be useful. Infants with formula-induced enterocolitis can have fever, elevated white blood cell counts, and fecal leukocytes, which may mimic an acute infectious problem. Eosinophilia in both peripheral blood as well as in stool smears (Wright's stain) is highly suggestive of allergic gastroenteritis. Stool cultures will eliminate bacterial enteritis.

Symptoms resolve within 48 hours after withdrawal of the formula and recur if the formula is reintroduced.

Infants with milk- or soy-induced colitis are treated with an elemental formula, such as nutramagen or pregestamil.

Infectious Colitis

Infectious colitis is a common cause of lower gastrointestinal bleeding worldwide. It can appear from early infancy through adulthood. Certain bacterial organisms are strongly linked to bloody diarrhea, although viruses can also cause heme-positive stools. Infectious colitis usually presents with vomiting and diarrhea. Patients are often febrile. Older children may complain of colicky abdominal pain, but the abdomen is usually nontender on examination. Microscopic examination of the stools usually reveals red blood cells and polymorphonuclear leukocytes. The subject of infectious colitis is covered extensively in the section on gastroenteritis.

Lymphonodular Hyperplasia

Lymphonodular hyperplasia is a benign disorder seen in infants and preschoolers. It can be associated with bright red rectal bleeding, which is rarely severe. Diagnosis is made by sigmoidoscopy or air-contrast radiography. There is no treatment, and the disorder usually resolves within 3 months of onset.

Meckel's Diverticulum

Meckel's diverticulum is the result of incomplete obliteration of the omphalomesenteric duct, usually located within 10 cm of the ileocecal valve. The condition can result in massive, painless rectal bleeding, obstruction, perforation, and peritonitis or may remain totally silent. Rectal bleeding results from acid secreted by ectopic gastric tissue that causes ulceration and erosion of tissue. Sixty percent of complications from Meckel's diverticulum, including hemorrhage and obstruction, occur in patients <2 years of age. The diverticulum is confirmed by performing a technetium-99m scan that identifies ectopic gastric tissue. When symptomatic, the diverticulum is removed surgically.

Intussusception, malrotation, and Hirschsprung's disease are other surgical causes of rectal bleeding (Chap. 53).

Preschool (2 to 5 Years of Age)

In the preschool age group, lower gastrointestinal bleeding can result from a focal lesion of the gastrointestinal tract or result from an infectious or systemic process. Meckel's diverticulum can also present in this age group.

Juvenile Polyps

In preschoolers with painless rectal bleeding, a juvenile polyp is a likely possibility. Juvenile polyps account for 90 percent of all polyps found in children. They are found primarily in children <8 years old, with a peak at 3 to 4 years. They have no malignant potential. Rectal bleeding is usually minor, but in some cases can be severe. Diagnosis is made by colonoscopy, and treatment consists of polypectomy.

Hematochezia can also be a manifestation of systemic diseases such as hemolytic uremic syndrome and Henoch-Schonlein purpura.

School Age (Over 5 Years of Age)

In children >5 years of age, lower gastrointestinal bleeding is most commonly the result of an infectious diarrhea. Juvenile polyps can also cause bleeding, although they are more likely to present in younger children. In older children, major considerations are the inflammatory bowel diseases, ulcerative colitis and Crohn's disease. Due to the predilection of both to cause toxic megacolon, they are covered in Chapter 53.

COLIC

Colic is an imprecise term used to describe a combination of symptoms that occur in infants between the ages of 1 and 4 months. Symptoms include episodes of excessive crying, fussiness after feeding, and paroxysms of irritability. Colic has been reported to affect between 16 to 30 percent of infants. The severity of symptoms varies greatly from patient to patient and may be relieved by the passage of stool or gas. Episodes of colic often occur in the evening and can last several hours, resulting in extremely frustrated or worried parents and an emergency department visit.

In many cases, persistent crying is the only manifestation of colic. Infants appear well and are afebrile. It is important to exclude serious manifestations of inconsolable crying before making the diagnosis of colic. These include sepsis, meningitis, entrapment of the penis or a digit by a hair, occult fracture, incarcerated hernia, or corneal abrasion.

Though the etiology of colic is unknown, studies highlight the importance of intolerance to milk protein as the cause. These studies report that 20 to 40 percent of infants with colic respond to a milk-exclusion diet and show other features of cow's milk protein intolerance when challenged 3 to 6 months after initial diagnosis. Infants may benefit from a change in formula. For persistent problems, simethicone (Mylicon), an inert chemical that reduces intestinal gas, may provide some relief. Sedatives and anticholinergic medications are not indicated.

SPECIFIC DISEASE ENTITIES

Gastroesophageal Reflux

Gastroesophageal reflux refers to the regurgitation of stomach contents into the esophagus. It is a common condition, with an incidence estimated at 18 percent in the infant population. While it is a multifactorial disorder, the increased frequency in infants <4 months of age suggests developmental immaturity of the lower esophageal sphincter. Although complications may occur, most infants and children have physiologic reflux with no clinical consequences. Distal esophagitis is by far the most common complication. Severe GER can result in failure to thrive, esophageal strictures, Barrett's esophagus, gastrointestinal bleeding, recurrent aspiration pneumonia, reactive airway disease, and iron deficiency anemia.

Parents frequently seek medical attention because infants "spit up" after feedings. The regurgitated contents are not bile stained, but they often contain partially digested formula and, in severe cases, can be bloody. In the emergency department, it is important to distinguish reflux from true vomiting, which in infants can result from an obstructive lesion such as a volvulus or pyloric stenosis.

In the majority of cases, an extensive work-up is not indicated. Infants with refractory regurgitation or those with associated symptoms require more extensive evaluation. Studies performed vary among centers, but include barium swallow, esophageal pH monitoring, endoscopy, and scintiscanning with a ^{99}Tc-sulfur-colloid–labeled meal.

Studies have found an association between GER and cow's milk allergy, as well as resolution of symptoms of persistent GER and eosinophilic esophagitis within weeks of the start of feeding with amino-acid–based formulas.

In cases of milk-tolerant GER, feeding smaller amounts at more frequent intervals and thickening the formula with cereal may improve symptoms. Parents are encouraged to "burp" babies frequently during feeding. Placing infants in the prone position at 45° to 60° after feeding may help more severe regurgitation. Medical management includes histamine-blocking agents such as ranitidine (Zantac), which reduces gastric acid secretion; bethanechol, which increases gastric motility; and metoclopramide, which increases tone in the lower esophageal sphincter and relaxes pyloric sphincter tone. In older children, symptomatic management includes antacids and sucralfate. There is some evidence that high-osmolality formula may worsen reflux.

Patients who do not respond to medical management may require surgical intervention, most commonly a Nissan fundoplication, in which the body of the stomach is wrapped around and sutured in front of the esophagus.

Gallbladder Disease

Diseases of the gallbladder are rare in children because gallstones are extremely uncommon before puberty. However, certain disorders can predispose children to gallstones and cholecystitis. Hemolytic anemias, especially sickle cell disease and the thallasemias predispose patients to the formation of pigmented stones. Patients with cystic fibrosis also have a relatively high incidence of gallstones, as do patients with ileal Crohn's disease.

Cholelithiasis in children has a similar presentation to that of adults. Intermittent, colicky right upper quadrant pain that may radiate to the scapula is characteristic. Vomiting may occur. The presence of nonremitting pain accompanied by fever and leukocytosis indicates cholecystitis. Ultrasonography will demonstrate stones and can define the anatomy of the gallbladder wall and the width of the common bile duct. For patients with cholecystitis, antibiotic therapy and surgical consultation are indicated.

Certain illnesses in children are associated with non-calculous distension of the gallbladder, known as hydrops. These include leptospirosis, scarlet fever, and Kawasaki's disease. Patients are often jaundiced and complain of right upper quadrant pain. The gallbladder can be massively distended, and there may be a right upper quadrant mass. In most cases, management is expectant, but on occasion cholecystectomy is necessary.

Pancreatitis

Pancreatitis results when an inflammatory process causes a cascade of events that eventually lead to autodigestion of the pancreatic tissue by various pancreatic enzymes, including lipase, amylase, elastase, and phospholipase.

It is uncommon in children, especially before the age of 10 years.

Blunt abdominal trauma is a relatively frequent cause of pancreatitis in children. In some cases the injury may appear relatively trivial; it can also result from child abuse. Viral illnesses, especially mumps, can cause pancreatitis, as can a multitude of drugs. It is also associated with congenital anomalies of the biliary tree and infrequently with gallstones that obstruct the pancreatic duct.

Pancreatitis causes epigastric pain that may radiate to the back. In many cases the onset of pain is gradual. Vomiting is usually present. Patients with severe disease or who develop hemorrhagic pancreatitis may be hypotensive. The abdominal exam may reveal tenderness in the epigastrium, but the severity of the patient's pain may be out of proportion to the abdominal findings. Affected children tend to lie still, with their hips slightly flexed. Bluish discoloration around the umbilicus (Cullen's sign) or flank (Grey Turner's sign) imply severe disease. Low-grade fever is present in 50 to 60 percent of cases, but high fever is uncommon. In severe cases, mental status changes can occur.

The laboratory work-up includes measurement of liver function tests, a complete blood cell count, and electrolyte, BUN, creatinine, glucose, and calcium levels. The quantitative amylase level is useful as a screening for pancreatic disease but does not correlate with the severity of illness and can be elevated in other diseases, including diabetic ketoacidosis and pelvic inflammatory disease. Somewhat more specific is an elevation in the amylase:creatinine clearance ratio. Serum lipase level may also be elevated. An abdominal radiograph may show a sentinel loop sign or localized ileus. An ultrasound evaluation of the pancreas or a computed tomography of the abdomen may be useful.

Most pediatric patients with pancreatitis recover. Therapy consists of fluid resuscitation and maintenance of serum electrolyte level. Nasogastric suction may help to diminish pain. Analgesics are usually necessary for pain relief. Meperidine is the drug of choice; morphine or codeine should not be used because they increase spasm at the sphincter of Oddi. Complications include the formation of a pancreatic abscess or pseudocyst and the development of pleural effusion.

Hepatitis

Hepatitis is a common viral infection with clinical manifestations that range from asymptomatic infection to fulminant liver failure. Several distinct viral etiologic agents have been identified and are currently labeled hepatitis A, B, C, D, and E. Of these, hepatitis B is the most problematic.

The hepatitis A virus is a ribonucleic acid virus of the picornavirus group. Transmission in humans is usually via contact with infected fecal material. This is particularly problematic for children who attend day care or are institutionalized. The incubation period is usually 2 to 4 weeks.

Hepatitis A infection in children is usually mild and self-limited, although occasionally severe infection can occur. In young children the illness is frequently asymptomatic and is usually not associated with jaundice. Symptomatic patients usually suffer an acute febrile illness characterized by nausea, anorexia, and fatigability. There may or may not be icterus or jaundice apparent on physical examination. If present, it generally does not appear until several weeks after exposure.

Laboratory findings include elevation in serum transaminase levels that reflect liver injury. Both conjugated and unconjugated fractions of bilirubin are elevated. IgM antibody to hepatitis A is usually detectable 6 to 8 weeks after the illness. IgG develops later and persists for years.

Treatment of hepatitis A is supportive. Hospitalization is indicated for patients who are unable to tolerate oral nutrition. Serum immune globulin treatment is indicated in household contacts of affected patients to prevent the spread of clinical hepatitis. Families are encouraged to promote good hand-washing and stool precautions during the course of the illness. Hepatitis A in pregnant patients does not infect the fetus. There is no carrier state in hepatitis A. There is now a vaccine available against hepatitis A, especially recommended for travelers to endemic countries.

Hepatitis B virus (HBV) is a deoxyribonucleic acid virus with multiple components, including the surface antigen (HbsAg), the core antigen (HbcAg), and the hepatitis B e antigen (HbeAg). It is transmitted through body secretions such as semen, cervical secretions, saliva, and exudative wound secretions. It can also be transmitted by infected blood or blood products, where even a minute quantity of infected blood can produce active infection. Hepatitis B virus can be transmitted from an infected mother to the newborn, perhaps at delivery. About 90 percent of infected newborns become chronic carriers of the infection. The incubation period of HBV is 2 to 5 months. Rarely, HBV results in severe, fulminant hepatitis.

In many patients, especially infants and young children, infection with HBV is asymptomatic. Symptomatic infection produces nausea, vomiting, and malaise.

It may also cause extrahepatic symptoms such as arthralgia and arthritis and can result in a papular acrodermatitis on the face, buttocks, and extensor surfaces of the arms and legs. Some patients can develop immune-mediated glomerulonephritis. Hepatomegaly or splenomegaly may be present. By the time jaundice appears, children will probably be afebrile. The classic description of clay-colored stools may not be present in children.

Laboratory findings reveal elevated serum transaminase levels and both conjugated and unconjugated bilirubin values. Testing for the HBV is through a series of serum tests for antigen and antibody detection.

Treatment of HBV infection is supportive. Hospital admission is indicated for patients in whom nausea and vomiting preclude adequate hydration and nutrition and for the rare patient with fulminant hepatitis.

Infection with HBV is now preventable due to the development of a highly effective synthetic vaccine. Passive immunization is possible with hepatitis B immune globulin (HBIG).

Previously described non-A non-B hepatitis is now identified as two separate etiologic agents. Parenterally acquired non-A non-B is now called hepatitis C. It is usually a mild infection of insidious onset, manifested by malaise and jaundice. It is more common in adults. The incidence of developing chronic liver disease approaches 50 percent. Enterically transmitted non-A non-B is now called hepatitis E. Transmission of hepatitis E closely resembles that of hepatitis A. Malaise and jaundice are presenting signs, with arthralgias, fever, and abdominal pain additional associated symptoms. There are no serologic markers for HEV and, therefore, it is a diagnosis of exclusion.

Hepatitis D virus can only multiply in the presence of hepatitis B. It is usually transmitted parenterally. Infection with hepatitis D results in an increased incidence of chronic liver disease.

Fulminant Hepatic Failure

Fulminant hepatic failure is a syndrome characterized by severe hepatic dysfunction and encephalopathy. It usually evolves over a period of <8 weeks and affects all organ systems. Any infectious cause of hepatitis can result in fulminant hepatic failure, though it is uncommon in hepatitis A. Hepatic failure can also result from toxic exposure, especially from acetaminophen or the mushroom amanita phalloides. Severe hypotension can result in hepatic necrosis and liver failure. Depending on the etiology, hepatic failure may be reversible or irreversible.

A predominant manifestation of hepatic failure is encephalopathy, which usually begins with lethargy and can progress to confusion and combative behavior. In later stages, coma can develop. Cerebral edema may develop and may result in death. Associated complaints include anorexia, vomiting, and abdominal pain. Tachypnea may be present and may result in a respiratory alkalosis. On abdominal examination the liver may be small, and there may be ascites. Failure to synthesize liver-dependent coagulation factors results in a bleeding diathesis.

Laboratory findings reveal elevated transaminase and serum ammonia levels. The prothrombin time is increased. Serum albumin may be decreased. In the vast majority of cases, serum bilirubin level is increased. An exception to this is Reye's syndrome, in which the serum bilirubin level is usually not significantly elevated. Hyponatremia may be present, but is usually dilutional. In some patients, renal failure develops.

Management consists of support of respiration, circulation, electrolyte balance, and nutrition. Hypoglycemia is especially common and may necessitate the administration of $D_{10}W$ or $D_{15}W$. The administration of fresh frozen plasma may help correct the coagulopathy. Gastrointestinal hemorrhage may be averted by the administration of H_2 blockers. Oral lactulose causes watery diarrhea of a low pH and may decrease serum ammonia levels. Oral neomycin also may decrease the formation of ammonia.

Jaundice

Jaundice is the clinical manifestation of hyperbilirubinemia. It is relatively common in newborns, where some degree of hyperbilirubinemia is virtually universal. However, the appearance of jaundice beyond the immediate neonatal is virtually always a manifestation of pathology.

Pathophysiology

Bilirubin is largely formed by the destruction of red blood cells and the catabolism of heme proteins. Bilirubin is transported to the liver, where it undergoes enzymatic-mediated conversion from an insoluble unconjugated form to a water-soluble conjugate. The insoluble form of bilirubin is indirect reacting, the water-soluble form direct reacting. After conjugation, bilirubin is excreted in the bile and from there into the intestinal tract. In the intestinal tract, some of the conjugated bilirubin is reconverted to the unconjugated variety, which undergoes enterohepatic reabsorption. At elevated levels, the unconjugate form is neurotoxic.

The newborn is especially vulnerable to hyperbilirubinemia for several reasons. Increased hemolysis secondary to shortened red blood cell survival time or fetal-maternal blood group incompatibility can result in increased formation of bilirubin. Impaired hepatic uptake and inadequately developed enzymes delay its conjugation, and increased enterohepatic circulation results in inefficient excretion.

Hyperbilirubinemia is especially common in newborns and young infants, and it is helpful to consider this age group separately.

Unconjugated Hyperbilirubinemia

Newborns and Young Infants

In the immediate neonatal period, unconjugated hyperbilirubinemia is of great concern largely because of its association with kernicterus, an irreversible neurologic disorder that occurs when unbound bilirubin is deposited in the brain. In its early phases, kernicterus is characterized by lethargy, poor feeding, and, in some cases, opisthotonus. In its full-blown form, it ultimately results in choreoathetosis, extrapyramidal signs, and mental retardation. In full-term newborns, kernicterus is associated with levels of unconjugated serum bilirubin levels >20 mg/dL. In premature infants, lower levels can cause kernicterus. Because of the danger of kernicterus, the presence of hyperbilirubinemia can signify the presence of serious underlying disease.

Physiologic Jaundice

The most common cause of unconjugated hyperbilirubinemia in the neonatal period is physiologic jaundice. It is thought to result from transiently impaired conjugation and excretion of bilirubin. Jaundice becomes visible on the second to third day of life and peaks around the fourth day. The maximum elevation is usually <6 mg/dL. In premature infants, jaundice both peaks and resolves somewhat later, and peak levels can reach 12 mg/dL. Physiologic jaundice is a nonpathologic condition, with no neurologic sequelae.

Breast Milk Jaundice

In general, jaundice is more common in breast-fed infants than it is in bottle-fed infants. This may, in part, be due to substances contained in breast milk that antagonize the conjugation and excretion of bilirubin. Rarely, breast-fed infants can develop elevations of unconjugated bilirubin starting in the first week of life that can reach 15 to 27 mg per 100 mL by the second or third week. The hyperbilirubinemia resolves with the cessation of breast-feeding and does not recur when it is resumed. A diagnosis of breast-milk jaundice assumes that other pathologic causes of hyperbilirubinemia have been considered.

Increased Hemolysis

Increased hemolysis in newborn infants is the most common cause of hyperbilirubinemia severe enough to warrant phototherapy or exchange transfusion. It is usually secondary to maternal-fetal blood group incompatibility in either rhesus or ABO antigens. Jaundice usually appears in the first 24 hours of life. Severe bruising or cephalohematoma secondary to trauma during delivery can also result in increased metabolism of heme proteins and unconjugated hyperbilirubinemia. Other causes of hemolysis include congenital diseases such as hereditary spherocytosis and glucose-6-phosphate dehydrogenase deficiency.

Miscellaneous

Unconjugated hyperbilirubinemia can result from a variety of unusual causes. These include hypothyroidism, Down's syndrome, and pyloric stenosis or other high intestinal obstructions. Bacterial infections, including those from the urinary tract, can cause unconjugated hyperbilirubinemia, although there may also be a component of conjugated bilirubin (see later).

Evaluation and Management

The evaluation of unconjugated hyperbilirubinemia depends on the time at which jaundice is noted and the rate of rise of bilirubin. Infants with unconjugated bilirubin >5 to 6 mg/dL after 2 to 3 days of life merit investigation. Laboratory evaluation includes a complete blood cell count, reticulocyte count, and Coomb's test. If a bacterial infection is a consideration, cultures of blood, cerebrospinal fluid, and urine are obtained, in addition to a urinalysis. In infants with vomiting, a bowel obstruction must be ruled out. The diagnosis of breast-milk jaundice is made after pathologic causes of hyperbilirubinemia are excluded and serum bilirubin level decreases after breast-feeding is stopped.

The majority of newborns with unconjugated hyperbilirubinemia do well with expectant management, with particular attention paid to maintaining adequate hydration. For patients with moderate to severe elevation, phototherapy is the treatment of choice. Indirect hyperbilirubinemia is reduced by exposure to high-intensity light. The criteria for the initiation of phototherapy are not completely clear and vary according to gestational age and birth weight. Consultation with a neonatologist is indicated in full-term infants with values nearing 20 mg/dL. Infants with rapidly rising serum bilirubin who do not respond to phototherapy may require exchange transfusion.

Older Children

In older children, unconjugated hyperbilirubinemia is most likely the result of a hemolytic process or an inherited defect in the conjugation of bilirubin. Hemolytic anemia can be congenital, as in the case of sickle cell disease, thallasemia, or hereditary spherocytosis, or can be acquired, as in drug-induced hemolysis. The work-up for hemolytic anemia includes a complete blood cell and reticulocyte count and a serum haptoglobin level. A common genetic defect in conjugation is Gilbert's syndrome, a deficiency in glucuronyl transferase that is associated with normal hepatic function.

Conjugated Hyperbilirubinemia

Newborns and Infants

Conjugated hyperbilirubinemia is far less common in newborns and young infants than is the unconjugated variety. Conjugated hyperbilirubinemia is present when the conjugated fraction of bilirubin exceeds 20 percent of the total. It most commonly occurs secondary to intrahepatic cellular damage and is less often due to obstruction of biliary flow. Conjugated hyperbilirubinemia is always pathologic. Most infants with conjugated hyperbilirubinemia will present within the first month of life.

Infectious Causes

Neonatal cholestasis can occur secondary to hepatic injury from a multitude of infectious causes. Cytomegalovirus, rubella, herpes simplex, varicella, coxsackie, and hepatitis B are common viral etiologies. Syphilis and toxoplasmosis are also implicated. Most of these result from intrauterine involvement and are often associated with congenital anomalies and hepatosplenomegaly.

Bacterial sepsis can result in conjugated hyperbilirubinemia, although the unconjugated fraction is also usually increased. The urinary tract is a common site of infection and can involve gram-negative organisms such as *Escherichia coli.* Jaundice often starts at 3 to 4 days of age and, in some instances, can be the only manifestation of infection.

Metabolic Causes

Metabolic disorders that can cause conjugated hyperbilirubinemia include alpha$_1$ antitrypsin deficiency, cystic fibrosis, and galactosemia. Most metabolic disorders will have clinical manifestations other than jaundice that will lead to the diagnosis.

Extrahepatic Diseases

The major extrahepatic cause of conjugated hyperbilirubinemia in infancy is biliary atresia, a syndrome characterized by absence of the bile ducts anywhere between the duodenum and hepatic ducts. Patients present with jaundice, dark urine, and often with acholic stools. Mild hepatomegaly may be present. The evaluation of patients with suspected biliary atresia usually includes a liver biopsy, which may help to exclude neonatal hepatitis, a disorder of unknown etiology in which there is diffuse hepatocellular destruction. Depending on the location of the lesion in the biliary tree, surgical anastamosis of the remaining bile ducts to the bowel may be successful. For patients in whom atresia extends to the portahepatis, the Kasai procedure, a hepatoportoenterostomy, may allow drainage of bile. A major complication of the Kasai procedure is the risk of ascending cholangitis.

Another cause of extra-hepatic biliary obstruction is choledochal cyst, a congenital saccular dilatation of the common bile duct. It can present with jaundice and a right upper quadrant mass or with symptoms of cholangitis, including fever and leukocytosis.

Most patients with conjugated hyperbilirubinemia require referral to a pediatric gastroenterologist for definitive evaluation.

Older Children

Conjugated hyperbilirubinemia in older children most commonly results from infectious hepatitis. Drug-induced liver injury is also fairly common. Less commonly, genetic or metabolic disorders can present with jaundice and conjugated hyperbilirubinemia. Relatively common metabolic defects include alpha$_1$ antitrypsin deficiency and Wilson's disease.

BIBLIOGRAPHY

Baker SS, Liptak GS, Colletti RB, et al: Constipation in infants and children: Evaluation and treatment. *J Pediatr Gastroenterol Nutr* 29:612–626, 1999.

Braden B, Posselt H, Ahrens P, et al: New immunoassay in stool provides an accurate noninvasive diagnostic method of Helicobacter pylori screening in children. *Pediatrics* 106:115–117, 2000.

Dennery PA, Seidman DS, Stevenson DK: Neonatal hyperbilirubinemia. *N Engl J Med* 344:581–590, 2001.

Gupta R, Gernsheimer J, Golden J: Acute abdominal pain and vomiting in a 10-year-old girl. *Ann Emerg Med* 30:322–328, 1997.

Hardy S, Keel SB: Weekly clinicopathological exercises: Case 35-1999: A five-month-old girl with coffee-grounds vomitus. *N Engl J Med* 341:1597–1603, 1999.

Hill DL, Heine RG, Cameron DJS, et al: Role of food protein intolerance in infants with persistent distress attributed to reflux esophagitis. *J Pediatr* 136:641–647, 2000.

Hill D, Hosking CS: Infantile colic and food hypersensitivity. *J Pediatr Gastroenterol Nutr* 30(suppl):S67–S76, 2000.

Matsumoto T, Goto Y, Miike T: Markedly high eosinophilia and an elevated serum IL-5 level in an infant with cow milk allergy. *Ann Allergy Asthma Immunol* 82:252–256, 1999.

53

Acute Abdominal Conditions That May Require Surgical Intervention

Jonathan Singer

HIGH-YIELD FACTS

- Infants with an abrupt onset of bilious vomiting are likely to have a midgut volvulus complicating malrotation.

- In the first few months of life, infants with persistent, painless, and forceful vomiting should be evaluated for upper intestinal tract obstruction. Pyloric stenosis is far more common than are congenital bands, antral webs, intestinal duplication, or annular pancreas.

- Failure to remove the diaper of infants with deceptively benign vomiting may preclude the diagnosis of incarcerated inguinal hernia.

- Enterocolitis is a potentially deadly complication of Hirschsprung's disease. It can develop before the diagnosis of Hirschsprung's disease is established or present years after surgical repair.

- Inflammatory bowel disease should be suspected in any infants or children with prolonged gastrointestinal symptoms. This is especially true when stomatitis or perianal disease is present.

- The most likely diagnosis of an abdominal catastrophe presenting as peritonitis is appendicitis.

A large number of gastrointestinal disease states can lead to an emergency department (ED) visit. It is the responsibility of the emergency physician to accurately assess these patients, establish a working diagnosis, and promptly initiate treatment for those patients with an abdominal emergency. A detailed inquiry that characterizes the nature and course of recent events and elicits the contributing symptoms, as well as past medical history, will usually lead to an appropriate provisional diagnosis for those children beyond infancy. For younger patients without a wide verbal repertoire, observations of the caretaker are of no less importance, but may be misinterpreted. Thus, the essential tetrad of the abdominal examination (inspection, auscultation, percussion, and palpation) assumes greater importance in preverbal children. Radiologic laboratory parameters may confirm clinical suspicion and provide baseline parameters for surgical consultants.

In this chapter, nontraumatic abdominal disease states are discussed where emergent recognition and expeditious surgical intervention are essential. An expansion of these entities is found under the general headings of "The Obstructions," "Intraabdominal Sepsis," "Gastrointestinal Foreign Bodies," and "Megacolon."

THE OBSTRUCTIONS

Malrotation With Midgut Volvulus

An arrest of the normal embryonic rotation of the alimentary tract may result in suspension of sections of bowel, including the vascular supply, by a narrow pedicle. Three outcomes are possible. Least likely is the lifelong absence of symptoms. More likely, a rotational anomaly will create a vague gastrointestinal symptom such as failure to thrive, chronic recurrent abdominal distension, pain-free episodic vomiting, or persistent unexplained diarrhea. Most likely, especially with malrotations about the duodenum, small bowel, and colon up to the midtransverse portion (the midgut), a strangulating twist affects dramatic symptomatology. In >75 percent of cases, this precipitous event occurs within the first month of life. Males are affected twice as often as females.

Patients who develop midgut volvulus experience sudden abdominal discomfort and vomiting. The pain is intense and unremitting. The vomiting becomes repetitious and bile stained. If the volvulus is not recognized within hours, viability of the gut may be compromised and bloody vomiting or bloody stools with or without shock may occur.

Affected children are acutely ill, pale, and distressed, and may have poor perfusion. If the obstruction is high, and effectively decompressed by repeated vomiting, abdominal distension is absent. Abdominal distension becomes more prominent with obstruction of the distal small bowel or colon. In advancing cases, gangrenous bowel loops may be transabdominally visualized as a discolored mass. A newborn with malrotation and midgut volvulus evaluated shortly after onset of the vomiting may have a soft, nontender abdomen. However, in older children and with longer standing ischemia in all age groups, children will voluntarily guard an abdomen that is diffusely tender. Distended bowel loops may be appreciated. Bowel sounds are diminished. Stool from the rectal exam may be positive for occult blood.

Plain radiographs of the abdomen, with two views, will demonstrate the presence and general level of obstruction. Duodenal obstruction yields air-fluid levels in the dilated stomach and duodenum with little air (doubled bubble) or no gas in the remainder of the bowel. More distal complete obstruction typically creates numerous loops of dilated bowel and air-fluid levels with a paucity of intraluminal air beyond the obstruction. With incomplete obstructions, the bowel gas pattern may appear relatively normal and further imaging is required. Ultrasonography of the abdomen may provide supporting evidence of obstruction such as bowel wall edema and intraluminal fluid. However, contrast studies provide conclusive diagnostic evidence. Since the cecum may be upwardly or medially displaced in early infancy, a barium enema may not differentiate a normally mobile cecum from malrotation. Thus, the upper gastrointestinal series is preferred. The findings of midgut volvulus include obstruction of the duodenum at its third portion and an associated inability to locate the normal ligament of Treitz to the left of the spine. Intestinal obstruction of the descending duodenum, just over the right of the spine, is pathognomonic. Also, with midgut volvulus the intestine distal to the obstruction wraps around the superior mesenteric vessels and creates a corkscrew appearance.

Obstructed children require intestinal intubation and decompression. Volume depletion necessitates fluid resuscitation. In selected circumstances, blood replacement may be needed in the preoperative period. Prophylactic antibiotics are preferred in toxic patients. Prompt laparotomy, the definitive care, is necessary to preserve the bowel.

Pyloric Stenosis

Pyloric stenosis is the most common cause of intestinal obstruction after the first month of life. Affected patients may present as early as 1 week or as late as 3 months of age. The typical infant becomes symptomatic between the second and sixth week of life. Symptoms in preterm infants are delayed. Males are four times more likely to be affected than are females, with first-born males being especially prone to develop pyloric stenosis. Symptoms of gastric outlet obstruction are produced by hypertrophy of circular fibers about the pylorus.

The initial symptom is intermittent nonprojectile vomiting. The vomiting becomes more frequent, more forceful, and eventually incessant. Within a week, nonbilious, postprandial, projectile vomiting is uniformly encountered. Anorexia is absent. Stools are generally small and infrequent in nature. Urination may decrease in frequency secondary to dehydration. The antecedent history of a steady weight gain is replaced by weight deceleration as formula retention is compromised.

The physical examination generally reveals alert infants with good nutritional status. However, adipose tissue may be reduced and there may be decreased elasticity of the skin, particularly if dehydration is present. The hydration status may be severely compromised if vomiting has been of a prolonged duration. Unless significantly electrolyte or volume depleted, infants suck eagerly and, if fed, swallow without difficulty. A midabdominal peristaltic wave may be seen prior to the eventual regurgitant event. An epigastric, rounded mass, traditionally described as olive-like, is found in 80 to 90 percent of cases. Gastric distension may displace the pyloris posteriorly and prevent palpation of the mass, which may be more successful after children vomit, following decompression of the stomach with a feeding tube or by placing infants in a decubitus position. In circumstances where an abdominal mass cannot be palpated, radiography or imaging may establish the diagnosis.

A plain abdominal radiograph may demonstrate a dilated stomach and hypertrophic walls. An ultrasound study will reveal an elongated and hypertrophied pyloric sphincter, and thickened mucosa may be seen protruding into the gastric antrum (antral nipple sign). If ultrasonography is not available, then an upper gastrointestinal study can be performed. A barium feeding reveals curvature, elongation, and narrowing of the pyloric channel (string sign). Loss of both potassium and hydrogen ions from vomiting can result in a characteristic hypokalemic, hypochloremic, metabolic alkalosis.

When infants have pyloric stenosis, a nasogastric tube should be placed and volume and electrolyte replacement initiated. Once a diagnosis is confirmed, surgical intervention with a pyloromyotomy constitutes definitive care.

Intussusception

Intussusception is an invagination of a proximal portion of the intestine into a distal adjacent part. Intussusception is the most frequent cause of intestinal obstruction between the ages of 3 months and 5 years. More than 60 percent of cases occur in the first year of life, with most of those occurring between the fifth and ninth month. Classically, it occurs in well-nourished children. Males are affected twice as often as females, and this difference becomes more pronounced in children over 4 years of age, rising to an 8:1 ratio.

Intussusception classically creates a triad of clinical symptoms: colicky pain, vomiting, and bloody stools. In a typical case, there is a sudden onset of severe abdominal pain that may last several minutes. After an asymptomatic interval, repeated paroxysms will cause children to cry out again. Children may be impossible to console or may seem comfortable only in a knee-chest position on the floor or in the arms of an attendant. The intermittent nature of the pain with the children appearing quite well between bouts is a significant clue that should be given weight when considering the diagnosis. Pain is the initial manifestation of intussusception in over half of the patients. Vomiting may occur either with the initial painful episode or soon after. Concurrent with vomiting, children typically have several bowel movements, which vary from formed stools to thin liquid. Within 12 to 24 hours, mucus, blood, or both may be passed per rectum, creating the classic "currant jelly" stool.

The classic triad is found in less than one-third of all patients and only 85 percent of children have classic colicky abdominal pain. Only 75 percent of patients experience vomiting. Rectal bleeding may be found in as few as 40 percent of patients. Currant jelly stools, which are bloody, maroon-colored, mucus-laden stools, are typically seen late in the course of the disease.

Associated findings can occur in combination with the classic triad, or they may occur alone, contributing to diagnostic error. Anorexia is an almost universal but nonspecific symptom. Diarrhea may be seen in about 7 to 10 percent of cases where there is complete intestinal obstruction and may be found in up to 40 percent of cases where there is an incomplete bowel obstruction. There is increasing appreciation that apathy or listlessness may occasionally be the dominant manifestation. This altered sensorium with intussusception may be seen in the context of prolonged symptomatology or as the initial complaint. Mental status changes may be accompanied by pronounced pallor, mimicking shock.

The general appearance of children may vary from cheerful and interactive to lethargic and poorly perfused. Not uncommonly, those with advanced disease complicated by either fluid or electrolyte imbalance or blood loss may appear less responsive. However, children with a very brief history of enteric manifestations may be obtunded at presentation. Unless patients have an underlying disease such as anaphylactoid purpura or cystic fibrosis, positive physical findings are typically limited to the abdominal examination. On inspection, the abdomen may appear scaphoid and the right lower quadrant may seem empty (Dance's sign). Guarding or distension is uncommon. Bowel sounds may be normal, decreased, or absent. A sausage-shaped mass may be found. The advancing mass, typically ill-defined and variably tender, may be palpated in any quadrant or on rectal examination. Grossly bloody stool may be found on the withdrawn examining finger, or normal-appearing stool may be positive for occult blood.

Plain abdominal radiographs, in two views, should be obtained. Depending on the time course, the age of patients, and the presence of a lead-point, films may be normal (30 percent) or may reveal nonspecific findings, such as localized air-fluid levels, dilated small bowel loops, reduced intestinal air, or minimal fecal content in the colon. The intussusception itself may be visible in up to one-half of patients. Ultrasonography has been reported to be nearly 100 percent sensitive. Sonographic findings include a large sonographic target, bull's eye, or doughnut sign on the transverse or cross-section, and a sleeve or pseudokidney sign on the longitudinal section. The rim in either case represents the head of the intussusception.

Nontoxic, hydrated children with a provisional diagnosis of intussusception should be given nothing by mouth (NPO). Those who appear dehydrated are given a normal saline bolus, followed by polyionic intravenous fluid pending serum electrolytes. A nasogastric tube may be inserted.

Both an air insufflation or barium enema reduction is performed with the consent, and in the presence, of the surgeon who accepts the responsibility for operating if the reduction is unsuccessful. Attempted reduction with barium enema is contraindicated if there is evidence of intestinal perforation or peritonitis, due to the risk of barium peritonitis.

Incarcerated Hernias

Hernias are protrusions of tissue through an abnormal opening. In children, they occur with descending frequency at the umbilicus, inguinal and scrotal regions, midline epigastrium, and lateral border of the rectus sheath. Due to attenuation of musculofascial layers, preperitoneal fat, abdominal, or pelvic viscus (including small bowel, large bowel, ovary, fallopian tube, testicle, or testicular appendages) may become entrapped. When the incarcerated sac contents cannot be reduced nonoperatively into the peritoneal cavity, strangulation and necrosis of tissues may result. Male children with hernias outnumber female children by an 8:1 to 10:1 ratio. Both sexes have the greatest risk for incarceration during the first 6 months of life. With advancing age, incarceration becomes less likely. There is a very low incidence of incarceration after 8 years of age.

The hallmark of childhood hernias is an asymptomatic bulge that becomes more prominent with increased abdominal pressure, such as straining at defecation, crying, coughing, or laughing. Usually the hernia has been long-standing and recognized both by the parent and primary physician prior to incarceration. On rare occasion, the initial clinical presentation is one of abrupt appearance of the hernia with incarceration.

The first symptom of incarceration in infancy is the abrupt onset of irritability. Expressive children indicate crampy abdominal pain that does not necessarily localize to the hernia site. Poor rooting and refusal to feed is seen in infancy shortly after incarceration. Anorexia or nausea may be expressed in older children. Infrequent nonbilious vomiting may rapidly progress to bilious vomiting. If the incarceration is long-standing, feculent vomiting may be seen as the bowel strangulates.

The diagnosis of incarcerated hernia is not difficult if children are completely undressed. All children with incarceration appear uncomfortable. The abdominal findings vary depending upon the site of incarceration. The omental, reproductive, or intestinal masses are usually nontender and fluctuant at onset. They become firm and tender with passage of time and when viability of the viscus is compromised.

The diagnosis of incarcerated hernia is obvious upon inspection. Radiographic confirmation is rarely necessary. Plain films of the abdomen may reveal partial or complete bowel obstruction. With inguinal hernias, gas-containing soft tissue masses may be noted within the scrotum. Ultrasonography may be used in infants born prematurely to discriminate the contents of an incarcerated sac.

Nonoperative reduction of a strangulated hernia can often be achieved by the emergency physician. Greatest success follows a period of withheld oral intake and application of ice to the hernia sac. Sedation is usually necessary. Suspected strangulation or unsuccessful reduction by the emergency physician mandates surgical consultation.

INTRAABDOMINAL SEPSIS

Acute Appendicitis Without Perforation

Appendicitis is a disease of all ages, but the late elementary school age population has the highest incidence of appendicitis in childhood. There is a gradual reduction in frequency of acute appendicitis in younger children, with a precipitous drop ($<$2 percent of all patient encounters) in children younger than 2 years of age. Acute appendicitis without perforation is encountered equally in both sexes. Transmural bacterial invasion of the appendix may begin as an intraluminal infection or result from obstruction of the appendiceal lumen by enlarged lymphatic tissue, intestinal parasites, foreign bodies, or fecalith. Irrespective of the precipitating factor, the inflammatory process gives rise to a clinical picture that is "classic" in 60 to 75 percent of cases.

The triad of abdominal pain, vomiting, and low-grade fever is highly suggestive of appendicitis. Abdominal pain is the first manifestation of the disease. The pain is epigastric or periumbilical. At onset, the pain is described as a dull, aching sensation. As the obstruction in the appendix maximizes, pain becomes more intense and constant. As the inflammation proceeds to include the parietal peritoneum of the cecum over a 1- to 12-hour time frame, pain migrates and localizes. In most cases the pain is maximal at 3 to 5 cm from the anterosuperior iliac spine on a straight line drawn from that process to the umbilicus (McBurney's point). Pain may radiate to the flank or back with retrocecal appendicitis or the suprapubic region with a pelvic appendicitis, and to the testicle with a retroileal appendicitis. The inflammatory process causes reflex pylorospasm, and patients will vomit. At least one to two episodes of nonbilious vomiting occur in over 90 percent of cases. On occasion, parents may not be aware of the abdominal pain that precedes the vomiting or they may not consider their child's discomfort significant until vomiting ensues. Temperature elevation is a noted feature in 75 to 80 percent of patients. Review of systems may be positive for upper respiratory tract symptoms, anorexia, nausea, or constipation in 15 to 50 percent of affected children. An inflamed appendix, particularly if retrocecal, may cause fecal urgency, tenesmus, and frequent passage of a small volume of stool in approximately 15 percent of children. Dysuria may be experienced by 5 to 15 percent of children with an inflamed appendix in proximity to the ureter. The latter two atypical symptoms are more often clinical features in misdiagnosed cases.

With the exception of low-grade fever, typically in a 38°C (100.4°F) to 39°C (102.2°F) range, patients with nonperforated appendicitis will have minimal alteration of their vital signs. They are ambulatory, but they may walk slowly or limp favoring the right leg and climb upon the examining table only with assistance. If the appendix is in a retrocecal position or in contact with pelvic musculature, elevation and extension of the right leg against pressure of the examiner's hand causes pain (iliopsoas sign). Alternately, when the flexed right thigh is held at right angles to the trunk and internally rotated, hypogastric pain may result (obturator sign). Increased abdominal pain with a heel strike is variably present. Bowel sounds may be normal or diminished. Abdominal distension is absent. Patients may voluntarily guard the entire abdomen or only the right lower quadrant. Exquisite tenderness is often noted directly over McBurney's point. Pressure applied to the descending colon may cause referred pain at the McBurney's point (Rovsing's sign). No abdominal masses are palpated. A rectal examination reveals right lower quadrant tenderness but no masses.

Radiological studies and other imaging techniques are not necessary with clear-cut appendicitis. However, imaging studies may be helpful in equivocal cases. Flat plate and upright abdominal radiographs are frequently the first imaging studies obtained. Plain radiographic findings suggestive, but not pathognomic, of appendicitis include protective scoliosis of the lumbar spine, localized air-fluid levels in the region of the cecum and terminal ileum, obliteration of the right properitoneal fat stripe, haziness over the right sacroiliac joint, and loss of the right-sided psoas shadow and fecalith. In puzzling cases, barium enema may resolve the confusion. A contrast enema in which the appendix fails to fill with barium is highly suggestive of appendicitis. However, ultrasonography has largely replaced the use of contrast material. Sounding has reported sensitivity between 75 and 89 percent and specificity between 86 and 100 percent. With ultrasonography, the appendix is visualized on longitudinal imaging as a hypoechogenic, tubular structure in continuity with the cecum and having a blind distal end. The appendix appears as a target lesion on transverse sections. With appendicitis, the organ is enlarged, exhibiting >2-mm thickness or an outer wall-to-wall diameter >6 mm.

Conventional computed tomography (CT) utilizing intravenous and oral contrast is another technique that may be employed for patients in whom the diagnosis of appendicitis is uncertain. Sensitivity ranges from 87 to 100 percent and specificity from 83 to 100 percent. The highest accuracy has been achieved with focused appendiceal CT. For this imaging, a water-soluble contrast is administered rectally and followed by contiguous 5-mm cuts of the right lower quadrant.

Surgical consultation should be obtained immediately when appendicitis is the primary diagnosis after completion of the history and physical examination. When the emergency physician is in doubt regarding the diagnosis, nonoperative diagnostic modalities may be chosen and consultation delayed. In all circumstances, appendectomy prior to rupture is the treatment of choice for acute appendicitis.

Acute Appendicitis With Perforation

Age is the single most important factor in determining the likelihood of perforation in the course of acute appendicitis. In younger patients, particularly in those <2 years of age, the anticipated sequence of migratory and advancing abdominal pain may not occur. Symptoms in the very young also may be misleading. Irritability, lethargy, refusal to be handled, apparently painless vomiting, or unexplained abdominal distension may overshadow the anticipated symptoms of acute appendicitis. As a result of these ambiguous features, nearly 100 percent of patients in the first year of life will have perforated appendixes at the time of diagnosis, 94 percent of those >2 years of age, 60 to 65 percent of those <6 years of age, and 30 to 40 percent of those >6 years of age. Younger patients have an appendix that is relatively thin walled and the cecum may fail to distend and ineffectively decompress an inflamed appendix. Necrosis, gangrene, and perforation may therefore result with greater rapidity than they will in those who are older. Rapid progression with perforation has been described in preschool-age children in as little as 6 to 12 hours from onset of symptoms.

Classically, patients experience increasingly severe abdominal pain until the appendix perforates. Pain may then lessen or cease. Once the perforation has occurred, age may also influence the subsequent clinical course. After the appendix ruptures, a small amount of pus is extruded. In the first year of life, a short, thin omentum has little capacity to wall off infection. Diffuse peritonitis within hours to days is anticipated rather than focal abscess. Older children tend to isolate an expanding collection of pus. Children who have appendixes that have perforated may encounter vague abdominal complaints for days to weeks after the intraperitoneal event. There may be periods of remissions interspersed with exacerbations. The abscesses that develop are most common in the periappendiceal region, although subphrenic abscess or empyema has been described. The specific signs with perforated appendicitis may therefore vary.

Patients with perforated appendicitis appear acutely ill and their vital signs are abnormal. Tachycardia and fever are common. The temperatures tend to be higher with perforation, typically in the range of 39°C (102.2°F) to 40°C (104°F). Extreme tachycardia, hypotension, and altered tissue perfusion may be found with severe dehydration or superimposed sepsis. Patients with perforation experience great discomfort with all bumps in the road en route to the ED. They plead to be carried from their vehicle to the examining table. If forced to ambulate, the children will shuffle forward, severely bent at the waist. They cannot climb onto the examining table, and when placed supine, they will remain motionless with the right leg flexed. Abdominal distension may be prominent, especially in infancy. Bowel sounds are diminished or absent. Children will voluntarily and involuntarily guard the abdomen. A mass, even if present, may therefore be difficult to discern. Palpation of the abdomen in any quadrant may be painful. Rebound tenderness is most prominent in the right lower quadrant. Iliopsoas and obturator signs are variable. Rectal tenderness is noted, but a mass is an inconstant finding.

Imaging studies may be performed as long as they do not impede the preparation of patients for exploratory laparotomy. Scoliosis, appendicolithiasis, obliteration of the right psoas margin, interruption of the properitoneal fat line, and abnormal intestinal gas patterns may be seen on plain films as in nonperforated appendicitis. Signs that suggest appendicitis with perforation include a focal increase in thickness of the lateral abdominal wall, the presence of a single gas bubble at the inferior portion of the right lower abdominal quadrant, free intraperitoneal fluid, or pneumoperitoneum. Results of barium enema may mimic an ileocecal intussusception or pathonomically demonstrate extravasation of contrast near the cecum. Ultrasonography, in addition to revealing an enlarged, edematous appendix, may demonstrate a periappendiceal fluid collection. An oral, intravenous, or focused rectal contrast CT may be equally satisfactory in diagnosing complications associated with perforated appendix, including the extent and progression of an abscess. Abdominal CT may have equal ability for diagnosing complications associated with perforated appendicitis, including the extent and progression of an abscess.

The preferred preoperative management of patients with perforated appendicitis includes the following:

- 45° to 60° elevation of the head of the bed
- NPO status

- Nasogastric suction
- Sedation
- Intravenous hydration
- Antibiotics
- Blood
- Supplemental oxygen (as necessary)
- Mechanical reduction of fever, with tepid water sponging, fans, or cooling blanket

Spontaneous Peritonitis

The most common childhood conditions leading to peritonitis, in descending order, are the following:

- Perforated appendicitis
- Intestinal obstruction
- Incarcerated hernia
- Inflammatory bowel disease
- Hirschsprung's disease
- Posttraumatic (including instrumentation and foreign body)
- Spontaneously ruptured viscus (including Meckel's diverticulum, bile duct, and inflamed colon or ileum)
- Necrotizing enterocolitis

In cases with the preceding conditions, the normally sterile peritoneal cavity is contaminated from an intraabdominal source. In 10 to 15 percent of cases, pyoperitoneum results from a focus outside of the abdominal cavity. The bacterial access is postulated to result from bacteremia or extension of a urogenital infection. This spontaneous peritonitis may occur in previously healthy children, but patients with ventriculoperitoneal shunt, immunodeficiency (including splenectomy and HIV infection), and ascites from cirrhosis or nephrosis are at increased risk. Rarely, a spontaneous bacterial peritonitis may be the presenting feature of unrecognized nephrotic syndrome. Whatever the inciting condition, primary peritonitis tends to occur more often in females, with peak incidence between the ages of 5 and 10 years.

Patients with spontaneous peritonitis have insidious onset of diffuse abdominal pain. The pain does not localize and increases in intensity over hours to days. Nonbilious vomiting, diarrhea, and fever follow the abdominal pain.

Affected children are anxious and acutely ill. Vital signs are typically abnormal. Temperature elevations are noted in the 39°C (102.2°F)-40.5°C (104.9°F) range; tachycardia is prominent. The respirations are rapid and shallow and may be accompanied by a terminal expiratory grunt. Bowel sounds are diminished. The abdomen is diffusely distended, and when ascites is present, evidence of free fluid will be evident. The abdomen is diffusely tender and guarded. Rebound tenderness may be generalized. Rectal examination reveals tenderness without mass.

Plain radiographic features of peritonitis include marked gaseous distension of the large and small intestines. Multiple air-fluid levels may be present. Intestinal loops may become separated, and the more dependent portions become more opaque. In circumstances where peritoneal exudate localizes into a large abscess, intestinal coils may be displaced away from the inflammatory mass.

If a spontaneous peritonitis is suspected preoperatively, abdominal paracentesis with Gram's stain and culture of the fluid may obviate the need for exploratory laparotomy. If the diagnosis cannot be established preoperatively, laparotomy is necessary.

Necrotizing Enterocolitis

Diverse events in the perinatal period may lead to gastric dilatation, functional ileus, and erosive intestinal mucosal injury, all of which are characteristic of necrotizing enterocolitis (NEC). The terminal ileum and colon are the most common sites of histologic changes. The pathologic findings range from mucosal edema to full-thickness necrosis with perforation. Premature infants who have sustained any of multiple stresses to their cardiovascular system such as acute blood loss, transient hypotension, and birth asphyxia or who require central vascular instrumentation are at increased risk for NEC. Approximately 10 percent of cases occur in term infants. Most infants are diagnosed prior to their initial hospital discharge, but the emergency physician may encounter infants affected with NEC within the first month of life.

Necrotizing enterocolitis represents a spectrum of illness that varies from a self-limited, transient process to a potentially fatal disease. The symptoms range from isolated gastrointestinal upset to systemic manifestations. Anorexia and gastric distension, followed by non-bilious vomiting, abdominal distension, or diarrhea are seen at the onset. Hemochezia may develop. Those who do not spontaneously recover may develop altered mental status and profound alteration of all vital signs. Apnea, bradycardia, hypotension, and vascular instability may all occur.

Affected infants are pale and often septic-appearing. Abdominal distension may be generalized, or a single segment of colon may dilate to striking proportions. Multiple dilated loops of bowel or a localized dilated loop of bowel may be palpated. Abdominal tenderness and guarding are highly variable. Bowel sounds are diminished. Rectal exam reveals grossly bloody stool or seedy stool that is guaiac positive.

On abdominal flat plate, bowel distension is the most common finding. The dilatation may occur in an isolated, diseased, unobstructed colonic segment. Alternately, multiple loops of distal small and large bowel exhibit dilatation suggesting partial obstruction. Concentric loops, centrally located, and associated with increased opacity in the flanks may be seen with ascites. Intraluminal air (pneumatosis intestinalis) may be limited to scattered colonic segments or be generalized. Intrahepatic portal vein gas and pneumoperitoneum are ominous findings. The documentation of either is enhanced with cross-table lateral, decubitus, or erect views. When the clinical picture or radiographic signs are ambiguous, barium enema may provide evidence of colitis, including small ulcerations, mucosal irregularity, and intraluminal extravasation of barium. Ultrasonography in NEC has proved to be of benefit only to detect and track the passage of air through the portal vein system.

Treatment includes withholding feedings, initiating parenteral nutrition, nasogastric decompression, and parenteral as well as intraluminal antibiotics. In the absence of perforation, obvious peritonitis, and gangrenous bowel, surgery is withheld.

Hirschsprung's Disease

Hirschsprung's disease is characterized by the absence of intramural ganglion cells. The histologic deficit is usually limited to a segment of bowel in the rectosigmoid region. The functional abnormality with Hirschsprung's disease is an increase in muscular tone and contractility of the aganglionic segment. Relaxation needed to facilitate the onward movement of stool does not occur. This disease is four times more frequent in males than females.

The pattern of presentation of Hirschsprung's disease is extremely variable. The diagnosis may be suspected within the first few days of birth or not entertained until late childhood. Newborns with aganglionosis may have delayed passage of the first meconium stool. Infants have diminished stool frequency. If undiagnosed, the clinical course in the first year of life is one of gradually increasing fecal retention, obstipation, constipation, and sporadic abdominal distention. Diminished appetite and extended periods of failure to thrive are often noted. Intermittent vomiting and unexplained bouts of nonbloody diarrhea may be encountered. Patients with previously undiagnosed Hirschsprung's disease may present with rectal prolapse.

Parents frustrated by repeated therapeutic failures for chronic constipation are likely to seek ED attention. Examination of affected children reveal a variable nutrition status. There may be mild to moderate abdominal distention. The abdomen is soft, and nontender, mobile fecal masses may be palpable in the left lower quadrant. Children's underwear is not soiled from overflow, as is typically the case with children who have functional constipation. Rectal examination reveals an empty vault that is not dilated. Withdraw of the examining finger may result in an explosive release of stool. This "squirt" in the correct historical context suggests the diagnosis of aganglionosis. If the diagnosis is not entertained, patients may precipitously develop a potentially fatal enterocolitis.

Enterocolitis with Hirschsprung's disease is more common in the newborn period, but can occur at any age. The enterocolitis is characterized by sudden abdominal distention, generalized abdominal discomfort, and explosive diarrhea that rapidly becomes bloody. Temperature elevation, volume depletion, and altered mental status are typically noted. With the most severe cases, a denudation of the intestinal mucosa predisposes to colonic perforation, peritonitis, and Gram-negative septicemia.

Progressively confirmatory steps for diagnosing Hirschsprung's disease in children with chronic constipation include plain abdominal films, barium enema, anal rectal manometry, and pathologic examination of rectal tissue. The latter two diagnostic modalities require equipment and personnel that are typically unavailable in an ED. With aganglionosis, the abdominal flat plate may be normal or demonstrate dilated colon proximal to the aganglionic segment. Barium enema confirms a normal caliber of the rectum and dilatation of the proximal colon. A cone-shaped transition zone in between is pathognomonic.

In the presence of enterocolitis, plain abdominal radiographs show variable distention of multiple intestinal loops and air-fluid levels. The sigmoid or descending colon may be massively dilated. Pneumoperitoneum may be present if spontaneous perforation of the colon has occurred.

Emergency department intervention for enterocolitis includes gastric decompression, use of a rectal tube, fluid resuscitation, parenteral antibiotics, and keeping patients NPO.

GASTROINTESTINAL FOREIGN BODIES

The size, configuration, consistency, and chemistry of an ingested object, when coupled with children's age and personal anatomy, determines whether the children remain asymptomatic or if they develop clinical manifestations. Small (<15 to 20 mm), round, oval, and cuboid objects without sharp edges or projections cause the least difficulty. Rigid, elongated, slender objects may also traverse the intestinal tract without difficulty, but are more inclined to cause complications. Medicamental concretions or repeated ingestion of hair or vegetable matter, such as seeds, leaves, roots, stems, and fiber, can lead to bezoars. These compact masses of foreign material can create havoc anywhere within the intestinal tract. Ingested batteries retained within the esophagus, stomach, or lodged in the appendix or a Meckel's diverticulum can lead to tragedy. Children with underlying congenital, anastomotic, or inflammatory diseases of mediastinal structures are at increased risk of gastrointestinal foreign body impaction. Children <1 year of age, those most likely to inappropriately mouth objects, are at increased risk for complications due to the diminutive caliber of their digestive system.

Complications of gastrointestinal foreign bodies may occur rapidly after inadvertent ingestion or be delayed for months. They include obstruction within the gastrointestinal tract and perforation anywhere within the gut, with subsequent peritonitis, intraperitoneal, hepatic, or extraperitoneal abscess. Other gastrointestinal complications include gut fistulization or hemorrhage. Less common, but with higher mortality, are complications of prolonged esophageal foreign bodies that include obstruction of the airway, mediastinitis, and erosion into the major vessels.

The symptoms exhibited by individual patients who have ingested a foreign body are therefore myriad. Those who become obstructed typically do so at the hypopharynx, thoracic inlet, and the cardioesophageal junction. Patients with a hypopharyngeal foreign body have persistent gagging and pooling of oral secretions, extreme pain localized to the superior neck, and are unable to swallow or speak. Those who have a foreign body lodged at the aortic arch may localize pain to the area of the sternal notch. They too have dysphagia and drooling, but lack dysphonia. Foreign bodies retained at the distal esophagus create vague chest discomfort as well as dysphagia and odynophagia. Obstruction lower down in the intestinal tract causes intermittent abdominal pain with or without vomiting. Distal problem sites include the pylorus, the loop of the duodenum, the ligament of Treitz, and the ileocecal valve.

Physical findings are limited when an ingested foreign body has caused isolated obstruction in the gastrointestinal tract. Vital signs are normal, the abdomen is generally soft and nontender, and, with the exception of bezoars, a mass is absent. Bowel sounds are normal or high-pitched; crescendo sounds may be heard coincident with colicky abdominal pain and separated by periods of silence. A metal detector (used by even a novice examiner) is an effective, radiation-free diagnostic tool for locating ingested metallic bodies. If patients are found to have a metallic foreign body below the diaphragm, there is no need for radiography. If a hand-held unit is unavailable, the mainstay for locating metallic foreign bodies remains anteroposterior films of the chest and abdomen. A lateral neck film should be reserved for children with retained esophageal coins in order to determine the number of coins present. Sounding or CT is of benefit only in patients who have perforated organs.

Children without underlying esophageal disease who have a single coin lodged for <24 hours in any portion of the esophagus are likely to have spontaneous passage of the coin into the stomach. If there is no respiratory compromise, they may be kept NPO and provided intravenous hydration for 12 hours while awaiting spontaneous passage. Children with proximal or middle esophageal impaction may require sedation while waiting for passage of the object. Alternative management to watchful waiting includes balloon extraction and esophagoscopy. One of these active methods should be employed for batteries with corrosive potential regardless of the level point of esophageal impaction. Active retrieval may also be required for objects that are pointed or elongated.

In cases where patients with a history of foreign body ingestion are discharged from the ED, the parents should *not* be instructed to examine fecal contents. This recommendation is unnecessarily burdensome and typically unrewarding. Parents *do* need to be advised of the potential for delayed obstruction anywhere in the gastrointestinal tract and made aware of the signs and symptoms of obstruction.

MEGACOLON

Inflammatory bowel disease in late childhood or early adolescence may be due to ulcerative colitis, primarily a disease of the rectal and colonic mucosa, or Crohn's disease, a transmural disease primarily restricted to the distal ileum. The risk of acquiring either disease is similar in both sexes. Extraintestinal manifestations such as growth retardation, fever, anemia, arthritis, arthralgia, mouth ulcerations, erythema nodosum, pyogenic gangrenosa, liver dysfunction, and uveitis are common to both disorders and may precede the onset of the gastrointestinal complaints. In most children with these two conditions, the overriding concern is persistent diarrhea followed by the appearance of mucus and blood admixed in the stools. In the majority of cases the diarrhea begins insidiously, but a small percentage may have an acute, fulminant course with apparent bacterial sepsis and profuse, bloody diarrhea.

Either as an exacerbation of long-standing disease or as the precipitating event of the disease, patients with either condition may develop a toxic dilatation of the colon (megacolon). The transverse colon is typically involved. A transmural inflammatory process occurs, and the segment of colon massively dilates. Peristalsis ceases. Significant hemorrhage and multiple areas of microperforation may be preludes to peritonitis and overwhelming sepsis.

Patients with megacolon develop a temperature spike and experience malaise and anorexia. Abdominal pain and distension will occur over a period of a few hours to a day. Abundant, grossly bloody stools will be passed. Lethargy may develop.

Physical examination is remarkable for toxicity and apparent volume depletion. Temperature elevation and tachycardia are noted. Bowel sounds are diminished. The abdomen is distended, tympanitic, and tender. Guarding and rebound may occur with frank perforation. Rectal examination is painless and reveals no masses, sinuses, or fistulas unless the inflammatory bowel disease has been long-standing. Stool is grossly bloody.

The hallmark radiologic feature of toxic megacolon, seen on a supine abdominal film, is dilatation of the transverse colon ≥6 to 7 cm in diameter. As perforation may complicate megacolon, an upright or decubitus view should be obtained to search for free air. Ultrasonography is more useful following perforation. However, edema and inflammatory infiltration of the colon wall may be determined by sounding the transverse colon.

Initial treatment for toxic megacolon involves fluid resuscitation, with added albumin or blood as necessary. High-dose corticosteroids are required for patients on maintenance steroids. Pending surgical consultation, a nasogastric tube should be passed and parenteral antibiotics begun.

BIBLIOGRAPHY

Heller RM, Hernanz-Schulman M: Applications of new imaging modalities in the evaluation of common pediatric conditions. *J Pediatr* 135:632–639, 1999.

Irish MS, Pearl RG, Caty MG, et al: The approach to common abdominal diagnoses in infants and children. *Pediatr Clin North Am* 45:729–772, 1998.

Markinson DS, Levine D, Schacht R: Primary peritonitis as a presenting feature of nephrotic syndrome: A rare case report and review of the literature. *Pediatr Emerg Care* 15:407–409, 1999.

McLario D, Rothrock SG: Understanding the varied presentation and management of children with acute abdominal disorders. *Pediatr Emerg Med Rep* 111–122, 1997.

Nance ML, Adamson WT, Hedrick HL: Appendicitis in the young child: A continuing diagnostic challenge. *Pediatr Emerg Care* 16:160–162, 2000.

Rothrock SG, Pagane J: Acute appendicitis in childhood; Emergency department diagnosis and management. *Ann Emerg Med* 36:39–51, 2000.

Seikel K, Primm PA, Elizondo BS: Handheld metal detection localization of ingested metallic foreign bodies: Accurate in any hands? *Arch Pediatr Adolesc Med* 153:853–857, 1999.

Singer JI: Altered consciousness as an early manifestation of intussusception. *Pediatrics* 64:93–95, 1979.

Winesett M: Inflammatory bowel disease in children and adolescents. *Pediatr Ann* 26:227–234, 1999.

54

Disorders of Glucose Metabolism

Elizabeth E. Baumann
Frank Thorp
Robert L. Rosenfield

HIGH-YIELD FACTS

- In diabetic ketoacidosis (DKA), a lack of insulin prohibits intracellular utilization of glucose by somatic cells, and, in response to intracellular starvation, the levels of counterregulatory hormones—glucagon, epinephrine, cortisol, and growth hormone—rise. Gluconeogenesis and glycogenolysis occur in the liver, proteolysis occurs in peripheral tissues, and lipolysis occurs in fatty tissues.

- In DKA, mental status ranges from normal to lethargy and (in severe cases) coma. Virtually all patients have signs of significant dehydration, including tachycardia, dry mucous membranes, and poor skin turgor.

- A bedside glucose oxidase test can quickly confirm the presence of hyperglycemia, which in DKA is almost always >300 mg/dL. The patient's urine can also be tested at the bedside for the presence of ketones, and acid-base status can be rapidly evaluated with an arterial blood gas or venous pH and bicarbonate level.

- The initial fluid resuscitation is with either normal saline or Ringer's lactate at a dose of 20 mL/kg. In stable patients, the bolus is given over 1 to 2 hours; patients in shock require administration as fast as possible.

- As soon as the diagnosis of DKA is made and fluid resuscitation instituted, supplemental insulin is administered. Current recommendations are for low-dose, continuous, intravenous insulin infusion at a starting dose of 0.1 U/kg/h.

- Virtually all patients with DKA are potassium-depleted. Replacement therapy is started once a normal or low serum potassium is ensured and urine output is established, usually at a dose of 3 to 4 mEq/kg/24 hr provided as 40 mEq/L in the IV fluids, with half as potassium chloride and half as potassium phosphate.

- Cerebral edema is the most feared and most lethal complication of DKA, accounting for at least half of DKA-related deaths. Factors implicated but not proved to be associated with cerebral edema include a rapid fall in blood glucose, hypoglycemia, fluid volume replacement, a failure of the actual serum sodium to rise during treatment, and the use of bicarbonate.

- Hypoglycemia is defined as a decrease in the plasma glucose level below 55 mg/dL in children and below 35–45 mg/dL in neonates. The actual glucose level at which obvious signs and symptoms of hypoglycemia are manifested is variable.

- Newborns and young infants with hypoglycemia may be asymptomatic or may manifest nonspecific symptoms such as irritability, pallor, cyanosis, tachycardia, tremors, lethargy, apnea, or seizures. Older children exhibit more classic symptoms of hypoglycemia, including diaphoresis, tachycardia, tremor, anxiety, tachypnea, and weakness.

- Glucose is administered to symptomatically hypoglycemic patients in a dose of 0.5 g/kg/dose. Dextrose 25 percent at a dose of 2 to 4 mL/kg is appropriate therapy, but in neonates and preterm infants, dextrose 10 percent at a dose of 5 to 10 mL/kg/dose is used to avoid sudden hyperosmolarity; in older children and adolescents, dextrose 50 percent at a dose of 1 to 2 mL/kg/dose is used.

DIABETIC KETOACIDOSIS (DKA)

DKA, an endocrinologic condition caused by an absolute or relative lack of insulin, is characterized by hyperglycemia, dehydration, and metabolic acidosis. It is due to severe, uncompensated diabetes mellitus and requires immediate, careful therapeutic management. DKA is more often seen as the initial presentation of diabetes in young children. In young patients, DKA accounts for 70 percent of diabetes-related deaths.

Epidemiology

Diabetes is one of the most common diseases occurring in teenagers. The annual incidence of DKA in the United States ranges from 4.6 to 8 episodes per 1000 patients with diabetes. Recent epidemiologic studies show that hospitalizations for DKA during the past two decades have increased. Treatment of DKA is estimated to represent >1 of every 4 health care dollars spent on direct medical care for adults with type 1 diabetes or 1 of every 2 dollars in those experiencing multiple episodes. It is therefore imperative that we prevent DKA from occurring, that we treat patients efficiently, and that we educate those who repeatedly present with this metabolic emergency.

Pathophysiology

In DKA, a lack of insulin prohibits intracellular utilization of glucose by somatic cells. In response to intracellular starvation, the levels of counterregulatory hormones—glucagon, epinephrine, cortisol, and growth hormone—rise. Gluconeogenesis and glycogenolysis occur in the liver and proteolysis occurs in peripheral tissues. Lipolysis occurs in fatty tissues, forming the ketoacids, β-hydroxybutyrate, and acetoacetic acid. The combination of hyperglycemia and ketoacidosis causes a hyperosmolar diuresis that results in loss of fluids and electrolytes. The severity of the episode depends on the degree of insulin deficiency, length of prodrome, and nature of the underlying stressor. The combination of ketonemia and hypoperfusion can result in a severe anion gap metabolic acidosis.

Diabetic ketoacidosis is precipitated by a variety of causes. In adolescents, noncompliance with insulin is a major problem. Particularly in adolescents with diabetes, DKA may be the clinical correlate of "glycemic chaos" resulting from insulin omission due to behavioral or psychological problems. In young female patients, psychological problems complicated by eating disorders may contribute to the development of recurrent DKA in up to 20 percent of cases. Insulin doses may be omitted because of fear of weight gain, fear of hypoglycemia, rebellion against authority, and stress related to the presence of chronic disease. Most DKA is precipitated by infection or inadequate insulin supplementation during intercurrent illness. The recent use of short-acting insulins, especially in pumps, has increased the number of episodes of DKA. In the Diabetes Control and Complications Trial (DCCT), the incidence of DKA in patients on insulin pumps was double that in the multiple-injection group. This was suspected to be due to exclusive use of short-acting insulins by the patients on the pump. Although the pump has fewer technical problems now than in the past, if it is interrupted, there is no reservoir of insulin for tonic control of basal blood glucose. Severe emotional stress may also be a precipitating factor.

Clinical Manifestations

The clinical manifestations of DKA depend primarily on the severity of metabolic imbalance and the degree of intravascular volume depletion. Mental status ranges from normal to lethargy and (in severe cases) coma. Virtually all patients have signs of significant dehydration, including tachycardia, dry mucous membranes, and poor skin turgor. Poor peripheral perfusion is indicated by cool extremities with delayed capillary refill. Especially in young children, blood pressure can remain normal despite severe dehydration. The metabolic acidosis induces hyperventilation in order to decrease Pco_2; therefore most patients are tachypneic. Patients with severe acidosis may demonstrate Kussmaul breathing, characterized by deep, sighing respirations and fruity odor to their breath. Some patients may develop vomiting, which can be accompanied by abdominal pain severe enough to resemble an acute abdomen. The physical examination always includes a careful search for an infection that may have precipitated DKA.

Laboratory Studies

Initial laboratory studies include a complete blood count, serum electrolytes, glucose, calcium, phosphorus, and serum acetone. A bedside glucose oxidase test can quickly confirm the presence of hyperglycemia. In DKA, the serum glucose is almost always >300 mg/dL. The patient's urine can also be tested at the bedside for the presence of ketones. The patient's acid-base status can be rapidly evaluated with an arterial blood gas or venous pH and bicarbonate level. An initial electrocardiogram should be performed and compared with a follow-up study 6 to 8 hours after the start of therapy.

During the resuscitation (approximately the first 12 hours), serum glucose levels are monitored every hour. Serum glucose and acetone are monitored every 2 hours and serum electrolytes and pH every 4 hours. Urine is monitored for ketones at every void. It is imperative that a flowsheet with accurate estimates of input and output be maintained.

Management

The fundamental management of DKA consists of replacing the patient's fluid and electrolyte deficit and reversing the pathophysiology by administration of exogenous insulin (Appendix 1).

Fluid Resuscitation

Most patients with DKA are at least 10 percent dehydrated. Patients with severe metabolic disturbance can lose enough fluids to develop cardiovascular collapse. The initial fluid resuscitation is with either normal saline or Ringer's lactate at a dose of 20 mL/kg. In stable patients, the bolus is given over 1 to 2 hours; patients in shock require administration as fast as possible. After the initial bolus, the patient's cardiovascular status is reevaluated. If perfusion is not adequate, a second bolus of 20 mL/kg is administered. After the initial resuscitation, rehydration is continued with 0.45 NS or 0.9 NS depending on state of hydration, serum sodium, and hemodynamic status of the patient. In patients with extreme hyperosmolarity, some recommend continuing therapy with isotonic fluids until serum osmolarity decreases below 320 mosm/L, and others advocate the use of hypotonic fluids after restoration of the intravascular volume. This aspect of care is controversial. In either case, corrected serum sodium should not be allowed to drop faster than 10 to 12 mEq/L/24 h, and hydration status must be monitored carefully. If significant hyponatremia is present, the first 6-8 hrs of corection should occur with 0.9 NS. Serum osmolality may be estimated using the following formula:

serum osmolality,(mosm/L)

= 2[serum Na (mEq/L)] + blood glucose (mg/dL)/18;

with normal being 297 ± 2 mosm/L.

Recommendations for continuing fluid resuscitation vary. We advocate use of the body surface area as the basis for calculating replacement of fluids and providing fluids evenly over 24 hours. If the corrected sodium is dropping too quickly; change to NS and recalculate fluid replacement over a 36- to 48-hour period. Total fluid volume for 5 percent dehydration is 3000 mL/m^2, 7.5 percent 3750 mL/m^2, and 10 percent 4000 mL/m^2 for a 24-hour period. We recommend that total fluid volume not exceed 4 L/m^2/24 h, including maintenance and deficit fluids. The volume of fluids used for shock should be subtracted from the total 24-hour fluid calculation and the remainder administered from the conclusion of shock therapy to the end of the first 24 hours. Do not actively replace ongoing losses as the surface area recommendation takes this into consideration.

Insulin Administration

As soon as the diagnosis of DKA is made and fluid resuscitation instituted, supplemental insulin is administered. Current recommendations are for low-dose, continuous, intravenous insulin infusion. This provides reliable, titratable absorption. An initial bolus of insulin is not necessary and can precipitate rapid fluid exchanges that may be dangerous. The starting dose is 0.1 U/kg/h. On occasion, the infusion may have to be increased to 0.15 to 0.2 U/kg/h to lower the serum glucose and reverse the ketosis if the patient's serum glucose is unresponsive to the initial starting dose of 0.1 U/kg/h after the first 1 to 2 hours of insulin therapy. The goal of therapy is to decrease the serum glucose by 75 to 100 mg/L/h. When the serum glucose reaches 250 mg/dL, 5 percent glucose is added to the infusing fluid (Appendix 1). If the serum glucose is dropping precipitously, a glucose solution of ≥10 percent may need to be administered. It is dangerous to discontinue the insulin infusion completely if the patient has moderate to large serum ketones, since this can worsen the ketoacidosis. It is necessary to decrease the insulin infusion to 0.03 to 0.06 U/kg/h only in situations in which acidosis is minimal and glucose is dropping excessively.

During the initial resuscitation phase the patient should be given nothing by mouth. As the patient improves, sips of water or ice may be provided and advanced to clear liquids as tolerated. When the serum glucose normalizes, metabolic acidosis improves, and serum ketones decrease to ≤trace, the insulin infusion is discontinued in concert with a switch to subcutaneous insulin and enteral intake of liquids or solids. Subcutaneous insulin is administered 30 minutes prior to discontinuing the insulin infusion to allow for absorption of the subcutaneous insulin dose. Not administering subcutaneous insulin prior to discontinuing the infusion can predispose to rebound hyperglycemia and ketoacidosis.

Children in mild DKA or "day after resuscitation" can be managed by providing subcutaneous insulin using their baseline or "home" dose. This typically amounts to 0.5 to 1.5 U/kg/d, depending on age and pubertal status. The ongoing presence of ketones may be managed by providing additional insulin at approximately 6-hour intervals, in the form of regular or Lispro at a dosage of 5 to 10 percent of the total daily requirement for small, 10 to 15 percent for moderate, and 25 percent for large ketones. Additional insulin may be administered as often as every 2 to 3 hours if rebound acidosis occurs. If ketones persist, doses are increased by 5 to 10 percent until improvement is evident.

Potassium

Virtually all patients with DKA are potassium-depleted. This is because the metabolic acidosis causes a process in which intracellular potassium is exchanged for extracellular hydrogen in an effort to buffer the metabolic acidosis. The extracellular potassium is then lost through the kidney. Depending on multiple factors, including the severity and acuity of acidosis and the degree of dehydration, the initial serum potassium can be low, normal, or high. Both severe hypo- and hyperkalemia can cause life-threatening cardiac arrhythmias; therefore it is essential that the patient's serum potassium be determined as soon as possible. Hypokalemia is most common several hours after rehydration is initiated. Replacement therapy is started once a normal or low serum potassium is ensured and urine output is established. The usual dose of potassium is twice-daily maintenance, or 3 to 4 mEq/kg/24 h provided as 40 mEq/L in the IV fluids, with half as potassium chloride and half as potassium phosphate.

Sodium

The osmotic diuresis usually induces sodium depletion in patients with DKA. However, laboratory studies do not reflect actual serum sodium concentration, since both the hyperglycemia and the hyperlipidemia of DKA cause fictitiously low values. It is prudent to calculate the true sodium concentration prior to initiation of therapy and to follow it over the resuscitation period. For each 100-mg/dL increment in plasma glucose above a "normal" of 100 mg/dL, there is an expected decrease of 1.6 mEq/L in serum sodium. Some of the depleted sodium is replaced during the initial resuscitation with normal saline or Ringer's lactate. During the continuing resuscitation, sodium levels are monitored every 4 hours. As the glucose falls, the reported level of serum sodium should rise. A fall in serum sodium during continued fluid resuscitation may indicate excess accumulation of free water and may be a risk factor for the development of cerebral edema.

Phosphate

In addition to depletion of potassium and sodium, phosphate is also depleted during DKA. This can cause impaired cardiac function and insulin resistance. The benefit of urgent replacement of phosphate during DKA is debatable; however, supplementation is indicated if the serum level is <2 mEq/L. Phosphate can be administered in conjunction with potassium replacement as a potassium salt. When phosphate is replaced, one must watch for hypocalcemia and attendant cardiac arrhythmias after the initial treatment period.

Bicarbonate

The use of sodium bicarbonate in the treatment of DKA remains extremely controversial. Clinical studies have failed to demonstrate improved outcome in patients treated with supplemental bicarbonate. Its use can be considered in patients with severe acidosis (pH <7.1 or serum bicarbonate <5 mEq/L), which is associated with insulin resistance or cardiovascular collapse. For a serum carbon dioxide level of 5 or less, plan correction to one-third of the total deficit rapidly as a resuscitation procedure only (assume total CO_2 equals 25 mEq/L; total deficit = [normal CO_2 − actual CO_2] × 0.5 × weight in kg), and then discontinue bicarbonate therapy when CO_2 reaches 7 to 10 mEq/L. Do not complete correction to normal. Close laboratory follow-up of acid-base status is mandatory.

Complications

Complications in the management of DKA include hypoglycemia, electrolyte imbalance, cardiac arrhythmias, and cerebral edema.

Hypoglycemia is common, especially in young diabetics, who tend to be labile. It often occurs 6 to 8 hours after the initiation of therapy for DKA. Treatment consists of adjusting the insulin infusion and providing supplemental intravenous and oral glucose according to the principles outlined above. Toddlers appear to be unusually sensitive to insulin, requiring lower initial insulin infusion doses and greater vigilance regarding hypoglycemia. This is thought to be secondary to suboptimal counterregulatory hormone responses during DKA.

Hypokalemia is the most common electrolyte abnormality and occurs within several hours of initiation of therapy. Since it can lead to arrhythmias, cardiac monitoring is essential until metabolic parameters have stabilized. Treatment is with supplemental potassium, as discussed above.

Cerebral edema is the most feared and most lethal complication of DKA, accounting for at least half of DKA-related deaths. It usually occurs as the patient's metabolic parameters are improving and is often heralded clinically by complaints of headache, dizziness, changes in behavior, incontinence, and alterations in pulse and blood pressure, all of which can indicate increased intracranial pressure. It seems to be more common in young diabetics and in cases of new-onset diabetes.

At present, the etiology of cerebral edema is unknown and its occurrence unpredictable. Factors implicated but not proved to be associated with cerebral edema include a rapid fall in blood glucose, hypoglycemia, fluid volume replacement, a failure of the actual serum sodium to rise during treatment, and the use of bicarbonate. A recent study confirmed that children with cerebral edema had lower initial pCO_2 levels and higher blood urea nitrogen levels than controls. Also, treatment with bicarbonate was associated with cerebral edema. However, this study did not answer the question of whether cerebral edema results from the severity of metabolic disturbance before presentation to the ED or the requisite intensive treatment during the resuscitation period. Treatment with bicarbonate nevertheless must be done with close monitoring and conservatively.

The treatment of cerebral edema consists of hyperventilation, mannitol, and fluid restriction, all of which decrease intracranial pressure. Given the unpredictable nature of cerebral edema, careful attention to neurologic status with hourly mental status checks in a critical care setting is mandatory in the treatment of all patients with DKA.

Disposition

All patients presenting with DKA as the initial presentation of diabetes are hospitalized. Patients with severe acidosis are best treated in an intensive care unit, although criteria for this vary among institutions.

Outpatient management of DKA has been advocated for a selected group of patients, including those with stable vital signs, the ability to tolerate oral fluids, established physician follow-up, and a competent family setting. If after 3 to 4 hours of ED treatment the serum pH has risen to ≥7.35 and the serum bicarbonate is >20 meq/L, the patient is discharged. Both the patient's family and the physician should be in agreement with the decision to send the patient home. It is mandatory that the patient receive explicit instructions for additional insulin, increase the frequency of blood sugar testing, and be instructed as to how to contact the diabetes team regarding ketosis. It is mandatory to have access to a health professional should the patient be discharged directly from the ED. In all cases of DKA in the established diabetic patient, a clear understanding of why the patient developed DKA needs to be established first in the ED, taken into consideration for discharge planning, and conveyed to the patient's physician or health care team, so that patient education may ensue.

HYPOGLYCEMIA

Hypoglycemia is defined as a decrease in the plasma glucose level below 55 mg/dL in children and below 35–45 mg/dL in neonates. A plasma glucose level <45 mg/dL (blood glucose <40 mg/dL) in association with symptoms requires intervention. A plasma glucose 25–35 mg/dL requires intervention in an asymptomatic infant only if the infant is at risk of hypoglycemia (e.g., infant of diabetic mother or fetal malnutrition) and the glucose value does not rise to 45 mg/dL or more with feeding. The actual glucose level at which obvious signs and symptoms of hypoglycemia are manifest is variable. The clinical diagnosis of hypoglycemia involves demonstrating a cause-and-effect relationship between symptoms, laboratory evidence of hypoglycemia, and a demonstrable resolution of symptoms following the administration of glucose.

Pathophysiology

Glucose is the main energy substrate for the central nervous system and most other organs in the body. There must be an exogenous supply of glucose by food intake. The endogenous supply of glucose from liver and muscle stores is regulated by a complex interaction of hormones, including insulin (inhibitory) and glucagon, epinephrine, cortisol, and growth hormone (stimulatory).

In the presence of an adequate supply of glucose, insulin promotes the uptake of glucose and amino acids into muscle and adipose tissue, where they undergo anabolic conversion, including the formation of glycogen and protein. Insulin lowers blood glucose levels. Glucagon, epinephrine, cortisol, and growth hormone oppose the effects of insulin in an attempt to increase the serum level of glucose. They stimulate glycogenolysis in the liver as well as the mobilization of amino acids (especially alanine and glycine) for gluconeogenesis, and they promote lipolysis, generating free fatty acids and glycerol, which can be used in limited amounts as energy substrates. The cumulative effect is to maintain glucose levels in the normal range.

Signs and Symptoms

The wide variety of signs and symptoms of hypoglycemia usually results from the sympathetic stimulation driven by the insulin-antagonizing hormones that function to increase serum glucose. Newborns and young infants may be asymptomatic or may manifest nonspecific symptoms such as irritability, pallor, cyanosis, tachycardia, tremors, lethargy, apnea, or seizures.

Older children exhibit more classic symptoms of hypoglycemia, including diaphoresis, tachycardia, tremor, anxiety, tachypnea, and weakness. Parodoxically, refusal of food and vomiting may be present. Prolonged hypoglycemia can cause confusion, stupor, ataxia, seizures, and coma. In the early phase, many patients will complain of headache. Particularly after insulin misadventures or lack of substrate, prolonged, severe hypoglycemia may present as a stroke-like state with a Todd's paralysis. This condition, termed neuroglycopenia, takes several hours to resolve even after the glucose is restored to normal. The etiology of this particular presentation of hypoglycemia is not known.

Differential Diagnosis

Hypoglycemia can be due to inadequate substrate supply, accelerated glucose utilization, toxic ingestion, and disorders of endogenous glucose storage, release, and synthesis.

Hypoglycemia secondary to lack of exogenous glucose is common in acutely ill infants and children, since oral intake is often decreased during an acute illness. Diarrheal diseases may cause malabsorption of substrate and result in hypoglycemia. Deliberate fasting due to anorexia in an older child may present as hypoglycemia.

Idiopathic ketotic hypoglycemia is an entity usually seen in a previously healthy, slender young child, between the ages of 2 and 7 years (typically male) with normal growth and development who presents with an episode of symptomatic fasting hypoglycemia and an appropriate degree of ketosis without hepatomegaly. There is often a history of normal to low birth weight. Idiopathic ketotic hypoglycemia is the most common cause of hypoglycemia beyond infancy. This disorder is characterized by episodic bouts of hypoglycemia associated with fasting and ketonuria. It may also be associated with an intercurrent illness. The pathogenesis is unknown, but it is thought to be due to an exaggeration of the normal childhood inefficiency of gluconeogenesis. Hepatic glycogen stores are depleted at presentation, so there is no glycemic response to glucagon. In the acute phase, patients respond promptly to glucose. Avoidance of prolonged fasting is the only treatment necessary. The disorder is outgrown by late childhood.

Conditions leading to hyperinsulinemia can result in hypoglycemia. This most commonly occurs in a diabetic patient who has taken insulin but does not ingest sufficient calories. In children seen in the ED, the most common cause of hypoglycemia is an adverse reaction to insulin therapy in a known diabetic. Hypoglycemia is the most common acute problem suffered by patients with diabetes. With the DCCT results demonstrating the benefits of stringent control in decreasing the prevalence of complications of diabetes, hypoglycemia can be expected to become more prevalent in the ED setting. Other causes of hyperinsulinemia are not so easily recognized. These include the autosomal recessive persistent hyperinsulinemic hypoglycemia of infancy (formerly known as nesidioblastosis), infant of the diabetic mother, and the β-cell hyperplasia of Beckwith-Wiedemann syndrome. Particularly in older children, one might consider islet cell adenomas and "Munchausen by proxy syndrome," i.e., exogenous insulin administration by a caregiver; the earliest reported case involved an infant 2 months of age.

Inborn errors of metabolism can result in hypoglycemia by disrupting endogenous glucose metabolism. These include a wide array of defects in amino acid metabolism, glycogen storage diseases, fatty acid oxidation (FAO) disorders, enzyme deficiencies in gluconeogenic pathways, and activating mutations of glucose transporters.

The most common FAO disorder is medium chain acyl-CoA dehydrogenase deficiency (MCADD). It can be asymptomatic or present as unexplained death during infancy. It is inherited as an autosomal recessive disease. The allele frequency varies in different populations ranging from 1:40 in Northern Europeans to 1:15,000 in Caucasian Americans. Recent data show that MCADD accounts for 1 percent of sudden infant death syndrome; 19 percent of children with MCADD are diagnosed after death. For this reason it has been recommended for newborn screening and must be considered when entertaining the diagnosis of ketotic hypoglycemia.

Hormonal disorders such as hypopituitarism and adrenal insufficiency can also cause hypoglycemia.

Diagnosis

A rapid screen for the serum glucose level at the bedside is possible using a glucose oxidase reagent strip. More accurate confirmation is achieved by direct measurement done on an initial venous sample. This is the "critical sample" and should include not only a sample for glucose obtained in a gray top tube and placed on ice but important additional studies: insulin, C-peptide, growth hormone, cortisol, and glucagon levels. Urine is tested stat for ketones. The presence or absence of ketonuria is important for the differential diagnosis of hypoglycemia; negative ketones indicate hyperinsulinism or fatty acid oxidation abnormalities, whereas the presence of ketones is characteristic of ketotic hypoglycemia, adrenal insufficiency, growth hormone deficiency or other inborn errors of metabolism. Measurements of urinary amino acids, ammonia and energy substrates, lactate, pyruvate, and ketone bodies should be obtained if the etiology of hypoglycemia remains obscure.

Management

Treatment of hypoglycemia should be started while awaiting laboratory results.

Intravenous glucose is the first line of therapy. Glucose is administered to symptomatically hypoglycemic patients in a dose of 0.5 g/kg/dose. Dextrose 25 percent at a dose of 2 to 4 mL/kg is appropriate therapy. In neonates and preterm infants, dextrose 10 percent at a dose of 5 to 10 mL/kg/dose is used to avoid sudden hyperosmolarity. In older children and adolescents, dextrose 50 percent at a dose of 1 to 2 mL/kg/dose is used. If hypoglycemia persists, a continuous infusion of D5W or D10W at 5 mg/kg/min is indicated. The amount of intravenous glucose required to elevate blood glucose levels and to ameliorate symptoms may provide clues to the etiology of hypoglycemia. If glucose needs in an infant exceed 12 mg/kg/min, the diagnosis is most likely hyperinsulinemia.

If time permits prior to the administration of intravenous glucose, or in the event that intravenous access is not possible, glucagon at a dose of 0.3 mg/kg is given. A glucagon challenge is useful for both diagnosis and treatment: a negative challenge (blood glucose rise <40 mg/dL over baseline), suggests poor glycogen stores, as occurs in undernutrition, ketotic hypoglycemia, liver failure, or glycogen storage disease. A positive challenge (glycemic increment rising ≥40 mg/dL over baseline), suggests hyperinsulinism.

Patients with mild hypoglycemia who are capable of eating or drinking are treated with orange juice or some other age-appropriate source of calories.

After an episode of hypoglycemia, glucose levels are monitored every 1 to 2 hours until the patient is alert and capable of eating and drinking.

Disposition

When the cause of hypoglycemia is not known, hospital admission for further evaluation is indicated. Insulin-dependent diabetics who experience hypoglycemia can be discharged after a thorough review of the episode and when the patient/family fully understands where the care regimen deteriorated. Insulin should be adjusted to prevent further hypoglycemia. Typically, a 20 to 30 percent reduction in insulin dosage over the next 12 hours is indicated. If the diabetic patient has been experiencing recurrent or unexplained episodes of hypoglycemia, hospitalization may be warranted to adjust the insulin dose under supervision of a health care team and to investigate the nature of the medical or psychological issue underlying the problem.

BIBLIOGRAPHY

Diabetic Ketoacidosis

Bonadio W: Pediatric diabetic ketoacidosis: Pathophysiology and potential for outpatient management of selected children. *Pediatr Emerg Care* 8:287, 1992.

Glaser N, Barnett P, McCaslin I, et al: Risk factors for cerebral edema in children with diabetic ketoacidosis: The Pediatric Emergency Medicine Collaborative Research Committee of the American Academy of Pediatrics. *N Engl J Med* 344: 264–269, 2001.

Kaufman FR, Halvorson M: The treatment and prevention of diabetic ketoacidosis in children and adolescents with type I diabetes mellitus. *Pediatr Ann* 28:576–582, 1999.

Kitabchi AE, Umpierrez GE, Murphy MB, et al: Management of hyperglycemic crises in patients with diabetes. *Diabetes Care* 24:131–153, 2001.

White NH: Diabetic ketoacidosis in children. *Endocrinol Metab Clin North Am* 29:657–682, 2000.

Zangen D, Levitsky LL: Diabetic ketoacidosis, in Lifshitz F (ed): *Pediatric Endocrinology.* New York: Marcel Dekker, Inc., 1996, pp 631–643.

Hypoglycemia

Aquilar-Bryan L, Bryan J, Nakazaki M: The focal form of persistent hyperinsulinemic hypoglycemia of infancy. *Recent Prog Horm Res* 56:47–68, 2001.

Becker DJ, Ryan CM: Hypoglycemia: A complication of diabetes therapy in children. *Trends Endocrinol Metab* 11:198–202, 2000.

Cornblath M, Hawdon JM, Williams AF, et al: Controversies regarding definition of neonatal hypoglycemia: Suggested operational thresholds. *Pediatrics* 105:1141–1145, 2000.

Edidin DV, Farrell EE, Gould VE: Factitious hyperinsulinemic hypoglycemia in infancy: Diagnostic pitfalls. *Clin Pediatr (Phila)* 39:117–119, 2000.

Koh THH, Aynsley-Green A, Tarbit M, et al: Neural dysfunction during hypoglycemia. *Arch Dis Childhood* 63:1353–1358, 1988.

APPENDIX 54-1. MANAGEMENT OF PEDIATRIC DIABETIC KETOACIDOSIS

1. History, physical examination, weight determination, and estimation of percent dehydration.

2. Initial tests: electrolytes, pH, glucose, acetone, and electrocardiogram.

3. Start intravenous line and initiate fluid resuscitation. Treat hypovolemic shock with normal saline, 20 mL/kg bolus(es).
   If not in shock, administer normal saline, 20 mL/kg over 1 to 2 hours.

4. After the initial resuscitation, rehydration is continued with 0.45 NS or 0.9 NS depending on state of hydration, serum sodium, and hemodynamic status.
   Continue with calculated maintenance and replacement fluids, not to exceed 4 L/m^2/24 hr.

5. Add potassium chloride, 20 mEq, and potassium phosphate, 20 mEq, to each liter of fluid, after the patient has urinated.

6. Piggyback solution of insulin: 100 mL NS with 1.0 U/kg regular insulin (0.1 U/kg/10 mL) piggybacked via pump into the IV line at a rate of 0.1 U/kg/h (10 mL/h). Flush IV tubing with 50 mL of this solution before use.

7. Periodic biochemical monitoring for the first 12 hours.
   Every hour: bedside glucose determination by glucose oxidase reagent strip technique
   Every 2 hours: serum glucose and acetone
   Every 4 hours: electrolytes and pH

8. Maintain flow sheet to follow vital signs, biochemical markers, input and output, weight, and hydration status.

9. When plasma glucose decreases to 250 mg/dL, change IV fluids to include glucose and change insulin dosage as follows:

	Plasma glucose stable at 200 to 250 mg/dL	Plasma glucose dropping rapidly to below 200 mg/dL
Acidosis (pH < 7.2) and ketonemia still present	D5/0.45 NS Insulin infusion at 0.1 U/kg/h.	D10/0.45 NS Insulin infusion at 0.1 U/kg/h
Acidosis improved (pH 7.2 to 7.4) and only mild ketonemia persists	D5/0.45 NS Insulin infusion at 0.03 to 0.06 U/kg/h	D10/0.45 NS Insulin infusion at 0.03 to 0.06 U/kg/h

10. Plasma glucose will usually fall at a rate of 80 to 100 mg/dL/h. If there is no change in plasma glucose by 2 to 3 hours, increase insulin infusion rate to 0.2/U/kg/h.

11. Stop infusion when serum acetone decreases to <1:2 dilution.

12. Give first dose of regular insulin subcutaneously 30 minutes before stopping insulin infusion. Dose depends on clinical condition, size of patient, and last blood glucose or home insulin dose, including some regular insulin, may be resumed.

13. Contact primary physician or diabetes specialist to arrange for admission or outpatient follow-up as appropriate.

55

Adrenal Insufficiency

Elizabeth E. Baumann
Robert L. Rosenfield

HIGH-YIELD FACTS

- The symptoms of adrenal insufficiency (AI) result from deficiencies of two classes of hormones secreted by the adrenal cortex:
  - glucocorticoid deficiency results from lack of cortisol
  - mineralocorticoid deficiency results from lack of aldosterone
- Glucocorticoid deficiency impairs gluconeogenesis and glycogenolysis, resulting in fasting hypoglycemia. It also resets the "osmostat" and causes dilutional hyponatremia via the syndrome of inappropriate secretion of antidiuretic hormone (SIADH).
- Aldosterone deficiency results in decreased sodium retention by the kidney, resulting in osmotic diuresis, hyponatremia, hypovolemia, and vascular collapse. In addition, it causes a decreased distal renal tubular exchange of potassium and hydrogen ions for sodium ions, leading to hyperkalemia and acidosis.
- AI is classified into primary (adrenocortical failure itself), secondary (pituitary), or tertiary (hypothalamic) types. Primary and tertiary AI, due to withdrawal from exogenous steroid administration and suppression of cortisol synthesis, are the two most common causes of adrenal crisis presenting to a pediatric emergency facility.
- The onset of primary AI is usually gradual, resulting in partial corticoid deficiencies and vague symptoms of fatigue, anorexia, occasional mild postural hypotension, or polyuria. However, primary AI in the presence of intercurrent illness or stress can present as shock, especially in infants.
- The most common cause of primary AI in infants is congenital adrenal hyperplasia (CAH) which, in the female newborn, presents with genital ambiguity secondary to virilization in utero. Hypotension, hyponatremia, hyperkalemia, natriuresis, and shock typically do not develop until about 7 to 14 days postnatally, and may be the presenting symptoms, especially in boys.
- Acquired causes of primary AI in children are less common than congenital disorders. Acquired AI results from autoimmune, infectious, infiltrative, hemorrhagic, or ablative disorders.
- Acute cardiovascular collapse is the most common presentation of AI. In impending AI, patients may complain of anorexia, nausea, vomiting, abdominal pain, weakness, fatigue, or lethargy.
- Laboratory findings in primary AI include hyponatremia, hypochloremia, hyperkalemia, and metabolic acidosis (low serum bicarbonate levels). An increased blood urea nitrogen:creatinine ratio occurs as the result of dehydration.
- If the patient's condition permits, synthetic ACTH (Cosyntropin) 0.15 mg/m^2 is administered to rapidly assess adrenal function by obtaining cortisol levels 30 to 60 minutes later, but treatment of individuals in adrenal crisis with steroids should never be delayed inordinately to perform diagnostic tests. However, the rapid ACTH test can usually be completed in the first 30 to 60 minutes of treatment while fluid resuscitation is occurring and, at the very least, a baseline level of cortisol and ACTH should be obtained in anyone presenting with unexplained shock (critical sample).

Addisonian crisis is a life-threatening emergency. Adrenal insufficiency (AI) results from inadequate adrenocortical function as a result of disruption of the hypothalamic-pituitary-adrenal axis at any point in the system. Two of three adrenal cortical hormones (cortisol and dehydroepiandrostenedione sulfate) are controlled by this system via adrenocorticotropin (ACTH). The third, aldosterone, is controlled by the renin-angiotensin system.

The symptoms of AI result from deficiencies of two classes of hormones secreted by the adrenal cortex.

- Glucocorticoid deficiency results from lack of cortisol.
- Mineralocorticoid deficiency results from lack of aldosterone.

Glucocorticoid deficiency impairs gluconeogenesis and glycogenolysis, resulting in fasting hypoglycemia. It also resets the "osmostat" and causes dilutional hyponatremia via the syndrome of inappropriate secretion of antidiuretic hormone (SIADH). Glucocorticoid deficiency also contributes to dysfunction of the mineralocorticoid system by decreasing the sensitivity of the vascular system to angiotensin II and norepinephrine, resulting in vascular instability manifesting as tachycardia and mild hypotension.

Aldosterone deficiency results in decreased sodium retention by the kidney. The resulting osmotic diuresis causes hyponatremia, hypovolemia, and vascular collapse. In addition, it causes a decreased distal renal tubular exchange of potassium and hydrogen ions for sodium ions, leading to hyperkalemia and acidosis.

Adrenal androgen deficiency is associated with poorly developed sexual hair in pubertal and postpubertal females only.

In primary AI, ACTH [a peptide derived from proopiomelanocortin (POMC) in the pituitary gland] oversecretion occurs due to lack of cortisol-negative feedback. Large quantities of ACTH, which has weak melanotropic activity, results in hyperpigmentation, as does beta lipotropin, another POMC-derived peptide that is secreted along with ACTH. Lack of aldosterone feedback on the renin-angiotensin system results in hyperreninemia.

ETIOLOGY

AI is classified into primary (adrenocortical failure itself), secondary (pituitary), or tertiary (hypothalamic) types. Primary and tertiary adrenal insufficiency, due to withdrawal from exogenous steroid administration and suppression of cortisol synthesis, are the two most common causes of adrenal crisis presenting to a pediatric emergency facility. They present in different ways; only the primary type is characterized by hyperpigmentation, hyperkalemia, and severe vascular collapse.

Primary AI results from congenital or acquired adrenal gland dysfunction. Clinical signs and symptoms do not become manifest until at least 90 percent of the adrenocortical tissue from both glands is destroyed. The onset of primary AI is usually gradual, resulting in partial corticoid deficiencies and vague symptoms of fatigue, anorexia, occasional mild postural hypotension, or polyuria. However, primary AI in the presence of intercurrent illness or stress, can present as shock, especially in infants.

The most common cause of primary AI in infants is congenital adrenal hyperplasia (CAH). The female newborn presents with genital ambiguity secondary to virilization in utero. Hypotension, hyponatremia, hyperkalemia, natriuresis, and shock typically do not develop until about 7 to 14 days postnatally. Boys, therefore, characteristically present at this time in cardiovascular collapse. 17-Hydroxyprogesterone is usually elevated on the neonatal screen; this identifies infants who escape diagnosis at birth and prior to acute presentation in the emergency department. CAH results from a block in the enzymatic activity of one of five enzymes in the cortisol biosynthetic pathway. Each enzyme deficiency results in a characteristic alteration in steroidogenic precursors, resulting in a particular clinical syndrome. Of the several types of CAH, 21-hydroxylase deficiency accounts for over 90 percent of cases. This type causes cortisol and aldosterone deficiency with androgen overproduction. The incidence varies from 1 in 12,000 in the general population to 1 in 600 in Alaskan Yupik Eskimos. Not all states screen for 21-hydroxylase deficiency, so it must be in the differential diagnosis of the shocky infant in the first month of life.

Congenital adrenal hypoplasia is a rare cause of primary AI in infancy; it has been reported to occur as an isolated defect with or without a familial tendency. There are two hereditary forms. The cytomegalic form is an X-linked disease in which the normal adrenal architecture is replaced by large, vacuolated cells. This X-linked form classically presents in the first 6 months of life with AI and is caused by DAX-1 mutation or contiguous gene deletions that are associated with hypogonadotropic hypogonadism, Duchenne's muscular dystrophy, and/or mental retardation. The "miniature" form occurs as an autosomal recessive disorder and may be secondary to isolated ACTH deficiency.

Congenital primary AI can also result from adrenal aplasia or hemorrhage associated with a traumatic delivery.

Familial isolated glucocorticoid deficiency appears to be caused by a heterogeneous group of autosomal recessive disorders. A rare form is the syndrome of familial unresponsiveness to ACTH, which results from an autosomal recessive genetic defect. In familial glucocorticoid deficiency, 50 percent of the cases have inactivating mutations of the ACTH receptor. The remaining patients have defects in one or more unidentified genes unlinked to the ACTH receptor. The pathologic defect results in degeneration of the zona fasciculata-reticularis. The "triple A syndrome," is a distinct clinical syndrome consisting of AI, alacrima, and achalasia of the esophagus, often associated with various neurologic defects, plus ACTH insensitivity or resistance. The defect has been localized to chromosome 12 in the region of the 12Q13 locus. The mineralocorticoid system is usually intact, thus cardiovascular collapse is rare, except in 15 percent of patients in which mineralocorticoids are deficient as well.

Progressive granulomatous, degenerative, or storage diseases involve the adrenal gland, such as tuberculosis, histoplasmosis, or lysosomal acid lipase deficiency (Wolman's disease), and occur in infancy. Wolman's disease is a disorder of abnormal storage of triglycerides and cholesterol esters that cannot be degraded by the adrenal, spleen, liver, or other affected organs. It is inherited in autosomal recessive pattern. Patients present with vomiting, diarrhea, failure to thrive, hepatosplenomegaly, and adrenal calcification. They invariably die at a few months of age despite corticosteroid therapy.

Adrenoleukodystrophy (ALD) is a rare cause of childhood primary AI. It is an X-linked recessive familial disorder, involving a gene encoding a peroxisomal integral membrane protein located on Xq28, characterized by fatty acid accumulation in adrenocortical and neural cells secondary to the inability of peroxisomes to degrade them. It is associated with progressive central demyelination, resulting in blindness, deafness, dementia, quadriparesis, and death. A neonatal form of ALD caused by defects in peroxisome assembly due to a mutation in the PEX gene has autosomal recessive inheritance and presents during the first year of life with hypotonia, seizure disorder, and severe developmental delay. Adrenomyeloneuropathy, a more slowly progressive form, presents in adolescence with weakness, spasticity, and distal polyneuropathy. It is an X-linked recessive disorder that must be considered in boys presenting with primary AI. Analysis of serum very long-chain fatty acids (C-24 and longer) levels is diagnostic.

Acquired causes of primary AI in children are less common than congenital disorders. Acquired AI results from autoimmune, infectious, infiltrative, hemorrhagic, or ablative disorders.

Autoimmune adrenalitis, which accounts for 80 percent of all cases of acquired primary AI, is often associated with immune destruction of other glands and is encountered in both types of polyglandular autoimmune syndromes. The autoimmune polyendocrinopathy-candidiasis-ectodermal dystrophy syndrome (type I, or APECED) is more commonly found during childhood, with a mean age at diagnosis of 12 years. It consists of AI with chronic mucocutaneous candidiasis and hypoparathyroidism and two or three of the following: insulin-dependent diabetes mellitus, primary hypogonadism, autoimmune thyroid disease, steatorrhea (malabsorption), alopecia, pernicious anemia, chronic active hepatitis, or vitiligo. Type I (APECED) has a high incidence in Finland, and may be inherited in an autosomal recessive fashion. The major autoantigens are the steroidogenic enzymes, particularly 21-hydroxylase (cytochrome P450c21), but presence of autoantibodies to these antigens does not necessarily predict adrenal failure. The mutated gene responsible is an "autoimmune regulator" or AIRE and located on chromosome 21q22.3. Females are affected more often than males. Type II (primary AI, hypothyroidism, and diabetes mellitus) is more common and typically occurs in middle life (mean age of onset 30 years). It has an autosomal dominant transmission pattern linked with the human leukocyte antigen (HLA)-B8 allele.

Acquired adrenal failure can occur secondary to infection of the adrenal gland with tuberculosis or fungi (e.g., coccidiomycosis, blastomycosis, histoplasmosis, and torulosis). Human immunodeficiency virus infection (HIV) has been reported as a cause of primary AI.

Infiltrative diseases, such as sarcoidosis, hemochromatosis, or malignancy, may affect the adrenal cortex, leading to destruction.

Primary AI may result from an acute adrenal hemorrhage in fulminating sepsis (the Waterhouse-Friderichsen syndrome). Surgical removal of the adrenal glands causes AI iatrogenically.

Isolated abnormality of the renin-angiotensin-aldosterone system leads to isolated hyponatremia, hyperkalemia, and failure to thrive. Causes of primary isolated mineralocorticoid deficiency include isolated aldosterone deficiency resulting from defects in the terminal steps of the aldosterone biosynthetic pathway or pseudohypoaldosteronism type I, a salt-wasting syndrome resulting from end-organ resistance to aldosterone at the distal renal tubule. Renin and aldosterone levels are elevated due to aldosterone receptor or postreceptor defects. Pseudohypoaldosteronism type II is accompanied by hyperkalemia and hyperchloremic acidosis (type IV renal tubular acidosis), low renin and aldosterone levels, and hypertension. This is an autosomal dominant disorder mapped to two loci on chromosomes 1q31-42 and 17p11, due to isolated increase in chloride reabsorption from the renal tubules. Either type of pseudohypoaldosteronism can be acquired as the result of obstructive or renal tubular uropathy, sickle cell or lead nephropathy, amyloidosis, or urinary tract infections. Hyporeninemia secondary to an abnormality in the juxtaglomerular apparatus of the kidney is another rare cause of aldosterone deficiency.

Secondary and tertiary AI result from pituitary or hypothalamic underfunction, respectively. Both lead to isolated cortisol deficiency. In corticotropin-releasing hormone (CRH) deficiency, the pituitary is intrinsically normal in its ability to secrete ACTH. In both, a picture of isolated glucocorticoid deficiency (and in females, androgen deficiency) prevails. Because ACTH is decreased, hyperpigmentation does not occur. In both secondary and tertiary AI, the mineralocorticoid system is intact. Thus, hyperkalemia and shock do not occur. Dilutional hyponatremia may be encountered, however, secondary to SIADH.

Secondary AI also results from any process that interferes with the pituitary's ability to secrete ACTH, such as tumors, craniopharyngioma, infections, infiltrative diseases of the pituitary, lymphocytic hypophysitis, head trauma, and intracranial aneurysms, or in association with cerebral malformation. Extremely low birth weight newborns may experience transient glucocorticoid deficiency due to a sluggish HPA axis. Neonatal ACTH deficit also occurs as part of the congenital hypopituitarism syndrome of hypoglycemia and cholestatic jaundice, with micropenis in males. Isolated ACTH deficiency is rare and may be congenital or due to a POMC mutation. The POMC mutations yield a syndrome resulting from lack of POMC-derived ligands for the melanocortin receptors: ACTH deficiency (ACTH receptor or melanocortin 2 receptor); red hair pigmentation due to α-melanocyte–stimulating hormone deficiency (melanocortin 1 receptor); and severe early-onset obesity due to α-melanocyte–stimulating hormone deficiency (melanocortin 4 receptor). However, most cases of ACTH deficiency are attributable to an autoimmune process.

Tertiary AI is most commonly caused by withdrawal from chronic administration of glucocorticoid pharmacotherapy, which suppresses the hypothalamic-pituitary-adrenal axis. Hyponatremia and hyperkalemia do not occur. It also occurs after cure of Cushing's syndrome, trauma, or any process that disrupts hypothalamic CRH secretion (e.g., intracranial tumor or its treatment).

Secondary and tertiary AI have been reported in HIV-infected individuals but less commonly than primary AI.

CLINICAL PRESENTATION

Crisis is typically encountered in a child with newly diagnosed primary AI who has been subjected to the stress of an acute illness. It may occur in a patient with previously established AI who has not increased the prescribed steroid dose appropriately during the stress of an intercurrent illness.

Acute cardiovascular collapse is the most common presentation of AI. In impending AI, patients may complain of anorexia, nausea, vomiting, abdominal pain, weakness, fatigue, or lethargy. Diffuse myalgia and arthralgias may occur.

Hypoglycemia may be the presenting symptom. In the most severe cases, a child may present in coma or suffer from severe mental confusion. Fever may be present.

Signs of primary AI include hyperpigmentation, most notably in areas exposed to the sun (face, neck, and hands), areas subject to friction (elbows, knees, and knuckles), the buccal mucosa, areolae, and anal mucosa. Vitiligo secondary to melanocyte destruction suggests an underlying autoimmune disorder. Moniliasis is associated with the AI of polyglandular autoimmune syndrome type I. Severe or long-standing AI has associated psychiatric abnormalities, including organic brain syndrome, depression, or psychosis.

Laboratory findings in primary AI include hyponatremia, hypochloremia, hyperkalemia, and metabolic acidosis (low serum bicarbonate levels). Urinary sodium excretion is elevated, approaching the osmolality of serum. An increased blood urea nitrogen:creatinine ratio occurs as the result of dehydration. Mild to moderate eosinophilia, lymphocytosis, and anemia are common. The electrocardiographic abnormalities that occur as the result of hyperkalemia include peaked T waves, low P waves, and wide QRS complexes. Rarely, asystole or intraventricular heart block results. Low cortisol levels, elevated ACTH levels, low aldosterone, increased plasma renin activity, and low dehydroepiandrosterone-sulfate levels (in pubertal children) are confirmatory.

Hypoglycemia is the primary finding in pure glucocorticoid deficiency, as is characteristic of unresponsiveness to or deficiency of ACTH. Seizures or coma may occur. Shock is a rare finding. Hyperpigmentation does not occur in secondary or tertiary AI. Dilutional hyponatremia may be present secondary to SIADH. If AI is due to hypopituitarism, symptoms and signs of other pituitary hormone deficiencies usually are present, and there may be central nervous system abnormalities, visual field disturbances, or papilledema.

DIFFERENTIAL DIAGNOSIS

Findings on physical examination that help to make the diagnosis of AI include decreased pubic and axillary hair in adolescent females, moniliasis, vitiligo, or hyperpigmentation.

The hyponatremia of AI must be distinguished from other causes of low serum sodium.

- states of excessive intake of free water (e.g., overzealous parenteral fluid therapy, neurogenic polydipsia, or tap water enemas)
- diminished water output (cardiac, liver, or renal failure, or SIADH)
- sodium deficiency states (inadequate intake or excessive gastrointestinal, urinary, or skin losses, or cerebral salt wasting)
- states in which extracellular sodium is redistributed into a "third space" (severe malnutrition, burns, or trauma)

A renal ultrasound may be useful for detecting obstructive nephropathy as the cause of hyponatremia. It is important to distinguish the cause of hyponatremia because management plans differ dramatically, depending on the etiology of low serum sodium.

Other causes of hypoglycemia may be confused with AI. AI is a cause of ketotic hypoglycemia, so it is in the differential diagnosis of substrate-limited hypoglycemia, which includes ketotic hypoglycemia, growth hormone deficiency, liver disease, and inborn errors of carbohydrate metabolism.

AI is in the differential diagnosis of shock. Two of the most common causes of shock in infants and children are sepsis and hypovolemia secondary to dehydration. However, in the management of unexplained shock, the clinician must not only empirically evaluate and treat for sepsis as well as replenish fluid deficits, but also must evaluate and treat for AI.

MANAGEMENT

It is critical to recognize adrenal crisis immediately and treat it aggressively. Therefore, a high index of suspicion is warranted in children with unexplained shock.

First, if sepsis is suspected, blood, urine, and cerebrospinal fluid cultures must be obtained. Then, it is advisable to obtain one blood sample for cortisol and another in an EDTA (ethylenediaminetetraacetic acid) tube, for ACTH levels, and promptly place it on ice. In addition, urine electrolytes, serum electrolytes, glucose, blood urea nitrogen, and creatinine levels, as well as a urinalysis must be obtained. An aldosterone level and plasma renin activity (also in EDTA tubes, on ice) may prove to be helpful for later diagnosis.

If the patient's condition permits, synthetic ACTH (Cosyntropin) 0.15 mg/m^2 is administered to rapidly assess adrenal function by obtaining cortisol levels 30 to 60 minutes later. Treatment of individuals in adrenal crisis with steroids should never be delayed inordinately to perform diagnostic tests. However, the rapid ACTH test is recommended at first presentation and can be completed in the first 30 to 60 minutes of treatment while fluid resuscitation is occurring. At the very least, a baseline level of cortisol and ACTH should be obtained in anyone presenting with unexplained shock (critical sample).

Fluid therapy should begin by giving a 20 mL/kg bolus of 5% dextrose/normal saline or colloid rapidly by the intravenous route. Because children in adrenal crisis are undergoing an osmotic diuresis, after the initial resuscitation, normal saline is usually required at a rate appropriate for severe dehydration. An appropriate rate is twice the normal maintenance rate (200 mL/kg/day for children weighing less than 10 kg and 2250 to 3000 mL/m^2/day for older children) to replenish sodium stores and keep up with ongoing losses of salt and water. Input and output must be monitored closely, with close attention to sodium losses in the urine. Hypoglycemia should be treated with 0.5 to 1.0 g/kg/dose (using boluses) of 50% dextrose in water, and 10% glucose should be included in replacement fluids as needed.

Specific treatment requires initiating glucocorticoid therapy with cortisol (hydrocortisone, Solu-Cortef), 50 mg/m^2/dose, intravenously every 6 hours. Mineralocorticoid need not be given in acute adrenal crisis, as high-dose hydrocortisone has mineralocorticoid-like action.

Diagnosis and treatment of the underlying stressor, such as infection, should be addressed. Antibiotics should be initiated intravenously if septic shock is suspected.

DISPOSITION

All patients presenting to an emergency department in acute adrenal crisis must be admitted to the hospital for continued parenteral fluid and corticosteroid therapy. Once the crisis is over, parenteral cortisol is discontinued and the patient is switched to oral cortisol. Mineralocorticoid therapy is then initiated with fludrocortisone (Florinef), 0.1 mg daily. In calculating the fluid replacement, it should be kept in mind that ongoing renal sodium losses continue for up to approximately 48 hours. Oral salt supplements in the range of 1 to 2 g daily are advisable. After the patient has been stabilized, efforts to further establish the cause of adrenal failure must ensue.

BIBLIOGRAPHY

Clark AJ, Metherall L, Swords FM, Elias LL: The molecular pathogenesis of ACTH insensitivity syndromes. *Ann Endocrinol (Paris)* 62:207–211, 2001.

Eledrisi MS, Verghese AC: Adrenal insufficiency in HIV infection: A review and recommendations. *Am J Med Sci* 321: 137–144, 2001.

Keffer JR: Endocrinology, in Siberry GK, Iannone R (eds): *The Harriet Lane Handbook: A Manual for Pediatric House Officers,* 15th ed. St. Louis: Mosby, 2000, pp 207–228.

Loke KY, Larry KS, Lee YS, et al: Prepubertal diagnosis of X-linked congenital adrenal hypoplasia presenting after infancy. *Eur J Pediatr* 159:671–675, 2000.

Muglia LJ, Mazoub JA: Disorders of the posterior pituitary, in Sperling MA (ed): *Pediatric Endocrinology.* Philadelphia: Saunders, 1996, pp 195–227.

New MI, Rapaport R: The adrenal cortex, in Sperling MA (ed): *Pediatric Endocrinology.* Philadelphia: Saunders, 1996, pp 195–227.

Rosenfield RL, Qin K: Adrenocortical disorders in infancy and childhood, in Becker KL (ed): *Principles and Practice of Endocrinology and Metabolism,* 3d ed. Philadelphia: Lippincott, 2001, pp 806–816.

Tabarin A: Congenital adrenal hypoplasia and dax-q gene mutations. *Ann Endocrinol (Paris)* 62:202–206, 2001.

Thakker RV: Genetic developments in hypoparathyroidism. *Lancet* 357:974–976, 2001.

Werbel SS, Ober KP: Acute adrenal insufficiency. *Endocrinol Metab Clin North Am* 22:303, 1993.

56

Hyperthyroidism

Elizabeth E. Baumann
Robert L. Rosenfield

HIGH-YIELD FACTS

- Thyrotoxicosis results from thyroid hormone excess due either to overproduction of thyroid hormone by the thyroid gland itself or by administration of exogenous synthetic hormone.

- Thyroid hormones activate the adrenergic system by inducing β-adrenergic receptors. Symptoms of sympathetic nervous system overactivity, including hyperthermia, may be present in thyrotoxicosis and these manifestations of thyroid hormone excess can be blocked by β-adrenergic antagonists.

- Specific conditions are known to precipitate thyroid storm in a patient with hyperthyroidism. They include thyroid surgery, withdrawal of antithyroid medications, radioiodine therapy, vigorous palpitation of a generous goiter, iodinated contrast dyes, or states in which thyroid hormone levels drastically increase, such as emotional distress, general surgery, infection, or other conditions that produce a high degree of stress.

- The most common disorder causing thyrotoxicosis in children, as in adults, is the autoimmune disorder Graves' disease. This accounts for 10 to 15 percent of all childhood thyroid diseases.

- Autonomously functioning thyroid nodules, typically single (toxic adenoma), are sometimes encountered in children. Multinodular goiters with thyrotoxicosis are unusual in childhood.

- Children who present with thyrotoxicosis complain of nervousness, palpitations, weight loss, muscle weakness, and fatigue. A history of declining school performance,

due to a decreased attention span, can usually be elicited.

- A goiter, although nonspecific, is the most common physical finding in Graves' disease. The eye signs are usually subtle in children.

- Signs of sympathetic overactivity are common and include tremor, brisk deep tendon reflexes, tachycardia, supraventricular tachycardia, flow murmur, overactive precordium, and a widened pulse pressure. Other cardiac disturbances may occur, such as atrial fibrillation, atrioventricular block, sinoatrial block, or congestive heart failure (CHF) due to the inability of cardiac function to meet metabolic demands.

- Thyroid storm is suggested by severe hyperpyrexia, atrial dysrhythmia, CHF, delirium or psychosis, severe gastrointestinal hyperactivity, and hepatic dysfunction with jaundice. A key feature in thyroid storm is a precipitating event, illness, or major stress, which should be sought and identified.

- Complete blockade of new hormone synthesis can be accomplished by the administration of propylthiouracil (PTU) at a dosage of 175 mg/m^2/day or 4 to 6 mg/kg/day at 6- or 8-hour intervals. To block release of thyroid hormone from the gland in thyroid storm, inorganic iodine therapy (as Lugol's solution or SSKI) is started 1 hour after antithyroid medication is initiated.

The most common disorder of thyroid gland function presenting to a pediatric emergency facility is thyrotoxicosis. The term thyrotoxicosis refers to the clinical complex that results from exposure to excessive thyroid hormone. The clinical manifestations of thyrotoxicosis depend on the severity of thyroid hormone excess, the patient's age, and whether or not disease of other organs coexists.

PATHOPHYSIOLOGY

Thyroxine (T_4) exerts its action primarily by selective binding to nuclear thyroid hormone receptors as triiodothyronine (T_3), in which form it binds to cellular receptors with up to 10 times the affinity of T_4. The actions of thyroid hormone at the cellular level include calorigenesis, acceleration of substrate turnover, amino acid and lipid metabolism, stimulation of water and ion transport, and growth and development of cells.

The free (unbound) thyroid hormone level is the bioavailable fraction in serum. The vast majority of the serum total T_4 is bound to thyroxine-binding globulin (TBG). Approximately 0.02 percent of the total is estimated to be free T_4. The standard method of estimating free T_4 is the free T_4 index, which can be expressed as the product of the fraction of thyroid hormone adsorbed by resin (proportional to the free fraction of endogenous T_4 in the patient's serum) and the total serum T_4 concentration. The free T_4 index remains normal when the serum total T_4 varies due to primary (e.g., hereditary) TBG abnormalities. In the last few years, the ability to measure free T_4 directly by analogue radioimmunoassay or by electrochemical luminescence has become widely available.

Thyrotoxicosis results from thyroid hormone excess due either to overproduction of thyroid hormone by the thyroid gland or by administration of exogenous synthetic hormone. Specifically, an increased concentration of serum free thyroid hormone is almost always found in thyrotoxicosis. Occasionally, only blood levels of T_3 are elevated (T_3 toxicosis).

Thyroid hormones activate the adrenergic system by inducing β-adrenergic receptors. Symptoms of sympathetic nervous system overactivity, including hyperthermia, may be present in thyrotoxicosis. These manifestations of thyroid hormone excess can be blocked by β-adrenergic antagonists. Why some individuals with hyperthyroidism have few symptoms and others develop the most extreme clinical manifestation of thyroid hormone excess, "thyroid storm," is poorly understood. No clear distinction between uncomplicated hyperthyroidism and symptomatic thyrotoxicosis can be made on the basis of circulating levels of free thyroid hormones alone. It is postulated that the rapidity with which free hormone concentrations change contributes to the symptom complex.

Thyrotoxicosis may occur in previously asymptomatic hyperthyroid patients during an acute or subacute non-thyroidal illness. In this case, the clinical manifestations of thyroid hormone excess are thought to be due to an uncoupling of oxidative phosphorylation secondary to the illness, resulting in an enhanced rate of lipolysis, with fatty acid oxidation, increased oxygen consumption, calorigenisis, and hyperthermia. Alternatively, heightened sensitivity to thyroid hormone during acute illness (secondary to decreased TBG levels) could lead to increased hormone entry, increased binding to receptors, or increased activation of gene response elements.

Specific conditions are known to precipitate thyroid storm in a patient with hyperthyroidism. They include thyroid surgery, withdrawal of antithyroid medications, radioiodine therapy, vigorous palpitation of a generous goiter, iodinated contrast dyes, or states in which thyroid hormone levels drastically increase. Emotional distress, general surgery, infection, or other conditions in which the patient encounters a high degree of stress may also precipitate storm.

ETIOLOGY

The causes of thyrotoxicosis may be partitioned into conditions in which endogenous or exogenous sources of thyroid hormone are in excess.

Autoantibodies against the thyrotropin-stimulating hormone (TSH) receptor are usually the cause. These antibodies have thyroid-stimulating activity (TSA). They act at the TSH receptor on thyroid cells and stimulate cAMP production in a manner similar to that of TSH itself. The end result is overstimulation of the thyroid gland, resulting in hyperthyroidism. The fundamental problem is one of defective cell-mediated immune surveillance. Lymphocytic infiltrates are found in the thyroid gland and extraocular muscles.

The most common disorder causing thyrotoxicosis in children, as in adults, is the autoimmune disorder Graves' disease. This accounts for 10 to 15 percent of all childhood thyroid diseases. Genetic predisposition (related to specific HLA haplotypes) and environmental factors are involved in its pathogenesis. Many patients have a family history of goiter, thyroid dysfunction (hyper- or hypothyroidism), or other autoimmune diseases. Graves' disease is more common in girls than boys, and its incidence increases with age. Its hallmark is Graves' ophthalmopathy.

In 5 to 10 percent of thyrotoxicosis, the disorder is due to a variant type of chronic autoimmune thyroiditis called hashitoxicosis. Patients present with goiter without ophthalmopathy.

In an even smaller percentage of patients, subacute thyroiditis can cause thyrotoxicosis due to destruction of thyroid tissue. This process is usually due to viral or granulomatous diseases, classically presents with a painful thyroid gland, and is self-limiting.

Autonomously functioning thyroid nodules, typically single (toxic adenoma), are sometimes encountered in children. Multinodular goiters with thyrotoxicosis are unusual in childhood.

Rarely, hyperthyroidism is secondary to TSH oversecretion from a pituitary tumor or to isolated pituitary resistance to negative feedback control by thyroid hormones on a genetic basis. Signs of an intracranial mass may be present with the former. Goiter is present with both.

A less common condition is neonatal thyrotoxicosis. It is caused by transplacental passage of TSA from a mother with Graves' disease to her fetus.

The possibility of a molar pregnancy, which may elaborate a thyroid stimulator, must be considered in adolescent females with thyrotoxicosis to guide appropriate therapy. Oversecretion of T_4 from ectopic thyroid tissue lying within a teratoma of the ovary (struma ovarii) can cause thyrotoxicosis.

Administration of iodine-containing medications, such as dyes, to patients with a nodular goiter may rarely induce hyperthyroidism in children (Jod-Basedow phenomenon). It occurs in patients with a variety of goitrous states, including Hashimoto's thyroiditis, endemic goiter, multinodular goiter, burnt-out Graves' disease, and nontoxic diffuse goiter. The pathogenesis is thought to be secondary to defective autoregulation of intrathyroidal iodide concentration.

Finally, thyrotoxicosis without glandular overproduction of hormone can occur as the result of excess thyroxine or triiodothyronine intake, intentionally or iatrogenically.

CLINICAL PRESENTATION

Children who present with thyrotoxicosis complain of nervousness, palpitations, weight loss, muscle weakness, and fatigue. A history of declining school performance, due to a decreased attention span, can usually be elicited. Other symptoms include tremulousness, anxiety, excessive sweating, temperature intolerance, and emotional lability. Gastrointestinal overactivity with symptoms of frequent stools are common. An increased appetite is classically present. However, an apathetic state, including decreased appetite, occasionally occurs. The only symptoms of exophthalmos may be sleeping with the eyes open and a resultant chronic conjunctivitis.

A goiter, although nonspecific, is the most common physical finding in Graves' disease. The eye signs are usually subtle in children. Decreased accommodation is more common than exophthalmos. Stare and lid lag are eye signs resulting from sympathetic overactivity.

Graves' dermopathy of the shins is uncommon in children.

Signs of sympathetic overactivity are common. These include tremor, brisk deep tendon reflexes, tachycardia, supraventricular tachycardia, flow murmur, overactive precordium, and a widened pulse pressure. Other cardiac atrioventricular conduction disturbances may occur, such as atrial fibrillation, atrioventricular block, or sinoatrial block.

Congestive heart failure (CHF) may develop due to the inability of cardiac function to meet metabolic demands. It is a classic cause of forward failure. Venous pressure is normal. Except in neonates and unless there is underlying cardiac disease, CHF is uncommon in childhood thyrotoxicosis. Mitral valve prolapse is common in the absence of CHF.

In thyroid storm, signs and symptoms of thyrotoxicosis are accentuated. Storm is suggested by the following: severe hyperpyrexia, atrial dysrhythmia and CHF, delirium or psychosis, severe gastrointestinal hyperactivity, and hepatic dysfunction with jaundice. A key feature in thyroid storm is a precipitating event, illness, or major stress, which should be sought and identified.

DIFFERENTIAL DIAGNOSIS

Conditions that cause tachydysrhythmias (atrial flutter, atrial fibrillation, and ventricular tachycardia) must be differentiated from hyperthyroidism. These include electrolyte disturbances and cardiac disease. The murmur of mitral valve prolapse in association with tachycardia may lead to a mistaken diagnosis of CHF and cardiac valvular disease. The added presence of tremor and fever may suggest rheumatic fever. The patient who is flushed and febrile may appear "toxic," mimicking an acute bacterial infection. Drug ingestions may also mimic the hypermetabolic state seen in thyrotoxicosis. Gastrointestinal hyperactivity may imitate an acute abdomen in thyroid storm.

MANAGEMENT

Treatment of severe thyrotoxicosis or impending thyroid storm is aimed at preventing further thyroid hormone synthesis and secretion, alleviating the acute peripheral effects of excess thyroid hormone if the patient is very symptomatic, supporting with general measures, and identifying the cause.

Initial laboratory tests should include the measurement of total and free T_4, T_3, and TSH levels. Antithyroid antibody levels help confirm the presence of autoimmune thyroid disease.

Complete blockade of new hormone synthesis can be accomplished by the administration of propylthiouracil (PTU) at a dosage of 175 mg/m^2/day or 4 to 6 mg/kg/day at 6- or 8-hour intervals. Alternatively, methimazole or carbimazole (which is converted to methimazole) may be given at a dosage 1/10 that of PTU. However, PTU is preferred because, in addition to blocking new hormone synthesis, it inhibits peripheral conversion of T_4 to T_3. Antithyroid therapy is extremely efficient at inhibiting new hormone synthesis, but it has little effect on glandular release of preformed thyroid hormone.

To block release of thyroid hormone from the gland in thyroid storm, inorganic iodine therapy is started 1 hour after antithyroid medication is initiated. Iodide in large doses not only inhibits thyroid hormone release but also blocks iodothyronine synthesis (Wolff-Chaikoff effect). The recommended dose of iodide in children is not established. However, 0.1 mg/kg/day orally or by nasogastric tube in orange juice divided every 8 to 12 hours, in the form of Lugol's solution (5 percent iodine), or as a saturated solution of potassium iodide (SSKI, 10 percent iodide) inhibits thyroid hormone release. Adults typically receive 3 drops of SSKI 3 times daily; therefore, children should receive 1 to 3 drops 3 times daily, depending on size. Iodine must always be given after blockade of new thyroid hormone synthesis has been initiated by PTU administration. Use of iodide alone will ultimately augment thyroid hormone stores, thereby increasing the risk of exacerbating the thyrotoxic state. Lithium carbonate can alternatively be used for patients with a history of iodine-induced reactions. This also impairs thyroid hormone release. Because the dose of iodide used for thyroid storm is large, the clinician must observe for signs of adverse reaction to iodide, such as rash, drug fever, or anaphylactic shock. Iodine therapy is useful for short-term management of severe thyrotoxicosis or storm, but long-term use of these agents alone results in escape from their antithyroid effects.

Beta-adrenergic antagonists are useful in the management of severe thyrotoxicosis or thyroid storm. They are most clearly indicated for tachyarrhythmias. Propranolol, in addition to its antiadrenergic effects, modestly decreases the conversion of T_4 to T_3. In neonates, it is administered as 2 mg/kg/day orally in 4 divided doses. In adolescents and adults, 10 to 40 mg every 6 hours orally is adequate. Beta-adrenergic blockade must be given cautiously to patients with cardiac failure or asthma, or to diabetics who suffer from hypoglycemic unawareness. Beta-adrenergic blockade must be avoided

in patients with evidence of atrioventricular conduction disturbances since it may aggravate this state.

Glucocorticoids are indicated in thyroid storm to inhibit peripheral conversion of T_4 to T_3 and for their immunosuppressive effect. Hydrocortisone should be used in stress doses of 50 mg/m^2 IV every 6 hours.

If metabolic decompensation has occurred as the result of thyroid storm, management must include a measure to reverse hyperthermia, such as acetaminophen or cooling blankets. Salicylates must be avoided because they can displace thyroid hormone from binding sites, potentially worsening the hypermetabolic state. If gastrointestinal and insensible fluid losses are excessive, normal saline, 20 mL/kg, is administered; then the fluid deficit is calculated and replaced in the form of 0.45 normal saline over the next 24 to 48 hours. Because hepatic glycogen stores are usually depleted, dextrose (5 to 10 percent) is used in the replacement fluids. Generalized supportive care must be instituted until the patient can be transported to a critical care unit.

Cardiovascular complications, such as arrhythmias and congestive heart failure, are treated with antiarrhythmics, digoxin, and diuretics. Finally, the precipitating event causing severe thyrotoxicosis must be sought and treated.

Plasmapheresis has been used for the physical removal of thyroid hormone. This should be reserved for cases of thyroid storm or thyroid hormone poisoning refractory to conventional treatment.

DISPOSITION

Patients who present in severe thyrotoxicosis or thyroid storm and those with cardiovascular compromise should immediately be transported to an intensive care unit. Patients with a milder presentation may be discharged home after baseline thyroid function studies are obtained and propranolol is initiated, as needed. It is important to emphasize that this is not curative therapy, and specific treatment must be instituted on obtaining confirmatory laboratory results.

BIBLIOGRAPHY

Burch HB, Wartofsky L: Life-threatening thyrotoxicosis: Thyroid storm. *Endocrinol Metab Clin North Am* 22:263, 1993.

Forest JC, Masse J, Lane A: Evaluation of the analytical performance of the Boehringer Mannheim Elecsys 2010 immunoanalyzer. *Clin Biochem* 31:81–88, 1998.

Iitaka M, Kawasaki S, Sakurai S: Serum substances that interfere with thyroid hormone assays in patients with chronic renal failure. *Clin Endocrinol* 48:739–746, 1998.

Kadmon PM, Noto RB, Boney CM, et al: Thyroid storm in a child following radioactive iodine (RAI) therapy: A consequence of RAI vs withdrawal of antithyroid medication. *J Clin Endocrinol Metab* 86:1865–1867, 2001.

Keffer JR: Endocrinology, in Siberry GK, Iannone R (eds): *The Harriet Lane Handbook,* 15th ed. St. Louis: Mosby, 2000, pp 207–228.

Kraiem Z, Newfield RS: Graves' disease in childhood. *J Pediatr Endocrinol Metab* 14:229–243, 2001.

Kramer MR, Shilo S, Hershko C: Atrioventricular and sinoatrial block in thyrotoxic crisis. *Br Heart J* 54:600–602, 1985.

Maciel LM, Rodrigues SS, Dibbern RS, et al: Association of the HLA-DRB1*0301 and HLA-DQA1*0501 alleles with Graves' disease in a population representing the gene contribution from several ethnic backgrounds. *Thyroid* 11:31–35, 2001.

Roti E, Vagenakis AG: Intrinsic and extrinsic variables; effect of excess iodide: Clinical aspects, in Braverman LE, Utiger RD (eds): *Werner and Ingbar's, The Thyroid: A Fundamental and Clinical Text.* Philadelphia: Lipincott, 1996, pp 316–327.

Woeber KA: Iodine and thyroid disease. *Med Clin North Am* 75:169–178, 1991.

57

Fluids and Electrolytes

Susan A. Kecskes

HIGH-YIELD FACTS

- Fluid therapy is guided by knowledge of the composition, distribution, and movement of body water.
- Fluid requirements are divided into three parts:
  - maintenance fluids
  - deficit replacement
  - replacement of ongoing losses
- Correction of circulatory failure with isotonic crystalloid or appropriate colloid is the first step in fluid management.
- Hypernatremia should generally be corrected gradually to avoid the complication of cerebral edema.
- Aggressive treatment of hyponatremia may lead to the osmotic demyelination syndrome.
- Therapy for hyperkalemia is aimed at halting intake, stabilizing cellular membranes, intracellular translocation, and enhancing elimination.
- Hypokalemia should be corrected orally, if possible. Extreme caution should be exercised during intravenous replacement to avoid hyperkalemia.

The initial approach to acutely ill children includes an assessment of their fluid and electrolyte status. The ability to maintain homeostasis and correct disturbances requires knowledge of the composition of the fluid spaces of the body and their changes with age and disease. This chapter discusses the physiologic basis of fluid management, some of the common disturbances, and an approach to management.

FLUIDS

Fluid Compartments

Total body water (TBW) is divided into the intracellular and extracellular compartments, with the extracellular compartment subdivided into intravascular and extravascular compartments. The relative size of these compartments varies with age. TBW is approximately 75 percent of body weight at birth, decreasing to the adult proportion of 55 to 60 percent over the first year of life. This primarily relates to a drop in extracellular fluid (ECF). Postnatal diuresis, as well as growth in cellular tissue, are responsible for the majority of the change. Additionally, blood volume decreases from 80 mL/kg at birth toward the adult value of 60 mL/kg. By the time the child is 1 year of age, TBW comprises approximately 60 percent of body weight and is approaching the adult distribution of one third in the extracellular compartments and two thirds in the intracellular compartments (Table 57-1).

Body water exists as a complex solution of salts, organic acids, and proteins. The exact composition varies with body compartment (Table 57-2).

Movement of Fluid

Cellular membranes form the barrier between the extracellular and intracellular spaces. They are freely permeable to water, but impermeable to electrolytes and proteins, except by active transport. Although the specific osmoles differ in the two compartments, the osmolality is equal. Water distributes across this barrier by osmotic pressure. A rise in extracellular osmolality, as occurs with a sodium load, results in movement of water from the intracellular space to the extracellular space. Conversely, water intoxication leads to a movement of water from the extracellular space to the intracellular space.

The vascular endothelium forms the barrier between the intravascular and interstitial spaces. It is permeable to water and electrolytes, but not to protein. Two forces regulate fluid movement. Hydrostatic pressure, created by the propulsion of blood through vessels, favors movement of fluid from the intravascular space to the interstitial space. This pressure falls as blood travels from the arterioles through the capillary bed to the lower pressure veins. Oncotic pressure, exerted primarily by albumin found in the vascular space, favors water movement from the interstitium into the vascular space. Under normal conditions, there is a balance in the movement of water and electrolytes from the vascular space to the endothelium at the arteriolar side and in the reverse direction at the venous side.

Table 57-1. Distribution of Body Water Between Extracellular and Intracellular Fluid as a Percent of Body Weight

Age	Total Water, %	Extracellular Water, %	Intracellular Water, %	Extracellular Water/ Intracellular Water
0–1 Day	79.0	43.9	35.1	1.25
1–10 Days	74.0	39.7	34.3	1.14
1–3 Months	72.3	32.2	40.1	0.80
3–6 Months	70.1	30.1	40.0	0.75
6–12 Months	60.4	27.4	33.0	0.83
1–2 Years	58.7	25.6	33.1	0.77
2–3 Years	63.5	26.7	36.8	0.73
3–5 Years	62.2	21.4	40.8	0.52
5–10 Years	61.5	22.0	39.5	0.56
10–16 Years	58.0	18.7	39.3	0.48

Source: As modified from Holliday MA: Body fluid physiology during growth, in Maxwell MH, Kleeman CR (eds): *Clinical Disorders of Fluid and Electrolyte Metabolism,* 2d ed. New York, McGraw-Hill, 1972, p 544, with permission.

These factors guide the selection of fluid to be administered to a patient. Free water added to the vascular space will distribute proportionally to all three compartments. Isotonic crystalloid distributes throughout the extracellular space. Isooncotic fluid will remain in the vascular space, with the exception of a small distribution to the interstitial space because of the increase in hydrostatic pressure.

Table 57-2. Electrolyte Composition of Body Compartments

Electrolytes	Extracellular Fluid (Plasma), mEq/L	Intracellular Fluid (Muscle), mEq/kg H_2O
Cations		
Sodium	140	±10
Potassium	4	160
Calcium	5	3.3
Magnesium	2	26
Anions		
Chloride	104	±2
Bicarbonate	25	±8
Phosphate	2	95
Sulfate	1	20
Organic acids	6	
Protein	13	55

Source: Modified with permission from Hill LL: Body composition and normal electrolyte concentrations. *Pediatr Clin North Am* 37:244, 1990.

Fluid Requirements

Fluid requirements can be divided into three categories:

- Maintenance fluids, which replace routine daily fluid losses
- Replacement of a fluid deficit, if needed
- Ongoing excessive losses

Maintenance fluids include insensible losses and routine outputs of urine and stool. These are proportional to the body surface area (BSA). Since infants and children have a higher body surface area per kilogram, they also have proportionally higher fluid requirements. There are four common methods to calculate maintenance fluids (Table 57-3). Common maintenance fluids are D_5 0.2 NaCl with 20 mEq/L of KCl in infants and young children and D_5 0.45 NaCl with 20 mEq/L of KCl in older children and adults. Patients in renal failure should have maintenance fluids calculated as insensible loss plus urine replacement.

Many patients have fluid deficits that require replacement. In pediatrics, the most common cause is gastrointestinal disease associated with vomiting and diarrhea. The first priority in patients with fluid deficits is to restore circulation. To begin, the adequacy of the patient's perfusion is determined (Table 57-4). Mental status, urine output, skin character, capillary refill, and vital signs are assessed. Serum electrolytes, blood urea nitrogen, creatinine, acid-base status, urinalysis, and urine sodium concentration may be useful. If the patient's perfusion is inadequate, fluid resuscitation should be initiated. An initial bolus of 20 mL/kg of isotonic crystalloid

Table 57-3. Four Methods for Maintenance Fluid Calculations

Body Surface Area Method

1500 mL/BSA (m^2)/day

100/50/20 Method

Weight	Fluid
0–10 kg	100 mL/kg/day
11–20 kg	100 mL + 50 mL/kg/day for every kg >10 kg
>20 kg	1500 mL + 20 mL/kg/day for every kg >20 kg

4/2/1 Method

Weight	Fluid
0–10 kg	4 mL/kg/h
11–20 kg	40 mL + 2 mL/kg/h for every kg >10 kg
>20 kg	60 mL + 1 mL/kg/h for every kg >20 kg

Insensible + Measured Losses Method

400–600 mL/BSA (m^2)/day + urine output (mL/mL) + L
other measured losses (mL/mL)

[0.9% NaCl or lactated Ringer's (LR) solution] is given intravenously over <20 minutes. The patient is reassessed and further boluses are given until perfusion is adequate. Pediatric patients commonly require >60 mL/kg of resuscitation fluid to restore perfusion. If required, blood products may be substituted for some of the bolus fluid. Additional therapy, such as inotropes or pressors, may be added if the circulatory failure is not solely related to fluid deficit.

Once circulation has been stabilized, the remaining deficit needs to be replaced. The magnitude of dehydration is divided into mild (water loss <5 percent TBW), moderate (water loss 5 to 10 percent TBW), and severe

(water loss >10 percent TBW). Fluid deficit can also be estimated from changes in body weight (assuming all loss is due to fluid loss):

$$[\text{premorbid body weight (kg)} - \text{morbid body weight (kg)}] \times 1000 = \text{fluid loss (mL)}$$

Resuscitation fluids may be subtracted from the calculated deficit and the remainder replaced over 24 hours if the patient is in a normal osmotic state. Typically, the remaining deficit would be replaced with a hypotonic fluid, such as D$_5$ 0.2% NaCl with 20 mEq/L of KCl or an oral rehydration solution. Replacement solutions should be adjusted to the electrolyte status of the individual patient.

Table 57-4. Signs and Symptoms of Dehydration

	Mild (5% TB Wt)	Moderate (10% TB Wt)	Severe (15% TB Wt)
Mental status	Alert	Irritable; drowsy	Lethargic
Skin turgor	Brisk retraction	Mild delay	Prolonged retraction
Anterior fontanel	Normal	Minimally sunken	Sunken
Eyes	Moist; + tears	Dry; − tears	Sunken; − tears
Mucous membranes	Moist	Dry	Very dry
Pulses	Normal	Rapid; weak peripherally	Rapid; weak centrally
Capillary refill	<2 sec	2–5 sec	>5 sec
Respiration	Normal	Rapid	Deep and rapid
Urine output	>1 mL/kg/h	<1 mL/kg/h	Minimal or absent
Blood pressure	Normal	Low normal	Hypotension

Table 57-5. Adjustments to Maintenance Fluids

Fever	Increase maintenance fluids by 10% for each degree $>37.8°C$.
Tachypnea (nonhumidified environment)	Increase maintenance fluids by 5–10%.
Vomiting and gastric loss	Replace with 0.45% NaCl with 10 mEq/L KCl.
Stool loss	Replace with LR with 15 mEq/L KCl or 0.45% NaCl with 20 mEq/L KCl and 20 mEq/L NaHCO$_3$.
Cerebrospinal fluid	Replace with LR or 0.9% NaCl.
Pleural fluid, peritoneal fluid, wound drainage (serous)	Replace with LR or 0.9% NaCl; may need to replace albumin periodically— base replacement on measured serum albumin levels.
Blood	$≤25\%$ TBV[a]: Replace with LR or 0.9% NaCl; assess hematocrit and physiologic status for administration of blood.
	$>25\%$ TBV[a]: Replace one-half to two-thirds of loss as whole blood and reassess. Alternatively, use "3-for-1" and replace $3\times$ the blood loss with LR or 0.9% NaCl.
Third-space losses	Estimate based on patient's physiologic status. Replace with LR or 0.9% NaCl.

[a]TBV = Total blood volume

Some patients may require replacement of ongoing fluid losses not included in normal maintenance requirements (Table 57-5). Continuing emesis and diarrheal losses require replacement along with losses through external drains. Fever increases the water requirement by 10 percent for each degree elevation over 37.8°C. Ongoing third space loss should be estimated and replaced. The type of fluid should be tailored to the content of the fluid lost. A standard solution with a composition close to the fluid being replaced is usually adequate to maintain homeostasis in patients with intact renal function. If more precision is required, the electrolyte content of the fluid being lost may be measured and replaced.

SODIUM

The concentration of sodium reflects the total body store of sodium and its relation to total body water. In both hyponatremia and hypernatremia, the total body store of sodium may be high, low, or normal. It is the amount of total body water relative to total body sodium that determines sodium concentration. Sodium is found in highest concentration in the extracellular compartment and is normally maintained between 135 and 145 mEq/L.

One of the primary regulatory mechanisms is antidiuretic hormone (ADH). ADH is secreted by the posterior pituitary gland in response to stimulation of osmoreceptors residing in the anterior hypothalamus, baroreceptors in the great vessels, and volume receptors

in the left atrium. The release of ADH results in increased water absorption by the renal tubule. Osmoreceptors detect increasing osmolarity, with sodium being the primary ion responsible for extracellular osmolarity. Baroreceptors and volume receptors regulate the intravascular volume. In cases of decreasing intravascular volume and diminishing osmolarity (due to body water in excess of body sodium), the volume receptors will override the osmoreceptors, resulting in ADH secretion and water retention, despite decreasing concentrations of sodium.

Hypernatremia

Hypernatremia is defined as serum sodium >150 mEq/L. It may result from intake of sodium in excess of water or, more commonly, from loss of water in excess of sodium (Table 57-6). Primary sodium excess is usually associated with iatrogenic causes, such as inadequately diluted infant formula, excessive sodium bicarbonate administration, or intravenous hypertonic saline administration. More frequently encountered is hypovolemic hypernatremia, in which water loss exceeds sodium loss. The most common cause in pediatrics is gastroenteritis with diarrhea and vomiting. Other causes include increased insensible water loss (i.e., fever, use of radiant warming devices, burns), diabetes mellitus (solute diuresis), or inadequate access to free water.

Diabetes insipidus (DI) is a less common cause of hypovolemic hypernatremia. The essential feature is a functional lack of ADH, resulting in urinary water loss

Table 57-6. Causes of Hypernatremia

Sodium excess
   Inadequately diluted infant formula
   Excessive administration of sodium bicarbonate
   Excessive administration of hypertonic saline
Water deficit
   Vomiting and diarrhea
   Increased insensible water loss
   Inadequate access to water
   Diabetes mellitus (osmotic diuresis)
   Diabetes insipidus
      Central
         Brain tumors (i.e., craniopharyngioma)
         Head trauma
         Hypoxic-ischemic brain injury
      Nephrogenic
      Congenital (X-linked recessive)
      Renal disease (renal dysplasia, reflux, polycystic
         disease)

despite increasing osmolarity and hypovolemia. It may be caused by insufficient production and release of ADH (central DI) or end-organ unresponsiveness to ADH (nephrogenic DI). Disruption of the hypothalamic-pituitary axis by tumors, head trauma, hypoxic-ischemic brain injury, or neurosurgical procedures, results in central DI. It is frequently seen in children near brain death. Nephrogenic DI is a congenital (X-linked recessive) disorder in which the ADH receptors in the renal tubules are defective and unable to respond to ADH. It is present at birth and can be life-threatening if unrecognized. Very dilute urine (osmolarity <150 mOsm/L or specific gravity <1.005), serum hyperosmolarity (osmolarity >295 mOsm/L), and hypernatremia characterize both central and nephrogenic DI. In acute situations, they may be differentiated by their responsiveness (central DI) or lack thereof (nephrogenic DI) to vasopressin.

As the serum sodium rises, ECF becomes relatively hyperosmolal compared to intracellular fluid (ICF). Water moves from the intracellular space to the extracellular space to equilibrate the osmolality. Assessment of decreased intravascular volume status is associated with a greater total body water deficit in hypernatremia than in isotonic or hypotonic states. The brain attempts to conserve water by an increase in glucose, electrolytes, and idiogenic osmoles. This process occurs over approximately 48 hours. Thus, although the intracellular space is relatively volume-depleted in hypernatremia, the brain preserves its volume status.

Clinical manifestations of hypernatremia depend on the volume status of the patient. In primary sodium excess, the skin is often described as "doughy." In hypovolemic hypernatremia, the signs and symptoms of dehydration are manifest. In both, the central nervous system is adversely affected. Irritability and lethargy can progress to coma and seizures. Hyperreflexia and spasticity may occur. Concomitant laboratory findings may include hyperglycemia and hypocalcemia.

Initial therapy of hypovolemic hypernatremia is focused on correction of circulatory failure, if present. Subsequent restoration of total body water should be gradual, over ≥48 hours. Fatal cases of cerebral edema have occurred with correction over 24 hours, as fluid enters the already volume-replete brain. A gradual correction allows the brain to reduce the idiogenic osmoles and equilibrate with the ECF. The goal is to reduce the serum sodium at a rate of 0.5 to 1 mEq/L/h. The higher the serum sodium, the slower the rate of correction should be. Typically, the correction is started with isotonic crystalloid for stabilization of the circulatory system and completed with hypotonic crystalloid, such as D_5 0.45 NaCl. Maintenance fluids and replacement of ongoing losses must be provided, in addition to the deficit correction. Plasma electrolytes and osmolality should be monitored frequently.

In patients in whom DI is suspected, a trial of vasopressin may be attempted. The drug of choice is desmopressin (DDAVP). The initial dose is 0.05 to 0.1 mL (5 to 10 μg), delivered intranasally, once or twice per day. Alternatively, aqueous pitressin may be given by continuous infusion beginning at 0.5 mU/kg/h and titrated every 30 minutes (maximum dose 10 mU/kg/h) to produce urine osmolality greater than serum osmolality.

Primary sodium excess is treated by removal of excess sodium. First, sodium intake is curtailed. In patients with intact renal function, diuretics in combination with administration of hypotonic fluid diminish sodium concentration. Patients with renal failure require dialysis.

Hyponatremia

Hyponatremia is defined as a serum sodium concentration <130 mEq/L and reflects excess body water relative to body sodium. Depending on etiology, total body sodium may be decreased, increased, or normal (Table 57-7). Hyponatremia with decreased total body sodium occurs when sodium loss exceeds water loss. These losses may be extrarenal or renal. The most common extrarenal losses in children are vomiting and diarrhea. Other causes include burns, peritonitis, and pancreatitis.

Table 57-7. Causes of Hyponatremia

Decreased Total Body Sodium	Normal Total Body Sodium (excess water)	Increased Total Body Sodium
Extrarenal sodium loss	SIADH	Congestive heart failure
Vomiting and diarrhea	CNS disorders (i.e., meningitis)	Renal failure
Burns	Pulmonary disease	
Peritonitis	Post-operative states	
Pancreatitis	Malignancies	
Renal sodium loss	Glucocorticoid deficiency	
Diuretics	Hypothyroidism	
Osmotic diuresis	Water intoxication	
Salt-losing renal disease	WIC syndrome	
Nephritis		
Obstructive uropathy		
Renal tubular acidosis		
Adrenal insufficiency		

Extrarenal etiologies are associated with renal sodium conservation (urine sodium <20 mEq/L). Renal losses include diuretic use, osmotic diuresis, and salt-losing renal disease. Thiazide diuretics are more common culprits in hyponatremia than loop diuretics. Osmotic diuresis may be produced iatrogenically with mannitol or glucose administration. It is also associated with glucosuria in diabetes mellitus. Hyperglycemia and mannitol induce urinary sodium and water loss along with osmotic water movement from ICF to ECF, further lowering serum sodium. Salt-wasting renal diseases include nephritis, obstructive uropathy, renal tubular acidosis, and adrenal insufficiency (congenital adrenal hyperplasia, Addison's disease). Renal causes of hyponatremia with decreased total body sodium are associated with ongoing urinary sodium loss (urine sodium >20 mEq/L).

Hyponatremia with increased total body sodium occurs when the increase in TBW exceeds sodium retention. Common etiologies include congestive heart failure (CHF) and renal failure. In CHF, decreased cardiac output leads to decreased GFR. The kidney then conserves water and sodium in an attempt to increase intravascular volume and improve renal perfusion. Water is conserved in excess of sodium. In renal failure, decreased urine output is unable to maintain sodium balance in the face of excess water intake.

Hyponatremia with normal total body sodium is commonly associated with two etiologies in children. First, the syndrome of inappropriate antidiuretic hormone (SIADH) leads to a dilutional hyponatremia. ADH is excreted in the absence of a physiologic stimulus for its secretion, leading the kidney to retain water. This syn-

drome is associated with diverse causes including central nervous system disorders, pulmonary disease, postoperative states, malignancies, glucocorticoid deficiency, and hypothyroidism. The most frequent etiology in the pediatric emergency room is meningitis. Urinary osmolarity (>200 mOsm/L) and sodium concentration (>20 mEq/L) are inappropriately elevated for the hypotonicity and sodium concentration of the serum. The second common etiology of hyponatremia with normal total body sodium is water intoxication. WIC syndrome occurs when small infants are fed overly dilute formula or excess water. Inappropriately hypotonic replacement of fluid losses is an iatrogenic cause of water intoxication. In both, the intake of free water exceeds the ability of the body to eliminate it.

The clinical manifestations of hyponatremia depend on the volume status of the patient, the rapidity of development, and degree of hypoosmolality. In hypovolemic hyponatremia, the symptoms of dehydration and acute circulatory failure prevail. Hyponatremia produces a decrease in the osmolarity of the ECF. Water flows into the ICF to maintain homeostasis. Rapid changes result in brain edema and CNS pathology. Symptoms range from lethargy to coma. Brain herniation may occur in the most severe cases. Hyponatremia is the most common cause of afebrile seizures in children <6 months of age. More gradual onset of hyponatremia allows the brain to extrude electrolytes and other osmoles to prevent brain swelling and diminish the CNS pathology.

Treatment of hyponatremia begins with an assessment of the patient's volume status and correction of hypovolemic shock, if present. Correction of the hyponatremia requires a loss of water in excess of sodium. This must be undertaken with care, as aggressive correction may lead to the osmotic demyelination syndrome. Just as the brain can generate idiogenic osmoles to maintain cellular volume in hyperosmolal states, it can rid itself of osmoles in hypoosmolal states to prevent brain edema. Once rid of these osmoles, too rapid a correction of sodium can result in cell desiccation and myelinolysis. Gradual correction allows the brain time to equilibrate with a reduction in neurologic sequelae. In hyponatremia of acute onset (<48 hours), it appears safe to correct the sodium over 24 hours. In hyponatremia of more gradual onset, sodium correction should not exceed a rate of 0.5 mEq/L/h. Therapy can be initiated with isotonic crystalloid at rates determined by the volume status of the patient. In euvolemic or hypervolemic patients, this may be at maintenance or fluid-restricted rates. Fluid restriction to two-thirds maintenance, or even insensible fluid loss, is the mainstay of therapy for SIADH. In hypovolemic patients, the deficit needs to be assessed and the correction timed to the desired rise in sodium concentration (approximately 10 mEq/L/24 h). Although most patients will correct gradually with isotonic crystalloid, more aggressive partial correction may be desired in patients with severe neurologic symptoms, such as seizures. A rise in serum sodium of 5 mEq/L can be produced by intravenous infusion of 6 mL/kg of 3 percent sodium chloride over 20 to 60 minutes. A single bolus is usually sufficient to reduce acute symptoms and the remainder of the correction can be undertaken more gradually. Loop diuretics, such as furosemide, have been used as an adjunct to therapy to increase free water clearance. In all types of hyponatremia, the underlying pathology should be identified and appropriate treatment initiated.

POTASSIUM

While only 2 percent of total body potassium is in the ECF, potassium is the main cation in ICF. Normal potassium concentration in the ECF is 3.5 to 5.5 mEq/L, compared to approximately 150 mEq/L in the ICF. The sodium-potassium ATPase pump in the cell membrane maintains this large concentration gradient.

Potassium homeostasis is managed through the use of both translocation and excretion. The majority of potassium excretion occurs in the kidney. The kidney can adjust urinary potassium excretion from <5 mEq to >1000 mEq/24 h. Approximately 10 percent of daily potassium intake is lost through the gastrointestinal tract in stool.

As only 50 percent of a potassium load is excreted in the first 4 to 6 hours, translocation allows the body to maintain stable ECF potassium. In the first hours after ingestion, potassium is translocated into cells, primarily in the liver and muscle. Potassium uptake is regulated by insulin, epinephrine, aldosterone, and acid-base balance. Insulin stimulates the sodium-potassium ATPase pump to promote potassium uptake in the liver and muscle. Catecholamines cause an initial rise in serum potassium as it is released from the liver. Subsequently, serum potassium falls as catecholamines promote movement to ICF. Aldosterone acts through both renal and extrarenal mechanisms to reduce serum potassium. Acid-base changes may result in potassium shifts. Acidemia promotes movement of potassium to the ICF, whereas alkalosis favors movement of potassium to the ECF.

Hyperkalemia

Hyperkalemia is defined as serum potassium >5.5 mEq/L and can result from increased potassium intake, decreased potassium loss, or from redistribution from the ICF. Increased potassium intake rarely results in an elevation of serum potassium unless iatrogenic or simultaneously associated with decreased excretion. Iatrogenic causes include excessive intravenous administration of potassium, administration of large quantities of cold stored blood, large doses of the potassium salts of penicillin, or oral intake of potassium-containing salt substitutes.

Acute renal failure is the primary cause of decreased excretion. Less commonly, adrenal insufficiency may result in hyperkalemia due to decreased mineralocorticoid activity. Use of potassium-sparing diuretics is also associated with decreased potassium excretion.

Redistribution of potassium from the ICF to the ECF may occur via cell destruction or translocation from intact cells. In patients with trauma, burns, rhabdomyolysis, massive intravascular coagulopathy, or tumor necrosis, injured cells release stores of intracellular potassium into the circulation. Hematomas in the newborn and gastrointestinal bleeding may result in large volumes of hemolyzing cells and elevated potassium levels. Potassium can be quickly shifted from the ICF to the ECF in response to metabolic acidosis. The ICF is a major part of the body's buffering system, with extracellular hydrogen ions being exchanged for intracellular potassium ions.

Pseudohyperkalemia is a common occurrence and must be considered in the differential diagnosis of hyperkalemia. It is associated with hemolysis from the blood draw. Causes include prolonged tourniquet use, heel squeezing, or use of small-gauge needles. When pseudohyperkalemia is suspected, specimens should be repeated with attention to avoiding such mechanical factors.

Most patients with hyperkalemia are relatively asymptomatic. Neuromuscular symptoms begin with paresthesias and progress to muscle weakness and, ultimately, flaccid paralysis. Cardiac abnormalities are much more likely to produce life-threatening situations. Characteristic changes in the electrocardiogram (ECG) include peaked T waves, prolongation of the PR interval, and progressive widening of the QRS complex. As potassium continues to rise (typically, >8 mEq/L), the classic "sine wave" of hyperkalemia appears (Fig. 57-1). This may rapidly degenerate to asystole or ventricular fibrillation.

An ECG should always be obtained when hyperkalemia is suspected, to confirm the clinical severity. Serum electrolytes, renal indices (BUN, creatinine, and urinalysis), a complete blood count (CBC), and acid-base status should be obtained. Urinary potassium levels may help evaluate the cause of the hyperkalemia. All patients with serum potassium levels >6.5 mEq/L should have continuous ECG monitoring and frequent laboratory follow-up.

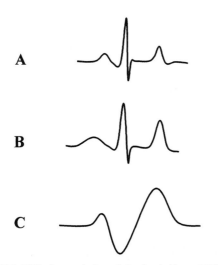

Fig. 57-1. ECG changes in hyperkalemia. *A.* Normal ECG. *B.* ECG with peaked T waves, prolonged PR interval, and widened QRS, seen in moderate hyperkalemia (potassium >7.0 mEq/L). *C.* "Sine wave" ECG seen at potassium levels >8 mEq/L.

Treatment of hyperkalemia depends on the level of serum potassium, along with the clinical symptoms and renal status of the patient. In all cases, intake of potassium and potassium-sparing medication should be halted. In asymptomatic patients with intact renal function and modest (<7 mEq/L) levels of serum potassium, halting intake and follow-up of serum potassium levels may be all that is required (Table 57-8). For patients with renal dysfunction, the addition of the potassium-binding agent, sodium polystyrene sulfonate (Kayexalate, 1 to 2 g/kg PO, NG, or PR), or dialysis should be considered to enhance elimination.

Those patients with serum potassium levels >7 mEq/L or who are symptomatic require aggressive intervention to stabilize the cellular membrane, shift potassium intracellularly, and increase potassium elimination. Membrane stabilization is effected by intravenous administration of calcium. Calcium gluconate, 10 percent, in a dose of 50 to 100 mg/kg, or calcium chloride, 10 percent, in a dose of 10 to 25 mg/kg, may be administered over 2 to 5 minutes with continuous ECG monitoring. Onset of action is immediate and the stabilizing effects last 30 to 60 minutes. Potassium may be shifted intracellularly to temporarily reduce serum potassium levels. Administration of sodium bicarbonate (1 to 2 mEq/kg intravenously over 5 to 10 minutes) has an onset of action of 5 to 10 minutes and a duration of 1 to 2 hours. The dose may be repeated if necessary. Insulin administered in conjunction with glucose effectively shifts potassium to the ICF as well. Dextrose (1 g/kg) may be combined with insulin (0.25 units/kg) and infused over 2 hours. Inhalation of β_2-agonists is an attractive alternative for patients with delayed intravenous access. Nebulized albuterol, in a dose of 2.5 mg for patients <25 kg and 5 mg for patients >25 kg, has been reported to reduce potassium in adult patients with chronic renal failure and is likely to have a similar effect in pediatric patients. It should not be a substitute for appropriate intravenous therapy, but may be used while access is obtained. None of these methods alter total body potassium, so the time they buy should be utilized to enhance elimination of potassium from the body. In the absence of renal failure, loop diuretics and/or thiazides will enhance renal elimination of potassium. Sodium polystyrene sulfonate is a resin that exchanges sodium for potassium at a 1:1 ratio. It is administered through the gastrointestinal tract and may be used in patients with and without renal failure. In patients with renal failure or severely symptomatic cases, dialysis is the definitive therapy. Although hemodialysis is more effective than peritoneal dialysis, the

Table 57-8. Treatment of Hyperkalemia

Halt potassium intake
    Eliminate high potassium food and drink
    Discontinue intravenous potassium-containing solutions
    Discontinue medications high in potassium or which cause increased potassium
Stabilize cell membranes
    Calcium chloride, 10%, 10–25 mg/kg, IV, over 2–5 min *or* calcium gluconate, 10%, 50–100 mg/kg, IV, over 2–5 min
Translocate potassium intracellularly
    Sodium bicarbonate, 1–2 mEq/kg, IV, over 5–10 min
    Regular insulin, 0.25 units/kg, with dextrose, 1 g/kg, administered as a continuous infusion over 2 h
    Albuterol, 2.5 mg for patients <25 kg and 5.0 mg for patients ≥25 kg, nebulized with 2.5 mL 0.9% NaCl
Eliminate potassium
    Sodium polystyrene sulfonate, 1–2 g/kg, PO, NG, or PR
    Diuretics
        Furosemide, 1–2 mg/kg, IV or PO
        Hydrochlorothiazide, 1 mg/kg (maximum 200 mg), PO
    Dialysis

peritoneal route is more readily available and may be instituted more quickly in many locations.

Hypokalemia

Hypokalemia is defined by a serum potassium level <3.5 mEq/L and can result from decreased intake, increased renal excretion, increased extrarenal losses, or a shift of potassium from the ECF to the ICF. A low-potassium diet, eating disorders such as anorexia nervosa, and prolonged administration of intravenous fluids without potassium, may all lead to hypokalemia. Increased renal excretion may result from use of diuretics, osmotic diuresis, hyperaldosteronism, Bartter syndrome, magnesium deficiency, and renal tubular acidosis. Extrarenal losses occur primarily through the gastrointestinal system. Vomiting and nasogastric losses may lead to hypokalemia, both from the direct loss of potassium and from secondary hyperaldosteronism associated with hypovolemia. Diarrhea is associated with large potassium losses. Movement of potassium into the cells from the ECF can occur with correction of acidosis, alkalosis, administration of insulin, administration of β_2-agonists, or familial hypokalemic periodic paralysis.

Clinical manifestations of hypokalemia are related to its rapidity of onset and degree of severity. Muscle contraction is dependent on membrane polarization and requires a rapid influx of sodium into cells and a comparable efflux of potassium. Hypokalemia impairs this process. The result is alteration of nerve conduction and muscle contraction. Clinical symptoms include muscle

weakness, ileus, areflexia, and autonomic instability, often manifested as orthostatic hypotension. Respiratory arrest and rhabdomyolysis can occur. The ECG can show flattening of the T wave, ST segment depression, U waves, premature atrial and ventricular contractions, and dysrythmias, especially in patients who are on digitalis. The kidney has a reduced ability to concentrate urine in hypokalemia, resulting in polyuria.

Laboratory data should include serum electrolytes, including magnesium, serum pH, and urine potassium. Urine potassium concentration of <15 mEq/L indicates renal conservation and suggests extrarenal loss. An ECG should be done looking for the alterations just noted.

Since serum potassium levels only measure extracellular potassium concentration, total body concentration may be decreased or normal. Also, potassium must cross the smaller extracellular space to the larger ICF, where the majority of potassium is stored. Both of these factors lead to concern of "overshoot hyperkalemia" during correction. In the patient without life-threatening complications, hypokalemia should be corrected gradually with oral supplementation or, in those patients with a contraindication to oral intake, an increase in the maintenance potassium concentration in the intravenous fluids. Underlying conditions that accompany the hypokalemia, such as alkalosis or hypomagnesemia, should be corrected. Sources of ongoing potassium loss are identified. The loss is measured and replaced. An effort should be made to determine the cause of the loss and, if possible, treat it. If hypokalemia is associated with digoxin use or life-threatening complications, such as cardiac dysrythmias, rhabdomyolysis, extreme muscle weakness, or respiratory arrest, intravenous therapy is required. Extreme care should be exercised in the ordering, preparation, and administration of intravenous potassium. Recommendations for dosage in pediatric patients range from 0.5 to 1 mEq/kg/dose (maximum dose: 30 mEq) to infuse at 0.3 to 0.5 mEq/kg/h (maximum rate: 1 mEq/kg/h). Potassium must be diluted prior to intravenous administration. In peripheral lines, the maximum concentration is 80 mEq/L. The maximum recommended central line concentration is 200 mEq/L (usually reserved for severely fluid restricted patients). Continuous ECG monitoring, along with frequent assessment of serum potassium levels, is essential during intravenous correction of hypokalemia.

CALCIUM

Calcium is one of the most abundant and important minerals in the body, with 99 percent of body calcium stored in bone. Of the 1 percent present in the circulation, 40 percent is bound to proteins such as albumin, 15 percent is complexed with anions such as phosphate and citrate, and 45 percent is physiologically free and ionized. Parathyroid hormone, vitamin D, and calcitonin interact to regulate calcium in a narrow range by controlling intestinal absorption, renal excretion, and skeletal distribution. Calcium is responsible for cellular depolarization, muscle excitation/contraction, neurotransmitter release, hormonal secretion, and the function of both leukocytes and platelets.

A serum calcium level measures both ionized and protein-bound calcium. Since approximately half of serum calcium is bound to albumin, the serum calcium level may need to be adjusted for alterations in the albumin level. For every 1 g/dL decrease in serum albumin, true serum calcium may be estimated by adding 0.8 mg/dL. Alternatively, ionized calcium levels are widely available.

Hypercalcemia

Hypercalcemia is defined as a serum calcium level >10.5 mg/dL. Although often asymptomatic, complaints may include constipation, anorexia, vomiting, abdominal pain, or pancreatitis. Rarely, lethargy, depression, psychosis, or coma may occur. ECG changes may include QT segment shortening, bradycardia, heart block, and sinus arrest. Nephrolithiasis can be an important consequence of hypercalcemia.

The conditions in adults that are commonly associated with hypercalcemia (hyperparathyroidism and malignancies of the breast, lung, kidney, and head and neck) are rare in children. In children, hypercalcemia with malignancy is associated with bone metastasis or tumor lysis syndrome. Other causes in children include primary or tertiary hyperparathyroidism, hyperthyroidism, vitamin D intoxication, immobilization, thiazide diuretics, milk-alkali syndrome, and sarcoidosis. Williams syndrome, consisting of peripheral pulmonic stenosis, aortic stenosis, and elfin facies, is associated with idiopathic infantile hypercalcemia. It is related to hypersensitivity to vitamin D and usually resolves by 2 years of age.

Laboratory investigation should include total and/or ionized serum calcium, serum albumin and total protein, electrolytes (including magnesium and phosphorus), BUN, creatinine, CBC, ECG, and urinalysis. Hyperchloremic metabolic acidosis suggests primary hyperparathyroidism.

In symptomatic patients or those with levels >14 mg/dL, therapy is aimed at expansion of ECF, calcium excretion, increased bone storage, and definitive treatment of the underlying cause. Volume expansion is begun with normal saline and followed by diuresis with furosemide to promote calcium excretion. Hemodialysis may be required in the setting of renal insufficiency or life-threatening dysrythmias. Calcitonin, glucocorticoids, mithramycin, and indomethacin have all been used to suppress bone resorption, although the onset of action is >24 hours.

Hypocalcemia

Hypocalcemia is defined as serum calcium <9 mg/dL. Major etiologies are hypoparathyroidism and vitamin D deficiency. Hyperphosphatemia and magnesium deficiency may lead to hypocalcemia. Additional etiologies are massive transfusion of citrated blood, phosphate enema toxicity, pancreatitis, and sepsis.

Nonspecific symptoms, including nausea, weakness, paresthesias, and irritability, are typical. Classic physical findings of neuromuscular irritability are Chvostek's and Trousseau's signs. In more severe cases, tetany, seizures, larygospasm, and psychiatric manifestations may be seen.

The ECG may show prolongation of the QT interval, bradycardia, and dysrythmias. Laboratory tests include ionized and total calcium, magnesium, phosphorus, albumin and total protein, BUN, creatinine, and alkaline phosphatase. Vitamin D and parathyroid hormone levels may help elucidate the etiology, as may urine calcium and phosphorus levels.

For significant or symptomatic hypocalcemia, intravenous calcium may be administered cautiously with continuous ECG monitoring. Calcium gluconate, 10 percent (50 to 100 mg/kg/dose), or calcium chloride, 10 percent (10 to 20 mg/kg/dose), may be administered at a maximum rate of 12 min/dose. Intravenous calcium is very irritating to tissues, and veins should be diluted prior to administration. The maximum concentration of calcium gluconate should be 50 mg/mL and calcium chloride, 20 mg/mL. It is preferably given through a central line or very secure peripheral venous access. It should never be given intramuscularly, subcutaneously, or via an endotracheal route, as tissue necrosis and sloughing will occur. Intravenous calcium predisposes to digitalis toxicity and precipitates when mixed with bicarbonate. Hyperphosphatemic patients are at risk of metastatic calcium deposition with calcium administration and require treatment aimed at lowering phosphorus levels. When hypomagnesemia is present, oral or intravenous correction should be undertaken. Magnesium sulfate may be administered intravenously at a dose of 25 to 50 mg/kg, diluted to a maximum concentration of 200 mg/mL, over 2 to 4 hours.

BIBLIOGRAPHY

Adelman RD, Solhaug MJ: Pathophysiology of body fluids and fluid therapy, in Behrman RE, Kliegman RM, Jenson HB (eds.): *Nelson Textbook of Pediatrics,* 16th ed. Philadelphia: Saunders, 2000, p 197, p 201.

Adrogue HJ, Madias NE: Hyponatremia. *N Engl J Med* 342:1581, 2000.

Farrar HC, Chande VT, Fitzpatrick DF, et al: Hyponatremia as the cause of seizures in infants: A retrospective analysis of incidence, severity and clinical predictors. *Ann Emerg Med* 26:42, 1995.

Gennari FJ: Current concepts: Hypokalemia. *N Engl J Med* 339:451, 1998.

Hill LL: Body composition and normal electrolyte concentrations. *Pediatr Clin North Am* 37:244, 1990.

Keating JP, Schears GH, Dodge PR: Oral water intoxication in infants: An American epidemic. *Am J Dis Child* 145:985, 1991.

Lee JH, Arcinue E, Ross BD: Brief report: Organic osmolytes in the brain of an infant with hypernatremia. *N Engl J Med* 331:439, 1994.

Lynch RE: Ionized calcium: Pediatric perspective. *Pediatr Clin North Am* 37:373, 1990.

Taketomo CK, Hodding JH, Kraus DM: *Pediatric Dosage Handbook,* 7th ed. Hudson, Ohio: Lexi-Comp, 2000.

58

Metabolic Acidosis

Margaret Paik
Marshall Lewis

HIGH-YIELD FACTS

- The normal range of pH of body fluids is between 7.35 and 7.45. Modification of two buffering systems, used by the lung and the kidney, helps to restore the pH toward the normal range when a disturbance occurs in the acid-base system.

- In general, for every 1 mEq/L fall in the serum bicarbonate, the P_{CO_2} should decrease 1 to 1.5 mmHg. If the P_{CO_2} is greater than expected, another acid-base disturbance, respiratory acidosis, should be considered; primary respiratory alkalosis should be considered if the P_{CO_2} is lower than expected.

- The serum anion gap (AG) is defined as the difference between the measured serum cations and anions. The formula for the AG is

$$AG = Na^+ - (Cl^- + HCO_3^-)$$

- The normal AG is between 8 and 12 mEq/L and represents serum anions other than chloride and bicarbonate, mostly negatively charged plasma proteins. In the presence of an acid, bicarbonate decreases as it is consumed as a buffer and an unmeasured acid is generated.

- Metabolic acidosis with a normal or near normal AG results from loss of bicarbonate, either through the gastrointestinal tract or the kidney, or from failure of the kidney to excrete an appropriate amount of hydrogen ion. A relative or absolute compensatory increase in chloride, along with sodium, preserves a normal AG.

- The finding of an elevated AG in the presence of a metabolic acidosis implies the presence of either an endogenously created or an exogenously ingested acid. In children, likely causes of acute endogenous production of acid are diabetic ketoacidosis, with the production of β-hydroxybutyric acid and acetoacetic acid, and processes that result in the accumulation of lactic acid.

- Another cause of elevated AG acidosis virtually unique to the pediatric patient is inborn errors of metabolism (IEM). Although these diseases are quite rare individually, as a group their incidence approaches 1 in 5000 live births.

- The diagnosis of an IEM depends on a high degree of suspicion. The typical emergency department (ED) presentation is a neonate with vomiting, lethargy, poor feeding, and failure to thrive.

- In pediatric patients, acute diarrhea is the most common cause of non-AG metabolic acidosis. Intestinal fluid, high in HCO_3^- and K^+ but low in Cl^-, is lost in the diarrheal fluid.

- Aside from the non-AG hyperchloremic metabolic acidosis, laboratory values in distal renal tubular acidosis may reveal hyponatremia, hypokalemia, and a urine pH of 6.5 to 7.5 in spite of the systemic acidosis. Hypokalemia can be severe enough to result in severe muscle weakness.

Regulation of the acid-base balance is a fundamental component of physiology. In clinical practice, acid-base status is reflected in the measurement of pH, defined as the negative log of the hydrogen ion concentration $[H^+]$. Fundamental acid-base kinetics for biologic fluids are described by the Henderson-Hasselbalch equation:

$$pH = 6.1 + \log_{10}[HCO_3^-]/[(0.03 \times Pa_{CO_2})]$$

The normal range of pH of body fluids is between 7.35 and 7.45. Modification of two buffering systems, used by the lung and the kidney, helps to restore the pH toward the normal range when a disturbance occurs in the acid-base system. The carbonic acid-bicarbonate system modifies the partial pressure of CO_2 (P_{CO_2}) to the concentration of HCO_3^-:

$$H_2O + CO_2 \leftrightarrow H_2CO_3 \leftrightarrow H^+ + HCO_3^-$$

Several types of acid-base disorders are encountered in the emergency department (ED), metabolic acidosis being one of the most common disturbances seen in children. Metabolic acidosis results from an increase in the concentration of hydrogen (H^+) or a decrease in the concentration of bicarbonate (HCO_3^-) or other buffers in the extracellular fluid. Despite the presence of compensatory mechanisms, either process can result in abnormally low pH. Metabolic acidosis in children differs in etiology and in some cases in presentation from that in adults. The emergency physician must be aware of the differential diagnosis and management of metabolic acidosis in children in order to initiate appropriate and timely therapy.

Acid production in the body is largely the result of the oxidation of nutrients. In general, the average child produces 1.5 to 2.5 mEq/kg/day of acid, whereas adults produce about 1 mEq/kg/day. The body must also cope with the addition of any nonphysiologic acids. A variety of buffer systems are available in the extracellular (ECF) and intracellular (ICF) fluid compartments. The initial defense is through buffering systems, which accept free H^+ and mitigate severe changes in pH; this is almost instantaneous in the ECF. The carbonic acid-bicarbonate system is the major buffering system in the ECF. Systemic acidosis stimulates the respiratory center to increase the excretion of CO_2, which increases pH and compensates for the acid load. The integrity of the bicarbonate-carbonic acid buffer system relies on the ability to maintain an open system for excreting CO_2; thus any factor that impedes ventilation will produce a rapid drop in pH. The system is also dependent on the kidney's ability to resorb HCO_3^- and excrete H^+, which is a slower process but essential in chronic compensation. In the ICF, HCO_3^-, proteins, phosphates, hemoglobin, amino acids, and bone carbonate are used as buffers.

It is important to recognize that values for pH, P_{CO_2}, and HCO_3^- will vary during childhood (Table 58-1). These differences are attributed to the relatively higher production of acid secondary to the increased metabolic demands in children and to an inability of the developing kidney to excrete acid and resorb bicarbonate. This "normal" tendency toward acidosis may predispose children to more severe disturbances in acid-base balance than adults.

In general, for every 1 mEq/L fall in the serum bicarbonate, the P_{CO_2} should decrease 1 to 1.5 mmHg. If the P_{CO_2} is greater than expected, another acid-base disturbance, respiratory acidosis, should be considered. A primary respiratory alkalosis should be considered if the P_{CO_2} is lower than expected.

Table 58-1. Normal Acid-Base Values for Pediatric Patients

Group	pH	P_{CO_2}	tCO_2
Preterm infant	7.35 ± 0.04	32 ± 3	17.9 ± 2.2
Term infant	7.34 ± 0.03	37 ± 1	20.2 ± 0.8
Children	7.41 ± 0.04	39 ± 3	25.2 ± 1.6
Male adults	7.39 ± 0.01	41 ± 2	25.2 ± 1.0

Source: From Edelman CM (ed): *Pediatric Kidney Disease.* Boston: Little Brown, 1992.

METABOLIC ACIDOSIS WITH ELEVATED ANION GAP

Calculation of the anion gap (AG) will help to elucidate the etiology of metabolic acidosis. The serum AG is defined as the difference between the measured serum cations and anions. In practice, sodium is the only cation used in calculating the AG, because the other extracellular cations, potassium, calcium, and magnesium, are present in relatively small quantities. The measured serum anions are chloride and bicarbonate. Thus, the formula for the AG is

$$AG = Na^+ - (Cl^- + HCO_3^-)$$

The normal AG is between 8 and 12 mEq/L and represents serum anions other than chloride and bicarbonate, mostly negatively charged plasma proteins. In the presence of an acid, bicarbonate decreases as it is consumed as a buffer, and an unmeasured acid is generated. This is distinctive from metabolic acidosis resulting from the loss of bicarbonate, in which the kidney actively reabsorbs NaCl, and the added chloride, when combined with the remaining bicarbonate, preserves a normal AG.

The finding of an elevated AG in the presence of a metabolic acidosis implies the presence of either an endogenously created or an exogenously ingested acid (see Table 79-4). In children, likely causes of acute endogenous production of acid are diabetic ketoacidosis, with the production of β-hydroxybutyric acid and acetoacetic acid, and processes that result in the accumulation of lactic acid. Lactic acid is an end product of anaerobic metabolism. Causes of lactic acidosis include seizures, hypoxemia, hyperthermia, and septic, cardiogenic and hypovolemic shock. Many ingestions cause metabolic acidosis, especially salicylates, alcohols, and iron.

Another cause of elevated AG acidosis virtually unique to the pediatric patient is inborn errors of metabolism (IEM). Although these diseases are quite rare individu-

Table 58-2. Inborn Errors of Metabolism Producing Acidosis

Organic acidemias
    Methylmalonic acidemia
    Propionic acidemia
    Isovaleric acidemia
Amino acidurias
    Maple syrup urine disease
Citrullinemia
Argininosuccinic aciduria
Glycogen storage disease
    Type I
    Type III
Fatty acid oxidation defects

Source: From Burton B: Inborn errors of metabolism: The clinical diagnosis in early infancy. *Pediatrics* 79:359, 1987.

ally, as a group their incidence approaches 1 in 5000 live births. Of the IEMs that cause metabolic acidosis, the most common are methylmalonic, propionic, and isovaleric acidemia. A more complete list is included in Table 58-2.

The diagnosis of an IEM depends on a high degree of suspicion. The typical ED presentation is a neonate with vomiting, lethargy, poor feeding, and failure to thrive. Such nonspecific findings make it difficult to distinguish IEM from more common diseases such as sepsis. Information that increases the possibility of an IEM includes a family history of such a disorder, an unexplained early death in a sibling, and a strong sweaty odor noted on physical exam.

Although the diagnosis of a specific IEM is unlikely to be made in the ED, helpful ancillary studies that are readily available include serum lactate, pyruvate, and ammonia.

NON–ANION GAP METABOLIC ACIDOSIS

Metabolic acidosis with a normal or near normal AG results from loss of bicarbonate, through either the gastrointestinal tract or the kidney, or from failure of the kidney to excrete an appropriate amount of hydrogen ion. A relative or absolute compensatory increase in chloride, along with sodium, preserves a normal AG. The clinical presentation of non-AG or hyperchloremic metabolic acidosis depends on the etiology but in general is unlikely to be as acute and fulminant as that of metabolic acidosis with an elevated AG.

Causes of non-AG or hyperchloremic metabolic acidosis include the following:

- Gastrointestinal loss of HCO_3^- from such causes as diarrhea, intestinal drainage or fistula, or ingestion of calcium chloride or magnesium chloride
- Renal loss of HCO_3^- through such factors as renal tubular acidosis, hypoaldosteronism, carbonic anhydrase inhibitors (e.g., acetazolamide), and potassium-sparing diuretics
- Miscellaneous causes such as dilutional acidosis, hyperalimentation, and recovery from ketoacidosis

DIARRHEAL DISEASE

In pediatric patients, acute diarrhea is the most common cause of non-AG metabolic acidosis. Intestinal fluid, high in HCO_3^- and K^+ but low in Cl^-, is lost in the diarrheal fluid. Because there is also contraction of the ECF, the remaining Cl^- has a smaller volume of distribution. In the ED, many infants appear well hydrated despite electrolyte profiles demonstrating serum bicarbonate between 16 and 20 mEq/L. The condition resolves with resolution of the diarrhea, although mild acidosis may continue until the total sodium deficit is corrected. Infants with diarrhea that results in severe dehydration may develop metabolic acidosis accompanied by an increased AG.

RENAL TUBULAR ACIDOSIS

The different types of renal tubular acidosis (RTA) are classified as type I or distal, type II or proximal, and type IV, which is associated with hypoaldosteronism and hyperkalemia. There are primary and secondary causes of RTA. The usual finding is a metabolic acidosis in which hyperchloremia preserves a normal AG. The hyperchloremia seen may be a result of renal loss of HCO_3^- without the concomitant loss of Cl^-.

Distal type I RTA is a defect in the ability of the kidney to secrete H^+, with renal HCO_3^- wasting and an inability to acidify the urine in response to an acid challenge. Patients with distal type I RTA usually cannot lower their urine pH below 5.5 despite severe acidosis. The acidification of urine takes place in the collecting tubules and is an active process by which H^+ is pumped into the tubular lumen in exchange for Na^+. Defects reported with distal RTA also include a relative paucity of luminal sodium and an inability to maintain a H^+ gradient, with a back-diffusion of H^+ ions.

Distal type I RTA is further divided into primary and secondary types. In the primary group, both permanent and transient varieties have been described. The permanent form, or Butler-Albright syndrome, results from a genetic defect that affects girls more often than boys. Clinically, findings are often subtle, with polyuria, occasional vomiting, mild dehydration, and constipation. Most often the syndrome is detected in the second or third year of life, when it presents with failure to thrive. If it remains undetected into early adulthood, it may present with nephrocalcinosis secondary to increased calcium secretion as bone is resorbed in an attempt to buffer the ongoing acidosis. The transient type was apparently common in Britain in the 1940s and 1950s but is now rare. Most patients present with anorexia, vomiting, and occasionally nephrocalcinosis. The syndrome usually resolves around 2 years of age.

The secondary type of distal RTA is associated with several disorders. The most common is obstructive uropathy. Other associated conditions include hypercalcemic and hypercalciuric states and complement-fixing immune disorders. Certain drugs, especially lithium and amphotericin B, can also produce distal type I RTA.

Aside from the non-AG hyperchloremic metabolic acidosis, laboratory values in distal RTA may reveal hyponatremia and hypokalemia. Hypokalemia can be severe enough to result in severe muscle weakness. Most importantly, despite a systemic acidosis, urine pH will typically be 6.5 to 7.5, reflecting the inability to excrete H^+.

Proximal type II RTA can be thought of as a defect in resorbing bicarbonate. Normally, virtually all filtered bicarbonate is resorbed, mostly in the proximal tubules. Carbonic anhydrase deficiency has been noted in some but not all cases. Hypokalemia is commonly seen.

Clinically the disorder is divided into primary and secondary syndromes. The primary form most often affects boys younger than 18 months of age. Initially affected patients may suffer from excessive vomiting, but the usual presentation is growth retardation or failure to thrive. Although proximal type II RTA can be an isolated finding, it more often occurs with Fanconi's syndrome. The secondary form is also associated with other disease processes, including hereditary fructose intolerance, cystinosis, galactosemia, and glycogen storage disease. In addition, heavy metals (e.g., cadmium and lead) and the use of outdated tetracycline have been implicated in proximal RTA.

Unlike patients with distal type I RTA, these children retain the ability to secrete hydrogen into the distal tubule and therefore can acidify the urine. In addition, patients with proximal RTA do not develop nephrocalcinosis and osteomalacia. It is postulated that the ability to acidify the urine protects the acid-base balance and reduces bone resorption, despite the ongoing loss of bicarbonate.

Type IV RTA is associated with hyperkalemia. The disorder is associated with hypoaldosteronism and in some cases with decreased responsiveness of the distal tubules to aldosterone, leading to impaired K^+ and H^+ secretion. There may also be hyponatremia and volume depletion. Patients are able to make a mildly acidic urine. Type IV RTA is common in adults and is associated with renal insufficiency, volume contraction, and potassium-sparing drugs.

The diagnosis of RTA is unlikely to be made in the ED, but a high degree of suspicion will lead to an appropriate evaluation, which is usually made in consultation with a pediatric nephrologist. The fundamental treatment of all types of RTA is directed at maintaining a normal or nearly normal pH. Most patients can be managed with a supplemental alkali at a dose of 1 to 10 mEq/kg/day, depending on the type of RTA. Some patients may require supplemental potassium. Patients with type IV RTA may benefit from therapy with mineralocorticoid, furosemide, and supplemental NaCl. Successful treatment can prevent some of the complications of RTA and permit normal growth and development.

CLINICAL PRESENTATION

The clinical presentation of metabolic acidosis depends on the underlying disease process and the rapidity with which it developed. Because the primary compensatory mechanism causes a decrease in P_{CO_2}, tachypnea is a universal finding in the acutely ill patient. Severe alterations in pH affect mental status; patients may be agitated, lethargic, or in extreme cases comatose. Alteration in mental status is especially severe for patients in whom acidosis develops quickly. In situations in which hypovolemia is an associated problem, as in diabetic ketoacidosis, hemorrhage, or gastroenteritis with dehydration, poor perfusion is usually clinically evident. Common gastrointestinal complaints include nausea, vomiting, and abdominal pain. Patients with chronic, well-compensated metabolic acidosis can have a more insidious presentation, as in the infant with RTA, who may present with failure to thrive.

The necessary laboratory evaluation of the patient with metabolic acidosis depends on the suspected etiology. The presence of acidosis is confirmed by obtaining an arterial blood gas. In addition to confirming acidosis, the arterial gas should demonstrate adequate respiratory compensation. Serum electrolytes (with calculation of the AG), blood urea nitrogen, creatinine, and serum glucose are also tested. If ingestion is suspected, a toxicology screen is indicated. A lactic acid level and serum osmolality may also be helpful. If the osmol gap, the difference between the measured plasma osmolality and the calculated value, is >10, an osmotically active particle, such as methanol or ethylene glycol, should be suspected. Osmolality is calculated using the following formula:

$$Osm = 2[Na^+] + [glucose]/18 + [BUN]/2.8 + [ethanol]/4.6$$

TREATMENT

The treatment of an elevated AG acidosis is primarily based on the treatment of the underlying disease. Many severely ill patients require aggressive fluid resuscitation. Patients with severe alteration of mental status may require intubation and mechanical ventilation. For patients requiring intubation, it is important to maintain hyperventilation in order to avoid the precipitous fall in pH that will occur with a rise in the P_{CO_2}. Chapter 3 discusses the management of low-perfusion states, which result in lactic acidosis. Chapter 54 discusses the management of metabolic acidosis secondary to the formation of ketoacids, and Section XVII discusses the management of toxicologic emergencies.

Controversies focus on the role of bicarbonate therapy as well as that of other buffering agents such as tromethamine (Tham) and Carbicarb (an equimolar solution of $NaHCO_3$ and Na_2CO_3). In practice, therapy with bicarbonate is rarely indicated, especially as a bolus. The use of $NaHCO_3^-$ is associated with hyperosmolality, hypernatremia, hypokalemia, overcorrection with alkalosis, and cerebrospinal fluid acidosis. Therapy with buffering agents may play a role in the postresuscitative phase of asphyxial arrest. The treatment of inborn errors of metabolism is complex and requires consultation with a pediatric endocrinologist. Treatment for RTA is discussed above.

BIBLIOGRAPHY

Badrich T, Hickman P: The anion gap: A reappraisal. *Am J Clin Pathol* 98:249, 1992.

Cronan K, Norman ME: Renal and electrolyte emergencies, in Fleisher GR, Ludwig S (eds): *Textbook of Pediatric Emergency Medicine,* 4th ed. Philadelphia: Lippincott Williams & Wilkins, 2000, pp 811–858.

Jospe N, Forbes G: Fluids and electrolytes—clinical aspects. *Pediatr Rev* 17:395, 1996.

Kurtzman NA: Renal tubular acidosis syndromes. *South Med J* 93:1042–1052, 2000.

Lolekha PH, Vanavanan S, Lolekha S: Update on value of the anion gap in clinical diagnosis and laboratory evaluation. *Clin Chim Acta* 307:33–36, 2001.

Mizok BA, Falk JL: Lactic acidosis in critical illness. *Crit Care Med* 20:80, 1992.

Salem MM, Mujuis SK: Gaps in the anion gap. *Arch Intern Med* 152:1625, 1992.

Shapiro JI, Kaehny WD: Pathogenesis and management of metabolic acidosis and alkalosis, in Schrier RW (ed): *Renal and Electrolyte Disorders,* 5th ed. Philadelphia: Lippincott-Raven Publishers, 1997, pp 130–171.

Swenson ER: Metabolic acidosis. *Respir Care* 46:342–353, 2001.

Zaritsky A: Pediatric resuscitation pharmacology. *Ann Emerg Med* 22:445, 1993.

59

Male Genitourinary Problems

Marianne Gausche-Hill

HIGH-YIELD FACTS

- Epididymitis is caused by urinary tract infections in young children, but by sexually transmitted disease in older children and adolescents. Antibiotic selection should be based on the likelihood of each, based on age and presentation.

- Testicular torsion is the most common cause of acute scrotal pain in children. Prompt urologic consultation must be obtained in each case.

- Color Doppler ultrasound is the diagnostic test of choice for evaluation of the acute scrotum in children.

- A genitourinary exam should be performed on all children with abdominal or genitourinary complaints, as signs and symptoms may be nonspecific and abdominal pain may be caused by testicular torsion, inguinal hernia or, rarely, by testicular tumor.

- The emergency department can reduce 85 to 95 percent of cases of inguinal hernia.

- Most varicoceles are benign and 85 percent of them are left sided; however, persistent scrotal swelling and a "bag of worms" appearance indicates possible obstruction from tumor.

- With normal growth and stretching of the prepuce, it will become retractable in 90 percent of children by the age of 6 years.

- The evaluation of children with paraphimosis must begin by establishing that the children have been circumcised and by determining that the cause is not secondary to hair tourniquet syndrome. Treatment is manual reduction of the prepuce over the glans penis.

- Pathophysiology of priapism can be divided into two mechanisms:
  1. Low flow or ischemic mechanism (sickle cell disease or polycythemia)
  2. High flow or engorgement mechanism (trauma)

  Treatment is targeted at resolution of these factors.

TESTICULAR PAIN/SCROTAL MASSES

The causes of the painful scrotum in children are varied. The emergency physician (EP) must distinguish these causes by considering the age of the patient, the history of symptoms, the physical findings, and the results of the diagnostic evaluation. One may separate the cause of scrotal swelling as painful or painless testicular swelling (Table 59-1). In all cases, the possibility of a surgical emergency must be considered and the evaluation and management must proceed accordingly.

Epididymitis

Epididymitis is not as common in young children as it is in adolescents and adults. The EP in evaluating young patients for epididymitis must always consider the possibility of testicular torsion as the cause of the scrotal pain and swelling because the consequences of a missed diagnosis can be devastating.

Pathophysiology

In young children, <6 years of age, urinary tract anomalies such as posterior urethral valves with vesicoureteric

415

Table 59-1. Causes of Scrotal Swelling in Children

Painful	Painless
Epididymitis	Testicular tumor
Testicular torsion	Idiopathic scrotal edema
Torsion of the appendix testis	Henoch-Schönlein purpura
Incarcerated hernia	Inguinal hernia
Idiopathic scrotal edema	Hydrocele
Trauma (testicular rupture)	Varicocele
Scrotal cellulitis or inflammation	Anasarca

reflux may be present and predispose to infection. Urinary tract infection (UTI), commonly caused by pathogens, such as *Escherichia coli, Klebsiella pneumoniae,* and *Pseudomonas aeruginosa,* can lead to local inflammation and swelling of the epididymis. In the adolescent, anatomic abnormalities are rare and epididymitis is often caused by sexually transmitted diseases, such as *Neisseria gonorrhoeae* and *Chlamydia trachomatis.*

Signs and Symptoms

A careful history must be obtained:

- Previous scrotal pain or surgeries
- History of trauma
- History of sexual activity
- History of urinary symptoms
- Vomiting
- Fever
- Time course for the onset of symptoms

Symptoms in young children may be vague and nonspecific. Fever and vomiting may be present followed by swelling of the epididymis and the hemiscrotum. The caregivers may note scrotal swelling and bring infants or children in for evaluation. In the older child, the onset is often insidious with pain isolated to the hemiscrotum and later becomes diffuse. Fever and urinary symptoms may also be present.

Physical examination reveals an erythematous, warm, swollen epididymis, testicle, and scrotum. A careful examination should note that tenderness is more posterior and lateral to the adjacent testis and can be separated from actual testicular tenderness. Prehn's sign, or relief upon elevation of the scrotum, may be present but is not reliable in distinguishing epididymitis from testicular torsion.

Diagnostic Evaluation

In prepubescent children, epididymitis is difficult to distinguish clinically from testicular torsion. A urinalysis may be helpful in showing signs of urinary tract infection with increased white blood cells (WBCs) and bacteria; but pyuria is present in only half the cases of epididymitis. A complete blood cell count may reveal an elevated white blood cell count and left shift, however it is often normal in epididymitis. Because the consequences of a missed testicular torsion are dire, the EP should obtain prompt urologic consultation when the cause of the scrotal pain is unclear. Nuclear medicine imaging (testicular scan using technetium pertechnetate) or color Doppler ultrasonography (US) should be performed on all children in whom the diagnosis of the scrotal swelling is unclear. Both the nuclear scan and the color Doppler US will reveal normal or increased flow to the affected testis if the patient has epididymitis. There may be a higher rate of indeterminate studies in infants and young children. Once the diagnosis of epididymitis is confirmed, the evaluation for young children or adolescents in whom a UTI is suspected includes a urine culture. An intravenous pyelogram (IVP) or computed tomography (CT) of the abdomen without contrast may be performed to look for urinary tract anomalies or obstruction from renal stones in the adolescent, and renal ultrasound and voiding cystourethrogram performed on prepubescent children who may have a preexisting urologic abnormality. In sexually active adolescents, a urethral swab for *N. gonorrhoeae* and *Chlamydia* cultures and blood for VDRL or RPR should be sent.

Management

Management is dependent upon the age and toxicity of children. Children under 1 month of age with associated UTI should be admitted to the hospital and receive IV antibiotics. This approach should be considered for infants 3 months of age or younger as well. Older infants and children under 2 years of age may also require admission depending on the level of toxicity and associated signs and symptoms.

Inpatient antibiotic therapy for infants and children with a suspected urinary source should include ampicillin and an aminoglycoside or cefotaxime (Table 59-2). The majority of children can be managed as outpatients. For the nonsexually active child, although drug resistance is

Table 59-2. Antibiotic Therapy for Epididymitis in Children

Antibiotic	Dose	Route
Outpatient Management		
Nonsexually active		
Trimethoprim-sulfamethoxazole	8–10 mg/kg/24 h	PO bid for 10–14 days
Or cephalexin	25–50 mg/kg/24 h	PO qid for 10 days
Sexually active		
Ceftriaxone	250 mg	IM
plus (if patient ≥9 years of age)		
doxycycline	100 mg	PO bid for 10 days
or tetracycline	500 mg	PO qid for 10 days
plus (if patient <9 years of age)		
erythromycin	50 mg/kg/24 h	PO qid for 10 days
Inpatient Management		
Ampicillin	100 mg/kg/24 h	IV q 6 h
plus gentamicin	7.5 mg/kg/24 h	IV q 8 h
or cefotaxime	50–150 mg/kg/24 h	IV q 6 h
or ceftriaxone	50–100 mg/kg/24 h	IV q 12–24 h

PO, nothing by mouth; bid, twice daily; qid, 4 times daily; IM, intramuscularly.

on the rise, trimethoprim (TMP)-sulfamethoxazole orally for 10 to 14 days is the drug of choice. Cephalexin may also be used in this age group. For the sexually active adolescent, especially if there is urethral discharge, antibiotic treatment should include ceftriaxone, 250 mg intramuscularly, followed by doxycycline, 100 mg orally twice a day for 10 days. Patients <9 years of age should be treated with erythromycin, 50 mg/kg/day divided 4 times a day. Prompt urologic consultation and subsequent follow-up is recommended for all of these patients.

Testicular Torsion

Testicular torsion may occur in children of any age, from infancy to adulthood. The peak incidence of torsion in the pediatric age group occurs in adolescence. Torsion of the testes is a urologic emergency and results in a significant amount of legal action against EPs for missed diagnosis. The EP must suspect this diagnosis in any child with complaint of scrotal pain or signs of scrotal swelling on physical examination.

Pathophysiology

The classic description of the anatomic abnormality associated with torsion is the "bell-clapper" deformity that

is often bilateral and causes the testes to have a horizontal lie within the scrotal sac (Fig. 59-1). The testicular attachments to the intrascrotal subcutaneous tissue of the tunica vaginalis are incomplete, allowing the testis to twist within the scrotal sac along with the spermatic cord and associated testicular artery. If the torsion is complete, vascular compromise ensues and eventually the testis will necrose and atrophy. Intermittent torsion may

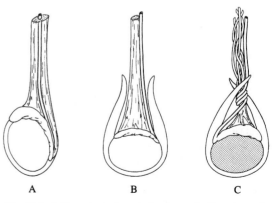

Fig. 59-1. *A.* Normal attachment of tunica vaginalis to the testis. *B.* Abnormal attachment resulting in horizontal lie of the testis. *C.* Resultant torsion of the spermatic cord.

occur sparing the testes for a longer time interval. Therefore, the actual duration of symptoms may not necessarily predict the viability of the testis. After 4 hours of pain, the salvage rate is 96 percent, but drops to 20 percent after 12 hours of pain and to <10 percent at 24 hours. Patients with symptoms for >24 hours are unlikely to have a viable testis.

Signs and Symptoms

History may be variable and include sudden onset of unilateral scrotal or testicular pain, followed by vomiting. Patients may also relate a history of previous symptoms on the other side, and the EP should be alerted to the possibility of bilateral testicular torsion. Many times the history is less clear and 6 percent of the time includes a history of trauma. Associated symptoms of nausea, vomiting, and abdominal or flank pain are common. Unilateral lower abdominal pain may indicate an undescended testis that has torsed, and indeed undescended testes are 10 times more likely to torse than fully descended ones.

Physical examination often reveals a swollen, tender, and erythematous hemiscrotum. The testis may be high riding or lying horizontally within the scrotum. Tenderness of the affected testis is diffuse, and the cremasteric reflex may be absent. Elevating the testis will cause further pain (Prehn's sign) instead of the relief that can be seen in epididymitis; however, Prehn's sign cannot reliably include or exclude torsion as the diagnosis.

Diagnostic Evaluation

In equivocal cases, a urinalysis should be performed looking for signs of UTI that are sometimes seen in cases of epididymitis. Other laboratory studies such as complete blood cell counts and chemistries are not helpful and could delay definitive management. Scrotal Doppler for testicular artery flow is rarely helpful because of the high (20 percent) false-positive and -negative rates. Once the diagnosis of testicular torsion is considered, urologic consultation should be obtained. Further diagnostic evaluation is reserved for those patients in which the diagnosis of torsion is in question and in which any delay in obtaining studies will not result in increased morbidity.

The nuclear medicine scan with 99^m technetium pertechnetate has been the diagnostic test of choice in the past, but many clinicians are opting to evaluate testicular artery flow with color Doppler US. Neither test should delay the urologic consultation. The radionuclide testicular scan requires that IV access be obtained, which can cause added pain for children. This test is otherwise simple and fairly rapid (25 min). Testicular scans may not be available 24 hours a day in some hospitals, causing delay in management. A unilateral "cold" defect on the side of the testicular pain indicates lack of blood flow to the testis and indicates possible torsion. Accuracy is excellent and ranges from 86 to 100 percent, but false-positive and -negative scans occur. Gray scale US alone is useful in the evaluation of many scrotal disorders, however it may not reliably distinguish between cases of epididymitis and torsion.

Color Doppler US is very accurate in adults, with reported sensitivity of 86 to 100 percent, specificity of 100 percent, and accuracy of 97 percent. Color Doppler US involves no radiation exposure and can be easily performed. Prospective studies in small numbers of children demonstrate that while accurate there are false-positive studies in prepubescent children because of the small testis and the low volume of arterial flow. Additional limitations to its general use include variability in experience of the physician interpreting the test.

Management

Rapid urologic consultation should be obtained on all patients with suspected torsion. Manual detorsion of the torsed testes may be attempted by the EP to reduce the ischemic time while awaiting the arrival of the urologist. Patients are sedated, and the testicle is detorsed by turning the testicle outward toward the thigh like "opening a book." Patients must then undergo intraoperative bilateral orchiopexy to avoid recurrence. In all cases of torsion, the affected testicle is untwisted and the contralateral testis is pexed. Orchidectomy of the affected testicle is often recommended. However, leaving the testicle in the scrotum did not result in autosensitization in 17 of 18 patients in one study.

Torsion of the Appendix Testis

Appendices are common and may occur on the testicle, the spermatic cord, or the epididymis. The hydatid of Morgagni or appendix testis is the most common of the types of vestiges to torse. Torsion of the appendix testis is often difficult to distinguish from torsion of the spermatic cord. Torsion of the appendix testis frequently occurs between 10 and 14 years of age, an age group in which testicular torsion also occurs.

Signs and Symptoms

Signs and symptoms of torsion of the appendix testis may be less severe than those of testicular torsion, but may be indistinguishable. Systemic symptoms such as nausea and vomiting are rare, and the physical exam may reveal focal tenderness in the upper pole of the testis or diffuse testicular enlargement and pain. A "blue dot" sign is occasionally noted in young children when the necrotic appendage casts a blue hue under the scrotal skin.

Diagnostic Evaluation

Laboratory evaluation is not helpful, and the urinalysis is normal. Testicular scan or color Doppler US is normal or reveals increased flow to the testicle.

Management

Once the diagnosis of torsion of the appendix testis is made, bed rest, urologic follow-up, and analgesia are recommended. Surgical intervention is sometimes indicated in cases in which the diagnosis of testicular torsion cannot be reliably excluded. Most patients are much improved within days and complications are rare.

Scrotal and Testicular Trauma

Trauma to the scrotum can occur by many mechanisms including child abuse. Most often, the mechanism is blunt, a result of play or motor vehicle accident. The resulting injury is scrotal hematoma and, rarely, testicular rupture.

Testicular rupture occurs when the testis is crushed against the bony pelvis. Patients have a painful, swollen testis after a traumatic incident. If the mechanism was minor, consider the possibility of a tumor, as tumors may rupture after minimal trauma. Bleeding into the scrotum occurs, and the scrotum may be ecchymotic or tense with blood. The testis may be difficult to palpate and may have an irregular border or is ill defined. If testicular rupture is suspected, prompt evaluation of the integrity of the testis by US is essential. Ultrasonography can also locate a dislocated testicle that was displaced after major trauma. Urologic consultation should be done immediately once the diagnosis of testicular rupture is made.

Scrotal hematomas and testicular contusions are treated with bed rest, scrotal support, ice packs (if tolerated), and analgesics. Testicular rupture is treated by surgical exploration and repair, although testicular salvage rates are poor.

Testicular Tumors

Testicular tumors are rare in childhood. They are more common in whites and less common in African Americans. The types of testicular tumors include teratomas, embryonal carcinomas, yolk sac, choriocarcinomas, Leydig cell, and Sertoli cell. Lymphoma and leukemia can metastasize to the testis and present as a testicular mass as well. The undescended testis is at increased risk to contain a tumor, especially if the testis is located intraabdominally (50 times).

Signs and Symptoms

Most often children (and adults) have a feeling of fullness, tugging, or increased weight to the scrotum. Patients or patients' caregivers may have felt a mass. On physical examination, the mass is firm, smooth, or nodular and will not transilluminate. Generally the tumor is painless, but bleeding into the tumor can cause sudden onset of testicular pain or referred pain to the abdomen or flank. A thorough physical examination should be performed including examination for lymphadenopathy, abdominal mass, or hepatosplenomegaly, petechial rash, and gynecomastia.

Diagnostic Evaluation

A urinalysis should be performed, as well as a complete blood cell count. The urine should be tested for the presence of human chorionic gonadotropin by a rapid urine pregnancy test as this hormone is often produced by germ cell tumors. Ultrasonography may be performed in cases where the presence of a tumor mass is unclear.

Management

Urologic consultation and prompt biopsy or removal of the mass is necessary to establish tumor type and subsequent treatment options for patients.

Inguinal Hernia

Pathophysiology

Inguinal hernia repair is the most common surgery performed on children. It occurs when peritoneal or pelvic contents herniate through a patent processus vaginalis into the scrotal sac. Boys are 5 times more likely to have an inguinal hernia than are girls.

Signs and Symptoms

Inguinal hernias often present in the first year of life when parents note an intermittent bulge into the scrotal sac when the infant cries or coughs. Some parents report that the infant is fussy. Children may note a pulling feeling or a heaviness in the groin and also note a bulge with increases in intraabdominal pressure. Systemic signs of fever, abdominal pain, and nausea and vomiting should alert the clinician to the possibility of incarceration of the hernia. Other signs of incarceration include a firm, painful, nonreducible mass in the scrotum.

Diagnostic Evaluation

In most cases, a diagnostic evaluation is not needed since inguinal hernia can be diagnosed from history and physical examination. An inguinal hernia should transilluminate, distinguishing it from the tumor. If the diagnosis is in question, US can be performed to establish the diagnosis.

Management

Most reducible inguinal hernias can be referred to a surgeon for repair. Incarcerated hernias can be reduced 85 to 95 percent of the time with firm finger pressure on the internal inguinal ring, analgesics, ice pack to the area, and placement of patients in the Trendelenburg position. If the hernia is reduced easily, then patients can be discharged home with close follow-up with a surgeon for definitive repair. Patients with hernias that do not reduce easily, but still can be reduced, should be admitted for observation and delayed surgical repair. Patients with hernias that remain incarcerated or patients that demonstrate signs of peritonitis or bowel perforation must be taken immediately to the operating room. In these cases, stabilization of patients with fluid resuscitation and antibiotics should be initiated in the ED.

Henoch-Schönlein Purpura

Henoch-Schönlein purpura (HSP) is a systemic vasculitis that often results in abdominal pain, gastrointestinal bleeding, purpuric rash, nephritis, and arthritis. Patients may also complain of testicular pain, scrotal edema, and swelling, or purpuric rash on the scrotum. In some cases, it is impossible to clinically distinguish HSP from testicular torsion. The EP must then assume that the patient has testicular torsion; consult a urologist; and obtain color Doppler US or nuclear scan. If the diagnostic evaluation is negative and the patient has other features of HSP, surgical exploration may not be necessary.

Hydrocele

A hydrocele is formed from a patent processus vaginalis that normally regresses to form the tunica vaginalis. The hydrocele may communicate with the peritoneal cavity and can be associated with an indirect inguinal hernia. Fluid is noted adjacent to the testis and may result in a swollen and bluish-appearing scrotum. Transillumination of the swelling reveals that the mass is fluid filled, but it may be difficult to distinguish hydrocele from indirect inguinal hernia. If the hydrocele becomes or presents as a painful swelling, then the physician must consider intraperitoneal pathology, such as a ruptured appendix, or testicular torsion as the primary cause, otherwise a nonpainful hydrocele may be observed for 6 months to 1 year of age for spontaneous resolution. If the hydrocele persists past the first year of life, a patent processus vaginalis is surgically repaired.

Varicocele

Varicocele often presents in the adolescent male as painless scrotal swelling. Incompetent valves in the veins of the pampiniform plexus result in venous dilatation and a scrotum that feels like a "bag of worms." Approximately 85 percent of varicoceles are left-sided and are usually benign in nature, but could represent obstruction at the level of the renal vein from a tumor. Right-sided varicoceles may indicate obstruction by tumor at the level of the inferior vena cava (IVC). Patients should all be examined in the standing position, which often exaggerates the findings of scrotal enlargement and "bag of worms" appearance, as well as in the supine position in which these findings are minimized or absent. Patients in whom the scrotal swelling persists in the supine position should be evaluated for obstruction at the level of the renal vein on the left or the IVC on the right by renal ultrasound, IVP, or angiography. Surgical repair may be necessary for cases of testicular atrophy and signs of proximal obstruction.

Other Causes of Scrotal Pain or Swelling

Other causes of scrotal swelling with and without pain include scrotal cellulitis, idiopathic scrotal edema, and lymphadenitis.

Fournier's Gangrene

There have been 56 cases of Fournier's gangrene in children reported. This rare entity of infectious origin that results in necrotizing fascitis may present initially as cellulitis, balanitis, balanoposthitis, or scrotal pain and swelling. Patients may appear relatively nontoxic even when obvious gangrene appears in the perineum. Although staphylococcal and streptococcal organisms are the most common organisms to be cultured, management includes broad-spectrum antibiotic therapy to cover anaerobic and aerobic, gram-positive and -negative organisms. Prompt surgical consultation and operative incision and drainage of infected tissue with excision of necrotic tissue is paramount. Generally the prognosis in children is better than it is in adult patients, and more conservative surgical debridement is recommended.

PENILE EMERGENCIES

Phimosis

Pathophysiology

Phimosis occurs when the distal prepuce is unable to be retracted over the glans penis. Normally, the prepuce cannot be retracted over the glans in infants and it should not be forced. With normal growth and stretching of the prepuce, it will become retractable in 90 percent of children by the age of 6 years. Local irritation or infection (balanoposthitis) can cause an abnormal constriction of the prepuce, preventing its ability to retract normally.

Signs and Symptoms

Phimosis may be noted on routine physical examination or may be reported by parents. Pain and swelling can occur with associated infections of the glans. Urinary stream in some cases may be diverted to one side or children may have hematuria.

Physical examination generally establishes the diagnosis. The EP will find a constricted distal prepuce that is unable to be retracted over the glans penis. Patients will sometimes have concomitant balanitis or balanoposthitis.

Diagnostic Evaluation

The diagnosis is established clinically; however, examination of the urine for UTI may be warranted in rare cases. If patients demonstrate signs of urinary tract obstruction, such as inability to urinate, abdominal fullness, or increased frequency of urination but with small amounts, then renal function studies should be obtained

to assess renal function. Renal US may be obtained to better define the degree of obstruction.

Management

As most cases are not a result of a pathologic condition but a result of normal growth and development, reassurance and an explanation of the natural course of this condition to parents is needed. Betamethasone valerate 0.6% cream applied twice daily for 2 weeks has been used to treat phimosis and may be prescribed in cases in which the phimosis is not anatomic but pathologic. Patients with recurrent balanitis, balanoposthitis, UTI, or obstruction should be referred to a urologist for circumcision.

Paraphimosis

Pathophysiology

Paraphimosis is a condition in which the prepuce in the uncircumcised male is retracted over the glans and then is unable to move into normal position. The prepuce, once retracted over the glans, causes venous congestion that further prevents the prepuce from movement into a normal position.

Signs and Symptoms

Patients have pain, swelling, and edema of the distal penis and prepuce. The physician must establish whether or not children have been circumcised; if not, a thorough examination to look for possible hair tourniquets and penile foreign bodies must follow.

Management

The management of this condition focuses on retracting the prepuce over the head of the glans. Without anesthesia, most children poorly tolerate ice packs to the groin. The physician may place a penile block by injecting lidocaine 1% without epinephrine around the base of the penis. This will effectively reduce the pain. Ice packs can then be placed for 10 minutes after which manual reduction should be attempted (Fig. 59-2). The physician's index fingers are placed on the leading edge of the edematous foreskin, and the thumbs are placed on the glans. Thumb pressure is directed inward toward the body as the prepuce is pushed back over the glans. Once reduction is complete, the prepuce should lie over the end of the glans and the urethral opening should not

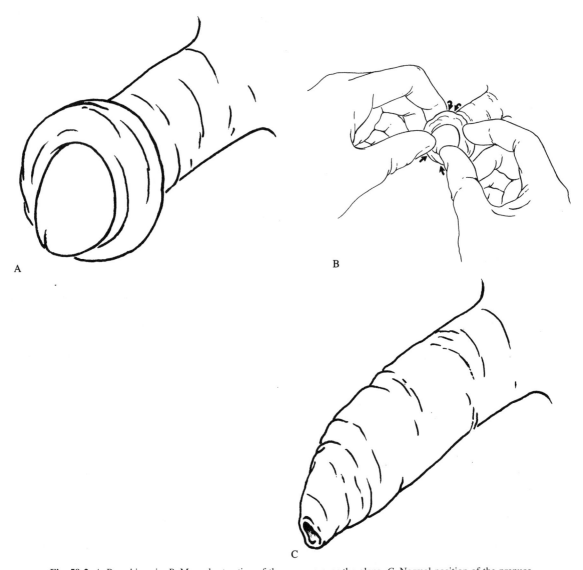

Fig. 59-2. *A.* Paraphimosis. *B.* Manual retraction of the prepuce over the glans. *C.* Normal position of the prepuce.

be visible (Fig. 59-2). If retraction of the prepuce is successful and the child is able to urinate spontaneously, then the child can be discharged with urologic follow-up. If the prepuce cannot be retracted, then emergent urologic consultation is needed for circumcision.

Balanitis and Balanoposthitis

Balanitis and balanoposthitis are infections of the glans and foreskin. Both are relatively more common in the uncir-

cumcised male (6 percent) but may also be found in circumcised children (3 percent). It frequently presents during the preschool age years and rarely prior to toilet training.

Pathophysiology

Balanitis may be caused by entrapment of organisms under a poorly retractable foreskin. Gram-negative or positive bacterial organisms may be causative, and Group A beta hemolytic streptococcus has been implicated. Monilial infections are also associated with balanoposthitis in infants (Fig. 59-3). In adolescents, syphilis as a cause must also be considered. Chronic balanitis or phimosis may result in balanitis xerotica obliterans, a sclerotic disease of the prepuce noted histologically.

Signs and Symptoms

Signs and symptoms include swelling, erythema, penile discharge, dysuria, bleeding, and, rarely, ulceration of the glans. Phimosis can occur, but is uncommon. A careful examination of the base of the penis should be performed to look for a strand of hair that may cause strangulation and edema.

Diagnostic Evaluation

Balanitis is diagnosed clinically. In selected cases, the clinician may wish to obtain a urinalysis and send bacterial and chlamydial cultures of the penile discharge.

Management

Local care with soaks (Sitz baths) and topical antibiotic ointment are recommended. The addition of oral antibiotics, such as cephalexin, for 5 to 7 days, may be reserved for the more severe cases. Patients should be followed within two days to assure that symptoms have resolved. Children with repeated episodes may be referred to a urologist for elective circumcision.

Priapism

Priapism is a prolonged painful erection unaccompanied by continued sexual stimulation. It is relatively uncom-

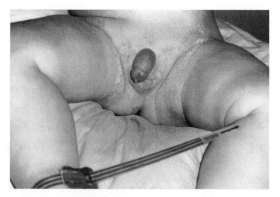

Fig. 59-3. Balanoposthitis in an infant with monilial diaper rash.

mon in childhood except in patients with sickle cell disease. In this group, priapism occurs in about 3 to 10 percent of patients. Priapism is exceedingly rare in the neonatal period. Polycythemia and trauma are presumed etiologies in this latter group.

Pathophysiology

Pathophysiology of priapism can be divided into two mechanisms:

1. Low flow or ischemic mechanism (sickle cell disease, polycythemia)
2. High flow or engorgement mechanism (trauma)

Either mechanism results in engorgement of the corpora cavernosum with a flaccid corpora spongiosum and glans. This engorgement leads to inflammation, increased stasis of blood, deoxygenation, further sludging, thrombosis, fibrosis, and impotence if unrelieved. Drugs of abuse such as cocaine, amphetamine, alcohol, and marijuana have also been implicated. Fortunately, most cases of priapism can be treated medically and do not result in impotence.

Factors that may precipitate priapism in patients with sickle cell anemia are infection, trauma, acidosis, hypoxia, sexual intercourse, and masturbation. Other etiologies of priapism include trauma, drugs, leukemia, Kawasaki's disease, and polycythemia.

Signs and Symptoms

Patients often have delayed presentation, possibly a result of embarrassment. Patients are noted on physical examination to have an erect penis, which is firm on the dorsal surface (corpora cavernosum) and soft on the ventral surface (corpora spongiosum) and the glans. Patients should be asked about placement of urethral and penile foreign bodies and the bladder palpated for enlargement. Urinary retention may be associated with priapism and can be easily relieved by placement of a urinary catheter.

Diagnostic Evaluation

Priapism is a clinical diagnosis based on physical examination. However, the physician may wish to order a complete blood cell count, looking for evidence of leukemia or anemia; a hemoglobin electrophoresis, looking for possible sickle cell disease; renal functions, if there has been significant urinary retention; and, if patients have suffered perineal trauma, a retrograde cystourethrogram may be indicated. Color Doppler US may be used to determine if the priapism is secondary to a low flow or a high flow state.

Management

Treatment is based on the presumed etiology. Providing oxygen, hydration, and analgesics to patients with sickle cell disease may alleviate the priapism. If not, an exchange transfusion of the patient's blood with 30 mL/kg of packed cells is performed in an effort to get the patient's hemoglobin above 10 g/dL. Patients with leukemia may receive hydration and analgesics and appropriate treatment for their cancer. A urinary catheter should be inserted to relieve bladder distension. Once medical management is initiated, patients should be admitted for observation. Urologic consultation is recommended in all cases. The timing of surgical management of priapism is controversial. Some clinicians recommend waiting no longer than 24 hours for medical management, followed by intracavernous injection of a vasoconstrictor (epinephrine, ephedrine, or phenylephrine) and, if unsuccessful, by surgical shunting of blood from the cavernosum to the spongiosum or the glans. Intravenous ketamine hydrochloride has been used to treat priapism in the newborn. Parenteral vasodilators, including hydralazine or terbutaline (0.25 to 0.5 mg IV every 4 hours), have been used to treat priapism but with varying success.

BIBLIOGRAPHY

Cornel EB, Karthaus HF: Manual derotation of the twisted spermatic cord. *Br J Urol* 83:672–674, 1999.

Gahukamble DE, Khamage AS: Early versus delayed repair of reduced incarcerated inguinal hernias in the pediatric population. *J Pediatr Surg* 31:1218, 1996.

Herberner TE: Ultrasound in the assessment of the acute scrotum. *J Clin Ultrasound* 24:405–421, 1996.

Kadish H, Bolte R: A retrospective review of pediatric patients with epididymitis, testicular torsion, and torsion of testicular appendages. *Pediatrics* 102:73–76, 1998.

Klein BL, Ochsenschlager DW: Scrotal masses in children and adolescents: A review for the emergency physician. *Pediatr Emerg Care* 9(6):351–361, 1993.

Langer J, Coplen D: Circumcision and pediatric disorders of the penis. *Pediatr Clin North Am* 45:801–812, 1998.

Mulhall JP, Honig SC: Priapism: diagnosis and management. *Acad Emerg Med* 3:810–816, 1996.

Niedzielski J, Paduch D, Racynski P: Assessment of adolescent varicocele. *Pediatr Surg Int* 12:410–413, 1997.

Paltiel HJ: Acute scrotal symptoms in boys with an indeterminate clinical presentation: Comparison of color Doppler sonography and scintigraphy. *Radiology* 207:223–231, 1998.

Van Howe R: Cost-effective treatment of phimosis. *Pediatrics* 102:1–4, 1998.

60

Urinary Tract Diseases

Marianne Gausche-Hill

HIGH-YIELD FACTS

- Signs and symptoms of urinary tract infection may be nonspecific in young infants, and even older children may not complain of dysuria.
- In the evaluation of infants and children with fever without a source, approximately 5 to 7 percent of patients will be found to have a urinary tract infection.
- Urinary catheterization is the method of choice for obtaining the urine specimen in febrile infants and young children.
- Seventy-five percent of infants <3 months of age with fever and a urinary tract infection are bacteremic. This number drops to 5 percent in older infants and children.
- About 90 percent of renal stones will be radiopaque.
- Computed tomography (CT) scan of the abdomen without contrast is the test of choice for the evaluation of children with renal stones.

URINARY TRACT INFECTION

Urinary tract infection (UTI) is a frequent cause of fever in infants and children. In a meta-analysis of children from 0 to 36 months of age with fever of no identifiable source on physical examination, 7 percent of male infants <6 months of age and 8 percent of female infants <1 year of age had UTI. The prevalence of UTI in children >2 months of age but <2 years of age is about 5 percent, even without a fever or other localizing signs. Girls are affected 4 times as often as are boys, and the rate in uncircumcised boys is 5 to 20 times higher than it is in circumcised boys.

Pathophysiology

UTIs are caused by a number of bacteria including *Escherichia coli*, *Proteus* spp., *Klebsiella* spp., *Staphylo-* *coccus epidermidis, Pseudomonas aeurginosa,* and *Enterococcus* spp. Bacteria enter the urinary tract from the bowel, retrograde from the urethra or, more commonly, from the bloodstream in infants. In fact, 50 percent of infants <3 months of age with a UTI are septic. After 3 months the risk of sepsis drops to <5 percent. Finally, approximately 75 percent of children <5 years of age with a UTI and fever have pyelonephritis documented on a renal cortical scan.

Signs and Symptoms

Signs and symptoms vary with the age of the patient. They may be nonspecific in the infant, including fever, vomiting, and irritability; and more localized in the older child, including frequency, urgency, dysuria, and hematuria.

Patients with abdominal or flank pain, high fever, vomiting, or other systemic signs must be evaluated for pyelonephritis.

Diagnostic Evaluation

Urine culture from an adequate urine sample is the most important diagnostic test to establish the diagnosis of UTI. Results of a urinalysis are helpful, but can be misleading. Although >50 percent of patients with UTI have pyuria, many other entities can cause pyuria including vaginitis, masturbation, trauma, appendicitis, gastroenteritis, renal tuberculosis, acute glomerulonephritis, and bubble bath soap or other causes of local inflammation. Approximately 20 percent of young children with a documented UTI have a normal urinalysis or reagent strip for leukocytes and nitrites. There are a number of methods of obtaining a urine sample that include "bagging" the perineum, clean catch, urinary tract catheterization, and suprapubic aspiration. Although bagging the perineum is easy and noninvasive, it is the least reliable method. With this method, the false-positive rate varies between 85 to 99 percent. Circumcised boys >1 year of age are less likely to have a UTI and are far less likely to have reflux. Therefore, the American Academy of Pediatrics (AAP) recommends that, in this age group, a bagged specimen may be obtained to assess the urine for a cause of fever. If the urine is then positive, urine obtained by catheterization or suprapubic aspiration should be sent to the laboratory for culture.

In infants <1 year of age of either gender, uncircumcised boys <2 years of age, and girls <2 years of age, a urinary specimen obtained by catheterization should be used. If infants are sufficiently ill to warrant immediate administration of antibiotics, the specimen may be collected by suprapubic aspiration. If bagged urine is sent and positive for possible UTI in this age group, the AAP recommends that only catheterized specimens or those obtained by suprapubic aspiration be sent to the laboratory for culture. Older children with adequate instruction and/or supervision may be able to provide a clean catch specimen. Overall, the most reliable methods of obtaining a urine specimen without contamination are urinary catheterization and suprapubic aspiration.

Suprapubic aspiration is a simple, but invasive, procedure that relies on the fact that the bladder is an intraabdominal organ in infants and children <2 years of age. It is best to perform the procedure when the bladder is full. Landmarks for aspiration are one fingerbreadth above the symphysis pubis and in the midline. The infraumbilical abdomen is prepped with povidone solution, and a small wheal of 1% lidocaine is injected subcutaneously with a 27-gauge needle. A 22-gauge, 1 1/2″ needle, with a 10 mL syringe, is then placed at a 60° to 90° angle cephalad, in the midline, above the symphysis pubis. The physician exerts negative pressure on the syringe as the needle is inserted and continues until urine is obtained. The needle is withdrawn and the abdomen cleaned of the povidone solution after which a bandage is placed over the aspiration site. Complications of the procedure are uncommon and include hematuria, bowel perforation, cystitis, and abdominal wall hematoma or infection.

Other studies, such as electrolytes and renal function tests, should be obtained on all patients with signs of dehydration or toxicity and on all infants, all males, and patients with signs of upper tract infection.

Management and Radiologic Evaluation of the Urinary Tract

Neonates, females with recurrent UTI or with pyelonephritis, and males of any age should undergo radiologic evaluation for urinary tract abnormalities. As many as 50 percent of these patients will show congenital anatomic abnormalities on radiologic evaluation.

The radiologic evaluation of the urinary tract has become more sophisticated in recent years. Table 60-1 summarizes the types of diagnostic tests and their indications.

The most common anatomic abnormality of the urinary tract is vesicoureteral reflux (VUR). It is usually diagnosed in the first decade of life and resolves spontaneously in most cases. Voiding cystourethrogram (VCUG) is the diagnostic test of choice for boys and girls with suspected urethral pathology. Otherwise girls can be evaluated for VUR with isotope cystography (IC).

Renal cortical scintigraphy (RCS) is displacing intravenous urography (IVU) as the diagnostic test of choice in the diagnosis of upper tract infections. With RCA, dimercaptosuccinic acid (DMSA) labeled with technetium-99m (^{99m}Tc) is injected intravenously and patients are scanned with a gamma camera approximately 2 hours later. Renal cortical scintigraphy has many advantages over IVU, including the following:

- RCS is not obscured by bowel contents as with IVU.
- RCS does not use highly osmotic agents.
- Allergic reactions are rare with RCS.
- RCS is more sensitive in patients with poor renal function.
- RCS delivers a lower radiation dose to the gonads.

Table 60-1. Diagnostic Tests and Their Indications

Diagnostic Test	Indication(s)
Renal cortical scan	Pyelonephritis; UTI; fever
Voiding cystourethrogram	Vesicoureteric reflux: *Initial* evaluation of boys with UTI; initial evaluation of girls with UTI (in some centers)
Isotope cystography	Vesicoureteric reflux: *Initial* evaluation of girls with UTI without suspected urethral pathology
Renal ultrasonography	Hydronephrosis; nephrolithiasis
Diuretic renography	Obstructive uropathies
Intravenous pyelogram	Nephrolithiasis; isolated renal or ureteral trauma
Computed tomography	Nephrolithiasis; renal and abdominal trauma

UTI, urinary tract infection.

Renal cortical scintigraphy should be performed on patients with fever and UTI to determine upper tract involvement. Clinical signs and symptoms, laboratory evaluation, or sonography are not reliable in determining pyelonephritis. An algorithm for the radiologic evaluation of children with their first UTI is summarized in Fig. 60-1.

Antibiotic therapy is directed at the presumed infecting organism until results of the urine culture are obtained. Almost 80 percent of community-acquired organisms causing UTI are resistant to ampicillin and amoxicillin, and many are now resistant to trimethoprim-sulfamethoxazole (TMP-SMX). While TMP-SMX remains the drug of choice in the treatment of outpatient UTI, some centers prefer alternate therapy. Other antibiotic regimens include sulfisoxazole (Gantrisin), 120 to 150 mg/kg per 24 hours orally every 6 hours, or cephalexin (Keflex), 50 to 100 mg/kg per 24 hours orally every 6 hours (Table 60-2). Older children (>6 years of age) may benefit from the addition of phenazopyridine (Pyridium) to the treatment regimen. Pyridium can be given 10 mg/kg/day in 3 divided doses for 2 to 3 days or until patients are less symptomatic.

Criteria for admission are listed in Table 60-3. All neonates or infants <3 months of age, infants with pyelonephritis, immunocompromised patients, and those with known urinary tract obstruction should be admitted for intravenous antibiotics. Intravenous antibiotic therapy that includes an aminoglycoside, such as genta-micin, 7.5 mg/kg per 24 hours divided every 8 hours, continues until the sensitivity of the organism is known and patients' clinical statuses are improved. Patients, once stable, may be discharged on the appropriate oral antibiotic and treated for a total of 14 days. Rapid diagnosis and appropriate antibiotic therapy will reduce the risk of complications, including renal scarring, hypertension, nephrolithiasis, and renal failure.

UROLITHIASIS

Urolithiasis refers to stone formation in the bladder, ureter, or kidney. It is less common in children than it is in adults, but nevertheless occurs in approximately 1 case per 7500 pediatric hospital admissions. The incidence of urolithiasis varies by geographic location. The southeastern and western United States are areas in which the incidence of stones is highest (1/1380 hospital admissions). In the United States, most urinary calculi are calcium oxalate or calcium phosphate (58 percent). Urolithiasis is rare in blacks but equally as common in girls as in boys, with a mean age of 9 years at presentation.

Pathophysiology

Urinary stasis from anomalies of the urinary tract, concentration of solute (calcium, oxalate, uric acid, and cys-

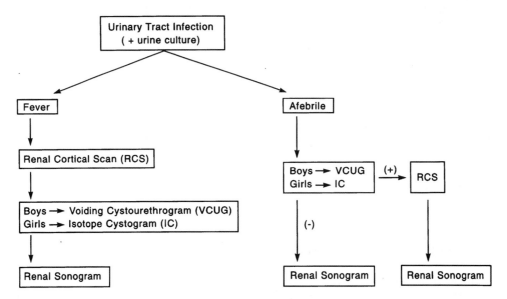

Fig. 60-1. Algorithm for the radiographic evaluation of children with their first UTI. (Adapted from Andrich MP, Majd M: Diagnostic imaging in the evaluation of the first urinary tract infection in infants and young children. *Pediatrics* 90:436, 1992.)

Table 60-2. Antibiotic Therapy for Treatment of Urinary Tract Infections in Children

Outpatient Management	
Cotrimoxazole (trimethoprim in combination with sulfisoxazole)	8 to 10 mg/kg/24 h divided bid
Or cefixime	8 mg/kg/24 h divided bid
Or cephalexin	50 to 100 mg/kg/24 h divided qid
Or cefpodixime	10 mg/kg/24 h divided bid

Inpatient Management	
Ampicillin *plus*	100 mg/kg/24 h divided qid
Cefotaxime	150 mg/kg/24 h divided qid
Or cetriaxone	75 mg/kg/24 h
Or ceftazidime	150 mg/kg/24 h divided qid
Or gentamicin	1.5 mg/kg/24 h divided tid
Or tobramycin	5 mg/kg/24 h divided tid

bid, twice daily; qid, 4 times daily; tid, three times daily.

tine) in the urine, presence of urinary infection (struvite), and concentrated urine promote stone formation. There are many causes of urolithiasis in children. The most common causes are a metabolic disorder and idiopathic and developmental anomalies of the urinary tract (Table 60-4).

Signs and Symptoms

Patients may present with abdominal or flank pain (44 percent), hematuria (38 percent), fever (15 percent), and other urinary tract complaints (18 percent). Flank pain is not as common in children, especially in those <5 years of age, as compared to adults. The emergency physician should assess for history of recurrent UTIs, frequent bouts of abdominal pain, family history of stones, history of microscopic or gross hematuria, passage of stones or gravel

Table 60-3. Admission Criteria for Children With Urinary Tract Infection

Neonate
Pyelonephritis (Infants)
Known urinary tract abnormality
Urinary tract obstruction (stone)
Ureteral stents or other urinary tract foreign bodies
Immunocompromised state
Intractable vomiting and dehydration
Renal insufficiency
Toxic-appearing infant or child

in the urine, intake of vitamins C and D, hydration status, recent trauma, and genitourinary surgery. A routine physical examination should be performed including evaluation of the blood pressure and normal growth parameters.

Diagnostic Evaluation

Urinalysis, urine culture, and renal function studies should be obtained on all children with possible urinary tract stones. Urinalysis may reveal hematuria (gross or

Table 60-4. Causes of Urolithiasis in North American Children

Cause	Number (%)
Metabolic	162 (32.9)
Idiopathic hypercalciuria	
Cystinuria	
Myeloproliferative disorders	
Hyperoxaluria	
Renal tubular acidosis	
Primary hyperparathyroidism	
Hypercortisolism	
Other	
Endemic (urate)	10 (2.2)
Developmental anomalies of the genitourinary tract	160 (32.5)
Infection	21 (4.3)
Idiopathic	139 (28.3)

microscopic) or be entirely normal. A complete blood cell count, renal function tests, and levels of electrolytes, uric acid, total protein, and albumin may also be obtained. Once the diagnosis is suspected from history, physical exam findings, and laboratory analysis, a CT of the abdomen without contrast should be performed. Since as many as 90 percent of renal stones in children are radiopaque, they will be visible on plain radiographs. Computed tomography, however, delineates underlying congenital abnormalities and degree of obstruction. Renal ultrasound or an intravenous pyelogram (IVP) may be performed if CT is not available. Renal ultrasound may be useful in those patients who are pregnant, have renal insufficiency, or are allergic to contrast media. Ultrasound cannot distinguish obstructive from nonobstructive causes of hydronephrosis.

Management

In the emergency department, patients are evaluated for signs of infection and given adequate hydration. Morphine sulfate, 0.1 mg/kg IVP or IM, or other narcotic agents are given to control pain. A nonsteroidal anti-inflammatory agent may be given to older children intravenously or orally as tolerated. Further diagnostic studies will need to be initiated but are not emergent and should be done in consultation with a pediatric urologist.

Patients with complete urinary obstruction, intractable pain, dehydration, a solitary kidney, renal insufficiency, or inability to keep fluids down may need to be admitted. In the past, most children with urinary tract stones required surgical removal. Today, with extracorporeal shock wave lithotripsy, medical management for urolithiasis may predominate. Sixteen percent of pediatric patients with urinary stones will have a recurrence, so close follow-up and outpatient dietary management are critical.

BIBLIOGRAPHY

American Academy of Pediatrics: Practice parameter: The diagnosis, treatment, and evaluation of the initial urinary tract infection in febrile infants and young children. *Pediatrics* 103:843–852, 1999.

Andrich MP, Majd M: Diagnostic imaging in the evaluation of the first urinary tract infants and children. *Pediatrics* 90:436–441, 1992.

Hoberman A, Chao HP, Keller DM, et al: Prevalence of urinary tract infection in febrile infants. *J Pediatr* 123(1):17–23, 1993.

Jakobsson B, Esbjorner E, Hansson S: Minimum incidence and diagnostic rate of first urinary tract infection. *Pediatrics* 104:222–225, 1999.

Nelson DS, Gurr MB, Schunk JE: Management of febrile children with urinary tract infections. *Am J Emerg Med* 16: 643–647, 1998.

Palinsky MS, Kaiser BA, Baluarte HJ: Urolithiasis in childhood. *Pediatr Clin North Am* 34:683–710, 1987.

Shaw KN, Gorelick MH: Urinary tract infection in the pediatric patient. *Pediatr Clin North Am* 46:1111–1124, 1999.

61

Specific Renal Syndromes

Roger Barkin

HIGH-YIELD FACTS

- Edema, hematuria, and oliguria suggest acute glomerulonephritis.
- Children with nephrotic syndrome are considered immunocompromised and are at risk for life-threatening infection.
- Patients with hemolytic uremic syndrome are at risk for hypertension and seizures.
- Hemodialysis may be needed for fluid overload in patients with acute renal failure who are refractory to medical management.

ACUTE GLOMERULONEPHRITIS

Glomerulonephritis is a histopathologic diagnosis acutely associated with clinical findings of hematuria, edema, and hypertension. It commonly follows infection with group A beta-hemolytic streptococcus in children between 3 and 7 years of age. Patients <2 years are rarely affected.

Glomerulonephritis probably results from the deposition of circulating immune complexes in the kidney. These immune complexes are deposited on the basement membrane, reducing glomerular filtration.

Diagnostic Findings

There is usually a preceding streptococcal infection or exposure 1 to 2 weeks before the onset of glomerulonephritis. An interval of less than 4 days may imply that the illness is an exacerbation of preexisting disease rather than an initial attack. Fever, malaise, abdominal pain, and decreased urine output are often noted.

The physical findings reflect the duration of illness. Initial findings may be mild facial or extremity edema only, with a minimal rise in blood pressure. Patients uniformly develop fluid retention and edema and commonly have hematuria (90 percent), hypertension (60 to 70 per-

cent), and oliguria (80 percent). Fever, malaise, and abdominal pain are frequently reported. Anuria and renal failure occur in 2 percent of children. Circulatory congestion, as well as hypertensive encephalopathy, may be noted.

Ancillary Data

An abnormal urinalysis with microscopic or gross hematuria is noted. Erythrocyte casts are present in 60 to 85 percent of hospitalized children. Proteinuria is generally under 2 g/m^2 per 24 hours. Hematuria (Fig. 61-1) and proteinuria (Fig. 61- 2) may present independently and require a specific evaluation. Leukocyturia and hyaline and granular casts are common.

The fractional excretion of sodium as a reflection of renal function may be reduced (Table 61-1). The blood urea nitrogen (BUN) level is elevated disproportionately to the creatinine level.

Total serum complement and specifically C3 is reduced in 90 to 100 percent of children during the first 2 weeks of illness, returning to normal within 3 to 4 weeks. Ongoing low levels suggest the presence of chronic renal disease. The antistreptolysin (ASO) level is elevated, consistent with a previous streptococcal infection. Anemia, hyponatremia, and hyperkalemia may be present.

Management

Fluid and salt restriction is essential to normalize intravascular volume. Diuretics are often required. Elevated blood pressure may require specific pharmacologic management. Specific complications, such as congestive heart failure, renal failure, and hyperkalemia, must be anticipated and treated.

Recovery is usually complete. Over 80 percent of patients recover without residual renal damage. Children without evidence of hypertension, congestive heart failure, or azotemia may be followed closely at home. A nephrologist is usually consulted.

NEPHROTIC SYNDROME

Historically known as lipoid nephrosis, childhood nephrosis, foot process disease, nil disease, minimal change nephrotic syndrome, and idiopathic nephrotic syndrome, nephrotic syndrome is associated with increased glomerular permeability, which produces massive proteinuria. Hypoalbuminemia results, producing a

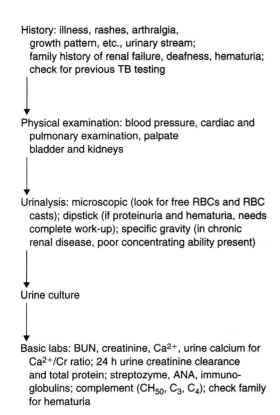

History: illness, rashes, arthralgia,
   growth pattern, etc., urinary stream;
   family history of renal failure, deafness, hematuria;
   check for previous TB testing

Physical examination: blood pressure, cardiac and
   pulmonary examination, palpate
   bladder and kidneys

Urinalysis: microscopic (look for free RBCs and RBC
   casts); dipstick (if proteinuria and hematuria, needs
   complete work-up); specific gravity (in chronic
   renal disease, poor concentrating ability present)

Urine culture

Basic labs: BUN, creatinine, Ca^{2+}, urine calcium for
   Ca^{2+}/Cr ratio; 24 h urine creatinine clearance
   and total protein; streptozyme, ANA, immunoglobulins; complement (CH_{50}, C_3, C_4); check family
   for hematuria

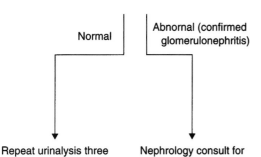

| Normal | Abnornal (confirmed glomerulonephritis) |

Repeat urinalysis three   Nephrology consult for
times; if blood persistent,   probable biopsy; also exclude
     needs IVP   TB, VDRL, Hepatitis B antigen

Fig. 61-1. Evaluation for hematuria. TB, tuberculosis; RBC, red blood cell; BUN, blood urea nitrogen; Ca, calcium; Cr, creatinine; ANA, antinuclear antibody; CH, ; IVP, intravenous pyelogram; VDRL, . [From Barkin RM, Rosen P (eds): *Emergency Pediatrics:A Guide to Ambulatory Care,* 5th ed. St. Louis, MO: Mosby–Year Book, p 266, 1999, with permission.]

decrease in the plasma osmotic pressure. The shift of fluids from the vascular to interstitial spaces shrinks the plasma volume, thereby activating the renin-angiotensin system and enhancing sodium reabsorption. Edema develops.

The etiology is generally idiopathic, but has been associated with glomerular lesions. Intoxications, allergic reactions, infection, and other entities have also been associated with the syndrome (Table 61-2). It may be a primary pathologic process, or associated with a systemic disease. Males have a higher incidence of primary nephrotic syndrome.

The renin-angiotensin-aldosterone system produces increased reabsorption of sodium chloride and worsens the edema state. Serum cholesterol levels rise and remain high even after resolution of urinary protein loss.

Diagnostic Findings

Patients frequently have edema, often with a history of a preceding flu-like syndrome. Edema initially is present periorbitally and may become generalized, associated with weight gain. Ascites may be caused by edema of the intestinal wall, often associated with abdominal pain, nausea, and vomiting. Pleural effusion or pulmonary edema may occur. Malnutrition may be noted secondary to protein loss.

Blood pressure may be decreased if the intravascular volume is depleted or increased in the presence of significant renal disease. Blood pressure is elevated in approximately 5 to 10 percent of these patients. Renal failure may develop.

Infection is probably the most common complication, related to the increased risk of peritonitis and concomitant immunosuppression due to the steroid therapy. Immune protein levels, including IgG, are low due to urinary losses. Children's blood is hypercoagulable, leading to an increased risk of thromboembolism. Renal vein thrombosis is probably underrecognized but should be suspected if hematuria, flank pain, and decreased renal function occur.

Hypoalbuminemia is common, as well as proteinuria and hyperlipidemia. A 24-hour urine collection reveals a protein excretion of >3.5 g /1.73 m^2 per 24 hours. A spot protein:creatinine ratio of >3.0 is noted, and BUN and creatinine levels are elevated in 25 percent of children. Serum complement is decreased. Plasma cholesterol carriers (low-density lipoprotein and very-low-density lipoprotein) are increased. Elevated lipids result from increased synthesis, as well as catabolism of phos-

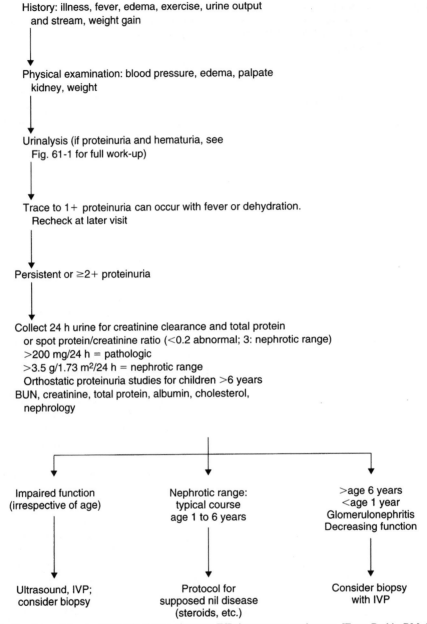

History: illness, fever, edema, exercise, urine output
   and stream, weight gain

↓

Physical examination: blood pressure, edema, palpate
   kidney, weight

↓

Urinalysis (if proteinuria and hematuria, see
   Fig. 61-1 for full work-up)

↓

Trace to 1+ proteinuria can occur with fever or dehydration.
   Recheck at later visit

↓

Persistent or ≥2+ proteinuria

↓

Collect 24 h urine for creatinine clearance and total protein
   or spot protein/creatinine ratio (<0.2 abnormal; 3: nephrotic range)
   >200 mg/24 h = pathologic
   >3.5 g/1.73 m²/24 h = nephrotic range
   Orthostatic proteinuria studies for children >6 years
BUN, creatinine, total protein, albumin, cholesterol,
   nephrology

Impaired function (irrespective of age)	Nephrotic range: typical course age 1 to 6 years	>age 6 years <age 1 year Glomerulonephritis Decreasing function
Ultrasound, IVP; consider biopsy	Protocol for supposed nil disease (steroids, etc.)	Consider biopsy with IVP

Fig. 61-2. Evaluation for proteinuria. BUN, blood urea nitrogen; IVP, intravenous pyelogram. [From Barkin RM, Rosen P (eds): *Emergency Pediatrics: A Guide to Ambulatory Care,* 5th ed. St. Louis, MO: Mosby–Year Book, p 267, 1999, with permission.]

Table 61-1. Evaluation of Renal Failure

Prerenal	Intrarenal	Postrenal
Ultrasound: normal	Ultrasound: Can have increased renal density or slight swelling	Ultrasound: Dilated bladder or kidney
Serum BUN:creatinine ratio >15:1		History and exam may be diagnostic
Urine Na$^+$ <15 mEq/L	Urine Na$^+$ >20 mEq/L	Indexes not helpful
Urine osmolality >500 mOsm/kg H$_2$O	Urine osmolality <350 mOsm/kg H$_2$O	
Urine:plasma creatinine ratio >40:1	Urine:plasma creatinine ratio <20:1 (often <5:1)	
Fractional excretion of Na$^+$ <1 (<2.5 in neonates)	Fractional excretion of Na$^+$ >2 (>2.5 in neonates)	

$$\text{Fractional excretion of Na}^+ = \frac{\text{Urine Na}^+ \text{ (mEq/L)}}{\text{Plasma Na}^+ \text{ (mEq/L)}} \times \frac{\text{Plasma creatinine (mg/dL)}}{\text{Urine creatinine (mg/dL)}}$$

Source: From Barkin RM, Rosen P (eds): *Emergency Pediatrics: A Guide to Ambulatory Care,* 5th ed. St. Louis, MO: Mosby–Year Book, p 811, 1999, with permission.

pholipid. Imaging studies, especially ultrasound, should document normal renal structure.

A renal biopsy should be considered if the following poor prognostic signs are present:

- Age over 10 years
- Azotemia
- Decreased complement
- Hematuria
- Persistent hypertension
- No response to steroids

Differential Diagnosis

Other causes of edema should be excluded, including congestive heart failure, vasculitis, hypothyroidism, starvation, cystic fibrosis, protein-losing enteropathy, and drug ingestions (such as steroids or diuretics).

Management

Management should focus on assuring hemodynamic stability and a balanced intake and output. Subsequent evaluation is described in Fig. 61-3. The majority of patients should be hospitalized initially, usually in consultation with a nephrologist. Treat hypovolemia with albumin and fluids. Monitor closely and treat hypertension if it occurs.

After diagnosis and stabilization, patients without complications (<10 years, normal complement, no gross hematuria, no large protein loss) are started on prednisone at a dose of 2 mg/kg per 24 hours up to 80 mg per 24 hours and tapered once a response is noted. Nearly 75 percent of patients will respond within 14 days. Treatment continues for about 2 months but is reinstituted if relapse is noted. Other pharmacologic agents may ultimately be needed. Salt and water restriction should be initiated.

Diuretics may be needed if there is pulmonary edema or respiratory distress. However, they must be used judiciously to avoid vascular volume depletion and electrolyte abnormality. Salt restriction is required.

Watch for signs of infection since these patients are considered immunocompromised. Avoid deep vein punctures if possible to avoid triggering a deep vein thrombosis.

HEMOLYTIC-UREMIC SYNDROME

Nephropathy, microangiopathic hemolytic anemia, and thrombocytopenia are found in patients with hemolytic uremic syndrome (HUS). This syndrome commonly occurs in children under 5 years of age following an episode of gastroenteritis or respiratory infection. Siblings may also develop the disease due to a familial genetic component. The illness has an acute onset with rapid progression to renal failure and thrombocytopenia.

Hemolytic uremic syndrome results from endothelial damage of the renal microvasculature. A microangiopathic hemolytic anemia develops as a result of mechanical damage and sequestration of red blood cells. Platelet aggregation may produce microthrombi and hy-

Table 61-2. Nephrotic Syndrome: Etiology

Primary renal disorders	Nil or minimal change disease
	Focal glomerulosclerosis
	Membranoproliferative glomerulonephritis
	Membranous glomerulonephritis
Intoxication	Heroin
	Mercury
	Probenecid
	Silver
Allergic reaction	Poison ivy or oak, pollens
	Bee sting
	Snake venom
Infection	Bacterial
	Viral: Hepatitis B, cytomegalovirus, Epstein-Barr virus
	Protozoa: Malaria, toxoplasmosis
Neoplasm	Hodgkin's disease, Wilms' tumor, etc.
Autoimmune disorder	Systemic lupus erythematosus
Metabolic disorder	Diabetes mellitus
Cardiac disorders	Congenital heart disease
	Congestive heart failure
	Pericarditis
Vasculitis	Henoch-Schönlein purpura
	Wegener's granulomatosis

poxia in the kidney. Decreased C3 may result from deposition of complement in the lumina of the glomeruli.

Etiology

Associated infections can be found. *Escherichia coli* serotype 0157:H7 is the most commonly found organism, producing a cytotoxin that inhibits protein synthesis leading to cell death in gastrointestinal organs.

Shigella and *Salmonella* and group A streptococcus may be associated with HUS, as well as coxsackievirus, influenza, and respiratory syncytial virus (RSV).

Diagnostic Findings

Patients usually have a history of gastroenteritis with vomiting, bloody diarrhea, and crampy abdominal pain within 2 weeks of the onset of HUS. Children who develop HUS without a prodrome of gastroenteritis have a poor prognosis. Low-grade fever, pallor, hematuria, oliguria, and gastrointestinal bleeding occur. Central nervous system deterioration can occur with a spectrum from irritability to seizures or coma.

There is a tremendous spectrum of severity of clinical disease ranging from mild elevation of BUN with ane-

mia to total anuria due to acute nephropathy with severe anemia and thrombocytopenia.

Ultimately, patients may develop hypertension; anemia with pallor, petechiae, and easy bruising; h patosplenomegaly; and edema. Hypertension occurs in up to 50 percent of patients. Irritability or lethargy may develop. Seizures occur in 40 percent of the cases. Hyponatremia and hypocalcemia are common. Acute abdominal conditions including intussusception, bowel perforation, and toxic megacolon can occur. Hepatic and pancreatic injury can occur in HUS. There may be cardiac involvement with cardiomyopathy, myocarditis, or high-output failure. Recurrences may occur, often without a prodrome, and may be associated with a high mortality rate.

Laboratory evaluation should include assessment of renal function including electrolyte, BUN, and creatinine levels and urinalysis. Hematologic studies reveal low hemoglobin with a microangiopathic, hemolytic anemia. Burr cells are common. Platelets are usually decreased below 50,000/mm^3. Coagulation studies are usually normal.

Management

Initial stabilization is followed by admission to an appropriate medical center. Volume overload may occur sec-

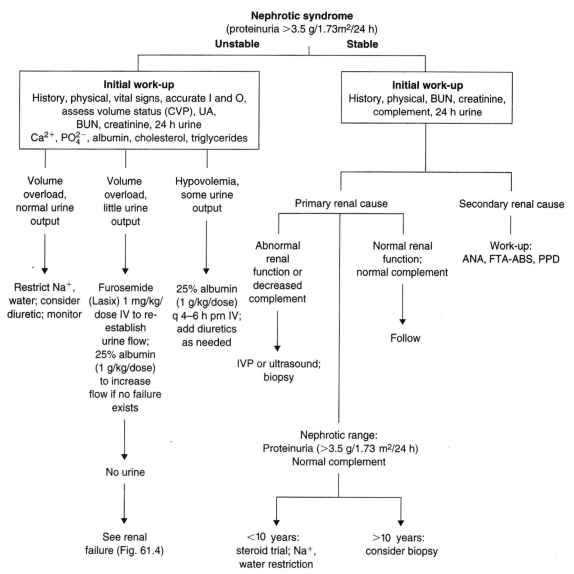

Fig. 61-3. Management of nephrotic syndrome. I, input; O, output; CVP, central venous pressure; UA, ; BUN, blood urea nitrogen; Ca, calcium; PO, ; Na, sodium; IV, intravenous; ANA, antinuclear antibody; FTA-ABS = Fluorescent Treponema Antigen-Antibody; PPD = Purified Protein Derivative for T.B.; IVP, intravenous pyelogram. [From Barkin RM, Rosen P (eds): *Emergency Pediatrics: A Guide to Ambulatory Care,* 4th ed. St. Louis, MO: Mosby–Year Book, p 735, 1994, with permission.]

ondary to anemia. Hypertension may occur and appears to be caused by increased renin levels. Treatment is recommended, if the diastolic pressure is above 120 mmHg. A variety of agents may be used, including nifedipine, labetolol, captopril, and hydralazine. Renal failure requires meticulous balancing of intake and output with specific treatment of hyperkalemia, acidosis, hypocalcemia, hyper-

phosphatemia, and other metabolic abnormalities. Peritoneal dialysis may be required, especially when the BUN is over 100 or when congestive heart failure, encephalopathy, or hyperkalemia are pres-ent. Peritoneal dialysis is also indicated when anuria has been present for 24 hours.

A serum hemoglobin <5 g/dL or hematocrit <15 percent generally requires treatment with packed red blood cells, infused slowly. Platelet survival is shortened and platelet infusions may be required in children with active bleeding. Seizures require specific management and are usually caused by hypertension or uremia. Acute treatment includes stabilization and anticonvulsants, as well as a consideration of emergency dialysis. Heparin and streptokinase have been tried without significant success.

ACUTE RENAL FAILURE

Impairment of the kidney's ability to regulate urine volume and composition produces problems with hemostasis. This is usually associated with a decreased glomerular filtration rate (GFR).

The etiology of acute renal failure may be categorized on the basis of the type of renal injury. It may be prerenal (decreased perfusion of the kidney), intrarenal (damage to the actual nephron), or postrenal (downstream obstruction of the urinary tract; Table 61-1).

Prerenal patients have decreased perfusion of the kidney. Dehydration is usually the cause and may be secondary to vomiting, diarrhea, diabetic ketoacidosis, or decreased intravascular volumes associated with nephrotic syndrome, burns, or shock.

Intrarenal failure results from direct, intrinsic damage to the nephrons caused by glomerulonephritis (hematuria, proteinuria, edema, and hypertension), HUS, nephrotoxic exposures, crush injuries, sepsis, or disseminated intravascular coagulation.

Obstruction leads to postrenal failure and may be accompanied by symptoms, although blockage may be insidious and without symptoms. Causes of postrenal obstruction include posterior urethral valves, ureteropelvic junction abnormalities, renal stones, and trauma. Abdominal pain and an abdominal mass due to hydronephrosis may be noted.

Diagnostic Findings

The history may reflect the underlying disease and the category of renal failure. The physical examination will help determine the mechanism. It is essential to evaluate for hypovolemia, volume overload, hypertension, or obstruction.

Patients may have oliguria with urine output under 1 mL/kg/h or be nonoliguric with an output excessive for the volume status. Azotemia may be noted.

Laboratory evaluation should include electrolytes, studies of renal function, and a search for the underly-

ing pathology. The creatinine clearance is a good measure of GFR and is useful in initial assessment and ongoing monitoring. A 24-hour urine is normally needed.

$$\text{Creatinine clearance (mL/min/1.73 m}^2) = \frac{UV}{P} \times \frac{1.73}{SA}$$

Where U = urinary concentration of creatinine (mg/dL);

  V = volume of urine divided by the number of minutes in collection period (24 hours = 1440 min) (mL/min);

  P = plasma concentration of creatinine (mg/dL);

 SA = surface area (m^2)

A rapid approximation can be made using the formula:

$$\text{Creatinine clearance (mL/min/1.73 m}^2) - \frac{0.55 \times ht \text{ (cm)}}{P}$$

Normal values are the following:

- Newborn and premature: 40 to 65 mL/min/1.73 m^2
- Normal child: female, 109 mL/min/1.73 m^2 or male, 124 mL/min/1.73 m^2
- Adult: female, 95 mL/min/1.73 m^2 or male, 105 mL/min/1.73 m^2

A single voided urine in adults has been of some use in assessing renal function. In patients with stable renal function, a spot protein:creatinine ratio of >3.0 represents nephrotic range proteinuria (a ratio of <0.2 is normal). Ultrasonography is also important in the evaluation of these patients. Combining data from serum, urine, and ultrasonography helps differentiate among prerenal, intrarenal, and postrenal failure (Table 61-1).

Management

Initial management must focus on stabilization with correction of fluid imbalance (Fig. 61-4). If the intravascular volume is adequate or overloaded, urine output may be enhanced with furosemide, usually in an initial dose of 1 mg/kg increased up to 6 mg/kg/dose. Mannitol may be administered if there is no response to furosemide. The dose is 0.5 to 0.75 mg/kg/dose IV. Do not utilize these agents if obstruction is present.

In oliguric or anuric patients with decreased intravascular volume, fluid may be administered slowly, often in conjunction with monitoring of the central venous pressure. Low-dose dopamine occasionally may be utilized to increase renal blood flow and GFR. Those with high

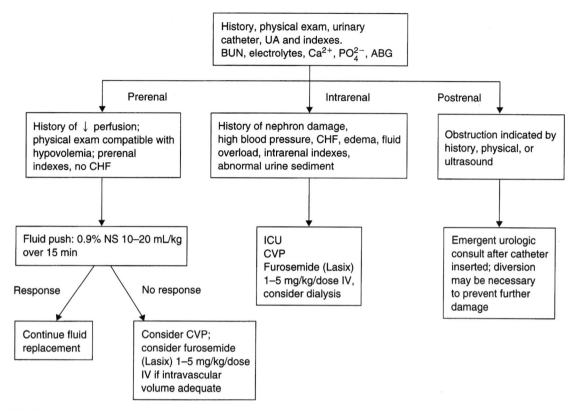

Fig. 61-4. Acute renal failure: initial assessment and treatment. UA, urine analysis; BUN, blood urea nitrogen; Ca, calcium; PO, ; ABG, arterial blood gas; CHF, congestive heart failure; NS, normal saline; ICU, intensive care unit; CVP, central venous pressure; IV, intravenous. [From Barkin RM, Rosen P (eds): *Emergency Pediatrics: A Guide to Ambulatory Care,* 5th ed. St. Louis, MO: Mosby–Year Book, p 812, 1999, with permission.]

urine output must receive a significant amount of fluid to avoid hypovolemia.

Hypertension may be caused by fluid overload or high renin secretion. Children having acute hypertension with a diastolic pressure over 100 mmHg should be treated parenterally because of the risk of seizures, encephalopathy, and other sequelae. Only a mild reduction is needed, usually to the diastolic range of about 100 mmHg. Nitroprusside and nifedipine are useful for reduction of pressure.

Hyperkalemia causes membrane excitability with possible cardiac dysrhythmias. A potassium level >6.5 mEq/L can cause elevation of the T wave. Specific and immediate treatment for a potassium level >7.0 mEq/L is required. Treatment may include calcium chloride, 20 to 30 mg/kg slowly; sodium bicarbonate, 1 to 2 mEq/kg/dose; or glucose and insulin infusion of 1 mL/kg of $D_{50}W$ followed by 1 mL/kg of $D_{25}W$ and 0.5 U/kg of regular insulin per hour to keep serum glucose between 120 to 300

mg/dL. Kayexalate at 1 g/kg/dose every 4 to 6 hours mixed with 70 percent sorbitol, orally or rectally, may be useful after initial stabilization. Other abnormalities that may need specific treatment include anemia, metabolic acidosis, hyponatremia, and hyperphosphatemia.

Dialysis may be required for unresponsive fluid overload, severe hyperkalemia, severe hyponatremia or hypernatremia, unresponsive metabolic acidosis, BUN >100 mg/dL, or altered level of consciousness secondary to uremia. Such patients obviously require hospitalization.

BIBLIOGRAPHY

Acute Glomerulonephritis

Roy S, Stapleton FB: Changing perspective in children hospitalized with post streptococcal acute glomerulonephritis. *Pediatr Nephrol* 4:585, 1990.

Wingo CS, Clapp WL: Proteinuria: Potential causes and approach to evaluation. *Am J Med Sci* 320:188–94, 2000.

Nephrotic Syndrome

Warshaw BL: Nephrotic syndrome in children. *Pediatr Ann* 23:495, 1994.

Hemolytic-Uremic Syndrome

Brandt JR, Fouser LS, Watkins SL, et al: *E. coli* 0157:H7–associated hemolytic-uremic syndrome after ingestion of contaminated hamburgers. *J Pediatr* 125:519, 1994.

Kelles A, Van Dyck M, Proeshan W: Childhood haemolytic uraemic syndrome: Long-term outcome and prognostic features. *Eur J Pediatr* 153:38, 1994.

Siegler RC, Milligan MK, Burningham TH, et al: Long-term outcome and prognostic indicators in the hemolytic uremic syndrome. *J Pediatr* 118:195, 1991.

Acute Renal Failure

Sehic A, Chesney RW: Acute renal failure: Diagnosis, therapy. *Pediatr Rev* 16:101, 137, 1995.

Thadhani R, Pascual M, Bonventre JV: Acute renal flow. *N Engl J Med* 334:1448, 1996.

62

Petechiae and Purpura

Julia A. Rosekrans

HIGH-YIELD FACTS

- Petechial rashes are the most serious dermatologic problem seen in the acute care setting because they may be symptomatic of significant life-threatening illnesses, which require rapid intervention.
- Child abuse should be considered if bruising occurs to nonbony prominences and the history does not match the physical findings in infants and toddlers.
- Children may present with abdominal pain, joint pain, or even seizures as a first symptom of Henoch-Schonlein purpura.

Petechial rashes are the most serious dermatologic problem seen in the acute care setting because they may be symptomatic of significant life-threatening illnesses, which require rapid intervention. Petechiae and purpura develop when small blood vessels in the skin rupture and bleed. They can occur because of increased capillary fragility, decrease in ability to clot, or because of traumatic injury (Table 62-1).

PETECHIAE DUE TO SEPSIS

Septic illnesses cause petechiae *both* by local vasculitis and through consumption of coagulation factors. These illnesses can be difficult to distinguish in the initial evaluation of patients. It is important to recognize the significance of the rash because treatment measures must be rapidly instituted. Petechial rashes in acute infections can range from a few scattered small petechiae to the pattern of widespread purpura and shock seen in purpura fulminans.

Etiology

The major cause of purpura fulminans is meningococcemia caused by the gram-negative bacteria *Neisseria meningitidis.* Other bacteria including gonococcus, *Salmonella typhi,* and *Escherichia coli* may also cause bacterial sepsis with petechiae. Rocky Mountain Spotted Fever is a rickettsial disease spread by tick bites in endemic regions. Many children with viral illnesses develop petechiae even though they are not severely ill.

Pathophysiology

Hemorrhagic skin lesions in sepsis are probably caused by several mechanisms. Infectious vasculitis results from direct bacterial invasion of capillary endothelial cells. An inflammatory response causes loss of integrity of the capillary wall. Consumption coagulopathy that may be initiated by cell wall endotoxins is also significant in production of petechiae.

Clinical Findings

Most children and adolescents with septic illnesses appear toxic with high fever, delirium, and, occasionally, hypotension. However, not all children "look sick" and occasionally bacteremic patients with a significant pathogen are not recognized until a blood culture is reported as positive.

Petechiae and purpura are hemorrhages in the skin that do not disappear when capillary blood is pressed out of the skin—they do not blanch. The rash may be identified before children are brought in for evaluation or before the rash develops during the exam. Small fresh lesions are red, while large lesions are blue to purple in appearance. Lesions darken and change color over several days as hemoglobin degrades and the hemorrhage resolves.

Petechiae above the nipple line suggest increased intravenous pressure in the superior vena cava and may

Table 62-1. Differential Diagnosis of Purpura

A. Infectious:
   Acute: Meningococcemia
                Rocky Mountain spotted fever
                Escherichia coli sepsis
                Gonococcemia
                Subacute bacterial endocarditis
                Atypical measles
                Echovirus 9, 4, 7
                Epstein-Barr virus
                Coxsackie A9
   Neonatal: Rubella
                Toxoplasma
                Cytomegalovirus
                Syphilis
B. Thrombocytopenic
   Idiopathic thrombocytopenic purpura
   Leukemia
   Systemic lupus erythematosus
   Hemangioma with platelet trapping
C. Nonseptic normal platelet count
   Henoch-Schonlein purpura
      (anaphylactoid purpura)
   Coagulation disorders
   Trauma including child abuse

result from vomiting or coughing. Petechiae seen in an acral distribution, on the hands and feet, suggest infectious vasculitis.

Diagnosis

Laboratory evaluation is essential to identify the organism causing the infection. A complete blood cell count to evaluate both total white cell and total platelet count is helpful in estimating severity of illness. Blood cultures are mandatory because some children with a normal clinical exam will be bacteremic. A lumbar puncture may be needed to diagnose meningitis.

Complications

Children with purpura fulminans run the risk of vascular compromise that can lead to loss of digits and sloughing of affected areas of skin if they survive the underlying infection. Meningitis frequently complicates septic illnesses.

HENOCH-SCHONLEIN PURPURA

Anaphylactoid purpura is a systemic vasculitis. Although the striking pattern of distribution of purpura may be the most obvious manifestation of the illness, most children also have visceral and joint involvement.

Etiology

Infectious illnesses such as mild viral respiratory infections and streptococcal pharyngitis have been implicated as agents that initiate an immune complex response. The immune complex reacts with blood vessel walls causing capillary leaking.

Pathophysiology

Skin biopsies show perivascular extravasation of blood probably caused by fibrinoid necrosis of dermal vein walls.

Clinical Findings

The presentation of this illness is quite variable. Children may present with abdominal pain, joint pain, or even seizures as a first symptom of Henoch-Schonlein purpura. In contrast, the typical rash may develop before any systemic symptoms. Some children have no difficulty beyond the rash.

Abdominal pain may resemble appendicitis; in addition, some children develop intussusception. In most children, abdominal pain lasts for only 24 hours, but it can be severe enough that children will refuse to eat or drink. Many children have microscopic intestinal bleeding and guaiac-positive stools.

Arthralgia or arthritis, especially of feet and hands, is seen in about 80 percent of children. This is usually mild and transient. Sometimes a complaint that children will not walk will not be recognized as Henoch-Schonlein purpura for several days if the rash is not present initially.

Renal involvement is common, and most children will have microscopic hematuria at some point during the illness. A few children develop nephrotic syndrome that can progress to chronic renal failure. Central nervous system involvement is a rare manifestation of Henoch-Schonlein purpura. Children with vasculitis of cerebral vessels may present with seizures, coma, or paralysis.

The rash may begin with urticaria, which progresses to palpable purpura over 24 hours. Frequently, the initial skin lesions are palpable purpura 1 or 2 mm in diameter. The acral distribution of the rash is its most characteristic finding. It is symmetrical and most prominent on the buttocks and thighs, although it can also be seen on hands and arms; genitalia are often involved. Most skin changes last for about 4 to 6 weeks and then resolve permanently.

Diagnosis

Clinical history and examination make the diagnosis. A complete blood cell count is necessary to evaluate the white blood cell count, with a platelet count to rule out thrombocytopenia. A urinalysis for hematuria and proteinuria should be done on initial diagnosis and at follow-up exams.

Complications

Ulcerations following cutaneous infarcts have been described but are extremely rare. Progression of renal disease, while rare, is the complication that must be followed most carefully.

Management

Most children can receive care at home with outpatient follow-up and no active treatment other than mild analgesics for pain control.

Inpatient treatment should be considered for children with significant joint pain, especially if they are too large for parents to carry. Children with abdominal pain may need intravenous fluids if they refuse to eat. Prednisone, 2 mg/kg/day, has been used to treat abdominal pain although studies of efficacy remain controversial. Corticosteroid therapy does appear to prevent nephritis, the most important long-term complication of this disease.

IDIOPATHIC THROMBOCYTOPENIC PURPURA

The sudden appearance of petechiae and ecchymosis in no particular distribution over the body may signal a decrease in the number of platelets. Idiopathic thrombocytopenic purpura is a common cause of an acute low platelet count in children.

Etiology

Easy bruising is usually preceded about 2 weeks earlier by a viral respiratory infection.

Pathophysiology

IgG antiplatelet antibodies develop in response to a viral infection. The antibodies fix to normal platelets that are then destroyed by reticuloendothelial phagocytic cells. The antibody titer is inversely related to the platelet count.

Clinical Findings

Many children have mild self-limited illnesses. Bruises appear spontaneously on areas of the body such as the abdomen and chest that are not areas where bruises from mild trauma usually appear. In severe cases, the skin findings may be accompanied by bleeding from the oral cavity and the gastrointestinal and genitourinary systems. The physical exam is otherwise normal with no significant lymphadenopathy and no enlargement of the spleen.

Diagnosis

A complete blood cell count is needed both to identify the low platelet count and to assess the total white blood cell count and hemoglobin. Antibody titers are not a necessary part of the initial evaluation.

Differential Diagnosis

Other illnesses in which platelets are destroyed rapidly include autoimmune collagen vascular disease, especially lupus. Some drugs, including thiazides, quinidine, and sulfa antibiotics can produce immunologic toxicity to platelets.

Diseases such as leukemia, lymphoma, and myeloma may cause thrombocytopenia by decreasing megakaryocytes in bone marrow so fewer platelets are produced.

Complications

In severe cases, bleeding into vital organs can occur. Intracerebral hemorrhage is the most serious potential complication.

Management

Most cases are mild and self-limited and require only close follow-up. When cases are more severe, prednisone has been used to decrease abnormal antibodies. Intravenous gamma globulin is also given to interrupt the process of platelet destruction. Splenectomy is a rare management strategy for patients whose illness does not remit spontaneously. Children with platelet counts below 50,000 require inpatient management.

CHILD ABUSE

Bruises that are caused by nonaccidental injury are important to recognize so appropriate supervision can be instituted. Children must be protected from further injury. See Chapter 118 for a comprehensive discussion of child abuse.

Etiology

Bruises due to maltreatment are often the result of attempts at discipline. They can be inflicted when an adult's anger becomes focused on a child and expressed with a beating. Some bruises can develop from an activity in which the child has been poorly supervised or neglected rather than from direct infliction. The pattern of injury and correlation of the pattern with the history of the injury are the best clues to etiology.

Epidemiology

Child abuse is a multifactorial problem seen in all socioeconomic groups. Bruising injuries tend to occur more frequently in toddlers and infants who are unable to divert violence and protect themselves or in adolescents who get into power struggles with their parents.

Physicians have an important role in identifying bruises caused by maltreatment. Failure to consider maltreatment has resulted in lack of investigation and prevention of ongoing abuse. In many fatal cases due to abuse, bruises had been seen on the child in previous encounters but were not recognized as nonaccidental.

Clinical Findings

Normal traumatic bruises occur over bony prominences. Toddlers commonly fall and bruise elbows, knees, and foreheads. It is unusual to bruise the abdomen or trunk during normal play. When adults slap children, the slap will typically hit a cheek or the buttocks. Abuse is often a chronic problem and bruises of various colors are often seen indicating injuries occurring on different occasions. Some bruises occur in obvious patterns such as bite marks, cord marks from being tied up, or belt shapes from a beating.

Diagnosis

One should consider abuse if there is a discrepancy between the appearance of bruises and the reported cause. A complete blood cell count is important to identify platelet abnormalities. In selected cases, further clotting studies may be needed.

A skeletal bone survey may be helpful for infants under 18 months with clear nonaccidental bruises to identify subtle unsuspected fractures.

Differential Diagnosis

Children with a large number of unexplainable bruises may have a problem with platelet number or activity such as idiopathic thrombocytopenic purpura, leukemia, or medication allergy. Other clotting disorders such as Wiskott-Aldrich syndrome may also be mild and only manifest as "easy bruising." Henoch-Schonlein purpura may be difficult to distinguish from maltreatment until the pattern of bruising develops beyond the buttocks.

Complications

The most important reason to identify bruises from child abuse is to alter adult behavior so that children will be protected from serious injury. Children with nonaccidental bruises often suffer from other types of maltreatment, such as neglect and emotional abuse, that are not immediately evident until in-depth investigation has been instituted.

Management

All states require physicians to report cases in which there is a suspicion of abuse to the appropriate investigative agency. Sometimes child abuse is obvious, but many more times it may be difficult to determine. Consultation with social service workers and physicians with experience in abuse may be needed.

An immediate assessment of the child's safety is an important part of the emergency department evaluation. Emergency placement should be considered for children whose safety cannot be assured. A plan for obtaining emergency assessments should be established as a department policy.

BIBLIOGRAPHY

Cohen B: *Pediatric Dermatology,* 2d ed. St. Louis, Mosby Year Book, 1999.

Edwards L: *Dermatology in Emergency Care.* WB Saunders, 1997.

Lilleyman J: *Pediatric Hematology.* Churchill Livingstone, 1999.

Monteleone J: *Child Maltreatment,* 2d ed. GW Medical Publishers, 1998.

Schachner LA, Hansen RC (eds): *Pediatric Dermatology* 2d ed. New York, Saunders, 1995.

Weston WL, Lane AT: *Color Textbook of Pediatric Dermatology.* St. Louis, Mosby Year Book, 1996.

63

Pruritic Rashes

Julia A. Rosekrans

HIGH-YIELD FACTS

- In infancy, cheeks and extensor surfaces of the legs are most commonly affected. Later in childhood, the antecubital and popliteal fossae are most affected.
- The skin of children with atopic dermatitis is colonized with *Staphylococcus aureus,* which can cause abscesses, cellulitis, and lymphangitis.
- Erythema multiforme is a fixed skin reaction. Individual lesions last for several days. Subcutaneous epinephrine can be given to clear urticaria, but it does not change erythema multiforme.

Parents frequently decide to see a physician if their child has a rash that causes itching and discomfort. Some rashes that present with itching as a primary symptom are acute problems that can be diagnosed and rapidly treated. Others are chronic problems for which control measures other than cure can be emphasized (Table 63-1).

ATOPIC DERMATITIS

This chronic relapsing condition appears in children who have a tendency to produce specific IgE when exposed to environmental antigens. It is associated with other atopic conditions including allergic rhinitis and asthma that may be seen in affected children or in family members.

Etiology

Atopic dermatitis appears to be an inherited disorder, although no particular patterns of inheritance or HLA typing have yet been useful in defining the familial pattern. If one parent has any atopic problem, there is a 60 per-

cent chance that a child will be atopic. If both parents are atopic, the child's risk increases to 80 percent. In comparison, the likelihood that a child whose parents are not atopic will develop atopic symptoms is about 20 percent.

Epidemiology

Atopic dermatitis is seen in all cultures; however, there are suggestions that it is more common in highly industrialized countries, and it may be increasing in incidence since the beginning of this century. This suggests that environmental pollutants may play a role in causing atopy.

Atopic dermatitis is more common in children than it is in adults and usually begins in infancy. It is equally prevalent in boys and girls. While the course of the disease is unpredictable, most children improve over time.

Pathophysiology

The exact pathogenesis is not known. Some clinicians believe that the clinical appearance is the result of scratching. Atopic dermatitis has been described as "an itch that rashes."

A common finding on skin biopsy is an inflammatory exudate in the epidermis with excessive numbers of lymphocytes and monocytes.

Although food allergies, house dust mite allergies, cellular immunodeficiency, and abnormal beta-adrenergic receptors have been hypothesized as triggers for the reaction, there is no convincing evidence for any of these as etiologic mechanisms.

Clinical Findings

In infancy, cheeks and extensor surfaces of the legs are most commonly affected. Later in childhood, the antecubital and popliteal fossae are most affected. Children with extensive atopic dermatitis are most likely to have problems as adults when there is a diffuse pattern of skin involvement.

The rash may range in severity from dry itchy skin to weeping open fissures. The most important and consistent symptom is itchiness that may be severe enough to interfere with sleep.

Associated physical findings include signs of scratching, rubbing, and other atopic problems. Some children show very shiny buffed fingernails from constant rubbing. Denny's lines on the lower eyelid and allergic shiners are commonly seen and may relate to rubbing the

Table 63-1. Pruritic Rashes

Chronic	Acute
Atopic dermatitis	Urticaria
Seborrhea	Scabies
	Insect bites
	Head lice
	Contact dermatitis

eyes or to venous stasis due to nasal congestion. Hypopigmented patches on the face may be quite pronounced in children with dark or tanned skin.

Diagnosis

Atopic dermatitis is a clinical diagnosis. The definitive features of the diagnosis are the following:

- Pruritus
- Flexural lichenification
- Chronic relapsing condition

Differential Diagnosis

The most commonly confused conditions are scaly or papulovesicular disorders such as seborrheic dermatitis, scabies, contact dermatitis, or tinea corporis. Some metabolic problems such as Hurler's syndrome and phenylketonuria may include eczematous rashes. Histiocytosis X may present with a rash that resembles atopic dermatitis but does not respond to appropriate treatment.

Complications

The most common acute complication is bacterial superinfection. The skin of children with atopic dermatitis is colonized with *Staphylococcus aureus,* which can cause abscesses, cellulitis, and lymphangitis.

Cataract formation is a possible chronic complication. Keratoconus, an abnormally shaped cornea, may develop in adolescents.

Management

Since there is no cure for atopic dermatitis, education of the family must be aimed toward relief of dryness, inflammation, and itching. Baths should be limited and soap should be mild and nonperfumed. Bath oils may be helpful in maintaining skin hydration. Topical moistur-

izers such as Eucerin and skin lotions are soothing after a bath.

Inflammation is treated with topical corticosteroid ointments. Care must be taken to avoid powerful fluorinated steroids that are systemically absorbed and can cause permanent thinning of the skin. Strong potency steroids may be used to briefly quell a severe flare; however, a rapid change to less powerful ointments is important.

H_1 antihistamines such as diphenhydramine hydrochloride (4 to 6 mg/kg per 24 hours, not to exceed 300 mg divided into 3 or 4 doses daily) and hydroxyzine hydrochloride (2 to 4 mg/kg per 24 hours divided into 2 or 3 doses) are commonly used to relieve the itch.

CONTACT DERMATITIS

Contact between the skin and irritating substances can cause a vesicular itchy rash. Some material will cause a contact dermatitis reaction in nearly all people. Other substances will cause reactions only in people who are sensitized to a specific chemical.

Etiology

Allergic contact dermatitis is a lymphocyte-mediated reaction to a particular allergen. Common allergens include metals such as nickel, chemicals from rubber in elastic or latex gloves, and chemicals found in tanning leather or dying fabric.

The most common cause of contact dermatitis in the United States is the *Rhus* group of plants, including poison ivy, poison oak, and poison sumac. Mango rind and cashew nut oil also contain similar chemical material.

Pathophysiology

A type IV immune response is produced primarily by the T-lymphocyte in response to direct physical contact of the skin with the sensitizing material. A reaction does not usually take place after the first exposure to a substance but only after the skin is sensitized. Initial sensitization can occur within 7 to 10 days after exposure; however, on subsequent exposures, a reaction can occur within 24 hours.

Clinical Findings

Erythema and a papulovesicular eruption develop on the skin that has been in contact with sensitizing material. When the reaction is to a contact with a plant, the rash may appear to be in lines like the edge of a leaf or a stem. An eruption in a discrete area such as ear lobes or the back of the wrist could indicate contact with a metal such as nickel found in earrings or a wristwatch.

Diagnosis

The diagnosis of contact dermatitis is made by recognizing the sudden development of a vesicular weeping eruption in a pattern suggestive of contact with a suspicious allergen. If it is necessary to identify a particular allergen, patch testing to elicit reactions in a controlled fashion may be useful.

Differential Diagnosis

Other pruritic vesicular rashes include atopic dermatitis, ichthyoses, and scabies.

Complications

In general, there are few complications once the offending material has been recognized and contact eliminated. Occasionally, reactions from plants such as wild parsnips can be deep enough to cause scarring.

Management

The first step in treating contact dermatitis is removing the sensitizing material. In the case of *Rhus* dermatitis, this includes washing the skin and washing clothes that may carry *Rhus* oleoresin. Once the reaction has begun, fluid from the blisters does not spread the reaction either to the patient or to other people. There may be some delay in the appearance of the rash on thicker areas of skin. If new lesions appear over several days, the child is probably being reexposed.

Topical corticosteroids may help to relieve some of the inflammation. However, the rash can last for several weeks. In severe cases, systemic steroids such as prednisone (1 to 2 mg/kg per 24 hours over 7 to 10 days) can be helpful. The medication must be tapered gradually because the inflammation often rebounds.

Systemic H_1 antihistamines such as hydroxyzine can help relieve itching. Cool compresses with tap water or Burow's solution are important in relieving discomfort.

PEDICULOSIS

Head lice are frequently discovered by school nurses or day care workers. This infestation can cause such anxiety that medical care is requested at any time of the day.

Etiology

Pediculus humanus capitus, the common head louse, is a wingless insect about 2 to 4 mm long, which feeds on human blood. The female louse attaches to a hair shaft and lays eggs along the hair. The eggs hatch in about 10 days.

Epidemiology

Head lice are most common on school age children and somewhat more prevalent in girls. They prefer to attach to fine straight hair. The presence of head lice is not related to poor hygiene, although good grooming will decrease the severity of an infestation.

Clinical Findings

Scratching the scalp may be the first sign of head lice. Nits are commonly found close to the scalp, especially behind the ears and at the nape of the neck. Nits may be confused with dandruff and can be identified because the egg cases are firmly stuck to the hair shaft. Head lice spread from child to child by direct contact. Combs and hats can act as fomites that spread the infestation.

Differential Diagnosis

Dandruff, seborrhea, and neurotic excoriation of the scalp can all be confused with head lice.

Complications

Bacterial superinfection of the scalp may develop as a result of scratching. While it is recognized that body lice can spread typhus and relapsing fever, there are no reports that head lice are implicated in spreading blood-borne diseases.

Management

Treatment requires education to prevent reinfection as well as eradication of the infestation. There are several insecticides available as shampoos or cream rinses that are effective at killing adult lice and nits. Permethrin 1% cream rinse (Nix) is available without prescription and has an excellent safety record.

All members of a household should be treated at the same time. A second treatment should be done after 7 days. Insecticides will usually kill the larva inside the egg case; however, it may be difficult to dislodge the nit. Diluted vinegar seems to soften nit cement and can be used with a fine-tooth comb to remove the nits. Because lice are very heat sensitive, clothing and bedding that are washed and dried in a hot air dryer will be effectively cleaned. Clothing or hats that cannot be heat-treated can be disinfected if sealed in a plastic bag for 4 weeks. Any lice that hatch will starve in this time. Parents need to be warned that pruritus can last for several weeks after successful treatment. Multiple treatments with insecticides can lead to contact dermatitis. Some lice have become resistant to insecticides. Barrier methods of suffocating the lice may be tried to eradicate the infestation; examples of this treatment method include Vaseline or mayonnaise applied thickly to the hair and left in place under a shower cap for at least 12 hours. Antihistamines by mouth and topical hydrocortisone cream may help alleviate itching.

SCABIES

Scabies, a very pruritic skin infestation, is caused by a mite, *Sarcoptes scabiei*. It is quite contagious and spreads readily from one person to the next.

Etiology

Mites are white transparent insects with four pairs of legs. Mites are very small, less than a half a millimeter in length, and they are host species specific.

Epidemiology

Transmission of scabies requires close human contact; however, adult mites can survive for several days off the human body so it is possible that scabies could be transmitted without skin-to-skin contact. Epidemics in nursing homes can be difficult to eradicate.

Pathophysiology

The female mite burrows into the stratum corneum and lays two to three eggs per day for about a month. Larvae hatch in 3 to 4 days and crawl off to make a new burrow either on the same person or someone in close contact.

Clinical Findings

The earliest symptom is itching, which may be present before any burrow or papule can be seen. In adults and older children, papules develop on the hands and wrists,

especially in the interdigital webs, elbows, belt line, and gluteal cleft. Infants, however, may develop papules and vesicles all over their body, including palms and soles. Infants often have scabies on the face and scalp while this area is rarely affected in older children. Because of intense scratching, burrows are frequently a site for bacterial superinfection, and impetigo may be the presenting chief complaint.

Diagnosis

Scraping papules and fresh vesicles may yield the mite itself or more often its stool pellets. However, the sudden onset of very pruritic papules in children with other affected family members is suggestive of scabies even if the mite cannot be found.

Differential Diagnosis

Atopic dermatitis, papular urticaria, and simple insect bites are often confused with scabies. Because it is so contagious, it is uncommon to find scabies in children without other affected family members. A family history of pruritic papules is an important diagnostic feature.

Complications

Secondary infection with streptococcus or staphylococcus is the most common complication of this dermatitis. Acute glomerulonephritis secondary to streptococcal skin infection related to scabies has been described.

Management

All close personal contacts, as well as the affected child, must be treated with an insecticide. Permethrin cream (Elimite) can be applied to the body overnight and then rinsed off. A second treatment after 7 days is suggested.

Clothing and bed linen should be washed with ordinary soap at usual temperatures to eliminate any mites that are present. Infestations can usually be controlled without insecticide sprays. Antihistamines by mouth may be necessary to control itching for several weeks after treatment is initiated.

PAPULAR URTICARIA

Young children frequently develop an intense hypersensitivity reaction to insect bites. The initial reaction to an insect bite or sting may begin as a typical wheal and flare but then progress to a hard papule that persists for several days.

Etiology

Animal fleas or sand fleas are common insects responsible for the hyperreaction; however, any insect including mosquitoes, gnats, and mites can cause the reaction.

Epidemiology

Papular urticaria is seen in preschool children, especially infants in the second summer season when they are exposed to insect bites. Usually only one member of a family is affected.

Pathophysiology

The papules represent a delayed-type hypersensitivity reaction. Since skin must be previously sensitized, the reaction is not usually seen in the first year of life. As time goes by and the child is repeatedly reexposed to the offending antigen, hyposensitization and resolution of the reaction develop.

Clinical Findings

Dome-shaped papules in crops on areas of the body that are exposed to insect bites develop acutely. The reaction may be severe enough to cause vesicles and bullae. In most cases, no discrete puncture wound can be seen. The papules last for up to 2 weeks.

Differential Diagnosis

Simple insect bites, viral exanthems, and sun sensitivity reactions may occur acutely in exposed skin areas and be quite itchy.

Complications

Scratching can lead to bacterial superinfection from impetiginization to cellulitis.

Management

Childen should be protected from further insect bites by wearing pants and long sleeves with insect repellent such as DEET applied to the clothes. If the bites are coming from fleas, treating infested pets is extremely important. Topical hydrocortisone cream applied to the papules may be helpful. Oral antihistamines may be necessary to control itching.

URTICARIA

Hives is a benign self-limited problem that causes alarm because the hives appear suddenly and cause itchy discomfort. Urticaria is the most common pediatric dermatologic problem seen in emergency departments.

Etiology

While urticaria may develop in response to a specific allergen, most cases of urticaria are not related to a diagnosable exposure. Most cases of urticaria have no known cause.

Medications, seafoods, strawberries, peanuts, and tomatoes are among the commonly recognizable causes of hives. Insect stings may cause local urticaria or progress to systemic anaphylactic reaction.

Many respiratory infections, including viruses and group A beta-hemolytic streptococci, are responsible for hives. If children develop hives while taking antibiotics for a respiratory infection, it may be difficult to decide whether they are actually allergic to the medication. It has been reported that with follow-up skin testing, greater than 90 percent of children who have hives while taking ampicillin have no evidence of ampicillin allergy.

Pathophysiology

Hives develop as a result of vasodilatation and enhanced vascular permeability caused by release of histamine. The immunologic reaction occurs when a specific lgE antibody is bound to a mast cell membrane. It should be noted that hives do not develop on exposure to a new substance. Prior sensitization to a substance is essential to produce an IgE-mediated reaction.

Clinical Findings

Urticaria occurs on all parts of the body. The condition is very pruritic and transient, lasting from a few minutes to several hours. Urticaria typically appears on areas of skin that are warm or which are under pressure, such as under waistbands. The hives are accentuated by heat and often develop after a bath or when children are wrapped in warm clothing.

Differential Diagnosis

Urticaria and erythema multiforme are frequently confused. Two clinical points can help to differentiate these conditions. Erythema multiforme is a fixed skin reaction. Individual lesions last for several days. Subcutaneous epinephrine can be given to clear urticaria, but it does not change erythema multiforme.

Complications

Some urticarial reactions may signal the potential to develop a future anaphylactic reaction. This is especially true for bee stings and significant food allergy reactions.

Management

If urticaria is severe, subcutaneous epinephrine (1:1,000) at a dose of 0.01 mL/kg (maximum 0.3 mL) will give some short-term relief. H_1 antihistamines can be used for long-term control of urticaria. Topical antihistamines and steroids do not help to control urticaria. Systemic corticosteroids have been used for chronic severe urticaria, but this is not needed for most cases.

ERYTHEMA MULTIFORME

The definition of this hypersensitivity reaction is controversial and includes a variety of skin problems from minor itching and urticaria-like lesions to severe blistering and desquamation.

Etiology

The agents most commonly responsible for erythema multiforme are infections and drug exposure. Sulfa products and phenytoin are medications commonly recognized as causing severe reactions. Penicillin and cephalosporins can also cause erythema multiforme.

Recurrent herpes simplex, as well as *Mycoplasma pneumoniae,* are infectious agents that can lead to erythema multiforme reactions. No specific inciting agent is identified for about 50 percent of cases.

Pathophysiology

The skin reactions result from an immune response to a foreign antigen. Circulatory immune complexes are often present in blood and may be found in skin lesions. This has been demonstrated in herpes-associated erythema multiforme.

Skin biopsies show evidence of epidermal damage with perivascular lymphatic infiltration and edema below the epidermis that produces the urticarial lesions.

Clinical Findings

There are several clinical syndromes within the erythema multiforme group. All have similar pathophysiologic findings.

Erythema multiforme minor is a condition of urticarial-like lesions with little systemic reaction. The lesions are different from common urticaria because they are fixed in the skin and fade slowly over a week's time. They do not blister, but they are usually pruritic. They can be differentiated from urticaria because they do not clear when subcutaneous epinephrine is given. The lesions may develop a characteristic target shape or they may remain as round-topped papules. They last for about 1 week and become darker as they start to resolve.

Stevens-Johnson syndrome is more severe with fever, general malaise, and blistering of mucous membranes. The epidermal lesions may blister and may look like varicella when the blisters are small. The mucous membranes of the mouth can become deeply eroded and crusted. Conjunctivae and urogenital mucous membranes also become inflamed.

Toxic epidermal necrolysis (TEN) is the most severe variant of erythema multiforme. Dramatic blisters develop rapidly over all areas of the body. High fever and severe mucous membrane involvement are common.

Differential Diagnosis

Urticaria and mild erythema multiforme are commonly confused but can be differentiated by the transient nature of urticaria that will clear with subcutaneous epinephrine. Vesicular rashes such as varicella may be confused with more severe erythema multiforme.

Severe reactions resemble staphylococcal scalded skin syndrome. A skin biopsy may be needed to differentiate the two. Biopsy of TEN will show a lymphocytic infiltrate with full-thickness necrosis of the epidermis, while staphylococcal scalded skin syndrome produces intraepidermal cleavage.

Complications

Mild cases resolve completely. Problems with maintaining fluid balance and adequate nutrition may develop in cases with oral blistering. Lesions that are severely blistered may be deep enough to produce scarring. There is a serious risk of mortality for patients with TEN who have significant disruption of the normal skin protective barrier.

Management

Mild cases need only symptomatic care with oral antihistamines. When mucous membranes become involved, intravenous fluids and hyperalimentation may be needed. The use of systemic corticosteroids is controversial. Mildly affected patients do well without them. For patients with TEN, the increased risk of complications such as gastrointestinal hemorrhage and sepsis outweigh the potential value of decreasing blistering; steroids should not be used. There is some suggestion that in moderate cases blistering may be diminished if steroids are initiated within the first 2 weeks of an eruption.

BIBLIOGRAPHY

AAP 2000 Red Book: *Report of the Committee on Infectious Diseases,* 25th ed. American Academy of Pediatrics.

Cohen B: *Pediatric Dermatology,* 2d ed. St. Louis, Mosby Year Book, 1999.

Edwards L: *Dermatology in Emergency Care,* New York, WB Saunders, 1997.

Schachner LA, Hansen RC (eds): *Pediatric Dermatology,* 2d ed. New York, Saunders, 1995.

Weston WL, Lane AT: *Color Textbook of Pediatric Dermatology,* St. Louis, Mosby Year Book, 1996.

64

Superficial Skin Infections

Julia A. Rosekrans

HIGH-YIELD FACTS

- Poststreptococcal glomerulonephritis has been seen when nephrogenic strains of streptococci cause skin infection.
- Staphylococcal scalded skin syndrome (SSS) is characterized by erythema, a generalized blistering and peeling of skin over the whole body. It is a serious systemic illness that has a risk of mortality.
- Most children with SSS are treated with intravenous antibiotics, such as cefazolin or nafcillin.

Children are brought to the emergency department for treatment when the parent recognizes that there is a rash that they are unable to treat at home. They often have questions about contagiousness of the rash, especially when children attend day care.

IMPETIGO AND ECTHYMA

The most common skin infection in children is impetigo. It develops as a secondary problem when the normal protective barrier of the skin is broken. Impetigo often complicates pruritic skin problems. Impetigo is superficial, involving the papillary epidermis, while ecthyma involves the entire thickness of the epidermis.

Etiology

There are two clinically distinguishable types of impetigo. Bullous impetigo is caused by *Staphylococcus aureus*. Both *S. aureus* and group A beta-hemolytic streptococci (GABHS) are involved in nonbullous impetigo and ecthyma.

Epidemiology

Superficial skin infections are more common during warm seasons of the year and in tropical climates. The infection spreads easily from child to child. If left untreated, a single lesion may heal spontaneously; however, new lesions crop up so that a single episode of impetigo may last for many weeks.

Pathophysiology

Microscopic breaks in the epidermis predispose to invasion by bacteria that are common environmental contaminants. The skin surface is often colonized with staphylococcal and streptococcal organisms before any infection is apparent. A wound or penetrating injury allows the bacteria to invade deeper epidermal tissues. Although biopsy is rarely used to diagnose this problem, it would show tiny vesicles within the epidermis containing bacteria and polymorphonuclear infiltrates.

Clinical Findings

Bullous impetigo begins as small papules that develop into 1- to 2-cm bullae. These thin-walled bullae rupture easily, and the shiny, wet, red base of the blister is usually all that is seen. The lesions are found most often on the buttocks and perineum or on the face, but can also occur anywhere on the body

Nonbullous impetigo forms a pustular reaction with a serous honey-colored crust. The lesions may be described as pruritic if the infection is a complication of an insect bite or other pruritic dermatitis. Sometimes the lesions spread leaving a central clear healed area. Regional lymph nodes may be enlarged if the infection is deep or has been present for a long period. Ecthyma, because it is deeper, is often painful and may involve lymphangitis or surrounding cellulitis.

Diagnosis

Laboratory studies are rarely needed to confirm the diagnosis.

Differential Diagnosis

Herpes simplex lesions often resemble impetigo, and a viral culture may be needed if identification is required. Varicella and contact dermatitis may resemble the vesicle stage of impetigo. Tinea capitus that has progressed to kerion formation looks as if it is impetiginized; however, the reaction is a response to the fungal infection.

Complications

Impetigo, because it is so superficial, rarely causes any scarring; however, ecthyma does tend to leave scars.

Poststreptococcal glomerulonephritis has been seen when nephrogenic strains of streptococci cause the skin infection. There have not been any reports of rheumatic fever or carditis due to impetigo.

Management

Treatment of impetigo depends on antibiotic therapy. In widespread cases, oral antibiotics active against staphylococci are needed. Dicloxacillin, 20 to 50 mg/kg per 24 hours divided in four doses, or cefadroxil, 30 mg/kg per 24 hours in two doses, work well. Mupirocin (Bactroban) 2% ointment is also effective in many situations, especially when the infection is localized.

STAPHYLOCOCCAL SCALDED SKIN SYNDROME

This superficial skin infection is characterized by erythema and generalized blistering and peeling of skin over the whole body. It is a serious systemic illness that has a risk of mortality.

Etiology

The illness is caused by an infection with a strain of *S. aureus* that produces an epidermolytic toxin. The infecting bacteria may be located in the nose, conjunctivae, or even an infected umbilical stump.

Clinical Findings

It is most often seen in children under 5 years of age. Children with this illness are usually febrile and often complain of painful skin. The rash begins with generalized erythema and quickly progresses to formation of large bullae with desquamation of large sheets of skin. Serous crusts may be seen around the nose and mouth.

Diagnosis

Cultures of the skin or bullae are often sterile. However, *S. aureus* may be recovered from cultures of the nose or any sores or wounds.

Differential Diagnosis

In the initial erythematous phase, scarlet fever, toxic shock syndrome, severe erythema multiforme, and even sunburn may be considered.

Complications

With early recognition and management, patients recover fully with no permanent sequelae or scarring.

Management

Fluid loss, electrolyte imbalance, heat loss, and pain control are problems that must be managed along with antibiotics to eradicate staphylococci. Most children are treated with intravenous antibiotics such as cefazolin or nafcillin. Analgesics such as acetaminophen are needed for pain. Mild lubricant creams may be helpful in the healing stages to reduce skin discomfort.

FUNGAL INFECTIONS

Fungi are simple plants that lack chlorophyll and obtain nourishment from other living or dead organic material. Superficial fungal infections of the epidermis, hair, or nails are caused by dermatophytes.

TINEA CAPITIS

Fungal infections of the scalp are most commonly seen in children between 2 and 10 years of age.

Etiology

Most cases in the United States are caused by *Trichophyton tonsurans*. *Microsporum audouinii* is seen in less than 10 percent of cases. *M. canis* can also cause infection, but is usually transmitted from an infected cat rather than a dog.

Epidemiology

Trichophyton tonsurans infections are found with equal frequency in girls and boys. The infection is quite contagious and will persist for years if not treated. Infections increase in frequency in hot humid climates and in crowded living conditions.

Pathophysiology

The most common pattern of fungal infections seen at the present in the United States is called endothrix. Fungal spores develop entirely within the hair shaft leading to fragile hairs that break easily and which do not fluoresce under ultraviolet light. Kerion formation develops in about one-third of cases of untreated tinea capitis. A kerion is a tender boggy crusted pustular mass caused by a vigorous cellular immune response to fungal antigen.

Clinical Findings

Typical patches of tinea capitis are round oval areas of alopecia about 1 to 5 cm in diameter. Stubby hair shafts broken off at the level of the scalp cause a "black dot" appearance.

Occasionally, tinea capitis can resemble flaky dandruff without any clear patches of alopecia. Close examination will still show black dots. If kerion formation occurs, occipital and cervical lymphadenopathy sometimes will be accompanied by low-grade fever.

Diagnosis

Hairs infected by *Microsporum species* will fluoresce yellow–green in the presence of long-wave ultraviolet light produced by a Wood's lamp. Unfortunately, this organism causes the minority of infections.

Potassium hydroxide (KOH) preparation of hair and scalp scrapings will show spores and hyphae, either along side or within the hair shaft. Fungal cultures should be obtained routinely because the course of therapy can be quite long.

Differential Diagnosis

Circumscribed areas of alopecia can result from noninfectious conditions such as alopecia areata and trichotillomania. Traction alopecia from tight braiding can cause hairs to break off close to the scalp. Seborrhea, dandruff, and psoriasis can be confused with the diffuse scaly form of tinea capitis. Kerion formation is most often confused with bacterial skin infections; however, the exudate of the kerion is sterile.

Complications

Complete destruction of the hair follicle with scarring and permanent baldness can result if untreated.

Treatment

Initial therapy for tinea capitis is oral griseofulvin at a dose of 15 mg/kg/day. This must continue for at least 6 weeks. Oral prednisone may be helpful in reducing the inflammatory kerion response.

Fungal spores remain viable for a long period. Barrettes, combs, and brushes must be washed frequently. All family members should be checked for infection since this is quite contagious. Children can be permitted to return to school after 1 week of griseofulvin therapy.

TINEA CORPORIS

Dermatophyte infections of the epidermis are superficial and less problematic than is tinea capitis. This condition can be found on any part of the body.

Etiology

Microsporum canis and *T. mentagrophytes* are responsible for tinea corporis. Any organism that can cause tinea capitis can also cause tinea corporis.

Epidemiology

Infected domestic and farm animals are a common source of infection. Tinea corporis is most common in children, and adults with tinea corporis are usually in contact with young children. Tinea corporis is seen worldwide but is more prevalent in warm climates.

Pathophysiology

The dermatophyte invades the stratum corneum and does not extend to deeper epidermal layers. Toxins released by the dermatophyte are thought to be responsible for the inflammatory response. Hair follicles are often invaded and may act as a reservoir for recurrent disease.

Clinical Findings

Lesions may appear as papules, vesicles, or eczematous plaques. However, the most recognizable pattern is the classic oval ringworm shape of an expanding inflammatory border with a clear central area.

The rash is often pruritic. Regional lymph nodes are usually not involved unless the lesion becomes impetiginized.

Diagnosis

Potassium hydroxide (KOH) prep of material from the scaly inflammatory border should be used to confirm the presence of hyphae. Cultures are not usually needed because topical treatment is usually effective.

Differential Diagnosis

Pityriasis rosea, granuloma annulare, and atopic dermatitis are sometimes confused with tinea corporis.

Complications

With treatment, infections usually clear completely without any scarring.

Management

Topical therapy may result in relief of itching within a week; however, therapy should continue for a minimum of 2 to 3 weeks after initial clearing.

There are several effective topical antifungal medications available without prescription, including tolnaftate (Tinactin), miconazole (Micatin), haloprogin (Halotex), and clotrimazole (Lotrimin). All are used by rubbing cream into the affected area twice a day. Failure to improve after 3 weeks of treatment is reason for further evaluation.

BIBLIOGRAPHY

AAP 2000 Red Book: *Report of the Committee on Infectious Diseases,* 25th ed. American Academy of Pediatrics.

Cohen B: *Pediatric Dermatology,* 2d ed., St. Louis, Mosby Year Book, 1999.

Edwards L: *Dermatology in Emergency Care,* New York, WB Saunders, 1997.

Schachner LA, Hansen RC (eds): *Pediatric Dermatology,* 2d ed. New York, Saunders, 1995.

Weston WL, Lane AT: *Color Textbook of Pediatric Dermatology,* St. Louis, Mosby Year Book, 1996.

65

Exanthems

Julia A. Rosekrans

HIGH-YIELD FACTS

- The most common problem for which children with measles require hospitalization is pneumonia. Encephalitis with neurologic sequelae can occur.
- Scarlet fever has the same risks as a group A beta-hemolytic streptococci (GABHS) infection without a rash.
- Acyclovir inhibits herpes virus deoxyribonucleic acid (DNA) polymerase. It can be given in intravenous form to immune-compromised children or children with significant complications of chickenpox.
- Neonatal herpes can disseminate and cause encephalitis or death.

Viral illnesses often produce characteristic skin rashes and a pattern of clinical symptoms that help to categorize the illness. Sometimes children are brought to the emergency department with a fever, and the rash is found only when the children are undressed. Contagiousness is the primary concern for some parents, especially when the child attends day care. At other times, parents may recognize the disease; however, the children are more ill than expected. Besides recognizing the rash, the physician should be prepared to discuss the course of the illness, risk to others, incubation period, and potential complications.

RUBEOLA (MEASLES)

The number of cases of measles has dropped precipitously since live attenuated virus vaccine was introduced in 1963. Today most cases occur as community epidemics when there are high rates of inadequately immunized children. To help control rubeola, some emergency pediatricians have suggested that measles immunizations should be given at emergency department visits.

Etiology

Measles virus is a single-stranded ribonucleic acid (RNA) paramyxovirus.

Epidemiology

The measles virus is transmitted by droplet spread and is highly contagious. There is an incubation period of about 9 to 12 days between exposure and the onset of symptoms. Patients with the illness are most contagious during the prodromal period, starting about 3 days before the onset of the rash, and are considered contagious for about 4 days after.

Pathophysiology

The measles virus enters the body through the respiratory tract. By the time symptoms appear, the virus is distributed throughout the body, and multinucleated giant cells can be recovered from urine, sputum, and nasal secretions.

Clinical Findings

Typical measles begin with a prodrome of respiratory symptoms. Cough, conjunctivitis, and coryza (nasal congestion) are usually present. Koplik's spots, tiny white spots on erythematous buccal mucosa opposite the lower molars, appear during the prodrome and last for about 24 hours. They are usually still present when the rash begins.

The exanthem appears about 14 days after exposure. It begins at the hairline behind the ears and then spreads from the head to the feet over about 3 days. It is erythematous and maculopapular. Although individual spots may be seen initially, these become confluent over time. Patients look most ill on the second or third day with high fever, brassy cough, and photophobia. In healthy children, the illness lasts for about 7 days.

Diagnosis

There are no specific laboratory tests that help identify the disease acutely. Serologic testing may be helpful for community surveillance.

Complications

Otitis media is the most common complication of measles. Respiratory complications include croup and

Table 65-1. Differential Diagnosis of Morbilliform Rashes

Viral	Drug-Induced Reaction
Measles	Ampicillin
Rubella	Nonsteroidal anti-inflammatories
Roseola	Barbiturates
Fifth disease	Phenytoin
Infectious mononucleosis	Sulfa antibiotics
Pityriasis rosea	Thiazides

Bacterial	Reactive Erythema
Scarlet fever	Urticaria
Toxic shock syndrome	Erythema multiforme
Kawasaki syndrome	Rocky Mountain Spotted Fever

laryngitis. The most common problem for which children with measles require hospitalization is pneumonia. Encephalitis with neurologic sequelae can occur.

Management

There is no treatment for measles other than symptomatic support with bed rest and analgesics. Live attenuated measles vaccine given within 72 hours of exposure can provide some protection by stimulating active antibody production. Immune serum globulin 0.25 mL/kg intramuscularly (IM), maximum 15 mL, will prevent or modify the disease if given within 6 days of exposure. Documented cases of measles should be reported to local public health authorities to reduce the possibility of an epidemic.

RUBELLA (GERMAN MEASLES)

Rubella, a mild viral illness, is significant because of its teratogenic effects.

Etiology

Rubella is a single-stranded RNA virus.

Epidemiology

The incidence of rubella disease has fallen since introduction of live attenuated viral vaccine in 1969. While some adolescents and young adults are not immune to rubella, a high rate of immunity among young children provides a protective level of herd immunity.

Droplet spread through the respiratory route results in a high rate of transmission among susceptible people. The incubation period is 14 to 23 days with a period of infectiousness from 1 week before to about 5 days after the rash appears. Infants with congenital rubella syndrome can spread infection because they shed the virus for months after birth. There is a high rate of subclinical infection and many adults are immune without a history of having the illness.

Pathophysiology

The cause of the rash is not fully understood. In a research setting, the virus can be recovered from papules on the skin as well as from skin that appears normal. The skin rash is probably due to an antigen-antibody reaction.

Clinical Findings

Rubella in children is a very mild disease, although parents sometimes describe children as being unusually fussy. Slight fever and marked lymphadenopathy with prominent postauricular and suboccipital lymph nodes usually occur at the same time that the rash is present. The rash itself is a nonspecific diffuse erythematous maculopapular eruption. Older children often complain of transient joint pain.

Diagnosis

Serologic tests can be done if it is necessary to reach a definitive diagnosis. This is not useful acutely.

Complications

Arthritis or arthralgia may begin during the prodrome or can follow the rash. This does not appear to predispose to arthritis later in life. Rare complications include thrombocytopenia or encephalitis.

The most significant complication is fetal malformation following a maternal rubella infection during the first or second trimester of pregnancy. The infection affects the organ system that is undergoing most rapid development of the time of the viremia. The only treatment is preventing maternal infection by maintaining a high rate of herd immunity among young children and by immunization of adults before pregnancy occurs.

Management

This self-limited disease requires only symptomatic treatment. Nonsteroidal anti-inflammatory medication may be needed to control symptoms of arthritis.

ROSEOLA (EXANTHEM SUBITUM)

Etiology

Human herpes virus C has recently been identified as the cause of roseola.

Epidemiology

Roseola, a common illness, rarely occurs before about 6 months of age or after 2 years. Clinical disease occurs in about 25 percent of all infants; however, antibody titers are present in most adults so subclinical infection must be common.

Most cases appear in spring and early fall. The illness is droplet respiratory spread with an incubation period of about 5 to 15 days.

Clinical Findings

The most characteristic feature of roseola is a well-looking child despite high fever. There does not appear to be a prodrome. The fever comes on suddenly and persists for 3 to 4 days. The rash appears as the fever vanishes and resolves within 48 hours.

Febrile seizures may occur with this illness. Some infants have a bulging fontanel without other meningeal symptoms, and results of lumbar punctures are unremarkable.

Diagnosis

There are no laboratory findings that are helpful in defining roseola. The diagnosis is based on the pattern of clinical symptoms and is usually made when the illness is over and the rash appears.

Complications

There are no known complications of roseola.

Management

Symptomatic care is all that is needed.

FIFTH DISEASE (ERYTHEMA INFECTIOSUM)

Fifth disease, a mild illness, is usually recognized in school age children.

Etiology

Parvovirus B19, a single-stranded DNA virus, was identified as the cause of Fifth disease in 1975.

Epidemiology

Fifth disease occurs in school age children in the spring and winter. It is probably droplet spread, but it is only mildly contagious. School-wide epidemics have been described.

Pathophysiology

Viremia occurs about 1 week after exposure and lasts for 3 to 5 days. By the time the characteristic rash develops, the virus is no longer recoverable.

Clinical Findings

The rash develops abruptly with bright red cheeks giving the "slapped cheek" appearance. A maculopapular faintly pink rash develops on the trunk and extremities then clears in a lacy pattern. The rash fades over several days but can reappear intermittently for several weeks, especially when skin is exposed to sun or a warm bath. Children occasionally have a low-grade fever but generally seem quite well.

Diagnosis

The diagnosis for Fifth disease is made on clinical evidence.

Complications

In a healthy person, there are no apparent complications. Adults may develop transient arthritis, although this is rare in children.

Parvovirus has been associated with bone marrow suppression and aplastic crisis in children with sickle cell anemia. Infection during pregnancy can result in fetal death or red blood cell aplasia with fetal hydrops.

Management

Fifth disease is self-limited in children and requires no therapy. Serologic testing is suggested for pregnant women who develop the disease or who are in close contact with children who have the illness.

SCARLET FEVER

Etiology

Scarlet fever is a result of a reaction to erythrogenic toxin produced by several strains of GABHS. It can develop in association with *Streptococcus* pharyngitis and can be seen with impetigo or cellulitis.

Pathophysiology

There are three different toxins that can produce scarlet fever, as well as several different strains of erythrogenic GABHS, so it is possible for an individual to have scarlet fever more than once.

Clinical Findings

A sandpaper rash begins in skin folds such as the groin, axillae, and antecubital areas. The area around the mouth and nose is not erythematous, giving an appearance of circumoral pallor. Generalized lymphadenopathy is common. The exanthem usually develops within 12 to 48 hours after onset of fever and chills. Desquamation progresses in the same pattern.

Diagnosis

The diagnosis for scarlet fever depends on culture documentation of GABHS infection, since viral illnesses may cause a similar rash.

Complications

Scarlet fever has the same risks as a GABHS infection without a rash. It is no more serious, although its name sounds worse to many parents. The risks of rheumatic fever and glomerulonephritis exist but at the same rate as streptococcal infections without rash.

Management

Oral penicillin VK 15 to 50 mg/kg per 24 hours divided in 3 doses, or erythromycin, 20 to 50 mg/kg per 24 hours in 3 to 4 divided doses is adequate to control disease spread. Children should not return to school until 24 hours after starting antibiotics.

CHICKENPOX

Chickenpox, a common childhood illness, is a primary viral infection with a typical clinical course and rash.

Etiology

Varicella zoster is a herpes-type virus. This group of viruses has the property of remaining latent in the body for years after a primary infection. The virus can be reactivated and produce a secondary recurrent illness.

Epidemiology

The incubation period for chickenpox is 14 to 21 days. Most cases occur in children under 14 years of age because the virus is so common. The method of viral spread is not clear and both direct contact and airborne spread has been documented.

Pathophysiology

Herpes viruses cause an intracellular infection. Because viral replication takes place within epidermal cells, antibodies cannot interact directly with the active virus. Epidermal multinucleated giant cells are produced either by fusion of several epidermal cells or by nuclear division without simultaneous cytoplasmic division.

Clinical Findings

Chickenpox begins with a mild 1- or 2-day prodrome of respiratory symptoms and low-grade fever. The rash appears on the trunk as small red papules that progress to tiny vesicles giving the "dew drop on a rose petal" appearance. Crops of vesicles develop for 3 to 5 days so that all stages of the lesions can be found at the same time on any part of the body. When the vesicles dry and crust, they are thought not to be infectious.

Subclinical infections are common, so many adults who are not known to have had the disease are actually immune. Although varicella usually gives lifelong immunity with the first infection, second attacks can occur. When one child starts a family epidemic of chickenpox, each subsequent child seems to develop a more severe illness.

Diagnosis

The clinical presentation is usually specific and no tests are needed. A Tzanck preparation to demonstrate multinucleated giant cells can be done to distinguish a herpes virus infection from other vesicular eruptions.

Differential Diagnosis

Typical chickenpox is rarely confused with other illnesses. Papular urticaria and hand-foot-and-mouth disease may be confused with early varicella. Disseminated herpes simplex could look like chickenpox, and a viral culture might be needed to distinguish these two viral illnesses.

Complications

The most common complications are bacterial superinfections of the skin lesions and otitis media. Since varicella is a systemic illness, all body systems can be involved. Adolescents are more at risk for complications than are young children. Inpatient care may be needed for children with cellulitis, pneumonia, or encephalitis.

Most adults have some shallow varicella scars. These occur most often in lesions that have become superinfected.

Management

For children with uncomplicated illnesses, treatment is symptomatic and supportive. Antihistamines such as diphenhydramine may help control itching. Oatmeal baths are also quite soothing.

Acyclovir inhibits herpes virus DNA polymerase. It can be given in intravenous form to immunocompromised children or children with significant complications of chickenpox. Oral acyclovir will decrease the duration of development of skin lesions in healthy children if it is given within the first 24 hours of rash appearance. It should be considered for therapy in household contacts and adolescents whose illness is often more problematic.

Children who are at high risk for severe or complicated infections should be given varicella zoster immune globulin if it can be given within 48 hours of varicella exposure. The dose is 125 U per 10 kg of body weight with a maximum dose of 625 U.

HERPES ZOSTER

After a primary varicella infection, the varicella zoster virus persists in a latent condition in spinal sensory nerve root ganglia. The virus can erupt years later.

Epidemiology

The incidence of zoster increases with age and is more common in people with immune suppression. Virus is present within these vesicles and a susceptible person can develop chickenpox from direct contact.

Tingling pain usually precedes the appearance of vesicles that occur in two or three crops within one dermatome. The most common area of involvement is the thoracic area where several adjacent dermatomes may be involved. The lumbosacral area is also commonly involved. The least commonly involved areas in children are the cranial nerves; however, since eruption here can involve the cornea, this pattern is the most medically worrisome.

Complications

Serious complications usually occur only in immunosuppressed patients. For most people, the eruption is troublesome and painful but self-limited. Postherpetic pain without any reappearance of skin lesions is more common in adults than it is in children. Acyclovir and varicella zoster immune globulin (VZIg) are useful in managing this type of herpes virus eruption.

HERPES SIMPLEX

The clinical manifestations of infection with herpes simplex virus range from recurrent cold sores to encephalitis.

Etiology

Two types of herpes simplex virus are known to cause infection in humans, type 1 (HSV-1) and type 2 (HSV-2). Both types can cause similar clinical patterns, however HSV-1 is more common and tends to be found in oral infections. HSV-2 is usually associated with genital infections. Both viruses can cause subclinical infection and both remain latent within the body after initial infection.

Epidemiology

Herpes simplex virus is species-specific and affects only humans. It is passed by direct contact, either with another person who has an active infection or with droplets on fomites. Lesions that are clinically inapparent can shed the virus. The incubation period is variable and ranges from 1 day to 4 weeks.

Pathophysiology

At the time of an initial infection, the virus enters the epithelium and travels to regional nerve ganglia where it remains for the host's lifetime. Because it is intracellular, normal immune protection mechanisms do not work against these latent viruses. Current antiviral agents also do not eradicate the latent state.

Clinical Findings

Herpes gingivostomatitis is a primary infection usually caused by HSV-1. The peak incidence of this infection is seen in children less than 5 years of age. Children appear quite ill with high fever, painful vesicles on the tongue and mucous membranes, and regional lymphadenopathy. They frequently drool and refuse to eat. The fever may last for 1 week with sores persisting for up to 2 weeks.

Herpetic whitlow describes a painful inoculation of herpes virus onto a finger. This often happens in children who suck their fingers. It can also develop in medical personnel with a needle stick. A primary infection with fever, local pain, regional lymphadenopathy, and general malaise may develop.

Genital herpes usually results from sexual contact with an infected partner; however, it can also develop from self-inoculation from an oral infection with virus spread on the patient's hands or from contact with fomites. A primary reaction will include painful local vesicles, regional lymphadenopathy, and fever.

Not all patients develop recurrent local herpes after a primary infection. In addition, many primary infections are subclinical so patients with recurrent local eruptions may not have had a severe primary illness. When a local reaction begins, most people describe itching and burning in the region for a day before vesicles appear. Pain can last for a brief time or up to 1 week. There is no lymphadenopathy, and viral shedding rapidly decreases. While some people know that local reactions are triggered by exposure to sun, spicy foods, stress, or trauma, many patients cannot determine a specific trigger mechanism.

Neonatal herpes simplex infection has a serious risk of mortality or long-term morbidity. It is usually caused by HSV-2 and results from either intrauterine or intrapartum exposure. Infants, however, with postpartum infection can be infected by exposure to any adult with an active herpes infection, including cold sores. Infants may develop disseminated systemic illness, an infection limited to the skin or encephalitis without any skin lesions. Symptoms may develop as late as 6 weeks after birth.

Diagnosis

Performing a Tzanck smear can identify herpes simplex infections. Material from the base of a fresh vesicle is stained with Giemsa's stain. Multinucleated giant cells can be identified easily. Confirmation of infection with viral culture may be necessary, especially for genital lesions.

Differential Diagnosis

Other vesicular rashes can be confused with primary herpes infections. Hand-foot-and-mouth disease and herpangina resemble gingivostomatitis. Impetigo and herpes labialis are often confused since both have yellow serous crust with surrounding erythema. Gram's stain or Tzanck smear may help to distinguish them. Herpetic whitlow is often confused with bacterial cellulitis since the involved finger is usually swollen and erythematous. Herpes genital infection can be confused with other venereal problems. This condition may coexist with gonorrhea or syphilis.

Complications

Most cases of herpes infections resolve without scarring. Problems are related only to the pain of the eruption. Neonatal herpes can disseminate and cause encephalitis or death.

Management

Acyclovir inhibits DNA synthesis and will shorten the course of a primary infection if started early in the illness. This has not been approved for use in children with gingivostomatitis, and the long-term effects of acyclovir in children are not known. It has been used in genital herpes infections at a dose of 200 mg every 4 hours for 5 doses a day for 10 days.

Local acyclovir 5% ointment applied in a small amount 6 times a day may provide some relief of symptoms and shorten viral shedding for localized perioral or genital infections.

If no treatment is given, as many as 70 percent of infants will develop disseminated infection. There is a 50 percent chance of mortality with systemic illness. Infants with herpes encephalitis usually develop permanent long-term neurologic sequelae.

Intravenous acyclovir is recommended for neonatal herpes infections when systemic illness or encephalitis is present. Because infants with skin lesions may develop encephalitis as a late complication, some authorities recommend oral acyclovir during the first few months after birth.

Local symptomatic care includes analgesics, cool compresses, ice packs, and enforcement of fluids. Children with oral primary herpes infections may have so much pain that they refuse to drink and require intravenous fluids.

While local eruptions do shed virus, this virus is so common in children that isolation to prevent contagion is not practical.

ENTEROVIRUSES

Many viral exanthems occur that are not clinically significant enough for an exact etiology to be sought. Nonspecific viral rashes may be maculopapular, scarlatiniform, vesicular, or urticarial. A few clinical syndromes can be differentiated. Most of these rashes come to a clinician's attention because a child has fever, fussiness, or other systemic symptoms.

Clinical Findings

Hand-foot-and-mouth syndrome is caused by coxsackievirus A16 and occasionally by A5 and A10. It is seen most commonly in summer and fall. The incubation period is variable, usually a few days. A prodrome of low fever, malaise, and abdominal pain may precede the rash. Children may complain of a sore mouth or painful hands and feet. Vesicles about 5 mm in diameter are found on palms, soles of feet, buttocks, and sometimes on the trunk. Oral lesions usually appear later on the soft palate, gingivae, and tongue. The illness lasts about 3 to 6 days and resolves without problems. It is possible for cases to recur for several weeks. Occasional cases of myocarditis, pneumonia, and meningoencephalitis have been reported.

Herpangina is an enanthem of tiny vesicles on the soft palate, uvula, and tonsils. This can be produced by several enteroviruses, as well as by herpes simplex. Sore throat and pain with eating are the most common complaints. Fever, headache, myalgia, and vomiting may be present.

Management

Soft diet, bed rest if needed, and analgesics for pain are used for symptomatic care. Good hand washing may help to reduce viral spread. Many infections are subclinical and isolation from day care is impractical.

PITYRIASIS ROSEA

Pityriasis rosea, a self-limited disorder, is usually seen in adolescents and young adults who seek medical care because the rash is spreading.

Etiology

An infectious etiology is thought to cause the rash because it tends to appear in community-wide clusters; however, no specific virus has been identified.

Clinical Findings

The distribution of the rash is diagnostic. Most cases begin with a single, large, oval scaly patch about 2 to 5 cm in diameter. This "herald patch" may not be noticed until the secondary eruption develops. Crops of small oval scaly patches appear on the trunk parallel to skin cleavage lines creating a "Christmas tree" pattern. The herald patch fades quickly while the secondary patches may take several weeks to fade. Some patients report mild itching. Occasionally, patients may have pharyngitis and malaise.

Differential Diagnosis

Other scaly lesions may be confused with pityriasis rosea. Tinea corporis is often mistaken for the herald patch. The most important differential consideration is secondary syphilis, and a serologic test should be ordered in all sexually active teenagers.

Management

Most patients require only reassurance and education. Exposure to sunlight may hasten disappearance of the rash. Topical steroids do not seem to shorten the course, although moisturizers may stop itching. Whether or not treated, the rash resolves without sequelae.

BIBLIOGRAPHY

AAP 2000 Red Book: *Report of the Committee on Infectious Diseases,* 25th ed. American Academy of Pediatrics.

Cohen B: *Pediatric Dermatology,* 2d ed. St. Louis, Mosby Year Book, 1999.

Edwards L: *Dermatology in Emergency Care,* New York, WB Saunders, 1997.

Schachner LA, Hansen RC (eds): *Pediatric Dermatology,* 2d ed. New York, Saunders, 1995.

Weston WL, Lane AT: *Color Textbook of Pediatric Dermatology,* St. Louis, Mosby Year Book, 1996.

66

Infant Rashes

Julia A. Rosekrans

HIGH-YIELD FACTS

- *Candida* diaper dermatitis appears as reddened skin with sharply demarcated margins.
- Perianal streptococcal infection should be treated with oral antibiotics—either penicillin or erythromycin.

SEBORRHEIC DERMATITIS

This chronic condition with greasy scaly skin may also be seen in adolescents; however, it is most commonly a parental concern when it develops in a young infant.

Etiology

Overproduction of sebum leads to accumulation of scaly exfoliated skin on the scalp and eyebrows and in flexural areas behind the ears and in the axillae. The mechanism for overproduction of sebum is not known; however, seborrhea seems more common in warm weather. There does not seem to be a genetic predisposition to developing seborrhea. Numerous theories about etiologies of seborrheic dermatitis have been proposed including food allergy and autoimmunity to *Candida* or epidermal tissue; however, no theory has been clearly validated.

Differential Diagnosis

Minor problems such as dandruff and significant problems such as Letterer-Siwe disease may be confused with seborrhea. Psoriasis, yeast infections, and atopic dermatitis all share similarities in appearance.

Management

Low-potency topical corticosteroids are used to treat inflamed weeping areas. Scales on the scalp can be softened with mineral oil and washed off with mild sham-poo. Diaper rash often requires treatment with antifungal medication to eradicate superinfection with *Candida*.

The process is chronic and follows a relapsing course until it resolves spontaneously, usually before 1 year of age. Infants with seborrhea do not have increased problems with seborrhea or acne as adolescents.

DIAPER DERMATITIS

Many different skin problems occur in the diaper area. Almost every diapered infant will develop some diaper rash, but only about 10 percent of infants will have serious problems.

Etiology

There are several problems that commonly cause diaper rashes. The most important problem is chronically wet skin. Wet skin is vulnerable to injury from friction and any condition that irritates the skin will be accentuated in a moist environment. Ammonia, although easy to smell, does not occur in levels that are high enough to cause burns and probably does not contribute to increased diaper rash.

Candida albicans frequently causes a secondary infection of damaged skin, although it is not thought to be a primary cause of diaper rash. Perianal inflammation is often due to localized group A beta-hemolytic (GABH) streptococcus infection.

Clinical Findings

Diaper rash due to chafing occurs mainly on the thighs and around the waist where skin folds rub together. The skin is mildly erythematous, dry, and may be lichenified. This type of rash tends to appear quickly and resolve quickly.

Irritant diaper rash occurs on exposed skin surfaces and tends to spare intertriginous folds. Skin is reddened with papules, vesicles, and scaly lesions on the lower abdomen, buttocks, and inner thighs.

Candida diaper dermatitis appears as reddened skin with sharply demarcated margins. Pustules and vesicles may be present at the edges of the affected area.

A painful, bright, glistening red eruption around the anus is characteristic of GABH streptococcal infection.

Differential Diagnosis

Psoriasis may be localized only in the diaper area and will appear as irritant diaper dermatitis in an infant with a strong family history of psoriasis or with typical plaques on other areas of the body.

Infants with atopic dermatitis or seborrhea frequently have trouble with nonspecific diaper rash and may be more prone to *Candida* infection than children with normal skin.

Management

The mainstay of treatment of diaper dermatitis is keeping the skin as dry as possible. Frequent diaper changes and the use of cornstarch powder to reduce friction may help to reduce development of diaper rash.

When an inflamed rash is present, it is important to avoid rubbing the skin and it may be necessary to rinse the baby in warm water in a sink rather than cleaning with a wash cloth or premoistened wipe. Emollients containing zinc oxide provide good barrier protection and decrease friction. If a rash has started, hydrocortisone cream (1%) applied in a thin coat two or three times a day may help to reduce inflammation.

Candida diaper rash can be treated with topical imidazole or nystatin in combination with 1% hydrocortisone cream. It is important to avoid fluorinated steroids since they are absorbed excessively from occluded skin such as the diaper area. Perianal streptococcal infection should be treated with such oral antibiotics as penicillin or erythromycin.

Diaper dermatitis usually responds well to outpatient care. Follow-up evaluation should be suggested for infants who have not improved within 7 days' time.

BIBLIOGRAPHY

Cohen B: *Pediatric Dermatology,* 2d ed. St. Louis, Mosby Year Book, 1999.

Edwards L: *Dermatology in Emergency Care,* New York, WB Saunders, 1997.

Schachner LA, Hansen RC (eds): *Pediatric Dermatology,* 2d ed. New York, Saunders, 1995.

Weston WL, Lane AT: *Color Textbook of Pediatric Dermatology,* St. Louis, Mosby Year Book, 1996.

67

Ear and Nose Emergencies

John P. Santamaria
Thomas J. Abrunzo

HIGH-YIELD FACTS

- Malignant otitis externa, almost always caused by *Pseudomonas aeruginosa,* is refractory to conventional treatment.

- Pneumatic otoscopy is an essential component of the ear examination, especially in the crying child.

- Myringitis, typically associated with bullae, is an infection of the tympanic membrane caused by *Mycoplasma pneumoniae.*

- There is to date no conclusive evidence supporting the efficacy of topical or systemic steroids, decongestants, or antihistamines in the treatment of otitis media.

- Worsening otitis media, while on antibiotics, may be a sign of suppurative complication.

- Symptoms of sinusitis may vary from the more common, persistent, purulent rhinorrhea and cough to the less common symptoms of fever, headache, facial pain, and swelling.

ACUTE OTITIS EXTERNA

Acute otitis externa refers to any inflammatory condition of the external ear. It is a common childhood illness and often presents to the emergency department. It is important to determine the severity of the infection, recognize unusual presentations, prevent complications, and avoid pitfalls in management.

Anatomy and Pathophysiology

The ear canal is a cul-de-sac extending from the pinna to the tympanic membrane. The lateral third, or cartilaginous portion, has hair follicles, ceruminous glands, and tightly applied skin. This tissue tension contributes to the extreme pain of inflammatory conditions in this area. The medial two-thirds, or osseous portion, when inflamed, is even more painful to touch. The avascular cartilage of the pinna and external acoustic meatus does not maximally mobilize host resources in wound healing and infection control.

The development of acute otitis externa is dependent upon the presence of microorganisms in a moist, warm environment. Glands of the cartilaginous canal produce cerumen with a bacteriostatic effect. However, the blind, bony end of the cul-de-sac supports bacterial growth since it lacks such glands, traps moisture, and approximates body temperature. The importance of moisture retention as a predisposing factor is underscored by the common name for external otitis, *swimmers ear.*

Anything that interrupts the integrity of the epithelial lining can predispose to infection. Trauma, instrumentation, dermatitis, and draining otitis media can all affect the ear canal in this way. Itching causes patients to scratch and instrument the ear canal, which allows bacteria to enter the traumatized skin. Degradation byproducts raise the pH and form an exudate that further promotes moisture retention and bacterial proliferation.

Etiology

Pseudomonas spp. are the most common cause of acute otitis externa. Other bacteria, including *Staphylococcus* spp., *Streptococcus* spp., gram-negative organisms, and diphtheroids are less frequently isolated. *Aspergillus,* which causes approximately 90 percent of fungal cases, is more common in patients who are immunosuppressed or who have uncontrolled hyperglycemia.

Diagnostic Findings

Local itching and mild pain are common early symptoms. Edema and increased tissue tension develop as bacterial invasion progresses. Pain is exacerbated by traction to the pinna, pressure on the tragus, or movement of the jaw from side to side. If untreated, swelling of the ear canal will occur and an exudate may develop. For patients with a fungal etiology, white-, yellow-green-, or dark-pigmented masses composed of hyphae are seen. Acute otitis externa is characterized by local symptoms. Systemic toxicity suggests another diagnosis.

Stains and cultures of ear discharge for bacteria and fungi are necessary only when disease is unresponsive to usual treatment or when unusual microorganisms are suspected. There is no role for radiographic studies in the evaluation or management of uncomplicated otitis externa.

Differential Considerations

A retained foreign body can exactly mimic the presentation of acute otitis externa of infectious etiology, only becoming apparent after thorough cleansing of the ear canal.

A furuncle, or localized pyogenic infection, is most frequently caused by *Staphylococcus aureus.* If not fluctuant, treatment should be begun with warm compresses and systemic antibiotics such as a first generation cephalosporin, amoxicillin with clavulanic acid, dicloxacillin, or macrolide, depending on local sensitivities.

Eczematous changes of the pinna and ear canal include atopic dermatitis, seborrheic dermatitis, dyshidrosis, and contact dermatitis. When edema of the ear canal prevents adequate visualization of the tympanic membrane and exudate is present in the canal, it may be impossible to distinguish otitis externa from otitis media with perforation.

Management

Cleansing of the ear canal has several advantages. Examination is improved, the exudate removed from the canal can no longer cause an inflammatory response, and topical medications can better contact the diseased area. Suction, dry mopping, curetting, and irrigation have all been used with success.

When topical medication is instilled directly, enough should be used to completely fill the canal. The use of a wick is particularly advantageous when significant edema is present, so that medication is maintained in direct contact with the epithelial surface. Topical agents may be directly instilled into the external acoustic canal or applied to a wick. Wicks are removed within 2 days of placement to avoid a foreign body reaction.

Commonly used antibiotic-steroid topical preparations are effective against *Pseudomonas,* other gram-

negative bacteria, and staphylococci. They also have anti-inflammatory and antipruritic effects. Based on efficacy, cost, risk of allergic reaction, and development of bacterial resistance, antiseptic drops, such as boric acid or aluminum acetate, are recommended in early cases.

An otolaryngologist should evaluate fungal otitis externa. Several weeks of topical tolnaftate therapy are usually effective.

Malignant otitis externa, almost always caused by *P. aeroginosa,* is refractory to conventional treatment. It has a high mortality and typically occurs in adults with diabetes mellitus. Malignant otitis externa in children is rare, primarily affecting diabetic adolescents and others who are immunosuppressed. Deeper tissue invasion explains the necrosis, local thrombosis, and vasculitis that can occur. Similar involvement of contiguous structures such as cartilage, bone, the mastoid air spaces, lymph glands, and parotid gland is possible. Sequelae are generally limited to facial nerve paresis, stenosis of the external canal, and hearing loss. Malignant otitis externa requires prolonged intravenous antibiotic therapy and possible surgical debridement. The otolaryngologist should manage it.

OTITIS MEDIA AND MASTOIDITIS

Otitis media includes the clinical syndromes of acute suppurative otitis media and otitis media with effusion. Significant overlap exists in their pathology, pathophysiology, microbiology, clinical findings, and treatment. The incidence peaks between the ages of 6 and 13 months, when examination is most difficult. It is necessary to appreciate the wide range of normal tympanic and middle ear findings so that otitis media is not overdiagnosed and other more dangerous processes overlooked. Mastoiditis is an important and treatable, albeit uncommon, complication of acute suppurative otitis media.

Anatomy and Pathophysiology

Eustachian tube dysfunction is most important in the pathogenesis of otitis media. In health, the eustachian tube has three major functions: equilibration of the middle ear and atmospheric air pressures, protection from secretions of the nasopharynx, and clearance of middle ear secretions into the nasopharynx. The eustachian tube becomes congested as a result of allergy, infection, or anatomic predisposition. Accumulated secretions serve as a culture medium. Suppuration and rupture of the tympanic membrane may result. Supine positioning and shorter eustachian tube length in young children enhances reflux of nasopharyngeal pathogens into the middle ear, thus predisposing to otitis media. Hematogenous spread of bacteria into the middle ear is possible in newborns, but uncommon.

The posterior wall of the middle ear communicates with the mastoid antrum and air cells via the aditus. The mucous membrane lining the tympanic cavity and mastoid structures is continuous.

Etiology

Otitis media and mastoiditis have similar microbiologic origins. *Streptococcus pneumoniae* is the most common bacte-rial isolate in otitis media at all ages. *Haemophilus influenzae* also remains an important pathogen throughout childhood and adulthood, not just in preschool children. In most cases, otitis media due to *H. influenzae* is associated with nontypable strains. In approximately 10 percent of cases due to *H. influenzae,* type b is causative; this explains the limited effect of the conjugate polysaccharide vaccine for *H. influenzae* type b on the overall incidence of acute otitis media. *Branhamella catarrhalis* has increased in importance since the early 1980s. Group A streptococcus and *S. aureus* are isolated much less frequently. *Chlamydia trachomatis* is difficult to isolate but is known to cause otitis media in infants <6 months old. *Mycoplasma pneumoniae* should be considered in cases unresponsive to initial therapy or when tympanic bullae are present. The role of viruses is poorly understood. The role of anaerobes is somewhat controversial. During the first 2 weeks of life, there is significant risk of infection with *S. aureus,* group B streptococcus, and gram-negative enteric bacteria.

Diagnostic Findings

Historic findings include local symptoms of ear pain, discharge, and hearing loss. Systemic symptoms such as fever, headache, malaise, gastrointestinal irritation, altered behavior, and anorexia may also be present.

Pneumatic otoscopy is an essential component of the ear examination, especially in crying children. After inspection of the pinna, postauricular area, and external auditory canal for inflammation, a pneumatic otoscope with a well-fitting speculum should be used to evaluate the color, lucency, light reflex, bony landmarks, and mobility of the tympanic membrane. Classic tympanic membrane findings in acute otitis media are redness, opacity, absence of landmarks, alteration of the light reflex, and lack of mobility. Tympanic membrane immobility is the only reliable sign of otitis media in crying children, since abnormalities of the color, lucency, light reflex, and landmarks can be false-positive findings.

Uncooperative children must be adequately immobilized before otoscopy is attempted. Foreign body and cerumen must be removed. Curettage, suction, and irrigation are most commonly used for cerumen removal and should be mastered by the emergency physician.

Redness and swelling over the mastoid area may be seen in more advanced cases of mastoiditis. Outward, downward protrusion of the pinna is suggestive of subperiosteal abscess.

There is no role for laboratory evaluation in the acute management of otitis media or mastoiditis. In mastoiditis, blood cultures are of low yield but still should be done. Culture of material from the mastoid mucosa or subperiosteal abscess cavity may provide a microbiologic diagnosis. Computerized tomography or magnetic resonance scanning may be helpful in the diagnosis of mastoiditis, brain abscess, or lateral sinus thrombosis.

Differential Considerations

Care must be taken not to overdiagnose otitis media, especially in young children who are at greater risk of having an unrecognized, more serious bacterial disease. Crying, otherwise normal children can have physical findings almost identical to one with acute otitis media. Partially treated meningitis, for example, can smolder and present later in a fulminant state.

Even when the diagnosis of otitis media is certain, other coexistent illnesses must be considered. Myringitis, typically associated with bullae, is an infection of the tympanic membrane caused by *M. pneumoniae,* bacteria, or viruses.

Dysbaric injury to the tympanic membrane can occur from diving, ascending to heights, and receiving a slap to the ear. In all of these conditions, tympanic membrane mobility should be preserved and careful pneumatic otoscopy and history may be the only ways to distinguish them from acute otitis media.

Otitis externa and otitis media with perforation may be impossible to differentiate unless the ear canal is thoroughly cleansed.

Complications

Complications of acute otitis media include bacteremia, tympanic perforation, mastoiditis, cholesteatoma, facial paralysis, labyrinthitis, and infectious eczemoid dermatitis. Intracranial suppurative complications such as meningitis, brain abscess, encephalitis, and lateral sinus thrombosis may be heralded by symptoms as vague as worsening ear pain while taking antibiotics, persistent headache, intractable emesis, or behavior change. More specific symptoms such as meningismus, visual changes, papilledema, seizure, and focal neurologic findings may not be present, especially when patients are "partially treated" with oral antibiotics.

Management

An antimicrobial agent effective against *S. pneumoniae, H. influenzae,* and *B. catarrhalis* is indicated. *S. pneumoniae* causes 40 to 50 percent of acute otitis media and is less likely than *H. influenzae* or *M. catarrhalis* to resolve without treatment. Therefore, treatment of drug-resistant *S. pneumoneae* (DRSP) is the most important consideration when choosing optimal antibiotic management.

Amoxicillin is the best oral antibiotic for treating DRSP. Amoxicillin is the recommended first-line agent based on its combination of efficacy, cost, palatability, convenience, and low incidence of side effects and toxicity. For children <2 years old who attend day care with recent antibiotic exposure, higher-dose amoxicillin is recommended. This recommendation is appropriate for most communities, despite the current incidence of beta-lactamase–producing *H. influenzae* and *B. catarrhalis* or penicillin-resistant *S. pneumoniae.* If the experience of physicians in a particular community indicates that there are frequent treatment failures on amoxicillin, or there is a large proportion of beta-lactamase–producing strains, other drugs should be considered as first-line therapy.

For children with treatment failures after 3 days (persistent ear pain, otorrhea, or red, bulging tympanic membranes), second-line antimicrobial treatment is recommended. Suitable second-line agents include high-dose amoxicillin-clavulanate, cefuroxime, and intramuscular ceftriaxone.

Two studies indicate that single-dose intramuscular ceftriaxone (50 mg/kg) has been shown to be as effective as 10 days of oral amoxicillin. Antibiotic recommendations should be continually reevaluated based on current patterns of microbiologic resistance and availability of new drugs.

Much discussion has centered around the observation that most episodes of acute otitis media resolve without antibiotic treatment when managed initially by observation alone. Initial observation, followed by antibiotic use only for children with a complicated course or who are categorized as high risk, results in cost reduction, fewer side effects from medications, and less antimicrobial resistance. However, limited use of antibiotics may result in a higher incidence of complications, such as acute mastoiditis. Observation without initial antibiotic use, while predominant in some countries, remains controversial in the United States.

Symptomatic therapy, such as analgesics, antipyretics, and local heat, is usually helpful. Relief of acute pain with topical anesthetic otic drops may be dramatic, although inconsistent. When topical medication and over-the-counter analgesics are not enough, oral narcotic preparations may be helpful.

In neonates, the possibility of hematogenously spread disease, including that from gram-negative bacilli or *S. aureus,* requires a complete septic work-up, admission, and intravenous broad-spectrum antibiotics pending culture results. The rarity of this occurrence has prompted some authorities to recommend that in the otherwise well neonate >2 weeks old, otitis media without systemic toxicity can be treated on an outpatient basis with oral antibiotics. A cautious approach is recommended, especially if fever is present.

There is, to date, no conclusive evidence supporting the efficacy of topical or systemic steroids, decongestants, or antihistamines in the treatment of otitis media. Their use is not recommended. In particular, steroids should not be used when the risk of concurrent varicella infection exists.

An otolaryngologist should manage mastoiditis. Before microbiologic confirmation, a broad-spectrum intravenous cephalosporin, such as ceftriaxone, can be used. Alternatively, a penicillinase-resistant penicillin, such as oxacillin, in combination with an aminoglycoside, such as gentamicin, can be used. Breakdown of bony septae between mastoid air cells (mastoid osteitis) and subperiosteal abscess are indications for mastoidectomy. Tympanostomy tubes are placed if concurrent otitis media with effusion is present.

Patients with otitis media should be rechecked if symptoms worsen or if, in 3 days, no improvement occurs. Otherwise, reevaluation in 2 weeks is appropriate. Worsening on antibiotics may be a sign of suppurative complication. At least partial improvement is expected after 3 days of treatment. Follow-up is necessary after treatment to assess for persistent middle-ear effusion. Children with concomitant systemic bacterial infection or toxic appearance may require hospitalization and intravenous antibiotics.

FOREIGN BODY OF THE NOSE AND EAR

The removal of nasal and aural foreign bodies can be very difficult. Optimally, physical examination confirms the history and removal is uneventful. Often the history is vague, the examination difficult, and the foreign body not easily grasped. Removal attempts under suboptimal conditions may precipitate bleeding, edema, and movement of the foreign body to a less accessible location.

Only the volumes to which the normal structures of the nose and ear can expand limit the size and shape of nasal and aural foreign bodies. This is evidenced by innumerable case reports of large retained foreign bodies. Some go unnoticed for long periods of time.

Anatomy and Pathophysiology

Anatomic characteristics of the ear and nose predispose to foreign body retention. The external acoustic meatus is oval in transverse section, with one constriction near the medial end of the cartilaginous part and another in the osseous portion. Infants have a short cartilaginous canal with a more horizontally oriented tympanic membrane. The superior portion of the tympanic membrane, being very close to the lateral meatal opening, is prone to injury, especially during instrumentation.

Visualization and removal of foreign bodies in the nose may be impeded by the three anatomic elevations of the lateral nasal wall—the superior, middle, and inferior turbinates.

Foreign bodies are most commonly self-inserted, either in play or as a response to an itch or irritation. Animals, such as insects, worms, and larvae, can be deposited as eggs or enter as adults. Trauma, dental procedures, and endotracheal intubation have also been associated with foreign body retention. The position, movement, size, and antigenicity of the foreign body influence bleeding and tissue reaction.

Etiology

Not even the most fertile imagination could anticipate the variety of foreign bodies described in the literature. A teenager had a broken door handle over 7 cm. long lodged in his nose for 24 days before diagnosis; another teenage boy had an 8.5-cm. wood fragment lodged in his nose as a result of a bicycle accident 5 months before diagnosis.

Excessive cerumen is a ubiquitous problem with a variety of presentations, including a painful, itchy, or draining ear; headache; and hearing loss. Cerumen production and clearance may be influenced by ethnic, familial, and individual factors. Home cleansing of the ear canals with cotton swabs packs the cerumen into the canal, sometimes adding cotton fibers to the wax mixture. Dry, often impacted cerumen is often seen in the small, tortuous external ear canals of children with trisomy 21. Cerumen that impedes complete visualization of the tympanic membrane must be removed if otitis media is suspected.

Diagnostic Findings

In the absence of a clear history, helpful clues include epistaxis, pain, fever, discharge, and alteration of sense of smell or hearing. Bleeding and purulent discharge can impede the physical examination.

Both sides of the nose and both ears must be examined. Children who have one foreign body are a greater risk for several. Foreign bodies can masquerade as chronic infections, tumors, recurrent epistaxis, and generalized body odor (bromidrosis).

Plain radiographs will miss the many nonradiopaque objects. A rhinolith is a mineralized nasal foreign body. Gradually increasing in size, it is usually discovered as an incidental finding on plain radiograph. Although rarely indicated, more sensitive radiographic techniques can demonstrate the presence of a foreign body in the posterior portion of the nose that is not readily visualized on examination. In difficult cases, radiographic studies can be used prior to removal to demonstrate the size and position of a retained foreign body.

Complications

Complications occur as a result of the foreign body, examination, or removal. Blockage of the external auditory canal or nares can interfere with normal function. Infection can closely follow the presence of a foreign body in both the ear and the nose. Occlusion of the sinus ostia in the anterior part of the nasal cavity and the eustachian tube posteriorly can predispose to sinusitis and otitis media. Undiscovered nasal foreign bodies may present with recurrent epistaxis due to mucosal erosion and local irritation. An expanding rhinolith may impinge on contiguous structures, complicating removal or predisposing to infection. A case of meningitis and death secondary to a foreign body is reported in the literature.

Adequate restraint of children and careful use of conscious sedation before instrumentation will minimize potential complications. Overzealous restraint can cause vascular compromise or ecchymosis. Inadequate restraint can increase the risk of tympanic membrane trauma and perforation. Foreign bodies that are pushed into the nasopharynx can be swallowed or aspirated.

Management

First, no harm should be done. Any case with a low probability of successful removal in the emergency department should be referred to an otolaryngologist. It is true that the first attempt at removal is the most likely to be successful, since removal attempts may stimulate bleeding, mucosal edema, and movement of the object to a less accessible area. Although many cases will not require elaborate supplies, it is prudent to be prepared for complications before attempting removal (Table 67-1).

After explanation of the procedure to children and family, adequate immobilization should be ensured. Optimally this is achieved with children's cooperation; more often assisted immobilization with or without sedation is required. Adequate personnel will reduce the chance of injury to children and emergency department staff. One person assigned to each limb and a fifth to control the head may be necessary in larger, stronger children. Use of an immobilization device fashioned from sheets or a papoose board may reduce the number of holders required.

No attempts at removal should be made without a good light source. For most foreign bodies of the nose and ear, direct visualization and instrumentation through an otoscope is adequate. A nasal speculum and headlight are preferable for nasal foreign bodies. Vertical opening of the nasal speculum will avoid septal damage. Topical

Table 67-1. Equipment for Examination and Removal of a Nasal or Aural Foreign Body

Immobilization device (sheet or papoose board)
Sedative medications (see Chap. 24)
Otoscope for instrumentation under direct visualization
Nasal speculum
Headlight (optional)
Topical vasoconstrictor (phenylephrine 0.125%–0.5%, cocaine 4%, or epinephrine 1:1000)
Alligator or Hartman forceps
Wire loop or curette
Suction apparatus, including catheters of various sizes
Foley or Fogarty catheter No. 8 (optional)

vasoconstriction may reduce intranasal tissue edema and aid foreign body removal.

Foreign body shape, location, and composition, as well as physician preference, influences the removal technique and instrument employed. Insects are usually easier to remove and cause less trauma when they are not wiggling their bodies or flapping their wings. It is generally recommended that they be killed with alcohol before removal is attempted. Wood and other vegetable matter tends to swell when wet and is best removed before irrigating the ear canal. Mineral-based foreign bodies, such as round plastic beads, are difficult to grasp. When possible, forceps are used to grasp the foreign body. Round, fragile objects may be more successfully removed by placing a wire loop curette behind the foreign body or by using super-glue-type adhesive on a cotton-tipped applicator.

Familiarity with the use of a curette is particularly helpful in removal of excess cerumen deposits. A curette with a small loop with rounded, smooth edges and which is slightly bent at the juncture of the shaft and curette ring is best to facilitate cerumen removal. Otic drops can soften hard cerumen prior to removal attempts. After cerumen removal, the canal should be checked for trauma, which could predispose to infection. If the canal is traumatized, prophylactic therapy for acute otitis externa should be considered.

To avoid damage to the ear canal or tympanic membrane while using an otoscope, curette, or other instrument near the ear canal, part of that hand should be anchored against the child's head. If the child's head moves suddenly, the examining hand and instrument will then move with it.

Small aural foreign bodies close to the tympanic membrane may be removed with body temperature tap water irrigation. A 30- to 60-mL syringe attached to a plastic infusion catheter or, preferably, a butterfly needle tubing cut off about 3 cm from the hub will deliver adequate volumes for irrigation at adequate pressures. The soft, flexible butterfly tubing is inserted atraumatically into the external acoustic meatus, directing the water inflow around a partial obstruction, allowing the foreign body to be removed with lateral water outflow. The myriad of methods advocated for the removal of aural and nasal foreign bodies attests the fact that no single technique is universally successful. Some practitioners remove foreign bodies with suction apparatus or small-size Foley catheters.

Since children may pack a nose or ear with several objects at once, a thorough check for other objects is advisable after a foreign body is removed. Always check both ear canals and both nares with a known foreign body.

The successful management of foreign bodies in the ear and nose requires careful patient selection, proper equipment, and a planned, coordinated approach to each child. If emergency department removal is not possible and immediate removal is not necessary, children can usually be started on oral antibiotics to cover normal upper respiratory flora and be referred to an otolaryngologist on an outpatient basis.

EPISTAXIS

Nosebleeds tend to occur in the preteenage population and are almost exclusively anterior in location, either at the nasal vestibule or the plexus of vessels on the anterior, inferior portion of the nasal septum (Little's area, Kiesselbach's plexus). Much less commonly, occult bleeding from the respiratory and gastrointestinal tracts can present as epistaxis.

Etiology

Epistaxis digitorum, or "nose picking," is the most frequent cause of nosebleed in children. Granulation tissue forms as a result of repetitive trauma and when "picked off" causes bleeding. Dry air, forceful nose blowing, increased vascularity associated with local infection, systemic bleeding disorders, drug use, and deviated nasal septum are also predisposing factors to nosebleed. Although possible, it is unusual to see childhood epistaxis associated with barotrauma, tumors, and postsurgical changes. No association with hypertension has been proved.

Nasal foreign bodies and septal hematomas are easily overlooked; careful examination is important. After blunt trauma to the nose, septal hematoma can occur if the mucous membrane remains intact and underlying vessels bleed. Septal perforation or abscess is a possible sequelae if surgical drainage is not done.

Diagnostic Findings

History of recent trauma, upper respiratory illness, allergy, or exposure to dry air may be obtained. Prolonged bleeding or easy bruisability in patients or family members is an important clue to systemic disorders. In bilateral epistaxis, the history of which side bled first usually reveals the bleeding site. Ask how much bleeding occurred, but expect an overestimation.

History of behavior change, pallor, or orthostatic dizziness suggests significant blood loss. Altered mental status and delayed capillary refill may be the only physical findings to suggest hypovolemia. Sustained tachycardia and tachypnea may be noted. Hypotension is a late finding.

Supplies, including suction apparatus, should be readied before attempting evaluation of children with epistaxis, so that treatment can accompany examination. The head down position will lessen the risk of aspiration from swallowed blood. Careful physical examination usually will reveal the bleeding point. Positioning small children in their parent's lap with manual restraint is often helpful. Optimal examination is facilitated by the use of a headlamp and nasal speculum. The speculum should be opened in a rostrocaudal direction to avoid damage to the nasal septum. Removal of blood with a Fraser suction tip can aid localization of the bleeding point.

Demonstration of blood under the nails may be evidence of nose picking. Associated lymphadenopathy or evidence of other bleeding suggests systemic disease.

Stat. hemoglobin and type and cross-match are indicated if there is clinical evidence of hypovolemia. Epistaxis alone is usually self-limiting and does not warrant evaluation for a coagulation defect.

Management

No treatment is required for patients whose bleeding resolves spontaneously or with direct pressure. Number of recurrences, general health of patients, and hydration status should be considered when deciding whether or not to treat a nosebleed.

All equipment should be readied before immobilizing children. Yankaur suction tips for suction of particulate matter (emesis) and Fraser tips for removal of blood are especially important. The use of a headlamp leaves both of the physician's hands free to use the nasal speculum, suction apparatus, and other equipment.

Filling the anterior nasal cavity with topical thrombin followed by 10 minutes of firm, constant pressure is safe, effective, technically simpler, and better tolerated than is using silver nitrate cautery. It is helpful to remove as much fresh blood and clot as possible before attempting this procedure.

Cautery of the bleeding site and the immediately surrounding area may be helpful if packing with thrombin is ineffective. Children's thin nasal septum must be considered at risk for perforation when cautery is done. A cotton pledget can be soaked in Neo-Synephrine (0.125 to 0.5%), epinephrine (1:1000), or cocaine (4%) and placed in the nose for 10 min. Injection of the site with 1 to 2 mL of lidocaine with epinephrine (1:100,000) has both tamponading and vasoconstrictive effects. Systemic effects should be anticipated.

It is uncommon for childhood epistaxis to require nasal packing. Packing should be done in consultation with an otolaryngologist. Nasal sponges are easily inserted when dry, can be cut to size, and expand when moistened. Packing with petrolatum gauze is much more uncomfortable and is poorly tolerated by small children. Complications include syncope during packing, sinusitis, bacteremia, local infection, toxic shock syndrome, and iatrogenic sleep apnea if bilateral sponges or packs are placed. Packing should be removed within 2 days, and antibiotic coverage provided while the packing is in place. Recommended antibiotics cover normal nasal flora. Amoxicillin is usually adequate, but better staphylococcal coverage (cephalosporins, macrolides, and amoxicillin with clavulanate potassium) is prudent. Erythromycin is a good choice for the older child.

Posterior bleeds are suspected when a bleeding site cannot be visualized and anterior packs are not effective. Inhospital management by an otolaryngologist is indicated. Patients better tolerate Foley catheters and pneumatic nasal catheters than they do petrolatum gauze nasal packs. Eustachian tube obstruction and subsequent iatrogenic otitis media can occur. A posteriorly placed pack, arterial ligation, pterygopalatine fossa block, and embolization are rarely needed in a child.

Pediatric epistaxis, usually a result of local trauma and dry nasal mucosa, is likely to recur. Humidifiers and petroleum jelly rubbed onto the anterior nasal septum and the skin at the nasal orifice may be helpful. Fingernails should be kept short. Habitual nose-pickers may benefit from covering their hands with socks during sleep.

RHINITIS

Rhinitis is the single most frequent cause of nasal discharge. It is a major cause of school absenteeism and missed parental workdays. Incidence reflects children's age, contact with other children, and general state of health. Estimates have ranged between 6 and 21 episodes per year.

Etiology

More than 200 antigenically different viruses cause rhinitis. Rhinovirus, influenza, parainfluenza, respiratory syncytial virus (RSV), and adenovirus are common. Incomplete immunity and multiple viral serotypes partially explain frequent episodes.

Bacterial rhinitis may complicate viral rhinitis and is usually heralded by the development of a purulent discharge and persistence of symptoms. Sinusitis often coexists, explained by the anatomic continuity of the nasal and sinus mucous membranes. Pathogens include *H. influenzae, Staphylococcus* spp., *B. catarrhalis,* and *S. pneumoniae.* In contrast to school age children, in whom *Streptococcus pyogenes* presents as acute pharyngitis or tonsillitis, children <3 years old generally develop streptococcosis, a subacute condition characterized by rhinitis, prolonged course, low-grade fever, and adenopathy. Rhinitis can also result from pertussis, diphtheria, or congenital syphilis. In young infants, prodromal nasal congestion, discharge, and sneezing may herald pneumonia caused by *Chlamydia trachomatis, Ureaplasma urealyticum, Pneumocystis carinii,* or cytomegalovirus.

IgE-mediated allergic rhinitis peaks in late adolescence. Greater concentrations of environmental pollutants and dust mites in the home may contribute to an increasing incidence of allergic rhinitis. Infants and young children tend to have perennial symptoms associated with allergens to which they are consistently exposed early in life.

Topical toxin exposure (e.g., vasoconstrictor drops or cocaine) or systemic absorption (e.g., aspirin or estrogens) may cause rhinitis. Prolonged topical vasoconstrictor use can cause rhinitis medicamentosa, characterized by inflammation and chronic nasal congestion, which further encourages the use of the offending agent.

Diagnostic Findings

The emergency physician should ask about known precipitants; discharge quality, quantity, and timing; factors that improve or worsen the discharge; and associated symptoms. Previous episodes, known sensitivities, medications, and prior therapy are potentially important. History of topical decongestant use should be sought.

The nasal mucous membrane is best examined with a good light source and nasal speculum. A large caliber otoscope speculum can also be used.

Immobilization of uncooperative children is necessary. Swelling, erythema, and secretions are evidence of inflammation. Laboratory and radiographic evaluation are not needed in the acute management of infectious or allergic rhinitis.

Table 67-2. Response to Treatment of Infectious and Allergic Rhinitis

	Infectious	Allergic
Decongestants	Fair	Fair
Antihistamines	Poor	Good
Steroids	None	Excellent
Immunotherapy	None	Variable
Cromolyn	None	Fair
Antibiotics/Antivirals	Disease specific	None

Therapeutic Trial

Therapy is disease specific. Therapeutic options for patients with allergic and infectious rhinitis are outlined in Table 67-2.

Decongestants (vasoconstrictors) may be used orally or topically. Limit therapy with topical decongestants to 5 days to minimize rebound phenomena. A single injection of dexamethasone and oral decongestants for a few days may facilitate removal of topical therapy. Others advocate use of nasal decongestant spray on only one side. The unsprayed side improves in approximately 3 days.

Evidence of bacterial infection should prompt antibiotic use. Antibiotics effective against *S. pneumoniae* and *H. influenzae,* such as amoxicillin, trimethoprim-sulfamethoxazole, and cefaclor, are first-line agents.

When avoidance, decongestants, and antihistamines fail, steroids, cromolyn sodium, and immunotherapy may be tried. Inhaled steroids cause less adrenal suppression and are preferred to oral preparations.

SINUSITIS

Sinusitis is a bacterial inflammation of the paranasal sinuses associated with nasal mucosal inflammation and obstruction of the sinus ostia. The condition is most often manifested as a prolongation or complication of viral upper respiratory tract infection. With children averaging six to eight upper respiratory infections per year, it is estimated that 0.5 to 5 percent become complicated with sinusitis.

Symptoms may vary from the more common persistent, purulent rhinorrhea and cough to the less common symptoms of fever, headache, facial pain, and swelling. While there exists some controversy regarding the definition of sinusitis, consensus defines the condition as

acute (<4 weeks duration), subacute (4 to 12 weeks duration), or chronic (>12 weeks duration). Further, symptoms lasting <7 days, without recent antibiotic use, generally are viral upper respiratory infections, not requiring antibiotic therapy. Worsening or persistent symptoms lasting >7 days are usually treated with antibiotics as discussed later.

Anatomy and Pathophysiology

The paranasal sinuses are 4 paired structures:

- Maxillary
- Ethmoidal
- Sphenoidal
- Frontal

Maxillary and ethmoidal sinuses are aerated soon after birth, while the frontal sinuses appear radiographically by the seventh year and the sphenoidals by the ninth year. The presence of functioning sinuses at birth means that sinusitis can occur at any age, with the maxillary and ethmoidals being involved most frequently.

The sinuses drain beneath two of the three shelf-like turbinates of the lateral nasal wall. The sphenoidal and posterior ethmoidals drain into the ostium of the superior meatus. The maxillary, frontal, and anterior ethmoidals drain into the middle meatus, which can sometimes be directly visualized.

Normal function of the paranasal sinuses depends on patency of the sinus ostia, function of the ciliary apparatus, and the nature of sinus secretions. Abnormality of any of these will predispose to bacterial infection.

Etiology

Predisposing clinical problems include allergies, rhinitis, foreign bodies, choanal atresia, cleft palate, neoplasm, septal deviation, adenoidal hypertrophy, polyps (allergic, cystic fibrosis), dental infection, immunodeficiency, and immotile cilia syndromes (such as Kartagener's syndrome). Swimming, trauma, and rhinitis medicamentosa may also cause mucosal swelling and sinus ostium obstruction. The causative organisms of acute bacterial sinusitis are similar to those of acute otitis media (Brook).

Diagnostic Findings

The key to differentiating an uncomplicated upper respiratory infection from sinusitis is the unusual severity or protraction of symptoms found in the latter. Measures of severity may include fever >39.0°C (102.2°F), purulent nasal discharge, and periorbital swelling. Protracted (>10 days) findings are common, including nasal discharge (clear or purulent), cough that is frequently worse at night, bad breath, facial pain, and periorbital edema that is worse in the morning. Fatigue, malaise, decreased appetite, and weight loss are sometimes noted. As compared with adults, headache, dental pain, and facial tenderness are less common complaints in children.

Sphenoidal sinusitis is uniquely associated with frontal, temporal, or retroorbital pain, which may be the only symptom. It is rare in children. Since isolated sphenoid sinusitis can result in severe intracranial complications (extension to brain) in the absence of the typical respiratory prodrome, it is an important consideration in the differential diagnosis of headache.

On physical examination, the emergency physician should look for purulent drainage from the middle meatus, boggy nasal mucosa, postnasal drip, and cobblestoning of the posterior pharynx. Transillumination is of limited value in children because of the variable development of sinuses before age 8 to 10 years. In older children, it is useful if light transmission is normal or absent.

The white blood cell count may help in assessing patient response to infection. Blood cultures may occasionally be useful in toxic patients. If a sinus puncture is done, the material should be sent for Gram's stain and aerobes and anaerobes should be cultured.

Radiologic plain film examination of children has variable reliability. Normal sinus films are helpful. Abnormal sinus films are difficult to interpret, although after 6 years of age the interpretation can be more definitive. Sinusitis appears as clouding, mucoperiosteal thickening >4 mm, or as air fluid levels within the sinuses, the latter being most helpful in defining acute infection. Preferred plain views include the following:

- Occipitomental (Water's) for maxillary sinus
- Anteroposterior (Caldwell) for frontal and ethmoidal sinuses
- Submentovertex for sphenoidal sinus
- Lateral for sphenoidal sinus

For most small children, where maxillary sinusitis is suspected, a single Water's view may suffice. With equivocal plain radiographs, computed tomography scan is indicated as the definitive evaluation of acute or chronic infection. It is usually indicated if children are seriously ill, have had recurrent episodes, have chronic disease, or have suspected suppurative complications.

Differential Considerations

In evaluating patients with suspected sinusitis, other entities with comparable presentations must be excluded. An acute upper respiratory tract infection or allergy may initially have similar symptoms, while a foreign body, neoplasm, or polyp commonly causes unilateral drainage and obstruction, possibly as predisposing factors in the development of sinusitis. Functional and organic causes of headache should also be excluded.

Complications

Sinusitis can seed the systemic circulation resulting in bacteremia or septicemia. Local extension can result in facial cellulitis, facial abscess, periorbital and orbital cellulitis, osteomyelitis of the skull (Pott's puffy tumor), cavernous sinus thrombosis, epidural abscess, subdural empyema, meningitis, and brain abscess.

Management

Though sinusitis resolves spontaneously in 40 percent of cases, antibiotic therapy is indicated to hasten resolution of symptoms and to prevent complications. For non-toxic patients, a 14-day course is appropriate. A longer treatment period may be warranted if symptoms persist. The choice of antibiotic therapy depends on duration of symptoms and local drug-resistance patterns. Initial suggested treatment includes amoxicillin (40 mg/kg/day divided bid) or, in the penicillin sensitive, a macrolide such as clarithromycin (15 mg/kg/day divided bid), or azithromycin (10 mg/kg/day on day 1, and 5 mg/kg/day on days 2 through 5). For nonresponsive cases and suspected resistant organisms, amoxicillin doses of 80 to 90 mg/kg/day divided bid; cefuroxime axetil 30 mg/kg/day divided bid; amoxicillin clavulanate at 40 mg/kg/day divided bid; or a combination of amoxicillin and amoxicillin clavulanate each at 40 mg/kg/day are recommended. For the most difficult cases, intramuscular ceftriaxone or, with known penicillin-resistant *S. pneumoniae,* clindamycin is also used. The non-responders deserve otolaryngologist consultation for confirmation of diagnosis and consideration of surgical drainage. In toxic children and those with evidence of sphenoid sinusitis, inpatient admission and parenteral antibiotics are indicated initially.

The use of standard-dose antihistamines, decongestants, steroids, and cromolyn sodium, while sometimes helpful in adults, are controversial in the treatment of pediatric sinusitis. Input from the consultant pediatrician or otolaryngologist is useful in developing a specific, personalized therapeutic regimen.

Needle or surgical drainage is necessary for patients unresponsive to antibiotics. Antral puncture by an otolaryngologist is indicated if there is severe pain unresponsive to medical management; sinusitis in a seriously ill, toxic child; an unsatisfactory response; suppurative complications; or if patients are immunocompromised.

Recurrent or refractory sinusitis is sometimes further evaluated by antral lavage to establish a definitive bacteriologic diagnosis. Persistent infection, unresponsive to multiple antibiotics, is treated surgically, by the creation of an antral window, or by endoscopic enlargement of the osteomeatal unit.

Degree of toxicity, ability to tolerate oral fluids, complicated or serious disease, age, and reliability of follow-up will dictate whether inpatient management is necessary. Immunocompromised hosts will frequently require inpatient therapy.

BIBLIOGRAPHY

Barnett ED, Teele DW, Klein JO, et al: Comparison of ceftriaxone and trimethoprim-sulfamethoxazole for acute otitis media. *Pediatrics* 99:23, 1997.

Bluestone CD, Stool SE, Kenna MA: *Pediatric Otolaryntology.* New York, W.B. Saunders Co., 1996.

Clayton MI, Osborne JE, Rutherford D, et al: A double-blind, randomized, prospective trial of a topical antiseptic versus atopical antibiotic in the treatment of otorrhoea. *Clin Otolaryngol* 15:7, 1990.

Dowell SF, Butler JC, Giebink GS, et al: Acute otitis media: management and surveillance in an era of pneumococcal resistance—A report from the drug-resistant *Streptococcus pneumoniae* Theraputic Working Group. *Pediatr Infect Dis J* 18:1, 1999.

Farrior J: Complications of otitis media in children. *Southern Med J* 83:645, 1990.

Green SM, Rothrock SG: Single-dose intramuscular ceftriaxone for acute otitis media in children. *Pediatrics* 91:23, 1993.

Kadish, HA, Cornell, HM: Removal of nasal foreign bodies in the pediatric population. *Am J Emerg Med* (15):54, 1997.

Van Zuijlen DA, Schilder AG, Van Balen FA, et al: National differences in incidence of acute mastoiditis: Relationship to prescribing patterns of antibiotics for acute otitis media? *Pediatr Infect Dis J* 20:140–144, 2001.

Wald ER: Purulent nasal discharge. *Pediatr Infect Dis J* 10:329, 1991.

68

Emergencies of the Oral Cavity and Neck

Thomas J. Abrunzo
John P. Santamaria

HIGH-YIELD FACTS

- Dental examination includes a search for discoloration, fractures, swelling, fluctuance, and percussion tenderness. Gentle probing of the suspicious area may disclose tenderness or purulent discharge.

- Uncomplicated dental infection is usually treated on an outpatient basis; deep fascial space infections require hospitalization.

- Gingivitis is significantly improved with good oral hygiene. Children with stomatitis, ulcers, or severe sore throat may benefit symptomatically from gargling or careful oral administration of a combination of kaopectate, diphenhydramine, and viscous lidocaine.

- Suppurative pharyngitis can spread to contiguous tissue causing peritonsillar abscess (quinsy), Lemierre's postanginal sepsis (septic thrombophlebitis of the tonsillar vein), and Ludwig's angina (submandibular abscess). Hematologic spread may result in meningitis, endocarditis, and other serious bacterial infections.

- Nonsuppurative syndromes due to streptococcal infection include scarlet fever, rheumatic fever, and glomerulonephritis.

- Needle aspiration is sometimes used diagnostically to differentiate between cellulitis and peritonsillar abscess and can be employed for definitive treatment instead of incision and drainage in cooperative patients.

- With retropharyngeal abscess, there is usually a prodromal nasopharyngitis or

pharyngitis progressing to the abrupt onset of high fever, dysphagia, refusal of feeding, severe throat pain, hyperextension of head, and noisy respirations.

- "Hot" or suppurative nodes are most commonly caused by beta-hemolytic group A streptococci and penicillin-resistant *Staphylococcus aureus*.

DENTOALVEOLAR INFECTIONS

Infections originating from dental structures begin in the periodontium or in the dental pulp, the latter being more common. The periodontium is the tissue investing and supporting the tooth. Periodontal infections tend to localize to intraoral soft tissue and seldom extend to deeper structures of the face and neck. These infections include gingivitis, periodontitis, or periodontal abscess and pericoronitis. Periodontitis is a chronic inflammation and infection of the dental-gingival interface usually seen in adults, but also occurring in immunosuppressed children. Pericoronitis is an acute, localized infection caused by food particles and microorganisms that have become trapped under the gum flaps [opercula] of partially erupted or impacted teeth.

Anatomy and Pathophysiology

Dental pulp infections are usually the result of caries that result from bacteria-facilitated disintegration of enamel, dentin, and cementum. These infections can erode the periodontal membrane and extend into the mandible and maxilla. Infection of the pulp can also result from a fracture or a defect in the apical foramen or lateral canals resulting from periapical abscess or pericoronitis. Hematogenous seeding with bacteria may also occur. Once infected, pus may exit the pulp canal apically, forming a periapical or alveolar abscess or it may track laterally, through the alveolar bone and gingiva to form a parulis ("gum boil"). Dental infections can extend locally to involve deep fascial spaces of the mandible, causing Ludwig's angina. *Bacteroides, Peptostreptococcus, Actinomyces,* and *Streptococcus* are common pathogens of orofacial infections arising from odontogenic sources.

Diagnositic Findings

A history of recent restoration or extraction; tactile (lingual) sensation of a change in restoration surface; and thermal, percussion, or chemical sensitivity suggest failed dental therapy, dental fracture, or new caries as a cause of pain. Pain, fever, gingival swelling, and purulent gingival discharge suggest periodontal abscess, periapical abscess, pulpitis, pericoronitis, or gingivitis.

Dental examination includes a search for discoloration, fractures, swelling, fluctuance, and percussion tenderness. Gentle probing of the suspicious area may disclose tenderness or purulent discharge. Anterior cervical adenopathy may be present.

A panoramic radiograph of the dentition and mandible may reveal evidence of primary dental disease or secondary involvement of the maxilla or mandible. A computed tomography (CT) scan of the orofacial area may be necessary to diagnose deep fascial space infection. A complete blood cell count and cultures of the site and blood may be useful in toxic patients.

Management

Caries require analgesics and dental referral. Pulpitis and periapical abscess also require analgesia, with warm compresses and systemic antibiotics, usually penicillin or erythromycin. Incision and drainage may be necessary. Pericoronitis and periodontitis are treated similarly; irrigation and gentle debridement of opercula, with removal of retained debris, may obviate the need for incision and drainage. Uncomplicated dental infection is usually treated on an outpatient basis; deep fascial space infections require hospitalization.

GINGIVOSTOMATITIS

Gingivitis presents as tender, swollen, edematous, and sometimes friable gum tissue with or without vesiculation or ulceration. Gingivitis may be accompanied by stomatitis, which presents as either diffuse erythema or vesiculoulceration. Ulcers appear as circumscribed loss of epithelium or local tissue necrosis (Table 68-1). Poor oral hygiene and neutropenia may predispose to gingivitis, as can mouth breathing due to large adenoids or tonsils, nasal blockage and poor lip muscle tone. Gingivitis may accompany prepubertal and pubertal maturation. Phenytoin therapy causes gingivitis, yielding a painless, extensive, firm, lobulated gingival hypertrophy. Hypovitaminosis C (scurvy) may cause gingivitis as well as bone pain, irritability, petechial hemorrhage, poor wound healing, and the sicca syndrome of Sjogren. Primary dental disease, such as pulpitis, periapical abscess, and pericoronitis may cause localized gingival inflammation.

Table 68-1. Oral Ulcers: Diagnostic Considerations

Acute necrotizing gingivostomatitis
(trench mouth: Vincent's angina)
Aphthous stomatitis
Autoimmune
Candidiasis (oral thrush)
Chemical (antineoplastic)
Drugs (phenytoin)
Epstein-Barr virus
Erythema multiforme and Stevens-Johnson syndrome
Hand-foot-and-mouth disease
Herpangina
Herpes simplex
Herpetic gingivostomatitis
Malignancy (leukemia)
Radiation-induced
Syphilis (primary and secondary)
Traumatic
Varicella zoster
Vitamin deficiency (scurvy)

Histiocytosis X, a pathologic increase in the monocyte and macrophage line, may cause gingivitis, swelling of the palate and loss of teeth, associated with dermatitis, proctitis, vaginitis, and hepatosplenomegaly.

Diagnostic Findings

History of specific exposures frequently assists in diagnosis:

• Chemotherapy causes mucositis.

• Phenytoin causes gingival hyperplasia.

• Nutritional deprivation causes scurvy.

• Physical disability may predispose to poor hygiene.

Fever is a common symptom in most infections, except for those due to *Candida*.

The presence of posterior pharyngeal ulcers is likely to represent coxsackie virus. Buccal and lingual vesicles and maculovesicles on the hands and feet (hand-foot-and-mouth disease) are also caused by enterovirus (coxsackie A5, 10, and 16). Primary herpes simplex infection is usually manifested by high fever and swollen, red, friable gums with diffuse oropharyngeal mucosal lesions that may become confluent. It can be differentiated from trench mouth (Vincent's angina) by the latter's isolated gingival involvement. Syphilis may present in its primary stage as oral, lingual, and tonsillar chancres and, in its secondary stage, as mucous patches, which are superficial, excoriated, weeping, exudative lesions found anywhere in the oropharynx. Erythema multiforme is an exanthem of erythematous macules or papules with superimposed vesicles, primarily of the upper extremity and trunk that evolve into annular or target lesions. An enanthem of mucosal blistering occurs in the Stevens-Johnson form of erythema multiforme. The stomatitis of *Candida* appears as white, flocculent, confluent patches found diffusely over the tongue and oropharyngeal mucosa.

Laboratory evaluation is not helpful in most cases of gingivostomatitis. A complete blood cell count may be useful in the diagnosis of leukemia and Epstein-Barr virus (EBV) infection. "Monospot" is also helpful with EBV infection. The diagnosis of syphilis can be made by serologic studies and dark-field exam.

Management

Gingivitis is significantly improved with good oral hygiene (tooth brushing and mouthwashes). Children with stomatitis, ulcers, or severe sore throat may benefit symptomatically from gargling or careful oral administration of a combination of kaopectate, diphenhydramine, and viscous lidocaine. Overuse of lidocaine may, however, cause seizures. Systemic analgesics are sometimes necessary.

Candida infection usually responds to nystatin swabbing. Trench mouth (NUGMA) is thought to respond to penicillin. Syphilitic ulcers require benzathine penicillin, tetracycline, or erythromycin with serologic follow-up at specified intervals. Stevens-Johnson syndrome can be life threatening, and patients should receive prompt consultation and admission. Acyclovir is recommended for herpes simplex virus infections in immunocompromised hosts at a dose of 15 to 30 mg/kg/day in three divided doses for 7 to 14 days. Limited data suggest that acyclovir may also be useful in immunocompetent individuals.

PHARYNGITIS

After the common cold and otitis media, throat infection is the most common illness diagnosed by pediatricians in the United States. About 11 percent of all school age children seek medical care for pharyngitis annually.

Anatomy and Pathophysiology

The pharynx is the musculomembranous sac adjacent to the mouth, nares, and esophagus. It includes Waldeyer's ring of lymphoid tonsillar and adenoidal tissue, just caudal to the soft palate. Infectious, allergic, mechanical, and chemical processes can cause inflammation in the pharynx.

Etiology

Viruses, bacteria, spirochetes, *Chlamydia, Mycoplasma,* mycobacteria, fungi, and parasites can all cause pharyngitis. Viral infections are the most common infectious cause. The common viruses include adenovirus, parainfluenza virus, rhinovirus, herpes simplex, respiratory syncytial virus, Epstein-Barr virus, influenza virus, enterovirus (coxsackie virus and echo virus), coronavirus, and cytomegalovirus.

Group A beta-hemolytic streptococcus is the most common bacterial cause of pharyngitis in children >3 years of age. One must also consider groups C and G streptococci, *Neisseria gonorrhoeae,* and *Corynebacterium diphtheriae. Corynebacterium hemolyticum* causes pharyngitis accompanied by a scarletiniform rash. Pneumococcus, *Staphylococcus aureus, N. meningitides,* and *Haemophilus influenzae* are thought to cause pharyngitis, usually after a viral upper respiratory infection. Syphilis may present with diffuse pharyngeal inflammation and focal chancres primarily; gray mucous patches are noted secondarily. *Chlamydia trachomatis* and *Mycoplasma pneumoniae* are occasionally responsible for pharyngitis in adolescence. *Candida* may cause diffuse oropharyngeal erythema with thick white exudate in immunosuppressed patients and patients taking prolonged courses of antibiotics.

A "scratchy" throat may be due to sinusitis, posterior nasal drip, or respiratory irritants, such as tobacco smoke. Caustic ingestions can present with pharyngeal pain. Agranulocytosis, lymphoma, and lymphocytic leukemia, though rare, can present with pharyngeal inflammation. Uvular inflammation results from bacterial infection, trauma (usually medical instrumentation), and allergy. Thermal and chemical injuries are less common. Uvulitis is most worrisome when associated with epiglottitis or angioneurotic edema, both potentially life-threatening conditions. Bacterial pathogens that can cause uvulitis are group A hemolytic streptococcus, *H. influenzae* type B, and *Streptococcus pneumoniae.*

Diagnostic Findings

Infants and toddlers with pharyngitis may have nonspecific irritability, poor feeding, anorexia, and drooling or oral lesions. Older children can verbalize and localize pain to the throat. Epiglottitis in older children may present as the "worst" sore throat.

Respiratory symptoms, such as clear rhinorrhea, cough, hoarseness, or mucosal ulcers, suggest a viral etiology. Epstein-Barr virus and cytomegalovirus infection often have associated pharyngeal inflammation, diffuse lymphadenopathy, and hepatosplenomegaly. Herpangina causes small vesicular lesions and punched-out ulcers in the posterior pharynx. Hand-foot-and-mouth disease causes vesicles and ulcers in the areas noted. Low-grade fever, follicular conjunctivitis, sore throat, and cervical lymphadenopathy characterize pharyngoconjunctival fever.

Headache, vomiting, abdominal pain, and scarletiniform rash (fine, erythematous, sandpaper-like) are noted with streptococcal pharyngitis. Onset is typically acute, with fever, throat pain, and dysphagia. It most often occurs in late winter and early spring. Diphtheria presents as an adherent, grayish pharyngeal membrane with bull neck and toxic appearance. History of exposure to the tissue or secretions of infected small animals may suggest tularemia. Pharyngitis accompanied by rash, joint pain, and urethral or vaginal discharge may indicate gonorrhea. Asymptomatic carriage of gonorrhea is not unusual. Urticaria, wheezing, or stridor may indicate an allergic etiology.

Rapid streptococcus detection by latex agglutination or enzyme immunoassay is useful when positive. False-positives with latex agglutination are uncommon (specificity 88 to 100 percent), but false-negatives occur more frequently (sensitivity 72 to 95 percent). A negative rapid screening test should be confirmed by a routine streptococcal culture using aerobic culture technique and sheep blood medium with bacitracin disk. Specific swabbing of tonsillar tissue yields the most success in detection of streptococci.

Local suppurative complications, manifested by severe dysphagia, stridor, dysphonia, and odynophagia, may require more aggressive diagnostic testing, such as soft tissue radiographs of the lateral neck and CT of the neck. Surgical incision and drainage may be necessary.

A CBC, EBV titers (Monospot), syphilis screening tests, and cultures for *N. gonorrhoeae* are indicated for atypical presentations. The presence of a positive gonococcal culture in a young child is a marker for sexual abuse and must be reported to the appropriate social service investigators. Additional studies may be useful in seriously ill or immunocompromised patients in order to exclude nonsuppurative complications of streptococcal infection. These tests may include urinalysis, assessment of immunologic response to infection [antistreptolysin-O (ASO), "Streptozyme"], renal function tests, and electrocardiogram.

Complications

Suppuration can spread to contiguous tissue causing peritonsillar abscess (quinsy), life-threatening Lemierre's postanginal sepsis (aerobic or anaerobic bacteremia from septic thrombophlebitis of the tonsillar vein), and Ludwig's angina (submandibular abscess). Hematologic spread may result in mesenteric adenitis, meningitis, brain abscess, cavernous sinus thrombosis, suppurative arthritis, endocarditis, osteomyelitis, sepsis, and septic embolization to the lung.

Nonsuppurative syndromes due to streptococcal infection include scarlet fever, rheumatic fever, and glomerulonephritis. Unrecognized gonococcal or syphilis infections can disseminate systemically. Untreated diphtheria may progress to seizures or respiratory failure.

Management

Antibiotics for streptococcal pharyngitis should generally be administered for a total of 10 days. Optimal initial management in areas of low rheumatic fever prevalence includes oral penicillin, 250 mg twice a day for children <12 years of age and 500 mg twice a day for children >12. Where poor compliance and follow-up are issues, intramuscular benzathine penicillin is given, 600,000 U for children <60 lb and 1,200,000 U for children >60 lb. Penicillin-allergic patients can be treated with erythromycin ethylsuccinate, 40 mg/kg/day in 2 to 4 doses daily for 10 days. Sulfa and tetracycline are not effective. Indications for tonsillectomy for recurrent sore throats are controversial.

Other bacterial diseases require specific and supportive management. If diphtheria is suspected, diphtheria antitoxin is given along with penicillin or erythromycin. Tularemia requires streptomycin or gentamicin.

Allergic entities frequently require epinephrine, 1:1000, 0.01 mL/kg/dose, subcutaneously. Antihistamines, such as diphenhydramine, 1.25 mg/kg/dose, intramuscularly or orally and corticosteroids, such as prednisone, 2 mg/kg/dose, orally are also used.

PERITONSILLAR ABSCESS

Peritonsillar abscess (quinsy) is the most common deep infection of the head and neck. Usually a complication of bacterial tonsillitis, it can also occur with EBV infection. Peritonsillar abscess is rare in children <12 years of age.

Anatomy and Pathophysiology

The peritonsillar space contains loose connective tissue and is bordered by the capsule of the tonsil medially, the superior pharyngeal constrictor muscle laterally, and the anterior and posterior pillars. The palatoglossus muscle forms the anterior pillar. The posterior pillar is the palatopharyngeus muscle. Infections in this space may extend to the peripharyngeal space and tissues. Infection in the tonsil breaks through the tonsillar capsule and lies between the capsule and the muscle of the superior constrictor.

Etiology

Most peritonsillar abscesses are polymicrobial infections. Group A streptococci are predominant; *Peptostreptococcus, Peptococcus, Fusobacterium,* and other normal mouth flora, including anaerobes, may also be detected. Uncommonly, *H. influenzae, S. pneumoniae,* and *S. aureus* are cultured.

Diagnostic Findings

The history is usually of gradually increasing pharyngeal discomfort and ipsilateral otalgia, followed by trismus, dysarthria, and, less commonly, dysphagia and odynophagia. Drooling is not unusual. The voice has a muffled, "hot potato" quality. Patients are often toxic.

Examination of the oropharynx may sufficiently distinguish peritonsillar cellulitis from an abscess. Cellulitis is commonly associated with diffuse swelling and edema in the peritonsillar region. An abscess causes varying degrees of trismus due to a peritonsillar mass effect with displacement of the soft palate medially and the uvula contralaterally. Fluctuance can frequently be palpated. There is usually ipsilateral cervical adenopathy.

The white blood cell count may be elevated. The throat culture will often document a streptococcal infection. Blood and tonsillar aspirate cultures are useful for directing antibiotic therapy. A CT of the head and neck is vital for delineating the extent of involvement if extension from the peritonsillar space is suspected and patients are not responding to standard antibiotic therapy.

Differential Considerations

Peritonsillar abscess is sometimes difficult to distinguish from uncomplicated tonsillitis or peritonsillar cellulitis.

Peritonsillar abscess may be confused with peripharyngeal space infections, cervical adenitis and abscess, foreign bodies, dental infections, tetanus, salivary gland infections, and tumors.

Complications

Extension beyond the peritonsillar space produces complications. These may become evident after the pharyngitis has resolved. Spiking fevers, chills, neck stiffness and pain, torticollis toward the opposite side (from sternocleidomastoid spasm), and swelling around the parotid gland may herald peripharyngeal extension. Necrotizing fasciitis has been reported as a lethal complication. Airway obstruction, aspiration pneumonia, mediastinitis, lung abscess, thrombophlebitis, and sepsis have also been reported.

Management

Generally, patients will require hospitalization for hydration, intravenous antibiotics, analgesia, and surgical drainage, if indicated. Antibiotics usually include a third-generation cephalosporin, such as ceftriaxone (100 mg/kg per 24 hours q 12 hours IV) or cefotaxime (150 mg/kg per 24 hours q 8 hours IV). Many clinicians add penicillin G (25 to 50 mg/kg per 24 hours or 40,000 to 80,000 U/kg per 24 hours q 4 hours IV) initially if the children are toxic. If resolution is slow, nafcillin 100 to 150 mg/kg per 24 hours q 4 hours IV (or equivalent) is started.

Needle aspiration is sometimes used diagnostically to differentiate between cellulitis and abscess. Some otolaryngologists employ needle aspiration therapeutically instead of incision and drainage in cooperative patients. Tonsillectomy after the acute episode is advocated by many, but appears necessary only infrequently in childhood for recurrent problems or slow resolution of symptoms.

RETROPHARYNGEAL ABSCESS

Retropharyngeal abscess is a local accumulation of pus in the prevertebral soft tissue of the upper airway.

Anatomy and Pathophysiology

The retropharyngeal space is a pocket of connective tissue that extends from the base of the skull to the tracheal carina. It harbors two paramedian chains of lymphoid tissue that drain the nasopharynx, adenoids, and posterior paranasal sinuses. These lymphatic chains begin to atrophy around the third or fourth year of life. Fifty percent of cases of retropharyngeal abscess occur between 6 and 12 months of age, and 96 percent occur in children <6 years of age. Bacterial infections of the areas drained by the retropharyngeal nodes may result in suppuration of the nodes and abscess formation. Otitis media and nasopharyngeal infection may lead to the suppuration of nodes of the small lymph chains between the buccopharyngeal and prevertebral fascia. Less commonly, extension of infection from penetrating injuries or vertebral osteomyelitis may cause retropharyngeal abscess.

Etiology

S. aureus and group A hemolytic streptococci are the most common pathogens. *H. influenzae* and anaerobes (*Bacteroides, Peptostreptococcus,* and *Fusobacterium* spp.) are also pathogenic.

Diagnostic Findings

There is usually a prodromal nasopharyngitis or pharyngitis progressing to the abrupt onset of high fever, dysphagia, refusal of feeding, severe throat pain, hyperextension of head, and noisy respirations. Predisposing factors include previous trauma or associated infections. Respirations are usually labored; drooling and stridor may be present. A bulge in the retropharynx is frequently visible. Meningismus may result from irritation of the paravertebral ligaments. Pain in the back of the neck or shoulder may occur when patients swallow.

An elevated white blood cell count, with a shift to the left, is noted, but is usually not needed for a therapeutic decision. The discovery of neutropenia, however, especially in the immunocompromised host, may reflect decompensation and the need for more aggressive therapy. Cultures and Gram's stain of purulent material obtained from incision and drainage is essential. A soft tissue lateral neck radiograph will usually demonstrate the retropharyngeal mass in stable patients. The prevertebral space is normally <7 mm anterior to C2 and <5 mm anterior to C3 and C4 or <40 percent of the anteroposterior diameter of the C3 or C4 vertebral bodies. Adequate hyperextension of the head and neck is necessary in order to allow for proper interpretation of the film.

Differential Considerations

Airway obstruction by retropharyngeal abscess may mimic epiglottitis or croup, peritonsillar abscess, and infectious mononucleosis. Other considerations include cystic hygroma, hemangioma, and primary neurogenic neoplasms. Trauma to the retropharynx from foreign body ingestion, instrumentation, and cervical spine injury can cause localized swelling.

Complications

The most serious acute complications are airway obstruction and aspiration. The abscess may rupture into the esophagus, mediastinum, or lungs. Empyema and pneumonia can result. Blood vessels may be eroded, and hemorrhage can occur. Inadequate drainage can allow reformation of the abscess.

Management

A standard approach to airway maintenance is vital since airway obstruction and aspiration can occur at any time. Patients will require hospitalization for hydration, intravenous antibiotics, analgesia, and surgical drainage. Antibiotics usually include penicillin G 25 to 50 mg (40,000 to 80,000 U)/kg per 24 hours q 4 hours IV or nafcillin (or equivalent) l00 to 150 mg/kg per 24 hours q 4 hours IV. A third-generation cephalosporin such as ceftriaxone (l00 mg/kg per 24 hours q 12 hours IV) or cefotaxime (150 mg/kg per 24 hours q 8 hours IV) may also be added. Emergent surgical intervention and drainage is necessary with particular attention to the airway and ventilation.

CERVICAL LYMPHADENOPATHY

Lymphadenopathy is enlargement of one or more lymph nodes. Benign lymph node enlargement and lymphadenitis account for most childhood neck masses. Stimuli that precipitate node inflammation and enlargement include bacterial, viral, mycobacterial, fungal, and parasitic infections. Kawasaki's disease, cat-scratch disease, Kikuchi's lymphadenitis, sarcoidosis, and antigenic stimulation by drugs, bites, or stings also occur.

Etiology

S. aureus accounts for 60 percent and group A streptococcus accounts for 85 percent of primary lymphadenitis in children. Less common etiologic agents include *Mycobacteria tuberculosis,* nontuberculous mycobacteria, and anaerobic bacteria. Rare causes include *Francisella tularensis* (tularemia), *Yersinia pestis* (plague), *Brucella melitensis* (brucellosis), *Chlamydia* spp., *Mycoplasma* spp., *Treponema pallidum* (syphilis), *Actinomyces israelii, Streptococcus pyogenes, H. influenza,*

Pseudomonas aeruginosa, and *Toxoplasma gondii* (toxoplasmosis).

Viral pharyngitis or tonsillitis due to rhinovirus, adenovirus, or enterovirus causes transient lymphadenitis. Mononucleosis, caused by EBV, may have a necrotic gray tonsillar membrane, malaise, fever, and hepatosplenomegaly. Mumps, rubella, rubeola, chickenpox, and herpes simplex can also cause cervical lymphadenitis.

Mucocutaneous lymph node syndrome (Kawasaki's disease) is associated with aneurysmal dilatation of the coronary vessels (Chap. 49). Early recognition and treatment can reduce mortality from this complication. The presence of cervical adenitis and fever for several days should prompt examination for other clinical findings of this syndrome: stomatitis, conjunctivitis, polymorphous exanthem, peripheral edema, and desquamation of the hands and feet.

Kikuchi's disease (necrotizing lymphadenitis) is a benign condition of concern primarily for its variable association with fever and leukopenia, which can be confused with lymphoma.

Cat-scratch disease causes regional lymphadenitis and is usually diagnosed based on historic association with recent kitten scratch. An antigenic skin test (Hanger-Rose test) is now available. A "cat-scratch bacillus," *Bartonella henselae,* and noncaseating granuloma are demonstrable on biopsy material.

Noninfectious causes of lymphadenopathy include traumatic soft tissue swelling, malignancy, congenital muscular torticollis, branchial cleft cyst, thyroglossal duct cyst, cystic hygroma, lymphangioma, and vascular abnormalities. Some developmental abnormalities are detected only after secondary infection occurs.

Diagnostic Findings

Time of symptom onset and clinical course should be clearly defined. History should include information about the following:

- Upper respiratory infection
- Concurrent sore throat
- Duration of symptoms
- Skin lesions of the scalp or face
- Fever
- Dental problems
- Pets
- Exposure to tuberculosis or other infections

The most useful differentiating finding on examination of an enlarged lymph node is the presence or absence of inflammation. A hot node presents with erythema, warmth, tenderness, and sometimes fluctuance. Examination of the scalp, teeth, neck, and tonsils often reveals a primary infection. "Cold" or apparently uninflammed nodes require a thorough search for associated disease such as cat-scratch disease, tuberculosis, nontuberculous mycobacterial infections, and malignancy. A painless, firm neck mass should be considered malignant until proven otherwise. A thorough otolaryngologic and systemic examination with detailed notation of all lymph nodes, including the axilla and groin, should be noted. If malignancy is suspected, a CBC with manual differential may reveal anemia, thrombocytopenia, or abnormal white blood cell count with immature cells.

If tuberculosis is suspected, a 5 T.U. purified protein derivative (PPD) skin test should be placed intradermally on the volar aspect of the forearm. If anergy is suspected, a control skin test should be placed on the contralateral volar forearm. Nontuberculous mycobacteria may weakly react to PPD.

Spontaneously draining nodes provides an excellent opportunity for culture. In immunocompromised patients, neonates, or when antibiotic therapy has failed, the abscess material should be cultured for aerobic and anaerobic bacteria, mycobacteria, and fungi.

Differential Diagnosis

Regional lymph node enlargement can be a response to tonsillitis, peritonsillar abscess, dental pathology, scalp trauma or infection, ear disease, or other antigenic stimulation in the head and neck. Second, cervical lymphadenopathy may be a manifestation of systemic disease. Frequently mononucleosis and, less commonly, sarcoidosis, tuberculosis, or Kawasaki's disease and, rarely, toxoplasmosis, syphilis, and other systemic diseases can cause inflammatory changes in the cervical lymph nodes. If neither a site of inflammation in the head and neck nor evidence of systemic disease can be detected, primary lymph node enlargement should be suspected.

Management

As always, life-threatening respiratory and cardiovascular compromise should be treated first. If primary lymph node infection is suspected and the child has been in an endemic area or has been exposed to tuberculosis, a 5 T.U. PPD and a suitable control such as *Candida* to exclude anergy should be placed. Historic or clinical clues may suggest an unusual microbiologic etiology. Specific antigenic skin tests are available for some of the non-tuberculous mycobacteria, but culture is the only reliable means of confirming the diagnosis. Tuberculosis is treated by medical means, but nontuberculous mycobacterial infections usually require complete node excision.

Hot or suppurative nodes are most commonly caused by beta-hemolytic group A streptococci *(S. pyogenes)* and penicillin-resistant *S. aureus.* A majority of the staphylococcal species is resistant to penicillin. A semi-synthetic penicillin, such as dicloxacillin, is the drug of choice, but greater palatability of cephalexin and amoxicillin-clavulanic acid makes them superior choices. Erythromycin should be considered when cost is a concern. If the cause is cat-scratch fever, then patients should be treated with rifampin or trimethoprim-sulphamethoxazole.

Toxic appearance, advanced disease, young age, unreliable follow-up, unresponsiveness to oral therapy, immunocompromised host, or inability to tolerate oral medications may make outpatient therapy impractical. Inpatient management should include semisynthetic penicillin, such as intravenous oxacillin. A short course of intravenous antibiotics may improve patients enough to allow completion of therapy as outpatients. The disease process determines the therapy of cold lymphadenopathy.

Follow-up in 2 to 3 days is helpful to assess progress of therapy, read skin tests if placed, and observe for fluctuance. If fluctuance occurs or if patients are unresponsive to optimal medical management, surgical consultation should be requested. Incision and drainage of the nodes by the emergency physician should be avoided, since a persistent draining sinus can result, especially when the infection is caused by nontuberculous mycobacteria. Distinction between bacterial and mycobacterial disease is not reliable by physical examination. Total surgical excision of the node is curative, prevents a draining sinus, and allows a clear etiologic diagnosis. A surgeon should evaluate suspected embryonic remnants for possible excision.

An otolaryngologist should follow children with suspected malignancy. In a review of 178 pediatric cases of malignant head and neck tumors, 1 of 6 malignant neck masses had an associated nasopharyngeal tumor. If questions about follow-up exist or if patients appear toxic, further evaluation and treatment should be completed on an inpatient basis.

BIBLIOGRAPHY

Alvarez A, Schreiber JR: Lemierre's syndrome in adolescent children—anaerobic sepsis with internal jugular vein thrombophlebitis following pharyngitis. *Pediatrics* 96 (2, Pt 1):354–359, 1995.

Amsterdam JT: Dental emergencies: Part I—Pain and trauma. *Emer Med* 26:21–39, 1994.

Hoyt DJ, Fisher SR: Kikuchi's disease causing cervical lymphadenopathy. *Otolaryngol Head Neck Surg* 102:755, 1990.

Kureishi A, Chow AW: The tender tooth: Dentoalveolar, pericoronal and periodontal infections. *Infect Dis Clin North Am* 2:163, 1988.

Morrison JE, Pashley NRT: Retropharyngeal abscesses in children: A 10-year review. *Pediatr Emerg Care* 4:9, 1988.

Paradise JL: Etiology and management of pharyngitis and pharyngotonsillitis in children: A current review. *Ann Otol Rhinol Laryngol* 101:51, 1992.

Pickering LK (ed): Red Book 2000. Report of the Committee on Infectious Disease. *American Academy of Pediatrics,* 2000, p. 213.

69

Eye Emergencies in Childhood

Katherine M. Konzen
Ghazala Q. Sharieff

HIGH-YIELD FACTS

- Normal visual acuity is 20/40 in a 3 year old; 20/30 in a 4 year old; and 20/20 in a 5 to 6 year old.

- Steroids should not be used for patients with iritis or keratitis until herpes simplex is excluded.

- Glaucoma should be suspected in patients who have eye pain and nausea and vomiting. Bilateral eye pressures should be checked immediately.

- Neonates with suspected gonococcal conjunctivitis should undergo a complete septic work-up, including a lumbar puncture. These patients should be admitted for intravenous antibiotics.

- Physical examination of patients with iritis reveals a miotic pupil, perilimbal injection, and an aqueous flare and cells on slit lamp examination.

- Chemical alkali burns to the eye can result in liquefactive necrosis and should be irrigated until the eye pH is between 6 and 8.

Children with eye disorders often come to the emergency department. It is imperative that the emergency physician perform a complete eye examination in order to avoid overlooking potentially debilitating ophthalmologic injuries. The physician must remember certain important guidelines when facing patients with ocular disease:

- The cardinal rules of resuscitation are: *A*irway, *B*reathing, *C*irculation. In patients with multiple trauma or severe systemic disease, the life-threatening conditions must be evaluated and managed first. The eye must be protected from further damage. In patients with blunt head trauma, the mechanism of injury must be considered and treated appropriately. Problems should be anticipated ahead of time.

- A thorough and complete history must be taken. Have there been previous eye problems or surgeries? Are there underlying health problems? Does the patient wear glasses or contact lenses? If a traumatic injury, when and where did it occur? Who saw it? What type of instrument was involved? Who else was involved? What was done for the patient prior to arrival in the emergency department? In the absence of trauma, is eye pain present? Has there been eye discharge or exposure to others with similar conditions? Has there been use of systemic or topical medications?

- The visual acuity in both eyes must always be checked. Information about the unaffected eye can help guide one in the assessment of the affected eye.

- A general physical examination should be performed and rapport should be built with the child. Physicians should look for other underlying injuries or signs of systemic illness. The eye examination should be performed in a logical, methodical manner. Patients should be observed for any facial asymmetry. Toys or other objects that hold the interest of the child and allow proper evaluation of the visual fields should be used. The eye should be touched and dilated only after a thorough systemic examination, and only if indicated.

- If the possibility of a globe perforation exists, manipulation of the eye should not be performed.

A metal shield should be used to protect the eye; a pressure patch is contraindicated. If there is concomitant head trauma, the pupils should not be dilated.

- Physicians must know when to stop and when to consult an ophthalmologist.

PHYSICAL EXAMINATION OF THE EYE AND DIFFERENTIAL CONSIDERATIONS

A thorough and systematic eye examination is divided into six major categories: vision, lids and orbit, anterior segment, pupils and extraocular movements, posterior segment, and intraocular pressure.

Vision

Some method of testing visual acuity must be available for both preverbal and verbal children. For very young children, the ability to focus on an object such as a toy may give a rough assessment of visual acuity. A newborn can fixate on a close object, and a 1 month old should be able to follow a moving object. For older children, Snellen letters or Allen figures are useful to check visual acuity in both eyes. Normal visual acuity is 20/40 in a 3 year old; 20/30 in a 4 year old; and 20/20 in a 5 to 6 year old. Vision can be impaired from any obstruction of the visual pathway.

Lids and Orbit

The lids must be examined by testing the ability to raise and lower the eyes, note any erythema, edema, lacerations, or ecchymosis. Children with periorbital cellulitis will often have significant edema and erythema of both the upper and lower eyelids. The upper lid must be everted to rule out the presence of a foreign body by firmly grasping the lashes at the lid margin and everting the lid against countertraction at the superior tarsal margin using a cotton-tip applicator. Lacerations involving the medial canthus may result in a lacrimal duct injury and should be repaired by an ophthalmologist.

Examination of the orbit includes palpation for defects in the orbital bony structure or for subcutaneous emphysema. Orbital fractures are often accompanied by ecchymosis, lid swelling, proptosis, and limitation in extraocular movements. Herniation and entrapment of the inferior rectus muscle within the orbital floor fracture results in paralysis of upward gaze. Sinus fractures may be associated with subcutaneous emphysema. Physicians should note the presence of exophthalmos or enophthalmos.

Anterior Segment

Inspect the sclera and conjunctiva for swelling, erythema, foreign bodies, hemorrhage, or discharge. Diseases of the cornea and conjunctiva are divided into two main categories of infection or trauma. The history should lead one to the most likely problem. Infections are of bacterial, viral, or fungal etiologies. Conjunctival infections often begin unilaterally but may spread to the other eye within a few days. Crusting and exudate are usually present. In North America, the most common corneal infection causing permanent visual impairment is herpes simplex. Throughout the rest of the world, the most common agent is trachoma. Traumatic injuries to the cornea should be considered in even the youngest of children and can be the cause of a crying infant. Fluorescein examination for a corneal abrasion may be appropriate during the initial examination. Evaluate the corneal light reflex for both briskness and adequacy of response. Self-inflicted thermal wounds from curling irons, microwave popcorn bags, or other mechanism should be thoroughly evaluated.

The anterior chamber comprises the aqueous humor, iris, and lens. Acute iritis (anterior uveitis) is rare in children and may be associated with juvenile rheumatoid arthritis or sarcoidosis. One should consider the possibility of iritis in children who have unilateral, sudden onset of pain, photophobia, and redness. Physical examination reveals a miotic pupil, perilimbal injection, and aqueous flare and cells on slit lamp examination. Treatment includes early ophthalmologic consultation, cycloplegics, and steroid drops if recommended by the specialist. Infections of the uvea can be caused by bacteria, fungi, viruses, or helminths. Measles, mumps, and pertussis may be associated with a uveitis; however, this is not due to direct invasion.

Trauma can cause damage to the anterior chamber. A hyphema occurs when there is hemorrhage in the anterior chamber. Complications of hyphemas include rebleeding, increased intraocular pressure, glaucoma, and corneal bloodstaining. Optic nerve atrophy can occur in patients with sickle cell disease. Since these complications may result in permanent loss of vision, an ophthalmologist should be consulted. The iris should be evaluated for shape and contour. Under penlight or direct ophthalmoscopic examination, the lens should be clear. If opacification is present, cataracts should be considered. Depending on the type of trauma, cataract formation can occur within days or years from an injury. For further discussion of eye trauma, see Chapter 17.

Aniridia presents as an apparent absence of the iris but has many variations. The pupil appears as large as the cornea while the iris remains as a small residual structure. The visual acuity for patients with aniridia is extremely poor due to macular hypoplasia; nystagmus and photophobia are often present. Two-thirds of patients have a hereditary autosomal dominant condition, while one-third are sporadic cases. Approximately 20 percent of infants with sporadic aniridia develop a Wilms' tumor, other genitourinary defects, or mental retardation. Other ocular defects associated with aniridia include a displaced lens, cataracts, corneal epithelial dystrophy, and glaucoma.

Pupils and Extraocular Movements

Pupils should be black, round, symmetric, and equally reactive to light. Changes in the anterior chamber, lens, or vitreous may result in a pupil that is not black. A ruptured globe or intracranial process can lead to pupillary asymmetry. Assess extraocular movements in all visual fields and clearly document all deficits. Pupillary assessment includes evaluation for an afferent pupillary defect known as a Marcus Gunn pupil in which pupillary constriction is delayed and diminished in both eyes when light is shone in the affected eye as compared to the normal eye. A Marcus Gunn pupil is evidence of injury to the anterior visual system and is a poor prognostic sign.

A white spot on the pupil, leukocoria, can be due to congenital cataract, coloboma, retinopathy of prematurity, retinal dysplasia, congenital toxoplasmosis, old vitreous hemorrhage, retinoblastoma, or retinal detachment, in addition to a wide variety of other hereditary, developmental, inflammatory, and miscellaneous conditions. It is essential for patients with leukocoria to have a thorough funduscopic examination by an ophthalmologist.

Posterior Segment

The posterior segment comprises the vitreous, retina, and optic nerve. The direct ophthalmoscope can be used to examine for papilledema, hemorrhages, retinal detachment, and intraocular foreign bodies. Chronic conditions including uveitis can cause deposits in the vitreous. Endophthalmitis (infections inside the eye) may result from penetrating injury, worsening superficial infection, or surgery. Children will have unilateral severe pain in or around the eye and compromised vision. Pu-

rulent exudate in the vitreous will show up as a greenish color on the ophthalmoscopic examination. Often a hypopyon (pus in the anterior chamber) is seen.

Blunt or penetrating trauma to the eye can lead to a vitreous hemorrhage. Other causes of hemorrhage include diabetes mellitus, hypertension, sickle cell disease, leukemia, retinal tears, central retinal vein occlusion, and tumor. Presentation of these patients is usually due to sudden loss of vision.

Retinal artery and retinal vein obstruction are relatively uncommon in the pediatric population. Etiologies include trauma and other systemic entities. Retinal artery occlusion is a true ocular emergency and can be due to emboli in patients with endocarditis and systemic lupus erythematosus or result from hypercoagulability in patients with sickle cell disease. When central retinal artery occlusion occurs, there is sudden, painless loss of vision in one eye. Ophthalmoscopic examination reveals the cherry-red spot of the fovea, a pale optic nerve and markedly narrowed arteries. A Marcus Gunn pupil may be present. Ophthalmology consultation should be immediately obtained for possible paracentesis of the anterior chamber to decompress the globe. Temporizing measures include ocular digital massage, topical beta-blocker (Timoptic 0.5%), Diamox, and CO_2 rebreathing by having patients blow into a paper bag for 5 to 10 minutes.

Retinal vein obstruction also leads to sudden painless loss of vision that varies depending on the extent of the obstruction. Retinal hemorrhages and a blurred, reddened optic disk may be seen. These findings are often described as a "blood and thunder" fundus. Arteries are often narrowed, veins are distended, and there may be white exudates. Retinal vein obstruction can occur in trauma as well as leukemia, cystic fibrosis, and retinal phlebitis. An ophthalmologist should be consulted. Aspirin therapy may be initiated to inhibit further thrombosis.

Retinal tears can lead to vitreous hemorrhage causing diminished vision in the affected eye. Retinal detachment may take years to develop after a tear. As the detachment progresses, patients may have a visual field deficit or may complain of flashing lights or a "curtain" draping over the affected eye. Ophthalmoscopic examination will reveal a light-appearing retina in the area of detachment.

The optic nerve is responsible for the transmission of visual information to the cortex. Disruptions in this transmission can lead to visual loss. Optic neuritis is usually due to inflammation or demyelination. It is characterized by an abrupt, rapid, unilateral loss of vision while pain is variable. Rarely does optic neuritis present as a separate entity in children. Most often it is caused by meningitis, viral infections, encephalomyelitis, and demyelinating diseases. Lead poisoning and long-term chloramphenicol therapy are other known culprits.

Various toxins have been associated with impaired vision. Most act on the ganglion cells of the retina or optic nerve causing visual defects. Methyl alcohol can cause sudden, permanent blindness. Other recognized toxins include sulfanilamide, quinine, quinidine, and halogenated hydrocarbons.

Finally, one must consider that visual loss can result from impedance within the visual cortex of the brain. Head trauma, hypoglycemia, leukemia, cerebrovascular accidents, and anesthetic accidents can all be associated with cortical blindness.

Intraocular Pressure

Either infection or injury to the anterior chamber can lead to increased intraocular pressure. Glaucoma can manifest any time after an insult to the eye. Pain and blurred vision should alert one to the possibility of glaucoma. The pupil is nonreactive and dilated, and patients may complain of seeing halos around objects. Accurate measurement is accomplished by slit lamp tonometry or with a handheld tonometer. This should not be undertaken, however, if the possibility of a ruptured globe exists. In patients with acute glaucoma, rough tactile measurement of intraocular pressure can be made by gentle palpation of the globes with the fingers through the eyelids. An extremely firm eye can easily be detected. Normal eye pressure in children ranges from 10 to 22 mmHg. An ophthalmologist must be immediately involved in the care and treatment of children with suspected glaucoma. Immediate medical management includes a combination of topical pilocarpine 1 to 2% once the intraocular pressure is below 40 mmHg, adrenergic agents, mannitol 1 to 2 g/kg IV, and carbonic anhydrase agents. Diamox is most often used at an oral dose of 15 mg/kg/day.

ERRORS TO AVOID

In managing eye emergencies, physicians should avoid some common mistakes:

- Forgetting to examine the unaffected eye
- Not thoroughly examining the injured eye
- Failing to consider and recognize globe perforation
- Prescribing topical anesthetics and steroids

- Using eye drops or ointment when a perforation exists
- Failure to ensure proper follow-up for patients

COMMON EYE COMPLAINTS

The Red Eye

History is extremely important in differentiating the etiology of the red eye. Although conjunctivitis is common in childhood, other etiologies must be thoroughly considered prior to arriving at the diagnosis. Time of onset, exposure to chemicals or noxious stimuli, exposure to other children with similar problems, presence of systemic illness, history of trauma, photophobia, and excessive tearing are all important in the consideration of the differential diagnosis. The differential diagnosis for the red eye is listed in Table 69-1.

Eye Pain

Two fiber systems are involved in the transmission of eye pain. Myelinated fibers transmit the sharp transient pain while unmyelinated fibers transmit the dull aching sensations. Pain fibers innervating the eye and periorbital structures arise from the trigeminal or fifth cranial nerve. The first (ophthalmic) division is the most important one responsible for eye pain. It innervates the globe, forehead, lacrimal gland, canaliculi, and the lacrimal sac, as well as the frontal sinus, upper lid, and side of the nose. The second major branch (maxillary nerve) supplies the cheek, lower eyelid, and a small lower segment of the cornea, upper lip, side of the nose, maxillary sinus, roof of the mouth, and temporal region. The third division of the trigeminal nerve (mandibular) supplies sensation to other areas of the cheek in addition to the preauricular region. Referred pain can occur if the sensory pathway is stimulated in other regions. Interestingly, the cornea represents one of the areas of greatest density of pain nerve endings in the body.

Eye pain often can be difficult to characterize in the young child. Superficial eye pain is frequently associated with such epithelial abnormalities as a corneal abrasion, whereas deep eye pain is more often associated with increased intraocular pressure or uveitis. Eye pain associated with burning makes one consider dry eyes, allergies, or irritation secondary to chemicals or noxious stimuli. Pain caused by bright light is associated with iritis, uveitis, and glaucoma.

Eye pain in children results from a variety of causes including foreign bodies, corneal abrasions, conjunctivi-

Table 69-1. Differential Diagnosis of the Red Eye

Conjunctivitis
    Bacterial
    Viral
    Herpes simplex
    Chemical
    Allergic or seasonal
    Neonatal ophthalmia
Corneal abrasion and corneal ulcer
Foreign bodies
Glaucoma
Hordeolum or chalazion
Iritis
Keratitis, episcleritis, scleritis
Periorbital or orbital cellulitis
Systemic disorders
    Ataxia-telangiectasia
    Collagen vascular disease
    Infectious disease—mumps, measles, otitis media
    Inflammatory bowel disease
    Juvenile rheumatoid arthritis
    Kawasaki disease
    Lyme disease
    Leukemia
    Stevens-Johnson syndrome
Trauma
    Chemical burns and thermal burns
    Ruptured globe
    Subconjunctival hemorrhage
    Hyphema

tis, episcleritis, acute dacryocystitis, congenital glaucoma, uveitis, optic neuritis, hordeolum, herpes zoster, and a wide array of trauma. Physicians should attempt to characterize the pain and then thoroughly search for the underlying etiology. Eye pain secondary to chemical alkali burns (lye or ammonia) result in a liquefactive necrosis that can cause permanent damage to the iris and lens. Acid burns result in a coagulative necrosis, and, therefore, the depth of the burn is self-limiting. Immediate treatment for both types of injuries includes irrigation with a minimum of 1 to 2 L of normal saline. The irrigation should be continued until the eye pH, measured by litmus paper, is between 6 and 8. Fluorescein examination should then be performed. If there is no epithelial deficit, erythromycin ointment or drops can be initiated 4 times a day with ophthalmologic consultation within 48 hours. If there is a corneal epithelial deficit,

ophthalmology consultation and referral within 24 hours is warranted. These patients benefit from a cycloplegic agent, erythromycin ointment, and possibly eye patching for comfort.

Excessive Tearing

Usually noted in infants, excessive tearing can be due to nasolacrimal obstruction (dacryostenosis) or may be secondary to bacterial, viral, or allergic conjunctivitis. Sometimes infants with a corneal abrasion or glaucoma will have tearing.

Eye Discharge

Purulent eye discharge is most often associated with bacterial conjunctivitis. Viral and allergic conjunctivitis are more often associated with mucoid discharge. Patients with blepharitis have crusting in addition to the discharge.

NONTRAUMATIC EYE DISORDERS

Eyelid Infections

Eyelid infections are frequent throughout childhood. The glands of Zeis are sebaceous glands attached directly to the hair follicles; the Meibomian glands are sebaceous glands that extend through the tarsal plate. Eyelid infections (blepharitis) often involve one of these glands. The most common infections of the eyelid include chalazion, hordeolum, impetigo contagiosa, and herpes simplex.

Clinical Findings

An external hordeolum or stye is a suppurative infection of the glands of Zeis, whereas an internal hordeolum or chalazion is an acute infection of a Meibomian gland. A chalazion presents as a painless, hard nodule and is often located in the midportion of the tarsus, away from the lid border caused from obstruction of the gland duct. Chalazions are uncommon during infancy but frequently occur during childhood. Initially, the swelling may be diffuse but usually becomes localized to the lid margin. Impetigo contagiosa is a pyoderma usually presenting with vesicles; it then develops a yellowish crust, which occurs due to local invasion by staphylococci or streptococci. In patients with impetigo, there can often be an underlying seborrheic dermatitis. Herpes simplex can present on the eyelids of children and can lead to latent infection, which may persist throughout life and be re-activated. Recurrent infection often involves the cornea. Herpetic blepharitis is characterized by the formation of vesicles, which break down and form a yellowish-crusted surface.

Differential Diagnosis

The differential diagnosis of an external hordeolum includes contact dermatitis and allergic conjunctivitis. Itching is a more prominent feature in the latter two entities and is not usually associated with a hordeolum. The differential diagnosis of a chalazion includes rhabdomyosarcoma, capillary hemangiomas, dermoids, orbital cysts, molluscum contagiosum, sarcoidosis, fungal infections, foreign bodies, and juvenile xanthogranuloma. Differentiation is made by lack of response to local therapy and/or biopsy. Impetigo contagiosa and herpes simplex can be easily confused. Cultures should be obtained to ascertain etiology.

Management

The management of a hordeolum includes warm compresses and eyelid hygiene using baby shampoo on a washcloth. Twice-daily application of an antistaphylococcal antibiotic ointment (erythromycin ophthalmic ointment or polymyixin B sulfate) or ophthalmic drops should also be initiated. A chalazion is initially managed in the same manner, and antibiotic treatment should be continued for several days after rupture of the chalazion to prevent recurrence. If there is a lack of response to medical treatment, surgical incision and drainage under general anesthesia is recommended for young children. Recurrence commonly results from autoinoculation and inattention to good hygienic care.

Impetigo contagiosa should be treated with removal of crusts and topical antistaphylococcal and streptococcal antibiotics. A cotton-tip applicator soaked in baby shampoo can be used to clean the lid margins. Bacitracin ophthalmic ointment is often effective; however, topical erythromycin and gentamicin can be used. If systemic impetigo is present, oral antibiotics should be initiated.

Herpes simplex blepharitis should be treated with vidarabine ophthalmic ointment and trifluorothymidine topical drops. Topical and oral acyclovir should be considered but may be of limited value. Treatment of herpes simplex will be discussed in further detail in the following sections.

Cellulitis of the Periorbital and Orbital Region

Periorbital infections are common in childhood and usually resolve with appropriate therapy and without sequelae. A review of the sinuses and classification of this infection is helpful in considering the correct diagnosis. The anatomic development of the sinuses in children is thought to play a major role in the development of orbital and periorbital infections.

Periorbital infections, particularly sinusitis, may cause infection or severe inflammation in the orbital tissues leading to a preseptal or orbital cellulitis. The proximity of the paranasal sinuses to the orbital walls and the interconnection between the venous system of the orbit and the face allow infection to spread from the sinuses to the orbit either directly or via the bloodstream. The orbital venous system is devoid of valves so that two-way communication is allowed with the venous system of the nose, face, and pterygoid fossa. The superior and inferior ophthalmic veins drain directly from the orbit and empty into the cavernous sinus. Orbital and facial infections can lead to cavernous venous thrombosis.

The orbital periosteum and septum are important anatomic structures, which help to limit direct spread of infection. The orbital periosteum acts as a barrier to the spread of infection from the sinuses; however, it may become eroded if a periorbital abscess develops. The orbital septum may also limit the spread of infection from the preseptal space to the orbit. The following classification has been described for orbital infections:

- Class I: Periorbital or Preseptal Cellulitis
  Cellulitis is confined to the anterior lamella tissue due to a lack of flow through the drainage ethmoid vessels. Lid edema and erythema may be mild or severe. The globe ordinarily is not involved so that vision and function remain normal.

- Class II: Orbital Cellulitis
  Orbital tissue is infiltrated with bacteria and cells, which extend through the septum into the orbital fat and other tissues. Manifestations usually include proptosis, impaired or painful movement, and periocular pain. Visual acuity may be impaired and septicemia may be present.

- Class III: Subperiosteal Abscess
  Purulent material collects between the periosteum and the orbital wall. Medial wall involvement causes the globe to be displaced inferiorly or laterally. Symptoms include edema, chemosis, and tenderness with

ocular movement, while vision loss and proptosis vary in severity.

- **Class IV: Orbital Abscess**
  When pus accumulates within the orbital fat inside or outside the muscle cone, an orbital abscess has developed. The infectious process becomes localized and encapsulated, unlike orbital cellulitis, which tends to be more diffuse. Exophthalmos, chemosis, ophthalmoplegia, and visual impairment are generally severe; systemic toxicity may be impressive.

- **Class V: Cavernous Sinus Thrombosis**
  Thrombosis results from extension of an orbital infection into the cavernous sinus. Nausea, vomiting, headache, fever, pupillary dilation, and other systemic signs may be present. There is marked lid edema and early onset of third, fourth, and sixth cranial nerve palsies.

The bacteriology involved in orbital infections depends on the age of the patient and the underlying problem. In the newborn period and up to the age of 5 years, *Haemophilus influenzae* and *Streptococcus pneumoniae* are predominant, particularly in children with upper respiratory tract infections, conjunctivitis, sinusitis, or otitis media. In patients with a history of skin infections or trauma, *Staphylococcus aureus* and streptococcal species are the main offending agents.

Fungal orbital cellulitis is uncommon in children. A slowly progressive course of orbital swelling in children with vomiting or dehydration may indicate an underlying fungal infection; immunocompromised children may be at greatest risk. *Rhizopus* and *Mucor* are the most common fungal infections.

Clinical Findings

Most of the clinical findings are described with each class of infection. Preseptal or periorbital cellulitis is marked by periorbital edema, erythema, and tenderness but is not accompanied by proptosis, ophthalmoplegia, or loss of visual acuity. Chemosis and conjunctivitis may be present, as well as fever and leukocytosis. In young children who have fever and other systemic signs, a lumbar puncture and intravenous antibiotics should be considered because of the possibility of underlying meningitis. In young children, *H. influenzae* type B can produce a distinctive type of bluish-purple hue to the eyelid. It is often accompanied by fever, irritability, otitis media, and bacteremia.

Patients with orbital cellulitis present similarly but have further development of ophthalmoplegia, proptosis,

pain on eye movement, worsening chemosis, and changes in vision. Fever and leukocytosis are often seen. Blood cultures are positive in up to 25 percent of patients. If the orbital cellulitis is secondary to sinusitis, headache, rhinorrhea, and swelling of the nasal mucosa may also be present. At times, swelling of the eyelid may be so severe that further evaluation is necessary. Computed tomography (CT) has been useful in the delineation of periorbital cellulitis from orbital cellulitis. It, however, has its limitations in making a definitive diagnosis of a subperiosteal abscess from reactive subperiosteal edema.

Management

In patients with mild periorbital cellulitis and no history of fever or other systemic illness, a thorough physical examination is recommended but laboratory investigation may be unnecessary. Mild cases of preseptal cellulitis due to local trauma or conjunctivitis can be treated with oral antibiotics such as amoxicillin-clavulanate (20 to 40 mg/kg/day), to cover against *S. aureus*. For cellulitis secondary to bug bites, oral antihistamines and warm compresses may also be helpful. Close follow-up is mandatory.

For patients requiring hospitalization, a complete blood cell count, blood cultures, lumbar puncture, and CT of the head may be warranted. A lumbar puncture should be considered to rule out meningitis if patients appear toxic and are <2 years of age. The following management scheme has been recommended by several authors:

- All patients hospitalized for orbital inflammation should receive ophthalmologic and otolaryngology consultation.

- Broadspectrum antimicrobial therapy should be instituted at once while awaiting blood or intraoperative culture results. Children <5 years of age, without a history of trauma, should be placed on appropriate coverage against *H. influenzae* type B, *S. pneumoniae,* and group A streptococcus. A suggested initial regimen consists of ceftriaxone, 100 mg/kg/day, with the addition of vancomycin, 40 mg/kg/day in severe cases. Children >5, or those fully immunized with the *Haemophilus* vaccine, do not generally require coverage for *Haemophilus;* appropriate antimicrobials are similar to those used for treatment of severe sinusitis.

- Attempts must be made to delineate if the cellulitis is of preseptal or postseptal origin. Computed tomography of the head is a helpful diagnostic aid but may not differentiate between subperiosteal abscess and reactive periosteal edema.

- Surgical indications include diminishing visual acuity, lack of improvement despite adequate antibiotics, or spiking fevers suggesting possible development of orbital abscess or cavernous venous thrombosis.

Posttraumatic suppurative cellulitis is treated by early incision and drainage of the infected space, coupled with parenteral antibiotics. Tetanus prophylaxis should be considered. Sufficient coverage for *S. aureus* and *Streptococcus pyogenes* is necessary. Anaerobic coverage should be instituted following animal and human bites. Intravenous antibiotics are recommended for a minimum of 48 to 72 hours, and then consideration of oral therapy may be appropriate.

Orbital cellulitis secondary to sinusitis should be managed with the consultation of ophthalmology and otolaryngology. Intravenous antibiotics should consist of a third generation cephalosporin and a penicillinase-resistant penicillin. If the potential for an anaerobic infection exists, clindamycin may be substituted for the penicillinase-resistant penicillin. Frequent ophthalmologic examination with thorough clinical reassessment is warranted to determine response to treatment and need for surgical intervention.

Complications

In addition to the previously mentioned complications of cavernous venous thrombosis and meningitis, blindness has been associated with postseptal cellulitis. In the pre-antibiotic era, up to 20 percent of patients with postseptal inflammation developed blindness. Alarmingly, studies report a 10 percent incidence of blindness resulting from orbital complications of sinusitis. Clearly, broad-spectrum antibiotics and modern surgical techniques have not totally alleviated this devastating complication. In fact, negative or equivocal CT findings often contributed to an inappropriate delay in surgical intervention. Computed tomography of the head cannot solely determine patient management; clinical judgment must prevail.

Scleritis and Episcleritis

The sclera, made up mainly of collagen and connective tissue, is the thick vascular covering of the eye. Scleritis is uncommon but can be associated with juvenile rheumatoid arthritis or various infectious processes including herpes simplex, varicella zoster, mumps, syphilis, and tuberculosis.

The thin vascular membrane between the sclera and conjunctiva is called the episclera. Inflammation of this area produces some irritation but not the severe pain associated with scleritis. Episcleritis is also associated with a variety of diseases including varicella zoster, syphilis, Henoch-Schonlein purpura, erythema multiforme, and penicillin sensitivity. Episcleritis often presents as a distinct area of injected conjunctiva with dilated vessels in the involved layer of tissue. Differentiation may be helpful with the administration of topical phenylephrine, which constricts vessels dilated by conjunctivitis but not those vessels involved in scleritis or episcleritis. Management consists of treating the underlying disease and some combination of oral nonsteroidal anti-inflammatory agents, topical corticosteroids, and cycloplegics.

Conjunctivitis

Diagnostic Terms

A review of certain diagnostic terms is cardinal to this discussion. *Hyperemia* is due to an increase in the number, caliber, and the tortuosity of vessels in the conjunctiva resulting in a reddish appearance to the conjunctiva occurring in both acute and chronic conjunctival processes. Edema often accompanies hyperemia. *Congestion* is caused by diminished conjunctival drainage, producing a dusky red discoloration secondary to prolonged circulation time within the conjunctival vessels. Congestion is most often seen in allergic conjunctivitis where the conjunctiva takes on a jelly-like appearance. *Exudates* are the by-products produced from conjunctival inflammation and may be purulent, watery, catarrhal, ropy, mucoid, or bloody. They collect in the lid margin and corners of the eyes and are viewed best when the lids are pulled away from the eye. *Follicles* are collections of lymphocytes within the conjunctiva and are often associated with allergy, viral conjunctivitis, and toxicity to topical medications. Vessels are usually located on the outside of each follicle. *Papilla* are elevations of the conjunctiva that have a central vascular core; around the core is a clear area of conjunctival swelling. Small ones produce a velvety appearance on the surface of the conjunctiva. Large papillae are easily seen without magnification and are associated with contact lens wear, irritation from surgical sutures, and vernal conjunctivitis. *Membranes and pseudomembranes* are coagulum formed by inflammatory reaction to an infection. Pseudomembranes are very fine coagula covering the conjunctival surface and, when removed, do not damage the underlying conjunctiva and hence do not cause bleeding. Membranes differ in that they are coagula firmly attached to the underlying conjunctiva and, when removed, cause bleeding. Pseudomembranes are seen in epidemic keratoconjunctivitis, primary herpes simplex conjunctivitis, streptococcal conjunctivitis, alkaline burns, and erythema multiforme. Membranes are associated with diphtheria and less frequently with streptococcal conjunctivitis, adenovirus types 8 and 19, alkali burns, and erythema multiforme.

Ophthalmia Neonatorum

Conjunctivitis in the newborn period (first 28 days of life) is not uncommon (Table 69-2). Because of the potential complications from ocular infections in infancy, neonates with symptoms mandate a thorough evaluation. Important guidelines for evaluation include:

- Obtaining a detailed maternal history including prenatal care, history or exposure to venereal disease, duration of rupture of membranes, type of delivery, agent used for ocular prophylaxis at birth, recent exposure to conjunctivitis, and timing of onset of symptoms. History should also include a description of excessive tearing, type and amount of exudate, and elucidation of systemic signs of illness in the baby, such as fever, vomiting, irritability, or lethargy.

- Physical examination must be thorough including a comprehensive eye examination searching for evidence of eyelid erythema, edema, discharge, corneal ulceration, globe perforation, or foreign body. In addition, general physical examination must be complete; special attention must focus on the skin, respiratory, and genitourinary system for evidence of concomitant systemic involvement.

- Conjunctival scrapings should be obtained for Gram's stain, Giemsa's stain, and viral and bacterial cultures including *Neisseria*. A rapid antigen test is sensitive and specific for *Chlamydia* and can be obtained easily from the conjunctiva. Culture is usually not necessary.

Differential Diagnosis

Chemical Conjunctivitis

Chemical conjunctivitis caused from silver nitrate drops in the immediate newborn period occurs in almost 10 percent of newborns. Signs of this type of conjunctivitis include bilateral conjunctival hyperemia and mild discharge that begin in the first 24 hours of life and usually subside within 48 hours. Gram's stain reveals no organisms and only a few white blood cells. The inflammation is typically quite mild and does not require intervention.

Chlamydia Trachomatis

Chlamydia infections have a typical incubation period of 1 to 2 weeks, but can occur earlier if there was premature rupture of membranes. The overall incidence of chlamydial ophthalmia is approximately 20 to 40 cases per 1000 births annually. The prevalence of chlamydial infections in pregnant women ranges from 2 to 23 percent; transmission rates from infected mothers range from 23 to 70 percent. Typically, the conjunctiva becomes hyperemic and edematous with the palpebral conjunctiva more involved than is the bulbar conjunctiva. Unilateral, purulent involvement is characteristic. Neonates may also have evidence of a concomitant otitis media or afebrile pneumonia. Samples are obtained by scraping the palpebral conjunctiva of the lower lid. The diagnosis is confirmed by identification of chlamydial antigen, detection of intracellular inclusions from Giemsa's stain, or isolation of the organism. Antigen detection tests are rapid, sensitive, and specific and are the most efficient means of confirming the diagnosis. Gram's stain is not helpful in confirming the diagnosis.

Management

Systemic therapy is absolutely essential in the treatment of this condition. The treatment of choice is oral erythromycin (40 to 50 mg/kg/day) for a 2- to 3-week course to eliminate both conjunctival and nasopharyngeal colonization. Administration of a topical agent is unnecessary. Since chlamydia is the most frequent sexually transmitted disease, prevention by detection in the mother prior to delivery is essential. Early studies suggested that the administration of erythromycin ointment prophylaxis in newborns was effective in preventing chlamydia conjunctivitis but not in altering the rate of development of pneumonia or nasopharyngeal infection. Studies have revealed that neonatal ocular prophylaxis with erythromycin does not reduce the incidence of chlamydial conjunctivitis. Chlamydial conjunctivitis can lead to chronic changes of conjunctival scarring and micropannus formation. Fortunately, these long-term ocular sequelae are quite rare.

Table 69-2. Ophthalmia Neonatorum

	Chemical Conjunctivitis	Chlamydia	Bacterial	Neisseria	Herpes Simplex	Viral
Onset	0–2 days	1–2 weeks	1–4 weeks	0–30 days	2–14 days	0–30 days
Discharge	−	+	+	+++	+	+
Unilateral/bilateral hyperemia	B	U	U/B	B	U/B	U/B
Fever	−	±	−	±	±	−
Diagnosis	Negative Gram's stain, few WBCs	Rapid antigen, Giemsa's stain, or culture	Gram's stain, culture	Gram's stain, culture	Fluorescein staining, multinucleated giant cells, intranuclear inclusion cells, fluorescent antigen tests	History of contact exposure, negative Gram's stain, and viral culture
Treatment	None	Systemic oral erythromycin, 2–3 weeks	Topical antimicrobial	Intravenous third-generation cephalosporin	Intravenous acyclovir, topical trifluorothymidine	Topical antimicrobial
Associated findings	None	Pneumonia, otitis media	None	Rhinitis, anorectal infection, arthritis, meningitis	Skin lesions, septicemia	Upper respiratory tract infection
Long-term complications	None	Conjunctival scarring, micropannus formation	None	Blindness	Keratitis, cataracts, chorioretinitis, optic neuritis, others	None

Key: − = absent; ± = may or may not be present; + = mild; ++ = moderate; +++ = severe. WBC, white blood cells.

Bacterial Conjunctivitis

The role of other bacteria in the newborn period is not quite as clear and can be caused by *S. aureus, Haemophilus* spp., *S. pneumoniae,* and *Enterococci.* Many studies have also shown that these bacteria, in addition to *Corynebacterium, Propionibacterium, Lactobacillus,* and *Bacteroides* can be normal flora. Typically, the conjunctiva is red and edematous with some amount of exudate. Diagnosis is made by Gram's stain and culture. Broad-spectrum topical antimicrobial therapy is initiated, although there are no good studies in this population to document the necessity or efficacy of topical therapy. If cultures have been obtained, antimicrobial therapy can be tailored to treat the offending organism. Untreated cases of bacterial conjunctivitis could potentially progress to corneal ulceration, perforation, endophthalmitis, and septicemia.

Neisseria Gonorrhoeae

Historically, gonococcal ophthalmia neonatorum has been of greatest concern because of its serious complications. In the early 1900s, approximately 25 percent of children admitted to American schools for the blind acquired their disability from *N. gonorrhoeae.* By the late 1950s, <0.5 percent were blind as a result of *Neisseria.* With the onset of antibiotics and postnatal prophylaxis, the current incidence in the United States is thought to be 2 to 3 cases per 10,000 live births. The mean incubation period is 6.5 days with a range of 1 to 31 days. Gonococcal ophthalmia neonatorum classically presents as a purulent, bilateral conjunctivitis. Conjunctival hyperemia, chemosis, eyelid edema, and erythema may also be seen. This entity is diagnosed by Gram's stain, revealing gram-negative intracellular diplococci. Cultures should be sent immediately on blood and chocolate agar, because the organisms die rapidly at room temperature. Cultural growth usually occurs within 2 days. Infants with conjunctivitis may have other manifestations of localized disease including rhinitis, anorectal infection, arthritis, and meningitis. Neonates with suspected gonococcal conjunctivitis or any neonate with fever and conjunctivitis should have a sepsis evaluation, including a lumbar puncture.

Management

Treatment must be systemic; there is no role for oral or topical antibiotics. Neonates without meningitis should be treated for 7 days with either ceftriaxone or cefotaxime. If meningitis is present, treatment continues for 10 to 14 days. If the organism is sensitive to penicillin, penicillin G can be substituted. Treatment must also include frequent saline irrigation of the eyes. Parents should be screened for gonococcal disease. An infant born to a mother with known active gonococcal infection should receive one dose of ceftriaxone immediately after delivery.

Herpes Simplex

Most neonates with herpes simplex become colonized during the birth process. Neonatal herpes simplex may occasionally present first as conjunctivitis. The onset is generally 2 to 14 days after birth. Characteristics are not clinically distinctive; however, unilateral or bilateral epithelial dendrites are virtually diagnostic. Fluorescein staining reveals these defects. Parental history of herpes is important to obtain. Often conjunctivitis leads to further disseminated infections that carry a high morbidity and mortality rate. The conjunctivitis can be diagnosed with conjunctival scrapings looking for multinucleated giant cells and intranuclear inclusions. A fluorescent antibody test should be obtained followed by a viral culture.

Management

Treatment should consist of intravenous acyclovir for 10 days and topical trifluorothymidine. Parents must be aware of the high risk of recurrence of keratitis later in life; an ophthalmologist ought to follow these children closely. Recurrences are treated with topical therapy alone. Neonatal herpes simplex can lead to the development of keratitis, cataracts, chorioretinitis, and optic neuritis in addition to numerous other ocular problems. Long-term follow-up studies have shown that more than 90 percent of neonates with neurologic sequelae from herpes simplex infection also have some type of ocular abnormality.

Viral Etiologies (Nonherpetic)

Other viral causes of conjunctivitis in neonates are infrequent. Conjunctivitis in sibling or parents is the most likely source of infection. Hands or other fomites are the modes of transmission. Diagnosis is made by history of recent exposure and clinical findings. Usually infections are self-limited; often topical antimicrobials are prescribed to avoid secondary infection but are probably of limited value. Education regarding hand-washing and nonsharing of washcloths and towels is necessary.

Obstructed Nasolacrimal Duct

Congenital nasolacrimal duct obstruction, or dacryostenosis, is often only recognized when infants have a history of recurrent ocular infections. The blockage is frequently caused by failure to canalize a membrane called the *valve of Hasner*, which is located at the lower end of the nasolacrimal duct. Affected infants often have pooling of tears onto the lower lid and cheeks and maceration of the eyelids. Upon crying, tears fail to arrive at the external nares. It is important to differentiate nasolacrimal obstruction from congenital glaucoma. Congenital glaucoma presents with tearing, photophobia, and a cloudy, enlarged cornea. Redness is not a major feature. Conservative treatment consists of massaging the lacrimal sac, suppressive topical antimicrobials, and warm compresses. Probing of the nasolacrimal system is not recommended until after 1 year of age because 95 percent of children <13 months will experience spontaneous opening of the lacrimal duct.

Noninfectious Etiologies

The differential diagnosis of the red eye in neonates should also include noninfectious etiologies. Corneal abrasions can be detected in infants and may often be secondary to a scratch from their fingernail. Conjunctival hyperemia may be present; fluorescein staining is diagnostic. Linear abrasions on the superior aspect of the cornea should alert the physician to an upper eyelid foreign body. Trauma to the eye during delivery can also cause a corneal abrasion or laceration. Foreign bodies in the neonatal period are rare but should be considered in the evaluation.

Conjunctivitis Beyond the Neonatal Period

Conjunctivitis is a frequently encountered entity in children (Table 69-3). Considerations in management include the following:

- Age
- Onset of conjunctivitis (acute being <2 weeks, chronic lasting >2 weeks)
- Previous history of conjunctivitis
- Trauma
- Type of eye discharge
- Unilateral versus bilateral symptoms
- Photophobia
- Lacrimation

- Pain
- Change in visual acuity
- History of herpes simplex
- Exposure to conjunctivitis
- Associated systemic symptoms of fever, sore throat, or rash

It is crucial to identify conjunctivitis from more serious conditions. Conjunctivitis in older children is characterized by normal vision, a gritty sensation in the eye, diffuse injection, and exudate. Photophobia and lacrimation are not usually associated with conjunctivitis. Keratitis and iritis typically are associated with impaired vision, true pain, photophobia, and lacrimation.

Clinically, viral conjunctivitis is difficult to distinguish from bacterial conjunctivitis. Marked exudate, severe injection, and lid matting is more typical of bacterial or chlamydial infections. Preauricular adenopathy is often associated with viral infections. Follicles on the palpebral conjunctivae are more indicative of viral or chlamydial infections.

Bacterial Conjunctivitis

The bacteriology of conjunctivitis in children is expansive and includes *H. aegyptius, S. pneumoniae, S. aureus, N. gonorrhoeae* and *meningitides, Moraxella* spp., *Escherichia coli, Pseudomonas aeruginosa, Proteus* spp., *viridans streptococci, S. pyogenes, Corynebacterium diphtheria, Chlamydia trachomatis,* and *Moraxella catarrhalis*. Outbreaks of acute catarrhal conjunctivitis, also known as "pink eye," may occur in day care or among school-aged children. The offending organisms are most frequently *S. pneumoniae* or *H. aegyptius*. Outbreaks are more often seen in the winter months. Results from prospective studies indicate that the organisms most significantly associated with conjunctivitis in childhood are *H. influenzae, S. pneumoniae,* and adenoviruses. The role of *S. aureus* in nontraumatic conjunctivitis is difficult to determine because it occurs frequently in asymptomatic patients. In addition, *Haemophilus* has been associated with concomitant otitis media, and subsequent studies have coined the term *conjunctivitis-otitis syndrome* when the two occur together.

Pseudomonas is an infrequent pathogen that can cause an acutely advancing necrotizing picture, so it must be recognized and treated aggressively. Phlyctenular conjunctivitis is a rare manifestation of active primary infection with *Mycoplasma tuberculosis* associated with a high degree of hypersensitivity. Notably small grayish

Table 69-3. Conjunctivitis in Childhood

	Bacterial	Pharyngo-conjunctival	Acute Hemorrhagic	Herpes Simplex	Gonococcal	Allergic
Organism	See text	Adenovirus	Enterovirus 70, coxsackie A24	Herpes simplex	*Neisseria gonorrhoeae*	None
Discharge	++	+	+++	±	+++	−
Unilateral/bilateral hyperemia	U/B	U/B	B	U	U/B	B
Fever	−	+	+	++	±	
Diagnosis	History and Gram's stain, culture if necessary	History and associated symptoms, viral culture if necessary	Subconjunctival hemorrhages and viral culture	Antifluorescent test Gram's stain, culture	Gram's stain, culture	History, physical examination
Treatment	Topical antimicrobial	Topical antimicrobial to prevent secondary infection	Topical antimicrobial to prevent secondary infection	Topical vidarabine, trifluorothymidine -	Intramuscular ceftriaxone	Topical antihistamine, vasoconstrictors, and/or glucocorticoids
Associated findings	Otitis media with *Haemophilus*	Upper respiratory infection, regional adenopathy	Malaise, myalgias, upper respiratory infection	Eyelid vesicles, preauricular adenopathy	Periorbital inflammation	Atopy
Long-term complications	None	None	None	Corneal ulcerations, cataracts	Blindness, septicemia	None

Key: − = absent; ± = may or may not be present; + = mild; ++ = moderate; +++ = severe.

nodules are present on the bulbar conjunctiva accompanied by intense pain and photophobia. Skin testing is recommended and culture for other bacteria is important because of the high incidence of secondary bacterial infections.

Although most types of acute bacterial conjunctivitis are self-limited, the use of topical antibiotic therapy is thought to shorten the clinical course and more quickly eradicate the organism, thereby decreasing the amount of time patients are contagious. Routine Gram's stain and culture usually is unnecessary unless there is a history of copious mucopurulent exudate *(Neisseria)* or a chronic history of conjunctivitis.

Treatment is empiric with topical antimicrobial ointments or ophthalmic drops. Specific drugs include polymyxin B sulfate (Polysporin) ointment, which has a broad spectrum of activity including coverage for *H. influenzae,* erythromycin ointment or sodium sulfacetamide (Sulamyd), trimethoprim-polymixin (Polytrim), or gentamicin drops.

Contact lenses can cause conjunctivitis and corneal abrasions. Lens wear should be discontinued; storage and cleaning solutions must be replaced to prevent further contamination. Although patching is no longer recommended in these patients, topical antibiotics to avoid *Pseudomonas* or secondary bacterial infection may be initiated. An aminoglycoside such as tobramycin (Tobrex) drops or a fluoroquinolone such as ciprofloxacin (Ciloxan) or ofloxacin (Ocuflox) should be administered 4 times a day for 5 to 7 days. Corneal ulcers should always be considered in patients who wear contact lenses and have a red eye. These patients should be referred to an ophthalmologist.

Viral Conjunctivitis

Adenoviruses are the most common cause of viral conjunctivitis in children. There are a few clinical syndromes associated with this group of viruses including pharyngoconjunctival fever, epidemic keratoconjunctivitis, and nonspecific follicular conjunctivitis. Pharyngoconjunctival fever is most common in children and is associated with an upper respiratory tract infection, regional lymphadenopathy, and fever. The illness is usually self-limited, lasting 1 to 2 weeks, and is due to serotypes 3, 4, and 7. Spread can occur by droplet transmission although numerous epidemics have been linked to swimming pools. Epidemic keratoconjunctivitis is more common in the second to fourth decades of life and causes preauricular lymphadenopathy with diffuse superficial keratitis. Serotypes 3, 8, and 19 are associated. Instruments in eye clinics have been linked to its transmission.

Enteroviral infections from particular coxsackie viruses and echoviruses may cause conjunctivitis but are often associated with other clinical signs including rash or aseptic meningitis. Acute hemorrhagic conjunctivitis is caused by enterovirus 70 or coxsackie A24 and also occurs in epidemics. Transmission is by direct contact with an incubation of <2 days. Clinically, patients present with sudden onset of unilateral ocular redness, excessive tearing (epiphora), photophobia, pain, purulent discharge, and eyelid swelling, which develop in a span of 6 to 12 hours. Patients may complain of a burning pain often described as a foreign body sensation that is thought to be due to discrete patches of epithelial keratitis (diagnosed with fluorescein staining). In 80 percent of cases, the other eye becomes involved within 24 hours. Some patients develop subconjunctival hemorrhages, which are usually located beneath the superior bulbar conjunctiva. Malaise, myalgias, fever, headache, and upper respiratory tract symptoms may also accompany the conjunctivitis. Conjunctival scrapings for a viral culture yield identification of the virus. Ophthalmologic sequelae are rare: <5 percent of cases develop a secondary bacterial conjunctivitis.

Management

Treatment is symptomatic with cool compresses. Many physicians prescribe a topical antimicrobial to prevent secondary bacterial infection, but this practice has not been proven.

Herpes Simplex and Varicella-Zoster

Vesicular lesions on the eyelid can be due to herpes simplex, varicella-zoster, impetigo, or contact dermatitis. History and a general physical examination should aid in the diagnosis. Of all herpes simplex infections, <1 percent involve the eye. Infections are characterized by unilateral, follicular conjunctivitis with vesicles localized to the eyelids. Preauricular lymphadenopathy is commonly present. Fifty percent of the patients develop keratitis within 2 weeks. The virus remains latent in the sensory ganglion and lacrimal glands. Approximately 25 percent of all children will have recurrences; these usually begin with corneal involvement. Long-term complications include necrotizing stromal disease, diffuse retinitis, and scarring. Herpes simplex is the most common cause of severe corneal ulceration in children and is second only to trauma as a cause of corneal blindness in children.

Ocular involvement with varicella is relatively uncommon, occurring in <5 percent of cases. In chickenpox, the conjunctiva can become involved through two mechanisms: Eyelid vesicles can slough virus into the conjunctival cul-de-sac or vesicle formation can take place on the conjunctival surface. Occasionally, the cornea is involved. Fluorescein staining of the cornea and conjunctiva is necessary.

Zoster is uncommon in children, with only 5 percent of all cases occurring in children <5 years of age. Zoster infections of the eye notably follow the distribution of the first division of the trigeminal nerve. Lesions are usually located on the forehead and upper eyelid and can be located on the tip of the nose.

Trifluorothymidine is the preferred agent for treatment of herpes simplex because of its increased solubility, diminished toxicity, and lack of viral resistance. Approximately 95 percent of the corneal ulcers treated with it are cured within 2 weeks; however, treatment should be extended for 1 additional week after resolution of the lesions. For herpetic eye lesions, systemic acyclovir is not recommended because the drug does not penetrate the avascular cornea.

Neisseria gonorrhoeae

Gonococcal eye infections can occur in prepubertal children. A nonvenereal mode of transmission has been suggested. Certain patients have a negative history and physical examination suggestive of abuse. Some of these patients have occasionally shared a bed with a parent. Interestingly, isolates collected from selected patients have identical sensitivities to that obtained from a parent. Intravenous antibiotics are still recommended for this age group.

Gonococcal conjunctivitis can occur in sexually active children and adolescents; the mode of transmission is similar to adults. Treatment may consist of ceftriaxone, 1 g IM plus saline irrigation. Alternatively, ceftriaxone 1 g IM or IV may be administered for 5 days along with saline irrigation.

Allergic Conjunctivitis

Seasonal and Perennial Allergic Conjunctivitis

Itching is frequently the hallmark of allergic conjunctivitis. Seasonal allergic conjunctivitis has its onset of symptoms in either the fall or spring. Patients with sensitivity to grass have more symptoms in the spring, while individuals sensitive to ragweed have more symptoms in the fall. Patients often complain of bilateral itchy, watery eyes with a burning sensation. The conjunctiva is mildly inflamed with varying degrees of edema. Perennial allergic

conjunctivitis is a variant with symptoms on a year-round basis and often allergens such as dust, mites, animal dander, and feathers are responsible for it. This conjunctivitis represents a type I hypersensitivity reaction.

Management

Treatment consists of a combination of topical vasoconstrictors (naphazoline-antazoline and naphazoline-pheniramine), antihistamines (levocabastine 0.05% and olopatadine 0.1%), steroids, and anti-inflammatory agents (ketorolac 0.5%). Systemic antihistamines may be of some benefit. Cromolyn sodium 4% and lodoxamide tromethamine 0.1% eyedrops have also been shown to be effective when used as a prophylactic agent.

Vernal Conjunctivitis

Vernal keratoconjunctivitis is a rare condition mainly affecting children under the age of 10. It is common in warm, dry climates, and males have a 2:1 ratio of being affected. Often there is a significant history of atopy. Peak incidence is between April and August. Patients usually have a history of bilateral itching, foreign-body sensation, clear mucoid discharge, photophobia, and injection. The giant papillae involve the upper tarsal conjunctiva and consist of large "cobblestone" papillae. The pathophysiology is not entirely clear; IgE and IgG are thought to play a role. Treatment is the same as for seasonal allergic conjunctivitis.

Special Forms of Conjunctivitis

Patients with Stevens-Johnson syndrome may have severe conjunctival involvement. In the acute phase of the disease, the palpebral and ocular conjunctiva can scar together. Often goblet cells are lost in the conjunctival epithelium, and the mucous layer of tear film is lost. Since mucus allows tear film to stick to the surface of the eye, the dry-eye state of Stevens-Johnson syndrome is characterized by abundant tears that do not cover the surface of the eye because they are unable to adhere to it. Treatment consists of a combination of topical lubricants and antibiotics.

Kawasaki disease is associated with a bilateral bulbar, nonexudative conjunctivitis. This diagnosis should be suspected in patients who have fever for >5 days and have conjunctivitis, strawberry tongue, cervical adenopathy, fissuring of the lips, diffuse oral injection, erythema and induration of the hands and feet, and desquamation of the fingers and toes.

A chronic blepharoconjunctivitis can be caused by *Pthirus pubis* when the eyelashes are infected by nits or by the bug itself. The only recognized lice to infect the eyelashes are pubic lice. Family members should be screened. The type of conjunctivitis seen with lice results from a hypersensitivity reaction. Systemic treatment of the organism is necessary for successful eradication. Eye ointments have been used for treatment because they are thought to paralyze and smother the lice. A cotton-tip applicator should be used for debridement prior to the placement of the ointment.

Molluscum contagiosum can cause conjunctivitis when the virus is shed into the eye. Typically, it causes a chronic conjunctivitis that does not respond to topical antimicrobials. The problem results from the virus protein, which is toxic to the eye. One may see lesions on the eyelids that are often buried between the eyelashes. Eradication of the virus requires that the lesions be opened with a needle and the central core of the umbilicated region be removed. Bleeding into the core is considered definitive treatment.

Other viral syndromes can be associated with nonspecific conjunctivitis. These include rubella, influenza, mumps, measles, infectious mononucleosis, and cytomegalovirus. Papillomavirus can cause eyelid warts, which shed on the conjunctiva, causing a conjunctivitis similar to that described for molluscum contagiosum.

Other systemic diseases presenting with eye findings mimicking conjunctivitis include ataxia-telangiectasia, where large tortuous vessels are noted on the bulbar conjunctiva. Patients with Lyme disease may develop nonspecific conjunctivitis with or without eye pain.

CONCLUSION

Patients with a red eye should have a thorough history and physical examination. Appropriate testing should include fluorescein staining and culture swabs for leukocytes and other organisms depending on the circumstance. Patients with conjunctivitis should be instructed concerning good hygiene, and the physician should adhere to good hand-washing techniques as well as thoroughly cleaning instruments between patients.

BIBLIOGRAPHY

Ambati B, Ambati J, Azar N, et al: Periorbital and orbital cellulitis before and after the advent of *Haemophilus influenzae* type B vaccination. *Ophthalmology* 107:1450–1453, 2000.

Hart A: The management of corneal abrasions in accident and emergency. *Injury* 28:527–529, 1997.

Herpetic Eye Disease Study Group: Oral acyclovir for herpes simplex virus eye disease. *Arch Ophthalmol* 118:1030–1036, 2000.

Kaufman H, Varnell E, Thompson H: Trifluridine, cidofovir, and penciclovir in the treatment of experimental herpetic keratitis. *Arch Ophthalmol* 116:777–780, 1998.

Laskowitz D, Liu G, Galetta S: Acute visual loss and other disorders of the eyes. *Neurol Clin North Am* 16:323–353, 1998.

Mitchell J: Ocular emergencies, in Tintinalli J, Kelen G, Stapczynski (eds): *Emergency Medicine: A Comprehensive Study Guide.* New York: McGraw-Hill, 1999, pp 1501–1518.

Wallace D, Steinkuller P: Ocular medications in children. *Clin Pediatr* 37:645–652, 1998.

Wright K: *Textbook of Ophthalmology.* Baltimore: Williams & Wilkins, 1997.

70

Pediatric and Adolescent Gynecology

Geetha Gurrala
Michael VanRooyen

HIGH-YIELD FACTS

- The evaluation of prepubescent patients requires particular sensitivity to the emotional concerns of the patient and family. A complete history and careful explanation of the examination is important prior to the physical examination.

- The gynecologic evaluation of prepubescent patients includes examination of the external genitalia and specimen collection, if indicated. A standard speculum examination is not indicated in most children; it is necessary only in patients who are sexually active and those with suspected vaginal foreign bodies or bleeding from trauma.

- Infants with vaginal obstruction who develop hydrocolpos can present with a lower abdominal mass or a visible bulging membrane at the introitus. Difficulty with urination or urinary retention secondary to urethral impingement can also occur and, in severe cases, hydronephrosis can result.

- The treatment of labial adhesions in asymptomatic girls is expectant; no specific therapy is required since the condition is usually self-limiting. In children who appear to have local recurrent irritation and adhesions, estrogen cream applied to the adhesions at bedtime for 3 to 4 weeks will usually be sufficient to facilitate labial opening.

- The most common cause of vaginal bleeding in prepubertal girls is trauma.

- Urethral prolapse is most common in young African-American females. In most cases, warm compresses or sitz baths, combined with a 2-week course of topical estrogen cream can be used to shrink the swelling of urethral tissue but surgical management to excise redundant tissue may be required if the condition persists or the urethral tissue has become gangrenous.

- Precocious puberty is defined as the appearance of secondary sex characteristics before the age of 8 years or the appearance of menarche before the age of 9 years.

- In the premenarcheal child, the lack of estrogen makes the thin vaginal epithelium vulnerable to infection and inflammation. Most childhood vulvovaginitis is due to irritation of the vulva and secondary involvment of the lower third of the vaginal canal. Inadequate local hygiene in the young child is the most common predisposing factor in nonspecific vulvovaginitis, caused most frequently by the inoculation of bacteria from the anal region onto the vulva and vagina.

- DNA amplification techniques now make it possible to diagnose *Chlamydia* and *Neisseria gonorrhoeae* from endocervical swabs and first-void urine specimens.

- Emergency treatment is indicated for the prevention of pregnancy in women after unprotected sex or suspected contraceptive failure. Two oral contraceptive tablets, containing 50 μg of ethinyl estradiol and 0.25 mg of levonorgestrel, are taken within 72 hours of intercourse followed, 12 hours later, by 2 more tablets.

The emergency physician is occasionally confronted with gynecologic problems in prepubertal children and often treats adolescents with gynecologic disease.

Knowledge of normal childhood sexual development is important, as is an empathic understanding of sexual issues involving adolescents. It is also important to organize appropriate follow-up for patients with gynecologic problems.

EVALUATION OF PREMENARCHEAL PATIENTS

The evaluation of prepubescent patients requires particular sensitivity to the emotional concerns of the patient and family. A complete history and careful explanation of the examination is important prior to the physical examination. Continuous reassurance during the examination is necessary to address the concerns and fears of the child, particularly in cases of sexual assault. While infants and very young children have general fears of the examining physician, they are not as aware of the sexual nature of the gynecologic examination as are older children and adolescents.

The Physical Examination

The gynecologic evaluation of prepubescent patients includes examination of the external genitalia and specimen collection, if indicated. A standard speculum examination is not indicated in most children; it is necessary only in patients who are sexually active and those with suspected vaginal foreign bodies or bleeding from trauma. Children are best examined by placing them in either the frog-leg position or the prone knee-chest position, usually with the assistance of the parent. The child may be positioned on the mother's lap. The examiner can obtain a good view of the child's introitus by grasping the labia majora firmly and exerting gentle laterocaudal traction. In the frog-leg position, an assistant may help the examiner by supporting the buttocks from underneath so as to facilitate abdominal relaxation.

Inspection of the vagina focuses on identifying the normal perineal landmarks and evidence of congenital abnormalities, as well as signs of trauma, foreign bodies, lacerations, excoriation, skin lesions, or vaginal discharge. If necessary, an otoscope may be used as an adjunct to check for vaginal lacerations or foreign bodies. If abdominal pain or an abdominal mass is suspected, a rectal examination may be helpful. A bimanual examination in prepubescent girls is not routinely indicated.

Vaginal cultures are obtained by gently swabbing the vaginal introitus or by using a soft dropper with a small amount of saline to lavage the introitus and obtain a specimen. The type of vaginal specimen collected is determined by the differential diagnosis. In cases of suspected sexual misconduct, cultures for *Neisseria gonorrhoeae* and *Chlamydia trachomatis* are obtained, along with slide preparations for *Trichomonas*. Children with vaginal discharge may require a sample for wet mount and Gram's stain to test for candidal infections or bacterial vaginosis.

GYNECOLOGIC DISORDERS OF INFANCY AND CHILDHOOD

Congenital Vaginal Obstruction

Etiology

Congenital obstruction of the vagina is a relatively common disorder, often presenting in infancy or early childhood. Up to 0.1 percent of all full-term female infants are affected. The most common etiology of vaginal obstruction is imperforate hymen. Less commonly seen is vaginal atresia, also called transverse vaginal septum. In neonates with imperforate hymen, the hymeneal ring occludes the vaginal opening and impairs the normal flow of mucoid secretions from the uterus. If the disorder is not detected on the initial physical examination of the infant, vaginal obstruction and uterine distension, termed hydrocolpos, can develop.

Clinical Presentation

Infants with vaginal obstruction who develop hydrocolpos can present with a lower abdominal mass or a visible bulging membrane at the introitus. Difficulty with urination or urinary retention secondary to urethral impingement can also occur and, in severe cases, hydronephrosis can result. Occasionally, patients can develop edema of the lower extremities.

If congenital vaginal obstruction remains undiagnosed until puberty, the patient may present with the complaint of noncyclic lower abdominal pain and amenorrhea. The patient will have normal pubertal development, except for menses. The obstructed flow of menstrual blood, termed hematocolpos, often presents with abdominal distension, urinary complaints, and a dark-blue, bulging introitus.

Patients presenting with transverse vaginal septum or vaginal atresia may present in a similar fashion. Evaluation of the complaint of vaginal outlet obstruction includes a search for associated anomalies and a workup for renal dysfunction, since congential renal anomalies are associated with vaginal atresia.

The treatment of imperforate hymen or vaginal atresia is surgical intervention. Most operations are performed on an outpatient basis unless there are complicating problems, such as a hydronephrosis or renal failure.

Labial Adhesions

Etiology

Labial adhesions, also called labial agglutination, represent an acquired and potentially recurrent condition in which the epithelial tissue around the labia minora becomes fused to form labial syncytia. A thin midline film of tissue is seen that connects both sides of the labia minora. Adhesions occur in 3 to 7 percent of all prepubescent females, mostly between the ages of 1 and 6 years. The etiology of this disorder is unknown, but it is thought to be due to a combination of a child's normally low levels of endogenous estrogen and recurrent irritation and inflammation. It is postulated that recurrent perineal irritation may lead to the development of increased syncytial tissue and subsequent formation of labial adhesions.

Clinical Presentation

The child is usually brought to the physician by the parents with the concern that the vagina is "closing." Other presenting complaints include difficulty urinating or symptoms referable to a urinary tract infection. Upon initial examination, this disorder may resemble congenital absence of the vagina or ambiguous genitalia. Adhesions may be differentiated by the presence of a vertical connecting line that forms a central seam or raphe.

Management

The treatment of labial adhesions in asymptomatic girls is expectant; no specific therapy is required since the condition is usually self-limiting. In children who appear to have local recurrent irritation and adhesions, estrogen cream applied to the adhesions at bedtime for 3 to 4 weeks will usually be sufficient to facilitate labial opening. Estrogen should be used sparingly, since prolonged use can lead to breast growth in children. After the labia have separated, an inert cream, such as zinc oxide, Vaseline, or Desitin, is applied for an additional 2 weeks to keep the labia apart while healing. Surgical or manual separation is not necessary and is not effective, as adhesions will recur.

Prepubertal Vaginal Bleeding

Etiology

The most common cause of genital trauma in childhood is accidental injury due to a fall. Straddle-type injuries can lead to blunt or penetrating trauma to the vulvar region, depending on the particular mechanism of injury. Vaginal hematomas are commonly seen in blunt injuries to the perineum, particularly from bicycle accidents. Penetrating trauma to the perineum from falling on a sharp object requires careful evaluation to exclude injury to the urethra, rectum, and peritoneum. In any patient with unexplained vaginal trauma, sexual abuse must be excluded.

Clinical Presentation

Vaginal hematomas are common and readily diagnosed by physical examination. Penetrating pelvic injuries may present with or without substantial abdominal pain; a high clinical suspicion for pelvic penetration is necessary to exclude intraperitoneal injury.

Management

In managing a patient who has sustained pelvic trauma, it is imperative to exclude pelvic fracture and intraabdominal injury. Vaginal hematomas from trauma rarely require surgical intervention and are most appropriately treated conservatively with cool packs and sitz baths. Early gynecologic or surgical consultation should be considered in cases of vaginal laceration, or when there is a suspicion of pelvic penetration. Urinalysis and rectal examination are done to exclude the possibility of urethral or rectal involvement. General anesthesia may be required to fully explore the extent of a vaginal laceration.

Urethral Prolapse

Etiology

Urethral prolapse is the protrusion of the urethral mucosa outward through its meatus, producing red or purplish edematous mucosa at the meatus, which is soft and doughnut shaped; the central dimple indicates the urethral lumen. The etiology of urethral prolapse is unclear but may be precipitated by the Valsalva maneuver when the patient is crying, constipated, or agitated. Patients may present with painless vaginal spotting, dysuria, or hematuria. Most cases of urethral prolapse are found in African American children between the ages of 2 and 10 years. If left untreated, urethral prolapse may progress to mucosal thrombosis and necrosis.

Management

In most cases, warm compresses or sitz baths, combined with a 2-week course of topical estrogen cream, can be used to shrink the swelling of urethral tissue. Severe cases of urethral prolapse are infrequent. Surgical management to excise redundant tissue may be required if the condition persists or the urethral tissue has become gangrenous.

Precocious Puberty

Etiology

Normal puberty occurs over a wide range of ages. Precocious puberty is defined as the appearance of secondary sex characteristics before the age of 8 years or the appearance of menarche before the age of 9 years. True precocious puberty is premature maturation of the pituitary and it results in both menstruation and ovulation.

Pseudoprecocious puberty is not secondary to pituitary control, and menses may occur without ovulation. In up to 74 percent of cases, precocious puberty is idiopathic and simply represents early sexual development.

Clinical Presentation

Increased growth is often the first change in precocious puberty, followed by breast development and the appearance of pubic hair. Menarche may occur before the appearance of secondary sex characteristics in 10 to 15 percent of patients with precocious puberty. Patients may present to the emergency department with complaints of the appearance of secondary sex characteristics or vaginal bleeding with no history of trauma or injury. Familiarity with the Tanner staging criteria may be helpful to the emergency physician (Table 70-1).

Management

The most appropriate management of patients with suspected precocious puberty is referral to a pediatric gynecologist or endocrinologist for evaluation to rule out disorders such as McCune-Albright syndrome, ovarian tumors, and central nervous system tumors. The two major concerns of precocious puberty that warrant prompt recognition and referral are the social stigma of early growth and development of secondary sex characteristics and the ultimate diminished stature due to early closure of epiphyseal growth centers.

Genital Tract Infections in Children

Vulvovaginitis

Vulvovaginitis, or inflammation of the vaginal and vulvar region, is the most common gynecologic problem in childhood and adolescence. Vaginitis can be produced by a variety of infections and irritants. The differential diagnosis varies with age. Childhood vaginitis may be manifested by vaginal discharge with or without vaginal bleeding. Adolescents may have normal vaginal discharge and the presence of vaginitis may be heralded by a change in discharge or pruritus and vulvar irritation.

Historical considerations include an overview of nutritional and hygienic practices (irritating soaps, constrictive clothing), underlying medical disorders (diabetes, immunocompromised state), and the potential for sexual abuse. A careful history includes an assessment of the presence of pruritus and odor, the character and amount of discharge, and the patient's menstrual and sexual history.

Table 70-1. Tanner Stages

Stage 1 (prepubertal): Elevation of breast papilla; no pubic hair

Stage 2 (age 9.8–10.5 years): Elevation of papilla; areolar diameter enlarged; sparse hair on labia majora

Stage 3 (age 11.2–11.4 years): Enlargement without separation of breast and areola; dark, coarse, curled hair over mons

Stage 4 (age 12.0–12.1 years): Secondary mound of areola and papilla above the breast; adult-type hair, abundant, covers mons and extends about halfway out to inguinal regions

Stage 5 (age 13.7–14.6 years): Mature, with projection of papilla only because of recession of areola to contour of the breast; adult-type hair in quality and distribution

---

Nonspecific Vulvovaginitis

In the premenarcheal child, the lack of estrogen makes the thin vaginal epithelium vulnerable to infection and inflammation. Most childhood vulvovaginitis is due to irritation of the vulva and secondary involvment of the lower third of the vaginal canal. In the young child, inadequate local hygiene is the most common predisposing factor in nonspecific vulvovaginitis, caused most frequently by the inoculation of bacteria from the anal region onto the vulva and vagina. The inflammation is further aggravated by scratching and subsequent excoriation of the skin. Vaginal cultures yield mixed bacterial flora unrelated to a specific disease.

The approach to vulvovaginitis in children is to exclude medically treatable causes of vaginitis by history, physical examination, and microscopic examination, if necessary. This includes addressing the possibility of foreign bodies, pinworms, and sexual abuse. Treatment includes antimicrobial therapy, when indicated, and encouraging proper hygiene and preventive measures (Table 70-2).

Neonatal Leukorrhea

Neonatal leukorrhea is a physiologic vaginal discharge seen in female newborns. The discharge occurs in response to high levels of circulating maternal estrogens, which stimulate mucoid secretions and desquamation of cornified vaginal epithelial cells from the vagina and cervix of the newborn. This transient condition usually subsides within a few weeks as the influence of maternal estrogen subsides. Reassurance is given to caretakers that the condition is self-limited.

Vaginal Foreign Bodies

Vaginal foreign bodies may cause local irritation and secondary infection of the vagina. Discharge may be purulent and bloody. The foreign body may be any object small enough to be inserted into the vagina, including small toys, tissue paper, or crayons. In adolescents, retained foreign bodies include condoms, sponges, and tampons. The associated secondary irritation or infection usually subsides after removal of the foreign body.

Vaginitis Due to Upper Respiratory Infections

Bacterial upper respiratory infections can precede a vaginal infection by 3 to 5 days. Organisms can be transmitted from the nose or mouth to the genitalia. Cultures can confirm the presence of respiratory flora, including *Haemophilus influenzae,* hemolytic streptococci, or *Staphylococcus aureus.* Symptoms are typically acute and associated with severe vulvar irritation. Most cases of vaginitis related to upper respiratory infection involve instructing the patient to use proper hygiene. Specific bacterial infections are confirmed by culture before antimicrobial treatment is instituted; unnecessary use of antibiotics can lead to candidal vaginitis and is avoided.

Candidal Vaginitis

Vulvovaginitis due to *Candida albicans* is uncommon during infancy and childhood. This may be the first manifestation of occult diabetes in older children but may also be caused by the use of steroids or broad-spectrum antibiotics. Other predisposing factors include poor hygiene and the use of bath soaps or restrictive clothing. The most common presenting symptom is intense pruritus and a thick, whitish, nonodorous discharge. Diagnosis is made by preparing a wet mount with potassium hydroxide (KOH) preparation, which reveals branching spores and pseudohyphae. Effective treatment can be accomplished by a variety of antifungal agents, clotrimazole, or micanazole cream, applied locally after cleansing 3 to 4 times per day for 7 to 10 days.

Shigella Vaginitis

Chronic cases of vulvovaginitis may be caused by organisms from the intestinal tract. *Shigella* vaginitis presents

Table 70-2. Nonspecific Vulvovaginitis in Children

Causes
 Poor toilet hygiene following bowel evacuation
 Tight-fitting underclothing
 Lack of proper bathing
 Irritative agents: bubble baths, harsh soaps
 Vaginal foreign bodies
 Upper respiratory infections
Treatment
 Elimination of the irritative agents
 Improved local hygiene
 Sitz baths (2 tbsp baking soda and lukewarm
  bathwater)
 Aveeno oatmeal baths
 Loose-fitting underclothing
 Hydroxyzine or diphenhydramine for pruritus
 Antibiotics directed by culture and sensitivity

with whitish to yellow discharge in three quarters of cases and is unresponsive to antifungal agents. Cultures will reveal growth of *Shigella flexnerni,* which can be treated with trimethoprim-sulfamethoxazole for 5 days.

Parasitic Vulvovaginitis

Parasitic vulvovaginitis can occur in young children (see Chap. 50). Parasites, which can cause vulvar pruritus, irritation, and discharge, include pinworms *(Enterobius vermicularis),* roundworms *(Ascaris lumbricoides),* or whipworms *(Trichuris trichiura).* Diagnosis is best made by inspecting the anal and perineal skin with a flashlight at night while the patient is sleeping, or by performing a "tape test." The "tape test" is conducted by pressing a piece of cellophane adhesive tape against the perianal area in the early morning to recover the parasitic ova, which can then be identified by microscopic examination. The treatment of pinworms is albendazole, given to each family member as a single dose of 400 mg and repeated in 2 weeks. Roundworms and whipworms can also be treated with a single 400-mg dose of albendazole but may be more resistant to treatment and require treatment for up to 3 days.

GYNECOLOGIC DISORDERS OF ADOLESCENCE

The Gynecologic Examination

Adolescents who are sexually active require a complete sexual history and a full speculum and bimanual examination to evaluate for sexually transmitted illnesses and disorders relating to pregnancy. A complete and candid history may be difficult to obtain in the presence of a parent, and it is important to reassure the patient that the history will remain confidential. The patient is questioned about sexual activity, the use of contraception, and the potential for sexually transmitted diseases. All sexually active adolescents with urinary complaints, pelvic complaints, or abdominal pain, receive a pregnancy test to rule out the potential complications of pregnancy. The male physician examining a patient is accompanied by a female chaperone whenever possible.

The examination of the sexually active adolescent requires placing the patient in the lithotomy position on a standard gynecologic table. This will allow for proper visualization of the genitalia and facilitate bimanual examination, speculum examination, and specimen collection.

Dysmenorrhea

Etiology

Primary dysmenorrhea is pain with menstruation that is not associated with recognized pelvic pathology. It is due to uterine contractions induced by increased prostaglandin production by the normal endometrium in response to falling progesterone levels. This causes an increase in uterine tone and myometrial contractions, resulting in abdominal pain and associated symptoms. Secondary dysmenorrhea is pain occurring during menstruation that is caused by underlying pelvic pathology, such as endometriosis; chronic pelvic inflammatory disease; uterine pathology, such as myomas and polyps; and genitourinary anomalies, such as bicornuate uterus or cervical stenosis. Primary dysmenorrhea is much more common than secondary dysmenorrhea, particularly in adolescents.

Clinical Presentation

Patients most commonly complain of crampy lower abdominal pain prior to or at the start of menses. Symptoms typically last for the first 24 to 48 hours of the menstrual period. Associated symptoms may include headaches, backache, thigh pain, nausea, and vomiting. Migraine headaches can also occur and may present with the aura and other symptoms of a vascular headache, such as dizziness or visual changes.

Management

Adolescents with complaints consistent with dysmenorrhea are examined to rule out causes of secondary dysmenorrhea. This includes a bimanual examination in sexually active patients and one-finger vaginal-abdominal palpation in virginal patients. Initial treatment of mild dysmenorrhea includes the use of aspirin, ibuprofen, mefenamic acid, or naproxen to inhibit prostaglandin synthesis, which is effective in 80 to 90 percent of cases. Patients with refractory or incapacitating pain can be treated with oral contraceptives, which inhibit ovulation and, therefore, effectively abolish dysmenorrhea.

Dysfunctional Uterine Bleeding

Etiology

Dysfunctional uterine bleeding (DUB) is defined as vaginal bleeding that is irregular (metrorrhagia), excessive in duration and amount (menorrhagia), or both (menometrorrhagia). Dysfunctional uterine bleeding most commonly occurs within the anovulatory phase but can occur during ovulation. Although DUB can occur in adolescence, it is most commonly seen in older women at the end of their reproductive years.

Dysfunctional uterine bleeding results from the absence of progesterone release during the luteal phase. This allows recurrent endometrial proliferation due to follicular estrogen production. Subsequent sloughing of endometrial tissue and bleeding occurs when estrogen levels fall. Other causes of vaginal bleeding must be excluded in the evaluation of the patient with suspected DUB, including ectopic pregnancy, spontaneous abortion, pelvic inflammatory disease, and uterine pathology, such as endometriosis and carcinoma.

Clinical Presentation

Dysfunctional uterine bleeding can cause significant anxiety in adolescents and can be disruptive to the normal lifestyle of a teen. Patients usually present with complaints of excessive vaginal bleeding, which should be quantified by the examiner based on the number of pads used and the duration of menses. Since DUB occurs most commonly in the anovulatory state, accompanying dysmenorrhea is absent.

Physical examination is directed at ruling out potential life threats, such as hemorrhagic shock and coagulopathy. Vital signs include measurement of orthostatic blood pressure. The patient is evaluated for signs of blood loss, including pallor and decreased capillary refill. The evaluation of the patient includes a pelvic examination to exclude vulvar and cervical pathology or uterine masses. Laboratory testing includes pregnancy testing, hemoglobin, and a coagulation profile if the suspicion of coagulopathy exists.

Management

The management of patients with DUB is directed initially toward stabilization and subsequently toward searching for underlying pathology. Patients can be categorized into three groups to simplify the managment of DUB. Those with minimal bleeding may be reassured and observed. Patients with moderate bleeding may be treated with medroxyprogesterone 10 mg/day orally for 5 days. If bleeding persists, this regimen may be repeated for a total of three cycles, after which normal menses should occur.

Patients with severe vaginal bleeding and unstable vital signs are treated aggressively. Management of shock includes immediate stabilization and circulatory resuscitation, followed by laboratory evaluations to determine the etiology and degree of bleeding. After the patient is stabilized, treatment with high-dose estrogens, such as Premarin, 20 to 25 mg, every 4 hours until bleeding stops, with a maximum of 6 doses. This treatment is followed by medroxyprogesterone, 10 to 20 mg, orally for 5 to 12 days. Curettage may be necessary if estrogen is unsuccessful. Subsequent evaluation is important to rule out underlying pathology, and supplemental iron may be prescribed to prevent iron deficiency anemia.

Mittelschmerz

Mittelschmerz is pain on ovulation caused by peritoneal irritation from minor ovarian bleeding. This disorder, which presents with right or left lower abdominal pain in midcycle, is benign and resolves spontaneously. It should, however, be distinguished from other causes of lower abdominal pain, including ectopic pregnancy, ovarian torsion, and appendicitis.

Premenstrual Syndrome

Premenstrual syndrome (PMS) is a constellation of symptoms attributable to the luteal phase of the ovulatory cycle. It occurs up to 10 days before menses and is characterized by vague pelvic pain, weight gain, headaches, and variations in mood. Medications used in PMS are mefenamic acid, gamma-linoleic acid, GnRH agonists, danazol, alprazolam, fluoxetine, and diuretics.

Ovarian Cysts

Ovarian cysts are most commonly painless and are usually discovered on routine pelvic examination. A physiologic ovarian cyst can result from failure of the follicle to rupture or regress. Ovarian cysts can be associated with menstrual irregularities and are normally <6 cm in diameter. Cysts can rupture and cause lower abdominal pain and hemoperitoneum; they may, therefore, be confused with appendicitis or ectopic pregnancy.

Ovarian Torsion

Ovarian torsion, or twisting of the ovary and adnexa, is an uncommon but important cause of abdominal pain. Torsion may present with intermittent unilateral abdominal pain, low-grade fever, and a tender mass on pelvic examination. Predisposing factors include ovarian enlargement from pregnancy, ovarian cysts, and polycystic ovary disease. Although Doppler ultrasound may be helpful in excluding this diagnosis, laparoscopy is the most reliable diagnostic procedure.

Genital Tract Infections

Vulvovaginitis in Adolescents

Various factors affect the vaginal physiology in adolescents and adults and determine the types of infections that occur in this age group. Mechanisms that provide a defense against vaginal and vulvar irritation are produced by the increased estrogen production in the postmenarcheal female. These protective factors include an acidic vaginal pH, thick protective epithelium, commensal bacterial flora, and physiologic mucous secretion. Factors that predispose the adolescent to vaginal infections include pregnancy, menstrual blood acting as a culture medium, multiple sexual partners, the use of broad-spectrum antibiotics, and possible underlying medical problems, such as diabetes and immunosuppression.

Candidal Vaginitis

Vulvovaginitis due to *Candida albicans* is common in adolescence and adulthood. Predisposing factors include pregnancy, diabetes, oral contraceptives, antibiotics, steroids, and restrictive clothing. Most commonly, patients present with thick vulvovaginal discharge associated with intense pruritus and inflammation. A KOH preparation will reveal pseudohyphae and branching spores. Treatment may be accomplished by a variety of antifungal agents, including miconazole nitrate (vaginal suppository, 200 mg) intravaginally at bedtime for 3 days or 2 percent cream intravaginally at bedtime for 7 days. Other agents, such as clotrimazole or terconazole, may be used. It can also be treated with single dose of flucanazole, 150 mg orally. Preventive measures against recurrent candidal infections include discontinuing antibiotics and steroid therapy, avoiding constrictive clothing, and switching to lower-estrogen oral contraceptives.

Trichomonas Vaginitis

Trichomonas is typically sexually transmitted and is a common cause of vaginitis in sexually active adolescents. Patients may complain of pruritus, a frothy yellowish or greenish discharge that smells foul. The vaginal mucosa and the cervix may have a spotted "strawberry" appearance. The diagnosis can be confirmed by a wet mount, which may demonstrate motile, flagellated trichomonads. Treatment is most commonly accomplished with metronidazole, which may be given as a single dose of 2 g, or 500 mg twice daily for 7 days in adolescents. The sexual partner should be treated concurrently. The presence of *Trichomonas* in children indicates the possibility of sexual abuse.

Gardnerella Vaginitis

Gardnerella vaginitis, which is also known as nonspecific vaginitis or bacterial vaginosis, results from overgrowth of an organism that may be found in the normal vaginal flora. Patients often complain of white or grayish discharge with a "fishy" odor. KOH prep may reveal characteristic "clue" cells, which are vaginal epithelial cells that have been invaded by bacteria. Effective treatments include metronidazole 500 mg twice daily for 7 days or clindamycin 300 mg twice daily for 7 days.

Herpetic Vulvovaginitis

Herpetic vulvovaginitis is a sexually transmitted disease usually caused by the herpes simplex II virus. However, in up to 10 percent of cases, it is caused by herpes simplex I virus. Genital herpes most commonly presents with labial or perianal vesicles, which rupture and progress to painful ulcerations. Ulcerations may be surrounded by a variable inflammatory reaction, and inguinal lymphadenopathy may be present. The diagnosis is made by physical examination and can be distinguished from lymphogranuloma venereum, chancroid, fungal infection, or hypersensitivity dermatitis by viral cultures. Genital herpes infections are self-limiting but recurrent. The course of the disease may be shortened by administration of acyclovir, 200 mg every 4 hours for 10 days.

Bartholin Abscess

A Bartholin cyst is an enlargement of the Bartholin gland, located at 4 and 8 o'clock positions in the vestibule. The swollen gland usually occurs after an episode of vaginitis. Presenting symptoms include a red, tender mass on the lateral introitus and progressive pain. Treatment requires incision and drainage and can be accomplished in the emergency department, although general anesthesia for adequate surgical drainage is often required. After incision and drainage, iodoform gauze or a balloon catheter should be inserted to promote healing. Close follow-up is important and antimicrobial therapy for concurrent vaginal infections may be required.

Gonorrhea

Gonorrhea is a sexually transmitted disease that can present as pelvic inflammatory disease (30 percent), cervicitis (40 percent), or as an asymptomatic infection (30 percent). Symptoms of foul-smelling vaginal discharge, dysuria, and dyspareunia may occur from 3 days to a month or more after infection, although patients may present with a variety of symptoms ranging from minimal discomfort or discharge to severe pelvic inflammatory disease (see discussion that follows). During the last few years, nucleic acid amplification techniques using the polymerase chain reaction (PCR) and ligase chain reaction (LCR) have been developed that are highly sensitive and specific for *Neisseria gonorrhoeae* when used on urethral and cervicovaginal swabs and on first-void urine specimens. The diagnosis can also be made by endocervical cultures on Thayer-Martin media. These techniques allow simultaneous testing for *N. gonorrhoeae* and *Chlamydia trachomatis*. Positive DNA probe test results should be verified by culture in cases where a false positive result will have adverse medical, social, or legal consequences. Patients are most appropriately treated with single-dose therapy, to ensure compliance, by either a single dose of ceftriaxone 125 mg intramuscularly or cefixime given as a single oral dose of 400-mg tablets.

Chlamydial Infections

Infections due to *Chlamydia trachomatis* have become the most common sexually transmitted diseases in the United States. *Chlamydia trachomatis* can cause acute cervicitis, lymphogranuloma venereum, and pelvic inflammatory disease. Presenting complaints of vaginal discharge and dyspareunia are similar to those found in gonorrhea. The polymerase chain reaction (PCR) and ligase chain reaction (LCR) are useful for evaluating urine specimens from either sex. Endocervical cultures can confirm the diagnosis, but patients with suspected cervicitis or pelvic inflammatory disease are treated presumptively with doxycycline, 100 mg twice daily for 7 days, or with azithromycin, 1 g as a single dose. As infection due to gonorrhea and *Chlamydia* are clinically indistinguishable, treatment for both is indicated until cultures confirm this diagnosis.

Condyloma Acuminata

Condyloma acuminata, or "venereal warts," are found in both premenarcheal patients and adolescents. The causative agent is the human papillomavirus. Condylomatous lesions are acquired by close physical contact with an infected individual, either by digital transmission or genital contact. Often, a history of condyloma is found in one or more family members who care for the preadolescent child, although potential sexual molestation should be addressed. In adolescents with condyloma, the infection is usually sexually transmitted. Genital warts have a cauliflower-type appearance and are associated with pruritus. Cryotherapy is the most effective treatment for young children, and podophyllin 25 percent ointment used once weekly for 3 to 4 weeks is effective in adolescents and adults. Laser fulguration may be used on larger lesions.

Pelvic Inflammatory Disease

Etiology

Pelvic inflammatory disease (PID) is an acute infection of the endometrium and the fallopian tubes. It is usually a sexually transmitted disease caused most frequently by *N. gonorrhoeae, C. trachomatis,* and a variety of anaerobic pathogens. Predisposing factors include multiple sexual partners, recent menstrual period or abortion, douching, and use of an intrauterine device. The consequences of untreated or inadequately treated PID include recurrent infections, tubo-ovarian abscesses, infertility (>50 percent in women experiencing recurrent PID), and subsequent ectopic pregnancies. For a variety of physiologic and psychosocial reasons, adolescents are at increased risk of acquiring and experiencing complications from PID.

Clinical Presentation

Patients may present with a wide variety of symptoms, including dull, generalized lower abdominal pain beginning 2 to 5 days after menstruation. Associated complaints may include dyspareunia, vaginal discharge, and pain on ambulation. Fever may also be present. Physical examination may reveal tenderness of the uterine fundus, adnexal fullness and pain to bimanual manipulation, and marked cervical motion tenderness. An ultrasound evaluation may reveal a tubo-ovarian abscess.

Management

Indications for hospitalization include a toxic appearance, marked peritoneal findings, repeated vomiting, a failed course of outpatient therapy, and pregnancy. Admission may also be indicated for patients in whom a tubo-ovarian abscess is suspected. Admission should also be considered in cases where compliance is suspect, especially in adolescent patients.

Outpatient treatment should consist of antibiotic coverage for both gonorrhea and chlamydial infections, which consists of ceftriaxone, 250 mg IM or cefoxitin, 2 g IM with probenecid, 1 g PO, and doxycycline 100 mg twice daily for 14 days. Inpatient treatment may include clindamycin and gentamicin intravenously for 4 to 7 days and subsequent 14-day outpatient therapy with doxycycline and clindamycin.

DISORDERS OF PREGNANCY

Hypertension in Pregnancy

All pregnant patients presenting to the emergency department are screened for hypertension because of the high maternal and fetal mortality associated with preeclampsia.

Preeclampsia and Eclampsia

Preeclampsia is also called toxemia of pregnancy. Preeclampsia occurs in patients who are >20 weeks of gestation. It is seen in 5 percent of pregnant patients and is a leading cause of maternal death in the United States. Preeclampsia can be classified into mild or severe forms, depending on the severity of symptoms. Mild preeclampsia is defined as

- Systolic BP ≥140 mmHg or ≥30 mmHg above baseline
- Diastolic BP ≥90 mmHg or ≥15 mmHg above baseline
- Urine protein ≥300 mg or ≥2+ on dipstick

Severe preeclampsia is defined as:

- Systolic BP ≥160 mm Hg
- Diastolic BP ≥110 mm Hg
- Urine protein ≥2 g/24 hour
- Serum creatinine >1.2 mg/dL, unless known to be previously elevated
- Platelets <100,000/mm^3
- Elevated ALT and AST
- Increased LDH
- Persistent headache or other cerebral or visual disturbance
- Persistent epigastric pain

Clinical Presentation

Patients with mild preeclampsia may be asymptomatic or may complain of progressive edema and headache. Patients with severe preeclampsia may complain of progressive visual blurring or abdominal pain and may present with hyperreflexia, vaginal bleeding, or coagulopathies secondary to disseminated intravascular coagulation (DIC). Twenty percent of women with severe preeclampsia or eclampsia develop hemolysis, elevated liver enzymes, and low platelets (HELLP syndrome). Uteroplacental perfusion may be compromised and placental abruption can occur. Patients are at risk for hepatic or renal failure. Neurologic irritability may herald this onset of seizures. Cerebrovascular accidents can occur.

Management

If mild preeclampsia is suspected, the patient is admitted for evaluation and workup, including fetal monitoring and evaluation of renal and liver function. The most widely used antihypertensive agent in pregnancy is methyldopa.

Aggressive emergency department management of severely preeclamptic patients is essential, as is prompt obstetric consultation. In all patients who meet criteria for severe preeclampsia, 4 g of magnesium sulfate is given intravenously as a loading dose, followed by 1 to 2 g/h to prevent seizures. Serum magnesium levels are kept between 4.8 and 8.4 mg/dL while confirming the presence of deep tendon reflexes. If respiratory depression occurs with magnesium administration, 1 g of calcium gluconate may be given over 3 minutes. Hypertension is controlled emergently and is reduced to a diastolic blood pressure of 90 to 100 mm Hg. Hydralazine, 5 mg/30 minutes IV, is the drug of choice for control of hypertension. Alternatively, intravenous labetalol, 20 to 50 mg, may be used. The ultimate treatment for preeclampsia is delivery of the fetus.

Eclampsia

Etiology

Eclampsia is defined as preeclampsia with associated tonic-clonic seizures. This obstetric emergency occurs in 0.5 percent of all deliveries and carries a high risk of maternal and fetal mortality, as well as DIC and placental abruption.

Management

After establishment of an airway, the first priority in the management of the eclamptic patient is seizure control. Magnesium sulfate is the anticonvulsant of choice and may be given as a bolus dose of 6.0 g intravenously. The maximum dose should not exceed 8 g. Benzodiazepines are not routinely used. After seizures are controlled, arterial blood gas analysis and fetal and maternal monitoring is performed. Supplemental oxygen is used to ensure adequate tissue oxygenation. Laboratory testing includes CBC, electrolytes (including calcium and magnesium), coagulation profile, and liver function studies. Central venous monitoring may be beneficial and careful monitoring of fluid status, including Foley catheter placement to measure urinary output, is also important. Patients should be admitted for induction of labor or cesarean section.

Vaginal Bleeding in Pregnancy

Threatened Abortion

Etiology

Threatened abortion occurs in approximately 20 percent of all pregnancies. Of all patients diagnosed with threatened abortion, 40 to 50 percent progress to a complete spontaneous abortion. The underlying cause of spontaneous abortion in early pregnancy is most likely chromosomal aberration of the conceptus. Late abortions may be due to abnormalities in placental implantation, uterine myomas, or cervical incompetence. Maternal factors that may lead to spontaneous abortion include exacerbations of underlying illnesses, trauma, or acute intraabdominal pathology, such as appendicitis or pancreatitis.

Clinical Presentation

Patients commonly present to the emergency department with the complaint of vaginal bleeding with or without lower abdominal pain. Bleeding is usually mild, but in some cases, is severe. The lower abdominal pain is usually cramping in character.

Management

After pregnancy has been confirmed, the patient is examined for the presence of cervical dilatation and the passage of clots and products of conception, which indicates a spontaneous abortion. A complete spontaneous abortion may be diagnosed if the conceptus is expelled, the cervical os closes, and the uterus returns to normal size. A septic abortion is a spontaneous or induced abortion that is infected. Septic abortions carry the risk of septic shock and disseminated intravascular coagulation and should be suspected in patients with a nonviable pregnancy and fever. It is important to address the possibility of ectopic pregnancy in patients presenting with vaginal bleeding, as described as follows.

Spontaneous abortion carries a 2 percent risk of Rh isoimmunization. It is mandatory for the Rh-negative woman who aborts to be given Rh prophylaxis. Protection from first-trimester Rh immunizations can be accomplished by mini-doses of RhIG (50 μg) intramuscularly. Women who have antepartum bleeding (threatened abortion) should receive RhIG, 300 μg IM.

A patient with threatened abortion can be managed as an outpatient, with bed rest and instructions to return if bleeding worsens.

Ectopic Pregnancy

Etiology

An ectopic pregnancy results when a fertilized ovum implants outside of the uterus. The most common site of an ectopic pregnancy is the fallopian tube (95 percent). Ectopic pregnancies less commonly occur in the ovary, cervix, or peritoneal cavity. The overall incidence is 1 in 100 pregnancies, which has increased in the past two decades.

The most common predisposing factor for ectopic pregnancy is chronic salpingitis or PID. This leads to fibrosis and scarring of the fallopian tube, which obstructs the passage of the ovum. Other less common predisposing conditions include previous ectopic pregnancy, in utero DES exposure, IUD, documented tubal pathology, and douching.

Clinical Presentation

The most common symptom of ectopic pregnancy is vaginal bleeding, which occurs in 60 percent of patients and may be mistaken for normal menses. Unilateral lower abdominal pain is a relatively common finding. Few patients actually present to the emergency department with the classic findings of acute abdominal pain, vaginal bleeding, and hypotension. A high index of suspicion for ectopic pregnancy is necessary in any woman of childbearing age with abdominal complaints. Life-threatening hemorrhage is possible in any patient with an ectopic pregnancy.

Urine pregnancy tests are very reliable in excluding pregnancy (98 percent sensitivity). Serum β-hCG may be more helpful in defining the progression of the pregnancy and the rise in serum β-hCG can help distinguish ectopic from intrauterine pregnancy. In normal pregnancy, serum quantitative β-hCG levels should double approximately every 2 days.

Pelvic ultrasonography is extremely useful in excluding ectopic pregnancy in patients who have a definable gestational sac. An intrauterine pregnancy is generally detectable by 6 weeks of gestation by transabdominal ultrasound, and as early as 5 weeks of gestation by transvaginal ultrasound. The correlation of serum β-hCG with accurate visualization of an intrauterine pregnancy on vaginal probe ultrasound remains somewhat controversial, and given advances in ultrasound technology and operator training, is probably not static. In an unstable patient with a suspected ruptured ectopic pregnancy, culdocentesis is an option. The aspiration of nonclotting blood confirms intraperitoneal bleeding, and is highly suggestive of rupture.

Management

The treatment for ectopic pregnancy includes stabilization and immediate gynecologic consultation. Hypotension and shock are treated aggressively with initial infusion of normal saline, followed by packed red blood cells. Ultimately, surgical excision of the conceptus is essential. The most common surgical treatment is salpingectomy, although the unruptured ectopic pregnancy may be resected from the tube (salpingostomy) or milked from the fimbriated end of the tube while preserving the normal tubal anatomy. In the past decade, clinical trials demonstrate that low-dose methotrexate with a single IM dose of 50 mg/m^2, is a viable nonsurgical option for treating hemodynamically stable patients with ectopic pregnancy. Methotrexate is a folic acid antagonist that interferes with DNA synthesis and multiplication.

Hydatidiform Mole

Etiology

Hydatidiform mole is a proliferative abnormality of trophoblastic tissue. The trophoblast develops in the absence of a fetus, cord, or amniotic membrane, and has the potential for benign or malignant degeneration.

Clinical Presentation

Commonly, most patients with vaginal bleeding in the first trimester. Nausea and vomiting are common, and the uterus is often larger than expected. Preeclampsia in the first trimester is uncommon in normal pregnancy and is very suggestive of a molar pregnancy. The diagnosis should be considered if the serum β-hCG is greater than expected.

Management

Patients with molar pregnancies are most commonly managed by dilatation and suction curettage. Follow-up should include monitoring of β-hCG levels, which have a half-life of approximately 24 hours and should be eliminated in 8 to 10 weeks, depending on the initial level.

Abruptio Placentae

Etiology

Placental abruption is defined as the detachment of the placenta from the uterus prior to delivery of the fetus. Premature detachment can occur in varying degrees, from partial separation to complete abruption.

Clinical Presentation

Placental abruption must be suspected in patients who present to the emergency department with third-trimester vaginal bleeding and lower abdominal pain, although vaginal bleeding may be minimal in patients with partial separation and clot formation between the placenta and the site of implantation. On physical examination, the uterus is firm and tender, and fetal heart tones may be absent because of fetal demise.

Management

Patients with suspected placental abruption must be managed aggressively. Fetal and maternal vital signs are monitored and immediate obstetric consultation should be obtained. Laboratory studies include a coagulation profile to exclude potential coagulopathy. Pelvic examination must be delayed until the patient is in the operating room because of the potential for massive hemorrhage and fetal demise.

Placenta Previa

Etiology

Placenta previa is the implantation of the placenta in the lower pole of the uterus over or near the internal os. It is more commonly associated with advanced maternal age and nulliparity and is due to an abnormality in the implantation of the placenta. Vaginal bleeding may occur because of tearing of the placental attachments due to cervical effacement and dilatation.

Clinical Presentation

Placenta previa is often confused clinically with abruptio placentae, as each condition may present with preterm vaginal bleeding. Placenta previa can be distinguished from abruption by the absence of abdominal pain, a contracted uterus, and the presence of bright red blood instead of dark, clotted blood, as found in placental abruption. Placenta previa must be suspected in any patient presenting with third-trimester vaginal bleeding.

Management

The most important principle in the management of possible placenta previa is avoidance of vaginal examination of patients in whom this diagnosis is suspected. Although initial bleeding is rarely severe, pelvic examination may precipitate massive hemorrhage and fetal demise. Ultrasonic examination is necessary and immediate obstetric consultation is indicated.

EMERGENCY CONTRACEPTION

Emergency treatment is indicated for the prevention of pregnancy in women after unprotected sex or suspected contraceptive failure. The Preven Emergency Contraceptive kit contains a pregnancy test and four oral contraceptive tablets, each containing 50 μg of ethinyl estradiol and 0.25 mg of levonorgestrel. Two tablets are taken within 72 hours of intercourse followed, 12 hours later, by the second dose. Best results are seen if the pills are taken within 72 hours of intercourse. The major mechanism of action is inhibition or delay of ovulation. The efficacy rate is 75 percent. As estrogen in the pill causes nausea and vomiting, it is advisable to give an oral antiemetic 1 hour before each dose. Other oral contraceptive pills, such as Ovral or Triphasil, can also be used for emergency contraception.

BIBLIOGRAPHY

American Academy of Pediatrics: Diagnostic tests, in Pickering LK (ed): *2000 Red Book: Report of the Committee on Infectious Diseases,* 25th ed. Elk Grove Village, Il: American Academy of Pediatrics, 2000, pp 255.

Centers for Disease Control and Prevention: 1998 guidelines for treatment of sexually transmitted diseases. *MMWR* 1998; 47(No. RR–1):57–62, 79–84.

Dart RG: Role of pelvic ultrasonography in evaluation of symptomatic first-trimester pregnancy. *Ann Emerg Med* 1999; 33:310–320.

Embling ML, Monroe KW, Oh MK, et al. Opportunistic urine ligase chain reaction screening for sexually transmitted diseases in adolescents seeking care in an urban emergency department. *Ann Emerg Med* 2000;36;28–32.

Lowy G: Sexually transmitted diseases in children. *Pediatr Dermatol* 1992;9:329.

Molitch ME: Endocrine problems of adolescent pregnancy. *Endocrinol Metab Clin North Am* 1993;22:649.

Muram D: Vaginal bleeding in childhood and adolescence. *Obstet Gynecol Clin North Am* 1990;17:389.

Tay JI, Moore J, Walker JJ: Ectopic pregnancy. *BMJ* 2000;320:916–919.

71

Anemias

David F. Soglin
Jane E. Kramer

HIGH-YIELD FACTS

- The mean hemoglobin concentration for normal neonates is 18 g/dL, after which it falls to a nadir of 11.5 g/dL (mean concentration) at 2 to 3 months of life, with anemia defined as a hemoglobin level <9 g/dL. Although mean hemoglobin concentrations in children continue to vary somewhat by age, 11 g/dL defines the lower limits of normal for the prepubertal patient population.

- Anemias are most easily classified based on red blood cell (RBC) size and degree of bone marrow activity. The size of RBCs is measured as mean corpuscular volume (MCV), with the lower limit of normal for the MCV equaling 70 plus the age in years; bone marrow activity is reflected by the reticulocyte count.

- The vast majority of microcytic anemia in young patients is caused by iron deficiency, but thalassemia is also an important cause.

- Risk factors for iron deficiency anemia include age between 6 months and 2 years, decreased prevalence or duration of breast-feeding, lack of use of iron-fortified formulas, early introduction of whole cow's milk into the diet, and low socioeconomic status.

- Thalassemias are inherited defects resulting in the inability to synthesize sufficient quantities of various globin chains of the hemoglobin molecule that affect the production of β-chains most commonly. Thalassemia trait produces marked microcytosis out of proportion to the degree of anemia.

- Lead poisoning must be considered in the child with microcytic anemia. High levels of lead can interfere with hemoglobin production, but much of the anemia seen with lead poisoning is actually due to concomitant iron deficiency.

- If the corrected reticulocyte count is high in the presence of a normocytic anemia, blood loss must be considered. If there is no evidence of blood loss, a hemolytic anemia is likely.

- A low reticulocyte count in the face of significant anemia indicates bone marrow underproduction. If the abnormality is isolated to the RBC line, the primary considerations are transient erythroblastopenia of childhood (TEC) and an aplastic crisis complicating an underlying hemolytic anemia.

- Thrombocytopenia or white blood cell (WBC) abnormalities associated with normocytic anemia and poor reticulocyte response suggests marrow infiltration or acquired aplastic anemia.

- Macrocytic anemia is quite uncommon in pediatric patients. Folate and vitamin B_{12} deficiencies can result in megaloblastic anemia, but these are rare in otherwise healthy children.

Anemia is defined as a hemoglobin concentration more than 2 standard deviations below the mean for a comparable population. The normal hemoglobin concentration varies by age and, in the postpubertal population, by sex. The mean hemoglobin for normal neonates is 18 g/dL. Infants reach a nadir in hemoglobin concentration at 2 to 3 months of life, at which time the mean hemoglobin is only 11.5 g/dL, with anemia defined as a hemoglobin level below 9 g/dL. This nadir is deeper and occurs at a younger age in premature infants. Although mean hemoglobin concentrations in children continue to vary somewhat by age, 11 g/dL defines the lower limits of normal for the prepubertal patient population. After puberty, normative data for adult populations apply, and gender differences become apparent.

Patients with mild anemia are usually asymptomatic, and the anemia is most commonly discovered on a routine complete blood count (CBC). Even children with moderate to severe anemia may be asymptomatic if the problem develops slowly, since they are able to compensate remarkably well despite severely reduced hemoglobin levels. When the hemoglobin becomes low enough to produce symptoms, patients may present with fatigue, irritability, or shortness of breath on exertion. Physical exam may reveal pallor, tachycardia, and a systolic ejection murmur from increased cardiac output. However, physicians are not able to predict hemoglobin levels based on the appearance of pallor. When the hemoglobin drops rapidly, the child may develop dizziness, orthostatic hypotension, or high-output cardiac failure.

The history and physical examination play important roles in determining the etiology of anemia. A thorough diet history may reveal evidence suggesting nutritionally induced anemia. A family history of hemoglobinopathy or a hereditary membrane disorder would help guide a diagnostic workup, as would a history of chronic renal disease or an ongoing inflammatory process. Physical exam may reveal findings that aid in the evaluation of the anemia, such as jaundice, which suggests hemolytic anemia; hepatosplenomegaly and lymphadenopathy, which suggests marrow replacement from malignancy or suppression from viral infection; or evidence of an underlying disease process, suggesting anemia of chronic inflammation.

Anemias are most easily classified based on red blood cell (RBC) size and degree of bone marrow activity. The size of RBCs is measured as mean corpuscular volume (MCV), the normal values of which vary with age. As a rough guide, the lower limit of normal for the MCV equals 70 plus the age in years. Bone marrow activity is reflected by the reticulocyte count. Correcting the measured reticulocyte count for the degree of anemia allows an accurate determination of marrow activity. An estimate of the corrected reticulocyte count is obtained by multiplying the measured reticulocyte percent by the ratio of measured hematocrit to normal hematocrit [Retic $\times$ (Hct measured/Hct normal)].

The appearance of the RBCs on the peripheral smear, the total number of RBCs, and the red cell distribution width (RDW), which measures the variability in RBC size, are also helpful in determining the etiology of anemia.

MICROCYTIC ANEMIA

Microcytic anemia is defined by an MCV lower than 2 standard deviations below the population mean. The vast majority of microcytic anemia in young patients is caused by iron deficiency, but thalassemia is also an important cause (Table 71-1).

Iron Deficiency

Risk factors for iron deficiency anemia include age between 6 months and 2 years, decreased prevalence or duration of breast-feeding, lack of use of iron-fortified formulas, early introduction of whole cow's milk into the diet, and low socioeconomic status. Whole cow's milk is deficient in bioavailable iron but rich in calories. Excess intake produces iron deficiency by its inherent lack of iron, by reducing appetite and intake of iron-rich foods,

Table 71-1. Differentiating Microcytic Anemia

Parameter	Iron Deficiency	Thalassemia Trait
History	Prematurity or high milk intake	None or family history
Reticulocyte count	Low	Normal
MVC	Low	Very low
RDW	High	Low
Mentzer's index (MCV/RBC)	>13	<11

MCV, mean corpuscular volume; RDW, red cell distribution width; RBC, red blood cell.

and it can lead to occult gastrointestinal bleeding from the effect of unmodified cow's milk proteins on gastrointestinal mucosa. Fetuses absorb most of their total body iron during the last trimester, so premature infants are at greater risk for iron-deficiency anemia. They deplete their reduced iron stores early and have an even greater need than full-term infants for iron supplementation. Iron nutrition in infancy has been steadily improving, as demonstrated by a continuing decline in the prevalence of anemia among low-income children.

Iron deficiency anemia develops slowly, and patients rarely present with acute symptoms. Even with drastically reduced hemoglobin levels, patients are usually well compensated and hemodynamically stable. The diagnosis is usually made on the basis of the history and CBC results showing anemia, microcytosis, and a high RDW. The reticulocyte count is not elevated. Thrombocytosis is common in iron deficiency anemia, but thrombocytopenia has been reported. In the usual setting, a trial of iron therapy is both diagnostic and therapeutic. Ferrous sulfate is administered in an amount sufficient to provide 5 to 6 mg/kg of elemental iron per day in three divided doses for approximately 3 months. An increase in the reticulocyte count is typically seen in a matter of days, and the hemoglobin level increases in 1 to 2 weeks. Diagnostic tests useful in the evaluation of iron deficiency anemia include an elevated free erythrocyte protoporphyrin level, reduced serum iron, elevated total iron binding capacity (TIBC), and reduced ferritin level. Ferritin, however, is an acute-phase reactant and in the face of infection may be elevated despite the presence of iron deficiency anemia.

Thalassemia

Thalassemias are inherited defects resulting in the inability to synthesize sufficient quantities of various globin chains of the hemoglobin molecule. The production of β-chains is generally the most affected. The defect is most common in people of Mediterranean ancestry and is present in a small percentage of African Americans. In general, the disease is classified as thalassemia minor or major, corresponding to heterozygous and homozygous states, respectively. The heterozygous form of thalassemia is often referred to as thalassemia trait.

Thalassemia trait produces marked microcytosis out of proportion to the degree of anemia. There is typically a high total RBC count and narrow RDW, which helps differentiate thalassemia trait from iron deficiency anemia. Unlike iron deficiency, the reticulocyte count in tha-

lassemia trait should be normal or slightly elevated. Mentzer's index, obtained by dividing the MCV by the RBC count in millions, can also help to differentiate thalassemia trait from iron deficiency; values less than 11 suggest thalassemia trait. In β-thalassemia trait, the hemoglobin concentration is often 2 to 3 g/dL below normal values. A hemoglobin electrophoresis will demonstrate an elevated A^2 component and in some cases an elevated level of fetal hemoglobin (Hgb F). Patients with α-thalassemia trait have normal hemoglobin electrophoreses.

β-Thalassemia major produces severe hemolytic anemia with marked microcytosis and reticulocytosis. It usually presents within the first year of life. Pallor, jaundice, and hepatosplenomegaly are often present. Because patients require life-long transfusion therapy, the use of uncrossmatched blood is avoided except in the most dire circumstances. The major side effect of long-term transfusion therapy is iron overload, which adversely affects multiple organs, especially the pancreas, liver, and heart.

Lead Poisoning

Lead poisoning must be considered in the child with microcytic anemia. High levels of lead can interfere with hemoglobin production, but much of the anemia seen with lead poisoning is actually due to concomitant iron deficiency. Iron deficiency can increase pica and therefore lead absorption from the gastrointestinal tract. The history may include residing in or frequently visiting an older dilapidated home with peeling paint, recent renovation of an older home, pica, or a parent or sibling with a job or hobby that involves exposure to lead. Patients with elevated lead levels typically have nonspecific complaints such as abdominal pain, irritability, and subtle behavioral changes. Even relatively low levels of lead (>10 μg/dL) have been shown to interfere with intellectual growth and development. With very high levels of lead, patients can present with seizures, increased intracranial pressure, and frank encephalopathy.

NORMOCYTIC ANEMIA

Although normocytic anemia is less common than microcytic anemia, the differential diagnosis in childhood is extensive (Table 71-2). The primary determinant in establishing a differential is whether the anemia is due to decreased production (low reticulocyte count) or increased blood loss or destruction (high reticulocyte count).

Table 71-2 Differential Diagnosis for Normocytic Anemia

Blood loss (high reticulocyte count)
Hemolytic anemia (high reticulocyte count)
   Immune
      Autoimmune hemolytic anemia
      Neonatal-maternal blood group incompatibility
   Nonimmune
      Microangiopathic
         Disseminated intravascular coagulation (DIC)
         Hemolytic uremic syndrome (HUS)
      Macroangiopathic
         Artificial cardiac valve
      Membrane abnormalities
         Spherocytosis
         Elliptocytosis
         Stomacytosis
      Metabolic abnormalities
         G6PD deficiency
         Pyruvate kinase deficiency
         Hemoglobinopathies
Nonhemolytic anemia (low or normal reticulocyte count)
   Abnormality isolated to red cell line
      Chronic hemolytic anemia with concurrent aplastic crisis
      Transient erythroblastopenia of childhood (TEC)
      Chronic disease
         Renal insufficiency
         Diamond-Blackfan anemia
   Abnormality affecting other cell lines
      Bone marrow infiltration
         Leukemia
         Lymphoma
         Tumor metastasis
      Acquired aplastic anemia

Normocytic Anemia With High Reticulocyte Count

If the corrected reticulocyte count is high in the presence of a normocytic anemia, blood loss must be considered. If there is no evidence of blood loss, a hemolytic anemia is likely. The workup for a patient with hemolytic anemia includes a Coombs test to determine whether the hemolytic anemia is immunologic in nature. Immune hemolytic anemia may be the result of a drug reaction, infection, collagen vascular disorder, or malignancy, but commonly no etiology is determined.

Patients often present acutely with severe anemia, pallor, jaundice, and hemoglobinuria. Transfusions may be necessary with severe symptomatic anemia, but this can be difficult because the circulating antibody causes "incompatibility" in vitro and rapid destruction of transfused RBCs in vivo. Immunosuppression with prednisone is frequently adequate to diminish RBC destruction, so that the patient's brisk reticulocytosis can repair the anemia. Intravenous γ-globulin is also useful. In severe cases, plasmapheresis may be necessary.

The differential diagnosis for nonimmune hemolytic anemia includes micro- and macroangiopathic destruction, membrane disorders, metabolic abnormalities, and hemoglobinopathies. Sickle cell anemia is discussed in detail in Chapter 72.

Microangiopathic RBC destruction can occur with disseminated intravascular coagulation and hemolytic uremic syndrome. The peripheral smear will demonstrate schistocytes, burr cells, and other RBC fragments.

Membrane disorders such as spherocytosis and elliptocytosis are hereditary in nature. Hereditary spherocytosis results in a hemolytic anemia due to splenic destruction of red blood cells. The disease is often apparent in infancy, and although the degree of anemia varies widely, it rarely results in a hematologic emergency. Laboratory studies reveal anemia, reticulocytosis, and hyperbilirubinemia. Many patients develop pigmentary gallstones. The diagnosis is confirmed by osmotic fragility studies, in which the membrane defect causes the RBCs to rupture when challenged with a hypotonic medium. Splenectomy is curative. The major hematologic crisis is aplastic anemia, which is usually secondary to a parvovirus infection. Hereditary elliptocytosis is another inherited defect that can occasionally result in significant hemolytic anemia. The peripheral smear reveals the characteristic elliptocytes. As in hereditary spherocytosis, splenectomy is curative. Aplastic crisis can occur.

Inherited metabolic disorders, such as pyruvate kinase and glucose-6-phosphate dehydrogenase (G6PD) deficiencies, also cause chronic hemolysis. Pyruvate kinase deficiency may present because of an increase in hemolysis or an aplastic crisis. There are multiple variants of G6PD deficiency, some of which are asymptomatic. Others cause severe hemolysis with relatively minor exposure to oxidant challenges. The A variant is seen in approximately 10 percent of African-American males and becomes symptomatic only after a significant challenge from a drug or infection. Typically, aspirin in therapeutic doses does not pose a problem for these patients. Sulfonamides, antimalarials, and naphthalene can precipitate hemolysis. Enzyme levels are higher in young cells, so normal levels of G6PD may be obtained when assayed from G6PD-deficient patients during periods of brisk reticulocytosis. The assay may have to be repeated when the acute hemolysis has passed.

Normocytic Anemia With Low Reticulocyte Counts

A low reticulocyte count in the face of significant anemia indicates bone marrow underproduction. If the abnormality is isolated to the RBC line, the primary considerations are transient erythroblastopenia of childhood (TEC) and an aplastic crisis complicating an underlying hemolytic anemia.

An acquired red cell aplasia, TEC spares the white blood cells (WBCs) and platelets and, as the name implies, resolves after a number of weeks. It typically affects children between 1 and 4 years of age. There is seasonal clustering and an associated history of preceding viral illness, but no causative viral agent has been identified. Supportive therapy is usually sufficient because patients are typically hemodynamically stable and recover spontaneously. In a referral population of children undergoing bone marrow biopsy to determine the etiology of their anemia, 60 percent of cases were due to TEC. Transfusions may be necessary in symptomatic patients and those with no evidence of RBC precursors on examination of the marrow. Steroids have not been shown to speed recovery.

Other entities in the differential of normocytic anemia with low to normal reticulocyte counts and no abnormalities of other cell lines include anemia of chronic disease, inflammatory processes, and decreased erythropoietin from renal insufficiency. Diamond-Blackfan anemia is a congenital RBC aplasia that usually presents in the first year of life with severe anemia. Occasionally other congenital abnormalities are associated, such as cleft palate, skeletal anomalies, and congenital heart disease.

Thrombocytopenia or WBC abnormalities associated with normocytic anemia and poor reticulocyte response suggests marrow infiltration or acquired aplastic anemia.

Marrow infiltration is most commonly due to leukemia. Leukemia is the most common malignancy in childhood, with acute lymphoblastic leukemia being the most frequent type. Although the diagnosis can be made in the emergency department when the presentation is classic and the WBC count markedly elevated, with lymphoblasts apparent on peripheral smear, atypical lymphocytes from Epstein-Barr virus or other viral infections can appear similar to lymphoblasts.

Lymphoma and other tumors can also cause failure of production, with resultant decreases in all cell lines through metastases to the bone marrow.

Acquired aplastic anemia in the absence of an underlying hemolytic anemia has been associated with drugs and infections. Often no etiology is determined. The prognosis is quite poor, and bone marrow transplantation is often required. Blood transfusion is performed judiciously for patients who are candidates for bone marrow transplantation because of the dangers of sensitization.

MACROCYTIC ANEMIA

Macrocytic anemia is quite uncommon in pediatric patients. Aplastic anemia, although usually causing normocytic anemia, can result in macrocytosis. Due to the large size of reticulocytes, marked reticulocytosis can lead to a high MCV, although mature RBCs may be of a normal size. Folate and vitamin B_{12} deficiencies can result in megaloblastic anemia. These are rare in otherwise healthy children. Chemotherapy and malabsorption can lead to folate depletion, as can rapid turnover of RBCs. Many patients with sickle cell anemia are treated with folate supplementation for that reason. Some drugs, notably AZT, can cause macrocytosis.

BIBLIOGRAPHY

Farhi DC, Luebbers EL, Rosenthal NS: Bone marrow biopsy findings in childhood anemia: Prevalence of transient erythroblastopenia of childhood. *Arch Pathol Lab Med* 122:638–641, 1998.

Hung OL, Kwon NS, Cole AE, et al: Evaluation of the physician's ability to recognize the presence or absence of anemia, fever and jaundice. *Acad Emerg Med* 7:146–156, 2000.

Sherry B, Bister D, Yip R: Continuation of decline in prevalence of anemia in low income children: The Vermont experience. *Arch Pediatr Adolesc Med* 151:928–930, 1997.

72

Sickle Cell Disease

David F. Soglin
Jane E. Kramer

HIGH-YIELD FACTS

- Sickle cell anemia (SCA) is a chronic hemolytic anemia that is most common among African Americans, of whom approximately 1 in 600 are affected with homozygous hemoglobin SS (HbSS), the most severe of the sickle syndromes. Patients with a single abnormal gene for HbS have sickle cell trait and typically have a concentration of HbS that is about 40 percent, resulting in a large enough percentage of normal hemoglobin to remain asymptomatic except under the most severe hypoxic stress.

- The most common of the sickle cell crises, vasoocclusive pain, presumably occurs when sickled red blood cells (RBCs) obstruct blood flow and cause tissue ischemia. Dactylitis, or hand-foot syndrome, is vasoocclusion in the metacarpal or metatarsal bones and is often the earliest presentation of SCA.

- Older patients typically experience vasoocclusive pain crises in the long bones, back, joints, and abdomen. There is a great deal of individual variation in the number and severity of painful crises.

- Patients with SCA and pain should be evaluated for other disease processes such as traumatic injuries, osteomyelitis, septic arthritis, and surgical abdominal problems. A complete blood count and reticulocyte count is indicated.

- Typically, patients in the emergency department receive a narcotic analgesic and are observed for 3 or 4 hours. If the patient remains comfortable, he or she can be given an oral agent and observed for an additional

hour, after which discharge is appropriate if pain control is maintained.

- Patients with SCA presenting with chest pain, hypoxemia, and infiltrates on chest radiograph are said to have *acute chest syndrome* (ACS). Fever may be present, and the syndrome can result from pneumonia or pulmonary infarction due to vasoocclusion.

- Because the etiology of ACS is often elusive, most patients receive antibiotic therapy directed at *Streptococcus pneumoniae* or *Mycoplasma.* The mainstay of therapy for pulmonary infarction in patients with SCA is early blood transfusion, with consideration of exchange transfusion.

- Patients with SCA are at high risk for infection with encapsulated bacteria, especially *Pneumococcus.* Overwhelming pneumococcal sepsis is a common cause of mortality.

- Splenic sequestration crisis occurs when RBCs become entrapped in the spleen, resulting in a rapidly enlarging spleen and a sudden drop in Hb and hematocrit. The mainstay of therapy is rapid blood transfusion.

- Viral infections, especially with parvovirus, can result in marrow suppression in normal children and those with SCA. In normal children, a brief marrow suppression will not lead to significant drop in Hb, but children with SCA may not tolerate even brief bone marrow suppression due to the extremely short half-life of the sickle cell.

Sickle cell anemia (SCA) is a chronic hemolytic anemia that is most common among African Americans, of whom approximately 1 in 600 are affected with homozygous hemoglobin SS (HbSS), the most severe of the sickle syndromes. It is also seen in people of Mediterranean, Indian, and Middle Eastern descent. It is secondary to a hemoglobinopathy that occurs when valine is substituted for glutamic acid in the 6 position of the β-chain. In addition to patients with HbSS, the diagnosis of SCA is applied to patients who are heterozygous for HbS and heterozygous for another abnormal hemoglobin such as HbC or β-thalassemia. Although there is wide variability in individual severity of illness, patients with double heterozygous states such as HbSC, HbSB thalassemia, and HbSD are typically less seriously affected than those with HbSS.

Patients with a single abnormal gene for HbS have sickle cell trait. The concentration of HbS is typically 40 percent, and the large percentage of normal hemoglobin allows the patients to remain asymptomatic except under the most severe hypoxic stress. However, the hypoxic environment of the renal medulla can cause localized sickling even for patients with sickle cell trait, leading to hematuria and isosthenuria.

Patients with SCA experience a number of complications that are likely to bring them to the emergency department.

VASOOCCLUSIVE CRISIS

The most common of the sickle cell crises, vasoocclusive pain, presumably occurs when sickled red blood cells (RBCs) obstruct blood flow and cause tissue ischemia. Dactylitis, or hand-foot syndrome, is vasoocclusion in the metacarpal or metatarsal bones. This is often the earliest presentation of SCA. It is common in infants, who present with hand and foot swelling and tenderness, refusal to walk, and irritability. The swelling is most marked on the dorsal surface, and there may be radiologic evidence of avascular bony necrosis.

Older patients typically experience vasoocclusive pain crises in the long bones, back, joints, and abdomen. There is a great deal of individual variation in number and severity of painful crises. On average, patients with SCA experience 0.8 hospitalizations per patient-year, but 5 percent of patients have frequent pain crises and account for approximately one-third of all painful episodes. Fetal Hb seems to have a mitigating effect. Patients with high levels of fetal Hb typically suffer less severe and less common crises, as do patients with HbSC and HbSB thalassemia.

As there is no diagnostic test or clinical finding that will identify patients in vasoocclusive crisis, the diagnosis is made on the basis of history alone. Patients with SCA and pain should be evaluated for other disease processes such as traumatic injuries, osteomyelitis, septic arthritis, and surgical abdominal problems. A complete blood count and reticulocyte count is indicated. Typically, patients remain at baseline levels of Hb during a painful event. Although evidence documenting benefit from hydration is lacking, therapy typically con-

sists of hydration at approximately 1½ times maintenance. Oxygen has not been shown to be beneficial in the management of pain crises unless hypoxemia is a complicating factor.

Pain should be assessed frequently using standardized pain scales. Pain relief is achieved with a variety of analgesics, depending on the severity of the crisis and the typical responsiveness of the patient. Oral agents such as acetaminophen, nonsteroidal antiinflammatory drugs (NSAIDs), and codeine used separately or in combination are the mainstays of treatment for mild to moderate pain. Such management frequently allows the child with a painful vasoocclusive crisis to remain at home. Ketorolac tromethamine is an NSAID that can be given orally or intravenously for acute pain. Its use should not be extended beyond 3 to 5 days. Usually, patients have unsuccessfully tried these therapies at home prior to presenting to the emergency department (ED). Parenteral agents such as morphine are often necessary in the ED setting. Anxiety about giving children narcotics leads to undertreatment of pain, which should be avoided. Although meperidine has commonly been used in the past, the availability of other potent analgesics has reduced its use for SCA vasoocclusive pain. Use of meperidine on a regular basis many times a day results in buildup of normeperidine, a toxic metabolite with poor analgesic effect. Normeperidine can cause dysphoria and increases the risk of seizures.

Typically, patients in the ED receive a narcotic analgesic and are observed for 3 or 4 hours. If the patient remains comfortable, he or she can be given an oral agent and observed for an additional hour. If the pain is controlled with the oral agent, discharge is appropriate. If adequate pain relief is not achieved with the oral agent, the patient is admitted for parenteral analgesia. Analgesia should be provided at frequent regular time intervals to avoid breakthrough pain. PRN pain relief should be avoided. As pain recurs between doses, the patient must request pain medication, and pain behaviors are possibly increased. Patient-controlled analgesia (PCA) with a morphine drip allows baseline levels of pain relief, and the patient may titrate pain relief as needed for activity or other painful times.

ACUTE CHEST SYNDROME

Patients with SCA presenting with chest pain, hypoxemia, and infiltrates on chest radiograph are said to have *acute chest syndrome* (ACS). Fever may be present. ACS can result from pneumonia or pulmonary infarction due to vasoocclusion. It is difficult to differentiate vasoocclusion from pneumonia in patients with ACS, since both etiologies cause similar manifestations. Lung scans are not useful in establishing a diagnosis. In most patients with ACS, no infectious etiology is isolated. When the etiology is bacterial pneumonia, *Pneumococcus* is the most common organism. *Mycoplasma* and *Chlamydia* are frequent causes, as are viral pneumonias. Many adults and older children are demonstrated to have fat emboli as an etiology with or without infection. Chest pain from vasoocclusion may lead to splinting and hypoventilation. Regular use of incentive spirometry has been shown to reduce the incidence of ACS in SCA patients with chest pain.

Because the etiology of ACS is often elusive, most patients receive antibiotic therapy directed at *Streptococcus pneumoniae* or *Mycoplasma.* The mainstay of therapy for pulmonary infarction in patients with SCA is early blood transfusion, with consideration of exchange transfusion. Patients with severe anemia, hypoxia, or a rapidly progressing process should receive blood transfusions. Patients are often treated with blood transfusions and antibiotics because of the difficulty in determining an etiolgy. All patients receive hydration, oxygen, and pain relief, although analgesia-induced hypoventilation must be avoided. Bronchodilation has been demonstrated to be helpful in a significant minority of patients.

INFECTION

Patients with SCA are at high risk for infection with encapsulated bacteria, especially *Pneumococcus.* Overwhelming pneumococcal sepsis is a common cause of mortality. Although prophylactic penicillin and vaccines for pneumococci and *Haemophilus influenzae* type B have reduced the incidence of sepsis in this vulnerable population, it remains the major cause of death in the young patient with SCA. Children younger than 3 years are particularly susceptible to bacteremia, which can occur as commonly as eight bacteremic events per 100 patient-years. The fatality rate is high, even though many of these children appear well at initial presentation.

Children younger than 5 years with SCA who present to the ED with fever are at high risk for bacteremia. After obtaining a complete blood count and blood culture, children with SCA should be promptly treated with parenteral antibiotics effective against *Streptococcus pneumoniae* and, if unimmunized, *H. influenzae* B. Although hospital admission is generally recommended, some institutions use a long-acting cephalosporin such as ceftri-

axone along with close outpatient follow-up to reduce the number of hospitalizations for these chronically ill children. Older children, who are less susceptible to overwhelming sepsis, can be managed on an individual basis depending on the height of the fever, the appearance of the child, findings on physical exam, and results of laboratory tests.

In addition to overwhelming sepsis, children with SCA are susceptible to other infections such as pneumonia, meningitis, and osteomyelitis. The etiology is most frequently encapsulated organisms. Unlike the general population, the most common organism identified as the cause of osteomyelitis in patients with SCA is *Salmonella.*

CEREBROVASCULAR ACCIDENTS

Cerebrovascular accidents (CVAs) are common in children with SCA and are thought to be due to intimal damage and RBC sickling. As in adults with CVAs, the physical findings on presentation are dependent on the site of the lesion. Because simple blood transfusions increase the viscosity of the blood and are potentially detrimental in an SCA patient with a CVA, exchange transfusion to reduce the burden of sickle cells without increasing blood viscosity is the management of choice. These patients are at high risk for subsequent CVAs and are usually managed with long-term blood transfusions to maintain their percentage of HbS below 30 percent. Exchange transfusion is unnecessary in the chronic phase of transfusion therapy. Problems with iron overload may develop with chronic transfusions. Close monitoring and chronic subcutaneous deferoxamine are necessary.

SPLENIC SEQUESTRATION

Splenic sequestration crisis occurs when RBCs become entrapped in the spleen, resulting in a rapidly enlarging spleen and a sudden drop in Hb and hematocrit. Affected patients present with a history of decreased exercise tolerance. The physical examination reveals pallor, splenomegaly, and often signs of high-output heart failure. Laboratory studies demonstrate marked anemia and a high reticulocyte count. Among patients with SS hemoglobinopathy, splenic sequestration occurs almost exclusively in young children, because as the SCA patients age, they undergo "autosplenectomy." This usually begins no later than 6 years of age. Patients with double heterozygote states such as HbSC or HbSB thalassemia often have persistent splenomegaly and thus remain at risk for sequestration crises into adulthood.

Early recognition of splenic sequestration is important, and parents have been successfully taught to palpate their children's spleens. The mainstay of therapy is rapid blood transfusion. Fluid expansion should be used in the initial stages of resuscitation while waiting for blood to be available, but it must be used carefully because volume overload and congestive heart failure can result. However, rehydration can release RBCs from the spleen. Nonetheless, blood transfusions will be necessary in most cases. Sequestration can recur, and occasionally splenectomy is necessary.

APLASTIC CRISIS

Viral infections, especially with parvovirus, can result in marrow suppression in normal children and those with SCA. In normal children, a brief marrow suppression will not lead to significant drop in Hb, because the half-life of a normal RBC is 120 days. However, children with SCA may not tolerate even brief bone marrow sup-

pression due to the extremely short half-life of the sickle cell. In these cases, patients may present in a decompensated state, complaining of fatigue and shortness of breath. There will be a significant drop in Hb from baseline and little or no reticulocytosis. Some patients can be managed with supportive care and close observation, because the marrow often rebounds in a matter of days. Many patients, however, will require a transfusion of packed RBCs. Folate deficiency is common in patients with SCA and may be responsible for a small percentage of aplastic crises. Folate supplementation is provided for these patients.

BIBLIOGRAPHY

Steinberg MH: Drug therapy: Management of sickle cell disease. *N Engl J Med* 340:1021–1030, 1999.

Vichinsky EP, Neumayr LD, Earles AN, et al: Causes and outcomes in acute chest syndrome in sickle cell disease. *N Engl J Med* 342:1855–1865, 2000.

Yaster M, Kost-Byerly S, Maxwell LG: The management of pain in sickle cell disease. *Pediatr Clin North Am* 47:699–710, 2000.

73

Bleeding Disorders

David F. Soglin
Jane E. Kramer

HIGH-YIELD FACTS

- Signs and symptoms of intracranial bleeding in hemophiliacs with head trauma may be delayed and initial imaging studies may be normal. Parental vigilance and follow-up exams are in order.
- Current factor replacement products for the hemophilias are prepared from either plasma-derived, monoclonal antibody purified proteins or by recombinant DNA technology and have virtually eliminated HIV transmission.
- Management of bleeding in hemophiliacs with inhibitors remains challenging and should be handled in conjunction with the child's hemophilia specialist.
- Treatment of bleeding episodes in von Willebrand's patients may include DDAVP, cryoprecitate, or factor VIII concentrates.
- Young children with idiopathic thromobocytopenic purpura and platelet counts <30,000 may be treated with high-dose steroids, intravenous gamma globulin, or intravenous anti-Rh(D) immunoglobulin.

HEMOPHILIA

Hemophilia is an X-linked recessive disorder of coagulation caused by deficiency of factor VIII (hemophilia A) or factor IX (hemophilia B or Christmas disease). The percentage of factor present determines the severity of disease: 5 to 25 percent denotes mild disease with no tendency for spontaneous hemorrhage; 1 to 4 percent, moderate disease; and <1 percent, severe disease with proclivity to spontaneous hemorrhage. Two-thirds of American hemophiliacs have severe disease. In both hemophilia A and B, prothrombin time (PT) and bleeding

time are normal and partial thromboplastin time (PTT) is prolonged. The same types of bleeding occur in both diseases. Bruising, hemarthroses, and intramuscular hematomas predominate. Intracranial hemorrhage is less common but can be devastating when it occurs. It is important to remember that initial bleeding in these patients may not be dramatic but that prolonged oozing is to be expected. Emergency physicians who may not often deal with these patients need to listen to the patient and their parents, who generally have a great deal of insight into subtle presentations of bleeding.

Acute Hemarthrosis

Knees, elbows, and ankles are the most commonly affected joints. Older patients may describe a sensation of warmth preceding overt pain and swelling, whereas younger patients may develop a limp or limitation of motion. It is generally agreed that even if joint bleeding cannot be confirmed, treatment is indicated. This philosophy is based on the potentially crippling sequelae of hemarthrosis. Intraarticular bleeding provokes synovial inflammation, which, in turn, increases the likelihood of more frequent hemarthroses. Joint swelling that is persistent and associated with fever may indicate a septic joint. Aspiration, preceded by appropriate factor replacement, may be necessary. Joint aspiration is not recommended for clear cases of bleeding.

Symptomatic treatment of hemarthroses consists of splinting, ice, immobilization, elastic bandages, and analgesia with acetaminophen with or without codeine. A single factor infusion to raise levels to 25 to 30 percent is usually sufficient to terminate bleeding. A joint that has bled repeatedly may require several doses of factor. Range of motion and physical therapy are instituted as soon as possible. Hip bleeds are especially worrisome, because pressure within the joint can lead to aseptic necrosis of the femoral head. Factor replacement to 50 to 75 percent levels with subsequent daily replacement to 30 percent may be necessary.

Intramuscular Bleeds

Such hemorrhage is usually identifiable by pain, tenderness, and swelling in the muscle and is treated with factor replacement to 30 percent levels. Forearm, calf, and hand bleeding can result in a compartment syndrome. Vascular compromise or nerve paralysis from compartment syndrome requires fasciotomy. Iliopsoas hemorrhage, which can be massive, presents with flexion of the thigh, groin and abdominal pain, and paresthesias below the inguinal ligament from femoral nerve compression. Ultrasound or computed tomography (CT) can confirm the diagnosis. Compartment syndromes and psoas hemorrhages are treated with correction to achieve factor levels of 50 to 60 percent and require admission for observation and continued factor replacement.

Intracranial Hemorrhage

A potentially devastating complication, intracranial bleeding may be traumatic or spontaneous. Minor trauma may present with neurologic changes days after the event. Symptoms include headache, lethargy, vomiting, and seizures. Forceful blows to the head, regardless of symptoms, are empirically treated with factor replacement. Symptomatic children need immediate factor replacement to 100 percent levels even before imaging results are available.

Other Bleeding Manifestations

Subcutaneous hemorrhage, abrasions, and lacerations that do not require sutures do not require factor replacement. Painless gross hematuria can occur. An anatomic source of the bleeding is usually not found. Treatment with factor may not be necessary if the bleeding is spontaneous. Use of epsilon aminocaproic is probably contraindicated because of the risk of ureteral clot formation. Prednisone is advocated by some to decrease the duration and degree of hematuria. Factor replacement is necessary before laceration repair, lumbar puncture, surgery, and dental extractions.

Management Issues

Intramuscular injections, aspirin, and jugular and femoral venipuncture are to be avoided. Simple peripheral venipuncture is followed by at least 5 minutes of pressure to the site.

Factor replacement for hemophilia A is accomplished by transfusion with a variety of factor VIII concentrates. These products are made from either plasma-derived or recombinant proteins. The purest of the plasma-derived products are monoclonal antibody purified. Recombinant products have human albumin added and are not necessarily superior. Product selection is based on cost and purity. Hemophilia B is treated with factor IX complex concentrates, the older, least pure of which contain significant amounts of factors VII and X and prothrombin. These carry the risk of disseminated intravascular coagulation (DIC) or thrombosis. More recently, mono-

clonal and recombinant factor IX became available. Recombinant factor IX is entirely plasma free, the first such approved antihemophiliac factor.

As indicated above, the amount of factor to be delivered will be dependent on the nature and severity of the bleeding episode. For life- or limb-threatening bleeds, treatment with factor replacement is generally required every 12 hours or by continuous infusion until healing occurs.

The following formulas may be used to calculate factor replacement:

- Factor VIII (units) = weight (kg) $\times$ 0.5 $\times$ desired increment (percent) of factor VIII level (i.e., 1 U/kg of factor VIII raises the level by 2 percent).
- Factor IX (units) = weight (kg) $\times$ 1.0 $\times$ desired increment (percent) of factor IX level (i.e., 1 U/kg of factor IX raises the level by 1 to 1.5 percent).

Patients with hemophilia A who have developed inhibitors (IgG antibodies to the missing factor) present difficult problems. Some 10 to 20 percent of severe hemophiliacs form factor inhibitors that are capable of neutralizing infused factor VIII. Treatment of bleeding episodes in these children depends on inhibitor titer and the severity of the bleeding. Children with low titers and serious hemorrhage may respond to large doses (up to 100 to 200 U/kg) of factor VIII. Some children with inhibitors demonstrate an anamnestic response (high responders), with high titers of antibody appearing rapidly after factor VIII administration. Alternatives for treating patients with high titers of inhibitor include highly purified porcine factor VIII; prothrombin complexes (which bypass the need for factor VIII through the presence of factors II, VII, and X); and plasmapheresis followed by factor replacement. A recombinant DNA product, factor VIIa, is another option for high-titer inhibitors. It has a very short half-life and must be given every 2 hours. The response to most of these therapies is judged by the patient's clinical response, although with porcine factor VIII, the PTT and factor levels should improve.

The rare patient with factor IX inhibitor can be managed with prothrombin complex concentrates or by exchange transfusion followed by factor IX infusion, if hemorrhage is life threatening.

Purified factor VIII concentrate prepared from pooled plasma donations transmitted hepatitis virus and human immunodeficiency virus (HIV) to hundreds of hemophiliacs in the 1970s and early 1980s. Fifty-five percent of hemophiliacs became HIV positive during those years. Today's concentrates, through a combination of mandatory donor screening and viral attenuation techniques, have greatly reduced, but not eliminated, viral transmission. No cases of HIV-1 transmission from clotting factor concentrates have been documented since 1986.

Adjuncts to therapy in hemophiliacs are available in certain situations. Some centers use corticosteroids for the management of hematuria or recurrent joint bleeds. Epsilon aminocaproic acid (Amicar) and tranexamic acid (Cyklokapron) are clot stabilizers used for the prevention or treatment of oral hemorrhage. Both can be administered orally or intravenously. Desmopressin (DDAVP) increases factor VIII levels in patients with mild hemophilia. Useful for minor bleeds, DDAVP is administered intravenously over 30 minutes (0.3 μg/kg) or intranasally (150 μg or one metered dose for children <50 kg and 300 μg or two metered dose sprays for children >50 kg). A more concentrated solution for subcutaneous injection should be available in the future.

VON WILLEBRAND DISEASE

Factor VIII is composed of two noncovalently bound proteins, factor VIII procoagulant protein (factor VIII:C) and von Willebrand factor (vWf). Von Willebrand disease exists when there is decreased or defective vWf, which is necessary for platelet adhesion to blood vessel walls. The condition is heterogeneous with respect to its genetics, molecular biology, clinical manifestations, and laboratory values. Unlike the sex-linked hemophilias, von Willebrand disease is typically transmitted as an autosomal dominant trait, although double heterozygotes and autosomal recessive patterns have been described. Classification systems separate quantitative deficiencies of vWf and factor VIII:C (type 1, classic) from qualitative abnormalities (types 2A and 2B) and type 3 in which plasma vWf and factor VIII levels are not measurable or are <5 U/dL.

Clinical manifestations include epistaxis, easy bruising, menorrhagia, and bleeding after dental extraction. Posttraumatic and postsurgical hemorrhage can occur, but hemarthroses are uncommon. Many people exhibit no clinical problems with bleeding in spite of biochemical abnormalities. Typical laboratory findings include a normal PT and platelet count, with a prolonged bleeding time and a PTT that may be normal or prolonged. Measurement of antigenic vWf (vWf:Ag) and ristocetin cofactor (vWf R:Co) activity can usually confirm the diagnosis. Both are decreased in most von Willebrand patients.

Type I von Willebrand disease is often amenable to DDAVP therapy, which stimulates the endogenous release of vWf. The dose is 0.3 μg/kg intravenously in 30 to 50 mL of saline over 20 to 30 minutes. This corrects the bleeding time for 3 to 4 hours. Stimate (1.5 mg/mL) is a concentrated intranasal preparation of desmopressin that has demonstrated effectiveness. In teens and adults, the dose is 150 μg/nostril with a total dose of 300 μg. For children <50 kg, the dose is 150 μg.

The treatment for hemorrhage in these patients may include the administration of cryoprecipitate, which contains intact vWf, or of intermediate or high-purity factor VIII concentrate.

ACQUIRED COAGULOPATHIES

Acquired abnormalities of coagulation include vitamin K deficiency, liver disease, DIC, thrombocytopenia, and platelet dysfunctions.

Vitamin K deficiency leads to decreases in the vitamin K–dependent factors (II, VII, IX, and X) and prolongation of the PT. It can be seen in malabsorption syndromes, such as cystic fibrosis and celiac disease, biliary obstruction, and prolonged diarrhea. Children with poor nutrition who receive broad-spectrum antibiotics are also at risk. Vitamin K deficiency can also be caused by drugs, such as diphenylhydantoin, phenobarbital, isoniazid, and coumadin. Vitamin K deficiency can lead to hemorrhagic disease of the newborn unless supplementation is provided routinely at delivery. Administration of vitamin K is safest by the subcutaneous route. Rare but severe anaphylactoid reactions are described with intravenous infusion. This route should only be used when the risk is justified.

The liver is the site of production of the clotting factors, although factor VIII is produced elsewhere as well, and severe liver disease causes coagulation defects that can mimic DIC.

Disseminated Intravascular Coagulation

In DIC, there is simultaneous activation of coagulation and fibrinolysis. Microthrombi form in small blood vessels, leading to occlusion and tissue ischemia. Excessive bleeding occurs due to thrombocytopenia, consumption of clotting factors, and fibrinolysis. These abnormalities are mediated by cytokines, especially interleukin-6 and tumor necrosis factor-α. In pediatric patients, the leading cause of DIC is overwhelming infections. However, conditions that can precipitate DIC are diverse and include tissue injuries such as burns, multiple trauma, and crush injuries; severe head trauma; abruptio placenta and eclampsia; tumors; hemolytic transfusion reactions; myocardial infarctions; giant hemangiomas; respiratory distress syndrome; snake bites; and heat stroke or hypothermia. Although bleeding is the predominant symptom, thrombotic damage can occur in most organ systems. Common ischemic complications include hemorrhagic necrosis of the skin, renal failure, seizures and coma, hypoxemia, and pulmonary infarcts. Laboratory findings in DIC are variable but usually include hemolytic anemia with schistocytes, thrombocytopenia, prolonged PT and PTT, and decreased levels of factor V, factor VIII, and fibrinogen with increased fibrin split products. There is also usually a marked decrease in protein C, protein S, and antithrombin III.

Management rests on treating the underlying disorder. The patient is stabilized and transfused if significant bleeding has occurred. Therapeutic options include factor replacement, anticoagulants, and antifibrinolytics. Factor replacement may be accomplished with fresh frozen plasma (10 to 15 U/kg) to keep the PT in the normal range. Cryoprecipitate provides increased concentration of fibrinogen, factor VIII, and vWf. Platelet transfusion may be considered to keep platelet counts >50,000. Heparin therapy may be helpful in the presence of widespread thrombosis, but it remains controversial. It is usually administered by a relatively low dose, continuous infusion. It does not replace the use of fresh frozen plasma or platelets. Repeated measurements of the coagulation profile and blood and platelet counts are essential.

Platelet Disorders

Normally functioning platelets are a necessary component of the clotting process. Platelet activation, adherence, recruitment, and aggregation and binding of fibrinogen result in the cellular clot that is responsible for primary hemostasis following a disruption of a vessel wall. A deficit in platelet number or function can lead to excessive bleeding following injury. Platelet dysfunction can be congenital, resulting from defects in receptors, platelet-vessel wall adhesion (von Willebrand disease, Bernard Soulier syndrome), platelet-platelet interaction (Glanzmann's thrombasthenia), platelet secretion, and other miscellaneous syndromes. Acquired platelet dysfunction is caused most commonly by aspirin, which inhibits production of thromboxane A_2 and causes decreased platelet aggregation and vessel constriction. Patients with congenital platelet dysfunction typically present with severe bleeding diatheses early in life. Even minor platelet dysfunction can result in easy bruisability and significant bleeding from mucosal membranes.

Deficits in platelet number are much more common in pediatric patients. Thrombocytopenia is defined as a platelet count less than 150,000/μL, although it is rare to develop any abnormal bleeding with counts greater than 50,000/μL. Platelet counts below 20,000/μL indicate severe thrombocytopenia; in that range, particularly when counts drop below 10,000/μL, there is significant risk for life-threatening hemorrhage and intracranial bleeding.

In the emergency department, thrombocytopenia is often an unexpected finding on a complete blood count obtained for unrelated reasons. Symptomatic patients may present as well-appearing children with a petechial or purpuric rash. At times the extensive ecchymoses in the absence of a history of significant trauma can wrongly suggest child abuse. With lower counts, patients may develop significant bleeding and bruising from minor trauma, mucosal bleeding, hematuria, or hematochezia. In addition to the skin findings, the physical exam should focus on lymphadenopathy and liver and spleen enlargement, as these findings help establish the differential diagnosis. Involvement of other bone marrow elements also help guide the workup.

The differential diagnosis of thrombocytopenia is extensive, but the single most common cause in the well-appearing child is immune (idiopathic) thrombocytopenic purpura (ITP). Other causes include autoimmune diseases such as systemic lupus erythematosus, in which anemia and lymphopenia are usually seen, and secondary immune destruction of platelets from infectious agents such as hepatitis B and Epstein-Barr viruses. Sepsis can cause destruction of platelets with or without full-blown DIC.

Bone marrow infiltration from leukemia, lymphoma, and other malignancies may initially present with thrombocytopenia but will often have associated hepatosplenomegaly, anemia, and abnormalities of the white blood cells. Decreased production of platelets can also occur in aplastic anemia or from drug effects. Cancer chemotherapy agents typically depress production of all cell lines, and idiosyncratic immune reactions leading to thrombocytopenia may be seen following administration of various agents. In the pediatric population, this is particularly seen with valproic acid, phenytoin, and trimethoprim/sulfamethoxazole.

Wiskott-Aldrich syndrome is an X-linked disorder with thrombocytopenia, immunodeficiency, and eczema. Typically these patients are identified as newborns because of bleeding and petechiae. The immunodeficiency presents later in infancy. The eczema, which is frequently severe, worsens as the patient ages. Thrombocytopenia-absent radius syndrome (TAR) is autosomal recessive and presents in the neonatal period with petechiae and typical upper limb anomalies. Infection with HIV can result in thrombocytopenia, and this diagnosis should be kept in mind for patients with compatible presentations or high-risk histories.

Hemolytic Uremic Syndrome

Hemolytic uremic syndrome presents with a triad of acute renal failure, microangiopathic hemolytic anemia, and thrombocytopenia; it is discussed in more detail in Chapter 61. The thrombocytopenia is usually mild to moderate. The typical presentation is that of a pale, somewhat lethargic young child with a prodromal history of a gastrointestinal infection. Abdominal pain, vomiting, and bloody diarrhea are common, as are acute renal failure and neurologic manifestations. Laboratory examination typically reveals anemia with red blood cell fragmentation, thrombocytopenia, electrolyte and acid-base disturbances, and elevated blood urea nitrogen and serum creatinine. Management consists of early dialysis to treat the effects of renal failure and reduce the fluid overload and hyperkalemia associated with the frequent blood transfusions that are necessary.

Idiopathic Thrombocytopenic Purpura

Idiopathic thrombocytopenic purpura (ITP) is the most common cause of thrombocytopenia in a well-appearing young child. Children typically have a history of a preceding viral illness, although the link to the development of antiplatelet immunoglobulin is not clear. The platelet surface is covered with increased amounts of IgG and the spleen removes the affected platelets from the circulation. Platelet production is increased in the bone marrow, but not enough to offset the rapid destruction.

Patients present with the acute onset of bruising, petechiae, and purpura; they have normal physical examinations other than for skin findings. Mucosal or gastrointestinal bleeding can occur. The most serious complication, intracranial hemorrhage, occurs in less than 0.1 to 0.5 percent of patients and almost exclusively with platelet counts under 20,000/μL.

The diagnosis of ITP is likely when the complete blood count reveals thrombocytopenia in association with normal red and white blood cell numbers and mor-

phology. Definitive diagnosis by bone marrow aspirate is not necessary in cases with thrombocytopenia and absence of signs, symptoms, or blood count results suggesting another diagnosis. Such children usually do not require hospitalization and can be followed as outpatients. The natural history of the condition is that 80 percent of children make a full recovery within 6 months. Treatment of patients with ITP is controversial. High-dose steroids can hasten the rate at which patients recover but are not necessary in most patients, who have only skin manifestations and platelet counts above 30,000/μL. Intravenous gamma globulin has been shown to promptly increase counts in patients with profound thrombocytopenia even more predictably than steroids and may be useful during active bleeding or intracranial hemorrhage. Both modalities are presumed to block reticuloendothelial destruction of platelets. Transfused platelets will be rapidly destroyed due to the immune response and have no role in the management of these patients except in the circumstance of life-threatening hemorrhage, which most commonly occurs intracranially. In that circumstance, massive platelet transfusions along with intravenous gamma globulin or steroids are administered, and emergency splenectomy can be considered.

Intravenous anti-Rh(D) immunoglobulin (Winrho-SD) is another technique to increase platelet counts. Infusion in Rh-positive individuals results in immune clearance of the antibody-coated red cells and coincident prolonged survival of autoantibody-coated platelets. Anti-D appears to be as safe and effective as IVIG in Rh-positive patients. The cost is much less, and infusion takes minutes as opposed to hours for IVIG.

BIBLIOGRAPHY

Blanchette V, Imback P, Andrew M, et al: Randomized trial of intravenous immunoglobulin G, intravenous anti-D, and oral prednisone in childhood acute immune thrombocytopenic purpura. *Lancet* 344:703, 1994.

DiMichele D, Neufeld EJ: Hemophilia: A new approach to an old disease. *Hematol Oncol Clin North Am* 12:1315, 1998.

Mannucci PM, Tuddenham EGD: Medical progress: The hemophilias—from royal genes to gene therapy. *N Engl J Med* 344:1773–1779, 2001.

Scaradavou A, Woo B, Woloski BMR, et al: Intravenous anti-D treatment of immune thrombocytopenic purpura: Experience in 272 patients. *Blood* 89:2689, 1997.

74

Blood Components

David F. Soglin
Jane E. Kramer

HIGH-YIELD FACTS

- A common pitfall in the management of the bleeding patient is to underestimate the amount of the blood loss. Continuous monitoring of vital signs and repeated hematocrit checks are essential.
- The use of O-negative blood is reserved for life-threatening hemorrhage.
- Fever, chills, nausea, and vomiting during a blood transfusion may be the result of a hemolytic reaction to noncompatible transfused red cells, of recipient antibodies to donor white cells or platelets, or (rarely) of bacterial contamination of the blood product.

Transfusion of blood and blood components is often necessary in the emergency department. Whole blood, packed red blood cells (PRBCs), platelets, granulocytes, fresh frozen plasma, cryoprecipitate, specific clotting factors, albumin, and immunoglobulins each have specific indications and risks associated with their use. As blood for transfusion is a scarce commodity, the component that will specifically address the patient's need is generally transfused.

WHOLE BLOOD

Transfusion of whole blood is rarely performed but may be indicated for prompt restoration of red cells and volume after trauma or surgery. After 24 hours of storage, whole blood has lost platelet and granulocyte function. Activity of labile clotting factors V and VIII is also diminished greatly within 3 to 5 days. Furthermore, the risk of transfusion reactions is doubled because of the volume of foreign proteins and antibodies that is transferred in whole blood.

PACKED RED BLOOD CELLS

PRBC units contain approximately 30 to 50 mL of plasma and have a hematocrit ranging from 60 to 80 percent. They are stored in solution with anticoagulant and preservative for up to 35 days. There are no functional platelets or granulocytes in this preparation. For patients with a previous history of febrile reactions to transfusions or if the risk of cytomegalovirus (CMV) transmission is to be particularly avoided, filtered, leukocyte-poor red cells are recommended. Patients with recurrent or severe allergic reactions to transfusions should receive PRBCs that have been saline-washed. This removes virtually all plasma from the transfusion.

PLATELET CONCENTRATE

These preparations contain approximately 5.5×10^{10} platelets in 40 mL of plasma. They should be ABO- and Rh-compatible, but crossmatching is not necessary. In children, the dose is estimated at 0.1 to 0.2 U/kg of random donor platelets to raise the platelet count by 50,000 to 100,000/μL. Platelet transfusions are indicated for patients with thrombocytopenia or platelet dysfunction who are actively bleeding. Counts above 20,000/μL rarely result in spontaneous bleeding, but at counts below 10,000/μL, the risk is severe. Patients with immune thrombocytopenia rarely benefit from platelet transfusions, since the ongoing disease process destroys the transfused platelets rapidly.

GRANULOCYTE CONCENTRATES

Transfusion of white cells is indicated in a severely neutropenic patient with documented or strongly suspected sepsis.

FRESH FROZEN PLASMA

This product is plasma frozen within 8 hours of collection. It contains all clotting factors, including labile factors V and VIII, and the naturally occurring anticoagulants protein S, protein C, and antithrombin III. ABO compatibility is important, but crossmatching is not necessary. Fresh frozen plasma is used at a dose of 10 to 20 mL/kg to treat coagulopathies secondary to unknown factor deficiencies, disseminated intravascular coagulation (DIC), and chronic liver disease and to compensate for excessive warfarin or dicumarol treatment. The risk of disease transmission is similar to that of whole blood transfusion, and allergic reactions are possible. Fresh frozen plasma is not indicated for volume expansion.

CRYOPRECIPITATE

Cryoprecipitate is prepared by slow thawing of FFP at 4°C and subsequent refreezing of the protein precipitate, which is rich in fibrinogen, factor VIII:vWf, and factor XIII. Cryoprecipitate does not require crossmatching. It is indicated for treatment of hypo- or a-fibrinogenemia and of von Willebrand's disease.

FACTORS VIII AND IX

Highly purified concentrates of factors VIII and IX are now produced by monoclonal antibody techniques and by recombinant DNA technology. A number of such products are available and have replaced single donor products such as fresh frozen plasma in the treatment of hemophilia because they avoid or greatly diminish the risk of infectious disease transmission.

ALBUMIN

Available in both 5 and 25 percent solutions, albumin is most frequently used for blood volume expansion in shock, trauma, burns, and surgery. Heat and chemical treatment eliminates the infectious transmission risk, and it contains no blood group antibodies. Only the 5 percent solution is isosmotic with plasma, and the 25 percent solution is never used to treat shock without other fluids.

IMMUNE GLOBULINS

These antibody-rich preparations are occasionally used in the emergency department to treat conditions such as rabies, tetanus, or varicella, as postexposure disease prophylaxis.

INDICATIONS FOR TRANSFUSION

Transfusion of blood in the emergency department is usually performed because of shock secondary to acute blood loss. Most other anemic patients are hemodynam-

ically compensated, and transfusion can be carried out after admission. The history of blood loss in a given patient is often inaccurate and the initial hemoglobin may not reflect losses, so it is crucial to monitor heart rate and blood pressure for changes of early shock.

Blood typing (for ABO and Rh) takes about 5 minutes, and screening for antibodies and crossmatching takes 30 minutes or more. The use of O-negative (universal donor) blood is reserved for life-threatening hemorrhage. The accompanying risks of minor blood group incompatibility with hemolysis or recipient sensitization to red blood cell antigens are overshadowed in this situation. The use of group- and Rh type-specific blood is preferred over O-negative transfusions when time precludes complete crossmatching. The formula for calculating the volume (V) of PRBCs (in milliliters) to infuse is as follows:

$$V = \text{blood volume} \times (\text{desired hematocrit} - \text{observed hematocrit/hematocrit of PRBC})$$

$$\text{Blood volume} = \text{weight (kg)} \times 70 \text{ mL/kg}$$

These formulas assume a hematocrit for the PRBCs of approximately 60 to 80 percent.

COMPLICATIONS

There are several types of transfusion reactions, which range from mild to life threatening. In the event of a reaction, the transfusion is stopped and the blood bank notified. Care in collecting specimens for the blood bank and in labeling them is crucial.

Acute Hemolytic Transfusion Reactions

Acute hemolytic transfusion reactions (AHTR) occur when a patient's anti-A or anti-B antibodies bind to incompatible transfused red cells. These reactions are seen immediately and are almost always the result of errors in drawing, labeling, or processing of specimens. The transfused cells are lysed, releasing inflammatory mediators. Symptoms include fever, chills, back or chest pain, nausea and vomiting, dyspnea, flushing, tachycardia, and hypotension. Disseminated intravascular coagulation, shock, renal failure, and death may ensue. Aggressive fluid resuscitation should be initiated to maintain blood pressure

Delayed Hemolytic Transfusion Reactions

Delayed hemolytic transfusion reactions (DHTR) are caused by sensitization to non-ABO antigens from a previous transfusion. They are delayed for 3 to 10 days because an anamnestic immune response must develop to increase antibody production. Signs and symptoms include fever, back pain, anemia, jaundice, and, rarely, hemoglobinuria. No treatment is usually required.

Febrile Nonhemolytic Transfusion Reactions

Febrile or nonhemolytic transfusion reactions (FNHTR) are benign and self-limiting; they account for the great majority of transfusion reactions and occur most commonly in the multiply transfused patient. This condition is typically caused by recipient antibodies to donor leukocytes and platelets. Symptoms include fever and chills. This may be difficult to distinguish from AHTR; therefore if the patient is very uncomfortable, the transfusion should be stopped. Antipyretics may be given.

Allergic Transfusion Reaction

Allergic transfusion reactions are of two types, which have different etiologies:

- Urticarial reactions may involve cytokines or histamine in stored blood products. The transfusion must be interrupted and the patient watched closely for signs and symptoms of anaphylaxis. An antihistamine such as diphenhydramine, 1 mg/kg/dose, should be administered. Then, when the urticaria fades, transfusion can be resumed.

- Anaphylactic reactions occur in patients with congenital IgA deficiency who have high-titer IgG anti-IgA antibodies. Activation of a complement and chemical mediator cascade precipitates increased vascular permeability, resulting in angioedema, respiratory distress, urticaria, and shock. The transfusion is stopped, epinephrine is administered, and blood pressure is stabilized with crystalloid and vasopressive agents if necessary.

Complications of Massive Transfusions

This generally refers to the transfusion of ≥ 1 entire blood volume within 24 hours. Risks involved include hypothermia if a blood warmer is not used, hyperkalemia, hypocalcemia, and coagulation disorders from the dilution of platelets and clotting factors.

Infectious Complications

Donated blood is routinely screened for HIV-1 and -2, HTLV, hepatitis B surface antigen, hepatitis B core antibody (a surrogate marker for non-A, non-B hepatitis), hepatitis C virus, and syphilis. The current estimated risk of transmitting HIV through a blood transfusion is 1 in 493,000; hepatitis B, 1 in 63,000; and hepatitis C, 1 in 103,000.

Bacterial contamination of blood products can occur and accounts for other transfusion reactions and fatalities. Fever, chills, rigor, vomiting, and hypotension present soon after the transfusion is begun. Blood cultures should be sent from the patient and from the blood product. AHTR is in the differential if the patient is receiving red blood cells, and samples should be sent to the blood bank to check for hemolysis.

BIBLIOGRAPHY

Manno C: What's new in transfusion medicine? *Pediatr Clin North Am* 43:793, 1996.

Schreiber GB, Busch MP, Kleinman SH et al: The risk of transfusion-transmitted viral infections. *N Engl J Med* 334: 1685–1690, 1996.

75

Oncologic Emergencies

Brenda N. Hayakawa

HIGH-YIELD FACTS

- Acute leukemia is the most common childhood malignancy and may present with fever, fatigue, bleeding, adenopathy, or bone pain. These nonspecific symptoms often make the diagnosis of acute leukemia dependent on a high index of suspicion.

- Retinoblastoma most commonly presents with leukocoria or a "white pupil."

- Complications of childhood cancer result from tumor- or therapy-induced infectious or hematologic complications, metabolic derangement, or structural consequences of tumor compression.

- Infection is the leading cause of death in children with cancer, with the development of neutropenia being the most important factor. Fever may be the only sign and other findings associated with inflammation may be absent.

- Initial antibiotic coverage usually includes an aminoglycoside and a beta-lactam penicillin or cephalosporin. The advent of broad-spectrum antibiotics has made single drug therapy a growing option.

- Metabolic complications of childhood cancer include tumor lysis syndrome and syndrome of inappropriate antidiuretic hormone (SIADH). Structural complications include superior vena cava (SVC) syndrome, spinal cord compression, and raised intracranial pressure (ICP).

Approximately 10 percent of childhood deaths are related to cancer. The leukemias, central nervous system (CNS) tumors, and lymphomas account for more than one-half of all childhood malignancies (Table 75-1). Advances in cancer treatment have led to improvements in survival, particularly with acute lymphocytic leukemia and lymphoma. However, the overall incidence of cancer among children continues to increase, especially among children younger than 3 years of age. Although childhood cancer is infrequently diagnosed in the emergency department, it is important for the emergency physician to be aware of its possible occurrence and to be ready to treat the complications of cancer in previously diagnosed patients.

COMMON PEDIATRIC MALIGNANCIES

Acute Leukemias

Leukemia is a condition in which there is uncontrolled growth of immature white blood cells within the bone marrow, with subsequent suppression of normal hematopoiesis. Acute leukemia is the most common childhood malignancy, representing approximately 30 percent of newly diagnosed cancers; 75 percent of these are of the acute lymphoblastic leukemia (ALL). Acute myelogenous leukemia (AML) involves immature nonlymphoid cells (myeloblasts). It is much less common than ALL, accounting for 25 percent of acute leukemia.

The peak incidence of ALL occurs between the ages of 3 and 5 years, with a second peak around the third decade of life. Overall, about 60 to 70 percent of patients survive more than 5 years beyond diagnosis, with many patients considered cured of disease. Unlike ALL, the incidence of AML is relatively constant throughout childhood and has a much poorer prognosis. Although the exact cause of leukemia is unknown, certain genetic, environmental, viral, and immunologic risk factors have been implicated.

The signs and symptoms of acute leukemia reflect involvement of bone marrow by leukemic cells. Common presentations include pallor, fatigue, petechiae, purpura, bleeding, and fever. Lymphadenopathy, hepatomegaly, and splenomegaly reflect extramedullary involvement.

Table 75-1. Cancer Incidence Rates in Children Aged 0 to 14 Years: SEER*[a] 1974–1991

Cancer	Rate**[b]
Leukemia	41
Central nervous system tumors	29
Lymphoma	15
Neuroblastoma	−9
Rhabdomyosarcoma	−8
Wilms' tumor	−8
Bone	−6
Retinoblastoma	−4

*[a]SEER: Surveillance, Epidemiology and End Results program of the National Cancer Institute.
**[b]Annual incidence rates per million children aged 0 to 14.
Source: Adapted from Ries LAG, Gurney JG, Linet M, et al: Cancer incidence and survival among children and adolescents: United States SEER Program 1975–1995, National Cancer Institute, NIH Publication No. 99-4649; Bethesda, MD, 1999.

Bone pain results from leukemic involvement of the periosteum and bone, causing patients to limp or even refuse to walk. The cause of joint pain is uncertain, but may be related to leukemic involvement of the joint and may mimic nonmalignant disease, such as juvenile rheumatoid arthritis. Other nonspecific symptoms such as anorexia, lassitude, low-grade fever, and irritability may also be present in a variety of nonmalignant conditions, making the diagnosis of leukemia dependent on a high level of suspicion.

The leukocyte count is $>10,000/mm^3$ in approximately one-half of patients with ALL. However, neutropenia may be encountered and may predispose to serious infections. Most patients will be anemic and thrombocytopenic.

Despite hematologic abnormalities in the peripheral blood cell count, the diagnosis of leukemia must be confirmed by bone marrow aspirate and biopsy. Further characterization of the leukemic blasts determines the particular treatment regimen. Treatment consists of combination chemotherapy for induction of remission, CNS preventative therapy, consolidation, and maintenance therapy.

Complications of Leukemia

Complications of leukemia include CNS involvement, which may be present at the time of initial diagnosis or can occur with relapse. Patients may have headache, nausea, vomiting, irritability, papilledema, or other signs of raised ICP. Diagnosis is confirmed through the demonstration of leukemic blasts in the cerebrospinal fluid.

Leukemia may relapse in the testes, where it causes painless, usually unilateral, testicular enlargement. Testicular biopsy confirms leukemic infiltrate. Since testicular leukemia is often indicative of bone marrow relapse, treatment consists of reinduction with chemotherapy and irradiation.

Hematologic complications include anemia, hemorrhage, and hyperleukocytosis. Management of anemia includes transfusion therapy with packed red blood cells (pRBC). Patients who are symptomatic will often have a hemoglobin of <6 to 7 g/dL and experience malaise, decreased activity, or irritability due to reduced oxygen-carrying capacity. They warrant transfusion with 10 mL/kg pRBC, given over 3 to 4 hours. Those with a hemoglobin <5 g/dL receive multiple transfusions of 3 mL/kg pRBC, each given over 4 hours. In the absence of hemorrhage, the anemia most often develops gradually, with ongoing compensation of the plasma volume; thus a rapid blood transfusion could precipitate or aggravate congestive heart failure. Patients with signs of fluid overload may be given furosemide (1 mg/kg). Patients with hemoglobin between 7 and 10 g/dL should have blood typed and crossmatched and are generally transfused if they are symptomatic or if there is ongoing hemorrhage. Patients with a hemoglobin >10 g/dL usually do not require immediate therapy unless there is concurrent hemorrhage. If possible, blood products given to patients with chemotherapy-induced defective cell-mediated immunity or recipients of transplanted autologous bone marrow are irradiated to 1500 rad. Blood-product irradiation helps minimize the occurrence of posttransfusion graft-versus-host disease by inhibiting the mitotic activity of lymphocytes in donor blood products.

Hemorrhage is a complication of leukemia and is most often due to thrombocytopenia. Petechiae, bruising, and mucosal bleeding may be seen with platelet counts $<20,000/mm^3$, but significant spontaneous hemorrhage is more likely with platelet counts $<10,000/mm^3$. Most cases of spontaneous intracranial hemorrhage are associated with a platelet count $<5000/mm^3$. Platelet transfusions are warranted for patients who have a platelet count in the range of 20,000 to $50,000/mm^3$ and who have significant bleeding, such as epistaxis, gingival bleeding, or gross gastrointestinal hemorrhage. Platelets are administered at a dose of 0.2 U/kg or 6 U/m². Prophylactic use of platelet transfusions for nonbleeding patients with a platelet count $<20,000/mm^3$ is controversial but may be justified in the presence of infection, prior to an invasive procedure, or for a platelet count <5000/mm^3.

Hemorrhage can also be secondary to disseminated intravascular coagulation, which causes a prolongation of the prothrombin time and partial thromboplastin time, reduced fibrinogen level, thrombocytopenia, and elevated fibrin degradation products. Disseminated intravascular coagulation may occur in the setting of sepsis, newly diagnosed or relapsing acute nonlymphocytic leukemia, hyperleukocytosis, and disseminated neuroblastoma. Initial management includes treatment of the underlying condition and replacement of coagulation factors with fresh frozen plasma (10 mL/kg). Platelet and pRBC transfusions may be necessary, as well as vitamin K (5 mg IV for infants and young children; 10 mg IV for older children).

Hyperleukocytosis, with an initial white blood cell (WBC) count >100,000/mm^3, may be seen with acute leukemias and chronic myelocytic leukemia. Unlike RBCs and platelets, WBCs are larger and not easily deformed, and they contribute significantly to blood viscosity. Blast cells tend to aggregate and impair tissue perfusion, which can cause lactic acidosis. Patients may be asymptomatic but are more often dyspneic, confused, or agitated or experience blurred vision. Physical examination may reveal plethora, cyanosis, signs of right ventricular failure, papilledema, or priapism. The complete blood cell count (CBC) will confirm an elevated peripheral WBC count. Arterial blood gas values may show an acidemia. The chest radiograph may be normal or show a diffuse interstitial infiltrate. Patients with hyperleukocytosis are at risk for tumor lysis syndrome and are treated with intravenous hydration, alkalinization measures, and allopurinol; they are admitted for antileukemic therapy. Thrombocytopenia is corrected to a platelet count of at least 20,000/mm^3, as there is a significant risk of intracranial hemorrhage with hyperleukocytosis. Leukapheresis is an option prior to initiation of chemotherapy.

Neutropenia may occur at the time of diagnosis or after chemotherapy. Febrile neutropenic patients are at significant risk of serious infection (see "Common Complications of Childhood Cancer," later).

Although hypercalcemia, with a serum calcium >10.5 mg/dL, is more commonly associated with adult malignancies, it may occur with ALL, non-Hodgkin's lymphoma (NHL), neuroblastoma, and Ewing's sarcoma. Disruptions in calcium homeostasis, excessive bone resorption by tumor, and, rarely, ectopic parathormone production are the usual causes. Clinically, patients may experience nausea, vomiting, constipation, polyuria, and polydipsia, which may progress to dehydration, lethargy, seizures, and coma. Treatment begins with intravenous hydration with normal saline, followed by furosemide to promote calcium excretion. Other metabolic complications include hyperuricemia and syndrome of inappropriate antidiuretic hormone, which are discussed further later.

Hodgkin's Disease

Hodgkin's disease is a malignancy of the lymph nodes, which may spread to other local nodes and lymphatic channels. The malignant cell is the Reed-Sternberg cell; its origin has not yet been proved, but current theories propose a B lymphocyte lineage. Approximately 5 percent of pediatric malignancies are Hodgkin's disease. The first peak in incidence occurs from ages 13 to 35 years, with a late peak at 50 to 75 years. A familial preponderance has been recognized.

The majority of pediatric patients have painless supraclavicular or cervical lymphadenopathy. Nodes are rubbery, matted, and, unlike reactive nodes, do not decrease in size. A lymph node is considered enlarged if it is >10 mm at its greatest diameter, with the exception of an epitrochlear node, which is considered enlarged at 5 mm, and an inguinal node, at 15 mm. The abdominal examination may reveal hepatomegaly or splenomegaly, which indicates more advanced disease. Systemic symptoms occur in one-third of the patients and include unexplained fever, weight loss, and night sweats.

The differential diagnosis of Hodgkin's disease includes other causes of lymphadenopathy, such as infectious mononucleosis, mycobacterial infections, toxoplasmosis, or other metastatic malignancies. A screening CBC and chest radiograph are indicated, as well as a tuberculin skin test. Patients are referred for lymph node biopsy if the node is enlarging after 2 to 3 weeks, remains enlarged, and has not returned to normal size by 5 to 6 weeks, or is associated with an abnormal chest radiograph finding such as mediastinal enlargement.

Once the diagnosis of Hodgkin's disease is confirmed and histologically classified, patients undergo further work-up for staging, which may involve exploratory laparotomy and splenectomy. Treatment regimens include multidrug chemotherapy and/or radiation, with a cure rate of >80 percent.

Non-Hodgkin's Lymphomas

Non-Hodgkin's lymphomas are a heterogeneous group of malignancies of lymphatic tissue. They account for 10 percent of all childhood cancer and usually occur in children >5 years of age. Unlike adult lymphomas, childhood NHLs are rapidly proliferating and are often disseminated in extranodal tissues at the time of presentation. Although the etiology of NHL is unknown, Epstein-Barr virus and immunodeficiency diseases have been linked to this malignancy.

Clinically, NHL may rarely present as an isolated, painless adenopathy in the cervical, supraclavicular, or inguinal areas. Intrathoracic tumors may present with supraclavicular adenopathy, cough, wheezing, chest pain, or signs and symptoms of superior vera cava (SVC) obstruction. Mediastinal lymphomas are more commonly of the lymphoblastic (T-cell) type. Burkitt or non-Burkitt undifferentiated types can present with abdominal involvement causing pain, nausea, vomiting, distension, ascites, or bowel obstruction. Right lower quadrant pain reflects distal ileal, appendiceal, or cecal involvement and may mimic appendicitis. Abdominal lymphoma may be a leading point for an intussusception. Bone, bone marrow, and the CNS are common sites of metastasis.

Initial laboratory studies include a CBC to assess for leukemia. Chest radiograph may reveal a mediastinal mass. Other mediastinal tumors in children are listed in Table 75-2. Patients with isolated nodal enlargement suspicious of lymphoma are referred to an appropriate

facility for biopsy. Patients with an abdominal mass are evaluated with abdominal ultrasound or computed tomography (CT) scan. Multiagent chemotherapy is the mainstay of treatment, with up to 80 percent long-term disease-free survival.

Central Nervous System Tumors

The second-most common group of pediatric malignancies is those of the CNS, accounting for 20 percent of all pediatric cancers. Two incidence peaks occur, one in the first decade and the other beyond the fourth decade of life. Associations of CNS tumors with genetic diseases occur, such as neurofibromatosis with optic gliomas and tuberous sclerosis with giant cell astrocytomas.

Classification of CNS tumors is generally based on histologic type. Tumors arising in the supratentorial region include cerebral astrocytoma, optic glioma, and craniopharyngioma. These more commonly occur in the neonatal and infancy period. Infratentorial tumors such as cerebellar astrocytoma, medulloblastoma, ependymoma, and brain stem glioma are more commonly seen after 2 years of age. Cerebellar astrocytomas account for 40 percent of CNS tumors in childhood.

The clinical presentation depends on the site and ex-

Table 75-2. Mediastinal Tumors in Children

	Malignant	**Benign**
Anterior Mediastinum	Non-Hodgkin's lymphoma	Teratoma
	Hodgkin's disease	Cystic hygroma
	Teratocarcinoma	Thymic cyst
	Thymoma	Hemangioma
	Sarcoma	Bronchogenic cyst
		Lipoma
Middle Mediastinum	Non-Hodgkin's lymphoma	Bronchogenic cyst
	Hodgkin's disease	Granuloma
	Rhabdomyosarcoma	Teratoma
	Teratocarcinoma	Esophageal cyst
	Other sarcoma	Diaphragmatic hernia
Posterior Mediastinum	Neuroblastoma	Ganglioneuroma
	Ganglioneuroblastoma	Neurolemmoma
	Ewing's sarcoma	Neurofibroma
	Pheochromocytoma	Enterogenous cyst
	Lymphoma	

Source: Adapted from King RM, Telander RL, Smithson WA, et al: Primary mediastinal tumors in children. *J Pediatr Surg* 17:512–520, [year?]. Used with permission.

tent of involvement of the tumor. Supratentorial tumors may cause headache, seizures, or visual impairment. Truncal ataxia or incoordination is typical of infratentorial tumors. Impingement of the brain stem may lead to cranial nerve palsies or Horner's syndrome. Raised ICP in infants and toddlers may manifest as vomiting, anorexia, irritability, developmental regression, or impaired upward gaze ("sunsetting" sign). There may be excessive enlargement of the head circumference and persistently palpable cranial sutures. Parents may note a change in behavior or personality in their child. Older children may complain of headache, fatigue, or vomiting. Headaches are rarely due to a CNS malignancy. However, headaches that are recurrent, intense, incapacitating, changing in character, or that awaken patients from sleep raise the suspicion of a malignancy. In addition, patients may have back pain, bladder, or bowel dysfunction, or focal neurologic deficits that suggest spinal cord or cauda equina involvement.

Other conditions that may present with raised ICP or neurologic deficits include brain abscess, chronic subdural hematoma, and vascular malformations. Tumors of the CNS may be diagnosed by CT, which is relatively accessible and can detect up to 95 percent of CNS lesions. Magnetic resonance imaging (MRI) is more sensitive than CT in detecting tumors. Specific tissue diagnosis is achieved through biopsy. Treatment is multimodal, utilizing surgical resection, chemotherapy, and radiation therapy. Newer therapies include immunotherapy and gene therapy.

Wilms' Tumor

Wilms' tumor (nephroblastoma), the most common pediatric abdominal malignancy, arises from embryonal renal cells. Most Wilms' tumors occur in children <6 years of age and present with a nontender or tender abdominal mass. If present, hematuria is usually microscopic. Systemic symptoms, such as fever, anorexia, vomiting, and weight loss, are infrequent, and children may appear well. Hypertension may result from increased renin activity. There may be signs of venous obstruction, such as leg swelling, prominent veins over the abdominal wall, or varicocele. Rarely, associated congenital abnormalities such as aniridia, hemihypertrophy, and genitourinary tract defects may be present.

The differential diagnosis includes other conditions that present with abdominal or pelvic mass. Initial work-up includes a CBC, urinalysis, and renal functions, as well as plain radiographs of the chest and abdomen. Ultrasound is a noninvasive means of evaluating a renal mass. Patients suspected of having a Wilms' tumor are referred for further evaluation and management, which includes surgical resection and chemotherapy or radiation.

Neuroblastoma

Neuroblastoma is a malignant tumor arising from sympathetic neuroblasts in the adrenal medulla and sympathetic chain. It is the most common extracranial solid tumor in childhood, usually presenting within the first 4 years of life. Presenting signs and symptoms are most often related to the local effects of the primary or metastatic tumor. Two-thirds of neuroblastomas arise in the abdomen and pelvis and may present as abdominal mass, bowel obstruction, or edema of the lower extremities and scrotum due to compression of venous and lymphatic drainage. Impingement of renal vasculature may lead to renin-mediated hypertension. Other sites of origin include the posterior mediastinum and neck. Horner's syndrome, with unilateral ptosis, miosis, and anhidrosis, may occur with cervical or high thoracic involvement. Tumors of the paraspinal ganglia may grow around and through the intervertebral foramina, causing spinal cord or nerve root compression. This may cause radicular pain, motor and sensory deficits, bladder or bowel incontinence, or paraplegia. At the time of diagnosis, more than one-half of patients with neuroblastoma will have metastases involving the lymph nodes, bone marrow, cortical bone, liver, or skin. Lung or brain involvement is rare and usually represents end-stage or relapsing disease. Retrobulbar involvement can cause proptosis or periorbital ecchymosis. Bone pain and limping may be related to bone and bone marrow disease. Massive hepatomegaly due to liver involvement, more common in infants, can cause respiratory compromise or liver failure. Skin manifestations appear as bluish, nontender subcutaneous nodules. They rarely occur outside of infancy. Paraneoplastic syndromes seen with neuroblastoma include opsoclonus, myoclonus, and cerebellar ataxia. Tumor secretion of vasoactive intestinal peptide may cause an intractable secretory diarrhea that results in hypokalemia and dehydration.

A CBC may reveal neutropenia or pancytopenia due to marrow involvement. Chest radiography may show a posterior mediastinal mass that may cause impingement on the upper airway. Abdominal radiographs may reveal a mass displacing normal tissues. Abdominal ultrasound or CT scan may reveal a suprarenal mass. Lytic lesions and periosteal reaction may be seen on radiographs of painful areas of bone. All patients are referred to a pediatric oncologist.

Primary Bone Tumors

Common primary pediatric malignancies of the bone include osteosarcoma and Ewing's sarcoma. Osteosarcoma has a predilection for the metaphysis of long bones, particularly around the knee. Ewing's sarcoma may also arise in extraosseous tissues.

Local pain, the most common symptom, may be exacerbated with activity and may cause a limp. The pain may be intermittent, remit for several weeks, and later return with increasing severity. Other presentations include a palpable mass, fever, and pathologic fracture. Back pain may be an early symptom of spinal cord compression.

Plain radiographs of the affected bone reveal bony destruction and soft tissue swelling. Later, the tumor may extend through the periosteum, causing new malignant bone deposition, which results in the characteristic radiographic sunburst sign, or it may cause a multilaminar periosteal reaction that results in an "onion peel" appearance on a radiograph. Osteosarcoma may metastasize to the lung, causing pulmonary hemorrhage, pneumothorax or, rarely, SVC obstruction.

Patients with radiographic changes suggestive of a bone tumor are referred to an orthopedist for confirmational biopsy and further management.

Rhabdomyosarcoma

Rhabdomyosarcoma is a malignant solid tumor from mesenchymal tissue that normally forms striated muscle. It most often presents as a painless mass. The most common site of origin is the head and neck region. Orbital tumors may present with periorbital swelling, proptosis, or ophthalmoplegia. Parameningeal tumors arising around the nasopharynx and paranasal sinuses may cause nasal obstruction, pain, sinusitis, or epistaxis. Tumor extension toward the meninges may cause cranial nerve palsies, meningeal irritation, headache, and vomiting. Chronic otitis media and otalgia may be due to middle ear involvement. Genitourinary tract involvement may manifest with hematuria or urinary obstruction. Vaginal tumors may present with vaginal hemorrhagic discharge and may mimic a vaginal foreign body. Rhabdomyosarcoma of the extremities or trunk usually presents as an enlarging soft tissue mass. Common sites of metastasis include lymph nodes, lungs, bones, bone marrow, brain, spinal cord, and heart.

A CT scan is used to evaluate suspected head or neck lesions. Ultrasound is a useful initial tool to define a pelvic mass. Plain radiographs of the affected area of the limb or trunk should be obtained. Patients with a soft tissue mass must be referred for diagnostic biopsy. Treatment of rhabdomyosarcoma is multimodal, utilizing surgery, chemotherapy, and radiation.

Retinoblastoma

Retinoblastoma is the most common intraocular tumor of childhood. It is strongly linked to deletions of part of chromosome 13. In 30 percent of cases, the disease is bilateral. Infants and young children are most commonly affected. Retinoblastoma most commonly presents with leukocoria or strabismus. Other rarer findings include vitreous hemorrhage, microphthalmos, and orbital cellulites. The disease may be localized to the orbit, or it may metastasize to the brain, liver, kidneys, and adrenals. Plain radiographs or ultrasound of the orbits may reveal deposition of calcium. A CT scan or MRI is needed to determine the presence of choroidal or optic nerve spread and orbital, subarachnoid, or intracranial involvement. Unilateral disease is predominantly treated with enucleation. With bilateral or more extensive disease, other modalities include radiation, chemotherapy, thermotherapy, and cryotherapy.

COMMON COMPLICATIONS OF CHILDHOOD CANCER

The emergencies encountered in cancer patients result from tumor or therapy-induced infectious or hematologic complications, metabolic derangement, or structural consequences of tumor compression.

Infectious Complications

Infection is the leading cause of death in children with cancer. The single most important factor is the development of neutropenia due to replacement of healthy bone marrow by malignant cells or from myelosuppressive chemotherapy, which often produces granulocytopenia 8 to 16 days posttherapy. The best estimate of production of neutrophils is the absolute neutrophil count (ANC), calculated as the total WBC count multiplied by the sum of the percentages of band cells plus polymorphonuclear neutrophils. Patients are defined as being neutropenic if their ANC is $<500/mm^3$ or if it is $<1000/mm^3$ with predicted decline to $<500/mm^3$. These patients are at significant risk of bacteremia or fungemia; the risk decreases and plateaus as the ANC approaches $1000/mm^3$. There are also qualitative abnormalities of granulocyte function that result from chemotherapy or radiation therapy. Impairment in cell-mediated immunity is more commonly encountered with Hodgkin's disease, lymphomas, and after treatment with chemotherapy or corticosteroids. Impaired cell-mediated immunity results in a greater risk for fungal, mycobacterial, and viral infections. Impairment of humoral immunity more commonly occurs with chronic lymphocytic leukemia or chemotherapy and after splenectomy. Splenectomized patients are at greatly increased risk for sepsis with encapsulated bacteria such as pneumococcus and *Haemophilus influenzae*. In addition, mechanical barriers such as the skin and mucous membranes may be broken down by infection, chemotherapy, or iatrogenically from intravenous catheters and other long-term indwelling venous access devices. Patients are at risk of infection from their own endogenous flora, as well as nosocomial pathogens from previous recent hospitalizations. It is important to promptly evaluate and treat immunocompromised patients with fever, since their infections can be life threatening. The virulence of the infection depends on the extent of the host's immune defect. About 75 percent of neutropenic cancer patients with fever have an infection, most commonly bacterial. Of the nonneutropenic cancer patients with fever, approximately 17 percent have associated infection. The common pathogens are listed in Table 75-3.

Evaluation of children with cancer and fever includes a careful history and physical examination. Particular attention is paid to occult sites of potential infection, such as the oropharynx, axillae, groin, perineum, and sites of previous procedures, as well as along the tract of any indwelling venous access device. It is important to note that fever may be the only positive sign. Due to a decreased number of neutrophils, the inflammatory response is blunted; hence, other findings, such as exudates, adenophathy, fluctuance, warmth, and swelling, may be absent. Children with early pneumonia may not have cough or sputum production. Rales are frequently absent on chest auscultation.

Initial investigations include a chest radiograph, urinalysis and urine culture, and CBC; in addition, two sets of blood cultures, obtained from different sites, are sent for bacterial and fungal cultures. If an indwelling catheter is present, one blood specimen is obtained from the line and one from a peripheral vein. An aspirate for Gram's stain and culture is sent from any other areas suggestive of focal infection. An arterial blood gas analysis is obtained for patients with suspected pneumonia or sepsis.

Prompt initiation of empiric antibiotic therapy in febrile neutropenic children have been associated with a

Table 75-3. Common Pathogens in Children With Cancer

Bacteria:
Gram-positive aerobes:
  Staphylococcus aureus
  Coagulase-negative staphylococci
  Alpha-hemolytic streptococci
  Enterococci
Gram-negative aerobes:
  Enterobacteriaceae (*Escherichia coli, Klebsiella pneumoniae*)
  Enterobacter, Citrobacter, Serratia
  Anaerobes
Fungi:
Candida species
Aspergillus species
Cryptococcus
Parasites:
Pneumocystis carinii
Cryptosporidium species
Strongyloides stercoralis
Viruses:
Herpes simplex virus
Varicella-zoster virus
Cytomegalovirus

Source: Adapted from Pizzo PA, Rubin M, Freifeld A, et al: The child with cancer and infection. I. Empiric therapy for fever and neutropenia and preventative strategies. *J Pediatr* 119:674–694, 1991.

reduction in morbidity and mortality. Traditionally, all patients are admitted to the hospital for intravenous antibiotics. However, there may be a select group of patients who may be treated as outpatients with parenteral antibiotics. This has been facilitated through newer, long half-life antibiotics, improved vascular access devices, and outpatient services. There have been attempts to elucidate factors to help identify those febrile neutropenic patients who carry a low risk of morbidity and mortality. These factors include an ANC $>100/mm^3$, solid tumor, absence of comorbid medical conditions, young age, absence of focus of infection, and initial monocyte count $>0.1 \times 10^3/mm^3$. Such low-risk patients may be eligible for outpatient parenteral antibiotic therapy. The decision to manage patients on an outpatient basis is best handled by a pediatric oncologist, as it requires careful patient selection and follow-up. The choice of antibiotic regimen must consider the microbial sensitivity patterns in the institution. Combination therapy has been the usual approach to provide broad-spectrum antibiotic coverage (Table 75-4), which includes an aminoglycoside and an antipseudomonal beta lactam. Once-daily dosing of antibiotics, such as aminoglycosides and ceftriaxone, has been shown to be effective. The development of broad-spectrum antibiotics has made monotherapy an increasingly popular option. Ceftazidime, imipenem, cefipime, and meropenem have good activity against *Pseudomonas aeruginosa,* and each has been shown to be as efficacious as the standard combination therapy. The routine use of vancomycin in the initial empiric regimen has not shown to be of added benefit. However, vancomycin is warranted if there is evidence of intravenous catheter-related infection, methicillin-resistant *Staphylococcus aureus* colonization, severe chemotherapy-induced mucosal damage, fluoroquinolone prophylaxis, or septic shock.

Modifications to Therapy

Infections related to indwelling intravenous catheters are frequently due to gram-positive bacteria, especially staphylococci, but may be caused by gram-negative organisms or fungi. For febrile neutropenic patients with an indwelling catheter, vancomycin should be included in the initial therapy. For those patients with fever without neutropenia, the decision of initiating empiric therapy is still in question. However, it is probably safest to start antibiotics (vancomycin and a third-generation cephalosporin) pending culture results.

Patients with a focus of infection may require modifications in therapy. Signs or symptoms suggestive of an infection along the gastrointestinal tract warrant extended anaerobic coverage with either metronidazole or clindamycin. The presence of a pulmonary infiltrate may represent a bacterial, viral, fungal, or parasitic infection. Patients with diffuse or interstitial infiltrates receive trimethoprim-sulfamethoxazole (TMP-SMX) for possible *Pneumocystis carinii* infection, as well as erythromycin for *Legionella* and *Mycoplasma* coverage. In the face of neutropenia, these antibiotics are added to the baseline broad-spectrum therapy. In neutropenic patients with a patchy or localized infiltrate, broad-spectrum antibiotic therapy should suffice initially.

Fungal Infections

Cancer patients who are febrile and neutropenic are at risk for fungal infections, particularly *Candida* species. In pediatric patients, the oral cavity is the most common site for fungal infection. It may present asymptomatically as punctate foci or diffuse erythematous mucosal plaques and ulcerations. Any patient with difficulty breathing, hoarseness, or stridor should be considered to have epiglottic or laryngeal candidiasis. A potassium hydroxide preparation of a scraping reveals hyphae. A scraping from the base of a lesion is sent for fungal and viral culture. Neutropenic patients who are afebrile and able to tolerate oral medication may be treated with topical antifungal agents such as clotrimazole (10 mg troche 5 times per day). If there has been minimal response with clotrimazole, ketaconazole (5 to 10 mg/kg/day divided qd or bid) or fluconazole (2 to 8 mg/kg once daily) may be tried. Patients with oral or esophageal candidiasis who have not responded to or are unable to tolerate topical therapy are candidates for intravenous antifungal agents such as amphotericin B. Those with suspected epiglottic or laryngeal involvement may require airway support and close observation. In the emergency department, empiric intravenous antifungal therapy is usually not indicated for febrile patients.

Viral Infections

Herpes simplex virus (HSV) infections tend to be localized, even in the immunocompromised patient, and commonly involve the mouth, nares, esophagus, genitals, and perianal region. Pain is the predominant presenting symptom. Disruption of the mucosa may promote secondary bacterial infection. Laboratory diagnosis is confirmed through viral culture or direct immunofluorescence studies on the inoculated tissue culture. Immunocompromised patients with mild mucocutaneous disease may be started on oral acyclovir (200 mg PO 5 times a day). Patients with moderate or severe HSV infection should be admitted for intravenous acyclovir therapy (250 mg/m^2 IV q 8 h).

Varicella-zoster virus (VZV) infections in immunocompromised patients are associated with significant morbidity and mortality, including potential dissemination to the lung, CNS, and liver. Patients with Hodgkin's disease, NHL, solid tumors, and bone marrow transplants are particularly at risk. Diagnosis of VZV infection is usually based on the characteristic vesicular lesions. Laboratory confirmation is by positive culture of the virus from scraping of the base of the lesions. Direct immunofluorescence staining of the vesicular fluid smear or tissue specimen is also rapid and accurate. A chest radiograph is obtained to assess for pneumonia. Liver transaminases may be elevated in varicella hepatitis. Cancer patients with VZV infection are usually admitted for intravenous acyclovir. Varicella-zoster seronegative patients who are seen within 96 hours of virus exposure

Table 75-4. Empiric Antibiotic Therapy for Febrile Neutropenic Patients

Regimen	Drug	Dose	Notes
Monotherapy	Ceftazidime Or	150 mg/kg/day IV, divided q 8 h	Poor coverage for coagulase-negative staphylococci, methicillin-resistant
	Imipenem/cilastin Or	40–60 mg/kg/day IV divided q 6 h (max 2 g/day)	*Staphylococcus aureus,* eneterococci, some strains of penicillin-resistant *Strepococcus pneumoniae* and viridans
	Meropenem Or	60–120 mg/kg/day IV divided q 8 h	streptococci; meropenem and cefipime have enhanced gram-positive and gram-negative coverage
	Cefipime	150 mg/kg/day IV divided q 8 h	
Duotherapy (without vancomycin): Aminoglycoside			Avoid if patients are receiving nephrotoxic, ototoxic, or neuromuscular blocking agents or have
	Gentamicin Or	5–7.5 mg/kg/day IV divided q 8 h	renal dysfunction, severe electrolyte disturbance, or suspected meningitis
	Tobramycin Or	5–7.5 mg/kg/day IV divided q 8 h	(poor blood-brain barrier)
	Amikacin	30 mg/kg/day IV divided q 8 h	
PLUS: Antipseudomonal penicillin	Ticarcillin Or	300 mg/kg/day IV divided q 6 h	
	Ticarcillin/clavulanate Or	300 mg/kg/day IV divided q 6 h	
	Mezlocillin Or	300 mg/kg/day IV divided q 6 h	
	Piperacillin	300 mg/kg/day IV divided q 6 h	
OR Aminoglycoside	As above	As above	
PLUS Antipseudomonal cephalosporin	Ceftazidime OR	As above	
	Cefipime	As above	
If immediate-type penicillin allergy	Aztreonam	75–150 mg/kg/day IV divided q 4–6 h	
	Plus aminoglycoside	As above	
Regimen with vancomycin for additional gram-positive coverage (viridans streptococci, enterococci)	Vancomycin	40–60 mg/kg/day IV divided q 6 h	Indications: Obvious catheter-related infection Severe mucositis Quinolone prophylaxis prior to fever Colonization with methicillin-resistant *S. aureus* or penicillin/cephalosporin-resistant *S. pneumoniae* Hypotension
PLUS Antipseudomonal cephalosporin	Ceftazidime	As above	
If suspect *Pneumocystis carinii*	Add trimethoprim/ sulfamethoxazole	15–20 mg/kg/day IV divided q 6 h (based on trimethoprim component)	

Source: Adapted from Hughes WT, Armstrong D, Bodey GP, et al: 1997 guidelines for the use of antimicrobial agents in neutropenic patients with unexplained fever. *Clin Infect Dis* 25:551, 1997. Used with permission.

receive varicella-zoster immune globulin at a dose of 125 U per 10 kg body weight IM with a maximum dose of 625 U.

Parasitic Infections

P. carinii is the most common parasitic infection in immunocompromised patients. Children with hematologic malignancies are most at risk. Typically, patients will have fever, dry cough, tachypnea, and intercostal retractions without detectable rales. The chest radiograph may be normal in early disease, but later progresses to bilateral alveolar infiltrates. Atypical radiographic findings include lobar consolidation and effusion. Arterial blood gas analysis reveals a decrease in Po_2, normal or decreased Pco_2, and increased pH. Diagnosis is confirmed by bronchoalveolar lavage or open lung biopsy. Immunocompromised patients should be started on empiric therapy with TMP-SMX pending definitive diagnosis, as well as erythromycin for empiric *Legionella* coverage.

Tumor Lysis Syndrome

Tumor lysis syndrome results from the rapid degradation of tumor cells and release of the intracellular metabolites, uric acid, phosphate, and potassium in excess of their renal clearance. The result is hyperuricemia, hyperphosphatemia, and, in some cases, hyperkalemia.

The syndrome occurs prior to or within several days after the initiation of cancer therapy. It is more commonly seen in patients with a large tumor cell load or rapidly growing tumors such as Burkitt's lymphoma and T-cell lymphoma leukemia. The syndrome is generally not seen with nonlymphomatous solid tumors, although it may complicate chronic myelogenous leukemia.

Uric acid, a product of purine catabolism from nucleic acids, usually exists as a soluble form. However, with excessive amounts and in an acidic environment, as with concurrent lactic acidosis, it may precipitate in the renal collecting ducts, leading to obstruction, oliguria, azotemia, and renal failure. The phosphate concentration in lymphoblasts is four times higher than it is in normal lymphocytes. Calcium phosphate crystals start to form when the calcium-phosphate product exceeds 60 mg/dL and becomes trapped in the renal microvasculature. The result is renal failure and hypocalcemia. Potassium is a major intracellular electrolyte, which, with tumor lysis syndrome, can cause hyperkalemia, as well as exacerbate existing hyperkalemia due to renal failure. Cardiac complications include ventricular arrhythmias and asystole.

Signs and symptoms of tumor lysis syndrome include nausea, vomiting, lethargy, abdominal or back pain, and change in urine color and amount. Hypocalcemia may manifest as muscle weakness, spasms, tetany, convulsions, altered level of consciousness, photophobia, or abdominal pain.

All patients with possible tumor lysis syndrome require studies disclosing the following values: CBC; renal function, electrolytes, glucose, calcium, phosphate, uric acid, urinalysis; and electrocardiogram.

Therapy is directed at treatment of hyperuricemia and hyperphosphatemia and prevention of renal failure. Hydration is important in facilitating uric acid and phosphate excretion. Intravenous fluid is administered at a minimum of twice the patient's maintenance rate, aiming at a urine specific gravity >1.010. To treat hyperuricemia, uric acid production may be reduced with allopurinol (age >6 years: 300 mg PO q6h; age <6 years: 150 mg PO q6h), which inhibits xanthine oxidase, the enzyme that promotes the degradation of purine to uric acid. In addition to hydration therapy, alkalinization of the urine increases uric acid solubility and excretion. This is achieved by adding one ampul (44 mEq) of sodium bicarbonate to each liter of D_5 0.2 normal saline to keep the urine pH around 7 or 7.5. Urine pH >7.5 may promote precipitation of hypoxanthine and calcium phosphate, while uric acid crystals tend to form at a pH <7. Calcium supplementation for hypocalcemia is indicated only in patients who are severely symptomatic with a normal serum phosphate. Giving calcium in the face of hyperphosphatemia may increase the precipitation of calcium phosphate. Hyperkalemia may be reduced by calcium gluconate (100 to 200 mg/kg/dose slowly by IV), sodium bicarbonate, and insulin, along with dextrose. Sodium polystyrene sulfonate (Kayexalate) per rectum in neutropenic patients may create a perirectal infection and is therefore to be avoided. Dialysis is indicated for persistent hyperkalemia, uric acid concentrations exceeding 10 mg/dL, creatinine >10 mg/dL, phosphate >10 mg/dL, and symptomatic hypocalcemia.

Syndrome of Inappropriate Antidiuretic Hormone

The SIADH results in excessive free water retention and subsequent fall in serum sodium concentration. It is associated with a variety of conditions, including CNS infection and trauma, malignancy, stress, pain, pneumonia, and drugs. In pediatric cancer patients, SIADH is often related to chemotherapeutic agents such as vincristine, cisplatinum, and cyclophosphamide.

The syndrome is characterized by ongoing secretion of antidiuretic hormone (ADH) in response to a perceived hypovolemia, irrespective of the plasma osmolality. Antidiuretic hormone acts on the distal renal tubules and collecting ducts, causing reabsorption of free water. The result is reduced plasma osmolality and sodium concentration and water intoxication.

Clinically, patients may have weight gain, fatigue, lethargy, confusion, seizures, or coma. Typical laboratory studies reveal hyponatremia, hypoosmolality (often <260 mOsm/L), and an increase in urine osmolality and urine sodium concentration. Asymptomatic patients may be treated with fluid restriction to about two-thirds of their usual maintenance needs. Those symptomatic patients with hyponatremia and seizures or coma require correction of the serum sodium concentration to approximately 125 mEq/L with 3% saline (see Chapter 57).

Superior Vena Cava Syndrome

SVC syndrome refers to the signs and symptoms resulting from obstruction of the SVC. Although usually due to extrinsic compression of the SVC and its branches, up to one-half of the cases may have concomitant intravascular thrombosis. In children, compression of the narrow, more compliant trachea poses an additional complication.

This syndrome is rare, but it occurs in about 12 percent of pediatric patients with malignant anterior mediastinal tumors, most commonly NHL and Hodgkin's disease. The presence of central venous catheters predisposes to vascular thrombosis and SVC syndrome. When structures surrounding the SVC and trachea enlarge, they cause compression and result in clotting and edema formation, impeding airflow and blood return from the head, neck, and upper thorax. Collateral vessels become enlarged but provide inadequate compensation. In children and adolescents, symptoms of SVC syndrome may progress rapidly over several days, unlike adults where the onset is more insidious.

Patients have edema and plethora of the face, conjunctivae, neck, and upper torso. Tortuous collateral veins appear on the chest and upper abdomen. Headache, papilledema, seizures, coma, cerebral hemorrhage, and engorgement of retinal veins are a result of cerebral venous hypertension. Compression of the tracheobronchial tree may cause tachypnea, wheezing, stridor, orthopnea, or cyanosis. Other presentations include vocal cord paralysis, Horner's syndrome, and, in extreme cases, lower cervical or upper thoracic spinal cord compression. Fatalities from SVC syndrome are related to airway obstruction, cerebral edema, or cardiac compromise.

Chest radiography reveals superior mediastinal widening and occasionally a pleural or pericardial effusion. The trachea may appear deviated or narrowed. Computed tomography scan or MRI allows for identification of the lesion causing obstruction and the anatomic level of obstruction. A CBC with differential may show evidence of leukemia or lymphoma.

The first priority in management is to protect and secure the airway. If SVC syndrome is due to central venous catheter thrombosis, a thrombolytic agent such as urokinase might avoid the need to remove the catheter. Radiation has been the traditional mode of therapy for tumor-induced SVC syndrome. Chemotherapy was an effective alternative, but side effects were significant and results were often suboptimal. More recently, treatment of SVC syndrome utilizes a combination of endovascular techniques, including thrombolysis, angioplasty, stent therapy and surgical bypass. Some patients will require empiric therapy prior to tissue diagnosis to reduce the compressive effects of the tumor.

Supportive therapy includes minimizing cerebral hypertension by elevation of the head of the bed. Intravenous hydration may be more efficient through a low-pressure lower extremity vein. Upper extremity phlebotomy should be avoided as these veins are under high pressure and may bleed excessively. Correction of electrolyte abnormalities and treatment of hyperuricemia should be initiated.

Spinal Cord Compression

Spinal cord compression due to a tumor occurs in approximately 4 percent of pediatric cancer patients. Extradural metastatic tumors such as soft tissue sarcomas, neuroblastoma, germ cell tumors, and Hodgkin's disease account for the majority of cases, while a few may be related to an intradural cord tumor or treatment-related myelopathy. Pain is the most common and usual initial presenting symptom. The pain is usually worse when supine and localized in the thoracic region; it is tender with percussion. Thoracic radicular pain is usually bilateral, but more often unilateral in the cervical or lumbar area. Muscle weakness, which is usually symmetric, is a later finding. Most patients with weakness will already have extradural spinal cord compression at the time of diagnosis. Sensory deficits are less common than is weakness and present with ascending numbness and paraesthesias. Changes in bladder or bowel function are also a common but late finding. Hydrocephalus may result from physical obstruction from a high cervical tumor or elevated cerebrospinal fluid protein levels. Most patients will usually have objective neurologic deficits at the time of presentation.

Plain spine radiographs will show an abnormality in <50 percent of patients with spinal cord compression. Contrast myelography or MRI provides a more definitive study.

Spinal cord compression is a true neurologic emergency. Treatment begins with dexamethasone to reduce tumor-related edema. Myelography or MRI should be done immediately in those patients with progressive neurologic deficit or within 24 hours in stable symptomatic patients without loss of function. Patients should be promptly referred for possible radiation therapy. Analgesics for pain management are appropriate. Epidural masses require immediate decompression with corticosteroids or radiation therapy. Chemotherapy is an option for chemotherapy-sensitive diseases such as Hodgkin's disease, NHL, neuroblastoma, or germ cell tumors.

Central Nervous System Emergencies

Children with cancer may have CNS abnormalities, such as altered mental status, intracranial hemorrhage, and seizures. Metabolic or structural insults to the reticular activating system or cerebral hemispheres may alter patients' level of consciousness and may or may not be accompanied by raised ICP. Electrolyte abnormalities, hypoxia, renal or hepatic failure, disseminated intravascular coagulation, and sepsis are some common metabolic derangements. Primary CNS tumors and metastatic lesions may present with acute mental status changes. CNS infections may be diffuse or localized. Hyperviscosity may present with headache, visual changes, lethargy, focal deficits, or coma; treatment includes plasmapheresis and chemotherapy. Cerebrovascular accidents may complicate acute leukemia as a result of thrombosis or hemorrhage. Occasionally, hemorrhage can occur at the site of intracerebral metastases. Unlike primary intracerebral hemorrhage, intratumor hemorrhage is treated with corticosteroids. Subdural and subarachnoid hemorrhage may occur due to thrombocytopenia or coagulopathy. Cerebral arterial or venous thrombosis may occur after CNS irradiation or chemotherapy. Leukemic cells are rich in procoagulants, which are released upon cell lysis and predispose to thrombus formation. Seizures may arise from a metabolic abnormality, infection, metastatic disease, or as a complication of CNS therapy. The initial evaluation includes the following values: CBC, electrolytes, glucose, creatinine, blood urea nitrogen, phosphate, calcium, uric acid, magnesium, and coagulation studies. Arterial blood gas analysis or oxygen saturation is obtained to evaluate for hypoxia. A CT scan of the head without contrast can assess for tumor or intracranial bleeding.

Treatment for patients with altered mental status begins with support and protection of the airway and breathing. If raised ICP is suspected, controlled ventilation to a P_{CO_2} of 30 to 35 mmHg will cause cerebral vasoconstriction and thereby help reduce cerebral blood flow. Dexamethasone is given to those patients with an intracranial tumor in order to decrease cerebral edema. Hyperosmolar agents, such as mannitol, may help to reduce cerebral edema by creating an osmotic gradient between the blood and the brain with an intact blood-brain barrier. Use of a diuretic (furosemide) in conjunction with mannitol may enhance the reduction in ICP. Prompt surgical consultation is recommended if a mass lesion or hemorrhage is demonstrated on CT scan. If meningitis is suspected, lumbar puncture is deferred but antibiotics are initiated prior to the CT scan. Thrombocytopenia and coagulopathy are corrected, especially in the presence of an intracranial hemorrhage.

Gastrointestinal Emergencies

In addition to the more common causes of acute abdominal pain, pediatric cancer patients with an acute abdomen are at risk for unique conditions, such as esophagitis, gastric ulcers, typhlitis (a severe necrotizing cecitis occurring in neutropenic patients), perirectal abscess, pancreatitis, and cholecystitis. Several different lesions that can occur at any site along the gastrointestinal tract have been identified in patients with leukemia. Leukemic infiltrates can accumulate in the stomach and small bowel, predisposing to intussusception and bowel obstruction. Hemorrhagic necrosis of the mucosal layer can occur and may be related to vascular insufficiency, coagulation abnormalities, or chemotherapeutic agents. Agranulocytic necrosis is a result of bacterial invasion of the bowel wall and is complicated by perforation. Fungal lesions can invade the gastrointestinal tract or solid organs. Perirectal cellulites and abscess result from anaerobic and gram-negative bacteria invading the perirectal area. Gastrointestinal hemorrhage can result from thrombocytopenia, coagulopathy, mucosal ulceration, or abnormal tumor vessels.

Determining the etiology of the abdominal pain may be difficult in neutropenic or immunosuppressed patients, since processes that are usually localized in a normal host are often more diffuse in patients with this complaint. In addition, the inflammatory response may be variable.

Evaluation of cancer patients with acute abdominal pain includes characterization of the pain and associated symptoms. The abdominal exam begins with careful observation, gentle palpation, and serial reexamination. Rectal examination is key in detecting pelvic and perirectal disease, and neutropenia is not a contraindication to this maneuver.

Laboratory work-up includes a CBC, blood and urine cultures, urinalysis, and values of electrolytes, glucose, and amylase. A chest radiograph is done to assess for pneumonia, while abdominal films may reveal bowel obstruction, perforation, or pneumatosis intestinalis.

Patients with an acute pain in the abdomen should be admitted and started on intravenous hydration. Nonneutropenic patients with esophagitis and presumptive gastric stress ulcers may benefit from H_2 antagonists. Thrombocytopenia and coagulopathies are corrected in the presence of hemorrhage. Patients with typhlitis must be started on broad-spectrum antibiotics. Early surgical consultation is recommended. Indications for laparotomy include evidence of perforation, persistent gastrointestinal hemorrhage despite correction of existing coagulopathies, and clinical deterioration.

BIBLIOGRAPHY

Abramson DH, Frank CM, Susman M, et al: Presenting signs of retinoblastoma. *J Pediatr* 132:505, 1998.

Barri YM, Knochel JP: Hypercalcemia and electrolyte disturbances in malignancy. *Hematol Oncol Clin North Am* 10:775, 1996.

Fisman DN, Kaye KM: Once-daily dosing of aminoglycoside antibiotics. *Infect Dis Clin North Am* 14:475, 2000.

Freifeld AG, Pizzo PA: The outpatient management of febrile neutropenia in cancer patients. *Oncology* 10:599, 1996.

Hughes WT, Armstrong D, Bodey GP, et al: 1997 Guidelines for the use of antimicrobial agents in neutropenic patients with unexplained fever. *Clin Infect Dis* 25:551, 1997.

Klaassen RJ, Goodman TR, Doyle JJ: "Low-risk" prediction rule for pediatric oncology patients presenting with fever and neutropenia. *J Clin Oncol* 18:1012, 2000.

Mullen CA, Petropoulos D, Roberts WM, et al: Outpatient treatment of fever and neutropenia for low risk pediatric cancer patients. *Cancer* 86:126, 1999.

Schiff D, Butchelor T, Wen PY: Neurologic emergencies in cancer patients. *Neurol Clin* 16:449, 1998.

Schinder N, Vogelzang RL: Superior vena cava syndrome: Experience with endovascular stents and surgical therapy. *Surg Clin North Am* 79:684, 1999.

76

Infectious Musculoskeletal Disorders

Gary R. Strange
Diana Mayer

HIGH-YIELD FACTS

- *Staphylococcus aureus* predominates as the cause of septic arthritis and osteomyelitis. Other bacteria commonly implicated, especially in younger patients, include pneumococcus and group A *Streptococcus.*

- Neonates and young infants are particularly vulnerable to infection of the hip. In older infants and children, the knee is more commonly affected.

- No single test or finding is sufficient to predict the presence of a septic joint, but, by using four clinical predictors, investigators have shown >99 percent accuracy in predicting the presence of a septic joint:

  - History of fever
  - Inability to bear weight
  - Elevated erythrocyte sedimentation rate (>40 mm/hr)
  - Elevated white blood cell count (>12,000/mm^3)

- The mainstay in the diagnosis of septic arthritis is analysis of joint fluid. Fluid is usually obtained by percutaneous aspiration, which, in the case of a suspected septic hip joint, is facilitated by sonographic guidance.

- Treatment of septic arthritis consists of antibiotic therapy directed at the likely bacterial organisms and drainage of the involved joint. Serial aspiration is generally indicated for joints that are easily accessible, with incision and drainage procedures preferred for joints that are more difficult to access for serial aspiration or when serial aspiration has not resulted in resolution of fluid accumulation.

- Ultrasound is able to detect subperiosteal abscesses accurately and simply early in the course of the disease and may be the only imaging test required in uncomplicated cases. Magnetic resonance imaging has the highest sensitivity and specificity for detecting osteomyelitis.

- Intervertebral diskitis is an acute infection of the vertebral disk usually seen in children younger than 5 years. The lumbar area is most commonly involved.

- Lyme disease is caused by the spirochete *Borrelia burgdorferi* and is transmitted by *Ixodes scapularis,* commonly called the deer tick. In the United States, most cases are seen in southern New England, the Middle Atlantic states, and the upper Midwest.

- The early localized phase of Lyme disease begins around 1 week after inoculation by the tick and is marked by a characteristic rash known as erythema migrans. The lesion starts as an erythematous papule or macule that spreads outward to form an enlarging circle with a red rim and central clearing.

- Treatment of early localized infection will stop progression of the disease, and the prognosis is excellent, even if treatment is not begun until the late phase. In contrast to studies in adults, long-term follow-up studies of children with Lyme disease do not show an increased risk of cognitive impairment.

Musculoskeletal diseases are frequently encountered in pediatric patients. They vary in significance from minor, self-limited illnesses to serious systemic diseases. Limb-threatening complications can occur. In the case of infants and young children, the evaluation of musculoskeletal complaints is complicated by the patient's inability to articulate the problem and the inherent difficulty of performing a sufficient physical examination in an uncooperative patient.

SEPTIC ARTHRITIS

Septic arthritis is an infection within a joint space. It occurs more commonly in children than in adults, and the frequency is greater in infants and toddlers than in older children. Half of all cases occur in the first 2 years of life, and three-fourths of all cases are in children younger than 5 years. For unknown reasons, males are more frequently affected than females. The infection involves a joint of the lower extremity in 75 percent of cases, with the knee and hip being the most frequently involved joints.

Etiology

A microbial etiology can be defined in about two-thirds of cases. Seeding of the joint with bacteria occurs either by hematogenous spread, direct inoculation of infected material into the joint capsule, or spread from an adjacent site of infection. Infection secondary to trauma most commonly affects the knee. Spread from a contiguous focus is uncommon, but, in neonates and small infants, metaphyseal osteomyelitis can spread to the joint via blood vessels that bridge the epiphysis. In otherwise healthy children, most cases of septic arthritis are thought to be of hematogenous origin.

The bacterial pathogen in septic arthritis depends largely on the age of the patient. In the first 2 months of life, *Staphylococcus aureus* and group B *Streptococcus* are the most common pathogens. However, infection with gram-negative organisms such as *Escherichia coli* can occur. From 3 months to 3 years, *Haemophilus influenzae* type B accounted for over half of cases until widespread use of vaccination for this pathogen essentially eliminated it. *Staphylococcus aureus* predominates as the cause of septic arthritis until adolescence, when *Neisseria gonorrhoeae* becomes a frequent pathogen. Other bacteria commonly implicated in septic arthritis, especially in younger patients, include pneumococcus and group A *Streptococcus*. Immunosuppressed patients are particularly vulnerable to infection with gram-negative organisms, including *Pseudomonas*.

Clinical Presentation

The clinical presentation of septic arthritis varies with age. Neonates and young infants are particularly vulnerable to infection of the hip. The first manifestation of disease may be nonspecific irritability. Parents may note that the baby appears to be in pain when its diaper is changed. As the disease progresses, the baby holds the hip flexed and abducted, which allows for maximum opening of the joint capsule and helps relieve pressure. These infants do not appear particularly ill, and fever is much less common than in older children. The presence of lethargy may indicate concomitant meningitis.

In older infants and children, the knee is more commonly affected. Patients old enough to ambulate may begin to walk with a limp or may refuse to walk altogether. Unlike the hip, where significant swelling may be absent, septic arthritis of the knee and most other joints is characterized by warmth, the presence of an effusion, and, in most cases, significant limitation in range of motion. Most patients in this age group are febrile.

Gonococcal arthritis is likely in any postpubertal patient with joint pain and fever. It usually accompanies asymptomatic disease of the genitourinary tract. In the early stages, patients may complain of fever, chills, and polyarthralgia. The knee, the ankle, and especially the joints of the wrist, hand, and finger are affected. Some patients develop tenosynovitis. A rash may develop that can consist of petechiae, papules, and pustular lesions with erythematous halos. Monoarticular arthritis can eventually occur.

Diagnostic Evaluation

The laboratory evaluation of suspected septic arthritis includes a complete blood count, erythrocyte sedimentation rate, blood culture, and joint fluid analysis. In most patients, the white blood count and the erythrocyte sedimentation rate will be elevated. Many patients, especially neonates and young infants, will have positive blood cultures.

No single test or finding is sufficient to predict the presence of a septic joint, but, by using four clinical predictors, investigators have shown >99 percent accuracy in predicting the presence of a septic joint:

- History of fever

- Inability to bear weight

- Elevated erythrocyte sedimentation rate (>40 mm/hr)

- Elevated white blood cell count (>12,000/mm^3)

The mainstay in the diagnosis of septic arthritis is analysis of joint fluid. Fluid is usually obtained by percutaneous aspiration. In the case of a suspected septic hip joint, aspiration is facilitated by sonographic guidance. The fluid from a septic joint is often turbid. Although there is considerable overlap in the cell count between bacterially mediated arthritis and other causes of joint inflammation, the white blood cell count in a septic joint is generally >50,000 to 75,000/mL and is associated with >75 percent neutrophils. The amount of glucose in an infected joint is often <50 percent of the serum value. Table 76-1 contrasts the characteristics of joint fluid under various conditions. Culture of the joint fluid is positive in up to 70 percent of patients except in the case of gonococcal arthritis, in which the culture is usually negative. Up to 50 percent of patients have a positive Gram's stain.

Radiographic studies may be useful in demonstrating the presence of a joint effusion and to rule out other etiologies, such as trauma, but normal plain films do not rule out a septic joint. Ultrasound is most useful in evaluating the potentially septic hip. Radionuclide scanning can be helpful in difficult cases. Magnetic resonance imaging (MRI) is highly sensitive in detecting signal intensity alterations in the bone marrow of septic hips and in differentiating septic arthritis from transient synovitis.

In infants, if clinical findings are indicative of or cannot exclude meningitis, a lumbar puncture is also indicated.

Differential Diagnosis

The differential diagnosis of septic arthritis includes transient synovitis, cellulitis, traumatic hemarthrosis, os-

teomyelitis, and a multitude of processes that can cause sterile joint inflammation, such as collagen vascular diseases and Henoch-Schönlein purpura. It is also common for children with acute leukemia to have bone or joint pain. In the hip, a number of problems specific to that joint must be considered. These include Legg-Calvé-Perthes disease, slipped captial femoral epiphysis, psoas abscess, obturator internus abscess, and diskitis. In the knee, the possibility of referred pain from the hip must be considered. Nonbacterial causes of infectious arthritis include viral, mycoplasmal, mycobacterial, and fungal etiologies. Fungal etiology is a greater consideration for premature infants and for those with central venous catheters. Reactive arthritides following streptococcal infections, gastrointestinal problems, and viral hepatitis may be especially difficult to diagnose since the interval between the inciting illness and the reactive arthritis may be 2 weeks or more.

Treatment

Treatment of septic arthritis consists of antibiotic therapy directed at the likely bacterial organisms and drainage of the involved joint. In neonates, antibiotic treatment usually consists of an antistaphylococcal penicillin, such as oxacillin (150 to 200 mg/kg/24 hr in 3 to 4 divided doses), and a broad-spectrum cephalosporin, such as cefotaxime (100 to 150 mg/kg/24 hr in 3 to 4 divided doses). Aminoglycoside antibiotics have reduced activity in joint infections and are not considered first-line choices. Older infants and children younger than 10 years of age can be treated with nafcillin (150 mg/kg/24 hr in 4 divided does) or a second- or third-generation cephalosporin, such as cefotaxime (150 mg/kg/24 hr in 3 divided doses) or ceftriaxone (50 mg/kg/24 hr given once daily). If *N. gonorrhoeae* is a possibility, ceftriaxone is the drug of choice. With drainage and appropriate antibiotic therapy, improvement should be rapid. Shorter

Table 76-1. Analysis of Joint Fluid

Characteristic	Normal	Bacterial	Inflammatory
Appearance	Clear	Turbid, purulent	Clear or turbid
Leukocytes (cells/mL)	<100	>50,000	500–75,000
Neutrophils (%)	25	>75	50
Glucose (synovial/blood)	>50%	<50%	>50%

Table 76-2. Treatment of Septic Arthritis and Osteomyelitis

Age or Condition Group	Organisms	Initial Antibiotics

Neonates	Group B *Streptococcus*
	Staphylococcus aureus
	Gram-negative enteric bacilli
	Candida[a]
	Neisseria gonorrhoeae[a]
		Oxacillin,
		  150–200 mg/kg/24 hr in 3–4 divided doses
		  and
		Cefotaxime, 100–150 mg/kg/24 hr in 3–4
		  divided doses

Infants and children <5 years of age	*Staphylococcus aureus* Group A *Streptococcus* *Haemophilus influenzae* type B (HiB)—if unimmunized	Ceftriaxone, 50 mg/kg/24 hr given once daily

Children >5 years of age	*Staphylococcus aureus*	Nafcillin, 150 mg/kg/24 hr in 4 divided doses
		  or
		Cephalothin, 100–150 mg/kg/24 hr in
		  4 divided doses
		  or
		Vancomycin, 40 mg/kg/24 hr in 4 divided
		  doses—if suspicion of methicillin-resistant
		  staphylococcal infection

Children >5 years of age
  without HiB immunization
	Staphylococcus aureus
	Haemophilus influenzae type B
		Cefuroxime, 100–150 mg/kg/24 hr in 3
		  divided doses

Adolescents	*Neisseria gonorrhoeae* *Staphylococcus aureus*	Ceftriaxone, 50 mg/kg/24 hr given once daily

Immunocompromised	Gram-negative enteric bacilli
	Staphylococcus aureus
	Pseudomonas aeruginosa
		Ceftazidime, 100–150 mg/kg/24 hr in 3
		  divided doses
		  and
		Vancomycin, 40 mg/kg/24 hr in 4 divided
		  doses

Sickle cell disease	*Salmonella* spp.
	Gram-negative enteric bacilli
	Staphylococcus aureus
		Ceftriaxone, 50 mg/kg/24 hr given once daily
		
		  and
		Nafcillin, 150 mg/kg/24 hr in 4 divided doses
		  or
		Cephalothin, 100–150 mg/kg/24 hr in
		  4 divided doses

Puncture wounds of
  the foot
	Pseudomonas aeruginosa
	Staphylococcus aureus
		Ceftazidime, 100–150 mg/kg/24 hr in 3
		  divided doses
		  and
		Nafcillin, 150 mg/kg/24 hr in 4 divided doses

courses of antibiotic therapy are now used for these infections, but a minimum of 21 days of therapy is recommended for *S. aureus* and gram-negative infections; 14 days for group A *Streptococcus,* pneumococcus, and *H. influenzae* type B; and 7 days for *N. gonorrhoeae.* Table 76-2 summarizes the treatment.

The procedure used for drainage depends to some degree on the joint involved. Serial aspiration is generally indicated for joints that are easily accessible, such as the knee. Incision and drainage procedures are preferred in joints that are more difficult to access frequently for serial aspiration, such as the hip or shoulder, or when serial aspiration has not resulted in resolution of fluid accumulation.

OSTEOMYELITIS

Osteomyelitis is an infection of the bone. In the pediatric age group, it is most common between the ages of 3 and 12 years. Boys are more commonly affected than girls.

Pathophysiology

Seeding of the bone with bacteria occurs by hematogenous spread, direct inoculation, or extension from an adjacent septic joint. Neonates subjected to invasive procedures in the setting of the intensive care unit are especially prone to develop osteomyelitis.

The anatomy of the growth plate may contribute to the development of osteomyelitis. The metaphysis possesses a rich capillary network with loops that have few anastomotic connections. This may result in sluggish circulation that can promote seeding with bacteria. In addition, fenestrations present in metaphyseal cortical bone are potential sites for seeding by bacteria. Infection usually develops in the metaphysis and may spread along the bone. The incidence of adjacent joint involvement may be higher than previously reported, with up to one-third of patients having septic joint involvement.

Etiology

Overall, the most common etiology of osteomyelitis is *S. aureus.* In neonates, group B *Streptococcus* and enteric gram-negative organisms are also possible etiologies. *H. influenzae* should be considered in infants and toddlers if they have not been adequately immunized. *Pseudomonas aeruginosa* is often associated with osteomyelitis after puncture wounds of the foot. *Salmonella* is a consideration in sickle cell anemia patients.

Clinical Manifestations

The presentation of osteomyelitis varies according to age. Neonates may demonstrate few clinical findings other than irritability, fever, and some resistance to movement. Older infants and children may be able to localize discomfort over the affected site. Limp is a common finding in ambulatory patients. Most patients are febrile. In some cases, the physical examination reveals erythema, warmth, and swelling over the area of bone involvement, but more subtle presentations are common.

Diagnostic Testing

Laboratory assessment includes a complete blood count, erythrocyte sedimentation rate, blood culture, and radiograph of the affected area. The white blood cell count may be normal or elevated, but the erythrocyte sedimentation rate is usually increased. Blood cultures are positive about 50 percent of the time.

Radiographs are usually unremarkable during the first week of the illness. Mottling and demineralization are usually observed a week after the initial symptoms. New periosteal bone formation is often evident after 10 days of symptoms.

Radionuclear scanning with technetium-99m is often utilized because it is more sensitive than radiography early in the course of disease. Increased uptake is usually observed within 1 to 2 days after the onset of infection. However, false-negative studies occur up to 25 percent of the time, particularly in infants and young children. Other processes, such as cellulitis, trauma, and tumors, may also result in increased uptake, simulating osteomyelitis. Gallium-67 or indium-111 bone scan may be useful when technetium-99m scans are inconclusive.

Ultrasound is able to detect subperiosteal abscesses accurately and simply early in the course of the disease and may be the only imaging test required in uncomplicated cases. MRI has the highest sensitivity and specificity for detecting osteomyelitis. MR diagnosis is based on the bone marrow and surrounding soft tissue. Computed tomography is also useful and can be considered when MRI is unavailable or impractical.

The diagnosis is confirmed by needle aspiration of infected material. A steel needle is needed to penetrate the cortex. Aspiration of subperiosteal or metaphyseal pus confirms the diagnosis and provides an excellent specimen for culture.

Treatment

Treatment for osteomyelitis is directed at eradicating the infection. Antibiotic coverage for *S. aureus* is always indicated. Other antibiotic coverage depends on the age of the patient and the clinical situation. In general, hospitalization is warranted. Table 76-2 lists antibiotic coverage for osteomyelitis under various circumstances. If chronic osteomyelitis develops, surgery may be required to evacuate pus or to excise necrotic tissue.

INTERVERTEBRAL DISKITIS

Intervertebral diskitis is an acute infection of the vertebral disk occasionally seen in children. Affected patients are usually younger than 5 years old. The lumbar area is most commonly involved. The most common pathogen is *S. aureus*. Less commonly, pneumococcus and gramnegative organisms are involved. Rarely, the infection results from tuberculosis.

Most cases are preceded by an upper respiratory infection. Infants may become irritable and refuse to sit. Toddlers may refuse to walk. Older children may complain of back or leg pain and may develop a limp. If the lesion occurs at the lower thoracic or upper lumbar area, the child may have gastrointestinal symptoms.

The physical examination may show a loss of lordosis. If the cervical vertebrae are involved, torticollis can occur. Tenderness along the vertebrae, mild fullness of the paraspinal muscles secondary to irritation, and occasionally hip pain and stiffness can occur. Fever may be present.

The erythrocyte sedimentation rate is usually elevated. In about 40 percent of cases, blood cultures are positive.

Radiographs of the involved area may demonstrate a narrowing of the disk space and, eventually, erosion of the vertebral end plates. Technetium-99m bone and MRI scans are able to diagnose the disease early in the course.

Affected children can usually be managed as outpatients, with antibiotic therapy directed against *S. aureus*. Despite treatment, older children commonly develop spontaneous spinal fusion.

LYME DISEASE

Lyme disease is caused by the spirochete *Borrelia burgdorferi* and is transmitted by *Ixodes scapularis*, commonly called the deer tick. In the United States, most cases are seen in southern New England, the Middle Atlantic states, and the upper Midwest. A smaller number of cases are reported from the Pacific states. Many patients do not recall being bitten, probably due to the tick's small size.

The overall risk of acquiring Lyme disease is low even in endemic areas. Prevention efforts center around the use of protective clothing and insect repellants, followed by close checking for ticks after exposure. Recombinant Lyme vaccines are safe and effective but are not licensed for use in children younger than 15 years of age.

Lyme disease is divided into two stages: early and late illness. The early stage is further split into an early localized phase and an early disseminated phase. The early localized phase begins around 1 week after inoculation by the tick and is marked by a characteristic rash known as erythema migrans. The lesion starts as an erythematous papule or macule that spreads outward to form an enlarging circle with a red rim and central clearing. In some cases, the center of the lesion may become vesicular or necrotic. It often disappears within 4 weeks of the initial tick bite. In addition to erythema migrans, some patients experience flu-like illness.

Those with early disseminated disease will often develop secondary erythema migrans, presenting with several lesions that are smaller than the initial lesion. These lesions appear several days to weeks after the original lesion and are often accompanied by fever, myalgias, headache, malaise, conjunctivitis, and lymphadenopathy. Patients may develop aseptic meningitis, encephalitis, or radiculopathies. Cranial neuritis, such as facial nerve palsy, may also occur. Arthralgia is also seen in this stage, as is carditis.

The late stage of Lyme disease consists of arthritis and, rarely, fever and encephalopathy. Large joints are most commonly affected, especially the knee, although virtually any joint can be involved. The swelling observed is usually out of proportion to the discomfort experienced by the patient. The arthritis usually occurs months after the initial inoculation, lasts for 1 to 2 weeks, and may recur.

The differential diagnosis of Lyme arthritis includes septic joint, acute rheumatic fever, juvenile rheumatoid arthritis, and postinfectious virally induced arthritis.

Laboratory studies include a complete blood count, antinuclear antibody, rheumatoid factor, urinalysis, electrocardiogram, throat culture, and Lyme disease titers. Joint fluid in patients with active arthritis may contain up to 100,000 white blood cells/mL, with a preponderance of polymorphonuclear leukocytes. Joint aspiration for culturing *B. burgdorferi* is considered impractical at this time because the cultivation period can take up to 4 weeks. The culture medium is also expensive and not readily available. Confirmation of Lyme disease is based on demonstration of antibodies to *B. burgdorferi* that appear after about a month of disease.

Antibiotic treatment of Lyme disease shortens the course of disease and can prevent the development of chronic illness. In some cases it effectively treats established chronic arthritis and neurologic symptoms. Erythema migrans and disseminated early disease without focal findings are treated with oral doxycycline or amoxicillin for 21 days. Children younger than 8 years of age should not receive doxycycline. Erythromycin can be substituted for allergic patients. Cranial nerve palsies and arthritis are treated with the same medication, but for 30 days. Intravenous or intramuscular treatment is used for patients with carditis or neurologic disease other than cranial nerve palsy. Treatment is with ceftriaxone or penicillin for 14 to 21 days. Symptomatic arthritis may respond to therapy with nonsteroidal antiinflammatory agents.

Treatment of early localized infection will stop progression of the disease, and the prognosis is excellent, even if treatment is not begun until the late phase. In contrast to studies in adults, long-term follow-up studies of children with Lyme disease do not show an increased risk of cognitive impairment.

ACUTE SUPPURATIVE TENOSYNOVITIS

The palmar surface of the hand is vulnerable to suppurative tenosynovitis, because the flexor tendons of the finger are surrounded by a synovial sheath that localizes an infection and, if treatment is delayed, can provide a conduit for spread to deep spaces of the palm. It usually occurs as an extension of a localized infection.

Physical examination of the hand reveals erythema and tenderness along the tendon sheath. Patients hold the affected finger in a flexed position, and active or passive extension provokes intense pain. The affected finger is diffusely swollen.

The most common bacterial etiologies are *S. aureus* and group A *Streptococcus*. In adolescents and sexually abused children, *N. gonorrhoeae* is a likely possibility.

Management consists of therapy with antibiotics and surgical drainage.

BIBLIOGRAPHY

Adams WV, Rose CD, Eppes SC, et al: Long-term cognitive effects of Lyme disease in children. *Appl Neurospsychol* 6:39–45, 1999.

Bachman DT, Srivastava G: Emergency department presentations of Lyme disease in children. *Pediatr Emerg Care* 14:356–361, 1998.

Fernandez M, Carrol CL, Baker CJ: Discitis and vertebral osteomyelitis in children: An 18-year review. *Pediatrics* 105:1299–1304, 2000.

Kaiser S, Jorulf H, Hirsch G: Clinical value of imaging techniques in childhood osteomyelitis. *Acta Radiol* 39:523–531, 1998.

Klein DM, Barbera C, Gray ST, et al: Sensitivity of objective parameters in the diagnosis of pediatric septic hips. *Clin Orthop* 338:153–159, 1997.

Kocher MS, Zurakowski D, Kasser JR: Differentiating between septic arthritis and transient synovitis of the hip in children: An evidence-based clinical prediction algorithm. *J Bone Joint Surg [Am]* 81:1662–1670, 1999.

Lee SK, Suh KJ, Kim YW, et al: Septic arthritis versus transient synovitis at MR imaging: Preliminary assessment with signal intensity alterations in bone marrow. *Radiology* 211:459–465, 1999.

Nelson JD: Osteomyelitis and suppurative arthritis, in Behrman RE, Kliegman RM, Jenson HB (eds): *Nelson Textbook of Pediatrics,* 16th ed. Philadelphia: WB Saunders, 2000, pp 776–780.

Perlman MH, Patzakis MJ, Kumar PJ, et al: The incidence of joint involvement with adjacent osteomyelitis in pediatric patients. *J Pediatr Orthop* 20:40–43, 2000.

Shapiro ED: Lyme disease *(Borrelia burgdorferi),* in Behrman RE, Kliegman RM, Jenson HB (eds): *Nelson Textbook of Pediatrics,* 16th ed. Philadelphia: WB Saunders, 2000, pp 911–914.

77

Inflammatory Musculoskeletal Disorders

Gary R. Strange
Diana Mayer

HIGH-YIELD FACTS

- In many inflammatory and infectious disorders, arthritis is an associated finding in which joint manifestations appear to be secondary to an immunologic reaction to the disease process.

- The treatment of reactive arthritis is with antiinflammatory agents. Antibiotic therapy has not been shown to be helpful once reactive arthritis has developed.

- Toxic synovitis of the hip is an inflammatory process that often follows an upper respiratory infection. The disorder is usually seen in children between the ages of 18 months and 7 years, with a presenting complaint of refusal to walk.

- Ultrasound is useful for detecting the joint effusion and guiding arthrocentesis. However, in the absence of fever and without elevated white blood cell count and erythrocyte sedimentation rate, septic joint is unlikely, and the diagnosis of transient synovitis can be made without obtaining joint fluid.

- In juvenile rheumatoid arthritis (JRA), polyarticular disease involves more than four joints, usually begins in large joints, and is often symmetrical.

- Pauciarticular JRA by definition involves four or fewer joints. Large joints are most commonly affected, although hip involvement is unusual.

- Systemic onset JRA occurs throughout childhood and is more common in boys. Intermittent spiking fever is especially common and is often the initial manifestation of disease.

- The treatment of JRA consists of aggressive therapy with nonsteroidal antiinflammatory drugs (NSAIDs). For pauciarticular disease, intraarticular steroids may be used, and for polyarticular and more severe cases, cytotoxic drugs or gold salts may be effective.

- Systemic lupus erythematosus (SLE) is an inflammatory disease of probable autoimmune etiology that affects multiple organ systems. About 20 percent of cases of SLE begin in childhood or adolescence.

- Therapy for SLE is directed primarily at ameliorating the underlying inflammatory process. In mild disease, NSAIDs may suffice, but most patients will require steroids.

- The diagnosis of rheumatic fever is made by utilizing a combination of clinical and laboratory findings, summarized in the modified Jones criteria.

- Patients with suspected ARF are admitted to the hospital. Penicillin is indicated to eradicate any residual carriage of group A *Streptococcus,* and patients with arthritis but without carditis are managed with high-dose aspirin.

- Ankylosing spondylitis is a rheumatic disorder that can present in later childhood or adolescence. The disorder is predominantly characterized by involvement of the sacroiliac joints and lumbar spine, but many patients have associated peripheral arthritis.

REACTIVE AND POSTINFECTIOUS ARTHRITIS

In many inflammatory and infectious disorders, arthritis is an associated finding in which joint manifestations appear to be secondary to an immunologic reaction to the disease process. Although this is considered a sterile synovitis, bacterial degradation products and even bacterial DNA have been isolated.

A number of enteric processes are associated with reactive arthritis. Both ulcerative colitis and Crohn's disease can be associated with arthritis, as can gastroenteritis caused by *Shigella, Salmonella, Yersinia, Giardia,* and *Campylobacter.* Many viral infections, including hepatitis and infections due to Epstein-Barr virus, adenovirus, and rubella, are also associated with arthritis. Infection with *Mycoplasma pneumoniae* is also occasionally associated with arthritis. Reiter's syndrome, which consists of urethritis, conjunctivitis, and arthritis, can follow infections caused by *Shigella* or sexually transmitted diseases, such as gonorrhea and chlamydia. The treatment of reactive arthritis is with antiinflammatory agents. Antibiotic therapy has not been shown to be helpful for full-blown reactive arthritis, but antibiotics probably are helpful in preventing the development of reactive arthritis when the primary problem is diagnosed prior to the development of arthritis.

TRANSIENT SYNOVITIS

A common cause of nontraumatic hip pain is transient synovitis, which is also referred to as toxic synovitis. It is presumed to be an inflammatory process and often follows an upper respiratory infection. The disorder is usually seen in children between the ages of 18 months and 7 years but is most common during the second year of life.

The presenting complaint in a toddler may be refusal to walk. Older patients may complain of hip or knee pain. Patients are usually afebrile, although a low-grade fever may be present. Physical examination reveals pain localized to the hip. Some resistance to range of motion is present.

Laboratory studies are mostly useful in distinguishing transient synovitis from a septic hip. In transient synovitis, the white blood cell count and erythrocyte sedimentation rate are usually normal or only slightly elevated, in contrast to septic arthritis, in which both are usually significantly elevated. Radiographic findings are negative but can help exclude other etiologies. Ultrasound is useful for detecting the joint effusion and guiding arthrocentesis. In the absence of fever and without elevated white blood cell count and erythrocyte sedimentation rate, septic joint is unlikely and the diagnosis of transient synovitis can be made without obtaining joint fluid. In older children with hip pain, Legg-Calvé-Perthes disease is a diagnostic possibility necessitating follow-up films.

The treatment of transient synovitis is bed rest and therapy with antiinflammatory agents. The prognosis is excellent.

JUVENILE RHEUMATOID ARTHRITIS

Juvenile rheumatoid arthritis (JRA) encompasses a spectrum of clinically distinct inflammatory diseases that have their onset in childhood and have in common the involvement of the joints. Among these clinical entities, there is no known cause. Juvenile rheumatoid arthritis is classified as polyarticular, which involves about 50 percent of patients; pauciarticular, which affects about 35 percent; and systemic-onset, affecting the remaining 15 percent.

Polyarticular disease involves more than four joints and is further categorized as rheumatoid factor-positive or rheumatoid factor-negative. Both types of disease are more common in girls, but rheumatoid factor-positive disease tends to develop later in childhood and is more likely to result in severe arthritis. The onset of illness may be insidious or fulminant. Arthritis often begins in large joints and is often symmetrical. Many patients note that symptoms are worse in the morning. Affected joints are swollen and warm, although erythema is unusual. Whereas discomfort on range of motion exists, joint pain is generally not severe. Many patients have significant involvement of the joints of the hand, and up to half have involvement of the cervical spine, which, in severe cases, can result in atlantoaxial instability. Some patients have involvement of the temporomandibular joint. Occasionally arthritis occurs in the cricoarytenoid joint, where it can result in hoarseness of the voice.

Systemic involvement in polyarticular disease includes fever, irritability, and occasional hepatomegaly. In severe cases, significant growth disturbances can occur.

Pauciarticular disease by definition involves four or fewer joints. It is categorized as type I or II. Type I is more common in girls, has its onset in early childhood, and is usually associated with the presence of antinuclear antibodies. Large joints are most commonly affected, although hip involvement is unusual. Even though some patients develop chronic arthritis, severe joint destruction is uncommon. However, up to 30 percent of patients with pauciarticular disease develop chronic iridocyclitis; therefore frequent ophthalmologic evaluation is essential. Other systemic manifestations of disease are generally mild.

Type II pauciarticular disease is more common in boys, has an onset in later childhood, and is not associated with antinuclear antibodies. There is a strong association with HLA B27, and patients often have a family history of arthritis. As is the case with pauciarticular disease type I, large joints are most commonly involved. Hip involvement and sacroiliitis can occur, as can Achilles tendinitis. These patients, unlike those with type I disease, may develop chronic spondyloarthropathies, especially of the lumbar area. Patients with type II disease are also at risk for acute iridocyclitis.

Systemic onset disease occurs throughout childhood and is more common in boys. Intermittent spiking fever is especially common and is often the initial manifestation of disease. The fever is often accompanied by a characteristic rash, which appears as pink, often coalescent macules that commonly develop on the trunk and extremities. The rash is transient and recurrent. Hepatosplenomegaly and lymphadenopathy are also common. Eventually, patients develop joint involvement, which tends to be polyarticular. The onset of joint disease may be significantly delayed, which can obscure the diagnosis of JRA.

Systemic-onset JRA is often associated with chronic, debilitating arthritis. Other complications include the development of pericarditis, which in some cases can result in a clinically significant pericardial effusion. Myocarditis and pleuritis are also observed. Some patients develop anemia, which can be severe. Episodes of severe disease can also be accompanied by abdominal pain.

The differential diagnosis of JRA includes acute rheumatic fever, systemic lupus erythematosus, bacterial arthritis, reactive arthritis, and neoplastic diseases, especially leukemia. In the emergency department, the workup of suspected JRA includes a complete blood count, renal function studies, and a rapid streptococcal screen. Tests for antinuclear antibodies and rheumatoid factors are indicated but not immediately available in the emergency department. If a pyogenic arthritis is suspected, analysis of joint fluid is indicated. Patients with systemic-onset disease with evidence of myocarditis or pericarditis require an electrocardiogram and echocardiogram. It may not be possible to make the diagnosis of JRA in the emergency department, and consultation with a pediatric rheumatologist may be necessary. Especially in the case of systemic-onset disease, hospitalization is likely to be necessary.

The treatment of JRA consists of aggressive therapy with nonsteroidal antiinflammatory drugs (NSAIDs). For pauciarticular disease, intraarticular steroids may be used. For polyarticular and more severe cases, cytotoxic drugs or gold salts may be effective. Patients with severe pericarditis or myocarditis, which can occur in systemic-onset disease, may respond to therapy with prednisone.

SYSTEMIC LUPUS ERYTHEMATOSUS

Systemic lupus erythematosus (SLE) is an inflammatory disease of probable autoimmune etiology that affects multiple organ systems. About 20 percent of cases of SLE begin in childhood and adolescence. After puberty, the disease is far more common in females.

Complaints in patients with SLE include fever, malaise, weight loss, and fatigue. Skin manifestations are common, including the characteristic erythematous rash extending from the malar regions across the bridge of the nose. Some patients develop alopecia. About half of pediatric patients will complain of joint pain. Most will eventually develop joint disease. Aside from pain, symptoms include morning stiffness and swelling. Clinically, the patient's pain may be disproportionately greater than the degree of swelling would suggest. This is in contrast to most patients with JRA, who often have markedly swollen joints but complain of mild discomfort. In SLE, joint involvement is usually symmetrical. Other musculoskeletal complaints include tenosynovitis and periostitis. Myalgia and diffuse muscle weakness can also occur. In approximately 15 percent of patients, avascular necrosis occurs, most commonly in the femoral head. Involvement of serosal membranes—including the pleura, peritoneum, and pericardium—is a prominent aspect of SLE and leads to complications that include pleuritis with or without pleural effusion, peritonitis, and pericarditis. Pericarditis can occasionally result in a clinically significant pericardial effusion. Cardiac complications include myocarditis and myocardial infarction. Pulmonary disease includes pneumonitis and, on occasion, pulmonary hemorrhage. Involvement of the central nervous system can result in alterations of mental status, seizures, or cerebrovascular accidents. Most patients develop renal disease, which is a predominant manifestation of the illness and can ultimately result in renal failure. Hematologic abnormalities include anemia, which may be from hemolysis but most commonly reflects the presence of chronic disease. Thrombocytopenia can occur, as can leukopenia.

The differential diagnosis of SLE is vast, and it is unlikely that the initial diagnosis will be made in the emergency department. To confirm SLE, it is necessary to integrate data from the history, physical, and laboratory results. Important disorders to exclude in the emergency department are malignancies, especially leukemia; acute rheumatic fever; JRA; and infectious processes.

In all patients with suspected SLE, a complete blood count, prothrombin time (PT), partial thromboplastin time (PTT), and erythrocyte sedimentation rate are indicated. The prevalence of renal involvement requires serum electrolytes, blood urea nitrogen, and creatinine. A urinalysis will often reveal microscopic hematuria and proteinuria. Antinuclear antibody, rheumatoid factor, complement studies, and quantitative immunoglobulins are indicated, but the results will not be available in the emergency department. If there is evidence of a coagulopathy, lupus anticoagulant and antiphospholipid antibody tests are indicated.

There is no definitive treatment for SLE. Therapy is directed primarily at ameliorating the underlying inflammatory process. In mild disease, NSAIDs may suffice, but most patients will require steroids. More severe manifestations or flare-ups of quiescent disease may respond to therapy with corticosteroids, which, in outpatients, usually involves the use of prednisone. For patients with acute, severe symptoms, high-dose pulse therapy with intravenous glucocorticoids may be necessary. In extremely severe cases, such as rapidly progressive renal disease, immunosuppressive agents such as cyclophosphamide or azathioprine are added to glucocorticoid therapy. The use of both glucocorticoid and immunosuppressive agents in patients with severe disease results in an increased risk of opportunistic infection.

RHEUMATIC FEVER

Acute rheumatic fever (ARF) is a systemic inflammatory condition that is a complication of group A β-hemolytic streptococcal pharyngitis. It does not occur following cutaneous infection. The exact pathology of the disease is unknown, but it is thought to be autoimmune in nature. The systemic manifestations of the illness involve the musculoskeletal, cardiac, central nervous, and cutaneous systems.

Acute rheumatic fever occurs most commonly in children between the ages of 5 and 10 years. Although it is now fairly uncommon in the United States, ARF remains a significant cause of morbidity worldwide. It is most common during the winter and spring and generally develops about 2 to 3 weeks following the pharyngitis.

The initial manifestations of ARF include fever, anorexia, and fatigue. Joint complaints are common and range from arthralgias to frank arthritis. The arthritis tends to move from joint to joint and is therefore termed migratory. It generally affects the large joints of the extremities, but any joint can be affected. The arthralgia associated with ARF is especially intense at night and can wake children from sleep. A predominant characteristic of the arthritis of ARF is the disproportionate severity of the pain compared with the clinical findings. The joint symptoms tend to resolve within a month and leave no permanent damage.

The cardiac involvement of ARF results in carditis, which can affect all layers of the heart, including the pericardium, and is responsible for most of the morbidity associated with the disease. The carditis can be clinically silent or severe enough to result in congestive heart failure. Involvement of the valves, especially the mitral and aortic, results in significant long-term morbidity. A common manifestation of rheumatic carditis is the development of a new murmur, which most commonly reflects mitral regurgitation.

Chorea occurs in up to 10 percent of patients, usually in preadolescent girls, and can be the only manifestation of disease. It consists of random, purposeless movements, most commonly involving the muscles of the extremities and face, that in some cases are preceded by behavioral changes. The duration of chorea varies, but it is a self-limited process.

The dermatologic manifestations of ARF include erythema marginatum, which is an intermittent, red, slightly raised rash that occurs most commonly on the trunk and extremities. Subcutaneous nodules are painless, movable lesions that may develop later during the course of illness. They are rare.

The differential diagnosis of ARF includes JRA, septic arthritis, bacterial endocarditis, leukemia, and SLE. In addition, postinfectious arthritis can mimic ARF.

The diagnosis of rheumatic fever is usually made by utilizing a combination of clinical and laboratory findings. These are summarized in the modified Jones criteria (Table 77-1). The presence of two major and one minor or one major and two minor criteria is highly correlated with ARF. In addition to the criteria, virtually all children have serologic evidence of an antecedent

Table 77-1. Diagnosis of Rheumatic Fever (Revised Jones Criteria)[a]

Level of Significance	Manifestation
Major	Carditis
	Polyarthritis
	Chorea
	Erythema marginatum
	Subcutaneous nodules
Minor	Fever
	Arthralgias
	Elevated erythrocyte sedimentation rate or C-reactive protein
	Prolonged PR interval

[a]For formal diagnosis of acute rheumatic fever, either two major or one major and two minor manifestations must be accompanied by supporting evidence of streptococcal infection (positive throat culture or elevated anti-streptolysin O titer).

streptococcal infection. A negative throat culture, however, does not rule out ARF. An electrocardiogram is indicated, as is an echocardiogram to assess heart size as well as the structural and functional integrity of the valves. A chest radiograph can exclude congestive heart failure.

Patients with suspected ARF are admitted to the hospital. Penicillin is indicated to eradicate any residual carriage of group A *Streptococcus*. Patients with arthritis but without carditis are managed with high-dose aspirin. Patients with evidence of significant carditis are treated with prednisone. Chorea may respond to haloperidol.

Patients who suffer one attack of rheumatic fever are especially vulnerable to recurrent attacks, which can exacerbate damage to previously affected heart valves. Recurrent attacks can be prevented by prophylactic administration of antibiotics, most commonly by injections of benzathine penicillin administered every 3 weeks. Alternatively, oral penicillin may be used if careful compliance can be ensured. First attacks can be prevented by prompt treatment of streptococcal pharyngitis, but care should be given to avoid inappropriate overtreatment of nonstreptococcal infections with antibiotics.

ENTHESOPATHIES

Enthesopathy, also known as enthesitis, is an inflammation of tendons, ligaments, and fascia at their sites of attachment. Enthesopathies are found in a variety of rheumatologic disorders, such as juvenile ankylosing spondylitis, psoriasis, inflammatory bowel disease, and seronegative enthesopathy and arthropathy (SEA) syndrome.

Tenderness from enthesopathy may be noted in the chest wall, iliac crest, ischial tuberosity, posterior or plantar surface of the heel, metatarsophalangeal area, and anterior tibial tuberosity. Pain resulting from enthesopathies is treated with NSAIDs.

ANKYLOSING SPONDYLITIS

Ankylosing spondylitis is a rheumatic disorder that can present in later childhood or adolescence. It is most common in males. Approximately 90 percent of patients are HLA B27 positive.

The disorder is predominantly characterized by involvement of the sacroiliac joints and lumbar spine. Many patients have associated peripheral arthritis. Affected patients often complain of hip, back, and thigh pain that is worse at night and improves with movement. Systemic symptoms include fatigue and low-grade fever. A significant percentage of patients develop acute iridocyclitis.

The physical examination may reveal tenderness over the sacroiliac joints and loss of range of motion of the lumbar spine. Ultimately, there is radiographic evidence of destruction of the sacroiliac joints. However, magnetic resonance imaging is able to identify sacroiliitis very early in the disease process. A complication of ankylosing spondylitis is vertebral fusion.

The primary treatment of ankylosing spondylitis is with NSAIDs. Cyclooxygenase 2 (COX-2) inhibitors show promise for use with this syndrome, but safety in pediatric patients has not been established. Physical therapy, along with education and exercise, plays an important role along with medical management.

BIBLIOGRAPHY

Arkachaisri T, Lehman TJ: Systemic lupus erythematosus and related disorders of childhood. *Curr Opin Rheumatol* 11:384–392, 1999.

Cron RQ, Sharma S, Sherry DD: Current treatment by United States and Canadian pediatric rheumatologists. *J Rheumatol* 26:2036–2038, 1999.

Eich GF, Superti-Furga A, Umbricht FS, et al: The painful hip: Evaluation of criteria for clinical decision-making. *Eur J Pediatr* 158:923–928, 1998.

Fendler C, Laitko S, Sorensen H, et al: Frequency of triggering bacteria in patients with reactive arthritis and undifferentiated oligoarthritis and the relative importance of the tests used for diagnosis. *Ann Rheum Dis* 60:337–343, 2001.

Saxena A: Diagnosis of rheumatic fever: Current status of Jones criteria and role of echocardiography. *Indian J Pediatr* 67(suppl):S11–14, 2000.

Toivanen A: Bacteria-triggered reactive arthritis: Implications for antibacterial treatment. *Drugs* 61:343–351, 2001.

Toivanen P: From reactive arthritis to rheumatoid arthritis. *J Autoimmun* 16:369–371, 2001.

Toussirot E, Wendling D: Therapeutic advances in ankylosing spondylitis. *Expert Opin Investig Drugs* 10:21–29, 2001.

Van Der Linden S, Van Der Heijde D: Clinical aspects, outcome assessment and management of ankylosing spondylitis and postenteric reactive arthritis. *Curr Opin Rheumatol* 12:263–268, 2001.

Visvanathan K, Manjarez RC, Zabriskie JB: Rheumatic fever. *Curr Treat Options Cardiovasc Med* 1:253–258, 1999.

78

Nonmalignant Tumors of Bone

Gary R. Strange
Diana Mayer

HIGH-YIELD FACTS

- Since benign bone tumors may be painless, they are often found incidentally on routine radiographs. Another common presentation is pathologic fracture.

- Osteoid osteoma is a relatively common benign tumor, most commonly affecting the femur and tibia in boys between the ages of 5 and 20 years. It frequently causes pain responsive to NSAIDs, especially at night.

- Nonossifying fibromas are extremely common fibrous lesions, seen in up to 40 percent of preadolescents and adolescents. While they are often incidental findings, they can also cause chronic pain.

- Osteochondromas may result in a nonpainful mass or pathologic fracture, but many are completely asymptomatic. Radiographs demonstrate sessile or pedunculated lesions that should be biopsied and usually require removal.

- Patients with enchondromas may present with a mass or pathologic fracture, but most are asymptomatic. The metacarpals, metatarsals, and phalanges are most commonly involved.

- Solitary bone cysts in the lower extremity are prone to associated fracture and require excision.

- Aneurysmal bone cysts commonly involve the femur, tibia, and vertebral bodies. They are associated with pain and swelling that may be rapidly progressive, leading to the consideration of malignancy.

A number of histologically benign tumors of bone present in childhood. Malignant bone neoplasms are much rarer (see Chap. 75). Since these tumors may be painless, they are often found incidentally on routine radiographs. Another common presentation is that of pathologic fracture. Pathologic fractures are treated as are traumatic fractures, followed by specific treatment of the bone tumor as indicated. Some benign tumors are associated with pain that is usually relieved by aspirin or other nonsteroidal antiinflammatory drugs (NSAIDs).

OSTEOID OSTEOMAS

Osteoid osteoma is a relatively common benign tumor. It frequently causes pain, especially at night, which is responsive to NSAIDs. The most commonly affected areas are the femur and tibia, but osteoid osteoma may involve the vertebral bodies as well. Osteoid osteoma occurs primarily in boys between the ages of 5 and 20 years. Point tenderness at the site is usual. Radiographs demonstrate a radiolucent center of osteoid tissue encircled by sclerotic bone. Surgical removal of the lesion is curative.

NONOSSIFYING FIBROMAS

Nonossifying fibromas are extremely common fibrous lesions, seen in up to 40 percent of preadolescents and adolescents. While they are often incidental findings, they can also cause chronic pain. Occasionally, pathologic fractures can occur. Radiographs reveal a characteristic scalloped lesion. Treatment is not required.

OSTEOCHONDROMAS

Osteochondromas, also called cartilaginous exostoses, are occasionally seen in children and adolescents. The most commonly affected areas are the proximal tibia, proximal humerus, and distal femur. The lesion may result in a nonpainful mass or pathologic fracture, but many are completely asymptomatic. Radiographs demonstrate sessile or pedunculated lesions. These lesions should be biopsied and usually require removal.

ENCHONDROMAS

Patients with enchondromas may present with a mass or pathologic fracture, but most are asymptomatic. The metacarpals, metatarsals, and phalanges are most commonly involved. Malignant transformation is rare. Radiographs show thinning bone with cortical bulging and stippled calcification. Orthopedic consultation is indicated since curettage and bone grafting may be considered for larger or symptomatic lesions.

SOLITARY BONE CYSTS

Solitary bone cysts start near the epiphyseal plate and extend toward the diaphysis during growth. Most often they are found incidentally. These lesions are prone to associated fracture and require excision, especially in the lower extremity, so orthopedic consultation is indicated. Steroid injection into the lesion is another possible treatment.

ANEURYSMAL BONE CYSTS

Aneurysmal bone cysts are filled with blood rather than fluid. They most commonly involve the femur, tibia, and vertebral bodies, and are associated with pain and swelling that may be rapidly progressive, leading to the consideration of malignancy. Radiographs show eccentric lytic lesions of the metaphysis. The usual treatment is curettage and bone grafting. These cysts may recur.

BIBLIOGRAPHY

Lefton DR, Torrisi JM, Haller JO: Vertebral osteoid osteoma masquerading as a malignant bone or soft-tissue tumor on MRI. *Pediatr Radiol* 31(2):72–75, 2001.

Shaughnessy WJ, Arndt CAS: Benign tumors, in Behrman RE, Kliegman RM, Jenson HB, (eds): *Nelson Textbook of Pediatrics,* 16th ed. Philadelphia: Saunders, 2000, pp 1567–1569.

79

General Principles of Poisoning: Diagnosis and Management

Timothy Erickson

HIGH-YIELD FACTS

- Many patients with ingestions have typical "toxidromes."
- Ipecac is rarely useful in pediatric ingestions.
- Activated charcoal is useful in the majority of toxic ingestions.
- Whole bowel irrigation is increasingly used for gastric decontamination.
- There are several antidotes available for specific toxic ingestions.

There has been a 95 percent decline in the number of pediatric poisoning deaths in children <6 years of age over the past few decades, with 450 reported deaths in 1961 and 24 in 1999. Child-resistant product packaging, heightened parental awareness of potential household toxins, and more sophisticated medical intervention at the poison control and emergency and intensive care levels have all contributed to reduce morbidity and mortality. Nonetheless, poisoning continues to be a preventable cause of pathology in children and adolescents. It is imperative that the pediatric emergency physician be familiar with the general approach to poisoned children, as well as the latest treatment modalities available.

EPIDEMIOLOGY

Two-thirds of poisonings reported to the American Association of Poison Control Centers (AAPCC) occur in individuals under the age of 20 years. Most exposures in this age group are accidental and result in minimal toxicity. The majority of these poisonings result from ingestions. They may also result from inhalation, intravenous, dermal, ocular, and environmental exposure. Nonaccidental causes of drug toxicity include recreational drug abuse, suicide attempts, and Munchausen-by-proxy.

Of the over 1.4 million exposures involving individuals <20 years of age reported to poison control centers in 1999, 2700 patients (0.2 percent) experienced a major outcome defined as a life-threatening effect or residual disability, with 85 fatalities (0.004 percent). Cosmetics, personal care products, cleaning substances, analgesics, and plants accounted for 40 percent of the reported exposures. Although responsible for the majority of pediatric poisonings, children <6 years of age comprised only 2.7 percent of the fatalities. Of these deaths, 83 percent were accidental, with 3 percent resulting from malicious intent from a parent or caregiver. Over half (58 percent) of the deaths were caused by nonpharmaceutical agents. One-third was environmental, with carbon monoxide the leading cause of fatal poisoning. In adolescents (13 to 19 years), 85 percent of these deaths were intentional. In addition, 23 percent of fatalities were from inhalants, and 19 percent from street drugs or stimulants. It is important to note that the AAPCC data underestimates the actual frequency of pediatric poisoning, since many of the cases are never reported to regional poison centers.

HISTORY

Although it may be difficult to obtain an accurate and complete history regarding an ingestion, this is an essential part of the proper evaluation of poisoned pediatric patients. All sources of information are explored in children who are comatose or too young to provide details. The history includes the toxin or medication to which the children were exposed, the time of the exposure or ingestion, what other medications were available to the children, and how much was taken. It is prudent to assume the worst-case scenario.

PHYSICAL EXAMINATION

A comprehensive physical examination may provide valuable clues regarding the ingestion or exposure. Since many

Table 79-1. Toxic Vital Signs

Bradycardia (PACED)
P Propranolol (beta blockers)
A Anticholinesterase drugs
C Clonidine, calcium channel blockers
E Ethanol and alcohols
D Digoxin, darvon (opiates)

Tachycardia (FAST)
F Free base (cocaine)
A Anticholinergics, antihistamines, amphetamines
S Sympathomimetics
T Theophylline

Hypothermia (COOLS)
C Carbon monoxide
O Opiates
O Oral hypoglycemics, insulin
L Liquor
S Sedative hypnotics

Hyperthermia (NASA)
N Neuroleptic malignant syndrome, nicotine
A Antihistamines
S Salicylates, sympathomimetics
A Anticholinergics, antidepressants

Hypotension (CRASH)
C Clonidine
R Reserpine (antihypertensive agents)
A Antidepressants
S Sedative hypnotics
H Heroin (opiates)

Hypertension (CTSCAN)
C Cocaine
T Theophylline
S Sympathomimetics
C Caffeine
A Anticholinergics, amphetamines
N Nicotine

drugs and toxic agents have specific effects on the heart rate, temperature, blood pressure, and respiratory rate, monitoring the vital signs may direct the clinician toward the proper diagnosis (Table 79-1). Additionally, the level of consciousness, pupillary size, and potential for seizures may be directly affected by the poison in a dose-dependent fashion. Other diagnostic clues are obtained in the skin exam and breath odor (Table 79-2). Several groups of toxins consistently present with recognizable patterns or signs. Recognizing these toxic syndromes or toxidromes may expedite not only the diagnosis of the toxic agent, but also its management (Table 79-3).

DIAGNOSTIC AIDS AND LABORATORY

In children with significant or unknown ingestion, baseline laboratory studies include a complete blood cell count, renal functions, and levels of electrolytes, glucose, and arterial blood gases. In patients with known ingestion demonstrating no overt signs of toxicity, a more selective approach to diagnostic studies is acceptable. If the arterial blood gas value reveals a metabolic acidosis, calculating the anion gap can assist in formulating a differential diagnosis. A metabolic acidosis with an increased anion gap results from the presence of organically active acids and is characteristic of several toxins and various other disease states (Table 79-4). Normal anion gap acidosis results from loss of bicarbonate (diarrhea and renal tubular acidosis) or from addition of chloride-containing compounds (NH_4Cl and $CaCl_2$). The anion gap can be calculated from serum electrolytes as follows:

$$Anion\ Gap\ Calculation = Na - (Cl + HCO_3)$$

The normal anion gap ranges from 8 to 12 mEq/L.

If ingestion of a toxic alcohol, such as methanol or ethylene glycol, is suspected, calculation of the osmolal gap is critical. The osmolal gap is the difference between the actual osmolality, best measured by freezing-point depression, and that calculated from major osmotically active molecules in the serum (sodium, glucose, and blood urea nitrogen).

$$Calculated\ Osmolality = 2(Na) + Glucose/18 + BUN/2.8 + ETOH/4.6$$

$$Osmolal\ Gap = Measured\ Osmol - Calculated\ Osmol\ (Normal < 10)$$

When a particular drug or toxin is known or highly suspected, blood or serum can be tested for specific drug

Table 79-2. Toxic Physical Findings

Miosis (COPS)

C	Cholinergics, clonidine
O	Opiates, organophosphates
P	Phenothiazines, pilocarpine, pontine bleed
S	Sedative hypnotics

Mydriasis (AAAS)

A	Antihistamines
A	Antidepressants
A	Anticholinergics, atropine
S	Sympathomimetics (cocaine, amphetamines)

Seizures (OTIS CAMPBELL)

O	Organophosphates	**C**	Camphor, cocaine
T	Tricyclic antidepressants	**A**	Amphetamines
I	INH, insulin	**M**	Methylxanthines (theophylline, caffeine)
S	Sympathomimetics	**P**	PCP
		B	Beta-blockers, botanicals
		E	Ethanol withdrawal
		L	Lithium, lindane
		L	Lead, lidocaine

Diaphoretic skin (SOAP)

S	Sympathomimetics	**Red Skin:**	Carbon monoxide, boric acid
O	Organophosphates		
A	ASA (salicylates)	**Blue Skin:**	Cyanosis, methemoglobinemia
P	PCP		

Breath odors

Bitter almonds	(Cyanide)
Fruity	(DKA, Isopropanol)
Oil of wintergreen	(Methyl salicylates)
Rotten eggs	(Sulfur dioxide, hydrogen sulfide)
Pears	(Chloral hydrate)
Garlic	(Organophosphates, arsenic, DMSO)
Mothballs	(Camphor)

INH, isonicotinic acid hydrazide (isoniazid); ASA, acetylsalicyclic acid; PCP, phencyclidine; DKA, diabetic ketoacidosis.

levels. These levels confirm the ingestion and often guide medical management. Commonly available tests are listed in Table 79-5.

Toxicology screening can be helpful in the diagnosis of the unknown ingestion if the clinician is aware of its limitations. Even when a drug has been ingested, blood toxicology screens may be negative if the drug has a short half-life and the specimen is not obtained immediately after the exposure. The urine toxicology screen may be of greater value, since the drug's metabolites continue to be excreted in the urine for 48 to 72 hours following the ingestion. Toxicology panels typically screen for drugs of abuse such as narcotics, amphetamines, cannabinoids, phencyclidine (PCP), and cocaine. However, since most of these screens are qualitative, the mere detection of a drug does not necessarily entail toxicity. A grave error can also occur if the physician assumes the child ingested nothing simply because the toxicology screen is reported as negative and the actual drug ingested has not been included in the screen.

Radiologic testing can prove valuable with certain ingestions, particularly those that are radiopaque or those that may induce a noncardiogenic pulmonary edema or chemical pneumonitis (Table 79-6).

Table 79-3. Toxic Syndromes

Anticholinergic (tricyclic antidepressants, antihistamines)

Hot as a hare	(hyperthermia)
Dry as a bone	(dry mouth)
Red as a beet	(flushed skin)
Blind as a bat	(dilated pupils)
Mad as a hatter	(confused delirium)

Cholinergic (organophosphates)

D	=	Diarrhea, diaphoresis
U	=	Urination
M	=	Miosis, muscle fasciculations
B	=	Bradycardia, bronchosecretions
E	=	Emesis
L	=	Lacrimation
S	=	Salivation

Sympathomimetic (cocaine, amphetamines)
  Mydriasis
  Tachycardia
  Hypertension
  Hyperthermia
  Seizures

Narcotic
  Miosis
  Bradycardia
  Hypotension
  Hypoventilation
  Coma

Withdrawal
  Alcohol
  Benzodiazepines
  Barbiturates
  Antihypertensives
  Opioids

MANAGEMENT

Stabilization

The cornerstone of management of patients with a suspected overdose is supportive care, with particular attention to the airway, breathing, and circulation. Resuscitative measures are instituted prior to antidotal therapy or gastric decontamination.

In children with an altered level of consciousness or in whom a bedside glucose oxidase test documents hypoglycemia, the physician should administer intravenous dextrose at 0.5 to 1.0 g/kg, given as 2 to 4 mL/kg of $D_{25}W$ in children or 50 mL (1 ampul) of $D_{50}W$ in the

Table 79-4. Metabolic Acidosis and Elevated Anion Gap

Methanol, **M**etformin
Ethylene glycol
Toluene, **T**heophylline
Alcoholic ketoacidosis
Lactic acidosis

Aminoglycosides (uremic agents)
Cyanide, **C**arbon monoxide
Isoniazid, **I**ron
DKA (diabetic ketoacidosis)

Grand mal seizures (toxic-related)
ASA (salicylates)
Paraldehyde, **P**henformin

Source: Adapted from Bryson PD: *Comprehensive Review of Toxicology,* 2d ed. Rockville, MD: Aspen Publishing, 1989.

adolescent. If intravenous access is difficult or unobtainable, glucagon, 1 mg, is administered intramuscularly.

In addition to dextrose, naloxone is given to children or adolescents with lethargy or coma. Naloxone is a specific opiate antagonist with minimal side effects. Agitation and signs of withdrawal may develop in opiate-dependent adolescents or in neonates whose mothers are narcotic addicts or on methadone during pregnancy. The initial dose is 0.1 mg/kg intravenously or 2 mg for children weighing >20 kg. Often, additional doses of naloxone are required for certain opiates, such as codeine, methadone, and propoxyphene, which have high potency and a prolonged half-life. If an intravenous line cannot be established, naloxone may be administered via the endotracheal tube, intramuscularly, subcutaneously, or intralingually.

Gastric Decontamination

Gastric decontamination is one of the more controversial topics in toxicology. Whether patients are managed with

Table 79-5. Serum Drug Levels

Acetaminophen	Lithium
Carbon monoxide	Methanol
Cholinesterase	Methemoglobin
Digitalis	Phenobarbital
Ethanol	Phenytoin
Ethylene glycol	Salicylate
Iron	Theophylline
Lead	

Table 79-6. Toxicology and Radiology

Noncardiogenic pulmonary edema (MOPS)
M   Meprobamate, Mountain sickness
O   Opiates
P   Phenobarbital
S   Salicylates

Toxins radiopaque on radiographs (CHIPES)
C   Chloral hydrate
H   Heavy metals
I   Iron
P   Phenothiazines
E   Enteric-coated preps (Salicylates)
S   Sustained release products (theophylline)

syrup of ipecac, gastric lavage, cathartics, or activated charcoal depends on the toxicity of the particular drug, the quantity and time of ingestion, and patients' conditions. If children ingest a nontoxic agent or a very small amount of a poison unlikely to cause toxicity, no gastric decontamination measures are necessary. However, if the ingestion is recent and the children are symptomatic, or the toxin ingested may cause delayed toxicity, gastric evacuation is recommended. Several clinical trials have been conducted to determine which of the gastric decontamination modalities are most efficacious. However, the investigations either involve adult volunteers who are taking subtoxic amounts and receive decontamination at a set postingestion time, or involve mild-to-moderately poisoned patients, excluding patients with significant overdoses. Additionally, few children have been included in these trials. Therefore, these studies must be critically interpreted prior to their definitive application in the clinical setting.

Gastric Evacuation

Induction of Emesis

Syrup of ipecac is the most commonly used emetic agent. However, its use has largely fallen out of favor in the emergency department setting. In 1983, it was administered in 13 percent of all oral exposures, but in 1999 it was administered in only 1 percent. Ipecac can be expected to induce vomiting within 20 to 60 minutes. The recovery of ingested material in the vomitus is approximately 30 percent if ipecac is administered within 1 hour of ingestion. Unfortunately, most children experience >3 episodes of vomiting, which delays the administration of activated charcoal in the emergency department setting. Ipecac is contraindicated in children <6 months

of age, in patients with evidence of a diminished gag reflex and potential for coma or seizures, and in the ingestion of most hydrocarbons, acids, alkalis, and sharp objects. The use of ipecac in the home immediately following ingestion is a matter of controversy in the toxicology literature. It may have some use in small children in whom gastric decontamination is indicated but technically difficult due to an oversized gastric lavage tube or in ingestion of large toxic plant parts, seeds, berries, or mushrooms. (See Table 79-7 for dosage.)

Gastric Lavage

Gastric lavage mechanically removes toxins from the stomach using a large-bore orogastric tube irrigated with aliquots of normal saline. This mode of gastric decontamination is preferred in intoxicated children with a depressed level of consciousness who present within 1 hour or have ingested a potentially life-threatening agent. In most cases, airway protection by endotracheal intubation prior to the lavage is indicated. Gastric lavage is contraindicated in ingestions of most hydrocarbons, acids, alkalis, and sharp objects. Although relatively safe when performed properly, complications including aspiration, esophageal perforation, bleeding, electrolyte imbalance, and hypothermia have been described. Gastric lavage is most effective if performed within 1 hour of ingestion and, at best, removes up to 40 percent of the ingested toxin. There may be some efficacy for lavage beyond 1 hour when the agent ingested slows gut motility, such as with anticholinergics or opioids, or when the toxin forms concretions, such as with iron and salicylates. However, this has never been substantiated in the toxicology literature.

Chemical Decontamination

Activated Charcoal

The majority of poisoned children who are not critically ill can be managed safely and effectively in the emergency department setting with charcoal alone. Activated charcoal is an odorless, tasteless, fine black powder that is effective in adsorbing many toxins. It has now become the most frequently used and most effective gastric decontamination agent. It is most beneficial when administered within 1 hour after the ingestion. The recommended initial dose of activated charcoal is summarized in Table 79-7.

For some drugs, such as theophylline, phenobarbital, and carbamazepine, multiple dosing of activated charcoal may enhance elimination due to enterohepatic or

Table 79-7. Doses for Gastric Decontamination

Syrup of Ipecac:	6–12 months of age: 5–10 mL with 15 mL/kg clear fluids
	12 months–12 years: 15 mL ipecac plus 8 oz of clear fluids
	>12 years: 30 mL ipecac plus 16 oz water
Activated Charcoal:	1–2 g/kg prepared as a slurry in water or sorbitol to achieve a 25% concentration.
	For repetitive dosing: 1 g/kg every 2–4 hours without sorbitol or cathartic.
Cathartics:	Sorbitol (35% solution): 4 mL/kg of commercial solution diluted
	1:1 Magnesium citrate (10% solution): 4 mL/kg
	Magnesium sulfate: (10% solution): 1–2 mL/kg

enteroenteric circulation of the drug. Repeated use of charcoal preparations premixed with cathartics such as sorbitol is to be avoided, since dehydration and electrolyte imbalance may result. Although charcoal is probably the safest method of decontamination, rare cases of vomiting, constipation, obstruction, and aspiration have been reported. Activated charcoal is neither effective nor indicated in heavy metal poisonings, such as with iron or lithium, or following ingestion of acids or alkalis where endoscopy may be required.

Cathartics

Cathartics are osmotically active agents that eliminate toxins from the gastrointestinal tract by inducing diarrhea. The most common agents are sorbitol, magnesium citrate, and magnesium sulfate. No studies have been conducted to evaluate cathartics as the sole decontamination modality in the overdose setting. However, studies investigating the use of sorbitol in combination with activated charcoal have found that it enhances charcoal's palatability. In the pediatric population, cathartic agents can result in hypermagnesemia, dehydration, and severe electrolyte imbalances if used excessively or repeatedly.

Whole Bowel Irrigation

Originally used as a preoperative bowel preparation, whole bowel irrigation is now used in the overdose setting to "flush" the toxin down the gastrointestinal tract

Table 79-8. Antidotes

Toxin	Antidote
Acetaminophen	*N*-acetylcysteine
Benzodiazepines	Flumazenil
Beta blockers	Glucagon
Calcium channel blockers	Calcium, glucagon, insulin, and glucose
Carbon monoxide	Oxygen
Cyanide	Amyl nitrate, sodium nitrate, sodium thiosulfate
Digitalis	F(AB) fragments
Ethylene glycol/methanol	Ethanol, (4-MP)
Iron	Deferoxamine
Lead	(EDTA), (BAL), (DMSA)
Mercury/arsenic	BAL, D-Penicillamine
Methemoglobinemia	Methylene blue
Opiates	Naloxone
Organophosphates	Atropine, (2-PAM)
Tricyclic antidepressants	Sodium bicarbonate

4-MP, 4-methylpyrazone; EDTA, calcium ethylenediamine tetraacetate: BAL, British antilewisite; DMSA, dimercaptosuccinic acid, 2-PAM, 2-pralidoxime.

and prevent further absorption. In theory, it may also produce a concentration gradient that allows previously absorbed toxins to diffuse back into the gastrointestinal tract. The solution used is a polyethylene glycol electrolyte solution that does not appear to create fluid or electrolyte disturbances. The dose is 0.5 L/h for small children and 1 to 2 L/h for adolescents. The irrigation process is continued until the rectal effluent is clear, which is usually in 2 to 6 h. Whole bowel irrigation has been used in the pediatric population with minimal to no side effects and has been effective in ingestions of lead chips, iron, button batteries, and cocaine packet ingestions.

Antidotes

Although the majority of poisonings in the pediatric population respond to supportive care and gastric decontamination alone, there are a few toxins that require antidotes (Table 79-8). The purpose of antidotal therapy is to reduce the agent's toxicity by inhibiting the toxin at the effector site or target organ, to reduce the toxin's concentration, or to enhance its excretion.

Hemodialysis and Hemoperfusion

Although hemodialysis is recommended for a wide variety of toxins, it is necessary in only a few severely poisoned patients. Drugs that may be adequately dialyzed include those with a low molecular weight, low volume of distribution, low protein binding, and high water solubility. Examples include isopropanol, salicylates, theophylline, uremia-causing agents, methanol, barbiturates, lithium, and ethylene glycol. Theophylline is also responsive to charcoal hemoperfusion. If children have a severe overdose that may require dialysis, early consultation with a nephrologist is critical.

DISPOSITION

Disposition of poisoned pediatric patients is not always straightforward and depends on the clinical condition of the children, as well as the potential toxicity of the agent. Clearly, all children demonstrating clinical instability are best monitored in an intensive care setting. Emergency department observation for 6 to 8 hours is adequate if patients demonstrate no overt signs of toxicity and the ingestion does not involve a sustained release formulation. However, if the children have ingested a potentially dangerous dose of a toxin, are manifesting mild-to-moderate toxicity, require antidotal therapy, or their home environment is not considered safe, a general pediatric admission is indicated. In the setting of any accidental overdose, the parents are counseled and educated regarding proper poison prevention in the home. In the case of adolescents with recreational drug abuse, drug rehabilitation programs are encouraged. If the adolescents are suicidal, psychiatric consultation is obtained once they are stabilized medically.

BIBLIOGRAPHY

Brent J, McMartin K, Phillips S, et al: Fomepizole for the treatment of ethylene glycol poisoning. *N Engl J Med* 340:832–838, 1999.

Ford M, Delaney KA: Initial approaches to the poison patient, in Ford M, Delaney KA, Ling L, et al (eds): *Clinical Toxicology.* Philadelphia, Harcourt-WB Saunders, 2001, pp 1–4.

Henretig FM: Special considerations in the poisoned pediatric patient. *Emerg Clin North Am* 12:549–567, 1994.

Koren G: Medications which can kill a toddler with one tablet or teaspoonful. *Clin Toxicol* 31:407–414, 1993.

Kulig K: Initial management of toxic substances. *N Engl J Med* 326:1677–1681, 1992.

Liebelt EL, Shannon MW: Small doses, big problems: A selected review of highly toxic common medications. *Pediatr Emerg Care* 9:292–297, 1993.

Litovitz TL, Schwartz-Klein W, White S, et al: 1999 Annual Report of the AAPCC Toxic Exposure/Surveillance System. *Am J Emerg Med* 18:517–574, 2000.

Position statements on gastric lavage, activated charcoal, syrup of ipecac, cathatrics and whole bowel irrigation. *J Toxicol Clin Toxicol* 35:711–762, 1997.

Yuan TH, Kerns WP, Tomaszewski CA, et al: Insulin-glucose as adjunctive therapy for severe calcium channel antagonist poisoning. *J Toxicol Clin Toxicol* 37:463–474, 1999.

80

Acetaminophen

Leon Gussow

HIGH-YIELD FACTS

- Acetaminophen toxicity is a potentially reversible cause of hepatic failure.
- Children are relatively resistant to the toxic effects of acetaminophen.
- *N*-acetylcysteine (NAC) is the antidote for acetaminophen toxicity.
- *N*-acetylcysteine should be utilized in any case of acetaminophen-induced hepatotoxicity, regardless of the time of ingestion.

In 1999, almost 64,000 cases of acetaminophen ingestion in patients <19 years of age were reported to poison control centers in the United States. Despite the large number of reports, only 6 deaths occurred, all in adolescents, some of which may have involved other toxins. Young children are relatively resistant to the hepatotoxic consequences of acetaminophen ingestion, an effect that may be due to early spontaneous vomiting or differences in drug metabolism. Although NAC is an effective antidote if given early, initial signs and symptoms of acetaminophen overdose are usually nonspecific, and the therapeutic window in which treatment is effective may be missed unless acetaminophen levels are routinely obtained when any drug ingestion is suspected.

PHARMACOLOGY AND PATHOPHYSIOLOGY

Acetaminophen (also called APAP or paracetamol) is a synthetic analgesic and antipyretic that lacks the anti-inflammatory effects found in salicylates and nonsteroidal agents. Clinical effects are most likely mediated by inhibition of prostaglandin synthesis.

The therapeutic dose of APAP in children is 15 mg/kg given every 4 to 6 hours, with a maximum recommended daily dose of 80 mg/kg. Therapeutic serum levels are 5 to 20 μg/mL. Acetaminophen is well absorbed after an oral therapeutic dose, with peak levels generally occurring at 1 to 2 hours. However, slowed gastric emptying may delay the peak level for up to 4 hours. Following gastrointestinal absorption, APAP is taken up by the liver, where tissue concentrations are high. Serum half-life is 1 to 3 hours after a therapeutic dose, but may be prolonged significantly following an hepatotoxic ingestion. Volume of distribution is 1 L/kg, and plasma protein binding is <50 percent.

Acetaminophen is eliminated primarily by hepatic pathways. After a therapeutic dose, 90 percent of the drug is metabolized to inactive sulfate and glucuronide conjugates. In young children, unlike in adults and adolescents, the sulfate conjugate predominates. Less than 5 percent is excreted unchanged in the urine. A small amount (2 to 4 percent) is metabolized by the cytochrome-P_{450}-mixed-function-oxidase (MFO) system to the toxic intermediate *n*-acetyl-*p*-benzoquinoneimine (NAPQI). In the presence of adequate hepatic stores of glutathione, NAPQI is rapidly converted to nontoxic mercapturic acid and cysteine conjugates. In the overdose setting, the sulfate and glucuronide pathways become saturated, and increased amounts of acetaminophen are shunted through the P_{450}-MFO system. Glutathione becomes depleted and free NAPQI forms covalent bonds with structures on the hepatocytes. Necrosis ensues, distributed in a centrilobular fashion, corresponding to the area of greatest MFO activity.

Acetaminophen can directly produce toxicity on organs other than the liver. Local metabolism to a toxic metabolite in the kidney can rarely cause proximal tubular necrosis and renal failure, even if the liver is relatively unaffected. Pancreatitis can also occur, particularly in the setting of severe hepatic necrosis. Such nonhepatic manifestations, however, are virtually never seen in children.

The toxic dose of acetaminophen is generally considered to be 140 mg/kg, but susceptibility to hepatotoxicity after acetaminophen overdose varies significantly. Children are more resistant than are adults. Certain drugs will induce cytochrome P_{450} enzymes, causing increased production of NAPQI. These include phenobarbital, phenytoin, carbamazepine, rifampicin, and isoniazid. Patients taking these medications can present relatively early after acetaminophen overdose with severe hepatotoxicity, even with serum levels generally considered nontoxic. Malnutrition may also predispose to more severe acetaminophen toxicity by depleting hepatic glutathione.

CLINICAL PRESENTATION: THE FOUR STAGES OF ACETAMINOPHEN TOXICITY

Stage 1 (0 to 24 Hours): Gastrointestinal Irritation

Patients may be asymptomatic, but young children frequently vomit after acetaminophen overdose, which may partially explain their relative resistance to severe toxicity. In massive overdose or in children on chronic therapy with enzyme-inducing medication, an anion-gap metabolic acidosis can rarely occur within hours of ingestion.

Stage 2 (24 to 48 Hours): Latent Period

As nausea and vomiting resolve, patients appear to improve, but rising transaminase levels may reveal evidence of hepatic necrosis. On physical examination, hepatic tenderness and enlargement may be apparent. Fortunately, the incidence of hepatotoxicity is significantly lower in children than it is in adults with similar acetaminophen levels.

Stage 3 (72 to 96 Hours): Hepatic Failure

Severe hepatotoxicity presents with jaundice, hypoglycemia, renewed nausea and vomiting, right upper quadrant pain, coagulopathy, lethargy, coma, hyperbilirubinemia, and markedly elevated transaminase levels. Renal failure may occur.

Stage 4 (4 to 14 Days): Recovery or Death

Patients who ultimately recover show improvement in laboratory parameters of hepatic function starting at about day 5 and recover completely. Follow-up histology is normal. Other patients show progressive encephalopathy, renal failure, bleeding diatheses, and hyperammonemia and will die unless a liver transplant is performed.

LABORATORY

An acetaminophen level is drawn 4 hours after an acute ingestion or immediately if >4 hours have elapsed since the ingestion. Levels drawn earlier than 4 hours may not represent the peak serum concentration and thus may be misleadingly low. In addition to the acetaminophen level, laboratory tests that influence management or indicate prognosis include testing for levels of liver enzymes, amylase, bilirubin, electrolytes, and creatinine, as well as prothrombin time.

MANAGEMENT

Gastric Decontamination

Induction of emesis with syrup of ipecac is contraindicated in known or suspected acetaminophen ingestion since it is only minimally effective and will delay administration of NAC. Standard doses of activated charcoal can be given if patients come in within 2 hours of ingestion of acetaminophen alone or if other toxic substances are also involved.

Antidote

A glutathione precursor, NAC restores the liver's ability to detoxify NABQI and prevents hepatonecrosis. It is most effective if started within 10 hours of ingestion and seems to have decreased efficacy if treatment is delayed beyond that time. However, there is now good evidence that NAC has some benefit even if started very late, possibly up to days after ingestion when hepatic failure has already ensued. It should not be withheld on the basis of an arbitrary time limit.

The Rumack-Matthew nomogram indicates which patients will require treatment with NAC. Any patient with a level that falls in the range of possible or probable hepatotoxicity is treated with a full course of NAC. Repeat levels are unnecessary and do not change management. If the time of ingestion is unknown, or if ingestion of significant amounts of acetaminophen occurred over a prolonged period, treatment is started and a repeat level is drawn 4 hours after the first. Elevated liver enzyme levels, elevated prothrombin time, or a serum half-life of acetaminophen >4 hours are indications to complete treatment with NAC. If there is any doubt, it is best to administer the full course of therapy.

If patients are chronically on medication that induces the P_{450} system, the threshold for treatment indicated on the Rumack-Matthew nomogram is reduced. Although the threshold for treatment in such patients is not clear, some advocate treating if the acetaminophen level is more than half that on the algorithm that indicates possible or probable toxicity.

The oral protocol approved by the United State Food and Drug Administration requires a loading dose of 140 mg/kg and then 17 additional doses of 70 mg/kg. The commercial 20% solution (Mucomyst, Mead Johnson &

Company) is unpalatable and is diluted with 3 parts fruit juice or soda. If vomiting occurs within 1 hour of treatment, the dose is repeated. Persistent vomiting that interferes with therapy can be suppressed with metoclopramide or ondansetron. If necessary, NAC can be infused slowly through a nasogastric tube. If activated charcoal has been administered, the usual dose of NAC does not need to be increased, but should be given at least 30 to 60 minutes after the charcoal.

Intravenous NAC is commonly used in Europe, but has not yet been approved by the United States Food and Drug Administration. In cases of significant overdose where oral NAC is either contraindicated or not tolerated despite all efforts mentioned earlier, the same NAC preparation used for oral dosing can be given intravenously. In such cases, a poison control center should be consulted for precise instructions and informed consent obtained from either the patient or a relative.

CHRONIC ACETAMINOPHEN POISONING

The Rumack-Matthew nomogram applies specifically to a single acute overdose taken at a known moment in time. It is now clear that children can develop hepatotoxicity after even moderately supratherapeutic doses of acetaminophen administered over several days. Doses >150 mg/kg/day can cause toxicity. These children often have lethargy and a history of fever. Liver enzymes are elevated. Renal failure and pancytopenia may also be seen. The differential diagnosis includes Reye's syndrome and hepatitis. These children should be treated with a full course of NAC.

BIBLIOGRAPHY

Anker A: Acetaminophen, *in* Ford MD, Delaney KA, Ling LJ, Erickson T (eds): *Clinical Toxicology.* Philadelphia, WB Saunders, 2001, pp 265–274.

Day A, Abbott GD: Chronic paracetamol poisoning in children: A warning to health professionals. *N Z Med J* 107:201, 1994.

Henretig FM, Selbst SM, Forrest C, et al: Repeated acetaminophen overdosing causing hepatotoxicity in children. *Clin Pediatr* 28:525, 1989.

Heubi JE, Barbacci MB, Zimmerman HJ: Therapeutic misadventures with acetaminophen: Hepatotoxicity after multiple doses in children. *J Pediatr* 132:22, 1998.

Kearns GL, Leeder JS, Wasserman GS: Acetaminophen overdose with therapeutic intent (editorial). *J Pediatr* 132:5, 1998.

Litovitz TL, Klein-Schwartz W, White S, et al: 1999 Annual report of the American Association of Poison Control Centers toxic exposure surveillance system. *Am J Emerg Med* 18:517, 2000.

Perry HE, Shannon MW: Efficacy of oral versus intravenous *N*-acetylcysteine in acetaminophen overdose: Results of an open-label clinical trial. *J Pediatr* 132:149, 1998.

81

Toxic Alcohols

Timothy Erickson

HIGH-YIELD FACTS

- Ethanol overdose in children often results in hypoglycemia.
- Methanol ingestion is associated with visual disturbance and metabolic acidosis.
- Ethylene glycol poisoning is associated with metabolic acidosis and renal failure.
- Isopropanol may cause CNS depression but does not usually cause metabolic acidosis.
- All of the toxic alcohols produce an osmolal gap.

ETHANOL

According to the American Association of Poison Control Centers (AAPCC), there were over 8000 exposures to alcohol in children <6 years of age in 1999, accounting for 2.5 percent of all reported exposures. There were two reported fatalities.

Sources

In addition to alcohol-containing beverages, such as beer, wine, and hard liquors, children have access to mouthwashes that can contain up to 75 percent ethanol, colognes, and perfumes (40% to 60% ethanol) and over 700 medicinal preparations that contain ethanol.

Pharmacokinetics and Pathophysiology

Ethanol undergoes hepatic metabolism via three metabolic pathways:

- Alcohol dehydrogenase
- Microsomal ethanol-oxidizing system (MEOS)
- Peroxidase-catalase system

The alcohol dehydrogenase pathway is the major metabolic pathway and the rate-limiting step in converting ethanol to acetaldehyde. In general, nontolerant individuals metabolize ethanol at 15 to 20 mg/dL/h and alcoholics metabolize at 30 mg/dL/h. Children often ingest large amounts of ethanol in relation to their body weight, resulting in rapid development of high blood alcohol concentrations. In children <5 years of age, the ability to metabolize ethanol is diminished due to immature hepatic dehydrogenase activity.

Clinical Presentation

Ethanol is a selective central nervous system (CNS) depressant at low concentrations and a generalized depressant at high concentrations. Initially, ethanol produces exhilaration and loss of inhibition, which progresses to lack of coordination, ataxia, slurred speech, gait disturbances, drowsiness, and, ultimately, stupor and coma. The intoxicated child may demonstrate a flushed face, dilated pupils, excessive sweating, gastrointestinal distress, hypoventilation, hypothermia, and hypotension. Death from respiratory depression may occur at ethanol levels >500 mg/dL. Convulsions and death have been reported in children with acute ethanol intoxication due to alcohol-induced hypoglycemia. Hypoglycemia results from inhibition of hepatic gluconeogenesis and is most common in children <5 years of age. It does not appear to be directly related to the quantity of alcohol ingested.

Laboratory

In symptomatic pediatric patients who have suspected ethanol intoxication, the most critical laboratory tests are the serum ethanol and glucose levels. Although blood ethanol levels roughly correlate with clinical signs, the physician must treat patients based on symptomatology and not the absolute level. If the ethanol level does not correlate with the clinical picture, consider other ingestions. If children have experienced fluid losses, serum electrolytes are monitored.

Management

The majority of children with accidental acute ingestions of ethanol respond to supportive care. Attention is directed toward management of children's airway, circulation, and glucose status. All obtunded patients should receive 2 to 4 mL/kg of $D_{25}W$ (1 ampul of $D_{50}W$ in older children and adolescents), after a specimen for blood glucose level is drawn. If no response is elicited, administration of naloxone 2 mg IV push is indicated to rule out opiate toxicity. If children respond to glucose administration, serial glucose levels are followed to avoid recurrent episodes of hypoglycemia. Unless children are comatose or coingestion of another drug is suspected, gastric decontamination is usually unnecessary unless performed within 1 hour of ingestion. Activated charcoal and cathartics can be administered but are probably not efficacious in isolated ethanol ingestions. Since hemodialysis increases ethanol clearance by 3 to 4 times, it may be indicated with ethanol levels >500 mg/dL or with evidence of deteriorating vital signs or hepatic function.

Disposition

Any young pediatric patient with significant altered mental status following acute ethanol ingestion is admitted for observation of respiratory status, fluid resuscitation, and glucose monitoring. Asymptomatic patients may be discharged home with reliable caretakers.

METHANOL

In 1999, there were 363 exposures to methanol reported to the AAPCC in individuals <20 years of age, with no reported deaths. Methanol is present in a variety of substances found around the home and workplace, including antifreeze, paint solvents, gasohol, gasoline additives, canned-heat products, windshield washer fluid, and duplicating chemicals.

Pharmacokinetics and Pathophysiology

Methanol is rapidly absorbed following ingestion. Peak serum levels can be reached as early as 30 to 90 minutes postingestion. As with ethanol, methanol is primarily metabolized by hepatic alcohol dehydrogenase. The half-life of methanol may be as long as 24 hours, but, in the presence of ethanol, can last for days. Methanol itself is harmless: however, its metabolites, formaldehyde and formic acid, are extremely toxic. Fatalities have been reported after ingestion of as little as 15 mL of a 40 percent methanol solution, although 30 mL is generally considered a minimal lethal dose. Ingestion of only 10 mL can lead to blindness. Adults have survived ingestions of 500 mL.

Clinical Presentation

The onset of symptoms following methanol ingestion varies from 1 to 72 hours. Patients commonly have the following classic triad:

- Visual complaints
- Abdominal pain
- Metabolic acidosis

Eye symptoms include blurring of vision, photophobia, constricted visual fields, snowfield vision, "spots before the eyes," and total blindness. The ophthalmologic examination may reveal dilated pupils with hyperemia of the optic disk, but it can be normal early in the clinical course. Although the blindness is usually permanent, recovery has been reported.

Patients also typically complain of epigastric pain, nausea, and vomiting and can experience gastrointestinal bleeding and acute pancreatitis. Unlike with the other alcohols, these patients often lack the odor of ethanol on their breath and can have a clear sensorium.

Laboratory

Baseline laboratory data include complete blood cell count; levels of electrolytes, glucose, amylase, and arterial blood gases; renal functions; and urinalysis. Classically, methanol-intoxicated patients have an elevated anion gap metabolic acidosis.

The anion gap is calculated using the equation

$$(Na) - (Cl + HCO_3)$$

The normal anion gap is 8 to 12 mEq/L.

Another valuable clue in establishing the diagnosis is the presence of an elevated osmolal gap. The osmolal gap is the difference between measured and calculated osmolarity. It shows that methanol, a highly osmotic compound not normally found in the serum, is present in a significant quantity. The normal difference is <10. Other causes of elevated osmolal gaps include ethylene glycol, ethanol, and isopropanol, all of which are highly osmotically active compounds. Though the osmolal gap is a useful clue, cases of significant methanol and ethylene glycol overdoses have been reported with normal osmolal gaps. The most accurate determination of the measured serum osmol is made using a freezing-point depression method, since the standard vapor pressure analysis merely volatilizes the alcohols, often producing erroneous results.

Measurement of methanol and ethanol levels is critical in managing these overdoses. However, since the measurement of serum methanol is often delayed, the clinician may have to rely on the history, clinical presentation, and the other laboratory data to establish the diagnosis. Generally, levels <20 mg/dL result in minimal to no symptoms. Central nervous system symptoms appear with levels >20 mg/dL and peak levels >50 mg/dL indicate serious toxicity. Ocular symptoms occur at levels >100 mg/dL, and fatalities have been reported in untreated victims with levels >150 mg/dL.

Management

Gastrointestinal decontamination may be efficacious for patients presenting within 1 hour of ingestion. However, since methanol is rapidly absorbed, gastric lavage may not be effective if it is delayed. Although the utility of activated charcoal and cathartics in preventing absorption of the toxic alcohols has not been well established, 1 g/kg can be administered, particularly if a coingestion is suspected.

If a significant ingestion of methanol is likely, empiric treatment with intravenous ethanol is recommended, even if laboratory tests are unavailable. Other indications for ethanol therapy include serum methanol levels >20 mg/dL or acidemia (pH <7.20). Ethanol competitively binds hepatic alcohol dehydrogenase 20 times greater than methanol and delays the formation of the toxic metabolites, formaldehyde and formic acid. To inhibit toxic metabolite formation, ethanol levels are maintained between 100 and 150 mg/dL. An intravenous solution of 10 percent ethanol in D_5W is optimal, with a loading dose of 0.6 g/kg. A simplified approximation of the loading dose is 1 mL/kg of 10 percent diluted absolute ethanol. Close monitoring of the ethanol level every 1 to 2 hours is necessary in order to adjust the maintenance infusion rate for each individual patient. If IV ethanol preparations are unavailable, oral ethanol therapy can be instituted. Continued therapy is recommended until methanol levels fall below 10 mg/dL. Since hypoglycemia is a complication of toxic ethanol levels in young children, serum glucose levels should be monitored.

The antidote for toxic alcohols, 4-methylpyrazole (4-MP), also slows the metabolism of methanol to its toxic metabolites. Unlike ethanol, it lacks CNS-depressant effects and is a direct inhibitor of alcohol dehydrogenase. In most cases, administration of 20 mg/kg of 4-MP adequately inhibits formate formation for 24 hours. Bicarbonate administration should be considered if the serum pH falls below 7.20.

Folate, the active form of folic acid, is a coenzyme in the metabolic step converting the toxic metabolite formate to CO_2 and H_2O and is indicated in the methanol-intoxicated patient. Up to 50 mg of folate can be given intravenously every 4 hours, until the acidosis is corrected and methanol levels fall below 20 mg/dL.

Hemodialysis effectively removes methanol as well as formaldehyde and formic acid. Indications for dialysis include the following:

- Any visual impairment
- Metabolic acidosis not corrected with bicarbonate administration
- Renal failure
- Methanol levels >50 mg/dL (with or without symptoms)

It is important to note that ethanol is readily dialyzed, so the rate of IV administration may have to be increased during dialysis.

Disposition

Any patients who are comatose and have abnormal vital signs, visual complaints, or high methanol levels need admission to an intensive care unit. Asymptomatic patients without evidence of acidosis and with levels <10 mg/dL may be discharged from the emergency department following a period of observation.

ETHYLENE GLYCOL

In 1999, there were 255 exposures to ethylene glycol reported to the AAPCC in individuals <20 years of age, with two reported deaths. Ethylene glycol is a colorless, odorless, sweet-tasting compound that is found in antifreeze products, coolants, preservatives, and glycerine substitutes.

Pharmacokinetics and Pathophysiology

Ethylene glycol undergoes rapid absorption from the gastrointestinal tract, and initial signs of intoxication may occur as early as 30 minutes postingestion. As with the other alcohols, it undergoes hepatic metabolism via alcohol dehydrogenase to form various toxic metabolites, including glycolaldehyde, glycolic acid, and oxalate, all of which are ultimately excreted through the kidney. The hallmark of ethylene glycol toxicity is a severe anion gap metabolic acidosis due to accumulation of glycolic acid and lactate, along with hypocalcemia, which results from the precipitation of calcium oxalate crystals in the kidney.

Clinical Presentation

The clinical effects of ethylene glycol toxicity can be divided into three distinct stages:

- Stage I occurs within the first 12 hours of ingestion, with CNS symptoms similar to that experienced with ethanol. It is characterized by slurred speech, nystagmus, ataxia, vomiting, lethargy, and coma. Patients may suffer convulsions, myoclonic jerks, and tetanic contractions due to hypocalcemia. As with methanol toxicity, patients can demonstrate an anion gap acidosis with an elevated osmol gap. In approximately one-third of cases, calcium oxalate crystals will be discovered in the urine, a finding considered pathognomonic for ethylene glycol poisoning.

- Stage II occurs within 12 to 36 hours after ingestion and is characterized by rapidly progressive tachypnea, cyanosis, pulmonary edema, adult respiratory distress syndrome, and cardiomegaly. Death is most common during this stage.
- Stage III occurs 2 to 3 days postingestion and is heralded by flank pain, oliguria, proteinuria, anuria, and renal failure.

Ethylene glycol poisoning is possible in any inebriated patient lacking an odor of ethanol, who has severe acidosis; calcium crystalluria, or renal failure.

Laboratory

Indicated laboratory studies include complete blood cell count; levels of electrolytes, glucose, calcium, creatine kinase, serum ethanol and ethylene glycol, and arterial blood gases; renal functions; serum osmolarity; and urine analysis for crystals, protein, and blood. Both anion and osmolal gaps are calculated. Due to the potential for severe cardiopulmonary effects in stage II, a chest radiograph and an electrocardiogram are recommended. Since fluorescein is present in many antifreeze products, fluorescence of the patient's urine when exposed to light from a Wood's lamp may be a valuable diagnostic clue, although the clinical efficacy of this test has been challenged in the recent literature.

Management

Gastric lavage may be useful in patients presenting within 1 hour of ingestion. Syrup of ipecac is contraindicated due to potential CNS depression, coma, and convulsions. Activated charcoal can be administered, although there are no good studies documenting its effectiveness in ethylene glycol toxicity. Patients who develop seizures are treated with standard doses of benzodiazapenes and phenobarbital.

If ethylene glycol poisoning is likely, patients are acidotic (pH <7.20), or the ethylene glycol level is >20 mg/dL, intravenous ethanol therapy is instituted. Ethanol competitively binds alcohol dehydrogenase with an affinity

Table 81-1. Toxic Alcohol Antidotes

Methanol	Ethylene Glycol
Ethanol drip	Ethanol drip
Folate	Thiamine
	Pyridoxine
Methylpyrazole	Methylpyrazole

100 times greater than ethylene glycol and slows the accumulation of toxic metabolites. If an intravenous preparation of ethanol is unavailable, patients can be loaded orally to achieve an ethanol level of 100 to 150 mg/dL. Since toxic ethanol levels result in profound hypoglycemia in small children, serial glucose measurements are monitored.

As with methanol, the alcohol dehydrogenase inhibitor 4-MP is an antidote for ethylene glycol toxicity. Bicarbonate administration is recommended for patients with pH <7.20.

Serum calcium levels are monitored and hypocalcemia is treated with 10 percent calcium gluconate. Additionally, thiamine and pyridoxine (vitamin B_6) are recommended in ethylene glycol poisonings in order to shunt or reroute the metabolism of ethylene glycol toward less toxic metabolites (Table 81-1).

Hemodialysis effectively removes ethylene glycol, as well as its toxic metabolites and is indicated in the setting of metabolic acidosis not responsive to bicarbonate administration, pulmonary edema, renal failure, and serum ethylene glycol levels >50 mg/dL, regardless of symptoms.

ISOPROPANOL

In 1999, there were 5800 cases of isopropanol exposure reported to the AAPCC in individuals <20 years of age. Of note, 90 percent of exposures occurred in children <6 years of age. Isopropanol is a common solvent and disinfectant with CNS-depressant properties similar to ethanol. Exposure from isopropyl alcohol occurs more frequently in children <6 years old than ethanol ingestions. Toxicity results from both accidental and intentional ingestions, as well as inhalation and dermal exposures in young children given rubbing alcohol sponge baths.

Pharmacokinetics and Pathophysiology

Isopropanol is rapidly absorbed from the gastric mucosa with acute intoxication occurring within 30 minutes of ingestion. It is metabolized by alcohol dehydrogenase, but, unlike the other alcohols, is metabolized to the CNS depressant, acetone. Respiratory elimination of the ace-tone causes a fruity-acetone odor on the patient's breath similar to diabetic ketoacidosis. Because 70 percent iso-propanol is a potent inebriant and twice as intoxicating as ethanol, a level of 50 mg/dL is comparable to an ethanol level of 100 mg/dL.

Clinical Presentation

Isopropanol-intoxicated patients are classically lethargic or comatose, hypotensive, and tachycardiac, with the char-acteristic breath odor of rubbing alcohol or acetone. Coma develops at levels >100 mg/dL. Hypotension results from peripheral vasodilation and cardiac depression. Gastroin-testinal irritation with acute abdominal pain and he-matemesis can also ensue. With isopropanol, unlike the other toxic alcohols, acidosis, ophthalmologic changes, and renal failure are classically absent. However, like ethanol, methanol, and ethylene glycol, isopropanol can produce a significant osmolal gap (Table 81-2).

Laboratory

Patients are tested for the presence of acetonemia and ace-tonuria. Unlike diabetic ketoacidosis, the acetone is typi-cally found in the absence of glucosuria, hyperglycemia, or acidemia. Indicated laboratory studies include a com-plete blood cell count; levels of electrolytes, arterial blood gas, glucose, and serum ethanol and isopropanol; serum osmolarity, and renal functions. Isopropanol levels >400 mg/dL correspond to severe toxicity.

Management

Patients are managed with particular attention paid to the integrity of the airway. Hypotension is treated with

Table 81-2. Comparison of Toxic Alcohols

Parameter	Methanol	Ethylene Glycol	Isopropanol
Anion gap acidosis	+	+	−
Osmolal gap	+	+	+
CNS depression	+	+	+
Eye findings	+	−	−
Renal failure	+/−	+	−
Ketones	−	−	+
Oxalate crystals	−	+	−

intravenous crystalloid. Since isopropanol is so rapidly absorbed from the gastrointestinal tract, gastric deconta-mination is only indicated if performed within 1 hour postingestion. Induction of emesis is avoided, due to the potential for the rapid development of coma. Activated charcoal may be administered particularly if a co-ingestion exists, although the efficacy in the setting of isopropanol alone is questionable. No ethanol drip is in-dicated since the metabolite acetone is relatively non-toxic and excreted through the lungs. Hemodialysis is effective in removing isopropanol, but is reserved for prolonged coma, hypotension, and isopropanol levels >400 to 500 mg/dL. Typically, patients progress well with supportive care alone.

Disposition

Isopropanol-intoxicated patients who are lethargic should be admitted, while asymptomatic children may be observed in the emergency department. Ingestion of >3 swallows (15 mL) of 70 percent isopropanol by a 10-kg child (1.5 mL/kg) is an indication for several hours of observation.

BIBLIOGRAPHY

Barceloux DG, Krenzelor E, Olson K, et al: American Acad-emy of Clinical Toxicology Ad Hoc Committee: Guidelines on the treatment of ethylene glycol poisoning. *J Toxicol Clin Toxicol* 37:537–560, 1999.

Brent J, McMartin K, Phillips S, et al: Fomepizole for the treat-ment of ethylene glycol poisoning. *N Engl J Med* 340: 832–838, 1999.

Burkhart KK, Kulig KW: The other alcohols: Methanol, ethyl-ene glycol and isopropanol. *Emerg Clin North Am* 8: 913–928, 1990.

Erickson T: Toxic alcohol poisoning: When to suspect and keys to diagnosis. *Consultant* 40:1845–1856, 2000.

Jacobsen D, McMartin KE: Antidotes for methanol and eth-ylene glycol poisoning. *J Toxicol Clin Toxicol* 35:127, 1997.

Litovitz TL, Schwartz-Klein W, White S, et al: 1999 Annual Report of the AAPCC Toxic Exposure Surveillance System. *Am J Emerg Med* 18:517–574, 2000.

Liu JJ, Daya MR, Carrasquill O, et al: Prognostic factors in patients with methanol poisoning. *J Toxicol Clin Toxicol* 36:175, 1998.

Saladino R, Shannon M: Accidental and intentional poisoning with ethylene glycol in infancy: Diagnostic clues and man-agement. *Pediatr Emerg Care* 7:93–96, 1991.

Woolf AD, Wynshaw-Boris A, Rinaldo P, et al: Intentional in-fantile ethylene glycol poisoning presenting as an inherited metabolic disorder. *J Pediatr* 120:421–424, 1992.

82

Anticholinergic Poisoning

Steven E. Aks

HIGH-YIELD FACTS

- Anticholinergics are found in diverse products ranging from plants to antihistamines and other drugs.
- The typical anticholinergic toxidrome can be remembered as: Hot as a hare, blind as a bat, dry as a bone, red as a beet, and mad as a hatter.
- Diphenhydramine overdose has caused QRS widening, and astemizole overdose has caused torsades de pointes.
- Most cases of anticholinergic overdoses can be treated with supportive care, along with benzodiazepines.
- Physostigmine should be reserved for patients with severe agitation and delirium. One must be sure that the QRS is normal and that a tricyclic antidepressant has not been ingested prior to using this antidote.

Anticholinergic poisoning results from both pharmaceutical agents and natural toxins. Common pharmaceuticals include antihistamines and decongestants, while natural toxins include plants and mushrooms. According to the American Association of Poison Control Center (AAPCC) data in 1999, there were a total of 56,807 anticholinergic and antihistamine exposures. There were 37,645 in children <6, 11,088 in children from 6 to 19, and there were a total of 32 deaths. Many of these products are widely available in over-the-counter preparations (Table 82-1).

PHARMACOLOGY AND PATHOPHYSIOLOGY

Anticholinergics act by inhibiting the action of the neurotransmitter acetylcholine, which is found at the sympathetic and parasympathetic ganglia, at parasympathetic nerve endings, at neuromuscular junctions, and in the central nervous system. These agents competitively block the action of acetylcholine at the effector site. The manifestations of toxicity can be broken down into central and peripheral effects. Central effects include agitation, disorientation, hallucinations, and seizures. Peripheral manifestations include mydriasis, tachycardia, tachypnea, flushing, dry mucous membranes, urinary retention, and loss of gastrointestinal motility.

CLINICAL PRESENTATION

The central and peripheral manifestations of anticholinergic substances (the anticholnergic toxidrome) are described by the following phrases:

- Hot as a hare
- Blind as a bat
- Dry as a bone
- Red as a beet
- Mad as a hatter

The major central nervous system manifestations of anticholinergic toxicity range from overstimulation, with nervousness, agitation, and delirium, to depression, with lethargy, drowsiness, and coma. Tremor may be present, and, in extreme cases, seizures. Cardiovascular effects include tachycardia and dysrhythmias. Syncope can occur, and either hypotension or hypertension may be present. Electrocardiogram changes secondary to anticholinergic poisoning include prolonged QT interval, QRS widening, ventricular dysrhythmias, and heart block. Torsades de pointes has been described after antihistamine (astemizole) overdose. Skin and mucous membranes will appear dry, and the former will appear flushed. Urinary retention is an important clinical finding to recognize. Hyperthermia can also occur and may be severe.

DIAGNOSIS

Diagnosis is generally based on the constellation of signs and symptoms of the anticholinergic toxidrome. Occasionally, unusual physical findings give clues to the diagnosis of anticholinergic poisoning. A unilaterally fixed and dilated pupil with an otherwise normal neurologic exam can be seen after the instillation of anticholinergic drops in the eye. This can also be seen as "corn picker's" pupil, where dust from the anticholinergic plant jimsonweed makes its way into a person's eye. In general, the history of ingestion will support the diagnosis.

Table 82-1. Common Examples of Anticholinergics

Pharmaceuticals
  Astemizole
  Atropine
  Cyprohepatidine
  Dimenhydrinate
  Diphenhydramine
  Hyoscyamine
  Pyrilines
Natural Products
  Deadly nightshade (belladonna)
  Jimson weed
  Mushrooms (*Amanita muscaria*)
Other Drug Categories With Anticholinergic Properties
  Antiparkinson agents
  Antipsychotics
  Antispasmodics
  Cyclic antidepressants
  Phenothiazones

Routine laboratory studies include complete blood cell count and levels of electrolytes, BUN, creatinine, and glucose. Creatine phosphokinase is useful to rule out rhabdomyolysis that may result from seizures or hyperthermia. A 12-lead electrocardiogram and continuous monitoring are essential for patients with anticholinergic poisoning. Routine urine toxicology screens may not include common antihistamines, which may need to be specifically requested.

MANAGEMENT

As with any toxin that can induce seizures or cause coma, strict attention must be paid to the ABCs. Patients have venous access secured and are given supplemental oxygen as needed. Continuous cardiac monitoring is essential. Decontamination by lavage is preferred, followed by the administration of activated charcoal. Lavage can be of value several hours after ingestion because of decreased gut motility seen with anticholinergic poisoning. Ipecac is contraindicated because of the potential of altered mental status and seizures. Multiple dosing of activated charcoal in the setting of anticholinergic poisoning is controversial because of the likelihood of toxin-induced gastric atony.

Supportive care is generally all that is needed to successfully treat anticholinergic poisoning. For agitation and seizures benzodiazepines can be of value. Hyperthermia is treated aggressively with cooling measures. Urinary retention is managed symptomatically.

Cardiac dysrhythmias are treated by standard measures. However, wide complex tachycardia after diphenhydramine has been treated successfully with sodium bicarbonate. This may work by reversing the local anesthetic properties of the drug. Magnesium has been used successfully to treat torsades de pointes after astemizole overdose.

Physostigmine has been used for years as an antidote to many poisons that alter mental status. However, it should probably be used only for pure anticholinergic poisoning. Physostigmine functions as an anticholinesterase and counteracts the effects of anticholinergic drugs. It is a tertiary amine that crosses the blood brain barrier and reverses both the central and peripheral effects of the anticholinergic poison. It has a half-life of only 90 minutes and repeat dosing may be necessary. The dose of physostigmine is 2 mg slow IV push in adults. In children, it is 0.02 mg/kg (not to exceed 0.5 mg) slow IV push over 2 minutes. The dose can be repeated after 20 minutes if no effect is noted.

The use of physostigmine should be reserved for those cases not manageable with supportive care and those that manifest profound agitation, persistent seizures, tachydysrhythmias, refractory hypotension, or malignant hypertension. It is indicated only in pure anticholinergic poisoning and not for drugs with mixed actions such as phenothiazines and cyclic antidepressants. Physostigmine has significant complications including nausea, vomiting, seizures, and worsening dysrhythmias. It has been reported to cause cardiac standstill in the setting of atrioventricular block with cyclic antidepressant overdose. Excessive administration of the drug will cause symptoms of cholinergic excess, including salivation, lacrimation, diarrhea, bronchorrhea, bronchospasm, and bradycardia. Cardiac monitoring is essential during its administration.

DISPOSITION

Any case of significant toxicity with alteration of mental status or dysrhythmias is observed overnight in an intensive care setting. If patients receive physostigmine, admission is also warranted. Children or toddlers who have had an accidental ingestion and exhibit only minor or no symptoms can be observed in the emergency department for at least 6 hours after decontamination and administration of activated charcoal and then be discharged to reliable caretakers.

BIBLIOGRAPHY

Burns MJ, Linden CH, Graudins A, et al: A comparison of physostigmine and benzodiazepines for the treatment of anticholinergic poisoning. *Ann Emerg Med* 35:374–381, 2000.

Clark RF, Vance MV: Massive diphenhydramine poisoning resulting in a wide-complex tachycardia: Successful treatment with sodium bicarbonate. *Ann Emerg Med* 21:318–321, 1992.

Farrell M, Heinrichs M, Tilelli JA: Response of life-threatening dimenhydrinate intoxication to sodium bicarbonate administration. *Clin Toxicol* 29:527–535, 1991.

Hasan RA, Zureikat GY, Nolan BM: Torsade de pointes associated with astemizole overdose treated with magnesium sulfate. *Pediatr Emerg Care* 9:23–25, 1993.

Hyers JH, Moro-Sutherland D, Shook JE: Anticholinergic poisoning in colicky infants treated with hyoscyamine sulfate. *Am J Emerg Med* 15:532–535, 1997.

Litovitz TL, Klein-Schwartz W, White S, et al: 1999 Annual Report of Poison Control Centers Toxic Exposure Surveillance System. *Am J Emerg Med* 18:517–574, 2000.

Mendoza FS, Atiba JO, Krensky AM, et al: Rhabdomyolysis complicating doxylamine overdose. *Clin Pediatr* 26:595–597, 1987.

Thompson HS: Cornpicker's pupil: Jimson weed mydriasis. *J Iowa Med Soc* 61:575–578, 1971.

Wiley JF, Gelber ML, Henretig FM, et al: Cardiotoxic effects of Astemizole overdose in children. *J Pediatr* 120:799–802, 1992.

Wyngaarden JB, Seevers MH: The toxic effects of antihistamininc drugs. *JAMA* 145:277–282, 1951.

83

Oral Anticoagulants

Jerrold B. Leikin

HIGH-YIELD FACTS

- After ingestion of "superwarfarin" agents, effects can be seen for weeks.
- Intervention may be required for warfarin ingestions >0.5 mg/kg or superwarfarin ingestions >0.05 mg/kg.
- Accidental single pediatric ingestions rarely require intervention.
- Vitamin K_1 is the specific antidote.

If the potential toxicity of anticoagulants is underestimated, disaster can result. These agents are commonly available in the home in the form of prescription medications, such as warfarin (Coumadin) and are the predominant agent in many rodenticides, which are often placed in areas accessible to small children (Table 83-1). Rodent baits and pellets are usually colored with water-soluble blue or green dye to facilitate recognition or oral exposures.

Some rodenticides contain newer, extremely potent and long-acting superwarfarin anticoagulants that can result in severe toxicity even when ingested in very small amounts. Of the 18,477 warfarin-based exposures called into poison control centers in 1999, 96 percent involved rodenticides and about 90 percent involved children <6 years of age. Vitamin K_1 was used in 370 cases. There were 3 reported deaths.

PATHOPHYSIOLOGY

While there are many substances that can be considered anticoagulants, it is the vitamin K antagonists that cause most of the problems in the pediatric age group. They can be categorized into either hydroxycoumarins, which include warfarin, and indandiones, which include pindone. The hydroxycoumarin group also includes difenacoum and brodifacoum, superwarfarin agents used in rodenticides, whose anticoagulant activity can last for weeks. Chlorphacinone is a powerful, long-acting inandione. The onset of anticoagulation is usually within 1 to 2 days. The serum half-lives of the anticoagulant rodenticides are 25 days for brodifacoum and 12 days for difenacoum.

Each category of anticoagulant inhibits the formation of vitamin-K–dependent clotting factors II, VII, IX, and X by inhibiting the action of K_1 reductase and depleting active vitamin K_1. Depletion of the vitamin-K–dependent clotting factors interrupts the coagulation cascade and can result in bleeding.

Acute exposure to >0.5 mg/kg of warfarin or about 0.05 mg/kg of the superwarfarins usually requires intervention. Patients who have chronic ingestions may require prolonged observation.

DIAGNOSIS

The clinical toxicity of anticoagulants is almost entirely restricted to bleeding diathesis. Spontaneous emesis, epistaxis, ecchymosis, soft tissue hematomas, gastrointestinal bleeding, hematuria, and hemoptysis can occur. Intracranial hemorrhage is a devastating complication and is possible in any patient with a history of anticoagulant exposure and a history of headache or who develops mental status changes.

For patients who ingest a rodenticide, it is essential to determine whether the compound contained a "normal" anticoagulant or one of the superwarfarins. Ingestion of the lower toxicity agents is more common, and usually does not require aggressive intervention, while ingestion of the superwarfarin compounds is cause for concern.

Laboratory Studies

In the acute ingestion, all laboratory studies are likely to be normal. In chronic exposures or in cases where a toxic dose has been ingested significantly prior to arrival to the emergency department, measurement of the prothrombin time (PT) or International Normalized Ratio (INR) correlates with the depression of the vitamin-K–dependent clotting factors. In cases where the PT is prolonged, baseline hemoglobin and platelet count are necessary. Additionally, the urine and stool should be checked for blood.

MANAGEMENT

Gastric Decontamination

Gut decontamination after ingestion of anticoagulants is controversial.

Table 83-1. Vitamin K–Antagonist Agents

Coumarin Derivatives

Difenacoum (Ratak®)	Phenprocoumon
Bromadiolone (Bromone®)	Acenacoumarin
Brodifacoum (Talan®)	Sodium warfarin
Coumatetralyl (Endox®)	Prolin (Eraze)
Discoumacetate	Coumafene
Zoocoumarin (Rodex®)	Fumarin
Valone (PMP Tracking Powder®)	Coumapuryl
Bishydroxy-Coumarin	Tomarin

Indandione Derivatives

Diphacione (Dipazin®)	Diphenadione
Pindone (Pival®)	Diphacin (Kill-ko Rat Killer)
Chlorphacione (Caid®, Drat®)	
Valone	Pival
Anisindione	Piraldione (Tri-Ban)
Phenindione	Radione

In chronic cases or in situations where arrival to the emergency department has been delayed, emesis or lavage is contraindicated due to the possibility of a coagulopathy and iatrogenically induced gastric hemorrhage. Activated charcoal is indicated in acute ingestions.

Vitamin K_1 is the specific antidote for anticoagulant toxicity and is indicated in the presence of a prolonged INR/PT or for patients who have bleeding. Vitamin K_3 and vitamin K_4 are not useful antidotes. Vitamin K_1 can be ad-

Table 83-2. Doses of Vitamin K_1

Oral dose	Adult: 15–25 mg
Larger daily amounts for superwarfarin poisoning	
For small ingestion	Child: 5–10 mg
Intravenous dose	Adult: about 10 mg
For rapid correction only; diluted in a saline or glucose at a rate not to exceed 5 percent of total dose per minute	Child 1–5 mg
Intramuscular dose	
Mild ingestions—where risk of hematoma is low	Child: 1–5 mg
Subcutaneous injection	Adult: 5–10 mg Child: 1–5 mg

ministered subcutaneously, intramuscularly, and intravenously. For patients with severe toxicity, the intravenous route is preferred. The major adverse reaction to intravenous administration is anaphylaxis. The intramuscular route is not recommended for patients with severe toxicity because of the risk of hematoma formation (Table 83-2).

Patients with severe bleeding or with evidence of intracranial hemorrhage require rapid reversal of coagulopathy and are treated with fresh frozen plasma (15 mL/kg) or pooled clotting factors.

Patients ingesting superwarfarin agents have been treated with phenobarbital, which potentially increases the hepatic synthesis of vitamin-K–dependent clotting factors. The efficacy of this is unknown. Likewise, cholestyramine has been utilized to increase clearance of warfarin, but this remains experimental.

DISPOSITION

Hospitalization is usually not necessary for children who ingest warfarin tablets or rodenticides that do not contain superwarfarin compounds. However, they require close outpatient follow-up with an INR or PT measurement at 48 hours, with observation for gastrointestinal bleeding and prolongation of PT for up to 5 days after the ingestion. After ingestions of >0.5 mg/kg of warfarin or >0.05 mg/kg of a superwarfarin compound and for patients with prolonged PTs or active bleeding, hospitalization is indicated until the coagulation profile normalizes. For patients who ingest superwarfarin compounds, observation and monitoring of PT continues for several weeks.

BIBLIOGRAPHY

Bruno GH, Howland MA, McMeeking A, et al: Long-acting anticoagulant overdose (bodifacoum) kinetics and optimal vitamin K dosing. *Ann Emerg Med* 35(3):262–267, 2000.

Hung A, Tait RC: A prospective randomized study to determine the optimal dose of intravenous vitamin K in reversal of over-warfarinization. *Br J Hematology* 109:537–539, 2000.

Litovitz TL, Klein-Schwartz W, White S, et al: 1999 Annual report of the American Association of Poison Control Centers toxic exposure surveillance system. *Am J Emerg Med* 18(5):517–574, 2000.

Mullins MF, Branda CL, Daya R: Unintentional pediatric superwarfarin exposures. Do we really need a prothrombin time? *Pediatrics* 105:402–404, 2000.

Sheperd G, Klein-Schwartz W, Anderson B: Acute pediatric brodificoum poisoning. *J Toxicol Clin Toxicol* 30(5):464, 1998.

Smolinske SC, Scherger DS, Kearns PS, et al: Superwarfarin poisoning in children: A prospective study. *Pediatrics* 84:490–494, 1989.

84

Antihypertensives, Beta Blockers, and Calcium Antagonists

Gary R. Strange
Kennethr Bizovi

HIGH-YIELD FACTS

- Due to the rapid absorption of many β-blockers, the onset of symptoms may be as rapid as 30 minutes after ingestion, but it most commonly occurs within 1 to 2 hours. Cardiovascular manifestations include hypotension, bradycardia, heart block, and congestive heart failure.

- Absorption of β-blockers can be decreased by gastric emptying and administration of activated charcoal. If the ingestion occurred less than 4 hours prior to presentation, gastric emptying is indicated.

- For patients with symptomatic bradycardia and hypotension, glucagon has been shown to reverse the toxic effects of β-blockers. It is a positive inotrope that appears to work by increasing cyclic AMP.

- Patients who do not respond to glucagon are treated with aggressive fluid resuscitation and sympathomimetics. Epinephrine is the catecholamine of choice, given as a continuous infusion, starting at a rate of 1 μg/min and titrating to perfusion parameters.

- A patient with a history of non–sustained-release β-blocker ingestion is observed on a cardiac monitor for 6 hours after ingestion. Patients with signs of cardiovascular, respiratory, or CNS toxicity are admitted to a monitored bed. A patient who ingested a β-blocker that is not a sustained-release product can be discharged home after the observation period if there is no suicidal ideation and there are no signs of toxicity

found by clinical examination, ECG, or cardiac monitoring.

- The different pharmacologic profiles of calcium channel blockers will cause various presentations, but in all cases, the cardiovascular effects predominate. Verapamil and diltiazem typically cause bradycardia and hypotension.

- For calcium channel blocker overdose with hypotension that persists despite the administration of fluids, calcium salts and glucagon therapy with vasopressors are indicated. Dopamine is a reasonable first-line option.

- High-dose insulin has been shown to be effective in the management of calcium channel blocker overdose, presumably by improving myocardial contractility and by improving conduction by lowering potassium concentrations. Insulin should be used early in the ED course and administered as a bolus of regular insulin, 1 U/kg, followed by 1 U/kg/h for the first hour, then 0.5 U/kg/h thereafter until no longer needed.

- Clonidine-induced bradycardia is treated with atropine if it is associated with hypotension. Hypotension is treated with aggressive fluid resuscitation. Moderate-dose dopamine may be useful for hypotension and may also ameliorate bradycardia.

- There may be a role for naloxone in reversing the opiate-like side effects of clonidine on mental status and respiration and there is some indication that it can reverse clonidine-mediated hypotension.

BETA-ADRENERGIC BLOCKING AGENTS

Beta blockers are a diverse category of drugs with multiple therapeutic uses and toxic effects. They are used in the treatment of hypertension, thyrotoxicosis, dysrhythmias, angina, migraine headaches, withdrawal states, and glaucoma. Frequently, children are exposed to these drugs by ingesting the medications of their parents or grandparents.

In 1999, the American Academy of Poison Control Centers (AAPCC) reported 9502 β-blocker exposures. Of these, 2556 (27 percent) exposures were in children

<6 years old and 972 (10 percent) were in children or adolescents aged 6 to 19 years. There were a total of 26 deaths (0.3 percent). The overall mortality of β-blocker overdose is much lower than that of overdose from calcium channel blockers or digoxin.

Pharmacology

Beta-blocker properties that determine the drug's effect are β_1-antagonist activity, β_2-antagonist activity, intrinsic sympathomimetic activity, and membrane-stabilizing activity. Labetalol is the only β-blocker that has α-antagonist activity. β_1-antagonist activity causes decreased cardiac contractility and conduction. β_2-antagonist activity causes increased smooth muscle tone, which manifests itself as bronchospasm, increased peripheral vascular tone, and increased gut motility. Although many β-blockers are β_1-selective at therapeutic doses, these drugs have both β_1- and β_2-effects in the overdose setting. The intrinsic sympathomimetic property of some β-blockers causes an agonist-antagonist activity, which may lead to paradoxical effects of hypertension and tachycardia in overdose. The membrane-stabilizing activity of β-blockers causes a quinidine-like effect, leading to decreased contractility. This effect is additive to the β_1- toxic effects. Membrane-stabilizing activity also causes central nervous system (CNS) depression. Those drugs that are lipophilic and have membrane-stabilizing activity, such as propranolol, acebutolol, and oxprenolol, have increased mortality in overdose. The α-antagonist activity of labetalol causes decreased peripheral vascular resistance. Sotalol is a β-blocker with class III antiarrhythmic properties. In overdose, this drug can lead to prolongation of the QT interval and ventricular arrhythmias, including torsades de pointes. Each different β-blocker preparation may have only some of the described activities and manifestations may vary.

Pharmacokinetics

The absorption, distribution, and elimination of β-blockers vary with the various drug preparations. Some β-blockers are available in extended-release preparations. As with all extended-release preparations, the onset of toxic effects may be delayed. Beta blockers are rapidly absorbed, with a 30 to 90 percent bioavailability. The elimination half-life varies from 2 to 24 hours, depending on the drug. In many cases, the half-life is significantly increased in overdose.

Pathophysiology

Suppression of the cardiovascular system is the hallmark of β-blocker overdose. β_1-blockade leads to negative inotropic and chronotropic effects. Membrane-stabilizing activity further exacerbates cardiotoxicity. Respiratory compromise during β-blocker overdose can result from cardiogenic shock, decreased respiratory drive, or β_2-antagonist effects. β_2-blockade causes bronchospasm and usually affects patients with previously diagnosed bronchospastic disease. Hypoglycemia may occur secondary to β_2-mediated decrease in glycogenolysis and gluconeogenesis. Central nervous system depression may be caused by direct toxicity, hypoxia, hypoglycemia, or shock. Those drugs with membrane-stabilizing properties cause direct CNS depression.

Clinical Presentation

Due to the rapid absorption of many β-blockers, the onset of symptoms may be as rapid as 30 minutes after ingestion, but it most commonly occurs within 1 to 2 hours. The cardiovascular manifestations include hypotension, bradycardia, heart block, and congestive heart failure. Aside from atrioventricular (AV) block, electrocardiographic manifestations of toxicity include prolongation of the PR interval, QRS complex, and QT interval, as well as bundle branch block. Respiratory toxicity includes noncardiogenic pulmonary edema, pulmonary edema, exacerbation of asthma, and decreased respiratory drive. Patients may also present with CNS depression or seizures.

Laboratory Evaluation

All patients with a history of β-blocker ingestion are placed on a cardiac monitor and receive an electrocardiogram (ECG). Laboratory tests for blood levels of β-blockers are available from reference laboratories but are helpful only in confirming the exposure. Serum electrolytes are obtained and abnormalities addressed. Serum glucose may be decreased and is evaluated. Arterial blood gas may be useful in the patient with respiratory signs or symptoms. Chest radiograph is obtained for patients who are admitted or have respiratory signs or symptoms.

Management

The patient with a history of β-blocker ingestion is placed on a cardiac monitor and intravenous access is established. If the patient is stable, he or she is monitored for signs of toxicity and measures are taken to decrease absorption.

Absorption can be decreased by gastric emptying and administration of activated charcoal. If the ingestion occurred less than 4 hours prior to presentation, gastric emptying is indicated. Ipecac is relatively contraindicated because rapid CNS depression may occur, leading to aspiration. In cases that present early, lavage is the preferred method of gastric decontamination. The airway is protected with endotracheal intubation in patients with altered mental status. Activated charcoal and sorbitol cathartic are administered (see Table 79-7).

The patient with respiratory compromise is evaluated for the presence of pulmonary edema or bronchospasm. Patients with pulmonary edema are supported with oxygen and, if necessary, intubation until cardiogenic shock is corrected.

For patients with symptomatic bradycardia and hypotension, glucagon has been shown to reverse the toxic effects of β-blockers. It is a positive inotrope that appears to work by increasing cyclic AMP. In adults, an initial bolus of glucagon is administered at a dose of 50 to 150 μg/kg, administered intravenously over 1 minute. If symptoms recur, a repeat bolus is given. If symptoms persist, an infusion may be started at 1 to 5 mg/h. Pediatric dosing has not been established. If glucagon is administered multiple times or as an infusion, it is mixed in normal saline or D_5W, since the package diluent contains phenol, which is cardiotoxic.

Patients who do not respond to glucagon are treated with aggressive fluid resuscitation and sympathomimetics. Epinephrine is the catecholamine of choice, given as a continuous infusion, starting at a rate of 1 μg/min and titrating to perfusion parameters. Dopamine or dobutamine may be helpful. Isoproterenol, a pure β-agonist, has at least theoretical use, but can cause hypotension and has been associated with myocardial ischemia when used in the treatment of asthma. It is reasonable to try atropine for patients with bradycardia, but it is frequently ineffective. For patients with bradycardia and hypotension refractory to pharmocologic intervention, temporary pacing is an option, but it too may not reverse the cardiac depression of severe β-blocker overdose.

Interventions such as extracorporeal membrane oxygenation (ECMO) or cardiac bypass are considerations for patients with toxicity refractory to all other therapy.

Hemodialysis and hemoperfusion are of limited use in the setting of β-blocker overdose. Most of the β-blockers have a large volume of distribution and are highly protein bound. A few drugs, such as nadolol, sotalol, atenolol, and acebutolol, can be dialyzed, but information is limited to case reports. The main indications for hemodialysis are renal failure and hemodynamic instability. Patients who are unstable often cannot tolerate the procedure, making their care difficult.

Disposition

A patient with a history of non–sustained-release β-blocker ingestion is observed on a cardiac monitor for 6 hours after ingestion. Patients who have signs of cardiovascular, respiratory, or CNS toxicity are admitted to a monitored bed. Patients with a history of ingestion of extended-release preparations are admitted and monitored for 24 hours. A patient who ingested a β-blocker that is not a sustained-release product can be discharged home after the observation period if there is no suicidal ideation and there are no signs of toxicity found by clinical examination, ECG, or cardiac monitoring.

CALCIUM CHANNEL BLOCKERS

The calcium channel blockers have various clinical uses centered around their ability to decrease peripheral and coronary vascular tone as well as to slow AV node conduction. They are used to treat hypertension, coronary artery disease and atrial fibrillation, and to prevent cerebral vasospasm. In 1999, the AAPCC reported 8844 exposures to calcium channel antagonists, of which 2304 (26 percent) were pediatric ingestions. There were 61 deaths (0.7 percent).

Pharmacology

Calcium channel blockers decrease contraction of vascular muscle and myocardium by inhibiting the influx of calcium into the cell. This action decreases activity of the calcium-dependent actin-myosin ATPase. The three calcium channel blockers, verapamil, diltiazem, and nifedipine, are structurally different. Each drug affects a different subset of calcium channels, leading to a unique set of physiologic effects. Verapamil affects both the myocardium and the peripheral arterioles, causing decreased contractility, AV node conduction, and peripheral vascular resistance. Diltiazem has less effect on peripheral vasodilatation and myocardial contractility than verapamil. Diltiazem slows AV node conduction and causes coronary artery dilatation. Nifedipine has the greatest effect on peripheral vascular resistance and also decreases contractility, with minimal effect on AV node conduction. The unique properties of each drug define their therapeutic and toxic effects; however, in overdose, any of these drugs can cause peripheral vasodilatation, decreased AV conduction, and decreased myocardial contractility.

Pharmacokinetics

The various calcium channel blockers have slightly different pharmacokinetic properties. They are >90 percent absorbed, with a significant first-pass metabolism. Verapamil and diltiazem have 20 to 30 percent bioavailability and nifedipine has a 60 percent bioavailability. The onset of action is <30 minutes. All three drugs have a large volume of distribution and are highly protein bound. They are metabolized by the liver. The half-life of calcium channel blockers varies from 3 to 7 hours but can be greatly increased in the setting of overdose. It is extremely important to be aware that sustained-release preparations can have life-threatening sequelae 24 hours after ingestion due to their prolonged absorption time.

Pathophysiology

In overdose, the pharmacologic effects of calcium channel blockers may lead to life-threatening physiologic sequelae. Slowing of the sinus node leads to bradycardia. Slowing of conduction leads to heart blocks and asystole. Decreased contractility can cause heart failure and shock. Lowered peripheral vascular resistance leads to hypotension, which may exacerbate the hypotension associated with bradycardia, bradyarrhythmias, and heart failure. Patients with cardiac disease and those on cardiosuppressant drugs may develop severe toxic effects in mild overdose or even at otherwise therapeutic doses.

Clinical Effects

The different pharmacologic profile of calcium channel blockers will cause various presentations, but in all cases, the cardiovascular effects predominate. Verapamil and diltiazem typically cause bradycardia and hypotension. Hypotension may be due to sinoatrial node depression, atrioventricular node depression leading to AV blocks, or decreased peripheral vascular resistance. Nifedipine primarily affects the arterioles, causing decreased peripheral vascular resistance, which leads to hypotension and reflex tachycardia.

Neurologic and respiratory findings are usually secondary to cardiovascular toxicity and shock. Respiratory effects include decreased respiratory drive, pulmonary edema, and ARDS. Neurologic sequelae include depressed sensorium, cerebral infarction, and seizures. Nausea, vomiting, and constipation can occur.

The most important gastrointestinal consequence to recognize is obstruction due to a concretion of sustained-release capsules. In addition to causing a bowel obstruction, the concretion can be a source of continued toxicity. Early recognition of sustained-release capsules in the gastrointestinal tract and their prompt evacuation can decrease morbidity and mortality.

Laboratory

Hypoperfusion, inhibition of insulin release, and electrolyte abnormalities are the metabolic consequences of calcium channel blocker overdose. Decreased insulin release can lead to hyperglycemia. Hypoperfusion may lead to profound lactic acidosis. Hypocalcemia is the most frequent electrolyte abnormality. Hypokalemia and hyperkalemia have also been reported.

Drug levels for calcium channel blockers are available by reference laboratories but are helpful only in confirming the presence of the agent. An ECG is obtained in any patient with a history of calcium channel blocker overdose and is assessed for blocks, bradycardia, and ischemic changes. When possible, the ECG is compared to previous ECGs. Electrolytes are evaluated, specifically Na^+, Ca^{2+}, Mg^{2+}, and K^+. Arterial blood gas is obtained in patients with signs or symptoms of toxicity and when co-ingestions are suspected to evaluate oxygenation and acid-base status. Chest radiographs are obtained for patients with respiratory signs or symptoms. Sustained-release tablets may be radiopaque. An abdominal radiograph may be useful for patients with signs of obstruction or history of ingesting sustained-release tablets.

Management

In the unstable patient, supportive care and antidotal therapy are instituted immediately. The patient is placed on a cardiac monitor, intravenous access is established, and fluid resuscitation with crystalloid is initiated in hypotensive patients. In the patient with altered mental status, oxygen and naloxone are administered and glucose is given if a bedside test indicates hypoglycemia. Intubation may be necessary for airway protection or for patients with respiratory failure secondary to pulmonary edema or ARDS.

If the patient is stable, he or she is monitored for signs of toxicity and measures are taken to decrease absorption. Absorption can be decreased by gastric emptying and administration of activated charcoal. If the ingestion was <1 hour prior to presentation, gastric emptying may be helpful. Ipecac is relatively contraindicated because rapid CNS depression may occur, leading to aspiration. In cases that present early, lavage is indicated.

For patients who have ingested sustained-release preparations, whole bowel irrigation is a consideration. The goal of whole bowel irrigation is to move the pills through the entire gastrointestinal tract prior to their being absorbed. Whole bowel irrigation is accomplished by administering polyethylene glycol solution at a rate of 25 mL/kg/h by mouth or nasogatric tube until the rectal effluent is clear. Polyethylene glycol is an isoosmotic solution. A dose of charcoal is administered prior to initiating whole bowel irrigation, as it can adsorb drug that is released while the pills remain in the GI tract.

For bradycardia, atropine is administered at 0.02 mg/kg/dose for two doses. The minimum dose of atropine is 0.1 mg.

The primary antidote for an overdose of a calcium channel blocker is calcium. Increasing the extracellular calcium increases the influx of calcium into the cell, thus augmenting the calcium reserve of the sarcoplasmic reticulum. This reserve makes calcium available to the calcium-dependent ATPase, increasing contractility. Calcium is indicated for patients with hypotension, bradycardia, or heart blocks.

Two calcium salts are available: calcium gluconate and calcium chloride. Both of these are supplied in 10 percent solutions, but each contains a different quantity of calcium. Calcium chloride contains 1.3 mEq/mL of calcium and calcium gluconate contains 0.45 mEq/mL of calcium. The recommended pediatric doses are calcium chloride, 10 percent solution, 10 to 20 mg/kg/dose (0.1 to 0.2 mL/kg/dose) or calcium gluconate, 10 percent solution, 0.2 to 0.5 mL/kg/dose by slow IV push. The dose is repeated in 10 to 15 minutes for persistent hypotension or bradycardia. Calcium chloride can contribute to acidosis; therefore, calcium gluconate is preferred for patients with acidosis.

The calcium salts primarily reverse hypotension due to vasodilation and may have little or no effect on heart rate or conduction. Although calcium is the first line of therapy, there have been several cases in which calcium salts failed to reverse toxic effects. For patients with symptomatic bradycardia or heart block, atropine administered at 0.02 mg/kg may be helpful. However, hypotension is often related to peripheral vasodilation and will not respond to an increase in heart rate. Conversely, in a patient with stable blood pressure despite bradycardia, atropine will be of no benefit.

Glucagon is another proposed antidote for calcium channel blocker toxicity. It stimulates adenylate cyclase, which increases the formation of cyclic AMP and promotes intracellular calcium influx. Currently, glucagon should be reserved for toxicity refractory to other measures. The adult dose is 150 µg/kg given by slow IV push over 1 minute. It can be infused at a rate of 1 to 5 mg/h. Pediatric dosing has not been established. If glucagon is administered multiple times or as an infusion, the package diluent should not be used, since it contains phenol. It can be mixed in normal saline or D_5W.

When hypotension persists despite the administration of fluids, calcium salts and glucagon therapy with vasopressors are indicated. Dopamine is a reasonable first-line option. If it is ineffective, therapy with norepinephrine or dobutamine may be helpful. Amrinone, a phosphodiesterase inhibitor used in treating congestive heart failure, has been reported in both case reports and animal models to be effective in reversing hypotension secondary to calcium channel blocker overdose. In adults, amrinone can be given as an initial bolus of 0.75 mg/kg over 2 to 3 minutes, followed by an infusion of 5 to 10 µg/kg/min. Pediatric dosing has not been established. Currently, clinical experience with amrinone is limited.

High-dose insulin has been shown to be effective in the management of calcium channel blocker overdose. Insulin is thought to improve myocardial contractility and may improve conduction by lowering potassium concentrations. Insulin should be used early in the ED course and administered as a bolus of regular insulin, 1 U/kg, followed by 1U/kg/h for the first hour, then 0.5 U/kg/h thereafter until no longer needed. Serum potassium and glucose must be monitored at least hourly during the infusion and dextrose administered to maintain euglycemia.

Hemodialysis and hemoperfusion are of limited usefulness in the setting of calcium channel blocker overdose. The calcium channel blockers have a large volume of distribution and are highly protein bound. Dialysis could be considered in a patient who has renal failure. There has been one case of clinical improvement after hemoperfusion in a patient with combined diltiazem and metoprolol ingestion.

Disposition

Children who have signs of cardiovascular, respiratory, or CNS compromise are admitted to an intensive care unit. Children with a history of sustained-release ingestion are observed with cardiac monitoring for at least 24 hours. Those patients with no signs of toxicity, no history of sustained-release ingestion, and no ECG abnormalities can be observed for 8 hours after the time of ingestion. If they do not develop any signs of toxicity or ECG abnormalities during this period, they may be discharged.

CLONIDINE

Clonidine is widely used as an antihypertensive agent and as a treatment for opiate withdrawal. It is available in tablets and in sustained-release patches. Both preparations can be ingested by children. Although clonidine is infrequently used to treat high blood pressure in children, they can be exposed to this agent by coming into contact with the medication of a parent or grandparent. Especially in young children, even small doses of clonidine can cause serious toxicity.

Pathophysiology

Clonidine is an α_2-agonist that functions at the level of the brain stem by blocking sympathetic flow. It decreases heart rate, cardiac output, and peripheral vascular resistance. At high doses, it can stimulate peripheral α_1-receptors and actually cause hypertension, although this effect is transitory and is usually followed by hypotension. Clonidine also functions as a CNS depressant by depressing noradrenergic activity. It is rapidly absorbed from the gastrointestinal tract, with a decrease in blood pressure noted 30 to 60 minutes after ingestion. Hypotensive effects can last up to 24 hours. Severe toxicity has been reported after an ingestion of as little as 0.1 mg by a child.

The effects of an overdose of clonidine are variable but largely reflect CNS toxicity. They include altered mental status, somnolence, respiratory depression, and, especially in children, recurrent apnea. Central nervous system depression can last for 24 hours. Miosis can occur, which, in combination with altered mental status and depressed respiratory drive, can appear exactly like opiate toxicity. In addition to miosis, the neurologic examination may reveal hypotonia and decreased reflexes. Seizures are rare. Some patients may develop hypothermia.

Bradycardia and hypotension are the predominant cardiovascular manifestations, although patients can initially be hypertensive. Cardiac arrhythmias can occur. The cardiovascular effects can develop hours after the onset of mental status changes; thus, initially normal vital signs do not exclude the possibility that cardiovascular instability will ensue.

Management

The initial management of clonidine overdose focuses on stabilizing the airway and breathing. Respiratory depression may require ventilatory support, although all patients receive naloxone prior to intubation. This is especially important given the difficulty in distinguishing clonidine ingestion from an opiate overdose. In addition, as discussed as follows, naloxone may actually be useful in reversing the effects of a clonidine overdose.

After ventilation is stabilized, gastric decontamination is indicated. Lavage is the preferred method, given the tendency of clonidine to cause CNS depression and seizures. Ipecac-induced emesis can potentially result in aspiration. Following lavage, activated charcoal is administered (see Table 79-7).

Clonidine-induced bradycardia is treated with atropine if it is associated with hypotension. Hypotension is treated with aggressive fluid resuscitation. For hypotension that does not respond to fluids, moderate-dose dopamine may be useful. Dopamine may also ameliorate bradycardia. For patients with hypertension, it is important to realize that this side effect is transient and should be treated only if there is evidence of end-organ compromise. A short-acting agent, such as nitroprusside, is used to avoid precipitating profound hypotension, which can occur if a longer-acting agent, such as nifedipine, is administered.

As mentioned previously, there may be a role for naloxone in reversing the opiate-like side effects of clonidine on mental status and respiration and there is some indication that it can reverse clonidine-mediated hypotension. However, data on this subject are conflicting and naloxone cannot be considered a specific antidote for clonidine overdose. Although there are no contraindications to its use, the administration of naloxone in the setting of clonidine overdose has been associated with hypertension, and blood pressure monitoring is necessary during its administration.

Tolazoline is an α-antagonist agent that has been reported to reverse clonidine-mediated hypotension. However, it is not the specific antidote for clonidine. Data on its use are conflicting. It can cause profound hypotension, and its use should be restricted to the most refractory cases.

BIBLIOGRAPHY

Beta Blockers

Brimacombe JR: Use of calcium chloride for propranolol overdose. *Anaesthesia* 47:907, 1992.

Litovitz TL, Manoguerra A: Comparison of pediatric poisoning hazards: An analysis of 3.8 million exposure incidents: A report from the American Association of Poison Control Centers. *Pediatrics* 88:999, 1992.

Love JN, Tandy TK: Beta-adrenoreceptor antagonist toxicity: A survey of glucagon availability. *Ann Emerg Med* 22:267, 1993.

Reith DM, Dawson AH, Epid D, et al: Relative toxicity of beta blockers in overdose. *J Toxicol Clin Toxicol* 34:273–278, 1996.

Calcium Channel Blockers

Kerns JA: Calcium channel antagonists, in Ford MD, Delaney KA, Ling LJ, Erickson T (eds): *Clinical Toxicology.* Philadelphia: Saunders, 2001, pp 370–378.

Kline JA, Raymond RM, Schroeder JD, Watts JA: The diabetogenic effects of acute verapamil poisoning. *Toxicol Appl Pharmacol* 145:357–362, 1997.

Kozlowski JH, Kozlowski JA, Schuller D: Poisoning with sustained release verapamil. *Am J Med* 85:127, 1996.

Litovitz TL, Klein-Schwartz W, White S, et al: 1999 Annual Report of the Amercan Association of Poison Control Centers Toxic Exposure Surveillance System. *Am J Emerg Med* 18:517–574, 2000.

Yuan TH, Kerns WP, Tomaszewski CA, et al: Insulin-glucose as adjunctive therapy for severe calcium channel antagonist poisoning. *J Toxicol Clin Toxicol* 37:463–474, 1999.

Clonidine

Maloney MJ, Schwam JS: Clonidine and sudden death. *Pediatrics* 96:1176–1177, 1995.

- A potentially lethal dose of arsenic is 1 to 3 mg/kg.
- Arsenic toxicity can be confused with Guillain-Barré syndrome.
- Brittle nails with transverse white striae (Aldrich-Mees lines) can be seen after 4 to 5 weeks of exposure.
- Arsenic is radiopaque.
- Chelation for arsenic is the therapy of choice, but is not effective for arsine gas exposure.
- Arsine gas is one of the most potent hemolytic toxins.

Arsenical pesticide exposures comprise more than two-thirds of arsenic exposures called in to regional poison control centers (Table 85-1). Eighty-five percent of exposures involve children <6 years old. Other sources of arsenic include flypapers (Orpiment), Fowler's solution (liquor arsenicalis), soil, well water, homeopathic preparations, wood preservative (chromium-copper-arsenate) and shellfish (usually organic arsenic). It is extremely rare for arsenic to be used in homicides.

PATHOPHYSIOLOGY

The toxicity of arsenic is twofold. Primarily, it combines reversibly with sulfhydryl groups of several enzymes of the Krebs cycle. In addition, arsenic can substitute as an anion for phosphate and disrupt oxidative phosphorylation. Trivalent inorganic arsenic is more toxic than pentavalent organic and inorganic arsenicals. Arsenic can deplete glutathione stores in red blood cells 6 hours postexposure, resulting in hemolysis. The blood half-life of arsenic is about 4 to 5 days. A potentially lethal dose of arsenic is 1 to 3 mg/kg or 20 mgm in young children.

CLINICAL MANIFESTATIONS

The initial manifestations of arsenic poisoning are dominated by gastrointestinal symptoms, which include nausea, abdominal pain, vomiting, and "rice water" diarrhea. Hypotension can occur from fluid losses as well as from decreased peripheral resistance. The patient may have a characteristic garlic odor to the breath or feces.

Other systemic manifestations are diaphoresis, renal failure, hepatic dysfunction, and cardiac rhythm disturbances, including torsades de pointes. In severe intoxication, seizures and coma can occur. A peripheral neuropathy can develop 10 days to 3 weeks after ingestion, characterized by paresthesias of the extremities, followed by motor disability. Due to the neuropathy, arsenic toxicity can be confused with Guillain-Barré syndrome. Hypoglycemia can result from inhibition of gluconeogenesis in the citric acid cycle.

Chronic arsenic toxicity can have a similar though less fulminant course, and is characterized by dermatologic manifestations. Hyperpigmentation in a configuration similar to raindrops can occur on the eyelids, temples, and neck region. Skin desquamation and brittle nails with transverse white striae (Aldrich-Mees lines) can develop after 4 to 5 weeks of exposure. Patchy and diffuse alopecia can develop. The mucosa are generally spared.

DIAGNOSIS

Laboratory findings in arsenic poisoning are generally nonspecific. Pancytopenia, elevated liver function tests, and elevated creatinine all may occur from arsenic poisoning.

While serum arsenic levels >7 μg/100 mL may be indicative of poisoning, urinary arsenic levels are more sensitive in demonstrating toxicity. Twenty-four-hour urinary arsenic levels >100 μg are consistent with poisoning. A mobilization test with a 24-hour urine collection during administration of D-penicillamine may be performed to aid in the diagnosis of subacute or chronic arsenic exposure, with levels >100 μg/24 h indicating a positive test. Arsenic exposure can also be diagnosed by segmental tissue testing of hair or fingernails. Arsenic is radiopaque, and in acute ingestions may be visible on plain radiographs.

MANAGEMENT

Initial therapy consists of stabilization of the airway and support of the circulatory system. Antiarrhythmic therapy

Table 85-1. Arsenical Pesticides

Type	Preparations
Inorganic—Trivalent	
Arsenic trioxide	Grant's Ant Control Stakes
Sodium arsenite	Weed control (aqueous solution)
Calcium arsenite	Used on fruit (powder)
Copper arsenite	Wood preservative (powder)
Copper acetoarsenite	Insecticide outside the United States
Inorganic—Pentavalent	
Arsenic acid	Defoliant/herbicide (aqueous)
Sodium arsenate	Ant insecticide
Calcium arsenate	Herbicide (powder)
Lead arsenate	Insecticide (powder)
Zinc arsenate	Used on potatoes/tomatoes (powder)
Organic—Pentavalent	
Cacodylic acid	Herbicide/defoliant
Methane arsenic acid	Herbicide
Monosodium methane arsenate	Herbicide/defoliant
Disodium methane arsenate	Herbicide/silvicide
Monoammonium methane arsenate	Postemergence herbicide
Calcium acid methane arsenate	Postemergence herbicide

may be required. If hemolysis is present, alkalinization of the urine is indicated.

Gastric decontamination is performed by gastric lavage within 1 hour of ingestion or, if abdominal radiographs are positive, whole bowel irrigation. Activated charcoal does not adsorb arsenic.

Chelation is indicated when the 24-hour urinary arsenic concentration exceeds 200 μg/L. Chelation probably needs to be performed during the first 24 hours after exposure to avoid the delayed neuropathy associated with arsenic toxicity. Each course of chelation is over a 5-day period, with 24-hour levels of urinary arsenic <50 μg/L as the endpoint. Hemodialysis is useful for enhancing arsenic elimination if renal failure develops. Other agents such as 2-3 dithioerythritol, N-acetylcysteine, steroids, and immunotherapy are investigational (Table 85-2).

The management of arsine gas, which like arsenic has a characteristic garlic odor, is radically different from that of arsenic ingestion. Toxicity from this nonirritating gas results in hemolysis, abdominal pain, jaundice, and hematuria. Chelation is not effective and the treatment consists of dialysis or exchange transfusion.

Table 85-2. Chelators of Arsenic

	Route	Dose	Dosing Interval
Dimercaprol	IM	3–5 mg/kg	4–12 h
D-Penicillamine	PO	25 mg/kg	4 times/day
2,3 dimercaptosuccinic acid (DMSA or succimer)	PO	10 mg/kg	Every 8 h for 5 d, then every 12 h for 14 d or until urinary arsenic <50 μg/L
2,3 Dimercaptopropaine-1-sulfonic acid (sodium salt-DMPS-Not FDA approved at present)	PO	5 mg/kg	Every 8 h
DMPS (not FDA approved at present)	IV	5 mg/kg	Every 2–6 h

Abbreviations: IM, intramuscularly; IV, intravenously; PO, orally.

BIBLIOGRAPHY

Angle CR, Centeno JA, Guha Maxumder DN: DMSA, DMPS treatment of chronic arsenicism. *J Toxicol Clin Toxicol* 36:495, 1998.

Flora SJS, Tripathi N: Treatment of arsenic poisoning; An update. *Indian J Pharmacol* 30:209–217, 1998.

Gebel TW: Arsenic and drinking water contamination. *Science* 283:1458–1459, 1999.

Gordon ME: Arsenics and old places. *Lancet* 356:170, 2000.

Henadez AF, Schiaffino S, Bullesteros JL, et al: Lack of clinical symptoms in an acute aresnic poisoning: An unusual case. *Veterinary Human Toxicol* 40(6):344–345, 1998.

Subramanian KS, Kosnett ML: Human exposures to arsenic from consumption of well water in West Bengal, India. *Int J Occup Environ Health* 4(4):217–230, 1998.

Szincz L, Mueckter H, Gelgehauer N, et al: Toxicodynamic and toxicokinetic aspects of the treatment of arsenical poisoning. *J Toxicol Clin Toxicol* 38(2):214–216, 2000.

Wax PM: Features and management of arsenic intoxications. *J Toxicol Clin Toxico* 39:235-236, 2001.

86

Aspirin

Michele Zell-Kanter

HIGH-YIELD FACTS

- Despite improvements in packaging, toxic ingestions of aspirin continue to occur.
- Children with aspirin toxicity can rapidly develop metabolic acidosis not preceded by respiratory alkalosis.
- Treatment of aspirin overdose consists primarily of supportive management and alkalinization of the urine.
- The decision to treat is predicated on symptomatology rather than the Done nomogram.

Acetylsalicylic acid (aspirin) is easily accessible and is commonly used in suicide attempts. Despite decreased incidence since the advent of improved packaging, accidental overdoses continue to occur. Patients taking high doses of aspirin for chronic inflammatory conditions such as juvenile rheumatoid arthritis can also suffer toxicity. Annual data from the 1999 American Association of Poison Control Centers reported more than 13,000 exposures to aspirin as a single agent, with one-third of these occurring in children less than 6 years of age.

PHARMACOKINETICS

At normal doses, aspirin is rapidly absorbed from the small intestine. If taken in large amounts, absorption can be delayed by the formation of concretions.

There is a very narrow therapeutic range for aspirin when it is used as an antiinflammatory agent. Toxicity can result due to enzyme saturable pharmacokinetics. In therapeutic doses metabolism is first-order, but with an overdose pharmacokinetics change to zero-order.

Ingestions of <150 mg/kg are generally nontoxic. With ingestions of 150 to 300 mg/kg mild to moderate toxicity occurs, and overdoses of >300 mg/kg can be lethal. It is crucial to know the concentration of the preparation ingested in order to estimate the potential for toxicity. Infant aspirin bottles are limited to 36 tablets of 81 mg each. Oil of wintergreen, on the other hand, contains 100 percent methylsalicylate, and can be lethal in extremely small amounts.

PATHOPHYSIOLOGY AND CLINICAL PRESENTATION

After an ingestion, children have a quicker onset of toxicity and exhibit more severe signs than adults. This can occur in part because salicylate is distributed more rapidly into organs such as the brain, kidney, and liver. Patients may complain of tinnitus and impaired hearing. Direct stimulation of respiratory centers causes tachy-pnea, which in turn results in an early respiratory alkalosis. Uncoupling of the Krebs cycle results in anaerobic metabolism and ketonemia, which causes the characteristic anion gap metabolic acidosis. The acidosis can be exacerbated by hypovolemia, which results from vomiting, increased insensible losses from tachypnea and perspiration, and an osmotic diuresis. Fluid losses are especially severe in young children. In pediatric patients, the onset of metabolic acidosis tends to occur more rapidly than in adults, and is often not preceded by a respiratory alkalosis as in adults.

An acidotic environment facilitates salicylate distribution into the brain, where it can cause agitation, delirium, seizures, and rarely coma. Rhabdomyolysis can occur and can cause acute renal failure.

Patients can develop noncardiogenic pulmonary edema, most likely due to a toxic effect of salicylates on pulmonary endothelium. Risk factors for this include central nervous system toxicity, metabolic acidosis, and chronic salicylate ingestion. Uncoupling of oxidative phosphorylation can result in hyperthermia, which generally indicates significant toxicity.

Commonly observed electrolyte abnormalities include hypo- and hypernatremia, hypokalemia, and hypocalcemia. In children, hypoglycemia is more common that hyperglycemia.

LABORATORY STUDIES

Required initial laboratory studies include complete blood count, electrolytes, and arterial blood gases. A toxicology screen is important, especially for patients with deliberate overdose.

Plasma salicylate levels are easily obtainable and are best drawn 6 hours postingestion, when they reflect peak concentration. However, since the history of ingestion is often incorrect, a plasma salicylate level should be drawn upon presentation, and repeated every 2 hours to ensure that the level is decreasing. Patients with toxicity from chronic ingestion generally have a worse prognosis and clinical findings are more predictive of toxicity than the plasma level.

MANAGEMENT

Goals in the management of the salicylate intoxicated patient are

- Correction of dehydration
- Correction of metabolic disturbances
- Prevention of further absorption of the toxin
- Enhancement of elimination

Treatment is based on symptomatology; the Done nomogram is no longer considered useful in predicating management.

Intravascular volume is restored by boluses of crystalloid at doses of 10 to 20 mL/kg until adequate perfusion is assured. After urine output is established, potassium is added to the intravenous fluid for patients who are hypokalemic.

For patients who present within 1 hour of ingestion and are alert and oriented, syrup of ipecac can be administered to induce emesis and evacuate gastric contents. Patients who have any alteration in mental status are best managed by gastric lavage, after stability of the airway is established. Large amounts of aspirin have a tendency to form concretions in the stomach. Patients with significant ingestion can potentially benefit from gastric evacuation for several hours after ingestion. Whole bowel irrigation can be considered for patients in whom a concretion is observed on radiograph or for patients who have ingested sustained-release preparations.

Activated charcoal is effective in adsorbing ingested aspirin and is administered as soon as gastric evacuation is accomplished. While studies evaluating multiple doses of charcoal are inconclusive, charcoal is indicated in significant ingestions. The efficacy of whole bowel irrigation with activated charcoal is unknown.

In conjunction with gastric decontamination, elimination of salicylate is enhanced by systemic alkalinization. Alkalemia increases the ionized fraction of salicylate and decreases its entry into the brain and other tissues. As the urine becomes alkaline, an increased fraction of salicylate in the tubular fluid becomes ionized and nonreabsorbable

and is excreted. The excretion of salicylate is influenced by urine pH far more than urine flow. As urine pH increases from 5 to 8, renal clearance of salicylate increases by a factor of 10 to 20. The goal of alkalinization is to increase the urine pH to 7.5 to 8. This is accomplished by administering sodium bicarbonate in an initial bolus of 1 to 2 mEq/kg, followed by a bicarbonate drip titrated to the urine pH. Serial arterial blood gases are obtained to assure that the patient is not overalkalinized.

Hypokalemia is common in salicylism and can impair attempts to alkalinize the urine since potassium is exchanged for hydrogen in the tubular fluid when serum potassium is low. In hypokalemic patients, potassium is added to the intravenous solution once urine output is adequate. Complications of alkalinization include congestive heart failure secondary to volume load, excessive alkalemia, and hypernatremia.

For patients with extreme toxicity, hemodialysis is an option. It removes salicylates 3 to 5 times faster than systemic alkalinization. Indications for its use include congestive heart failure, noncardiogenic pulmonary edema, central nervous system depression, seizure, metabolic acidosis refractory to alkalinization, hepatic failure, or coagulopathy. The salicylate level is not useful as a sole criterion for dialysis unless it is >80 mg/dL in an acute ingestion. The threshold for dialysis is lower for patients chronically on salicylates since toxicity is more severe.

An investigational approach to the management of salicylate poisoning involves the use of glycine, which may act as a substrate in enhancing the excretion of salicylate.

BIBLIOGRAPHY

Boldy D, Vale JA: Treatment of salicylate poisoning with repeated activated charcoal. *Br Med J* 292:136, 1986.

Donovan JW, Akhtar J: Salicylates, in Ford MD, Delaney KA, Ling LJ, Erickson T (eds): *Clinical Toxicology.* Philadelphia, Saunders, 2001, pp 275-280.

Litovitz TL, Klein-Schwartz W, White S, et al: 1999 annual report of the American Association of Poison Control Centers toxic exposure surveillance system. *Am J Emerg Med* 18:517, 2000.

Mayer AL, Sitar DS, Tenenbein M: Multiple-dose charcoal and whole bowel irrigation do not increase clearance of absorbed salicylate. *Arch Intern Med* 152:393–396, 1992.

Notarianni L: A reassessment of the treatment of salicylate poisoning. *Drug Safety* 7:292–303, 1992.

Patel DK, Ogunbona A, Notarianni LJ, et al: Depletion of plasma glycine and effect of glycine by mouth on salicylate metabolism during aspirin overdose. *Hum Exp Toxicol* 9:389–395, 1990.

87

Carbon Monoxide

Timothy Turnbull

HIGH-YIELD FACTS

- Carbon monoxide (CO) poisoning is most commonly due to smoke inhalation, but also occurs from exposure to malfunctioning or improperly vented heating and cooking appliances, automobile exhaust fumes, and methylene chloride, a component of paint strippers.

- The predominant toxic effect of CO poisoning is tissue hypoxia, since CO binds to hemoglobin with 250 times the affinity of oxygen and competitively displaces oxygen from the molecule.

- Clinical signs and symptoms of CO poisoning are notoriously nonspecific and correlate only roughly with the carboxyhemoglobin level.

- Any illness affecting more than one member of a family or group from a common environment requires that CO poisoning be ruled out.

- The cornerstone of treatment is high-flow oxygen. While the half-time of carboxyhemoglobin ranges from 4 to 6 hours in room air, it is decreased to 40 to 90 minutes at an F_{IO_2} of 100 percent.

Carbon monoxide (CO) is the most common cause of death due to poisoning, accounting for 3500 to 4000 fatalities annually in the United States. Age-specific death rates in unintentional exposures are lowest for children less than 15 years of age and highest in adults 75 years of age and older. Approximately 10,000 persons seek medical attention or miss at least 1 day of normal activity each year because of CO poisoning.

PATHOPHYSIOLOGY

Carbon monoxide is a colorless, odorless, tasteless, and nonirritating gas formed as a by-product of incomplete combustion of fossil fuels or materials such as wood or charcoal. CO poisoning is most commonly caused by smoke inhalation. It also occurs from exposure to malfunctioning or improperly vented heating and cooking appliances, automobile exhaust fumes, and methylene chloride, a component of paint strippers that is metabolized to CO by the liver.

The predominant toxic effect of CO poisoning is tissue hypoxia, since CO binds to hemoglobin with 250 times the affinity of oxygen and competitively displaces oxygen from the molecule. Carbon monoxide also alters the hemoglobin molecule in such a way that the remaining oxygen is bound with greater affinity, in effect displacing the oxyhemoglobin dissociation curve to the left. The result is a reduction in the oxygen-carrying capacity of the hemoglobin molecule and impairment of its ability to deliver oxygen to the tissues.

Carbon monoxide also binds to cytochrome enzymes, specifically cytochrome A3 oxidase, and in addition attaches to myoglobin. Binding of CO to cytochrome interferes directly with cellular respiration and may contribute to tissue hypoxia by causing myocardial dysfunction and adversely affecting tissue perfusion.

The most oxygen-sensitive organs of the body, the central nervous system and heart, are most susceptible to the effects of CO poisoning. Children, by virtue of their higher basal metabolic rates, are presumed to be more vulnerable to central nervous system damage at lower levels of CO than are adults. During pregnancy the developing fetus appears to be particularly vulnerable to CO toxicity. The fetal oxyhemoglobin dissociation curve normally lies farther to the left than the adult curve, and the normal oxygen content of fetal blood is quite low. During CO exposure, blood oxygen content decreases even further and the oxyhemoglobin dissociation curve is displaced even farther to the left, further exaggerating the effects of hypoxia. Furthermore, carboxyhemoglobin (CoHb) levels attained in the fetus are routinely 10 to 15 percent higher than in the maternal circulation and the elimination phase of CO in the fetus is markedly prolonged compared to that of the mother.

CLINICAL PRESENTATION

Clinical signs and symptoms of CO poisoning are notoriously nonspecific and correlate only roughly with the

CoHb level at the scene (Table 87-1). The longer the interval between exposure and evaluation, the more likely that the symptoms and level will be discordant.

The best clues to the diagnosis are found in the history, and a correct assessment relies on a high index of suspicion, especially in the winter months when CO poisoning is more prevalent. Many patients with occult CO intoxication complain of flu-like symptoms with headache, nausea, and fatigue. In more severe cases there may be a history of syncope, or the victim's recollection of events may differ from that of the individual bringing him to the hospital. In infants, the only suggestion of toxicity may be irritability or feeding difficulties. Other situations in which the possibility of CO poisoning should be considered include unexplained alterations of mental status, neurological abnormalities, and metabolic acidosis.

It is axiomatic that any illness affecting more than one victim of a family or group from a common environment requires that CO poisoning be ruled out.

As a rule, the physical examination is unrevealing and vital sign abnormalities are nonspecific. The cherry red skin commonly associated with CO poisoning is usually a postmortem finding. Retinal hemorrhages are suggestive of CO poisoning, but are infrequently present. Cardiac toxicity most commonly manifests as dysrhythmias, but in older patients CO can precipitate angina or an acute myocardial infarction. Neurological abnormalities vary widely, from a normal examination to deep coma. Pulmonary edema, rhabdomyolysis, and renal failure occur rarely.

Table 87-1. Relationship of Carboxyhemoglobin (CoHb) Level and Clinical Manifestations of Carbon Monoxide Toxicity

CoHb Level (%)	Signs and Symptoms
0–10	None
10–20	Mild headache, dyspnea on exertion
20–30	More severe headache, dyspnea
30–40	Severe headache, dizziness, nausea, vomiting, fatigue, poor judgement, dim vision
40–50	Confusion, tachypnea, tachycardia
50–60	Syncope, seizures, coma
60–70	Coma, hypotension, respiratory failure, death
>70	Rapidly fatal

LABORATORY STUDIES

The diagnosis of CO poisoning is confirmed by measurement of the CoHb level, which can be obtained from an arterial or venous sample. A normal CoHb level is less than 1 percent and is attributed to endogenous production during heme metabolism. Levels are as high as 5 percent in nonsmoking urban residents and heavy smokers can have levels between 5 and 15 percent.

In acute CO exposure, the CoHb level and the severity of toxicity correlate poorly. Some patients have severe toxicity despite relatively low CoHb levels, while others are asymptomatic at very high levels. The degree of toxicity seems to be related more to factors such as duration of exposure, environmental concentration of CO, and the activity level of the victim than to the actual level of carboxyhemoglobin.

Other diagnostic tests are occasionally indicated. Arterial blood gas analysis provides information concerning acid-base status, and in severe cases of CO intoxication may reveal a metabolic acidosis. It may also reveal a "saturation gap." Since CO does not affect the Po_2 its level will be normal, but measured oxygen saturation will be decreased. It is important to note that oxygen saturation as measured by pulse oximetry is essentially unaffected by CO. As such, this modality has no value in ruling out significant CO exposure.

An electrocardiogram may be useful for detecting ischemic changes in adults, but its value in children is unknown. Chest radiography is not indicated unless there is clinical evidence of pulmonary edema or a concern about related smoke inhalation injury. In selected cases, a hemoglobin may be useful to assess premorbid oxygen-carrying capacity. Urine myoglobin is indicated for patients with prolonged unconsciousness or who are otherwise at risk for rhabdomyolysis.

Computed tomography and magnetic resonance imaging may reveal characteristic changes in the globus pallidus and white matter in cases of CO poisoning. However, the utility of these tests in the acute phase of intoxication is unknown.

TREATMENT

The cornerstone of treatment is high-flow supplemental oxygen. While the half-time of CoHb ranges from 4 to 6 hours on room air, it is decreased to 40 to 90 minutes at an Fio_2 of 100 percent. Since short-term administration of high concentrations of oxygen is nearly risk-free, it is indicated as soon as the diagnosis of CO poisoning is entertained. In the awake patient an F_{IO_2} of 100 percent can be approached with a tight-fitting nonrebreathing mask with a reservoir. In children the mask may need to be secured by tape. Obtunded patients may require intubation to achieve adequate oxygenation.

In cases of mild to moderate intoxication, treatment with normobaric supplemental oxygen is sufficient. It can be terminated when the CoHb level falls below 5 percent and there are no clinical manifestations of toxicity. Pregnant women, regardless of time to delivery, must be treated 5 times longer than usual because of the more avid binding and prolonged elimination of CO by fetal hemoglobin.

In more severely intoxicated patients or those at high risk for central nervous system toxicity, hyperbaric oxygen (HBO) therapy may be indicated. HBO can reduce the half-time of CoHb to 20 minutes while increasing the amount of dissolved oxygen in the plasma by 2 volumes-percent for every atmosphere. HBO at 3 atmospheres increases the concentration of dissolved oxygen to 6 to 7 volumes-percent, an amount sufficient to support the oxygen demands of the body until the oxygen-carrying capacity of hemoglobin is restored. For patients with central nervous system toxicity and cerebral edema, HBO also seems to lower intracranial pressure. Advocates of HBO for the treatment of CO poisoning cite reduction in early morbidity and mortality, as well as the reduced incidence of delayed neuropsychiatric complications when compared to treatment with atmospheric oxygen. Recent data, however, are calling these benefits into question, making use of HBO for treating CO poisoning somewhat controversial, especially when transfer times to an HBO facility may be lengthy.

Specific indications for HBO vary among centers with hyperbaric chambers and are evolving. Generally accepted clinical indications include coma or other signs of neurological impairment, any period of unconsciousness including syncope, and evidence of myocardial ischemia. Also included is the pregnant patient with any evidence of significant exposure, especially when there is evidence of fetal distress. Aggressive use of HBO should also be considered in neonates and infants, given their greater vulnerability to the effects of CO intoxication and the difficulty in assessing symptoms. A useful strategy may be to treat these small children based on the symptoms of older victims of the same exposure. Use of the CoHb level to select patients with less severe manifestations of toxicity for HBO is a point of controversy.

If HBO is not available locally, consideration should still be given to transfer of patients who meet the clinical criteria for HBO. When in doubt as to whether a patient is in need of HBO to the extent that the potential benefit would justify the risk of transfer, it is best to consult with the nearest poison center or HBO treatment facility. The nearest HBO facility can be located by contacting Divers Alert Network at Duke University in North Carolina, telephone number (919) 684-8111.

DISPOSITION

Children with mild poisoning (CoHb level below 5 percent) who are no longer symptomatic can be discharged. Prior to discharge, every effort should be made to locate the source of CO, since reexposure can be extremely harmful. Parents and caretakers should be advised of the potential for delayed neuropsychiatric sequelae, including persistent headaches, memory lapses, irritability, and personality changes. Occasionally, gait disturbances or incontinence can occur. Since it is difficult to predict which children will develop sequelae, it may be useful to recommend psychometric testing in any patient with a history of significant toxicity 3 to 4 weeks after exposure.

Patients who require admission to the hospital include children with:

- CoHb levels greater than 20 percent
- Acidosis
- Requirement for HBO

Pregnant females with CoHb levels greater than 15 percent also require admission for more prolonged normobaric oxygen therapy.

PROGNOSIS

The mortality rate among patients with severe CO poisoning is about 30 percent. Most patients who die do so at the scene of exposure. Up to 11 percent of survivors have gross neurologic or psychiatric deficits. A larger number may develop more subtle pathology such as personality changes or memory impairment. These abnormalities occur more often in patients with a history of loss of consciousness or altered mental status, metabolic acidosis, or an abnormal ECG or CT. In addition, up to 25 percent of treated patients will experience delayed neurological deterioration following a period of apparent recovery. Although most delayed sequelae will resolve, the course may span years.

BIBLIOGRAPHY

Choi S: Delayed neurologic sequelae in carbon monoxide intoxication. *Arch Neurol* 40:433, 1983.

Cobb N, Etzel RA: Unintentional carbon monoxide-related deaths in the United States, 1979 through 1988. *JAMA* 266:659, 1991.

Ernst A, Zibrak JD: Carbon monoxide poisoning. *N Engl J Med* 339:1603–1608, 1998.

Myers RM, Snyder SK, Emhoff TA: Subacute sequelae of carbon monoxide poisoning. *Ann Emerg Med* 14:1163, 1985.

Rudge FW: Carbon monoxide poisoning in infants: Treatment with hyperbaric oxygen. *South Med J* 86:334, 1993.

Scheinkestel CD, Bailey M, Myles PS, et al: Hyperbaric or normobaric oxygen for acute carbon monoxide poisoning: A randomized controlled clinical trial. *Med J Aust* 170:203–210, 1999.

Tighe SQ: Hyperbaric oxygen in carbon monoxide poisoning. 100% oxygen is best option. *Br Med J* 321:110–111, 2000.

Turnbull TL, Hart R, Strange GR, et al: Efficacy of an emergency department screening program for unsuspected carbon monoxide exposure. *Ann Emerg Med* 16:521, 1987.

Thom SR, Keim LW: Carbon monoxide poisoning: a review of epidemiology, pathophysiology, clinical findings and treatment options including hyperbaric oxygen therapy. *Clin Toxicol* 27:141, 1989.

Van Hoesen KB, Camporesi EM, Moon RE, et al: Should hyperbaric oxygen be used to treat the pregnant patient with acute carbon monoxide poisoning? *JAMA* 262:1039, 1989.

88

Caustics

Bonnie McManus

HIGH-YIELD FACTS

- Alkali burns cause liquefaction necrosis, a deep penetration injury associated with a pronounced exothermic reaction. Tissue destruction continues until the compound is significantly neutralized by tissue or the concentration is greatly decreased.

- Acid burns cause coagulation necrosis with severe injury to superficial tissues, but penetration is avoided by the formation of an eschar that limits damage to deeper tissues. Unlike liquid alkali, which tends to produce injury very rapidly, acid injury may continue to evolve for up to 90 minutes after the ingestion.

- Induction of emesis in caustic ingestions is contraindicated. Increased tissue damage occurs as the esophagus is reexposed to the offending agent.

- The administration of charcoal and cathartics is contraindicated because caustics are poorly adsorbed by charcoal, the injury tends to occur prior to arrival in the emergency department, and charcoal creates a problem with visualization for the endoscopist.

- Endoscopy helps to define the extent of the injury and develop a prognosis. Because of the unreliability of clinical findings in predicting significant esophageal injury, the threshold for endoscopy is low.

- A battery lodged in the esophagus requires urgent removal. Burns have been reported as early as 4 hours after ingestion, and perforation as early as 6 hours.

Caustics are chemicals that cause injury on contact. They account for approximately 5 percent of all accidental toxic exposures, with small children most frequently af-

fected. Several thousand reports are made annually to poison control centers concerning childhood caustic ingestions. Lye is the most frequent reported exposure. Substances that are considered lye include sodium and potassium hydroxide, sodium and potassium carbonate, ammonium hydroxide, and potassium permanganate. The incidence and severity of alkali ingestions has decreased significantly in recent years due to changes in safety packaging, child-resistant caps, and a decrease in the concentration of commercially available sodium hydroxide. Acids are also frequently ingested, but the severe pain caused on initial contact usually limits accidental ingestion in small children.

PATHOPHYSIOLOGY

Regardless of whether the caustic is an acid or an alkali, the severity of injury depends on

- The nature, volume, and concentration of the agent
- Contact time
- Presence or absence of stomach contents
- Tonicity of the pyloric sphincter
- Esophageal reflux after the ingestion

Whether the caustic is a solid or liquid affects the nature of the injury. Solids tend to produce intense localized upper esophageal injury, while liquids, especially strong bases, tend to produce circumferential lesions in the distal esophagus. Areas of anatomical narrowing, such as at the cricopharyngeus or the carina, are subject to longer contact time and are associated with more severe injury. Theoretically, the presence of stomach contents will decrease tissue injury by exerting a buffering effect. Pylorospasm can increase contact time of the corrosive with the stomach and result in more severe gastric injury. Reflux of ingested material back into the esophagus can exacerbate tissue injury.

Alkali Burns

The pattern of injury differs for alkali and acid injuries. Alkali burns cause liquefaction necrosis, a deep penetration injury associated with a pronounced exothermic reaction. Tissue destruction continues until the compound is significantly neutralized by tissue or the concentration is greatly decreased. Chemicals with a pH >12.5 usually cause severe injury that frequently leads to esophageal strictures, while those with a pH <11.4 rarely cause more than superficial mucosal burns. Most household bleaches have a pH of 11 to 12 and only cause superficial burns.

Due to relatively prolonged contact time, solid alkalis tend to cause perioral, oropharyngeal, and upper esophageal injury. The injury may be severe with deep irregular linear burns. Clinitest tablets, although now less commonly used by diabetics, are of special concern. They usually cause minimal symptoms unless lodged in the esophagus, where they can cause catastrophic complications, including penetration into the aorta.

Liquid lye can cause severe esophageal injury with minimal oropharyngeal findings. The complications following liquid lye ingestion tend to be more severe than those from solid ingestions because the injury is circumferential and leads to stricturing. The stomach is involved about 20 percent of the time when there is esophageal injury. The incidence of stomach injury is relatively low because most of the lye is neutralized in the esophagus. Small quantities of ingested base can cause severe esophageal damage and never reach the stomach. The gastric acid in the stomach is insignificant in neutralizing a strong base.

There are three major phases of caustic esophageal injury:

- Phase 1 is an acute inflammatory stage in which vascular thrombosis and cellular necrosis peak at 1 to 2 days, followed by sloughing of the necrotic tissue at approximately 3 to 4 days, resulting in an area of ulceration.

- Phase 2 is the latent granulation phase, in which fibroplasia begins to fill in the ulcer with granulation tissue in the middle of the first week. By the end of the first week collagen starts to replace the granulation tissue. Perforation is most likely during the second week when the esophageal wall is the weakest.

- Phase 3 is the chronic cicatrization phase. It begins during weeks 2 to 4, producing variable degrees of scar formation and contractures.

Acid Burns

Acid burns cause coagulation necrosis with severe injury to superficial tissues, but penetration is avoided by the formation of an eschar that limits damage to deeper tissues. Unlike liquid alkali, which tends to produce injury very rapidly, acid injury may continue to evolve for up to 90 minutes after the ingestion. The nature of the injury is such that acid tends to reach the stomach without being buffered in the esophagus, and can cause severe

gastric injury, including perforation. Thus esophageal injury associated with severe gastric injury is rare, and esophageal perforation has not been reported. The major effect of acid seems to be on the columnar cells of the stomach, with the distal portions affected most severely. If the pyloric sphincter is relaxed at the time of ingestion, injury to the small bowel can occur.

PRESENTATION AND STABILIZATION

It is important to attempt to obtain an accurate history in a patient suspected of having ingested a caustic. Identification of the offending agent is crucial in determining the potential for harm. Caretakers who call the emergency department should be asked to bring the container, including labels, of the ingested substance.

The presentation of a child with a caustic ingestion varies from completely asymptomatic to fulminant respiratory distress or shock. Many caustics, including highly alkaline laundry detergents, can cause life-threatening airway edema which must be urgently addressed. Stridor, dyspnea, and dysphonia all indicate upper airway compromise that requires intervention. Patients with upper airway obstruction should be intubated under direct visualization or may need a surgical airway. Blind nasotracheal intubation is contraindicated.

Patients with a history of caustic ingestion, but without signs of airway compromise, are observed for excessive crying, drooling, or refusal to eat or drink, all of which indicate a significant injury. The mouth is examined for signs of intraoral burns and the chest for retractions, wheezes, or rhonchi that indicate potential aspiration. The abdomen is examined for tenderness, which in cases of acid ingestion suggests the possibility of gastric perforation. In cases of suspected perforation the patient is monitored carefully for the presence of intraabdominal hemorrhage and hypovolemic shock.

In patients with signs of respiratory distress, oxygen saturation or arterial blood gases are critical in assessing lung function. Many caustics are powerful emetics and if aspirated can cause severe pneumonitis or noncardiogenic pulmonary edema. Household bleach, when combined with acid or ammonia, produces chlorine or chloramine gas, respectively. Exposure to either in a closed area can result in severe respiratory compromise.

Laboratory studies should include a complete blood count, serum electrolytes, renal functions, coagulation profile, and glucose. A chest radiograph is indicated in patients with signs of a significant ingestion or respiratory distress. Patients with abdominal pain or tenderness require an abdominal radiograph to exclude the presence of free air, indicating perforation.

MANAGEMENT

Symptomatic patients require special attention to the airway. After the airway is secured, an intravenous catheter is placed for use in the event that volume resuscitation is required. In the event of a large acid ingestion, a nasogastric tube is placed in an attempt to remove pooled acid and reduce injury.

Diluents/Buffers

Some medical sources and product labels still advocate neutralization of caustics by giving acidic substances such as lemon juice or vinegar after an alkali ingestion, or sodium bicarbonate following an acid ingestion. The concern of some authorities was that attempting to buffer a strong acid or alkali would lead to an extraordinary exothermic reaction that could increase tissue destruction, but recently this concern has been called into question. Diluents may have a role in weak acid ingestion because injury is purely caustic and there is no risk of thermal injury; however, there are no controlled studies to support this. Milk or water may be indicated after the ingestion of solid alkali in an attempt to move particulate material out of the oropharynx and esophagus. The amount given should be easily tolerated by the child so as not to induce emesis. There is no value in administering diluents in the case of liquid alkali ingestion because the injury is complete in a very short time and the risk of inducing emesis is great.

Emesis

Induction of emesis in caustic ingestions is contraindicated. Increased tissue damage occurs as the esophagus is reexposed to the offending agent. With violent emesis there is an increased risk of both perforation and aspiration. In acid ingestion, emesis increases the overall contact time and worsens injury. In alkali ingestions the injury is usually complete prior to arrival at the emergency department.

Gastric Aspiration and Lavage

In general, gastric aspiration and lavage are not indicated in alkali injury because of the rapidity of the injury. Although there are no studies that show an advantage or disadvantage of gastric aspiration in strong acid ingestion, anecdotal reports suggest that potentially lethal acids should be removed through a soft catheter if the patient is seen within 90 minutes of ingestion. While concern may exist regarding the possibility of inducing a gastric perforation by placing a catheter, this is not supported by studies.

Charcoal and Cathartics

The administration of charcoal and cathartics is contraindicated because caustics are poorly adsorbed by charcoal, the injury tends to occur prior to arrival in the emergency department, and charcoal creates a problem with visualization for the endoscopist.

Endoscopy

The challenge in managing the child with a caustic ingestion is in identifying the patient who is at risk for a serious injury. Since many patients have minimal clinical findings, clinical criteria are not reliable in identifying the presence or severity of burns. In Gandreault's study of 378 children with caustic ingestion, 10 of 80 children who were asymptomatic had grade 2 lesions on endoscopy. Some studies suggest that there is a greater risk of a higher grade lesion if there are significant injuries to the oral mucosa. If two of the three symptoms of vomiting, drooling, or stridor are present, the likelihood of gastrointestinal burns is high. Of the three, vomiting is the most powerful predictor of severe esophageal injury.

Endoscopy helps to define the extent of the injury and develop a prognosis. Because of the unreliability of clinical findings in predicting significant esophageal injury, the threshold for endoscopy is low. Any child with a history of significant ingestion, with oral lesions, or who is otherwise symptomatic, warrants endoscopy. The optimal time for the procedure appears to be during the first several hours after the ingestion. Endoscopy is not indicated for asymptomatic ingestion of household bleach, ammonia, or nonphosphate detergents. Evidence of perforation or shock is a contraindication to endoscopy.

Steroids

Steroids are a controversial aspect of management of caustic ingestions. Theoretically, steroids decrease the incidence of esophageal strictures in patients with severe burns. Studies by Spain showed that glucocorticoids decrease fibroplasia and granulation tissue if given within

48 hours of the injury. However, results of Anderson's 18-year prospective study of 131 children did not support the use of steroids as a way to decrease stricturing. Potential adverse effects of steroids include the possibility of infection and perforation.

Steroids are not indicated for first-degree burns because they do not form strictures. Third-degree burns usually form strictures, but because steroids may significantly increase complications their use is not recommended. Steroids may or may not be helpful in second-degree burns. The potential benefit of steroids in this setting must be weighed against the risk of infection.

Special Concerns

Caustic Eye Injuries

Caustic eye injury can have devastating consequences, with blindness frequently resulting from extensive exposure. Management is discussed in Chap. 69.

Button Batteries

Button batteries are frequently swallowed by children. The batteries contain various combinations of zinc, cadmium, mercury, silver, nickel, or lithium in a concentrated alkaline medium, usually sodium or potassium hydroxide. Although the vast majority of patients do well, this ingestion poses a unique risk of caustic injury, and deaths have occurred. In Litovitz's study of 2382 cases of battery ingestion, only 2 patients had life-threatening symptoms; both had batteries lodged in the esophagus. The study also showed that 61 percent of the batteries passed spontaneously within 48 hours and 86 percent within 96 hours.

Injury may occur due to pressure necrosis at the site where the battery becomes lodged. Lodging is most likely to occur at sites of anatomic narrowing, such as the cricopharyngeus, where the aorta or carina cross the esophagus, or in gut malformations such as a Meckel's diverticulum. If the battery breaks open, the caustic contents may cause local injury and perforation. Mercuric oxide cells are most likely to fragment and batteries that come to rest in the stomach are likely to leak even though they may appear intact.

A battery lodged in the esophagus requires urgent removal. Burns have been reported as early as 4 hours after ingestion and perforation as early as 6 hours after. The preferred method of extraction is endoscopy, which allows direct visualization of any esophageal injury. Emetics are usually unsuccessful in assisting in expelling a battery.

If the battery is intact and has passed through the esophagus, it does not need to be retrieved unless there are indications of intraabdominal injury, which include abdominal pain, tenderness, and hematochezia. A large battery ingested by a small child may also require removal. If a battery greater than 15 mm in diameter ingested by a child less than 6 years of age has not passed the pylorus within 48 hours, it is unlikely to do so.

An asymptomatic patient with a gastrointestinal battery not lodged in the esophagus can be discharged and followed as an outpatient with serial radiographs to document passage of the battery. The parents can strain the child's stool until the battery has passed. Whole bowel irrigation is an alternative easily performed in the emergency department; it may promote passage of the battery in 4 to 8 hours. This can be especially useful in cases in which follow-up is unreliable.

Hydrofluoric Acid

Hydrofluoric acid is a weak acid found in some cleaning and rust-removing products. External contact can result in severe dermal or ocular injury. Death has been reported with exposures affecting as little as 2.5 percent of the body surface area. Severe pain and deep penetration despite minimal skin findings is the hallmark of a hydrofluoric acid burn. The mechanism of injury involves liquefaction necrosis and the formation of insoluble calcium and magnesium salts. Oral ingestions are frequently fatal. In cases of significant burns, systemic acidosis, hypocalcemia, hypomagnesemia, and hyperkalemia are common. Renal failure and hemolysis have been reported to occur.

En route to the emergency department, copious irrigation to decrease diffusion is indicated. A gel of 3.5 g of calcium gluconate and 5 ounces of water-soluble lubricant or a 25 percent magnesium sulfate soak (Epsom salt) will provide pain relief. Pain can also be alleviated by intradermal injection of calcium gluconate. In cases of oral ingestion, calcium and magnesium are given on a milliequivalent per milliequivalent basis.

BIBLIOGRAPHY

Anderson KD, Rouse TM, Randolph JG: A controlled trial of corticosteroids in children with corrosive injury of the esophagus. *N Engl J Med* 323:637–640, 1990.

Crain EF, Gershel JC, Mezey AP: Caustic ingestions: Symptoms as predictors of esophageal injury. *Am J Dis Child.* 138:863–865, 1984.

Ellenhorn MJ, Schowald S: *Medical Toxicology: Diagnosis and Treatment of Human Poisoning.* New York: Elsevier Science Publishing, 1997, pp 1083–1097.

Ford M, Delaney KA, Ling LJ, Erickson T (eds): *Clinical Toxicology.* Philadelphia: Saunders, 2001, pp 1002–1038.

Gaudreault P, Parent M: Predictability of esophageal injury from signs and symptoms: A study of caustic ingestions in 378 children. *Pediatrics* 71:767–770, 1983.

Homan CS, Singer A, Henry MC, et al: Thermal effects of neutralization and water dilution for acute alkali exposures in canines. *Acad Emerg Med* 4:27, 1997.

Howell JM: Alkaline ingestions. *Ann Emerg Med* 15:820–825, 1986.

Litovitz T, Schmitz BF: Ingestion of cylindrical and button batteries: An analysis of 2382 cases. *Pediatrics* 89:747–757, 1992.

Penner GE: Acid ingestion: Toxicology and treatment. *Ann Emerg Med* 9:374–379, 1980.

Previtera C, Giuisti F, Guglielmi M: Predictive value of visible lesions (cheeks, lips, oropharynx) in suspected caustic ingestion: May endoscopy reasonably be omitted in completely negative pediatric patients? *Pediatr Emerg Care* 6:176–178, 1990.

89

Cocaine Toxicity

Steven E. Aks

HIGH-YIELD FACTS

- Myocardial ischemia has been reported in patients with normal coronary arteries as young as 17 years old after the use of cocaine.

- Other causes of chest pain after cocaine use must be differentiated. Consider asthma, pulmonary infarction, pneumomediastinum, and aortic dissection pneumothorax.

- Patients presenting with headache or a neurological deficit after cocaine must receive computed tomographic imaging of the brain to evaluate for hemorrhagic or ischemic injury.

- Benzodiazepines are the first-line agents for agitation, tremulousness, mild hypertension, and tachycardia from cocaine use.

- Activated charcoal and whole bowel irrigation are indicated for orally ingested cocaine, as in the case of body stuffers.

Cocaine abuse and toxicity continue to be pervasive problems. Adolescents and adults predominantly use cocaine as a recreational drug. Children usually suffer toxicity when exposed to cocaine being used by others. Seizures have been reported in children who accidentally ingest cocaine, and toxicity has occurred in toddlers who inhale cocaine being "freebased" by nearby adults. Convulsions have been reported in a breast-fed infant whose mother abused cocaine. Cocaine, multiple drug ingestions, and tricyclic antidepressants are among the most prominent causes of cardiac arrest for patients younger than 40 years of age.

According to data obtained by the American Association of Poison Control Centers (AAPCC) in 1999, there were 4286 total exposures to cocaine. There were 91 exposures to children less than 6 years of age, 584 in children aged 6 to 19, and there were 70 total fatalities. In one study, 2.4 percent of children in a group of inner city preschoolers tested positive for the cocaine metabolite benzoylecgonine in their urine.

PHARMACOLOGY AND PATHOPHYSIOLOGY

Chemically, cocaine is benzoylmethylecgonine, a naturally occurring local anesthetic. It is derived from the plant *Erythroxylum coca* and is rapidly absorbed from mucous membranes, lung tissue, and the gastrointestinal tract.

Pharmacologically, cocaine is a sympathomimetic, whose primary target organs are the central nervous system (CNS), cardiovascular system, lungs, gastrointestinal tract, skin, and thermoregulatory center.

Clinically, cocaine causes CNS stimulation that can result in agitation, hallucinations, abnormal movements, and convulsions. Paradoxically, children may present with lethargy. Both ischemic and hemorrhagic strokes have been reported.

Cardiovascular manifestations of cocaine toxicity include sinus tachycardia and both supraventricular and ventricular dysrhythmias. Elevation in blood pressure can range from mild to fulminant hypertension associated with strokes. Myocardial ischemia, including myocardial infarction, has been described in otherwise healthy individuals as young as 17 years old having normal coronary arteries.

Multiple pulmonary effects from inhalation of cocaine have been described, including exacerbation of asthma, pulmonary infarction, pneumomediastinum, pneumothorax, and respiratory failure.

Orally ingested cocaine can cause ischemic complications in the gastrointestinal tract that include acute abdominal pain, hemorrhagic diarrhea, and shock.

In association with agitation and hypertension, cocaine-induced hyperthermia can occur. A potential complication of hyperthermia is acute rhabdomyolysis. Cocaine-induced rhabdomyolysis can also occur in the absence of hyperthermia. The mechanism causing this is unknown.

The dermatologic manifestations of cocaine abuse are primarily related to intravenous injection and "skin popping." These include localized areas of necrosis or infection.

DIAGNOSIS

Cocaine toxicity is likely in a patient who exhibits signs and symptoms consistent with sympathomimetic stimulation. Occasionally the sympathomimetic toxidrome is difficult to distinguish from that caused by anticholinergic toxicity. Both toxidromes are associated with CNS excitation, mydriasis, tachycardia, hypertension, and hyperthermia. Unlike sympathomimetic toxicity, however, anticholinergics will cause urinary retention and decreased bowel sounds. Also, sympathomimetic toxicity is often associated with diaphoresis, while anticholinergic overdose is associated with dry skin.

LABORATORY STUDIES

For patients in whom cocaine toxicity is suspected, a toxicology screen can confirm the ingestion and rule out co-ingestants. Blood levels of cocaine and cocaine metabolites correlate poorly with signs and symptoms. Cardiac monitoring is essential to evaluate the patient for dysrhythmias. Patients who complain of chest pain require a 12-lead electrocardiogram. For patients with chest pain, a radiograph is also useful to exclude pneumothorax, pneumomediastinum, or infiltrate.

Laboratory studies help establish a baseline and are useful for patients with significant toxicity. They include a complete blood count, serum electrolytes, glucose, blood urea nitrogen, and creatinine. If a urine dipstick is positive for blood but microscopy is negative for red blood cells, the patient is evaluated for rhabdomyolysis with a serum creatine kinase and urine myoglobin.

For patients with severe headache or neurological deficit, a computed tomographic (CT) scan of the brain is indicated to rule out the possibility of a cocaine-induced cerebrovascular accident.

MANAGEMENT

Mildly toxic patients generally require no specific therapy. Moderate to severe agitation responds to benzodiazepines, which are also the drugs of choice for seizures. Persistent seizure activity may require treatment with phenytoin or phenobarbital. Rarely, status epilepticus requires paralysis. Patients with persistent seizures may suffer from a structural CNS lesion or toxicity from a co-ingestant. Benzodiazepines are also effective treatment for most patients with mild to moderate hypertension. In more severe cases labetalol, which has both alpha- and beta-blocking characteristics, has been effective, as has sodium nitroprusside. Beta blockers are contraindicated, since unopposed alpha stimulation can exacerbate hypertension.

Patients with severe hyperthermia are treated with aggressive cooling and the urine is alkalinized in patients with rhabdomyolysis.

Activated charcoal adsorbs unpackaged orally ingested cocaine and is useful for the treatment of gastric contamination.

BODY STUFFERS

Body stuffers may swallow cocaine in an attempt to hide the drug to avoid prosecution when accosted by law enforcement officers. Often the cocaine is poorly wrapped, and even carefully packaged packets can rupture with fatal results. Types of packages that are likely to rupture are paper and poorly secured plastic bags. The physician may be able to gather enough information regarding the amount of cocaine ingested and the type of packaging to assess the potential for toxicity.

Abdominal radiographs may be useful if the ingested packets are radiopaque. Body packers package large amounts of drug with the intention of smuggling. These packets are more likely to be radiopaque. The packets ingested by body stuffers are rarely visible on a plain radiograph. A gastrograffin swallow or CT scan of the abdomen may reveal ingested packets in cases when plain radiographs are negative but the suspicion for ingestion is high.

In body stuffers, gastric decontamination with syrup of ipecac or gastric lavage is contraindicated, since both may cause rupture of the packets. Whole bowel irrigation with polyethylene glycol electrolyte lavage solution can be used to enhance transit through the gastrointestinal tract. All ingested packets should be passed before the patient is discharged. A gastrograffin swallow or abdominal CT may be required before discharge to make sure all packets have been passed. In symptomatic body stuffers, a surgical consultation is indicated since laparotomy may be necessary.

DISPOSITION

In asymptomatic or mild cases of cocaine toxicity, 4 to 6 hours of observation in the emergency department is adequate. Patients with moderate to severe symptoms are admitted to a monitored bed. Body stuffers are observed in a monitored setting until all packets have passed.

BIBLIOGRAPHY

Aks SE, Vanden Hoek TL, Hryhorczuk DO, et al: Cocaine liberation from body packets in an in vitro model. *Ann Emerg Med* 21:1321–1325, 1992.

Blaho K, Logan B, Winbery S, et al: Blood cocaine and metabolite concentrations: Clinical findings, and outcome of patient presenting to an ED. *Am J Emerg Med* 18:593–598, 2000.

June R, Aks SE, Keys N, et al: Medical outcome of cocaine bodystuffers. *J Emerg Med* 18:221–224, 2000.

Kharasch SJ, Glotzer D, Vinci R, et al: Unsuspected cocaine exposure in young children. *Am J Dis Child* 145:204–206, 1991.

Litovitz TL, Klein-Schwartz W, White S, et al: 1999 annual report of poison control centers toxic exposure surveillance system. *Am J Emerg Med* 18:517–574, 2000.

Minor RL, Scott BD, Brown DD, et al: Cocaine-induced myocardial infarction in patients with normal coronary arteries. *Ann Intern Med* 115:797–806, 1991.

Richman PB, Nashed AH: The etiology of cardiac arrest in children and young adults: Special considerations for ED management. *Am J Emerg Med* 17:264–270, 1999.

Riggs D, Weibley RE: Acute hemorrhagic diarrhea and cardiovascular collapse in a young child owing to environmentally acquired cocaine. *Pediatr Emerg Care* 7:154–155, 1991.

Seaman ME: Acute cocaine abuse associated with cerebral infarction. *Ann Emerg Med* 19:34–37, 1990.

Tomaszewski C, Vorhees S, Wathen J, et al: Cocaine adsorption to activated charcoal in vitro. *J Emerg Med* 10:59–62, 1992.

90

Cyanide Poisoning

Mark Mycyk
Anne Krantz

HIGH-YIELD FACTS

- Cyanide poisoning causes profound tissue hypoxia.
- Poisoning causes rapid onset of central nervous system and cardiovascular toxicity.
- Helpful laboratory clues include lactic acidosis and a diminished arterial-venous O_2 difference.
- Antidotal therapy with nitrites and sodium thiosulfate needs to be considered early.

Cyanide poisoning is unusual in the United States and very rare among children, although its contribution to toxicity and death may be underestimated in victims of smoke inhalation. In the 5-year period from 1995 through 1999, the annual reports of the American Association of Poison Control Centers (AAPCC) reported 174 pediatric cyanide exposures with one death.

There are a variety of sources of cyanide exposure in the pediatric population. In fires, hydrogen cyanide gas is formed as a combustion product of wool, silk, synthetic fabrics, and building materials. Cyanide exposure by this route is now recognized as a major cause of toxicity among fire victims previously thought to be poisoned by carbon monoxide. Acetonitrile, or methyl cyanide, is found in agents used to remove sculpted nails and is converted in vivo to hydrogen cyanide. Cyanide poisoning due to acetonitrile ingestion has occurred in children, resulting in at least one reported death. Poisoning has also occurred from accidental ingestion of cyanide-containing metal cleaning solutions imported from Southeast Asia. Amygdalin and other cyanogenic glycosides, found in the seeds and pits of certain plants such as apples, apricots, and peaches, are hydrolyzed in the gut to cyanide. Fruit pit ingestion has led to outbreaks of cyanide poisoning in children in Turkey and Gaza. These and other sources of cyanide exposure are summarized in Table 90-1.

TOXICOKINETICS

Hydrogen cyanide gas is rapidly absorbed in the lungs and may cause profound toxicity within seconds. Ingested cyanide salts, such as sodium cyanide and potassium cyanide, are also rapidly absorbed across the gastric mucosa and may result in toxicity within minutes. Ingestion of amygdalin and other cyanogenic glycosides requires hydrolysis to release cyanide, so toxicity may be delayed up to several hours after ingestion. Acetonitrile appears to release cyanide through oxidative metabolism by the hepatic cytochrome P450 system, thus delaying clinical manifestations of toxicity for 2 to 6 hours from the time of ingestion.

There are minimal data on the volume of distribution (Vd) of cyanide in humans. Pharmacokinetic data from one case of potassium cyanide ingestion suggested a Vd of 0.41 L/kg. Blood cyanide concentrates in the erythrocytes, with an RBC:plasma ratio of 100:1. Sixty percent of plasma cyanide is protein-bound.

Cyanide elimination occurs by four separate routes. The widely distributed endogenous enzyme rhodanase (sulfurtransferase) in the presence of thiosulfate converts cyanide to nontoxic thiocyanate. This accounts for the majority (80 percent) of elimination with thiosulfate availability being the rate-limiting factor. Some cyanide is converted in the presence of hydroxocobalamin (vitamin B_{12a}) to cyanocobalamin (vitamin B_{12}) which is also nontoxic. Clinically insignificant amounts of cyanide are excreted in expired air and in sweat. The reported elimination half-life in humans is variable, ranging from 20 minutes to 1 hour in nonlethal exposures, to a mean of 3 hours in fire victims treated with antidotes.

PATHOPHYSIOLOGY

The primary mechanism of toxicity in cyanide poisoning is cellular hypoxia. This is caused by cyanide binding with ferric iron (Fe^{3+}) in cytochrome a-a$_3$ of the mitochondrial cytochrome oxidase. Cyanide inhibition of cytochrome oxidase prevents efficient cellular oxygen use and disrupts ATP production. This shift to anaerobic metabolism results in a severe lactic acidosis. Cyanide also shifts the oxygen-hemoglobin dissociation curve to the left, further impairing oxygen delivery to the tissues. Cyanide inhibits a wide variety of other iron- and copper-containing enzymes, although their contribution to clinical toxicity is uncertain. The critical targets of cyanide are those organs most dependent on oxidative phosphorylation, namely the brain and the heart.

Table 90-1. Sources of Cyanide Exposure

Cyanogenic plants
  Prunus species (leaves, stem, bark, seed pits)
    American plum, wild plum
    Apricot
    Cherry laurel, Carolina cherry laurel
    Cultivated cherry
    Peach
    Wild black cherry
    Chokecherry
    Bitter almond
  Other
    Apple (seeds)
    Pear (seeds)
    Crabapple (seed)
    Elderberry (leaves and shoots)
    Hydrangea (leaves and buds)
    Cassava (beans and roots)
Household agents
  HCN-containing fumigants
  Rodenticides
  Insecticides (aliphatic thiocyantes: Lethane 60,
    Lethane 302, Thanite)
  Sculpted nail removers containing acetonitrile (e.g.,
    Nailene Glue Remover)
  Silver and metal polish
Combustion products
  Silk, wool
  Polyurethane
  Polyacrylonitrile
Other
  Nitroprusside

CLINICAL PRESENTATION

The clinical presentation depends on the route and dose of exposure. Inhalation of cyanide gas causes loss of consciousness within seconds, whereas symptoms from an oral exposure develop anywhere from 30 minutes to several hours from the time of ingestion. Since cyanide poisoning causes profound tissue hypoxia, it makes clinical sense that the central nervous system and the cardiovascular system (the two organ systems most dependent on oxygen) are affected the earliest.

Initial symptoms in victims not experiencing rapid loss of consciousness include headache, anxiety, confusion, blurred vision, palpitations, nausea, and vomiting. With progression of toxicity patients may experience a feeling of neck constriction, suffocation, and unsteadiness. Early clinical signs of cyanide poisoning are CNS stimulation or depression, tachycardia or bradycardia, hypertension, dilated pupils, bright red retinal veins on funduscopy, and declining mental status. Late signs of poisoning are seizures, coma, apnea, cardiac arrhythmias, and complete cardiovascular collapse. The characteristic smell of bitter almonds may be detected in some cases, but the ability to detect this is a genetically determined trait not possessed by every examiner. Although cyanide poisoning causes tissue hypoxia, the presence of cyanosis is a relatively late finding. Since cyanide poisoning typically causes a leftward shift of the oxygen dissociation curve, the absence of cyanosis in a patient with clinical evidence of severe hypoxia should prompt the examiner to consider the diagnosis of cyanide poisoning.

LABORATORY EVALUATION

Whole blood cyanide levels may be obtained, but these results are not available emergently and will therefore be of little value in guiding therapy. However, blood gas analysis and serum chemistries may be helpful in the acute setting. Arterial blood gases will typically show a marked metabolic acidosis. Obtaining a venous blood gas analysis for comparison may demonstrate a diminished arterial-venous O_2 difference ($AO_2 - VO_2$ approaching zero) since the tissues' ability to extract oxygen from the blood is severely impaired. Serum chemistries may demonstrate an elevated anion gap due to the presence of a lactic acidosis from anaerobic metabolism.

Numerous electrocardiographic changes may occur in cyanide toxicity. Sinus bradycardia may be noted early, and later sinus tachycardia may be seen, as well as atrial fibrillation, atrioventricular block, ventricular ectopy, and ventricular dysrhythmias. A shortened QT segment or T waves originating high on the R wave may be seen.

TREATMENT

The management of cyanide poisoning requires immediate supportive care as well as specific antidotal therapy. Airway management with 100 percent oxygen should be initiated and an intravenous line established in all patients. Fluid resuscitation should be administered to patients with hypotension, and sodium bicarbonate should be considered in profound acidosis. Mouth-to-mouth resuscitation by primary rescuers should be avoided because of the theoretical risk of secondary cyanide exposure. Contaminated clothing should be removed and skin and eyes should be copiously irrigated.

Cyanide Antidotes

Although some victims of cyanide poisoning have survived with supportive care alone, antidotal therapy clearly improves survival and shortens the recovery period. The only antidote currently approved for use in the United States is the Lilly Cyanide Antidote Kit, which contains amyl nitrite perles, sodium nitrite solution, and sodium thiosulfate.

The mechanism of action of nitrites in cyanide toxicity is not completely understood. It is understood that nitrites produce methemoglobin, which has a higher affinity for cyanide than does cytochrome oxidase. This combination of methemoglobin and cyanide forms cyanomethemoglobin. However, several experimental and clinical findings speak against methemoglobin formation by nitrites as the sole rescue mechanism. First, in animals pretreated with methylene blue where methemoglobin formation is inhibited, nitrites still effectively reduce cyanide toxicity. Second, clinical improvement following nitrite administration occurs within minutes, while peak methemoglobin levels occur later. Some authors suggest that the vasodilatory effect of nitrites allows for greater endothelial enzymatic degradation of cyanide. Indeed, in experimental models, some alpha-antagonists have also shown antidotal effects to cyanide.

Sodium thiosulfate provides a sulfur donor for the rhodanase-mediated conversion of cyanomethemoglobin to methemoglobin and thiocyanate. Thiocyanate is minimally toxic and is excreted by the kidneys.

The recommended regimen and pediatric doses for the Lilly kit components is summarized in Table 90-2. Amyl nitrite perles are administered first while establishing an intravenous line and preparing the sodium nitrite solution. The perles should be crushed in gauze and held near the nose and mouth for 30 seconds. Amyl nitrite administration will produce a methemoglobin level of 3 to 7 percent. Once an intravenous line is established and the sodium nitrite solution prepared, administration of amyl nitrite perles may be stopped.

Sodium nitrite (9 mg/kg, or 0.3 mL/kg of a 3 percent solution, not to exceed 10 mL) is administered at a rate of 2.5 mL/min. In an unstable or hypotensive patient, or when there is concomitant CO poisoning, the dose may be given more slowly, over 30 minutes. With the slower rate of infusion, the methemoglobin level peaks 35 to 70 minutes following administration and rises to roughly 10 to 15 percent. This level is lower than the 25 percent recommended as a goal of therapy in earlier literature, because it has been shown that these lower levels are equally therapeutic and avoid further impairment of tissue oxygen delivery from a high methemoglobin level. Methemoglobin levels should be monitored periodically after the infusion.

Side effects of nitrite administration include headache, blurred vision, nausea, vomiting, and hypotension. Methemoglobin levels of 20 to 30 percent are associated with symptoms of headache and nausea. Weakness, dyspnea, and tachycardia occur at levels of 30 to 50 percent, while dysrhythmias, CNS depression, and seizures occur at levels of 50 to 70 percent. Death occurs at methemoglobin

Table 90-2. Recommended Usage of the Lilly Cyanide Antidote Kit

Antidote	Quantity/Form	Pediatric Dose
Amyl nitrite	12 perles (0.3 mL/perle)	Crush 1–2 perles in gauze and hold under patient's nose or over ET tube for 15–30 seconds each minute[a]
Sodium nitrite	2 ampules of 3% solution (300 mg/10 mL)	0.3 mL/kg (9 mg/kg) not to exceed 10 mL (300 mg), intravenously at 2.5 mL/min, or over 30 minutes in smoke inhalation victims with carbon monoxide poisoning[b]
Sodium thiosulfate	2 ampules of 25% solution (12.5 g/50 mL)	1.6 mL/kg (400 mg/kg) up to 50 mL (12.5 g) at rate of 3–5 mL/min

[a]Check expiration date of all components. Shelf life for amyl nitrite is 1 year.
[b]Infuse more slowly when hypotension occurs. Monitor for blood pressure and be prepared to treat severe hypotension with fluids and vasopressors as needed. Monitor methemoglobin levels.

levels around 70 percent. A fatal methemoglobin level in a child treated with nitrites for cyanide poisoning has been described. That child received a cumulative dose of 21 mg/kg sodium nitrite.

Following the nitrite administration, sodium thiosulfate is given to enhance clearance of cyanide as thiocyanate. Alternately, the thiosulfate may be administered concurrently at a separate site. The pediatric dose is 1.65 mL/kg of a 25 percent solution up to 50 mL (12.5 g). Thiosulfate appears to have few if any side effects. Thiocyanate levels of greater than 10 mg/dL may be associated with nausea, vomiting, arthralgias, and psychosis, and may occur in the setting of renal failure and impaired thiocyanate excretion.

Typically, symptoms and signs of cyanide poisoning begin to respond within minutes of the administration of nitrites. When symptoms recur following antidote administration, both the sodium nitrite and sodium thiosulfate may be given again at half the original doses.

Because there is no diagnostic test for cyanide poisoning that can be obtained in a timely manner, the diagnosis in the acute setting needs to be made clinically. In a situation in which cyanide poisoning is being considered but the diagnosis is uncertain, the use of sodium thiosulfate alone may be considered. This approach avoids further compromise of the patient's oxygen-carrying capacity due to the nitrites. There are minimal published data on the efficacy of this approach. When a patient is treated with nitrites but shows no clinical response, the diagnosis of acute cyanide toxicity should be reconsidered.

Smoke Inhalation

Several studies suggest a correlation between elevated carboxyhemoglobin levels and cyanide levels in smoke inhalation victims. Thus, when an elevated carboxyhemoglobin level is found in a severely ill fire victim, cyanide poisoning is possible and it needs to be considered early and treated appropriately. This is particularly true in a fire victim who requires intubation or has a persistent metabolic acidosis, abnormal mental status, or cardiovascular instability not resolving with conventional therapy for carbon monoxide poisoning. Since nitrite-induced methemoglobinemia may further impair oxygen delivery, a patient with concomitant carbon monoxide and cyanide poisoning should be treated with 100 percent oxygen and thiosulfate therapy first. Some evidence suggests that hyperbaric oxygen therapy conventionally used for severe carbon monoxide poisoning is helpful in the treatment of cyanide toxicity as well. If the patient remains critically ill, sodium nitrite should be administered slowly while the blood pressure is monitored.

DISPOSITION

Patients who are asymptomatic and whose exposure has apparently been minimal are observed for 4 to 6 hours. Those who have ingested cyanogenic glycosides are observed for at least 6 hours for evidence of the onset of toxicity. Those ingesting acetonitrile-containing compounds are observed for 12 to 24 hours. Patients requiring antidotal treatment are cared for in an intensive care unit where vital signs, mental status, arterial blood gases, methemoglobin, and carboxyhemoglobin levels can be checked frequently. Following recovery, patients are observed for 24 to 48 hours. Rarely, late neurologic syndromes have been reported following cyanide toxicity, and periodic outpatient follow-up is advised.

BIBLIOGRAPHY

Baud FJ, Barriot P, Toffis V, et al: Elevated blood cyanide concentrations in victims of smoke inhalation. *N Engl J Med* 325:1761–1766, 1991.

Chin RG, Caldern Y: Acute cyanide poisoning: A case report. *J Emerg Med* 18:441–445, 2000.

Caravati EM, Litovitz TL: Pediatric cyanide intoxication and death from an acetonitrile-containing cosmetic. *JAMA* 260:3470–3473, 1988.

Clark CJ, Campbell D, Reid WH: Blood carboxyhemoglobin and cyanide levels in fire survivors. *Lancet* 1:1332–1335, 1981.

Delaney KA: Cyanide, in Ford MD, Delaney KA, Ling LJ, et al (eds): *Clinical Toxicology*. Philadelphia: Saunders, 2001, pp 705–711.

Hall AH, Rumack BH: Clinical toxicology of cyanide. *Ann Emerg Med* 15:1067–1074, 1986.

Johnson RP, Mellors JW: Arteriolization of venous blood gases: A clue to the diagnosis of cyanide poisoning. *J Emerg Med* 6:401–404, 1988.

Kirk MA, Gerace R, Kulig KW: Cyanide and methemoglobin kinetics in smoke inhalation victims treated with the cyanide antidote kit. *Ann Emerg Med* 22:1413–1418, 1993.

Kulis KW: Cyanide antidotes and fire toxicology. *N Engl J Med* 325:1801, 1991.

Yen D, Tsai J, Wang LM, et al: The clinical experience of acute cyanide poisoning. *Am J Emerg Med* 13:524–528, 1995.

91

Tricyclic Antidepressant Overdose

Steven E. Aks

HIGH-YIELD FACTS

- The quinidine-like effect of the tricyclic antidepressants produces QRS and QT abnormalities.
- A clinical hallmark of tricyclic antidepressant overdoses is that patients may appear to be clinically well, then suddenly deteriorate in the first 2 hours after presentation.
- Clinical signs and symptoms are the best way to diagnose tricyclic antidepressant toxicity. Blood levels are generally not helpful.
- One should have a low threshold to intubate patients who are drowsy in order to protect the airway.
- Alkalinization of the serum (pH 7.45 to 7.5) to overcome sodium channel blockade is the mainstay of treatment for tricyclic antidepressant toxicity.
- Seizures are particularly ominous because they can cause acidemia that may worsen the cardiac status.

Tricyclic antidepressants are commonly used by adults in suicide attempts. Children more commonly ingest these agents accidentally when they find them in the home. According to the American Association of Poison Control Centers (AAPCC), in 1999 there were 13,953 total ingestions. Of these 1850 were in children less than 6 years of age, 2061 were in children aged 6 through 19, and there was a total of 102 deaths out of all the ingestions. The greatest number of major effects were due to amitriptyline, followed by doxepin, and then imipramine.

PHARMACOLOGY

Amitriptyline and imipramine are the prototype tricyclic antidepressants. The newer generations of antidepressants have different chemical structures and different patterns of toxicity than the tricyclics. Newer antidepressants include amoxapine, maprotiline, trazodone, fluoxetine, and sertraline.

The effect of a given tricyclic antidepressant depends on its specific site of action. The major toxicities result from the effects of tricyclic antidepressants on the cardiovascular and central nervous systems. Toxic effects can be grouped as follows:

- A *quinidine-like effect* accounts for cardiac dysrhythmias by inducing conduction blocks that manifest clinically with a widened QRS interval and QT abnormalities.
- *Anticholinergic side effects* cause tachycardia and the anticholinergic overdose syndrome of mydriasis, dry mucous membranes, hyperthermia, decreased gastrointestinal motility, urinary retention, and mental status changes that can range from agitation to stupor and coma.
- *Blockade of norepinephrine reuptake* augments tachycardia and can cause hypertension. Upon depletion of norepinephrine stores, hypotension can occur.
- *Alpha blockade* causes hypotension by decreasing peripheral vasomotor tone.

In therapeutic doses, tricyclics are rapidly and almost completely absorbed. In toxic doses, absorption can be delayed because anticholinergic effects delay gastrointestinal motility. In addition, ionization of these compounds in gastric fluids can also delay absorption.

CLINICAL PRESENTATION

The clinical presentation of tricyclic antidepressant overdose is related primarily to the effects on the central nervous and cardiovascular systems.

Patients can present to the emergency department with mental status changes that range from anxiety and agitation to confusion, delirium, and coma. Seizures can occur, and are of ominous clinical significance. Tachycardia is the most common cardiovascular manifestation of tricyclic antidepressant toxicity. Other abnormal rhythms include ventricular dysrhythmias, bradydysrhythmias, and cardiac arrest. The patient's blood pressure can be high or low. Other possible manifestations of toxicity are hyperthermia, rhabdomyolysis, renal failure, pancreatitis, and hepatitis.

A patient who has taken an overdose of a tricyclic antidepressant is likely to arrive at the emergency department appearing clinically stable and may then suddenly deteriorate. The majority of patients who develop life-threatening problems do so within 2 hours of arrival in the ED.

DIAGNOSIS

Tricyclic antidepressant overdose is possible in any patient presenting with signs and symptoms of anticholinergic overdose.

When the diagnosis of tricyclic antidepressant overdose is entertained, cardiac monitoring is an essential first step. Persistent tachycardia is consistent with an overdose, and raises the suspicion that toxicity will progress. Several electrocardiographic parameters have been identified as markers of significant toxicity. The QRS duration has received much attention as a marker for overdose. In adults, a QRS duration less than 100 ms is correlated with a low risk of developing toxicity, while a QRS between 100 and 160 ms is sometimes associated with seizures and dysrhythmias, and a QRS greater than 160 ms with a high risk of seizures and dysrhythmias. However, in children the QRS duration has not been well studied. Likewise, in adults a frontal plane terminal 40 ms QRS with a rightward deviation is correlated with toxicity, but the significance of this parameter in children is unknown.

It is useful to obtain a qualitative drug screen in suspected cases of tricyclic antidepressant overdose to confirm the ingestion. Serum levels, however, are not always helpful in making clinical decisions. Because of the large volume of distribution of tricyclic antidepressants, the serum level does not accurately reflect clinical toxicity. Only when very high levels are present (>1000 ng/mL) do they correlate with life-threatening toxicity. Red blood cell antidepressant levels may give a more accurate indication of tissue levels, but work on this is still experimental.

In children, arterial blood gas monitoring is critical in the treatment of tricyclic antidepressant overdose. Acidemia may increase the proportion of drug released from binding sites, and contributes significantly to the propensity toward dysrhythmias.

MANAGEMENT

Stabilization

Proper airway management is the first step in managing a patient with tricyclic antidepressant overdose. Intubation is necessary for patients with depressed mental status and for those with an absent gag reflex. It is also justified for patients who appear to be deteriorating clinically or for patients with doubtful mental status in whom gastric lavage is necessary.

In intubated patients hyperventilation is indicated, since alkalemia can potentially reverse the cardiac toxicity of tricyclic antidepressant overdose. In all patients hypoxia should be avoided since it can worsen metabolic acidosis.

Hypotension is treated initially with boluses of crystalloid. If fluid resuscitation does not stabilize the blood pressure, pharmacological support is indicated. Norepinephrine has theoretical advantages over dopamine because of its potential to directly reverse the alpha blockade caused by tricyclic antidepressants, but dopamine has been shown to be similarly effective both clinically and in animal models comparing the two.

Gastric Decontamination

Induction of emesis with ipecac is contraindicated because of the potential for sudden deterioration, which can lead to airway compromise and aspiration if the patient vomits while unconscious. Activated charcoal is administered along with a single dose of sorbitol. Multiple doses are probably useful because charcoal binds to the drug still present in the gut and inhibits absorption. The contribution of multiple doses of activated charcoal to interruption of enterohepatic circulation is probably negligible.

Treatment of Severe Toxicity

If the QRS interval is greater than 100 ms, most authors agree that alkalinization is indicated. This can be accomplished by administering sodium bicarbonate as a 1 to 2 mEq/kg bolus, followed by an infusion of sodium bicarbonate in D_5W. If the child is intubated, alkalinization can be obtained by a combination of bicarbonate administration and hyperventilation. The goal of alkalinization is to achieve a pH between 7.45 and 7.50.

Alkalinization is believed to work by reversing the quinidine-like effects of tricyclic antidepressants. The administration of sodium bicarbonate has an effect on reversing sodium channel blockade. This has been demonstrated experimentally in animal studies, where improvement in cardiac rhythm occurs when concentrated saline solutions are administered. Alkalinization may increase the percentage of the drug that is protein-bound, and therefore may protect from toxicity.

Supraventricular dysrhythmias usually do not require intervention. Ventricular dysrhythmias unresponsive to boluses of bicarbonate are treated with lidocaine. Because of the quinidine-like effect of the tricyclic antidepressants, other type IA antidysrhythmics are contraindicated. Phenytoin, a type IB antidysrhythmic, may be of value but has not been shown to be uniformly effective. If the patient is hypotensive with a tachydysrhythmia, cardioversion is appropriate. Bradydysrhythmias may respond to overdrive pacing.

Seizures are an ominous sign in the setting of a tricyclic antidepressant overdose. While generally short, seizures have been associated with incipient cardiac dysrhythmias. Seizures usually require no treatment, but benzodiazepines are effective if needed. Phenytoin is useful in prolonged seizures, but has not been found to be useful prophylactically. Phenobarbital is also useful for prolonged seizures.

Physostigmine has been suggested as an antidote for anticholinergic toxicity. However, its use in association with AV blocks, QRS widening, and bradycardia has resulted in asystole and death. Physostigmine should be viewed as a last line of therapy in cases of uncontrolled seizures, supraventricular dysrhythmia, and severe hypotension.

DISPOSITION

Patients with signs and symptoms of overdose are treated aggressively. Patients who are symptomatic or who appear to be progressing are admitted to an intensive care unit. Patients who do not develop tachycardia, QRS widening, anticholinergic symptoms, or drowsiness can be discharged after 6 hours of monitoring in the emergency department.

BIBLIOGRAPHY

Boehnert MT, Lovejoy FH: Value of the QRS duration versus the serum drug level in predicting seizures and ventricular arrhythmias after an acute overdose of tricyclic antidepressants. *N Engl J Med* 313:474–479, 1985.

Borys DJ, Setzer SC, Ling LJ: Acute fluoxetine overdose: A report of 234 cases. *Am J Emerg Med* 10:115–120, 1992.

Callaham M, Kassel D: Epidemiology of fatal tricyclic antidepressant ingestion: Implications for management. *Ann Emerg Med* 14:1–9, 1985.

Callaham M, Schumaker H, Pentel P: Phenytoin prophylaxis of cardiotoxicity in experimental amitriptyline poisoning. *J Pharmacol Exp Ther* 245:216–220, 1988.

Goldberg RJ, Capone RJ, Hunt JD: Cardiac complications following tricyclic antidepressant overdose: Issues for monitoring policy. *JAMA* 254:1772–1775, 1985.

Kulig K: Management of poisoning associated with "newer" antidepressant agents. *Ann Emerg Med* 15:1039–1045, 1986.

Lavole FW, Gansert GG: Value of initial ECG findings and plasma drug levels in cyclic antidepressant overdose. *Ann Emerg Med* 19:696–700, 1990.

Litovitz TL, Klein-Schwartz W, White S, et al: 1999 annual report of poison control centers toxic exposure surveillance system. *Am J Emerg Med* 18:517–574, 2000.

McCabe JL, Cobaugh DJ, Menegazzi JJ, et al: Experimental tricyclic antidepressant toxicity: A randomized, controlled comparison of hypertonic saline solution, sodium bicarbonate, and hyperventilation. *Ann Emerg Med* 32:329–333, 1998.

McFee RB, Mofenson HC, Caraccio TR: A nationwide survey of the management of unintentional low dose tricyclic antidepressant ingestions involving asymptomatic children: Implications for the development of evidence-based clinical guideline. *Clin Toxicol* 38:15–19, 2000.

92

Digoxin Toxicity

Steven E. Aks
Jerrold B. Leikin

HIGH-YIELD FACTS

- Plants that contain cardiac glycosides include foxglove, oleander, lily of the valley, and red squill.
- Digoxin acts by poisoning the Na^+-K^+ ATPase pump in the heart. High serum potassium may be seen after acute overdose.
- A toxic dose of greater than 0.1 mg/kg may be an indication for antidotal therapy.
- Both hyperkalemia and hypokalemia can predispose to digoxin-induced cardiac dysrhythmias.
- Almost any cardiac dysrhythmia may be seen with digoxin toxicity. Accelerated junctional rhythms, premature ventricular contractions (PVCs), paroxysmal atrial tachycardia, and atrioventricular blocks are more commonly seen rhythms in this setting.
- Atropine is effective for digoxin-induced bradycardia.
- Calcium chloride, potassium, and bretylium should be avoided in treating digoxin toxicity.
- Digoxin immune Fab fragments are indicated in any patient exhibiting a life-threatening dysrhythmia, regardless of the digoxin level.

Digoxin is used today for the treatment of congestive heart failure and supraventricular dysrhythmias. In addition there are several plants that contain cardiac glycosides (digoxin-like substances), including foxglove, oleander, lily of the valley, and red squill.

Historically, mortality due to digoxin overdose has been related to the type of cardiac arrhythmia induced by toxicity, and the degree of associated hyperkalemia. Mortality rates of 68 percent for patients exhibiting digoxin-induced sustained ventricular tachycardia and

100 percent for ventricular fibrillation were noted prior to the development of digoxin immune Fab fragments. According to the American Association of Poison Control Centers, in 1999 there were a total of 2810 cardiac glycoside ingestions. Of these 812 were in children <6 years of age, 128 were in children between the ages of 6 and 19, and there were a total of 20 deaths.

PHARMACOLOGY/PATHOPHYSIOLOGY

Digoxin is a positive inotrope that increases the force and velocity of myocardial contractions. In the failing heart it can increase the cardiac output and decrease elevated end-diastolic pressures.

On the cellular level, digoxin presumably functions by binding to and inactivating the Na^+-K^+ ATPase pump in the heart. This results in increased intracellular sodium concentration. In addition, enhanced contractility depends on intracellular ionized calcium concentrations during systole. At toxic concentrations, it is felt that intracellular calcium concentrations are markedly increased, and that the membrane potential is unstable, which leads to dysrhythmias.

There are numerous factors that predispose the patient to digoxin toxicity, the most common of which is electrolyte imbalance. Both hypokalemia and hyperkalemia can increase the possibility of developing digoxin toxicity. Hyperkalemia in particular can result in significant conduction delays. Hypokalemia is common in patients on diuretic therapy and can predispose patients to the effects of chronic digoxin toxicity. Hypomagnesemia, hypercalcemia, renal insufficiency, and underlying heart disease all predispose to digoxin toxicity.

CLINICAL PRESENTATION

The presentation of digoxin toxicity is highly varied, and depends largely on whether it results from an acute overdose or is a manifestation of chronic toxicity.

In the acute setting patients tend to have more dramatic clinical and laboratory parameters than in chronic toxicity. Symptoms can be abrupt, with severe nausea, vomiting, and diarrhea. Associated complaints include weakness, headache, paresthesias, and altered color perception. Cardiovascular symptoms include palpitations and dizziness that may be secondary to hypotension.

Patients with chronic toxicity tend to have more vague complaints, though many of the symptoms of acute overdose also occur. Malaise, anorexia, and low-grade nausea and vomiting are common. Patients with chronic toxicity tend to be more symptomatic at lower levels than those with acute overdoses.

Cardiovascular toxicity is the most important factor in determining morbidity and mortality. Unfortunately, there are multiple dysrhythmias associated with digoxin toxicity, the most common being frequent premature ventricular beats. Other dysrhythmias can be supraventricular, nodal, or ventricular. Common disturbances are junctional escape beats and accelerated junctional rhythm, paroxysmal atrial tachycardia with AV block, and AV block of varying degrees. There is no single pathognomonic rhythm. Lethal cardiac disturbances rarely occur in children with normal hearts, but serious AV conduction disturbances can occur.

DIAGNOSIS

A history of the exact amount of digoxin ingested is extremely helpful. A dose greater than 0.1 mg/kg has been suggested as an indication for the use of digoxin-specific Fab fragments.

A digoxin level is indicated whenever there is clinical suspicion of toxicity. In an overdose situation, the level is most accurate if obtained ≥6 hours after the ingestion. The therapeutic digoxin range is between 0.8 and 1.8 ng/mL. Unfortunately, there is poor correlation between the digoxin level and clinical manifestations. In an acute overdose, a level as high as 2.6 ng/mL does not correlate well with toxicity. In a chronic overdose, toxicity can occur at lower levels. One author has recently suggested a cutoff level of 5 ng/mL alone as an indication for Fab therapy. The fatality rate approaches 50 percent when the serum digoxin level exceeds 6 ng/mL.

Other necessary laboratory studies include a complete blood count, serum electrolytes, calcium, magnesium, blood urea nitrogen, and creatinine. Cardiac monitoring is essential, as is a 12-lead electrocardiogram.

MANAGEMENT

Digoxin-intoxicated patients can be highly unstable. All patients require a secure airway, intravenous access, and cardiac monitoring.

Gastric Decontamination

Syrup of ipecac is relatively contraindicated in the asymptomatic child because of the potential for sudden hemodynamic instability, deterioration of consciousness, and the subsequent potential for vomiting and aspiration. It is absolutely contraindicated in any patient with abnormal vital signs or altered mental status. Gastric lavage is indicated after an adequate airway is assured, which may require intubation. Activated charcoal along with a cathartic is indicated as a single dose. Multiple doses of charcoal have been reported to be of value for digitoxin preparations in which there is avid enterohepatic circulation, but are probably of little value for digoxin.

Antidotal Therapy

Digoxin immune Fab fragments (Digibind) are specific antidigoxin antibodies derived from sheep. In order to decrease the risk of immunogenicity, only the Fab fragment is used. Specific indications include an ingestion of greater than 0.1 mg/kg, a digoxin level of greater than 5.0 ng/mL, or the presence of a life-threatening dysrhythmia. It has also been used successfully to treat cardiotoxicity from oleander poisoning. The antidote is indicated in any patient whose condition appears to be deteriorating. In the case of chronic toxicity, this can occur at relatively low levels. Hyperkalemia greater than 5.0 mEq/L is another indication to consider the use of Fab fragments. Standard modalities to treat hyperkalemia may also be used, with the exception of calcium salts. In the face of digoxin toxicity the administration of calcium may exacerbate the development of dysrhythmias.

The dose of Fab fragments is based either on the amount ingested or on the serum level. Guidelines are available in the package insert. Each vial of Fab fragments contains 38 mg of protein that will bind 0.6 mg of digoxin. Specific formulas for dosing Fab fragments are available on the package insert.

Allergic reactions to Fab fragments are rare. Skin testing can be performed, but is usually not necessary. In cases where Fab fragments have been effective, results have been achieved 30 minutes to 4 hours after administration. After administration of Fab fragments, subsequent digoxin levels will be falsely elevated for several days, because the bound digoxin is measured along with the free drug.

In addition to the administration of Fab fragments, standard treatment of dysrhythmias or AV blocks is indicated. Atropine or temporary pacing may be necessary to temporize while Fab fragments are taking effect. Cardioversion and lidocaine are appropriate in the event of ventricular tachycardia or fibrillation. Treatment with intravenous phenytoin or magnesium sulfate has been shown to be particularly useful in digoxin-induced tachydysrhythmias.

Drugs to avoid in the treatment of digoxin-induced cardiac toxicity include calcium, bretylium tosylate, sotalol, isoproterenol, and quinidine. Direct-current cardioversion should only be used as a last resort for life-threatening arrhythmia. If utilized, it should be dosed at the lowest energy possible.

Hemodialysis and hemoperfusion do not aid in the removal of digoxin or digitoxin. Plasma exchange is also not expected to be useful.

DISPOSITION

Children with trivial ingestions who are asymptomatic and have no detectable levels of digoxin 4 hours after the ingestion can be discharged from the emergency department after 6 hours of observation. Any child with signs or symptoms of toxicity is admitted to a monitored bed, preferably in a pediatric intensive care unit.

BIBLIOGRAPHY

Eddleston M, Rajapapakse S, Rajakanthan S, et al: Anti-digoxin Fab fragments in cardiotoxicity induced by ingestion of yellow oleander: A randomized controlled trial. *Lancet* 355: 967–972, 2000.

Kelly RA, Smith TW: Recognition and management of digitalis toxicity. *J Am Coll Cardiol* 17:590, 1991.

Kinlay S, Buckley NA: Magnesium sulfate in the treatment of ventricular arrhythmias due to digoxin toxicity. *J Toxicol Clin Toxicol* 33:55, 1995.

Lewis RP: Clinical use of serum digoxin concentrations. *Am J Cardiol* 69:97G–107G, 1992.

Litovitz TL, Klein-Schwartz W, White S, et al: 1999 annual report of poison control centers toxic exposure surveillance system. *Am J Emerg Med* 18:517–574, 2000.

Sekkul EA, Kaminer S, Sethi KD: Digoxin-induced chorea in a child. *Mov Disord* 14(5):877–879, 1999.

Valdes R Jr, Jortani SA: Monitoring of unbound digoxin in patients treated with anti-digoxin antigen-binding fragments: A model for the future? *Clin Chem* 44:183–185, 1998.

Wells TG, Young RA, Kearns GL: Age-related differences in digoxin toxicity and its treatment. *Drug Safety* 7:135–151, 1992.

Williamson KM, Thrasher KA, Fulton KB, et al: Digoxin toxicity: An evaluation in current clinical practice. *Arch Intern Med* 158:2444–2449, 1998.

Woolf AD, Wenger TL, Smith TW, et al: Results of multicenter studies of digoxin-specific antibody fragments in managing digitalis intoxication in the pediatric population. *Am J Emerg Med* 9:16–20(suppl), 1991.

93

Fish Poisoning

Timothy Erickson

HIGH-YIELD FACTS

- Classic findings in ciguatera poisoning include circumoral tingling, paresthesias, and reversal of heat and cold sensations.
- Scombrotoxin causes a histamine-like syndrome.
- Tetrodotoxin can cause death by inducing respiratory paralysis or cardiovascular collapse.

Hazardous marine life can be classified into four major groups:

- Venomous bites and stings, such as those inflicted by scorpion fish and the Portuguese man-of-war
- Shock injuries, as from electric eels
- Traumatogenic bites (sharks and barracudas)
- Toxic ingestions or fish poisoning

This final group of marine food-borne poisonings can be further divided into those induced by fish harboring ciguatoxin, scombrotoxin, paralytic shellfish saxitoxin, or tetrodotoxin. As a result of the wide availability of fresh and frozen fish, there is an increasing frequency of toxic ingestions in North America.

CIGUATERA

Pathophysiology

Ciguatera fish poisoning is a serious public health problem in the Caribbean and Indo-Pacific regions. Ciguatoxin is produced by a dinoflagellate, *Gambierdiscus toxicus,* and concentrated in the food chain of predator reef fish such as barracuda, grouper, red snapper, parrotfish, jacks, and moray eels. When humans ingest contaminated fish, poisoning can cause distinct neurological and gastrointestinal symptomatology, due to the toxin's anticholinesterase activity.

Clinical Presentation

In nonepidemic areas, the diagnosis of ciguatera poisoning is made only by a high index of suspicion combined with a recent history of ingestion of a specific fish. Within hours of ingestion, the patient may complain of neurologic symptoms such as circumoral tingling, headache, tremor, diffuse paresthesias, and classically, reversal of hot and cold sensations. Younger children may only present with discomfort and irritability. Other signs, such as miosis, ptosis, and muscular spasm are more objective but occur much less frequently. The patient also commonly suffers gastrointestinal symptoms, such as watery diarrhea, vomiting, and abdominal cramping, making it difficult to differentiate from typical pediatric gastroenteritis.

Because of their smaller size, children are potentially at a higher risk for greater concentration of the toxin. Potentially fatal cardiovascular manifestations such as severe bradycardia, hypotension, and respiratory depression are possible but uncommon. Mortality from poisoning is 0.1 percent. The neurological symptoms can become chronic and persist for several weeks to months.

Management

Treatment of ciguatera poisoning is primarily supportive. If the child presents within 1 hour of ingestion of the suspected fish and has not already vomited, decontamination with gastric lavage followed by activated charcoal is indicated. If the patient is already experiencing watery diarrhea, cathartics are not recommended, as they only exacerbate fluid losses and electrolyte disturbances. To date, specific treatment of ciguatera has been limited. Several agents such as amitriptyline and nifedipine have been advocated, but are of unproven efficacy. Recently there has been some success with mannitol administration. Its mechanism of action remains speculative, but may be due either to action as an osmotic agent or as a scavenger of hydroxyl radicals from the ciguatoxin molecule.

Disposition

If the child is experiencing significant fluid losses, electrolyte imbalance, or neurological manifestations, admission for observation and fluid resuscitation is recommended.

SCOMBROTOXIN

Pathophysiology

Scombroid poisoning is a food-borne illness associated with the consumption of improperly handled dark-meat fish, such as tuna, bonito, skipjack, mackerel, and mahi-mahi (dolphin fish). Unlike ciguatoxin, scombrotoxin is not contracted from the marine environment but rather directly from the flesh of the fish, which has undergone bacterial decomposition due to improper refrigeration. Although the symptoms of scombroid poisoning resemble an allergic reaction, this is a toxic phenomenon, since symptoms are a response to exogenous histamine rather than mast cell degranulation.

Clinical Presentation

Within minutes to hours following ingestion of a fish containing scombrotoxin, the patient experiences a histamine-like syndrome with diffuse erythema, pruritus, urticaria, dysphagia, and headache. Palpitations and dysrhythmias have been reported but are rare. The symptoms usually last about 4 hours, and occasionally may persist for 1 or 2 days.

Management

Although scombroid poisoning is typically self-limited, supportive measures and fluid resuscitation are indicated, as is gastric decontamination if the ingestion was recent. Antihistamines such as diphenhydramine have been reported to shorten the duration of symptoms, but the benefit is inconsistent, suggesting that the syndrome may be mediated by more than histamine alone. Intravenous infusion of a histamine H_2-receptor antagonist such as cimetidine has proven effective in patients with inadequate responses to diphenhydramine.

Disposition

If the vital signs are stable and there is good response to antihistamines, patients can be safely discharged home to take diphenhydramine and oral cimetidine for 2 to 3 days. If there is immediate threat of anaphylaxis or angioneurotic edema, aggressive therapy including proper airway management and admission is recommended.

PARALYTIC SHELLFISH POISONING

Pathophysiology

Specific neurotoxic species of the dinoflagellate *Gonyaulax* form red tides and concentrate the toxin saxitoxin in bivalve shellfish such as mussels, clams, and scallops. Humans who consume contaminated shellfish can develop profound muscle weakness via a curare-like effect mediated through blockage of sodium conduction channels.

Clinical Presentation

Gastrointestinal symptoms may develop within minutes to hours after ingestion, with vomiting, diarrhea, and abdominal cramping. Additionally, the patient may experience headache, ataxia, facial paresthesias, and on rare occasions muscle paralysis resulting in respiratory paralysis up to 12 hours after ingestion.

Management

Supportive measures include fluid resuscitation, and in recent ingestions gastric decontamination. If paralytic shellfish poisoning is suspected, the patient is admitted for a 24-hour period for observation for respiratory depression.

TETRODOTOXIN

Pathophysiology

Tetrodotoxin, one of the most potent poisons known, results in poisoning after the ingestion of the puffer fish, California newt, Eastern salamander, or blue-ringed octopus. Intoxication produces profound neurologic symptoms and muscle weakness due to its inhibition of the sodium-potassium pump and subsequent blockade of neuromuscular transmission. In some reported studies mortality rates have approached 60 percent.

Clinical Presentation

Symptoms following ingestion of fish or amphibians containing tetrodotoxin begin within 30 minutes of ingestion. Early manifestations include circumoral and throat paresthesias. These findings are followed by GI complaints of vomiting and abdominal cramping. If the patient has consumed a large amount of the toxin, within minutes to hours they may experience a "feeling of doom" heralding ascending paralysis, respiratory depression, dilated pupils, hypotension, bradycardia, and a classic "locked-in" or zombie-like syndrome. Death results from either respiratory paralysis or cardiovascular collapse. Typically, if the patient survives beyond 24 hours, recovery occurs.

Management

Treatment includes rapid stabilization and gastric decontamination with gastric lavage. Syrup of ipecac is contraindicated due to potentially rapid central nervous system and respiratory depression. Atropine has been recommended for bradycardia and hypotension. Edrophonium and neostigmine may be beneficial in restoring motor strength. Most importantly, the patient's airway and respiratory status should be supported aggressively.

Disposition

Any patient with suspected poisoning from tetrodotoxin is admitted to an intensive care unit for a minimum observation period of 24 hours.

BIBLIOGRAPHY

Herman TE, McAlister WH: Epiglottic enlargement: Two unusual causes. *Pediatr Radiol* 21:139–140, 1991.

Hughes JM, Potter ME: Scombroid fish poisoning. *N Engl J Med* 324:766–68, 1991.

McInerney J, Shagal P, Bogel M: Scombroid poisoning. *Ann Emerg Med* 8:235, 1996.

Senecal PE, Osterloh JD: Normal fetal outcome after maternal ciguateric toxin exposure in the second trimester. *Clin Toxicol* 29:473–478, 1991.

Shoff WH, Shepherd SM: Scombroid, ciguatera, and other seafood intoxications, in Ford M, Delaney K, Ling L, et al (eds): *Clinical Toxicology,* Philadelphia: Saunders, 2001, pp 959–969.

Swift AE, Swift TR: Ciguatera. *Clin Toxicol* 31:1–29, 1993.

Williams RK, Palafox NA: Treatment of pediatric ciguatera fish poisoning. *Am J Dis Child* 144:747–758, 1990.

94

Hydrocarbons

Bonnie McManus

HIGH-YIELD FACTS

- Young children most frequently ingest hydrocarbons accidentally, while adolescents are more likely to abuse volatile substances or deliberately ingest hydrocarbons in suicidal gestures or attempts.
- Fatal liver injury has been reported after ingestion of as little as 3 mL of carbon tetrachloride.
- Viscosity, volatility, and surface tension are physical properties that affect the type and extent of toxicity. Heavier compounds, such as mineral or baby oil, paraffin, and asphalt, have a minimal risk of toxicity.
- The principal concern after most hydrocarbon ingestions is pulmonary toxicity.
- In general, ingestion of most petroleum distillates in a volume of less than 1 to 2 mL/kg does not cause systemic toxicity.
- In any patient with a history of hydrocarbon ingestion, it is essential to try to identify the compound, since this information can have profound implications for management and prognosis.
- Most authors discourage the use of gastric decontamination procedures in the case of accidental ingestions.
- Activated charcoal is not indicated in the vast majority of hydrocarbon ingestions.
- Glucocorticoids do not affect outcome and their use is not indicated.

Hydrocarbons are organic compounds ubiquitous in daily life. Typical hydrocarbon products include gasoline, stove or lamp fuel, paints and paint thinners, glues, spot removers, degreasers, and typewriter correction fluid. In 1999 the National Data Collection System of the American Association of Poison Control Centers received 62,772 calls concerning hydrocarbons. Children <6 years of age accounted for 39 percent of these calls. The hydrocarbons most frequently ingested in accidental childhood poisonings include gasoline, kerosene, lighter fluid, mineral seal oil, and turpentine. The mechanism of exposure varies with age. Young children most frequently ingest hydrocarbons accidentally, while adolescents are more likely to abuse volatile substances or deliberately ingest hydrocarbons in suicidal gestures or attempts.

CLASSIFICATION AND PROPERTIES

Hydrocarbons are derived from petroleum distillation which generates compounds composed of chains of varying lengths. The terpenes, which are derived from wood distillation, are toxicologically considered with hydrocarbons because of the similarity of their clinical effects. The length of the chain affects the behavior of the hydrocarbon. At room temperature, short chains of carbons are gases such as methane and butane. Intermediate-length chains are liquids and account for most exposures seen in the emergency department. Solids, such as tar and paraffin, are long-chain hydrocarbons.

There are 3 major classes of hydrocarbons. The aliphatic, or straight-chain compounds, include kerosene, mineral seal oil, gasoline, solvents, and paint thinners. Aliphatic compounds include halogenated hydrocarbons, such as carbon tetrachloride and trichloroethane, which are typically found in industrial settings as solvents. The halogenated hydrocarbons are well absorbed by the lung and gut, making them particularly dangerous. Centrilobular hepatic necrosis and renal failure are associated with ingestion of halogenated hydrocarbons, especially carbon tetrachloride. Fatal liver injury has been reported after ingestion of as little as 3 mL of carbon tetrachloride.

The cyclic or aromatic compounds contain a benzene ring and are used in industrial solvents. The aromatics are highly volatile, and unlike the straight-chain hydrocarbons, benzene and its major derivatives toluene and xylene are well absorbed from the gastrointestinal tract. Of the aromatics, benzene is the most toxic, with death reported after ingestion of as little as 15 mL.

The terpene compounds consist mainly of cyclic terpene rings and include compounds such as turpentine and pine oil.

Viscosity, volatility, and surface tension are physical properties that affect the type and extent of toxicity. *Viscosity* is defined as the resistance to flow, and is the most important property in determining the risk of aspiration. *Volatility* describes the propensity of a substance to become a gas. *Surface tension* describes the propensity of a compound to adhere to itself at the liquid's surface. Low surface tension allows easy spread over a wide surface area. A substance with low surface tension may easily spread from the oropharynx to the trachea, promoting aspiration. Compounds that have low viscosity and low surface tension have the highest risk of aspiration. Mineral seal oil has very low volatility but surprisingly low viscosity, and when ingested is likely to cause aspiration and pneumonia. Heavier compounds, such as mineral or baby oil, paraffin, and asphalt have a minimal risk of toxicity.

Gaseous hydrocarbons such as methane and butane can act as asphyxiants by displacing air in the lungs and causing hypoxia. They are also capable of crossing the capillary membrane and directly causing central nervous system (CNS) depression. Gasoline and naphtha have relatively high volatilities and can cause primary CNS depression after inhalation of fumes with minimal pulmonary damage.

PATHOPHYSIOLOGY

The principal concern after most hydrocarbon ingestions is pulmonary toxicity. The lungs are spared unless there is direct contact with the hydrocarbon via aspiration. Gastrointestinal absorption by itself does not result in pulmonary toxicity. Very small amounts may be aspirated and result in chemical or lipoid pneumonitis.

Chemical pneumonitis may be due to direct destruction of lung tissue itself, depending on the type of hydrocarbon, or may be due to an aggressive inflammatory reaction. Later findings may be due to the destruction of surfactant, which results in decreased lung compliance and can cause significant atelectasis. Noncardiogenic pulmonary edema and bacterial superinfection can occur. Hemorrhagic pulmonary edema and respiratory arrest can occur within 24 hours. Following resolution of the acute insult, pulmonary dysfunction can persist for years.

Lipoid pneumonia is seen frequently with high-viscosity hydrocarbons, such as mineral oil and liquid paraffin. This lesion is more localized and less inflammatory than the reaction produced by low-viscosity petroleum distillates like kerosene. A hemorrhagic pneumonitis does not occur. Despite the less-aggressive inflammatory response, lipoid pneumonitis can take several weeks to resolve.

CNS compromise is frequently seen, but the factors responsible for this are unclear. Neurologic injury may be due to the direct effect on the CNS by the ingested hydrocarbon, but most authorities agree that asphyxiation and hypoxia are major contributors to CNS lesions. The aromatic hydrocarbons have a high potential for causing major CNS depression. The terpenes are easily absorbed and typically cause mild CNS depression. The halogenated and volatile hydrocarbons may produce a euphoric state similar to alcohol intoxication. These products rapidly attain high concentrations in the central nervous system, and can suppress ventilatory drive. This is most commonly seen in the adolescent glue sniffer who appears intoxicated.

Gastrointestinal symptoms include nausea, vomiting, abdominal pain, and diarrhea. These symptoms are frequent but usually mild. Vomiting increases the risk of aspiration pneumonitis; therefore it is important to limit emesis. Ingestion or chronic inhalation abuse can cause hematemesis. In general, ingestion of most petroleum distillates in a volume less than 1 to 2 mL/kg does not cause systemic toxicity.

When skin is exposed to hydrocarbons for an extended time, an eczematoid dermatitis develops due to the drying and defatting action of these compounds. This is typically seen in adolescents abusing volatile substances, and is known as "glue sniffer's rash" which is predominantly located in the perioral area or mid-face regions. There may be significant skin erythema, inflammation, and pruritus. Gasoline and other hydrocarbons can cause full-thickness burns. Renal failure has been reported after the use of diesel fuel as a shampoo, strongly suggesting cutaneous absorption.

Fever is seen on presentation in 30 percent of cases. It does not correlate with clinical symptoms and is possibly of central origin. Three-fourths of patients defervesce within 24 hours. If fever persists for more than 48 to 72 hours, bacterial superinfection should be considered.

Many anticholinesterase pesticides are combined with kerosene vehicles. A cholinergic crisis is likely in patients with excessive bronchorrhea, salivation, lacrimation, or urinary incontinence. The classic bradycardia and miosis may be obscured by the tachycardia and mydriasis from hydrocarbon-induced hypoxia.

CLINICAL PRESENTATION

On presentation, patients may be completely asymptomatic or may suffer severe respiratory distress and CNS depression. A history of coughing or gagging is consistent with aspiration. In addition to cough, early signs of pulmonary toxicity include gasping, choking, tachypnea, and wheezing. Bronchospasm may contribute to ventilation-perfusion mismatch and exacerbate hypoxia. Cyanosis may be present, and in the early stages cyanosis is usually due to replacement of alveolar air by volatilized hydrocarbon. In the later stages it is due to direct pulmonary toxicity. CNS symptoms range from irritability, which can be a sign of hypoxia, to lethargy and coma. After a significant oral ingestion, gastrointestinal disturbance is common.

In any patient with a history of hydrocarbon ingestion, it is essential to try to identify the compound, since this information can have profound implications for management and prognosis.

MANAGEMENT

The mainstay of treatment for hydrocarbon exposure is supportive care. It essential to realize that while the vast majority of patients will present with minimal if any symptoms, patients with respiratory compromise on presentation to the emergency department can suffer rapid deterioration.

Airway patency is evaluated and established. Intravenous lines and cardiac monitors are indicated in symptomatic patients. Any patient with respiratory symptoms, including grunting, tachypnea, or cyanosis is treated with humidified oxygen and requires an arterial blood gas evaluation. An abnormal alveolar-arterial gradient is frequently present in serious exposures. Nebulized β-2 agonists are the drugs of choice for patients with bronchospasm. Patients with respiratory failure require artificial ventilation. Because hydrocarbons solubilize surfactant, continuous positive airway pressure (CPAP) or positive end-expiratory pressure (PEEP) may be needed as a ventilatory adjunct in patients with significant respiratory distress. Extracorporeal membrane oxygenation (ECMO) has been reported to be successful in pediatric patients suffering hydrocarbon-induced pneumonitis who fail to respond to conventional ventilatory support.

Patients with altered mental status should have a bedside glucose test or be treated empirically with intravenous dextrose. The possibility of a concomitant opioid overdose is managed with naloxone.

Cyanosis is usually due to hypoxia, but may also be due to methemoglobinemia in cases where aniline or nitrobenzene has been ingested. Exposure to methylene chloride is a concern because it is frequently found in paint strippers, and after exposure is metabolized to carbon monoxide. Carbon monoxide poisoning must be considered in patients with persistent symptoms. Treatment consists of 100 percent oxygen, and depending on the degree of toxicity and the carboxyhemoglobin level, hyperbaric oxygen may be considered.

In the event of a cutaneous exposure, all clothing is removed and the skin is irrigated and washed twice with soap and water. Appropriate precautions should be taken by staff members to avoid becoming contaminated.

Gastric Evacuation

Most authors discourage the use of gastric decontamination procedures in cases of accidental ingestions. Usually the risk of aspiration is higher than the risk of systemic absorption in an accidental ingestion. Children are not likely to accidentally ingest sufficient quantities of hydrocarbons to cause significant systemic absorption. The Cooperative Kerosene Poisoning Study concluded that gastric lavage was neither harmful nor beneficial, and pulmonary complications correlated better with the quantity of petroleum distillate ingested (>1 ounce) or the fact that the patient vomited than they do to the use or omission of gastric lavage. Another study showed that in children in whom the time course of illness was known, 88 percent were symptomatic within 10 minutes of ingestion. Currently, gastric evacuation is not recommended in patients with minimal or no symptoms after ingestion of a pure petroleum distillate or turpentine. Gastric evacuation of most types of hydrocarbons is reserved for massive ingestions, which usually occur in adults or adolescents involved in a suicide attempt. While still controversial, ingestions of >4 to 5 mL/kg of naphtha, gasoline, kerosene, or turpentine should probably be removed. Other ingestions in which gastric evacuation is indicated are for those that contain dangerous additives such as benzene, toluene, halogenated hydrocarbons, heavy metals, camphor, pesticides, aniline, or other toxic compounds.

Currently there is no overwhelming support for either emesis with ipecac or gastric lavage as a superior mode of gastric evacuation. In the awake, alert patient with an intact gag reflex, ipecac is appropriate. Emesis is contraindicated if there is previous unprovoked emesis or any degree of neurologic, respiratory, or cardiac compromise. In these cases gastric lavage is indicated after endotracheal intubation with a cuffed tube. If the child is <8 years old, inflate the cuff only during lavage. A nasogastric tube may be adequate to remove liquids, but if there is concomitant ingestion of a solid, this would be insufficient. Orogastric tubes, without the added protection of the airway by an endotracheal tube, are extremely controversial because they usually induce gagging and vomiting, promoting aspiration.

Activated charcoal is not indicated in the vast majority of hydrocarbon ingestions. It does adsorb kerosene, turpentine, and benzene in vitro and in animal models, but because it may induce vomiting it is generally discouraged unless there is known to be an adsorbable co-ingestant. Its efficacy for other hydrocarbons is not documented.

Ancillary Therapy

Intravenous hydration may be indicated for patients with significant vomiting or diarrhea, and for patients with respiratory compromise who are unable to take oral fluids. Fluid replacement is restricted to a maintenance rate to diminish the risk of overhydration and the exacerbation of pulmonary edema.

Glucocorticoids do not affect outcome and their use is not indicated. Antibiotics are reserved for patients with definite evidence of infection. The use of commercially available surfactants in animal models has been evaluated, and at present no clear recommendations can be made for human exposures.

LABORATORY STUDIES

In about 90 percent of patients with respiratory symptoms on presentation, the initial chest radiograph will be abnormal. Radiographic abnormalities can occur as early as 20 minutes or as late as 24 hours after ingestion. Typical findings include increased bronchovascular markings and bibasilar and perihilar infiltrates. Lobar consolidation is uncommon. Pneumothorax, pneumomediastinum, and pleural effusions are rare. Pneumatoceles can occur and resolve over weeks.

Depending on the severity of the ingestion, the patient's acid-base status, electrolyte balance, complete blood count, and hepatic profile should be followed.

DISPOSITION

A patient who accidentally ingests a hydrocarbon and presents to the emergency department without symptoms should be observed for 6 hours. If during that time they remain asymptomatic and oxygen saturation and a chest radiograph are normal, discharge is appropriate. If symptoms develop during the 6-hour period of observation, hospital admission is indicated.

All patients who are symptomatic on presentation are admitted to the hospital. If respiratory compromise or hypoxia is present, admission to a pediatric intensive care unit is advised. Hospital admission is also indicated when there is risk of significant delayed organ toxicity, as in the case of ingestion of carbon tetrachloride or other toxic additives. When they are medically stable, psychiatric evaluation is needed for adolescents who acted with suicidal intent.

VOLATILE SUBSTANCE ABUSE

Among adolescents, inhalation abuse of volatile hydrocarbons is a significant health hazard. Typically, solvent-containing fluids such as typewriter correction fluid and adhesives, and other halogenated hydrocarbons, such as those found in gasoline and cigarette lighter fluid, are abused. These substances are inexpensive, easily obtained, and readily concealed by the adolescent.

Volatile substance abuse typically involves more than just sniffing. Multiple deep inhalations are taken after the substance is poured into a plastic bag, known as *bagging,* or a cloth is saturated and held to the face, known as *huffing.* Aerosolized products may be bubbled through water first to remove the unwanted product and then the gases captured and inhaled.

The predominant acute risk of inhalation abuse is "sudden sniffing death." It is believed that the myocardium is hypersensitized and a sudden outpouring of sympathetic stimulation leads to fatal cardiac dysrhythmias. There have been numerous case reports of patients abusing solvents and then collapsing shortly after beginning marked physical exertion or being startled. Indirect effects of volatile abuse include trauma due to impaired judgment, aspiration, and asphyxia associated with plastic bags.

As with alcohol, acute poisoning with volatile substances involves an initial period of euphoria and disinhibition, with further intoxication leading to dysphoria, ataxia, confusion, and hallucinations. There is rapid onset and recovery, but repeated inhalations can prolong the altered state. Because of the short half-life of these substances, patients rarely present acutely intoxicated. But if this should be the case, take care not to stress or excite the patient as this may stimulate cardiac dysrhythmias. Treatment of the intoxicated patient consists of supportive measures. If resuscitation is necessary, standard advanced cardiac life support measures are indicated.

BIBLIOGRAPHY

Anas N, Namasonthi V, Ginsburg CM: Criteria for hospitalizing children who have ingested products containing hydrocarbons. *JAMA* 246:840–843, 1981.

Dice WH, Ward G, Kelly J, et al: Pulmonary toxicity following gastrointestinal ingestion of kerosene. *Ann Emerg Med* 11:138–142, 1982.

Esmail A, Meyer L, Pottier A, et al: Deaths from volatile substance abuse in those under 18 years: Results from a national epidemiological study. *Arch Dis Child* 69:356, 1993.

Goldfrank LR, Kulgberg AG, Bresnitz EA: Hydrocarbons, in Goldfrank LR, Flomenbaum NE, Lewin NA, et al (eds): *Goldfrank's Toxicologic Emergencies.* Norwalk, CT, Appleton & Lange, 1998, pp 1383–1398.

Hart LM, Cobaugh DJ, Dean BS, et al: Successful use of extracorporeal membrane oxygenation (ECMO) in the treatment of refractory respiratory failure secondary to hydrocarbon aspiration (abstract). *Vet Hum Toxicol* 33:361, 1991.

Leikin JB, Kaufman D, Lipscomb JW, et al: Methylene chloride: Report of five exposures and two deaths. *Am J Emerg Med* 8:534, 1990.

Litovitz TL, Klein-Schwartz W, White S, et al: 1999 Annual report of the American Association of Poison Control Centers toxic exposure surveillance system. *Am J Emerg Med* 18(5):517, 2000.

Machado B, Cross K, Snodgrass WR: Accidental hydrocarbon ingestion cases telephoned to a regional poison center. *Ann Emerg Med* 17:804, 1988.

Subcommittee on Accidental Poisoning (SAP): Cooperative kerosene poisoning study: Evaluation of gastric lavage and other factors in treatment of accidental ingestion of distillate products. *Pediatrics* 29:648–674, 1962.

Widmer LR, Goodwin SR, Berman LS, et al: Artificial surfactant for therapy in hydrocarbon-induced lung injury in sheep. *Crit Care Med* 24:1524–1529, 1996.

95

Iron Poisoning

Steven E. Aks

HIGH-YIELD FACTS

- When calculating the amount of iron ingested one must convert to elemental content. More than 40 mg/kg is associated with significant toxicity and more than 60 mg/kg with death.

- Phase II of iron toxicity is the quiescent or danger phase of the overdose. The patient will appear to be better clinically, which may falsely reassure the clinician.

- Peak iron levels should be obtained between 2 and 6 hours after ingestion.

- The TIBC (total iron binding capacity) will be falsely elevated after iron ingestion and should not be relied upon.

- The "vin rose" urine occurs after deferoxamine treatment. It represents the ferrioxamine complex being excreted in the urine.

- Whole bowel irrigation should be considered if multiple radiopaque iron tablets are seen on abdominal radiography.

- The preferred route of deferoxamine administration is intravenously at a rate of 10 to 15 mg/kg/h.

Iron is one of the most important pediatric toxins. It is an extremely common cause of poisoning and has a high potential for morbidity and mortality. According to 1992 data from the American Association of Poison Control Centers, from 1983 through 1990 iron was the most common cause of pediatric unintentional ingestion death, accounting for 30.2 percent of reported cases. From 1985 through 1989, there were over 11,000 reported exposures to iron in children.

The FDA has required unit dose packaging (blister-packs) for most products containing more than 30 mg elemental iron per tablet. This new packaging of iron sup-plements is expected to decrease the frequency of pediatric iron overdose incidents.

PATHOPHYSIOLOGY

Iron is absorbed through the gastrointestinal mucosa in the ferrous (Fe^{2+}) state. It is oxidized to the ferric (Fe^{3+}) state and attaches to ferritin. Toxicity occurs when ferritin and transferrin are saturated, and serum iron exceeds the total iron binding capacity (TIBC). Circulating free iron can damage blood vessels and can cause transudation of fluids from the intravascular space, resulting in hypotension. Hypotension is potentiated by the release of ferritin, a potent vasodilator. Other target organs include the gastrointestinal tract, heart, and lungs. Autopsy findings include cloudy swelling, fatty degeneration, and necrosis of hepatocytes. Iron deposits can be found in hepatocytes and the reticuloendothelial cells of the liver and spleen. Fatty degeneration occurs in the heart and renal tubules. The lungs may reveal congestive changes.

CLINICAL PRESENTATION

Patients commonly present to the emergency department with a history of having ingested iron tablets or vitamins containing iron. It is useful to attempt to identify the exact preparation, since content of elemental iron, which is the toxic ingredient, varies. If the preparation is identified, the number of pills ingested is important information, since the ratio of elemental iron ingested to the weight of the patient is critical in estimating the potential for toxicity (Table 95-1). If the amount of elemental iron ingested cannot be closely approximated, a worst-case scenario is assumed. It is useful to describe iron overdose in terms of the known stages of toxicity. The stages are generally sequential, though there can be overlap.

Stage 1

This stage begins at the time of ingestion and lasts for about 6 hours. Mild cases demonstrate nausea and vomiting. More severe ingestions suffer vomiting, diarrhea, hematemesis, altered mental status, and possibly hypotension.

Stage 2

Stage 2 occurs from about 6 to 12 hours postingestion, and is referred to as the quiescent or "danger" phase because the patient can appear to be improving, or may

Table 95-1. Iron Preparations

Iron Preparation	Elemental Iron (%)
Ferrous sulfate	20
Ferrous fumarate	33
Ferrous gluconate	12

Ingested Dose (mg/kg)	Treatment Recommendation
<20	Dilute and observe
20–40 mg/kg	Ipecac at home and observe
>40 mg/kg	Refer to health care facility

even be asymptomatic. A meticulous history is vital to diagnosing a patient in this stage, with emphasis on stage 1 symptoms, especially vomiting and diarrhea.

Stage 3

The period, from about 12 to 24 hours postingestion, marks stage 3, in which the patient can exhibit major signs of toxicity. Gastrointestinal hemorrhage and cardiovascular collapse can occur. Patients may develop altered mental status ranging from lethargy to coma. Both renal and hepatic failure can occur, and patients can develop a severe metabolic acidosis, which is thought to result from an interruption of mitochondrial electron transport.

Stage 4

This is a latent phase in which the patient has recovered from the acute insult. It occurs 4 to 6 weeks after the ingestion when the patient develops symptoms due to strictures that develop in the gastrointestinal tract as a result of formation of scar tissue.

DIAGNOSIS

The easiest way to assess the potential of an iron ingestion to result in toxicity is to quantitate the amount ingested and determine if it is significant in the particular patient in question (Table 95-1). Certain laboratory tests are useful to support the diagnosis of iron toxicity. A white blood cell count (WBC) greater than 15,000 mm^3 and a serum glucose greater than 150 mg/dL have been correlated with serum iron levels greater than 300 µg/dL.

While more recent studies have cast doubt on the predictive value of these markers, they are considered suggestive of a toxic ingestion. Normal WBC and serum glucose do not rule out iron toxicity.

Iron levels can be obtained between 2 and 6 hours after ingestion, but are optimally drawn at 4 hours postingestion. A level greater than 300 to 350 µg/dL is considered toxic. Levels greater than 500 µg/dL suggest potentially life-threatening toxicity.

Measurement of the total iron binding capacity (TIBC) has been used to determine the presence of a toxic ingestion, based on the assumption that toxicity occurs when serum iron exceeds the TIBC. A recent study has indicated that this is not a reliable indicator, since ingesting iron will raise the measured TIBC level when it is done by standard colorimetric methods. The TIBC is not useful in the acute management of iron ingestion.

Abdominal radiographs can locate iron-containing tablets in the gut, and may reveal the presence of concretions. If pills are identified, the patient is at risk for delayed absorption of iron. Obtaining serial levels every 2 to 4 hours until the iron level peaks is appropriate. A positive radiograph after gastric lavage has recently been suggested as an indication for whole bowel irrigation.

Deferoxamine is a compound that chelates free iron. The deferoxamine challenge test can be administered to patients who have ingested an unknown or borderline quantity of iron. The challenge is conducted by administering 40 to 90 mg/kg intramuscularly of deferoxamine, up to a maximum of 1 g in children and 2 g in adults. Classically, a positive test is indicated by the patient's urine developing a "vin rose" color 4 to 6 hours after receiving deferoxamine. However, the classical appearance is seen in a minority of patients. A subtle change in the color of the urine may be more easily detected by obtaining a baseline urine specimen prior to administering the challenge. Even a slight change in color to an orange or red indicates a positive test. At present, there are no definitive data on the reliability of the test, and it must be correlated with the history and physical examination.

TREATMENT

Gastric Emptying

Since neither activated charcoal nor any other substance is capable of absorbing iron in the gastrointestinal tract, gastric emptying is the sole method of gut decontamination. While syrup of ipecac can be used in children older than 6 months of age, there is a trend toward gastric lavage for patients in whom it is technically feasible. Lavage is performed with saline. Previous recommendations included adding bicarbonate to the lavage solution, since it was felt it would bind iron and make it insoluble and easier to remove. This has not been shown to be effective in the clinical setting. In addition, both deferoxamine and phosphate have been suggested as additives to the lavage solution. Neither is currently recommended. Deferoxamine may actually enhance the absorption of iron, and phosphate may worsen the clinical course by causing significant hyperphosphatemia and hypocalcemia.

It is currently recommended that whole bowel irrigation with polyethylene glycol electrolyte lavage solution be initiated if pills are noted on abdominal radiographs after gastric lavage. The optimal regimen in children is not well established. The endpoint of therapy is clearing of the rectal effluent and disappearance of the pills seen on x-ray. Active gastrointestinal bleeding and ileus or bowel obstruction are contraindications to whole bowel irrigation. In the absence of pill fragments on x-ray, whole bowel irrigation is probably not helpful.

Chelation

Chelation with deferoxamine is used for significant iron ingestions. Standard indications for therapy include a peak iron level of 300 to 350 μg/dL or a patient who exhibits signs of toxicity in the absence of an available iron level.

Deferoxamine can be administered intramuscularly or intravenously. Intramuscular administration is appropriate for a deferoxamine challenge test or for patients who exhibit mild toxicity. Deferoxamine is administered at 6-hour intervals. The intramuscular dose is 90 mg/kg/dose, with a maximum single dose in children not to exceed 1 g.

Intravenous administration is indicated for patients with moderate to severe toxicity. Hypotension is the most common side effect of intravenous therapy, and can usually be treated by slowing down the drip or making the solution more dilute. Allergic reactions are rare. For patients undergoing chronic therapy, visual and hearing deficits have been reported.

The endpoint of chelation is reached when the color of the patient's urine returns to normal. Significant cases can require chelation for 12 to 16 hours or longer. Chelation should not exceed 24 hours, and in general the total dose of deferoxamine should not exceed 6 to 8 g. Delayed pulmonary toxicity with symptoms resembling those of acute respiratory distress syndrome has been reported in patients who received prolonged chelation.

Another proposed endpoint of chelation therapy that is not yet clinically available is the measurement of the urinary iron:creatinine ratio. This could allow a more reliable endpoint than the change in urine color. The dose of intravenous deferoxamine is 10 to 15 mg/kg/h.

DISPOSITION

Children with peak serum iron levels less than 300 μg/dL approximately 4 hours postingestion and without symptoms of toxicity may be discharged in the care of reliable caretakers. Children with symptoms of toxicity, iron levels greater than 350 μg/dL, or positive deferoxamine challenge tests require hospital admission. Mild overdoses can be managed on the floor. Any child who requires intravenous chelation is admitted to an intensive care unit.

BIBLIOGRAPHY

Burkhart KK, Kulig KW, Hammond KB, et al: The rise in total iron-binding capacity after iron overdose. *Ann Emerg Med* 20:532–535, 1991.

Chyka KA, Butler AY: Laboratory and clinical assessment of acute iron poisoning. *Vet Hum Toxicol* 34:325, 1992.

Curry SC, Bond GR, Raschke R, et al: An ovine model of maternal iron poisoning in pregnancy. *Ann Emerg Med* 19:632–638, 1990.

Klein-Schwartz W, Oderga GM, Gorman RL, et al: Assessment of management guidelines in acute iron ingestion. *Clin Pediatr* 29:316–321, 1990.

Ling LJ, Hornfeldt CS, Winter JP: Absorption of iron after experimental overdose of chewable vitamins. *Am J Emerg Med* 9:24–26, 1991.

Litovitz TL, Manoguerra A: Comparison of pediatric poisoning hazards: An analysis of 3.8 million exposure incidents: A report from the American Association of Poison Control Centers. *Pediatrics* 89:999–1006, 1992.

Morris CC: Pediatric iron poisonings in the United States. *South Med J* 93:352–358, 2000.

Tennebein M, Kopelow ML, DeSai DJ: Myocardial failure secondary to acute iron poisoning. *Vet Hum Toxicol* 28:491, 1986.

Tenenbein M, Kowalski S, Sienko A, et al: Pulmonary toxic effects of continuous desferioxamine administration in acute iron poisoning. *Lancet* 339:699–701, 1992.

Van Ameyde KJ, Tenenbein M: Whole bowel irrigation during pregnancy. *Am J Obstet Gynecol* 160:646–647, 1989.

96

Isoniazid Toxicity

Timothy J. Rittenberry
Michael Green

HIGH-YIELD FACTS

- The clinical triad of refractory seizures, metabolic acidosis unresponsive to bicarbonate therapy, and coma should alert the clinician to possible isoniazid (INH) toxicity.

- The initial signs of INH poisoning typically appear within 30 minutes to $2\frac{1}{2}$ hours of ingestion. Slurred speech, dizziness, ataxia, vomiting, and tachycardia may progress to seizures or coma.

- INH is metabolized in the liver and has a half-life of 2 to 4 hours in slow acetylators and 0.7 to 2 hours in fast acetylators.

- INH ingestion of as little as 20 mg/kg may produce seizures and death may occur at 50 mg/kg.

- The drug of choice for INH overdose is pyridoxine given in gram-for-gram equivalence to the amount of INH ingested. In unknown ingestions 70 mg/kg (up to a total of 5 g) of pyridoxine should be given IV and repeated if seizures or coma persist.

Isoniazid (INH) is an effective drug for the treatment of active tuberculosis (TB), as well as for prophylactic therapy in the face of positive tuberculin skin test reactions. As the incidence of tuberculosis cases and subsequent exposures increase, so does the potential for accidental or intentional ingestion in children. According to the 1999 annual report of the Poison Control Centers Toxic Exposure Surveillance System, there were 412 toxic INH exposures of which 86 were in children under the age of 6, 160 were in children between the ages of 6 and 19, and there was one pediatric fatality. The potential for immediate and severe morbidity or mortality requires a high degree of awareness on the part of the clinician, coupled with prompt, aggressive treatment.

PHARMACOLOGY

The chemical name of isoniazid is isonicotinic acid hydrazide. Its structure is similar to the metabolic cofactors nicotinic acid, nicotinamide adenine dinucleotide (NAD), and pyridoxine. Ninety percent of ingested INH is readily absorbed from the gastrointestinal tract, with peak serum concentrations reached in 1 to 2 hours. It is highly water soluble, with an apparent volume of distribution of 0.6 L/kg. Peak CSF levels reach approximately 10 percent of serum levels and INH is less than 10 percent protein bound, limiting the extent of drug interaction.

The metabolic degradation of INH is complex and occurs primarily via hepatic acetylation. The ability to inactivate INH via acetylation is genetically determined in an autosomal dominant fashion, resulting in two groups of patients: fast acetylators and slow acetylators, the latter being autosomal recessive for the acetylation gene. Fifty to sixty percent of the American population undergo slow acetylation, while this genetic predilection occurs in only 5 to 10 percent of persons of Japanese, Thai, Korean, Chinese, and Innuit lineage. The serum half-life in fast acetylators is 0.7 to 2 hours, and 2 to 4 hours in slow acetylators. Consequently, slow acetylators are more prone to toxicity. Following acetylation, the metabolites are excreted in the urine, with up to 95 percent of a single dose eliminated within 24 hours. The half-life in anephric patients ranges from 1 to 7 hours.

PATHOPHYSIOLOGY

INH is an inhibitor of several cytochrome P450-mediated functions, such as demethylation, oxidation, and hydroxylation. Its inhibition of pyridoxine phosphokinase impairs conversion of pyridoxine to the physiologically active pyridoxal phosphate, a necessary cofactor in the formation of the inhibitory brain peptide gamma aminobutyric acid (GABA). INH also combines with most active forms of pyridoxine, forming inactive INH-pyridoxal hydrazones, which undergo renal excretion. Pyridoxine depletion and reduced GABA levels in the brain lead to the lower seizure threshold seen in acute INH toxicity. INH is structurally similar to NAD, a necessary cofactor in the conversion of lactate to pyruvate in aerobic metabolism. INH blocks this conversion and leads to increased serum lactate levels, augmenting the lactate level and acidosis that is a by-product of seizure activity.

The toxic dose of INH is highly variable. Patients with an underlying seizure disorder may suffer toxicity at doses as low as 10 mg/kg. A case of fatal status epilepticus was reported after an ingestion of only 3 mg/kg in a patient with a known seizure disorder. Ingestion of as little as 20 mg/kg may induce seizures, while as little as 50 mg/kg may cause death. High mortality is associated with doses of 80 to 150 mg/kg.

INH can induce hepatotoxicity. This is more common when rifampin, carbamazepine, or ethanol is coingested. INH may inhibit the metabolism of phenytoin and contribute to toxicity when the two medications are concurrently administered. The coingestion of disulfiram may lead to ataxia and psychosis.

CLINICAL PRESENTATION OF ACUTE TOXICITY

Due to its rapid gastrointestinal absorption, symptoms can occur within 30 minutes of ingestion. Nausea, vomiting, dizziness, ataxia, slurred speech, and tachycardia may be quickly followed by metabolic acidosis, generalized seizures, and coma. Hyperpyrexia, hypotension, hyperglycemia, ketonemia, and ketonuria may also be seen. Suspicion of toxic INH ingestion in the pediatric patient is typically delayed until overt signs are apparent. The clinical triad of seizures, coma, and metabolic acidosis refractory to bicarbonate therapy should alert the emergency physician to the possibility of INH ingestion. INH toxicity should be strongly considered in any child or adolescent that presents with seizures who is undergoing treatment with or has access to INH.

In the acute ingestion, quantitative INH levels are typically unavailable. Any serum INH level of 10 μg/mL, >3.2 μg/mL 2 hours after ingestion, or >0.2 μg/mL after 6 hours should be considered toxic. Treatment of toxicity should never be withheld while awaiting confirmatory serum levels. The laboratory work-up must include evaluation for causes of coma, seizures, or anion gap acidosis.

TREATMENT

Stabilization

In the symptomatic patient with an INH overdose, aggressive supportive care and monitoring is necessary. In the patient presenting with protracted seizure or coma, endotracheal intubation is indicated.

Decontamination

Even in asymptomatic patients, the induction of emesis is not recommended, since seizures may occur abruptly and without warning. Gastric lavage performed within 1 hour of ingestion is useful in achieving gut decontamination, with the contents sent for toxicologic analysis. Activated charcoal and a cathartic such as sorbitol are then administered to further decrease absorption.

Antidotal Therapy

The mainstay of treatment in INH toxicity is pyridoxine. Commercially available in 1 g/10 mL vials, it is mixed in a 5 or 10 percent solution with D_5W. If the INH dose is known, an equal dose of pyridoxine on a gram-for-gram basis is administered over 5 to 10 minutes. If the dose of INH is unknown, pyridoxine is given initially at 70 mg/kg up to a total of 5 g and repeated in 15 minutes for the persistently comatose or convulsing patient. The therapeutic window for pyridoxine is large, and the cumulative dose is arbitrarily limited at 40 g in the adolescent and 20 g in the child. If the parenteral form of pyridoxine is unavailable or in inadequate supply, similar doses of crushed pyridoxine tablets may be given orally as a slurry. Given the prevalence of INH use in tuberculosis treatment and the potential for inadvertent or intentional overdose, a minimum of 10 g of pyridoxine (the upper limit necessary to treat an ingestion of a therapeutic 1-month supply of INH) should be readily available to the ED. The severe acidosis seen in INH overdose may require sodium bicarbonate administration, but in most cases control of seizures with anticonvulsants and pyridoxine and adequate fluid resuscitation will reverse acidemia. Bicarbonate therapy is reserved for severe, persistent acidosis and is guided by frequent reevaluation of arterial pH.

Commonly used anticonvulsants alone may be ineffective in controlling INH-induced seizures. However, there is evidence that benzodiazepines may act synergistically with pyridoxine and have a protective effect. If seizures continue despite appropriate use of pyridoxine and diazepam, short-acting barbiturates or inhaled anesthetics should be considered, in consultation with an anesthesiologist.

Hemodialysis, hemoperfusion, and exchange transfusion have all been described as useful, but are reserved for the most severe, refractory cases or for patients with renal failure.

Disposition

Patients with suspected INH poisoning who remain asymptomatic after 6 hours following ingestion or patients without a seizure disorder who have ingested <20 mg/kg may be discharged from the ED. Symptomatic patients require admission to a monitored bed.

CHRONIC TOXICITY

Chronic INH toxicity is extremely rare in the normal pediatric population and is usually restricted to children receiving active or prophylactic treatment. The appearance of nausea, vomiting, fever, abdominal pain, or pruritus may herald hepatic insult that, if not treated, can progress to fulminant hepatitis. Chronic INH use is associated with optic neuritis, optic atrophy, hepatitis, peripheral neuropathy, a pellagra-like syndrome of dermatitis, diarrhea, and dementia, and a variety of psychological reactions.

During treatment or prophylaxis of tuberculosis with INH, serum transaminase levels are examined periodically to screen for early signs of hepatic toxicity.

BIBLIOGRAPHY

Cash JM, Zawada Jr ET: Isoniazid overdose—successful treatment with pyridoxine and hemodialysis. *West J Med* 155:644–646, 1991.

Ellenhorn MJ, Barceloux DG: Anti-infective drugs, in Ellenhorn MJ, Barceloux DG (eds): *Ellenhorn's Medical Toxicology: Diagnosis and Treatment of Human Poisoning,* 2d ed. Baltimore, Williams & Wilkins, 1997, pp 240–243.

Litovitz TL, Klein-Schwartz W, White S, et al: 1999 Annual report of the American Association of Poison Control Centers toxic exposure surveillance system. *Am J Emerg Med* 8:517–574, 2000.

Osborn HH: Antituberculous agents, in Goldfrank LR, Flomenbaum NE, Lewin NA, et al (eds): *Goldfrank's Toxicologic Emergencies,* 6th ed. Stamford, CT: Appleton & Lange, 1998, pp 727–733.

Parish RA, Brownstein D: Emergency department management of children with acute isoniazid poisoning. *Pediatr Emerg Care* 2:88–90, 1986.

Rittenberry TJ: Antimicrobial agents, in Noji EK, Kelen GD (eds): *Manual of Toxicologic Emergencies.* Chicago: Year Book Medical Publishers, 1989, p 555.

Romero JA, Kuczler FJ: Isoniazid overdose. Recognition and management. *Am Fam Physician* 57:749–752, 1998.

Shah BR, Santucci K, Sinert R, et al: Acute isoniazid neurotoxicity in an urban hospital. *Pediatrics* 95:700–704, 1995.

Shannon MW: Isoniazid, in Haddad LM, Shannon MW, Winchester JF (eds): *Clinical Management of Drug Overdose,* 3d ed. Philadelphia: Saunders, 1998, pp 721–726.

Sullivan EA, Geoffrey P, Weisman R, et al: Isoniazid poisonings in New York City. *J Emerg Med* 16:57–59, 1998.

97

Lead Poisoning

Mark Mycyk
Yona Amatai
Daniel Hryhorczuk

HIGH-YIELD FACTS

- Lead poisoning causes multisystem clinical effects: headache, abdominal pain, constipation, vomiting, clumsiness, irritability, drowsiness.
- Laboratory evaluation may demonstrate anemia, basophilic stippling, elevated EP/ZPP, elevated BLL.
- Management requires identification and removal of the source of exposure.
- Chelation with CaNa$_2$EDTA, BAL, or Succimer is dictated by BLL and severity of symptoms.

The average blood lead level of American children has decreased by more than 80 percent since the 1970s because of early screening initiatives and hazard reduction. In spite of this progress, several long-term studies have shown an association of lead levels once thought to be nontoxic with impaired growth and behavioral and neurocognitive development. In 1991, the Centers for Disease Control and Prevention revised the 1985 blood lead intervention level of 25 μg/dL downward to 10 μg/dL. However, it is estimated that 1.7 million children (or 9 percent of American children) still have some degree of lead poisoning. Lead poisoning affects people of all ages and classes, but the prevalence of lead poisoning remains highest in inner-city underprivileged children.

SOURCES

Ingestion of leaded paint is the most common and clinically relevant source of lead poisoning in children. Most homes built before 1978 were painted with lead-based paint. A small paint chip containing 50 percent lead can produce acute lead poisoning in a toddler. Renovation of old buildings and poorly controlled lead abatement pose a risk for lead poisoning through inhalation and ingestion of contaminated dust and soil. Lead exposure can occur through ingestion of drinking water contaminated by lead in plumbing. Children living in close proximity to stationary air pollution sources such as lead smelters are at risk of lead poisoning. Other potential sources of toxicity include secondary exposure to lead brought home from workplaces, drinking from improperly fired lead-glazed pottery, some folk remedies, bullets lodged in joint spaces, and other unusual sources. The phase-out of leaded gasoline has had a major impact in reducing exposure to lead.

PHARMACOKINETICS/PATHOPHYSIOLOGY

The absorption rate of lead through the gastrointestinal tract in infants and children is about 50 percent. Iron deficiency and dietary calcium deficiency increase the absorption of lead in the gut. Lead dust and fumes can also be absorbed through the respiratory tract. Percutaneous absorption of lead is less than 0.1 percent of the applied quantity. Lead readily crosses the placental barrier, and fetal exposure is cumulative until birth. The distribution of absorbed lead in the body can be modeled using three compartments: blood, soft tissue, and bone. Under steady-state conditions, 99 percent of the lead in blood is attached to red blood cells. Under chronic exposure conditions, the bone serves as a storage organ and can release lead back into the blood and soft tissues. Absorbed lead is eliminated primarily in the urine and bile. In adults the elimination of lead is first-order and triphasic with elimination half-lives of 1 week, 1 month, and 10 to 20 years. Pediatric data are lacking, but some reports indicate that the biologic half-life of blood lead in 2-year-old children is about 10 months.

Lead toxicity results from interaction of lead with sulfydryl and other ligands on enzymes and other macromolecules. The major target organs of lead are the bone marrow, central nervous system, peripheral nervous system, and kidneys. Lead inhibits heme synthesis through inhibition of ALA-dehydratase, coproporphyrin utilization, and ferrochelatase, resulting in the build-up of aminolevulinic acid, coproporphyrins, and free erythrocyte protoporphyrin. Lead also inhibits the enzyme pyrimidine-5′-nucleotidase. Clinically, inhibition of heme synthesis is manifested as anemia. The pathophysiology of lead encephalopathy is demyelinization and precipitation of ribonucleoprotein with resulting cell death, tissue necrosis, vascular damage, and cerebral edema. There is an increase in cerebrospinal fluid protein and pressure. Lead can cause demyelinization of peripheral nerves. The central nervous system is the primary target in the fetus.

CLINICAL MANIFESTATIONS

Symptoms and signs of lead toxicity are often not noticeable or may be subtle and nonspecific. With the improvement in preventing childhood lead poisoning in the U.S., the most likely cause for ED referral in such children is a high blood lead level (BLL) found during a screening program. Since the effects of detrimental lead levels are often clinically silent, emphasis should be placed on periodic screening in preschool children. Symptomatic lead poisoning, on the other hand, is characterized by one or more of the following: decrease in play activity, irritability, drowsiness, anorexia, sporadic vomiting, intermittent abdominal pain, constipation, regression of newly acquired skills (particularly speech), sensorineural hearing loss, clumsiness, and slight attenuation of growth. It is not uncommon for some children to be seen by a health practitioner several times with these nonspecific symptoms before lead poisoning is even considered. Lead toxicity is grossly correlated with BLL (Table 97-1), but is more pronounced in young children and in those with prolonged exposure to lead.

Overt lead encephalopathy may ensue after days or weeks of symptoms and present with ataxia, forceful vomiting, lethargy, or stupor, and can progress to coma and seizures. Though this is seen less commonly than in the past, it represents a medical emergency. It may occur with a BLL >70 μg/dL, but is generally associated with BLLs in excess of 100 μg/dL. Permanent brain damage may result in 70 to 80 percent of children with lead encephalopathy, even with adequate treatment. Peripheral neuropathy is rare under the age of 5, and consists mainly of motor weakness in upper and lower limbs. In the upper limbs, weakness can result in wrist drop.

Lead nephropathy can result in Fanconi's syndrome and acute tubular necrosis, but is rare in children. Mild elevation in liver transaminases may occur. Microcytic anemia frequently coexists with lead poisoning.

Since lead poisoning is so frequent and may present with a variety of signs and symptoms, a high index of suspicion is required. This is particularly true among populations at risk, such as inner city dwellers, African Americans, all children from low socioeconomic classes, and those who live in old houses that have been recently renovated.

The differential diagnosis of lead poisoning includes iron deficiency, behavior and emotional disorders, abdominal colic and constipation, mental retardation, afebrile seizures, subdural hematoma, central nervous system neoplasms, sickle cell anemia, and Fanconi's syndrome. The definitive diagnosis of lead poisoning and assessment of its severity and chronicity depends on laboratory testing. The most important test is a venous BLL (Table 97-1). Periodic screening is important in all children aged 6 months to 2 years who live in houses built before 1960, who live near active lead smelters or other lead-related industries, in those who have siblings with lead poisoning, or with parents who have lead-related occupations or hobbies.

If screening done on capillary blood indicates a high BLL, a confirmatory venous BLL is obtained because of potential lead dust skin contamination in capillary samples. Since 99 percent of the lead in blood is in the red cells, lead assay is done on whole blood collected in tubes with heparin or EDTA. Definition of lead poisoning classes, the toxic effects of lead at various levels, and the recommended actions are outlined in Table 97-1. Elevation in BLL is followed by a rise in the free erythrocyte protoporphyrin (EP) or zinc protoporphyrin (ZPP). Since an elevated EP or ZPP reflects inhibited heme synthesis and affects only newly formed RBCs, this effect occurs at BLL >25 μg/dL and lags behind the initial rise in BLL by 2 to 3 weeks. Thus, low EP or ZPP and high BLL suggest recent acute exposure, whereas elevated EP or ZPP with high BLL suggests chronic exposure.

Radiographic evidence of lead poisoning consists of bands of increased density at the metaphyses of long bones that are best seen in radiographs of the distal femur and proximal tibia and fibula. The popular term "lead lines" is a misnomer, since the increased radiopacity is caused by abnormal calcification from the disrupted metabolism of bone matrix rather than actual deposition of lead in the metaphysis. The formation of lead lines requires a few months of BLLs >45 μg/dL, and their width grossly correlates with the duration of lead poisoning. Radiopaque foreign material seen in the intestine by a flat abdominal film suggests a recent (<48 hours previously) ingestion of lead-containing paint chips. However, a substantial recent ingestion of small particulate lead may not be seen in a flat abdominal film, such as in the case of lead-laden dust in old homes where renovation or deleading has been done by sanding and dry scraping of painted surfaces.

Other essential tests include measurement of hemoglobin and hematocrit, evaluation of the patient's iron

Table 97-1. Class of Child, Toxic Effect, and Recommended Action According to Blood Lead Measurement

Class	Blood Lead Level $(\mu g/dL)^a$	Toxic Effect	Recommended Action
I	0–5	No noticeable effect	
	5–9	Inhibition of ALAD	
IIA	10–14		Rescreen every 3 months; educate parents
IIB	15–19	Inhibition of ferrochelatase	Retest in 2 months, nutritional and educational intervention, environmental investigation
III	20–44	Reduced growth, hearing, nerve conduction, neuropsychological deficits, reduced heme synthetase, increased EP, urine d-ALA	All of the above plus pharmacological treatment: DMSA, penicillamine, or CaNa$_2$EDTA (following a positive lead mobilization test)
IV	45–69	Anemia, abdominal colic, reduced IQ, lead lines in x-ray	Immediate chelation: CaNa$_2$EDTA or DMSA
V	>70	Encephalopathy risk, nephropathy (>100 $\mu g/dL$)	Medical emergency: chelate with BAL plus EDTA, increased ICP precautions

^{a}Conversion factor: 1.0 $\mu g/dL$ = 0.04826 Mmol/L.
Abbreviations: ALAD, aminolevulinic acid dehydratase; EP, erythrocyte protoporphyrin; ALA, aminolevulinic acid.
Source: Adapted from Centers for Disease Control and Prevention: Screening young children for lead poisoning: Guidance for state and local public health officials. US Dept. of Health and Human Services, Public Health Service, *Federal Register,* February 21, 1997.

status, examination of the blood smear for basophilic stippling of the erythrocytes, and a urinalysis to exclude glycosuria or proteinuria. A spinal tap is avoided in children with lead encephalopathy due to the concern for herniation.

A new method for evaluating the total body lead burden by x-ray fluorometry (XRF) of bone lead has been introduced in adults and is being studied in children. With further reduction in radiation, this technique may eventually supersede blood lead screening in populations with low blood levels.

MANAGEMENT

The principles of management in lead poisoning include identification and removal of the lead source, correction of dietary deficiencies that enhance lead absorption, pharmacologic chelation, supportive therapy, and long-term follow-up.

For patients with lead levels between 10 and 20 $\mu g/dL$, treatment consists of environmental management, nutritional evaluation, and repeated screening. In many cases,

this involves removing the child from the home until the source of lead exposure is identified and removed.

Removal of lead-based paint from the home should be done by professional deleaders. Nutritional intervention consists of a review of the child's diet and correction of deficiencies of iron, calcium, and zinc. If there is evidence of recent ingestion of lead paint on an abdominal film, cathartics are given for several days.

For patients with BLLs between 20 and 44 $\mu g/dL$, environmental evaluation and remediation are required. Pharmacologic intervention may be indicated and is accomplished on an outpatient basis if the child is asymptomatic. The decision to treat may be aided by a CaNa$_2$EDTA immobilization test. CaNa$_2$EDTA is administered in a dose of 500 mg/m^2 in 5 percent dextrose infused over 1 hour, or the same dose may be given intramuscularly. The amount of lead is measured in urine collected over the next 8 hours. A ratio of lead excreted (in micrograms) to the CaNa$_2$EDTA dose (in milligrams) greater than 0.6 is considered positive.

Oral dimercaptosuccinic acid (DMSA) is currently the only treatment approved for oral chelation of childhood lead poisoning. DMSA is chemically similar to

British antilewisite (BAL) and produces a lead diuresis comparable to that produced by CaNa$_2$EDTA without depletion of other metals. It is given 30 mg/kg/d in three divided doses for the first 5 days, then 20 mg/kg/d in two divided doses for 14 more days. It has a bad odor and may cause nausea and vomiting, rashes, and transient elevation of liver enzymes. It is commonly used as an outpatient regimen for patients with lead levels higher than 20 μg/dL, only after environmental and nutritional interventions have also been initiated. Sending a child back to the source of lead exposure while actively on chelation therapy may be detrimental.

Outpatient treatment is also possible with oral d-penicillamine (Cuprimine). Currently it is not approved by the FDA for the treatment of lead poisoning, but is approved for other uses and has been successful in children not able to tolerate DMSA therapy. Side effects include leukopenia, thrombocytopenia, transient elevation of liver enzymes, vomiting, and, rarely, nephrotoxicity. It must not be given to patients allergic to penicillin. Iron supplements are avoided in patients treated with d-penicillamine, since they can block its absorption.

Children with asymptomatic lead poisoning and BLLs of 45 to 69 μg/dL are admitted to the hospital for chelation therapy with either CaNa$_2$EDTA or DMSA. Children with *symptomatic* lead poisoning with or without encephalopathy who have BLLs >45 μg/dL, and all patients with BLLs >70 μg/dL are treated with BAL at a dose of 25 mg/kg/d in six divided doses given by deep intramuscular injection. Once the first dose is given and adequate urine flow is established, CaNa$_2$EDTA is added as a continuous intravenous infusion at 50 mg/kg/d in dextrose or saline. When treating a child with encephalopathy, the intramuscular route for CaNa$_2$EDTA with procaine 0.5 percent is preferred to reduce the amount of fluid administered. This combined treatment is given for 5 days, with daily monitoring of blood urea nitrogen (BUN), creatinine, liver enzymes, and electrolytes. Side effects of CaNa$_2$EDTA include fever and transient renal dysfunction reflected in a rise in BUN, proteinuria, and hematuria. BAL may cause nausea and vomiting, transient hypertension, fever, transient elevation in liver enzymes, and hemolysis in G6PD-deficient patients. Iron can form a toxic complex with BAL and is not administered simultaneously.

Lead encephalopathy should always be considered in young children with mental status changes and no other clinical evidence of infection. Lead encephalopathy is treated with fluid restriction, mechanical hyperventilation, and furosemide. Mannitol is avoided because it may leak from the compromised vessels into the cerebellar interstitial spaces and cause a rebound of the intracranial pressure. Dexamethasone may have a salutary effect in improving vascular integrity. Seizures are controlled with diazepam. Patients with lead encephalopathy are best managed in an intensive care unit.

Lead poisoning is most commonly a consequence of chronic exposure, and a rebound elevation of BLL is expected after each course of chelation therapy as lead is mobilized from body stores. Repeat BLLs 2 weeks after the completion of chelation gives a reasonable peak rebound level. Since successful management of lead poisoning demands environmental, nutritional, and pharmacological intervention over a prolonged time course, these children should be followed by clinicians who are familiar with the multiple aspects of this disease and can provide a multidisciplinary team approach. The importance of removing the child from the source of lead exposure cannot be overemphasized.

BIBLIOGRAPHY

American Academy of Pediatrics, Committee on Drugs: Treatment guidelines for lead exposure in children. *Pediatrics* 96:155–160, 1995.

Angle CR: Childhood lead poisoning and its treatment. *Ann Rev Pharmacol Toxicol* 33:409–434, 1993.

Graef J: Lead poisoning, parts 1-3. *Clin Toxicol Rev* 14:8, 1992.

Liebelt EL, Shannon MW: Oral chelators for childhood poisoning. *Pediatr Ann* 23:616–626, 1994.

Manton WI, Angle CR, Stanek SL, et al: Acquisition and retention of lead by young children. *Environ Res* 82:60–80, 2000.

Pirkel JL, Brody DJ, Gunter EW, et al: The decline in blood lead levels in the United States—The National Health and Nutrition Examination Surveys (NHANES). *JAMA* 272: 284–291, 1994.

Rogan J, Dietrich KN, Ware JH, et al: The effect of chelation therapy with succimer on neuropsychological development in children exposed to lead. *N Engl J Med* 344:1421–1426, 2001.

Shannon M, Graef JW: Lead intoxication in infancy. *Pediatrics* 89:87–90, 1992.

98

Methemoglobinemia

Timothy Erickson
Michele Zell-Kanter

HIGH-YIELD FACTS

- Infants are more sensitive than adults to agents producing methemoglobinemia.
- Methemoglobinemia-producing agents include nitrites and nitrates.
- Methemoglobinemia can produce a "saturation gap."
- Methylene blue is the treatment for symptomatic methemoglobinemia.

Methemoglobin is formed when iron in hemoglobin is oxidized from the ferrous (Fe^{++}) state to the ferric (Fe^{+++}) state. Under normal physiologic conditions, methemoglobin is present in red blood cells at concentrations of 1 to 2 percent. The percentage of methemoglobin is the ratio of methemoglobin to hemoglobin. Because the oxygen in methemoglobin is so tightly bound, it is not available for tissue use, thus methemoglobin is not an oxygen-transporting pigment. The oxygen-hemoglobin dissociation curve is also shifted to the left, causing an increase in hemoglobin's affinity for oxygen, resulting in tissue hypoxia.

The methemoglobin formed is normally reduced by nicotinamide adenine dinucleotide (NADH) in the presence of NADH methemoglobin reductase. When methemoglobin levels rise above 1 to 2 percent, a second mechanism for reducing hemoglobin in normal erythrocytes is activated. This involves the formation of reduced nicotinamide adenine dinucleotide phosphate (NADPH). Under normal circumstances, this mechanism is not critical since no endogenous electron acceptor exists. Methylene blue can act as an electron donating cofactor to greatly accelerate this process, and is the basis for its use in treating severe methemoglobinemia.

Two forms of hereditary methemoglobinemia are deficiency in NADH-dependent methemoglobin reductase and hemoglobin M, which is a structural abnormality in hemoglobin. Acquired methemoglobinemia results from exposure to drugs or chemicals that accelerate the oxidation of hemoglobin beyond the cell's capacity to reduce it (Table 98-1). The exact mechanism by which these chemicals induce methemoglobinemia is unclear, but it involves the oxidation of ferrous hemoglobin to ferric methemoglobin by an oxidant drug or chemical.

Infants are more sensitive than adults to methemoglobin-producing agents, such as nitrites, nitrates, or contaminated foods. The infant's high gastric pH allows bacterial proliferation and increased production of nitrites. Also, the fact that hemoglobin reductase is not produced until 4 months of age makes the neonate particularly susceptible. Other populations with increased risk of developing methemoglobinemia include individuals with NADH-dependent methemoglobin reductase, uremic patients, and patients with underlying hypoxic states from disorders such as anemia, coronary artery disease, and underlying lung disease.

Most methemoglobin-producing substances are rapidly absorbed and slowly metabolized and eliminated. Methemoglobin formation may continue for up to 24 hours postexposure. The elimination half-life of methemoglobin averages 15 to 20 hours. Following methylene blue administration, the half-life is reduced to 40 to 90 minutes.

CLINICAL PRESENTATION

The clinical symptoms induced by methemoglobinemia are dependent on the amount of hemoglobin oxidized into methemoglobin. The classic chocolate brown coloration of blood is usually seen at concentrations of 15 to 20 percent. Although pediatric patients may have clinical signs of cyanosis at this level, they are typically asymptomatic. Concentrations ranging from 30 to 40 percent may produce generalized symptoms such as poor feeding, lethargy, and irritability. The older child may complain of fatigue, dizziness, headaches, and weakness. At levels above 55 percent, patients may experience respiratory depression, cardiac arrhythmias, seizures, and coma. Concentrations over 70 percent are potentially lethal.

Methemoglobinemia may be present in any child presenting with a history of exposure to any of the agents listed in Table 98-1 and in patients with central cyanosis that is unresponsive to oxygen therapy. A rapid bedside test that may help confirm a clinical suspicion of methemoglobinemia consists of placing a drop of the patient's blood on a filter paper alongside a normal control sample. If the concentration of methemoglobin exceeds 15

Table 98-1. Causes of Acquired Methemoglobinemia

Acetanilid	Lidocaine	Phenacetin
Aminophenols	Menthol	Phenols
Aniline compounds	Nitrates	Phenylazopyridine
Antimalarials	Nitrites	Phenylhydroxyamine
Benzocaine	Nitrofurans	Prilocaine
Bismuth subnitrite	Nitroglycerin	Pyridine
Chlorates	Nitrous oxide (contaminated)	Quinones
Cobalt preparations	Para-aminosalicylic acid	Resorcinol
Copper sulfate	Paratoluidine	Shoe polish
Dapsone	Pesticides (propham, fenuron)	Sulfonamides
Dinitrobenzene		Sulfones
Fuel additives		Trinitroluene

percent, the patient's blood will appear chocolate brown in color. Another screening test involves bubbling 100 percent oxygen through a sample of the patient's venous blood. Normal hemoglobin should turn bright red, while methemoglobin will be unaltered. In addition, an arterial blood gas may provide a diagnostic clue if a normal PO_2 is noted in the presence of decreased measured oxygen saturation. Finally, methemoglobin concentrations can be directly measured using a spectrophotometric method available to most hospital laboratories.

MANAGEMENT

Initial treatment of any drug- or chemically-induced methemoglobinemia involves supportive care consisting of airway control, supplemental oxygen, and removal of the patient from the source of exposure. Children with altered mental status, dyspnea, cyanosis, or unstable vital signs require immediate intervention. Oral exposure is managed with gastric emptying and charcoal administration. The skin is decontaminated if dermal absorption is suspected. If methemoglobin levels exceed 30 percent or the patient exhibits clinical signs of hypoxia, administration of methylene blue is recommended. The initial dose is 1 to 2 mg/kg of a 1 percent solution given intravenously over 5 minutes. If clinical signs persist, the dose is repeated in 1 hour and every 4 hours thereafter, to a maximum dose of 7 mg/kg. Above this dose, methylene blue can induce hemolysis and act as an oxidizing agent, thereby exacerbating the underlying methemoglobinemic state. During administration of methylene blue, the child's response is monitored by following the oxygen saturation. Patients with methemoglobin levels above 70 percent who are unresponsive to methylene blue are candidates for exchange transfusions or hyperbaric oxygenation.

DISPOSITION

Most authors concur that patients who have methemoglobin concentrations below 20 percent and are asymptomatic require only admission and close observation, as their hemoglobin levels should normalize within 24 to 72 hours. Any symptomatic pediatric patient with levels over 20 percent or those requiring methylene blue administration should be monitored in an intensive care setting.

BIBLIOGRAPHY

Coleman MD, Coleman NA: Drug-induced methemoglobinemia. *Drug Safety* 14:394–405, 1996.

Gilman CS, Veser FH, Randall DR: Methemoglobinemia from topical oral anesthetic. *Acad Emerg Med* 4:1011–1013, 1997.

Hanukoglu A, Danon PN: Endogenous methemoglobinemia associated with diarrheal disease in infancy. *J Pediatr Gastroenterol Nutr* 23:1–7, 1996.

Nakajima W, Ishida A, Arai H: Methemoglobinemia after inhalation of nitric oxide in an infant with pulmonary hypertension. *Lancet* 350:1002–1003, 1997.

Osterhoudt KC: Methemoglobinemia, in Ford M, Delaney K, Ling L, et al (eds): *Clinical Toxicology*. Philadelphia: Saunders, 2001, pp 211–217.

Wright RO, Lewander WT, Woolf AD: Methemoglobin: Etiology, pharmacology, and clinical management. *Ann Emerg Med* 34:646–656, 1999.

99

Mushroom Poisoning

Timothy J. Rittenberry
Jaime Rivas

HIGH-YIELD FACTS

- The timely identification of a mushroom responsible for a toxic ingestion is usually impossible.
- Mushrooms that present with delayed onset of symptoms are associated with greater morbidity and mortality and include the cyclopeptide, gyromitrin, and orellanine groups.
- The time from ingestion to onset of symptoms is an important clue to the mushroom group involved. However, the possibility of co-ingestion of another group makes this potentially unreliable in the acute care setting.
- The key to successful treatment is early gut decontamination, use of activated charcoal, and aggressive, supportive care. There are no mushroom-poisoning antidotes.
- There are no readily available laboratory tests that identify the type of mushroom ingestion.

Mushrooms are responsible for approximately 2 percent of all poisonings. Seventy percent occur in children. In 1999, there were 8996 cases of mushroom poisoning reported to the American Association of Poison Control Centers, of which, 7530 occurred in those <19 years of age and 5738 in children <6 years of age. There were no pediatric fatalities reported. Table 99-1 notes the frequency of ingestion by group. The frequency of toxic mushroom ingestions has remained relatively constant over the last 10 years. Compared to other toxic exposures, the incidence is low and fatalities are uncommon.

IDENTIFICATION

Exact mushroom identification is difficult or unlikely in most cases and is not critical to initiating emergency care. However, identification is possible if any of the specimens is available. Pertinent information includes the habitat in which the mushroom was found, the specific substrate on which it grew, and the season in which the ingestion occurred. Should a sample of the mushroom exist, it is examined for its pertinent anatomic structure, odor, texture, color, and in some cases, taste. A mushroom has seven basic anatomic components: the mycelia, the pileus or cap, the stipe or stem, the lamella or gills, the annulus or ring, and the volva or basal cap. The characteristics of any number of these may be useful in narrowing the identity of the ingestant. By placing a cap with gills down on a white paper in an area devoid of air currents, a characteristic spore print can be obtained as spontaneously released spores settle. The color of the spore print is a key factor in identifying the mushroom. When spores can be obtained, whether from an actual specimen or from a gastric sample, they may be examined microscopically after staining in Melzer's reagent, a solution of chloral hydrate, iodine, and potassium iodide. Spore morphology, coupled with the color reactions to Melzer's solution, assists further in mushroom identification. The key to success remains the inclusion of the local poison control center and an experienced mycologist. Carefully storing specimens in a paper container in a refrigerator until they can be examined by a mycologist is the most promising approach to prompt, accurate identification.

Even when identification is accomplished, toxin concentrations can be highly variable, depending on species, season, locale, and the specific part of the mushroom ingested. Toxicity may also depend on the particular mode of preparation or any accompanying nonfungal ingestion. Few actual antidotes exist. The prognosis of a patient is also dependent on age, with infants and small children most likely to suffer morbidity or mortality, time from ingestion to appearance of symptoms, and rapidity with which aggressive treatment is instituted.

CLASSIFICATION

Categorization based on the predominant toxin, conveniently groups North American mushroom ingestions into eight groups:

- Gastroenteric irritants
- Cyclopeptides
- Gyromitrin group
- Muscarine group

Table 99-1. 1999 Frequency of Mushroom Ingestion by Group

Mushroom Group	Age (years)	
	<6	6–19
Coprine	5	4
Cyclopeptide	13	7
Gastrointestinal irritant	74	40
Hallucinogenic	42	452
Ibotenic Acid	8	12
Monomethyhydrazine	3	2
Muscarine	0	3
Orellanine	1	0

Source: Adapted with permission from Litovitz TL, Klein-Schwartz W, White S, et al: 1999 Annual Report of the American Association of Poison Control Centers Toxic Exposure Surveillance System. *Am J Emerg Med* 2000;18:550, Table 22A.

- Coprine-containing group
- Those containing ibotenic acid and muscimol
- Hallucinogenic indole–containing mushrooms
- Orellanine group

Gastroenteric Irritants

Gastroenteric irritant mushrooms are the most commonly encountered mushroom ingestions in children. The grouping includes a myriad of mushroom species, which have in common the ability to cause marked gastrointestinal irritation without specific end organ injury or CNS manifestations. These include the "little brown mushrooms," found commonly in yards, and chlorophyllium molybdides, probably the most frequently reported toxic mushroom exposure in North America. Although severe hypovolemic shock has been reported with gastroenteric irritants, the course is typically benign in nature. Onset of symptoms in the gastroenteric irritants is rapid and provides a key characteristic to diagnosis. Symptoms begin in 30 minutes to 2 hours, with duration of 3 to 6 hours, and include nausea, vomiting, abdominal pain, and diarrhea, which can be bloody and can contain fecal leukocytes. Although the ingestion is self-limiting and rarely life-threatening, the clinician cannot ignore the possibility of a potentially lethal co-ingestion, since mushrooms of many species may be found at a single site. One should ensure gut decontamination with gastric lavage and early administration of activated charcoal. Further treatment consists of support of fluid and electrolyte status. Symptomatic patients are hospitalized for observation and, possibly, serial charcoal administrations until symptomatology and laboratory data can rule out a potentially lethal co-ingestion.

Cyclopeptides

This group of mushrooms is responsible for most North American deaths. It includes various members of the *Amanita, Lepiota,* and *Galerina* genera containing amatoxins, which cause severe hepatorenal dysfunction and gastritis. *Amanita phalloides,* known as "the death cap," is responsible for >50 percent of all serious mushroom poisonings, with several other *Amanita spp,* such as *A. virosa* ("destroying angel"), *A. vernal,* and *A. ocreata* also involved.

These mushrooms have in common the production of large amounts of cyclopeptide amatoxins, the most toxic of which is alpha-amanitin, capable of causing death in doses of 0.1 mg/kg, an amount which may be ingested in a single pileus. Toxicity is mediated by the amatoxin's ability to inhibit RNA polymerase II, thereby affecting RNA and DNA transcription and severely hampering protein production. Cells that display high rates of replication and protein synthesis, such as the liver, kidney, and gastrointestinal epithelium, are most vulnerable to amatoxin exposure. Probably due to the enterohepatic circulation of amatoxins, the liver is most profoundly affected.

Presentation, Diagnosis, and Treatment

The clinical presentation of ingestion of the cyclopeptide group of mushrooms occurs in four stages.

- The initial latent phase is characterized by a 6- to 12-hour asymptomatic period, during which time protein synthesis is being disrupted.
- A gastroenteritis-like phase follows, as phalloidin-induced nausea, vomiting, bloody diarrhea, and abdominal pain predominate. This phase may last up to 24 hours.
- The following latent phase is marked by an apparent remission of 6 to 24 hours, as overt symptomatology is absent but hepatocellular damage continues.
- The final hepatorenal phase follows, within 36 to 72 hours of ingestion, during which jaundice, hypoglycemia, confusion, coagulopathy, and hepatorenal failure develop.

The diagnosis of cyclopeptide-group ingestion relies on a high level of clinical suspicion supported largely by the characteristic symptom profile rather than by any available laboratory data. A delay in the development of gastrointestinal symptoms after mushroom ingestion is an ominous finding. In most cases, an actual sample of the ingested mushroom will be unavailable for identification. Although radioimmune assay and thin layer chromatographic analyses are available for identifying small amounts of alpha-amanitin, the typical lack of timely access to such methodology reduces them to clinical irrelevance, and the clinician must act presumptively. Even in the face of a gastroenteritis-like symptom profile immediately following ingestion, the prudent approach assumes the possibility of a mixed ingestion, with early symptoms masking the coingestion of an amatoxin-containing mushroom. Very early on, laboratory studies are normal. The severe gastroenteritis phase may cause electrolyte abnormalities, and the progressing subclinical hepatic injury will give eventual rise to elevated liver function tests. With increasing time, a rising serum ammonia level and deteriorating coagulation profile are harbingers of fulminant hepatic failure.

The key to treatment is early gut decontamination, but the typical latent phase preceding symptoms will often delay presentation and preclude effective removal of the toxin. The immediate home use of ipecac in the pediatric patient is important in all suspected mushroom ingestions and concerned parents who make immediate telephone contact are advised to give the appropriate dose of ipecac, followed by immediate medical evaluation. Gastric lavage is employed with the aspirate saved for possible use in identification. Activated charcoal is administered, with or without a cathartic, depending on the level of gastroenteric disturbance. Repeated doses of activated charcoal and duodenal drainage may be useful during the first 24 to 72 hours to enhance elimination and interrupt enterohepatic circulation of the amatoxins, thus ameliorating liver damage. Supportive care to maintain fluid and electrolyte balance is appropriate, as is the supportive treatment of any developing hepatic and renal insufficiency. Dialysis is only of use in the face of acute renal failure. Early forced diuresis, hemodialysis, hemofiltration, and plasmaphoresis have no clinical evidence or pharmacokinetic data to support their routine use.

Although several antidotes have been proposed for poisoning with the cyclopeptide group of mushrooms, there is no available agent recognized as clearly efficacious. The use of thiotic acid (a coenzyme of the Krebs cycle), penicillin G, silibinin (an extract of milk thistle), steroids, cimetidine, and kutkin (extracted from the root of *Picrorhiza kurroa*) have been reported useful in case studies and in animal models. However, there is no compelling data that any one of these agents can be relied on as an antidote and their use remains controversial.

Severe toxicity may require liver transplantation. The fatality rate in one case series was almost 50 percent for children <10 years of age, while age >10 was associated with 16 percent mortality.

Indole-Containing Mushrooms

Psilocybe semilanceata, Psilocybe coprophila, and *Paneolus* are the most commonly ingested mushrooms in this group, which contain psychoactive indoles that are similar to lysergic acid (LSD). Their resemblance to neurotransmitters leads to their characteristic CNS toxicity. These psilocybin/psilocin–containing mushrooms are sought out for recreational use and rarely cause direct toxicity in adults but may result in traumatic injury during intoxication. However, when ingested by children, more severe symptoms can result.

Presenting symptoms may include labile mood change, muscle weakness, panic, and hallucinosis. Laboratory findings are not useful in identification of indole-containing hallucinogenic mushroom ingestions. Although indoles can be identified by sophisticated techniques, these tests are not clinically useful.

Treatment consists of gut decontamination and supportive care. Hospitalization for observation in a low-stimulus environment, with repeated doses of activated charcoal, is appropriate. The severe complications of hyperpyrexia, seizures, and coma are treated with cooling, anticonvulsants, and supportive care.

Monomethylhydrazine Group

Gyromitrin is a toxic hydrazone, which is responsible for most of the effects of this group. It is a hemolysin, neurotoxin, and hepatotoxin that inhibits pyridoxal phosphate, requiring reactions in a manner similar to isoniazid and is toxic due to action at the level of gammaaminobutyric acid synthesis in the central nervous system. The mechanisms resulting in its renal and hepatic effects are unclear. *Gyromitrin esculenta* is the most likely source of this toxic mushroom ingestion. This mushroom was once a choice edible in Central Europe, where the heat labile *Gyromitrin* was rendered harmless by boiling prior to ingestion. The ingestion of this group by children is considered a serious toxic ingestion.

In severe cases, methemoglobinemia, hemolysis with hemoglobinuria, confusion, lethargy, seizures, acidosis, and hypoglycemia may develop. Laboratory findings are nonspecific. As with other fungal toxins, *Gyrometrin* can be identified by thin layer chromatography, which is typically not clinically available. Baseline laboratory studies, including complete blood count, electrolytes, renal functions, glucose, liver functions, urinalysis, and methemoglobin, are useful.

As in all mushroom ingestions, treatment is elimination and supportive care. Gastric lavage may be useful with an immediate presentation, but this scenario is unlikely in light of the typical 6- to 12-hour delay in onset of symptoms. Ipecac-induced emesis is potentially dangerous in light of an increased likelihood of seizures. Activated charcoal is indicated, and the clinical similarity to cyclopeptide ingestion suggests that repeated administration of activated charcoal and duodenal aspiration for the first 24 to 72 hours may be useful. Seizures are treated with pyridoxine in a manner similar to isoniazid toxicity. Pyridoxine is administered parenterally at an initial dose of 25 mg/kg, increasing to a maximum dose of 300 mg/kg or until seizures resolve. Anticonvulsants are indicated if seizure activity continues. Severe hypoglycemia, fluid loss, and electrolyte imbalance are the most likely cause of morbidity and are monitored and treated appropriately. Mortality approaches 10 percent in those patients developing symptoms.

Muscarine

Muscarine is found in the *Clitocybe, Inocybe,* and *Amanita* genera. Although *Amanita muscaria* has trace amounts of muscarine present, its toxicity is not due to this agent. Ingestion of mushrooms, such as *Clitocybe dealbata* or *Inocybe fastigiata,* results in a muscarine-induced cholingeric crisis.

Symptoms occur rapidly, usually within 15 to 60 minutes, and are those expected of cholinergic stimulation. Salivation, lacrimation, urinary frequency, increased gastroenteric motility, diarrhea, diaphoresis, miosis, blurred vision, bronchospasm, bronchorrhea, bradycardia, and even hypotension may occur. Symptoms are typically mild and short-lived, lasting up to 6 hours.

Treatment consists of gut decontamination using gastric lavage followed by activated charcoal. A cathartic is not necessary in the presence of increased gastroenteric motility. Cardiac monitoring is necessary due to the potential for bradyarrhythmias. The use of atropine in the face of severe cholinergic crisis is indicated with an initial dose of 0.01 mg/kg IV. The total dose of atropine is based on the drying of secretions, rather than pupillary dilation. Symptoms typically subside within 24 hours.

Coprine Group

The common alcohol inky *(Coprinus atramentarius)* is an edible mushroom without toxic effects when eaten in the absence of ethanol. However, when ethanol is co-ingested, a disulfiram-like reaction may occur. The biochemical events involved are not identical to that seen with Antabuse, but the clinical picture is similar. This is an unlikely symptomatic mushroom toxicity in very young children, who are unlikely to ingest alcohol, but is increasingly possible in adolescents. The prolonged effects of coprine may hinder any connection being made between mushroom and ethanol ingestion. Delayed or reingestion of ethanol for up to 48 hours may produce toxicity.

Patients presenting acutely after coprine exposure and ethanol use exhibit facial flushing, paresthesias, diaphoresis, headache, nausea, and vomiting. Severe reactions can result in hypotension or acidosis. Arrhythmias have been reported in adults. Gastric lavage may be useful in the event that mushroom ingestion was recent, or ethanol ingestion is recent and excessive. It is more likely that significant time will have elapsed since ingesting the alcohol inky, while violent vomiting immediate to the ethanol co-ingestion will have removed excess quantities of alcohol, making attempts at gastric lavage unnecessary. Activated charcoal is indicated only if toxicity from other mushrooms is entertained, since this disulfiram-like reaction will resolve spontaneously in a few hours as serum alcohol levels decrease. Severe reactions may require aggressive fluid resuscitation with normal saline, and supportive care to maintain fluid and electrolyte status is the cornerstone of treatment. Phenothiazine antiemetics may exacerbate hypotension and are avoided.

Ibotenic Acid and Muscimol

Amanita muscaria and *Amanita pantherina* contain the psychoactive isoxazoles, ibotenic acid and muscimol, which are responsible for the toxicologic profile of this ingestant. In spite of its name, *Amanita muscaria* carries insignificant amounts of muscarine and does not result in a syndrome of cholinergic excess. The pathway by which this predominantly central nervous system intoxication occurs is probably due to the isoxazoles activity at χ-aminobutyric acid (GABA) receptors.

Within 30 minutes to 2 hours of ingestion of mushrooms of this group, symptoms resembling ethanol intoxication occur, with ataxia, confusion, irritability, bizarre behavior, euphoria, and hyperkinetic activity.

Slurring of speech is common. With more severe ingestion, symptoms may progress to varying degrees of obtundation, hallucinosis, myoclonic jerking, or seizures. Vomiting is rare.

Supportive care is the mainstay of treatment. Gastric lavage followed by activated charcoal is followed by observation. The use of atropine is not indicated. Seizure activity is treated with anticonvulsants as necessary. Symptoms typically resolve in 4 to 6 hours.

Orellenine

Ingestion of *Cortinarius orellanus* causes tubulointerstitial nephritis, which can lead to acute or chronic renal failure. Although this is of greater importance in Europe and Japan, North American ingestions do occur. Delayed symptoms of anorexia, nausea, abdominal discomfort, headache, myalgia, polyuria, and thirst, may follow ingestion by 24 hours to several days. By the time of presentation, orellanine is not detectable in the blood or urine, and no laboratory tests, beyond those to establish baselines, are helpful. Toxicity from this group can be highly variable, probably due to differing individual susceptibility. Due to the prolonged latency period, the use of gut decontaminations and activated charcoal is of no benefit. Supportive care should center on fluid management and monitoring renal function. Renal function recovers in the majority of cases. Progressing renal failure may require the use of hemodialysis.

CONCLUSION

The incidence of mushroom ingestion is low and, except in the case of cyclopeptide ingestion, fatalities are uncommon. However, due to the inability to confidently identify the mushroom or mushrooms involved in a pediatric ingestion, an aggressive approach is prudent, hinging on gut decontamination, activated charcoal administration, observation, and compulsory supportive care. The assumption that a cyclopeptide mushroom may have been co-ingested warrants repeated activated charcoal doses every 4 hours until the clinical profile and laboratory data can comfortably rule out this possibility.

BIBLIOGRAPHY

Benjamin DR: Mushroom poisoning in infants and children: The *Amanita pantherina/muscaria* group. *Clin Toxicol* 1992;30:13–22.

Floersheim GL: Treatment of amatoxin mushroom poisoning—myths and advances in therapy. *Med Toxicol* 1987;2:1–9.

Gailer GW, Weisenberb E, Brositus TA: Mushroom poisoning: The role of orthotopic liver transplantation. *J Clin Gastroenterol* 1992;15:229–232.

Hanrahan JP, Gordon MA: Mushroom poisoning: Case reports and review of therapy. *JAMA* 1984;25:1057–1061.

Lampe KF, McCann MA: Differential diagnosis of poisoning by North American mushrooms with particular emphasis on amanita phalloides-like intoxication. *Ann Emerg Med* 1987;16:956–962.

Lehmann PF, Khuzan U. Mushroom poisoning by chlorophyllum molybdites in the Midwestern United States-cases and review of the syndrome. *Mycopatholgia* 1992;118:1–13.

Litovitz TL, Klein-Schwartz W, White S, et al. 1999 annual report of the American Association of Poison Control Centers toxic exposure surveillance system. *Am J Emerg Med* 2000;18:17–574.

Michelot D: Poisoning by *Coprinus atramentarius*. *Nat Tox* 1992;1:73–80.

Schneider SM: Mushrooms, in Ford MD, Delaney KA, Ling LJ, Erickson T (eds): *Clinical Toxicology*. Philadelphia: Saunders, 2001, pp 899–908.

Stenklyft PH, Augerstein LW: Chlorphyllum molybdites-severe mushroom poisoning in a child. *Clin Toxicol* 1990;28: 159–168.

100

Neuroleptics

Timothy Erickson

HIGH-YIELD FACTS

- Acute dystonia is an unpredictable side effect of neuroleptics.
- Overdoses of neuroleptics do not commonly cause serious cardiac dysrhythmias or severe respiratory depression.
- Phenothiazine levels correlate poorly with clinical effects.
- Neuroleptic malignant syndrome is characterized by hyperthermia, skeletal muscle rigidity, and altered mental status.

Neuroleptics or phenothiazines are a group of major tranquilizers or antipsychotic drugs that are therapeutically designed to treat schizophrenia and other psychiatric disorders. According to updated data from the American Association of Poison Control Centers (AAPCC), in 1999 there were 2017 exposures to phenothiazine/neuroleptic agents in individuals less than 20 years of age, with one reported death.

PHARMACOLOGY

There are five classes of neuroleptics, all of which have the same basic three-ringed structure. Although all classes exhibit similar therapeutic and adverse effects, modification of the basic structure results in variable degrees of toxicity.

PATHOPHYSIOLOGY

Neuroleptics act by blocking dopaminergic, alpha-adrenergic, muscarinic, histaminic, and serotonergic neuroreceptors. Blockade of the dopamine receptors results in the desired behavior modification, but also produces extrapyramidal side effects, such as dystonic reactions. Alpha-adrenergic blockade produces peripheral vasodilation and orthostatic hypotension. Muscarinic blockade results in anticholinergic properties such as sedation,

tachycardia, flushed or dry skin, urinary retention, and delayed GI motility. Neuroleptics also cause a membrane depressant action or quinidine-like effect that alters myocardial contractility, and can result in conduction defects. Although the mechanism of toxicity in neuroleptics resembles that of tricyclic antidepressants, serious cardiac dysrhythmias, refractory hypotension, respiratory depression, and seizures are uncommon.

DYSTONIC REACTIONS

Clinical Presentation

Acute dystonia is an unpredictable side effect of neuroleptics, and it occurs in approximately 10 percent of overdoses. It can also occur as an idiosyncratic reaction following a single therapeutic dose of a neuroleptic. Dystonic reactions are characterized by slurred speech, dysarthria, confusion, dysphagia, hypertonicity, tremors, and muscle restlessness. Other reactions or dyskinesias include oculogyric crisis (upward gaze), torticollis (neck twisting), facial grimacing, opisthotonos (scoliosis), and tortipelvic gait disturbances. Symptoms usually begin within the first 5 to 30 hours after ingestion. Dystonic reactions are relatively common in infants and adolescents. Of the neuroleptics, prochlorperazine most often causes acute dystonia. In recent years several new neuroleptic agents have become very popular, including clozapine, olanzapine, risperidone, and quetiapine. Several other agents are currently under investigation, including sertindole, ziprasidone, and remoxipine. This group of agents produces a lower incidence of extrapyramidal side effects than previous agents.

Management

If a child exhibits signs of acute muscular dystonia, intravenous diphenhydramine (2 mg/kg up to 50 mg over several minutes) is rapidly administered. Alternatively, the patient can be given benztropine intramuscularly in a dose of 0.05 to 0.1 mg/kg (up to 2 mg). Improvement usually occurs within 15 minutes. Doses exceeding 8 mg over a 24-hour period can result in severe anticholinergic symptoms.

ACUTE OVERDOSE

Clinical Presentation

Following an acute overdose of neuroleptics, mild CNS depression is common, usually occurring within 1 to 2 hours of the ingestion. Children are more susceptible to these sedative effects than adults. In the overdose setting, respiratory depression can occur, but rarely requires aggressive airway management. Phenothiazines tend to lower a patient's seizure threshold, though the actual incidence of seizures in acute overdose is low.

Like the tricyclic antidepressants, poisoning from neuroleptics can result in orthostatic hypotension and cardiac dysrhythmias, particularly with the piperidine and aliphatic phenothiazines. Sinus tachycardia is the most common dysrhythmia, but QT interval prolongation can sometimes be noted on electrocardiogram. Other clinical effects in the acute overdose setting include pupillary miosis, which in one study was observed in 72 percent of children with high-grade coma following ingestion of a phenothiazine. Due to the anticholinergic properties of the neuroleptics, the patient may also exhibit decreased GI motility, urinary retention, hyperthermia, and dry or flushed skin. Hypothermia can be noted but is rarely clinically significant. Therapeutic phenothiazine use has been associated with sleep apnea and sudden death in infants.

Laboratory Tests

Although serum phenothiazine levels can be obtained to confirm ingestion, levels correlate poorly with clinical effects, making their utility negligible. Baseline laboratory tests include complete blood count, electrolytes, renal function, and glucose. Urine should be collected for myoglobin, particularly if the patient is hyperthermic. The urine can be qualitatively tested with a 10 percent ferric chloride solution. Ten to fifteen drops of ferric chloride will change the urine to a deep burgundy color if phenothiazines are present. Due to potential neuroleptic-induced cardiotoxicity, an electrocardiogram is indicated.

Management

Initial management of an acute neuroleptic overdose includes stabilizing the airway and circulation. If the patient remains hypotensive despite adequate amounts of IV fluid, a vasopressor with alpha-agonist activity, such as norepinephrine, may be considered. Vasopressors with both alpha and beta agonist activity, such as dopamine, may actually exacerbate hypotension because of unopposed beta-adrenergic stimulation, during which alpha-receptors are being blocked by the neuroleptic. Because of the potential cardiotoxicity of phenothiazines, patients require close cardiac monitoring. Since pheno-

thiazine toxicity classically demonstrates central nervous system depression and pupillary miosis, adequate doses of naloxone are indicated to treat potential coexistent opioid toxicity. Gastric lavage may be considered if the patient presents within 1 hour of ingestion. Syrup of ipecac is relatively contraindicated in the setting of phenothiazine overdose since the patient has potential for CNS and respiratory depression. Activated charcoal may be administered following a recent ingestion. No specific antidote exists for acute neuroleptic poisoning and hemodialysis is not efficacious. Most children presenting after acute neuroleptic toxicity do well with supportive care alone.

NEUROLEPTIC MALIGNANT SYNDROME

Clinical Presentation

Less than 1 percent of patients exhibit the life-threatening extrapyramidal dysfunction known as the neuroleptic malignant syndrome, characterized by skeletal muscle rigidity, coma, and severe hyperthermia following the use of phenothiazines or haloperidol. This syndrome can occur following acute overdose, chronic therapy, or idiosyncratically following a single dose of a neuroleptic.

Management

The neuroleptic syndrome results in a high mortality rate and is treated aggressively with rapid cooling and administration of dantrolene at 0.8 to 3.0 mg/kg intravenously every 6 hours, up to 10 mg/kg/d. Dantrolene acts peripherally by treating skeletal muscle rigidity. Oral bromocriptine (a direct dopamine agonist) has been successfully used alone and in conjunction with dantrolene to successfully treat adult patients with neuroleptic malignant syndrome.

DISPOSITION

Any symptomatic child presenting with acute neuroleptic poisoning is admitted and observed for CNS and respiratory depression as well as for cardiotoxicity or thermoregulatory problems. Patients with minor, asymptomatic ingestions can be observed for up to 6 hours. If the patient is discharged, caretakers should be advised to watch for signs of delayed dystonic reactions. If the child has been treated successfully for acute dystonia with either diphenhydramine or benztropine, a 2- to 3-day course of oral diphenhydramine is indicated, since many of the neuroleptics have a long duration of action.

BIBLIOGRAPHY

Buckley P, Hutchinson M: Neuroleptic malignant syndrome. *J Neurol Neurosurg Psychiatry* 58:271–273, 1995.

Deroos FJ: Neuroleptics, in Ford M, Delaney K, Ling L, et al (eds): *Clinical Toxicology.* Philadelphia: Saunders, 2001, pp 539–545.

Gupta S, Mosnik D, Black DW, et al: Tardive dyskinesia: Review of treatments past, present, and future. *Ann Clin Psychiatry* 11:257–265, 1999.

Kane JM: Newer antipsychotic drugs. *Drugs* 46:585–593, 1993.

Litovitz TL, Klein-Schwartz W, White S: Annual report of the American Association of Poison Control Centers toxic exposure surveillance system. *Am J Emerg Med* 18(5):517–574, 2000.

Owens DGC: Adverse effects of antipsychotic agents: Do newer agents offer advantages? *Drugs* 51:895–930, 1996.

Raja M: Managing antipsychotic induced acute and tardive dystonia. *Drug Safety* 19:57–72, 1998.

Van Harten PN, Hoek H, Kahn RS: Acute dystonia induced by drug treatment. *BMJ* 319:623–626, 1999.

101

Nonsteroidal Anti-inflammatory Drugs

Michele Zell-Kanter

HIGH-YIELD FACTS

- In the overdose setting, NSAIDs are relatively devoid of toxicity.

- Typically, patients who ingest NSAIDs exhibit only central nervous system (CNS) or gastrointestinal (GI) toxicity.

- An exception to this is phenylbutazone, which has been associated with significant toxicity and death, especially in children.

- Long-term use of NSAIDs is associated with nephrotoxicity, including acute tubular necrosis, acute interstitial nephritis, and acute renal failure. Renal toxicity is not associated with acute overdose.

- Infrequently, overdose of NSAIDs has been associated with an anion-gap acidosis. For patients with severe clinical symptoms, an arterial blood gas is indicated.

- After the patient is stabilized, gastric decontamination is indicated. In a patient presenting within 1 hour of ingestion, syrup of ipecac or gastric lavage can be used in a patient with a stable airway and who has not ingested an NSAID known to cause seizures.

- Activated charcoal is administered after ipecac-induced emesis ceases, gastric lavage is terminated, or for the patient who presents more than 1 hour after ingestion.

There are many drugs in use today that are categorized as nonsteroidal anti-inflammatory agents (NSAIDs). These drugs function largely by inhibiting cyclooxygenase, the enzyme needed to convert arachidonic acid to prostaglandin. In the overdose setting, NSAIDs are relatively devoid of toxicity. The 1999 Annual Report of the American Association of Poison Control Centers

listed three deaths secondary to ibuprofen, although there were more than 54,000 ingestions. There were 18,000 ingestions of other NSAIDs, resulting in three deaths.

CLINICAL PRESENTATION

Typically, patients who ingest NSAIDs exhibit only central nervous system (CNS) or gastrointestinal (GI) toxicity. An exception to this is the pyrazolone compound phenylbutazone, which has been associated with significant toxicity and death, especially in children. In an overdose setting, patients who ingest phenylbutazone must be managed very aggressively.

Common symptoms of CNS toxicity can include drowsiness, dizziness, and lethargy. The mefenamic acid compound, Ponstel, has a propensity to cause seizures. Other NSAIDs associated with seizures include piroxicam, naproxen, and ketoprofen. Headache is more likely to occur after ingestion of indomethacin than other NSAIDs.

Symptoms of gastrointestinal toxicity include nausea, vomiting, and epigastric pain, all of which can occur at therapeutic doses. The gastritis associated with NSAIDs probably occurs secondary to inhibition of prostaglandin synthesis.

Cardiovascular complications of NSAID overdose are generally limited to tachycardia and hypotension, usually secondary to volume depletion. Rare respiratory complications are hyperventilation and apnea.

Long-term use of NSAIDs is associated with nephrotoxicity, including acute tubular necrosis, acute interstitial nephritis, and acute renal failure. Renal papillary necrosis has been reported in children being treated with NSAIDs for juvenile rheumatoid arthritis. Renal toxicity is not associated with acute overdose.

Other long-term complications of NSAID use include hepatocellular injury and cholestatic jaundice.

LABORATORY STUDIES

Assay procedures for measuring plasma ibuprofen levels are readily available. Although the assay can verify the presence of ibuprofen, at this time, there is a poor correlation between the absolute level and toxicity. Therefore, the clinical utility of an ibuprofen level is negligible.

In symptomatic patients, indicated laboratory tests include a complete blood count, electrolytes, glucose, creatinine, and coagulation profile. A toxicology screen can be useful.

Infrequently, overdose of NSAIDs has been associated with an anion-gap acidosis. For patients with severe clinical symptoms, an arterial blood gas is indicated.

MANAGEMENT

After the patient is stabilized, gastric decontamination is indicated. In a patient presenting within 1 hour of ingestion, syrup of ipecac or gastric lavage in a patient with a stable airway can be used. It is contraindicated in ingestions of NSAIDs known to cause seizures.

Activated charcoal is administered after ipecac-induced emesis ceases or gastric lavage is terminated, or for the patient who presents more than 1 hour after ingestion. At the present time, there are no data to support multiple doses of charcoal.

The high protein binding of NSAIDs renders extracorporeal methods of elimination ineffective. Likewise, forced diuresis is of no value.

BIBLIOGRAPHY

Hall AH, Smolinske SC, Conrad FL, et al: Ibuprofen overdose: 126 cases. *Ann Emerg Med* 15:1308, 1986.

Hall AH, Smolinske SC, Stover B, et al: Ibuprofen overdose in adults. *Clin Toxicol* 30:23, 1992.

Litovitz TL, Klein-Schwartz W, White S, et al: 1999 annual report of the American Association of Poison Control Centers toxic exposure surveillance system. *Am J Emerg Med* 18:517, 2000.

Martinez R, Smith DW, Frankel LR: Severe metabolic acidosis after acute naproxen sodium ingestion. *Ann Emerg Med* 18:1102, 1989.

McElwee NE, Veltri JC, Bradford DC, et al: A prospective, population-based study of acute ibuprofen overdose: Complications are rare and routine serum levels are not warranted. *Ann Emerg Med* 19:657, 1990.

Skeith KJ, Wright M, Davis P: Differences in NSAID tolerability profiles: Fact or fiction? *Drug Safety* 10:183, 1994.

Smolinske SC, Hall AH, Vandenburg SA, et al: Toxic effects of nonsteroidal antiinflammatory drugs in overdose. *Drug Safety* 5:252, 1990.

Vane JR, Botting RM: Anti-inflammatory drugs and their mechanism of action. *Inflamm Res* 1998; 47(Suppl 2): S78.

102

Opioids

Timothy Erickson

HIGH-YIELD FACTS

- The classical triad of central nervous system depression, respiratory depression, and pinpoint pupils characterizes opioid toxicity.
- Naloxone is a pure opioid antagonist.
- Some oral opioids—methadone, codeine, and diphenoxylate-atropine—can have delayed effects.
- Longer-acting opioid antagonists such as nalmefene may be effective in children.

Opioids are naturally occurring or synthetic drugs that have activity similar to that of opium or morphine. They are used clinically for analgesia and anesthesia and are widely available for illicit oral, inhalational, or parenteral abuse. According to the 1999 annual report of the American Association of Poison Control Centers, in children less than 20 years of age there were 770 exposures to codeine, 133 to meperidine, 187 to methadone, 271 to morphine, 298 to oxycodone, 32 to pentazocine, and 100 to propoxyphene. There were seven opioid-related deaths.

PHARMACOKINETICS/PATHOPHYSIOLOGY

Although most opioids have an onset of action within 1 hour, many of the oral agents, such as methadone, codeine, and diphenoxylate-atropine will demonstrate a delayed effect of up to 4 to 12 hours and half-lives as long as 24 hours. The toxic effects are mediated through the mu and kappa opioid receptors located in the central and peripheral nervous systems. Some specific agents such as propoxyphene can also cause cardiotoxicity and seizures.

CLINICAL PRESENTATION

Opioid poisoning classically presents with altered level of consciousness. The classic triad of acute toxicity consists of CNS depression, respiratory depression, and pupillary constriction (miosis). CNS depression ranges from mild sedation to stupor and coma. In massive overdoses, the respiratory toxicity can also cause noncardiogenic pulmonary edema. Patients are typically hypotensive, hypothermic, bradycardic, and hyporeflexic, with diminished bowel sounds. Less common effects of opioid toxicity include generalized seizure activity following overdose of propoxyphene, meperidine, or pentazocine. Neonates receiving continuous intravenous morphine can also have seizures following opioid withdrawal. Propoxyphene can cause cardiotoxicity via conduction system dysfunction.

MANAGEMENT

The primary management of opioid poisoning includes urgent stabilization of the airway and administration of the pure opioid antagonist naloxone. If adequate doses of the antidote are given in a timely fashion, intubation can be avoided, since the onset of action for naloxone is usually within 1 minute after administration. In addition to intravenous administration, naloxone can be given via the endotracheal tube subcutaneously, or intralingually with a comparably rapid onset of action. In the overdose setting, the dose of naloxone is 0.1 mg/kg in children aged from birth to 5 years or 20 kg body weight, at which time a 2-mg dose is given. If there is no response, repeat doses of 2 mg are given to older children and adolescents, up to a maximum of 10 mg. If no response occurs consider other causes for CNS and respiratory depression. Even with large doses of naloxone, minimal to no adverse side effects have been noted. An exception to this rule is in the chronic opioid abusing adolescent or dependent neonate, in whom a withdrawal syndrome can be precipitated. In this setting, the patient receives supportive care, since opioid withdrawal is not a life-threatening situation. Due to the short half-life of naloxone (20 to 30 minutes) repeated doses may be indicated, particularly when dealing with opioids with longer duration of action, such as codeine, methadone, and diphenoxylate-atropine. If repeat doses of naloxone are required, a continuous intravenous infusion of naloxone is instituted. The drip rate can be calculated by using two-thirds of the initial dose necessary to reverse the patient's respiratory depression and administering that amount hourly by continuous infusion. However, this infusion rate may vary depending on the specific opioid, and the patient's level of tolerance. The new longer-acting antagonist nalmefene may be used in the future, although studies of this agent in the pediatric population are limited.

Gastric lavage can be performed if the child presents within 1 hour after an oral ingestion. The airway must be protected since there is potential for CNS and respiratory depression. Additionally, an initial dose of activated charcoal with cathartic is advised following any oral ingestion.

DISPOSITION

Any pediatric patient presenting with CNS and respiratory depression from opioid poisoning that is responsive to naloxone is admitted for observation, since most of the opioids demonstrate longer duration of action than naloxone and require repetitive administration or continuous naloxone infusion.

BIBLIOGRAPHY

Chamberlain JM, Klein BL: A comprehensive review of naloxone for the emergency physician. *Am J Emerg Med* 12:650–660, 1994.

Chumpa A: Nalmefene hydrochloride. *Pediatr Emerg Care* 15:141–143, 1999.

Glick C, Evans OB, Parks BR: Muscle rigidity due to fentanyl infusion in the pediatric patient. *South Med J* 889:1119–1120, 1996.

Kaplan JL, Mark JA, Calabro JJ, et al: Double-blind, randomized study of nalmefene and naloxone in emergency department suspected narcotic overdose. *Ann Emerg Med* 34:42–50, 1999.

Kleinschmidt KC, Wainscott M, Ford M: Opioids, in Ford M, Delaney KA, Ling L, et al (eds): *Clinical Toxicology.* Philadelphia: Saunders, 2001, pp 627–639.

Litovitz TL, Schwartz-Klein W, White S, et al: 1999 Annual report of the AAPCC toxic exposure surveillance system. *Am J Emerg Med* 18:517–574, 2000.

McCarron MM, Challoner RR, Thompson GA: Diphenoxylate-atropine (Lomotil) overdose in children; an update. *Pediatrics* 87:694–700, 1991.

Sporer KA: Acute heroin overdose. *Ann Intern Med* 130:584–590, 1999.

103

Organophosphates and Carbamates

Jerrold Leikin

HIGH-YIELD FACTS

- Organophosphates permanently inactivate acetylcholinesterase, leading to an accumulation of acetylcholine at the neuromuscular junction.
- The early manifestations of organophosphate toxicity are primarily muscarinic signs.
- Inactivation of acetylcholinesterase by carbamates is temporary.
- Atropine and pralidoxime comprise the therapy of choice in treating organophosphate exposure, while atropine alone is the mainstay of treatment for carbamate toxicity.
- Nicotinic signs are common in organophosphate exposure, but uncommon in carbamate exposure.

The organophosphates, and to a lesser extent the carbamate compounds, are particularly toxic chemicals. They are widely distributed throughout industry, agriculture, and the home, where they are used predominantly as pesticides. Organophosphates are found in No-Pest Strips (Vapona) and roach killers. Pesticides account for 25 percent of exposures called in to animal poison centers, and for about 3 percent of total exposures called in to regional poison control centers. Over one-half of exposures involve children under the age of 6 years old.

PATHOPHYSIOLOGY

Organophosphate toxicity results from the linking with and inactivating of acetylcholinesterase, and this inactivation is essentially permanent. The inactivation of acetylcholinesterase leads to the accumulation of acetylcholine at cholinergic receptor sites. Excess acetylcholine initially stimulates, then paralyzes cholinergic transmission at parasympathetic nerve endings, certain sympathetic nerve endings, and the neuromuscular junction. Organophosphates penetrate the central nervous system (CNS), where they paralyze cholinergic transmission.

CLINICAL PRESENTATION

The initial signs and symptoms of cholinergic excess are usually muscarinic in nature. Gastrointestinal symptoms include abdominal cramps, vomiting, and diarrhea. Pulmonary findings include increased bronchial secretions, bronchoconstriction, dyspnea, and in some cases pulmonary edema. Lacrimation and salivation are increased. Miosis occurs, occasionally preceded by mydriasis. Bradycardia can occur, as can urinary incontinence. This constellation of findings is characterized by the mnemonic *SLUDGE:*

- *Salivation*
- *Lacrimation*
- *Urination*
- *Defecation*
- *Gastrointestinal cramps*
- *Emesis*

The mnemonic does not include the pulmonary findings, which can cause life-threatening hypoxia and require urgent intervention (Table 103-1).

Nicotinic manifestations include hypertension, pallor, and tachycardia. Striated muscle can be severely affected. Initially cholinergic excess stimulates fasciculations, which are followed by weakness that can range from very mild to full paralysis. The combination of increased airway secretions and weakness of the respiratory musculature can rapidly produce respiratory failure, often necessitating urgent intubation.

Central nervous system toxicity occurs with organophosphate toxicity and ranges from agitation to full delirium and coma. Seizures can also occur.

An intermediate syndrome has been described that is manifested by neck and extremity paralysis 12 hours to 7 days after exposure to certain organophosphate agents. The most common organophosphate compounds implicated in this syndrome include methylparathion, ethylparathion, fethion, and dimethoate. Cranial nerve palsies can also occur with the intermediate syndrome, which in some cases may be due to lack of administration of an oxime during treatment. An uncommon delayed neurologic manifestation reported after organophosphate exposure is a peripheral neuropathy that can result

Table 103-1. Clinical Effects of Organophosphate/Carbamate Intoxication

Muscarinic Effects (Organophosphates and Carbamates

Salivation	Bradycardia
Diaphoresis	Miosis (late finding)
Lacrimation	Bronchorrhea
Defecation	Bronchospasm
Abdominal cramps	
Rhinorrhea	

Nicotinic Effect (Organophosphates Only)

Fasciculations/twitching	Tachycardia
Weakness	Hypertension
Tremors	Pallor
Areflexia	Cramps

Central Nervous System Effects (Organophosphates Predominantly; Carbamates Rarely)

Headache	Seizures
Restlessness	Coma
Confusion	Respiratory depression
Bizarre behavior	Ataxia

Intermediate Syndrome (Organophosphates Only)

Paralysis of head, neck, extremity muscles 3.5–7 days after resolution of cholinergic synchrony

---

in permanent disability. This delayed syndrome (organophosphate-induced delayed neuropathy; OPIN) affects primarily the legs and may persist for months. Children appear somewhat more resistant to the development of OPIN than adults. The OPIN syndrome is thought to result from inhibition of a target esterase and has been described with methamidophos, trichlorfon, and leptophos. Neither the intermediate nor OPIN syndromes exhibit muscarinic symptomatology.

DIAGNOSIS

Organophosphate toxicity is part of the differential diagnosis of any patient presenting with the characteristic SLUDGE symptom complex. Muscle fasciculations with or without central nervous system abnormalities makes an organophosphate exposure highly likely. Patients exposed to agricultural or other occupational pesticides are at particularly high risk.

Laboratory Studies

In the acute phase there is no test that can identify organophosphate toxicity, and the initial management of the patient is based on clinical findings.

Organophosphates cause depression of red blood cell cholinesterase and plasma pseudocholinesterase. Red blood cell cholinesterase represents cholinesterase found in nerve tissue, brain, and erythrocytes. It is a better indicator of toxicity than plasma pseudocholinesterase, which is a liver protein. Reductions of 50 percent or more in red blood cell cholinesterase correlate with mild toxicity, while a 90 percent reduction indicates severe poisoning. In untreated organophosphate poisoning, regeneration of the enzyme takes 1 to 3 months.

Laboratory studies useful in the acutely ill patient include electrolytes for patients with vomiting and diarrhea, and in those with pulmonary symptoms, an arterial blood gas or percutaneous oxygen saturation is warranted. A chest radiograph is indicated for patients with evidence of pulmonary involvement.

TREATMENT

Stablization

The manifestations of organophosphate toxicity can range from isolated gastrointestinal involvement to fulminant respiratory failure. The most important aspect of stabilization is to assure adequate oxygenation and ventilation. In cases where there is severe bronchospasm, copious secretions, or marked weakness of respiratory muscles, urgent intubation and ventilation is indicated until antidotal therapy takes effect. Patients with marked central nervous system involvement may also require intubation to assure protection of the airway and reduce the risk of aspiration pneumonitis.

Fluid resuscitation may be required for patients who have suffered significant volume loss from the gastrointestinal tract. Boluses of crystalloid at doses of 10 to 20 mL/kg are adequate.

Decontamination

Decontamination is vital in a patient with organophosphate or carbamate toxicity. The patient is completely undressed, including removal of any jewelry, and the skin cleansed with soap and water. Contaminated clothing is discarded. The hospital staff must take care that they are not contaminated by contact with patients with dermal exposure.

Since emesis and diarrhea is common in organophosphate and carbamate intoxication, ipecac or lavage is rarely useful. In addition, many of these agents are combined with a hydrocarbon vehicle, thus induction of emesis or gastric lavage without first protecting the airway can result in aspiration pneumonitis. Pneumonitis can also occur from toxin-induced emesis and aspiration of gastric contents. Activated charcoal is indicated to adsorb toxin remaining in the gastrointestinal tract.

Antidotal Therapy

Atropine is the antidote for the muscarinic effects of organophosphate toxicity, and it also relieves the CNS manifestations. An initial dose of 0.05 mg/kg is indicated, and this may be doubled every 5 to 10 minutes until symptoms are relieved. The goal of therapy is the drying of airway secretions so that oxygenation and ventilation are maintained. Pupillary dilation can occur before the excessive secretions are alleviated; it is not an indication of adequate atropinization, and in some cases massive doses of atropine are required. Tachycardia is not a contraindication to its use. Treatment with atropine must usually continue for at least 24 hours. Endotracheal or nebulized administration of ipratropium bromide (0.5 mg every 6 hours) may also assist in drying secretions.

The specific antidote for the nicotinic manifestations of organophosphate toxicity is pralidoxime. It also relieves the central nervous system effects. Pralidoxime works by restoring the activity of acetylcholinesterase. It is most effective when administered early, but it should be used any time organophosphate poisoning with nicotinic or central nervous system manifestations is considered. Pregnancy is not a contraindication to its use.

Pralidoxime is administered at a dose of 25 to 50 mg/kg diluted to a 5 percent concentration in normal saline and infused over a 5- to 30-minute period. It is repeated at 6- to 12-hour intervals until there is relief of muscle weakness. Continuous infusion of 9 to 19 mg/kg/h following the loading dose of 25 to 50 mg/kg is indicated if breakthrough nicotinic symptoms occur or if there is continued absorption of poison. Treatment is generally necessary for at least 48 hours. Side effects of pralidoxime include nausea, tachycardia, lethargy, and diplopia. There may be mild elevation of liver enzymes.

Charcoal hemoperfusion is effective in removing parathion, demeton-S-methyl sulfoxide, dimethioate, and malathion. Exchange transfusion also has been utilized in parathion toxicity. Newer investigational modalities that may prove helpful in the management of organophosphate toxicity include exogenous plasma cholinesterase to act as a scavenger agent, and dextetimide or scopolamine which act as anticholinergic agents.

CARBAMATES

Carbamates are commonly found in flea and tick powders and in ant killers. Like organophosphates, carbamates inactivate acetylcholinesterase. Unlike organophosphates, however, inactivation is not permanent, and functional activity of the enzyme is often largely restored within 8 hours, and red blood cell cholinesterase is usually completely restored within 48 hours.

Toxicity with carbamates is primarily restricted to muscarinic effects, which are often the only manifestations of the poisoning (Table 103-1). They are much less likely than organophosphates to cause CNS effects, since they do not penetrate the blood-brain barrier well. Nicotinic manifestations are also uncommon. However, children with severe carbamate poisoning can develop CNS depression and occasionally seizures.

The initial management of the muscarinic effects of carbamate toxicity is the same as for organophosphates, with stabilization of the airway and breathing and complete decontamination of the patient. The skin is washed, although dermal exposure is less likely with carbamates than with organophosphates. Atropine is administered as antidotal therapy. Because the inactivation of acetylcholinesterase by carbamates is relatively short, pralidoxime is unlikely to be of benefit.

BIBLIOGRAPHY

Aaron CK: Organophosphates and carbamates, in Ford MD, Delaney KA, Ling LJ, et al (eds): *Clinical Toxicology.* Philadelphia: Saunders, 2001, pp 819-828.

Ekins BR, Geller RJ, Khasigian PA, et al: Severe carbamate poisoning caused by methomyl with clinical improvement produced by pralidoxime. *Veterinary Hum Toxicol* 35:358, 1993.

Fenske RA, Black KG, Elkner KP, et al: Potential exposure and health risks of infants following indoor residential pesticide applications. *Am J Public Health* 80:689–693, 1990.

Guven H, Tuncok Y, Gidener S, et al: The absorption of parathion by activated charcoal in vitro. *Veterinary Hum Toxicol* 35:359, 1993.

Kuffner E, Morasco R, Hoffman RS, et al: Human plasma cholinesterase protects against parathion toxicity in mice. *Veterinary Hum Toxicol* 35:332, 1993.

Litovitz TL, Schwartz-Klein W, White S, et al: 1999 Annual report of the American Association of Poison Control Centers toxic exposure surveillance system. *Am J Emerg Med* 18(5):517–574, 2000.

Mattingly JE, Sullivan JE, Spiller HA, et al: Intermediate syndrome after exposure of chlorpyrofos in a 16 month old female. *J Toxicol Clin Toxicol* 39(3):305, 2001.

Medicis JJ, Stork CM, Howland MA, et al: Pharmacokinetics following a loading dose plus a continuous infusion of pralidoxime compared with the traditional short infusion regimen in human volunteers. *J Toxicol Clin Toxicol* 34:289–295, 1996.

Rotenberg M, Shefi M, Dany S, et al: Differentiation between organophosphate and carbamate poisoning. *Clin Chim Acta* 234:11–21, 1995.

Senanayake N, Karalliedde L: Neurotoxic effects of organophosphorus insecticides. *N Engl J Med* 316:761–763, 1987.

104

Phencyclidine Toxicity

Steven E. Aks

HIGH-YIELD FACTS

- Phencyclidine (PCP) is a dissociative anesthetic structurally similar to ketamine.
- Street names of PCP include angel dust, peace pill, wickey weed, wacky weed, illy, Sherman, monkey tranquilizer, and embalming fluid.
- Bidirectional nystagmus is a classic finding of PCP intoxication.
- A urine dipstick positive for blood but negative for RBCs should prompt the diagnosis of rhabdomyolysis in PCP-intoxicated patients.
- Urinary acidification, while pharmacologically beneficial to eliminate PCP more rapidly, is contraindicated because it can cause precipitation of myoglobin in the renal tubules.

Phencyclidine (PCP) is a common drug that is used for recreational purposes by adolescents and adults. PCP is commonly used with marijuana, and is sometimes used along with alcohol, cocaine, or other substances. The ingestion of multiple drugs at the same time can confuse the clinical picture. Unfortunately, adolescents and adults are not the only patients at risk. Toddlers and infants have been exposed via passive inhalation, which has resulted in significant clinical toxicity. Indeed, these cases should alert health care workers to the possibility of abuse or neglect in the home. Phencyclidine should be included on every clinician's list of drugs that can cause altered mental status in children of all ages.

According to data in the 1999 annual report of the American Association of Poison Control Centers (AAPCC) there were a total of 465 cases of phencyclidine exposure. There were 21 cases in children younger than 6 years of age, 140 cases in children aged 6 to 19, and one death related to phencyclidine.

PHARMACOLOGY

Phencyclidine is a cyclohexylamine structurally related to ketamine. It was developed in the 1950s as a dissociative anesthetic. It fell out of favor for clinical use because of unacceptable neuropsychiatric effects.

Phencyclidine is commonly used via inhalation, although insufflation and intravenous administration are occasionally utilized. It has a pK_a of approximately 8.5, with a volume of distribution of 6.2 L/kg, and its serum half-life is in the range of 21 to 24 hours. The actual duration of action may be significantly longer in chronic PCP users. The drug undergoes significant enteroenteric recirculation and is subsequently resecreted into the stomach. Phencyclidine is hydroxylated in the liver and is excreted in the urine.

The mechanism of action of PCP is severalfold. It is thought to inhibit the uptake of dopamine and norepinephrine, and in addition has some anticholinergic and alpha-adrenergic properties.

Since naive users may not be aware of the nature of the substance they have ingested, health care workers need to be familiar with the many street names of PCP, which include angel dust, peace pill, wickey weed, wacky weed, Sherman, monkey tranquilizer, embalming fluid, cadillac, and rocket fuel. Some users soak marijuana with embalming fluid (formaldehyde and methanol) and then dust it with PCP. Terms for this combination are embalming fluid, illy, fry, amp, wet, clickers, and purple rain.

CLINICAL PRESENTATION

The neurologic effects of PCP overdose include excitation, hyperreflexia, blank stares, nystagmus, hallucinations, seizures, and psychosis. Phencyclidine can cause acute behavioral toxicity. A hallmark is its ability to cause a fluctuating level of consciousness, characterized by periods of lethargy and coma alternating with aggressive or assaultive activity. The combination of psychotic and aggressive behavior places the PCP user at great risk for traumatic injury. As with opioid toxicity, pupils are often pinpoint, although mydriasis may also be seen.

Young children exposed to PCP can present with the rapid onset of lethargy, coma, staring spells, ataxia, opisthotonos, and nystagmus. Side effects have been described in patients as young as 2 months of age. Cardiovascular side effects include hypertension that may be severe enough to create a hypertensive crisis, tachycardia, and dysrhythmias. The skin can be diaphoretic and flushed. Hyperthermia and muscle hyperactivity can occur, as can rhabdomyolysis and renal failure.

LABORATORY TESTS

Useful laboratory studies include CBC, electrolytes, and renal function tests. A blood glucose test is indicated to rule out PCP-related hypoglycemia, which has been described. A urinalysis is obtained, with particular attention paid to the presence of a dipstick positive for blood but a microscopic examination negative for red blood cells. This indicates the possibility of rhabdomyolysis and the presence of myoglobin in the urine. Measurement of serum creatine kinase and sequential monitoring of renal function is indicated. Calcium, phosphate, and uric acid levels are appropriate as well in cases of rhabdomyolysis. Liver function tests have also been noted to rise during the course of toxicity. Cardiac monitoring with attention to the development of sinus tachycardia and dysrhythmias is important. Urinary confirmation by toxicology screen for drugs of abuse will also be helpful when no clear history is known. Ketamine and phencyclidine are structurally related and false positive results for PCP on drug screening may be seen after ketamine use. However, a negative screen for PCP should not suggest the absence of ketamine; this requires specialized analysis. The clinical presentation of PCP and ketamine can be indistinguishable.

MANAGEMENT

The mainstay of management of the patient with phencyclidine intoxication is good supportive care. It is essential that health care providers take necessary measures to assure the safety of the patient and the emergency department staff. It is erroneous to view the psychosis and abnormal behavior as similar to that caused by the hallucinogens. Attempts to "talk the patient down" will be fruitless. Physical and appropriate chemical restraints should be used as necessary.

Initially, the patient's level of consciousness is assessed and the airway is secured. A determination of the degree of disorientation and intoxication is made. If multiple drugs are ingested, lavage with subsequent administration of activated charcoal is appropriate. However, in the vast majority of cases this will not be necessary, and the lavage procedure may only agitate the patient and increase the risk of injury to themselves or staff members. Nasogastric aspiration of gastric fluid has been

suggested as a means of removing PCP that is ionized in the stomach. This procedure is generally unrealistic when confronted with a wildly agitated patient. Placing the patient in a quiet room with dim lights will help control the violent behavior. However, appropriate monitoring of vital signs must take place.

Pharmacologic agents such as benzodiazepines and haloperidol have been used successfully in cases of PCP intoxication. They are titrated to effect, with meticulous attention paid to the integrity of the airway. Large doses of sedatives can induce respiratory depression. Phenothiazines are contraindicated in the setting of PCP intoxication because of their ability to lower the seizure threshold and the possibility of causing hypotension. Antihypertensives are generally not required in PCP overdose, but if necessary a short-acting agent such as nitroprusside would be of value.

Although acidification of the urine has been suggested to enhance elimination of PCP, it is contraindicated because of the potential to worsen renal insufficiency should rhabdomyolysis develop. In the event that rhabdomyolysis develops, the urine is alkalinized by adding sodium bicarbonate to the intravenous fluid.

DISPOSITION

Patients with severe toxicity and evidence of prolonged coma, seizures, hyperthermia, rhabdomyolysis, or unstable vital signs should be admitted to an intensive care unit for monitoring and supportive care. Patients with minor manifestations of toxicity can be observed in the emergency department for 6 to 8 hours and discharged in the care of responsible caretakers when the patient's mental state returns to baseline.

BIBLIOGRAPHY

Barton CH, Sterling ML, Vaziri ND: Rhabdomyolysis and acute renal failure associated with phencyclidine intoxication. *Arch Intern Med* 140:568–569, 1980.

Giannini AJ, Price WA, Loiselle RH, et al: Treatment of phenylcyclohexylpyrrolidine (PHP) psychosis with haloperidol. *Clin Toxicol* 23:185–189, 1985.

Litovitz TL, Klein-Schwartz W, White S, et al: 1999 Annual report of the American Association of Poison Control Centers toxic exposure surveillance system. *Am J Emerg Med* 18:517–574, 2000.

McCarron MM, Schulze BW, Thompson GA, et al: Acute phencyclidine intoxication: incidence of clinical findings in 1000 cases. *Ann Emerg Med* 10:237–242, 1981.

Moriarty AL: What's "new" in street drugs: "Illy." *J Pediatr Health Care* 10:41–42, 1996.

Patel R, Connor G: A review of thirty cases of rhabdomyolysis-associated acute renal failure among phencyclidine users. *Clin Toxicol* 23:547–556, 1985.

Schwartz RH, Einhorn A: PCP intoxication in seven young children. *Pediatr Emerg Care* 2:238–241, 1986.

Shannon M: Letter. *Pediatr Emerg Care* 14:180, 1998.

Strauss AA, Modaniou HD, Bosu SK: Neonatal manifestations of maternal phencyclidine (PCP) abuse. *Pediatrics* 68:550–552, 1981.

Weiner AL, Vieira L, McKay CA: Ketamine abusers presenting to the emergency department: A case series. *J Emerg Med* 18:447–451, 2000.

105

Poisonous Plants

Andrea Carlson
Kimberly Sing

HIGH-YIELD FACTS

- There is considerable overlap in the clinical manifestations of toxicity of many plants, and for most patients the treatment is supportive.
- Most toxic plants primarily cause nausea, vomiting, and diarrhea.
- During the Christmas holidays, children are often exposed to *mistletoe* and *holly.* The leaves are more toxic than the berries and mainly cause gastroenteritis, which is usually not very severe.
- The *Arum* spp., *Dieffenbachia* and *Philodendron,* are houseplants that toddlers tend to ingest and are the most common cause of symptomatic plant ingestions. They can cause severe oral and pharyngeal burns secondary to insoluble calcium oxalate crystals.
- Plants that contain cardiac glycosides inhibit the Na-K/ATP-ase pump, causing an increase in serum potassium and a decrease in intracellular potassium, thereby changing the membrane potential. Each of the following plants contains glycosides, in increasing potency: *lily of the valley* < *foxglove* < *oleander* < *yellow oleander.*
- Toxicity can consist predominantly of gastrointestinal symptoms, with vomiting and diarrhea. In severe cases, cardiac toxicity results, mainly in the form of arrhythmias that include first-, second-, and third-degree heart block.
- *Water hemlock* is easily confused with the wild carrot or Jerusalem artichoke. Patients may progress to status epilepticus, respiratory distress, rhabdomyolysis, and death.
- Plants that contain nicotine-like toxins cause a toxidrome consisting of nausea, vomiting, salivation, abdominal cramps, confusion,

tachycardia, mydriasis, and fever. Seizures may occur in this initial stimulatory stage.

- *Jimsonweed, black henbane,* and *mandrake* all contain varying amounts of both hyoscyamine and scopolamine. Decontamination is attempted even 12 to 24 hours after ingestion because there is delayed gastric emptying, but physostigmine is reserved for patients with seizures, severe hallucinations, hypertension, or arrhythmias.
- The stalk of the *rhubarb* is edible, but the leaves are toxic because of the high content of soluble calcium oxalate, which is concentrated in the kidneys and can cause renal failure. Symptoms usually begin 6 to 12 hours after ingestion but may be delayed for 24 hours.

Plants are commonly ingested by children. In 1999, plant ingestions accounted for 5.2 percent of all the calls to the poison control centers around the United States. Of the 113,864 calls, only 106 (0.09 percent) had a major outcome, and only 4 deaths were reported. Nearly 70 percent of plant ingestions are by children younger than 6 years. Infants ingest houseplants, whereas toddlers ingest both indoor and outdoor plants.

Although the vast majority of plants are nontoxic, a small number are mildly toxic and a few are harmful or fatal with even a small exposure. Plants vary in toxicity during stages of their growth cycle. In addition, some plant toxins are destroyed by heat and others are not.

Historical information to be elicited includes whether the plant is an indoor or outdoor variety and a description of the plant's flower, stem, leaves, height, location, and, if possible, name. There is considerable overlap in the clinical manifestations of toxicity of many plants, and for most patients the treatment is supportive. It is useful to consider certain plants according to the predominant and usually most serious manifestations of toxicity (Table 105-1).

GASTROINTESTINAL IRRITANTS

Most toxic plants primarily cause nausea, vomiting, and diarrhea. Children commonly ingest the red waxy berries of the *Taxus* spp. and do not develop symptoms because the berry lacks the taxine alkaloid. Death occurs with large ingestions. The *Solanum* spp. cause gastrointestinal symptoms and an anticholinergic syndrome. Children usually eat the brightly colored berries; two or three berries

Table 105-1. Poisonous Plants

Plant	Botanical Name	Toxin	Poisonous Section	Description	Symptoms	Treatment	Miscellaneous
Taxus spp.	*T. chinensis* *T. brevifolia* *T. baccata*	Taxine alkaloid Taxine alkaloid Taxine alkaloid	All except fleshy portion around the seed	Evergreen tree seed: waxy, red with open end	Latency of 1 to 3 h. Nausea, diffuse abdominal pain, decreased respiration, cardiac conduction changes, convulsions, coma.	Supportive; lavage; AC[a]	Common ornamental plant in gardens, seed is the usual part eaten by children
	Podocarpus macrophylla	Taxine alkaloid	All except fleshy portion around the seed	Evergreen shrub seed: blue and fleshy purple	Death (rare) with large ingestions within 30 min.		
Chinese yew Western yew English yew							
Japanese yew							
Solanum spp.	*S. nigrum*	Solanine alkaloid, ? atropine	Sprouts and stems concentrate toxin Unripe berries highest amount	Shrublike with small flowers (yellow, purple, white, blue) and red/black berries	Nausea, vomiting, abdominal pain, subnormal temp, dilated pupils, hallucinations; shock and circulatory collapse may occur in severe cases	Supportive; lavage vs ipecac; AC	
Nightshades							
	S. tuberosum	Solanine alkaloid	Green and spoiled potatoes, sprouts, and eyes of tuber	Potato			
Common potato							
Phytolacca	*P. americana*	Phytolaccine	All plant; mature plant more toxic Roots > leaves/ stem Green berries more toxic than mature berries	Shrublike plant Clusters of berries that ripen in July–Sept into dark dark purple	Delay of 2–3 h, then abdominal cramping, diaphoresis, emesis, dyspnea, lethargy, and convulsions	Supportive; lavage; AC	Delicacy in some areas of the US when cooked correctly: "poke salad"
Pokeweed							

(Continues)

Table 105-1. (*continued*) Poisonous Plants

Plant	Botanical Name	Toxin	Poisonous Section	Description	Symptoms	Treatment	Miscellaneous
Abrus Rosary pea or jequirty pea	*A. precatorius*	Abrin toxalbumin	Seed	Bright scarlet seed with black hilum	Severe gastroenteritis several hours after consumption; bloody diarrhea; symptoms may last as long as 10 days	Supportive; aggressive fluids; lavage vs ipecac; AC	Seed must be masticated to cause symptoms; commonly found as beaded jewelry
Ricinus Castor bean	*R. communis*	Ricin toxalbumin	Seed but also rest of plant		Mimic septic shock; leukocytosis, hypotension, dehydration	Supportive; aggressive fluids; lavage vs ipecac; AC	
Ilex Holly	*Ilex* spp.	Five toxins	Leaves > berries	Green leaves with red or black berries	Gastroenteritis with large ingestions	Supportive	
Phroradendron Mistletoe (U.S.)	*P. americana*	Alkaloid	All		Gastroenteritis in large quantities	Supportive	
Viscum album Mistletoe (European)	*Viscum album*	Viscotoxin	All		Gastroenteritis ?cardiotoxic	Supportive ipecac vs lavage; AC	
Cardiovascular Toxin							
Digitalis Foxglove	*D. purpurea*	Digitoxin	All	Tubular flowers in pink, white, purple, yellow	Gastroenteritis, cardiac conduction defects	Supportive; lavage vs ipecac; AC, watch K$^+$; Digibind[b]	Common ornamental flower in gardens
Convallaria Lily of the valley	*C. majalis*	Convallarin and convallamarin (less potent than digitoxin/digitalis)	All	Herbaceous perennial; long leaves; white, bell-shaped flowers; red berry	Gastroenteritis, cardiac conduction defects	Supportive; lavage vs ipecac; AC, watch K$^+$; Digibind[b]	Common ornamental flower in gardens

(*Continues*)

Table 105-1. (*continued*) Poisonous Plants

Plant	Botanical Name	Toxin	Poisonous Section	Description	Symptoms	Treatment	Miscellaneous
Nerium Oleander	*N. oleander*	Glycosides (× 5)	All	Ornamental shrub; flowers of white, pink, red in clusters	Gastroenteritis, cardiac conduction defects	Supportive; lavage vs ipecac; AC, watch K^+; Digibind[b]	Common ornamental shrub in mild climates
Thevetia Yellow oleander	*Thevetia peruviana*	Digoxin, digitoxin	All	As above; yellow flowers	Gastroenteritis, cardiac conduction defects	Supportive; lavage; AC, Digibind,[b] phenytoin	Seeds caused death in a 2½ year old
			Nicotinelike Toxins				
Conium Poison hemlock, poison fool's parsley	*C. maculata*	Coniine	All parts; increases with age of plant; with root containing most	Fernlike leaves; white umbel flowers in moist soils	Salivation, GI irritation, diploplia, bradycardia, decreased respiration, seizures; death through respiratory paralysis	Supportive; NO IPECAC, lavage, AC, benzo-diazepines ?Golytely	Rhabdomyolosis may occur and progess to renal failure
Nicotinia/ Lobelia Tobacco plants	*N. glauca*	Nicontine or nicontinelike alkaloids	All parts		Salivation, GI distress, diaphoresis, ataxia, confusion, weakness, convulsions, coma; miosis, lacrimation, bronchorrhea, fasciculations, paralysis may occur; transient hypertension and tachycardia, then hypotension and bradycardia may occur	Supportive; lavage, AC Atropine	Monitor BP but do not aggressively treat because of the depressive state that occurs after

(*Continues*)

Table 105-1. (*continued*) Poisonous Plants

Plant	Botanical Name	Toxin	Poisonous Section	Description	Symptoms	Treatment	Miscellaneous
Anticholinergics							
Datura spp.	*D. stramonium*	Hyoscyamine Scopolamine	All: 50–100 seeds = 3 – 6 mg atropine	Funnel-shaped white or purple flower; many-seeded fruit	Hallucinations, disorientation, mydriasis, hyperpyrexia, decreased bowel sounds, urinary retention, tachycardia; seizures uncommon but may occur	Decontamination even if 12–24 h after ingestion. AC; Physostigmine: for seizures/ hallucinations/ arrhythmias	"Blind as a bat, hot as a hare, dry as a bone, red as a beet, and mad as a hatter"; symptoms may be delayed for 2–6 h
Hyoscyamus	*H. niger*	Hyoscyamine Scopolamine	All	Yellowish flowers	As above	As above	As above
Mandragora	*M. offinarum*	Hyoscyamine Scopolamine	All	As above	As above	As above	As above
Renal Toxins							
Rhubarb		Soluble calcium oxalate crystals	Leaves	Large green leaves with reddish/ pink stalks	Sore throat, nausea, vomiting, anorexia, diarrhea, abdominal pain; may be delay of 24 h, but usually within 6–12 h; oliguria, anuria, proteinuria, and oxaluria; symptoms of hypocalcemia	Ipecac, AC,? lavage with 0.15% calcium hydroxide; calcium gluconate if hypocalcemic	Stalks are edible

(*Continues*)

Table 105-1. (*continued*) Poisonous Plants

Plant	Botanical Name	Toxin	Poisonous Section	Description	Symptoms	Treatment	Miscellaneous
			Miscellaneous				
Pitted fruits	Apricot seeds, bitter almonds, peach kernels, black/wild cherry seeds, elderberry	Amygdalin = benzaldehyde + cyanide	Seeds Leaves, stems, and roots		Dyspnea, cyanosis, vomiting, weakness, coma, convulsion, and cardiovascular collapse	Supportive; lavage AC; may require cyanide antidote kit	Large quantities must be ingested to cause symptoms

[a]AC = Activated charcoal.
[b]See text.

cause significant symptoms in adults. The phytolaccine alkaloid found in the *pokeweed* primarily causes irritation of the skin, mucous membranes, and gastrointestinal tract. The green berries contain more toxin than the purple berries, which are attractive to children: 10 uncooked berries are very toxic to adults. A 5-year-old child died after pokeberries were crushed into a pulp with water and sugar to simulate grape juice. The toxalbumins of the *rosary pea* and the *castor beans* inhibit protein synthesis and are the most toxic substances known. The bright scarlet seed of the rosary pea is very appealing to children. An Indian study of 57 children revealed that 22 displayed evidence of shock after ingestion of 4-5 seeds of the castor bean, with a maximum of 15 seeds eaten. The seed must be masticated to liberate the toxalbumin. Decontamination should be attempted even 4 hours after ingestion.

During the Christmas holidays, children are often exposed to *mistletoe* and *holly.* There are 300 to 350 species of holly, all having bright green leaves with red or black berries. The leaves are more toxic than the berries and mainly cause gastroenteritis, which is not very severe. The mistletoe, found primarily in the United States, contains an alkaloid that causes gastroenteritis. The European variety, also found in Sonoma County, California, contains a toxin that is similar to cobra venom and is reported to cause cardiotoxicity in animal studies. There are a few reports of death due to this variety, but the toxic effects are not well studied.

The *Arum* spp., *Dieffenbachia* and *Philodendron,* are houseplants that toddlers tend to ingest and are the most common cause of symptomatic plant ingestions. They can cause severe oral and pharyngeal burns secondary to insoluble calcium oxalate crystals. Usually the upper airway is the most affected. When there is severe exposure, the patient may need to be intubated to protect his or her airway. These plants do not cause gastroenteritis. Children who are not in extremis should be encouraged to drink milk or water. At home, application of oral numbing gels may be helpful. Respiratory obstruction usually progresses within the first 6 hours after exposure.

CARDIOVASCULAR TOXINS

Historically, plants that contain cardiac glycosides have been used for various cardiac ailments. These glycosides inhibit the Na-K/ATP-ase pump, causing an increase in serum potassium and a decrease in intracellular potassium, thereby changing the membrane potential. Each of the following plants contains glycosides, in increasing potency: *lily of the valley* < *foxglove* < *oleander* < *yel-low oleander.* Yellow oleander seeds have caused a death in a 2 ½-year-old child. Postmortem laboratory studies included a digoxin level of 11 ng/mL, digitoxin level of 17 ng/mL, and serum potassium of 9 mmol/L. Children have become symptomatic after using branches of this shrub for hot dog skewers.

Toxicity can consist predominantly of gastrointestinal symptoms, with vomiting and diarrhea. Some patients may complain of seeing yellow halos around lights. In severe cases, cardiac toxicity results, mainly in the form of arrhythmias that include first-, second-, and third-degree heart block.

For patients who have not vomited, gastric decontamination is indicated. For patients with bradydysrhythmias, atropine and cardiac pacing are indicated, although both may be ineffective because the myocardium may not be responsive. If cardiac instability is noted, a trial of Digibind is given. Although it has proved useful in dog studies, there is only one reported human case of Digibind being used in oleander toxicity.

Since not all the cardiac glycosides in plants are measured by the digitalis/digoxin assays in a normal laboratory, levels are not a reliable predictor of cardiac toxicity, and symptomatic patients are treated regardless of laboratory studies.

NEUROLOGIC TOXINS

Water hemlock is easily confused with the wild carrot or Jerusalem artichoke. Children tend to become toxic when experimenting with wild vegetation. Patients may progress to status epilepticus, respiratory distress, and death. Rhabdomyolysis may develop. Treatment is primarily supportive. Controversy exists over whether patients benefit from barbiturates. Patients who exhibit any central nervous system (CNS) symptoms (including spasticity) or cardiac instability require hospital admission. Patients who are asymptomatic are observed for 4 to 6 hours before discharge. Other plants thought to cause seizures are *podophyllum* resin, *trematol, pennyroyal oil, margosa oil, and eucalyptus oil.* Occasionally, *Aconitum (monkshood), Taxus* spp., and *Veratrum* spp. cause convulsions.

NICOTINE-LIKE TOXINS

Plants that contain nicotine-like toxins cause a toxidrome consisting of nausea, vomiting, salivation, abdominal cramps, confusion, tachycardia, mydriasis, and fever. Seizures may occur in this initial stimulatory stage, which progresses to CNS depression and may result in respiratory failure.

Poison hemlock contains coniine, which causes a curare-like paralysis at the neuromuscular junction and a strychnine-like convulsant activity. Death occurs from respiratory paralysis. In adults, ingestions of 100 to 300 mg are lethal. Whole bowel irrigation (Golytely 25 to 30 mL/kg/hr) may prove helpful if large amounts have been ingested. The *Nicotinia* and *Lobelia* spp. contain nicotine or nicotinic-like alkaloids. Mild intoxication may resolve in a few hours, with severe poisonings requiring 24 hours to resolve. When children ingest *cigarettes,* treatment is still controversial. Ingestion of one-half to one cigarette may cause symptoms, and two cigarettes will cause serious symptoms. Gastric decontamination is indicated in these children. Atropine may improve the bradycardia and hypotension but does not alter the neuromuscular weakness.

ANTICHOLINERGIC AGENTS

Atropine (a mixture of two isomers of hyoscyamine) has been known to be present in various plants for centuries. *Jimsonweed, black henbane,* and *mandrake* all contain varying amounts of both hyoscyamine and scopolamine. Decontamination is attempted even 12 to 24 hours after ingestion because there is delayed gastric emptying. Physostigmine is reserved for patients with seizures, severe hallucinations, hypertension, or arrhythmias. Physostigmine can be given 0.02 mg/kg up to 0.5 mg over several minutes. If there is no improvement, readministration after 5 minutes may be attempted, not to exceed 2 mg. Because of the short half-life, it may need to be readministered after 30 to 40 minutes. The *lowest* effective dose is utilized. This antidote cannot be given as an infusion. Symptoms usually resolve after 24 to 48 hours.

RENAL FAILURE

The stalk of the *rhubarb* is edible, but the leaves are toxic because of the high content of soluble calcium oxalate, which is concentrated in the kidneys and can cause renal failure. Symptoms usually begin 6 to 12 hours after ingestion but may be delayed 24 hours. Because of the precipitation of calcium, patients may develop hypocalcemia, resulting in electrocardiographic changes, paresthesias, tetany, hyperreflexia, muscle twitches, muscle cramps, and seizures. Calcium gluconate may be required to reverse the hypocalcemia. *Poison hemlock* has also been reported to cause renal failure, probably through the development of rhabdomyolysis.

MISCELLANEOUS PLANTS

About 150 species of plants contain cyanogenic glycosides. Amygdalin must be crushed to liberate the cyanide. Each species contains amygdalin in varying quantities. *Apple seeds* contain a very small amount of cyanide and require a large ingestion to cause toxicity. Symptoms usually start within a half hour after ingestion. Treatment involves supportive care, decontamination, and administration of the cyanide antidote kit, with adjustments made according to weight and hemoglobin content to avoid a fatal methemoglobinemia.

Ackee fruit (Blighia sapida) is often consumed in Jamaica. Jamaican vomiting sickness occurs when the unripe fruit is eaten. The unripe fruit contains the toxin hypoglycin A, which causes profound and persistent hypoglycemia, as well as liver damage that is pathologically indistinguishable from that of Reye's syndrome. Reports of this poisoning in the United States are extremely rare.

BIBLIOGRAPHY

Challoner KR, McCarron MM: Castor bean intoxication. *Ann Emerg Med* 19:159–163, 1990.

Harvey J, Colin-Jones D: Mistletoe hepatitis. *Br Med J* 282:186, 1981.

Haynes BE, Bessen HA, Wightman WD: Oleander tea: Herbal drought of death. *Ann Emerg Med* 14:350–353, 1985.

Hollman A: Plants and cardiac glycosides. *Br Heart J* 54:258–261, 1985.

Krenzelok EP: American mistletoe exposures. *Am J Emerg Med* 15:516–520, 1997.

Lampe KF, McCann MA: *AMA Handbook of Poisonous and Injurious Plants.* Chicago: American Medical Association, 1985.

Hung OL, Lewin NA, Howland MA: Herbal preparations, in Goldfrank LR, Flomenbaum NE, Lewin NA, et al (eds): *Goldfrank's Toxicologic Emergencies,* 6th ed. Stamford, CT: Appleton & Lange, 1998, pp 1221–1242.

Litovitz TL, Klein-Schwartz W, White S, et al: 1999 Annual Report of the American Association of Poison Control Centers Toxic Exposure Surveillance System. *Am J Emerg Med* 18:517–574, 2000.

Meda HA, Diallo B, Buchet J, et al: Epidemic of fatal encephalopathy in preschool children in Burkina Faso and consumption of unripe akee (Blighia sapida) fruit. *Lancet* 353:536–540, 1999.

Shih RD, Goldfrank LR: Plants, in Goldfrank LR, Flomenbaum NE, Lewin NA, et al (eds): *Goldfrank's Toxicologic Emergencies,* 6th ed. Stamford, CT: Appleton & Lange, 1998, pp 1243–1260.

106

Sedative Hypnotics

Timothy Erickson
Will Ignatoff

HIGH-YIELD FACTS

- In an overdose setting, sedative hypnotics produce CNS and respiratory depression.
- Urinary alkalinization can hasten the excretion of phenobarbital.
- Flunitrazepam ("roofies") are now a popular drug of abuse.
- Flumazenil is an antidote to benzodiazepines.
- Chloral hydrate overdose can result in CNS depression and cardiotoxicity.

This chapter will focus on those sedative hypnotic agents commonly encountered in the pediatric population, specifically, barbiturates, benzodiazepines, and chloral hydrate.

According to the 1999 American Association of Poison Control Centers annual report, there were 1238 toxic exposures to barbiturates, 8679 exposures to benzodiazepines, and 107 exposures to chloral hydrate in children under 20 years of age. There were no reported deaths.

BARBITURATES

Pharmacology/Pathophysiology

The barbiturates are classified as either ultra-short-acting (thiopental), short-acting (pentobarbital), or long-acting (phenobarbital). These agents are primarily used as anticonvulsants and for induction of anesthesia. Barbiturates are primarily central nervous system depressants that mediate their effect through inhibition of aminobutyric synapses of the brain. Toxicity can result in suppression of skeletal, smooth, and cardiac muscle, leading to depressed myocardial contractility, bradycardia, vasodilation, and hypotension.

Clinical Presentation

In the overdose setting, the pediatric patient will present with sedation and coma, often accompanied by respiratory depression. Vital signs may reveal hypotension, bradycardia, and hypothermia. Pupils are constricted early in the clinical course, but can be dilated in later stages of coma. As with most sedative hypnotic agents, noncardiogenic pulmonary edema has been described in severely toxic patients. After prolonged coma, the patient will rarely present with bullous skin lesions over dependent body parts. Cases of phenobarbital-induced hepatotoxicity have also been described in children.

Laboratory

In addition to baseline laboratory studies, a quantitative serum phenobarbital level is obtained to document the toxicity, but is not mandatory for definitive management. Therapeutic concentrations of phenobarbital range between 15 and 40 μg/mL. Patients with levels >50 μg/mL will exhibit mild toxicity, while those with levels >100 μg/mL are typically unresponsive to pain and suffer from respiratory and cardiac depression.

Treatment

The primary management of barbiturate toxicity is support and stabilization of the airway and circulation. Comatose patients may require intubation. Hypotensive patients are managed with fluid resuscitation, and if necessary, pressors. Gastric lavage may be useful up to 1 hour postingestion. Since most barbiturate ingestions cause CNS and respiratory depression, syrup of ipecac is contraindicated. Several investigations have demonstrated the efficacy of multidosing of activated charcoal in children, since the barbiturates, particularly phenobarbital, undergo enterohepatic circulation.

Urinary alkalinization with sodium bicarbonate to a pH of 7.5 to 8.0 can hasten the renal excretion of phenobarbital, which is a weak acid. This procedure is recommended in severe toxicity. Alkalinization is not effective for toxicity from shorter-acting agents. With alkalinization, fluid overload is avoided to prevent pulmonary and cerebral edema. In unstable patients not responsive to standard therapeutic measures, or in those with renal failure, hemodialysis is indicated for long-acting barbiturates. Charcoal hemoperfusion seems more efficacious for shorter-acting agents, which possess greater fat and protein binding.

BENZODIAZEPINES

Benzodiazepines are among the most commonly prescribed drugs in the world and they cause the majority of sedative hypnotic overdoses. They are used for their anxiolytic, muscle relaxant, and anticonvulsant properties. Benzodiazepines produce less CNS and respiratory depression than the barbiturates. Flunitrazepam is a potent benzodiazepine that has recently been popularized as a street drug of abuse and has been implicated as a date-rape drug. Flunitrazepam pills are often referred to as "roofies."

Pathophysiology

The benzodiazepines act by facilitating the neurotransmission of gamma-aminobutyric acid (GABA). Pure benzodiazepine overdoses result in a mild to moderate CNS depression. Deep coma requiring assisted ventilation is uncommon. In severe overdoses, benzodiazepines can induce cardiovascular and pulmonary toxicity, but fatalities resulting from pure benzodiazepine overdoses with adequate airway control are rare.

Clinical Presentation

Following an acute overdose, the patient classically presents with sedation, somnolence, ataxia, slurred speech, and lethargy. Profound coma is rare, and its presence should prompt a search for other coingestions or reasons for coma. The elderly and very young children are more susceptible to the CNS depression of these drugs.

Benzodiazepines can also induce paradoxical reactions, such as anxiety, delirium, combativeness, and hallucinations, particularly in children. Pupils are typically dilated and the patient may be hypothermic. As opposed to other sedative hypnotics, benzodiazepines rarely cause significant cardiovascular changes, although bradycardia and hypotension have been reported in severe overdoses.

Laboratory

Quantitative benzodiazepine concentrations correlate poorly with pharmacological or toxicological effects and are poor predictors of clinical outcome. However, qualitative screening determinations of benzodiazepines in the serum or urine can be useful in diagnosing patients with coma of unknown etiology.

Treatment

The most critical management intervention is stabilization of respiration. Ipecac is contraindicated due to the CNS effects of these agents. Gastric lavage is indicated for patients presenting within 1 hour of ingestion, and activated charcoal is recommended in all significant overdoses. Forced diuresis is not efficacious and, because benzodiazepines are highly bound to plasma proteins, hemodialysis or hemoperfusion are ineffective.

Flumazenil is an antidotal agent that reduces or terminates benzodiazepine effects by competitive inhibition at the central nervous system GABA sites. In comatose children, initial doses of 0.01 mg/kg intravenously have been recommended. If no response is elicited, this dose can be repeated. In neonates, an intravenous loading dose of 0.02 mg/kg is suggested, with a maintenance drip of 0.05 mg/kg/h, if indicated. Similar to naloxone, the duration of flumazenil is less than 1 hour. Subsequent doses or infusion drips are often required. Contraindications to flumazenil administration include seizure disorders, chronic benzodiazepine use (in order to avoid acute withdrawal), and coingestion of agents such as tricyclic antidepressants or isoniazid. As a result, it is not advised that flumazenil be given in cases of coma of unknown cause.

CHLORAL HYDRATE

Although uncommon in the overdose setting, chloral hydrate is frequently used in the pediatric population for sedation prior to procedures or radiologic testing.

Pathophysiology

Chloral hydrate is an effective sedative hypnotic that produces minimal respiratory and circulatory depression when given in therapeutic doses. Although most authorities recommend regimens of 25 to 50 mg/kg/dose, doses up to 80 to 100 mg/kg have been reported as safe and effective for pediatric sedation. Its structure is similar to that of the general anesthetic agent halothane. In large overdoses, chloral hydrate can depress myocardial contractility, resulting in dysrhythmias. The major active metabolites of chloral hydrate are trichlorethanol and trichloroacetic acid.

Clinical Presentation

Signs and symptoms of chloral hydrate toxicity are very similar to those seen in barbiturate overdoses, with respiratory, CNS, and cardiovascular manifestations. Pupils are typically miotic early in the clinical course but dilate in later stages of coma.

Following ingestion a child's breath may have a classic pear-like odor. Gastrointestinal upset with vomiting and abdominal pain is common, and occasionally elevation of hepatic enzymes is seen. Cardiac dysrhythmias can include atrial fibrillation, multifocal premature ventricular contractions, ventricular tachycardia, and ventricular fibrillation which may progress to torsades de pointes. Inadvertent intravenous administration has been reported and may irritate the surrounding skin, but seems no more toxic than oral exposure. In severe overdose, the pediatric patient can exhibit hypothermia, hypotension, and noncardiogenic pulmonary edema.

Laboratory

Chloral hydrate levels can assist in documenting the ingestion, but correlate poorly with clinical findings. Trichlorethanol levels may be a more reliable indicator of toxicity, but management is not delayed awaiting their result. If the ingestion is recent, an abdominal radiograph is obtained to confirm the diagnosis, since chloral hydrate may be radiopaque.

Treatment

As with the other sedative hypnotics, the child's airway is stabilized. Close attention is paid to the cardiovascular status due to the potential for cardiotoxicity. Gastric decontamination considerations are similar to those of the other sedative hypnotic agents. Ventricular dysrhythmias have responded to lidocaine, beta blockers, and magnesium administration; however, such cases have been anecdotal. If the patient is unstable, hemodialysis should be considered since this method effectively removes the active metabolite trichlorethanol.

Disposition

Any pediatric patient who is symptomatic following any sedative hypnotic overdose should be admitted and monitored for respiratory and cardiovascular stability.

BIBLIOGRAPHY

Amitai Y, Degan Y: Treatment of phenobarbital poisoning with multiple dose activated charcoal in an infant. *J Emerg Med* 8:449–450, 1990.

Frenia ML: Multiple dose activated charcoal compared to urinary alkalinization for the enhancement of phenobarbital elimination. *J Toxicol Clin Toxicol* 34:169–175, 1996.

Jones RD, Lawson AD, Andrew LJ, et al: Antagonism of the hypnotic effect of midazolam in children: A randomized, double-blind study of placebo and flumazenil administered after midazolam-induced anaesthesia. *Br J Anaesth* 66: 660–666, 1991.

Lacayo A, Mitra N: Report of a case of phenobarbital-induced dystonia. *Clin Pediatr* 31:252, 1992.

Lindberg MC, Cunningham A, Lindberg NH: Acute phenobarbital intoxication. *South Med J* 85:803–807, 1992.

Litovitz TL, Klein-Schwartz W, White S: 1999 Annual report of the American Association of Poison Control Centers toxic exposure surveillance system 2000. *Am J Emerg Med* 18(5):517–574, 2000.

Richard P, Auret E, Bardol J, et al: The use of flumazenil in a neonate. *J Toxicol Clin Toxicol* 29:137–140, 1991.

Sugarman JM, Paul RI: Flumazenil: A review. *Pediatr Emerg Care* 10(1):37–49, 1994.

Veerman M, Espejo MG, Christopher MA, et al: Use of activated charcoal to reduce elevated serum phenobarbital concentrations in the neonate. *Clin Toxicol* 29:53–58, 1991.

Waltzman ML: Flunitrazepam: A review of "roofies." *Pediatr Emerg Care* 15:59–60, 1999.

107

Theophylline

Frank P. Paloucek

HIGH-YIELD FACTS

- Important factors contributing to the toxicity of theophylline are its widespread use, narrow therapeutic index, the proliferation of dosage forms, its availability as a nonprescription product, and multiple drug-drug, drug-disease, and drug-food interactions.

- The clinical manifestations of acute theophylline toxicity are primarily gastrointestinal, cardiovascular, and neurological. Disturbances in serum electrolytes are also produced.

- Sinus and supraventricular tachycardias are, along with nausea and vomiting, the most common presenting features of acute theophylline toxicity, regardless of etiology. These are not life-threatening in the absence of other underlying cardiac disease.

- Status epilepticus can occur and is associated with more significant morbidity and mortality than other causes of status epilepticus in children. A predisposing factor for seizures in acute toxicity is a serum theophylline concentration >100 mg/L.

- Electrolyte disturbances are fairly typical in the acutely toxic patient and can include hypokalemia, hypophosphatemia, and hypercalcemia.

- Increased mortality is associated with age <2 years or serum theophylline concentrations >100 mg/L in acute pediatric overdoses.

- The single most important laboratory evaluation for suspected theophylline toxicity is serum theophylline concentration. The normal range is 10 to 20 mg/L and the toxic range is >20 mg/L, although toxic symptoms can occur at concentrations of 10 to 20 mg/L.

- Patients presenting with acute theophylline toxicity are managed with conventional supportive care and treatment of specific complications as they arise. There is no specific antidote for theophylline toxicity.

- Hemodialysis and charcoal hemoperfusion are indicated prophylactically for patients with theophylline concentrations >100 mg/L in an overdose. Withholding these modalities until toxicity occurs is undesirable, as severe toxicity can result in hypotension, seizures, and tachyarrhythmias, which can preclude initiation of these procedures.

- For chronic overdose patients with theophylline concentrations >30 mg/L, oral activated charcoal at 25 g every 2 hours is initiated and continued until concentrations are <30 mg/L or gastrointestinal complications occur. Either hemodialysis or charcoal hemoperfusion is indicated in the chronic patient when serum theophylline concentration is >60 mg/L, especially for patients >60 years of age, although there are fewer data supporting this recommendation than for acute ingestions and concentrations >100 mg/L.

Theophylline has been associated with several outbreaks of toxicity since its introduction as a medicinal agent. In the 1950s, fatalities occurred secondary to the use of adult-strength suppositories in children. In the 1960s, multiple episodes of morbidity and mortality occurred due to pharmacokinetic dosing of theophylline in elderly patients with heart failure or cirrhosis using dosing parameters derived from healthy or smoking volunteers. Finally, in the early 1980s, the introduction of sustained-release forms led to a significant increase in theophylline toxicity cases. In the early 1990s, according to the American Association of Poison Control Centers annual toxic exposure and surveillance summary, there were 3400 to 3700 pediatric exposures reported annually, with an average of 2 pediatric fatalities. Since 1995, these numbers have dropped to 500 to 1000 cases yearly with 1 to 2 deaths. Theophylline toxicity is one of the ten most frequent causes of reported fatalities for all age groups, and has an approximately fourfold increase in morbidity and mortality over the average accidental pediatric exposure.

Important factors contributing to the toxicity of theophylline are its widespread use, narrow therapeutic index, the proliferation of dosage forms, availability as a nonprescription product, and multiple drug-drug, drug-disease, and drug-food interactions. These all contribute to marked variation in presentation in the poisoned patient. It is therefore helpful to classify theophylline toxicity as either acute, acute-on-chronic, or chronic. While there is consensus on the need for this classification, there is no agreement on the definitions of the terms. For this discussion

- Acute toxicity refers to ingestion of ≥ 1 excessive dose within an 8-hour interval
- Acute-on-chronic toxicity refers to a single acute exposure in a patient ingesting therapeutic theophylline for >24 hours
- Chronic toxicity occurs in the presence of maintenance or therapeutic drug therapy for at least 24 hours

PHARMACOLOGY/PHARMACOKINETICS

The exact mechanism of action of theophylline is unknown. A majority of its effects appear to reflect its actions as a direct adenosine antagonist. It is known to possess the following pharmacodynamic properties:

- Central nervous system stimulation
- Medullary vomiting center stimulation
- Positive inotrope and chronotrope
- Reduction of peripheral arteriolar resistance
- Increase in renal blood flow and glomerular filtration rate
- Stimulation of secretion of gastric acid and pepsin

Many of these effects are mediated via stimulation of the β_2 adrenergic receptors, which is also responsible for theophylline-induced cellular shifts in electrolytes. Clinically, theophylline's toxicity results from direct extensions of some of these properties.

Theophylline is readily absorbed (80 to 100 percent). It is predominantly marketed and used in sustained-release dosage forms, which leads to significant delays in presentation or development of symptoms, and prolonged absorption times. Food and other drugs can affect the absorption processes, and the sustained-release products are known to form concretions or pharmacobezoars in the overdose setting. Peak serum theophylline concentrations have been reported 24 to 27 hours after referral to the emergency department. The volume of distribution is fairly consistent (0.5 L/kg), and remains unchanged in the overdose setting. This allows approximation of the peak concentration following an overdose. For most parenteral and immediate-release acute theophylline overdoses, the worst case scenario estimates peak serum concentration as twice the mg/kg exposure dose. Although the sustained-release products rarely act like the immediate-release forms, a more accurate estimation of the peak concentration following an overdose equals the mg/kg ingested dose.

Theophylline is hepatically metabolized by the mixed function oxidase system, specifically Cyp 1A2, with an average elimination half-life of 6 to 8 hours in adults. Multiple factors such as diseases, other drugs, age, sex, and diet can either enhance or impair its metabolism. Common factors contributing to chronic toxicity include age <2 or >60 years, symptomatic congestive heart failure, hepatic disease, acute viral infections, and concomitant treatment with erythromycins, H_2 histamine antagonists, fluoroquinolones, and allopurinol. In children <6 years old with parenteral overdose, nonlinear kinetics with significantly longer-than-expected metabolism has been reported. Other etiologies for chronic toxicity include the recent cessation of use of elimination-enhancing factors without concomitant theophylline dosage adjustment, such as smoking, barbiturates, carbamazepine, phenytoin, or rifampin.

ACUTE THEOPHYLLINE TOXICITY

The clinical manifestations of acute theophylline toxicity are primarily gastrointestinal, cardiovascular, and neurologic. Disturbances in serum electrolytes are also produced.

Gastrointestinal manifestations include nausea, vomiting, and gastrointestinal bleeding. Nausea and vomiting are nonspecific and can occur at therapeutic levels, with vomiting severe enough to limit the use of activated charcoal. Gastrointestinal bleeding, defined as hematemesis or heme-positive vomitus or stool, has been reported in acute pediatric overdoses of oral dosage forms. There have been no reports of clinically significant blood loss, so bleeding probably represents mild esophageal or gastric erosions. Concretions or bezoars should be suspected with markedly prolonged increases or unchanged serum concentrations for >24 hours.

Cardiovascular manifestations include tachyarrhythmias, hypotension, and cardiac arrest. Sinus and supraventricular tachycardias along with nausea and vomiting are the most common presenting features of theophylline toxicity, regardless of etiology. These are not life-threatening in the absence of other underlying cardiac disease. Specific to acute or acute-on-chronic toxicity, although not pathognomonic, are multifocal atrial tachycardias. Ventricular ectopy is reasonably common, but significant ventricular arrhythmias are very rare. Hypotension secondary to theophylline toxicity is unique to acute overdoses and is associated with serum concentrations >100 mg/L. It is due to peripheral β_2-receptor stimulation resulting in vasodilation. Cardiac arrests are exceedingly rare, can occur with acute or chronic toxicity, and are generally a terminal event.

Neurologic manifestations include mental status changes, tremor, seizures, and coma. Seizures are a very ominous event. Acute toxicity frequently presents with 1 to 3 generalized tonic-clonic seizures. Status epilepticus can occur and is associated with more significant morbidity and mortality than other causes of status epilepticus in children. A predisposing factor for seizures in acute toxicity is a serum theophylline concentration >100 mg/L. Literature summaries suggest that 20 percent of patients with reported theophylline-induced seizures die. Death may be a direct consequence of seizures, but more commonly secondary complications result in fatality. Coma has been reported in theophylline toxicity. This has always occurred post-ictally and is probably not a direct consequence of theophylline toxicity.

Electrolyte disturbances are fairly typical in the acutely toxic patient and can resemble common disorders such as diabetic ketoacidosis. They include hypokalemia, hypophosphatemia, and hypercalcemia. Potassium, phosphate, and calcium changes reflect transient cellular shifts associated with β_2 adrenergic stimulation. When due to theophylline effects alone, they are not associated with any significant pathology. They are concentration dependent. For potassium, the relationship to theophylline levels varies inversely and linearly correlates with theophylline concentrations >35 mg/L. All forms of acid-base disorders have been reported for theophylline, depending on underlying diseases and concomitant ingestant. Theophylline-induced lactic acidosis has been very rarely seen in severe acute toxicity.

Miscellaneous manifestations of theophylline toxicity include diuresis secondary to transient increase in renal blood flow in acute pediatric exposures, rhabdomyolysis, and tachypnea. Hyperglycemia can also occur.

Increased mortality is associated with age <2 years or serum theophylline concentrations >100 mg/L in acute pediatric overdoses.

The single most important laboratory evaluation for suspected theophylline toxicity is a serum theophylline concentration. The normal range is 10 to 20 mg/L and the toxic range is >20 mg/L, although toxic symptoms can occur at concentrations of 10 to 20 mg/L. Significant toxicity is likely with concentrations >100 mg/L for acute overdoses. Theophylline concentrations of 100 mg/L can be expected to occur with ingestion of 50 mg/kg of immediate-release tablets or 100 mg/kg of sustained-release tablets. Significant cross-reaction resulting in false reports of elevated theophylline levels occurs with caffeine, uremia, and hyperbilirubinemia, depending on the methodology used. It is critical, especially in known sustained-release overdoses, that serial concentrations be measured every 2 hours, until two consecutive decreasing theophylline concentrations are obtained. This allows for appropriate monitoring of the absorption phase of these products as well as potential concretion formation and identification.

Additional laboratory testing includes fingerstick glucose, serum electrolytes, arterial blood gas, and 12-lead electrocardiogram. An acetaminophen concentration is indicated in the overdose patient to rule out a concomitant ingestion. Both ultrasound and abdominal radiography (KUB) can identify intact sustained-release dosage forms or concretions in the gastrointestinal tract.

Management

Patients presenting with acute theophylline toxicity are managed with conventional supportive care and treatment of specific complications as they arise. There is no specific antidote for theophylline toxicity.

Gastric decontamination is indicated for the acute presentation. Ipecac is generally not indicated due to the emetogenic nature of theophylline and the need to administer activated charcoal. Use of ipecac is limited to the prehospital setting. Gastric lavage is indicated for diagnostic purposes, and should be performed within 1 hour after large ingestions (>50 mg/kg). The use of the largest bore tube available is critical, given the size of most sustained-release theophylline products. Activated charcoal is the gastric decontamination treatment of choice. The initial dose is calculated to deliver 10 grams of charcoal for every 1 gram of ingested theophylline, up to a maximum of 100 grams of charcoal. It is important to note that achieving a 10:1 ratio may require multiple doses. This initial therapy is separate from subsequent elimination enhancement achieved by gastrointestinal dialysis with multiple-dose activated charcoal. The initial dose is administered with sorbitol in a 1.5 g/kg dose for children and alert adults, and 3 g/kg in the obtunded adult. Charcoal can reduce apparent theophylline half-life to 2 hours, even in the absorption phase.

An alternative to gastric decontamination with charcoal is whole bowel irrigation with a high molecular weight polyethylene glycol dosed at 15 to 40 mL/kg/h in children and 1 to 2 L/h in adults. This is equally efficacious for acute ingestions when administered within 1 hour of ingestion, but is not effective in late presentations of acute ingestions, in which charcoal is the treatment of choice. There is to date no evidence of benefit from combining these two therapies.

Elimination enhancement is an important consideration for theophylline toxicity. Effective modalities include multiple-dose oral activated charcoal, hemodialysis, charcoal hemoperfusion, exchange transfusions, and plasmapheresis. For any significant ingestion (theophylline concentrations >30 mg/L), oral activated charcoal at 25 g every 2 hours is initiated and continued until concentrations are <20 mg/L or gastrointestinal complications occur. This can be administered as boluses or a continuous nasogastric infusion. In this setting it is critical to monitor concomitant sorbitol administration, especially with commercial preparations of charcoal in sorbitol. Inadvertent administration of such products has led to severe diarrhea, dehydration, electrolyte imbalances, and eventual permanent sequelae. Also, several of the initial doses of multidose regimens may be adsorbing theophylline from tablets still in the GI tract if the initial dose failed to achieve the preferred 10:1 dosing ratio.

Hemodialysis and charcoal hemoperfusion are indicated prophylactically in patients with theophylline concentrations >100 mg/L in an overdose. Withholding these modalities until toxicity occurs is undesirable, as severe toxicity can result in hypotension, seizures, and tachyarrhythmias, which can preclude initiation of these procedures. Hemoperfusion is preferred to hemodialysis because it achieves higher clearance rates. Practical considerations often lead to the use of hemodialysis rather than hemoperfusion due to staff familiarity and the speed of initiating treatment. Hemodialysis, if available, should not be withheld in favor of transfer for hemoperfusion or when the initiation of hemoperfusion would take significantly longer to be implemented. For adequate hemoperfusion, the charcoal cartridge should be exchanged every 2 hours to avoid saturation and loss of efficacy. Hemodialysis and charcoal hemoperfusion have been used simultaneously, although there are no comparative clinical data suggesting a benefit from this procedure.

There has been limited experience with exchange transfusion or plasmapheresis in neonatal and infant intoxications in which dialysis or hemoperfusion was not feasible. These cases suggest these methods are effective at enhancing elimination and should be considered in the pediatric population in whom more conventional modalities cannot be performed.

The treatment of choice for seizures is a benzodiazepine, with barbiturates being second-line therapy. Phenytoin is absolutely contraindicated as it lowers the seizure threshold in vitro and has not been effective clinically. The development of repetitive seizures or status epilepticus is an indication for barbiturate coma with or without paralysis. Single isolated seizures do not require long-term maintenance anticonvulsant therapy.

Arrhythmias are treated with beta blockade or calcium channel blockade. Verapamil is avoided, as it can inhibit theophylline metabolism. Short-acting agents such as esmolol are preferred. Ventricular arrhythmias and cardiac arrests are managed conventionally. Hypotension is initially managed by conventional supportive therapy. If the patient fails to respond, consider a trial with beta blockade to reverse the probable β_2-mediated hypotension. Again the shortest-acting agent available should be chosen.

Persistent vomiting may be treated by several methods, none of which has proven superior. First and foremost, avoid inducing emesis with syrup of ipecac. Slow charcoal administration over 15 to 20 minutes or infusion via gastrointestinal feeding tube systems has been effective. The preferred pharmacologic treatment is metoclopramide, 5- to 10-mg IV push, which is effective in approximately 50 percent of cases. If treatment fails, the dose can be increased to a maximum of 1 mg/kg or a 5-HT$_3$ antagonist (e.g., ondansetron) can be used.

Electrolyte disturbances in acute overdoses without other potential causes for the imbalance are managed expectantly. The cellular shifts of electrolytes are transient, usually resolve within 2 to 3 hours, and are nonpathologic. In cases of extreme values (K^+ <3.0 mEq/L), a single conventional replacement dose of the appropriate salt is indicated. Symptomatic overcorrection has occurred in patients with serial replacement doses without interval reassessment. Lactic acidosis is managed conventionally.

ACUTE-ON-CHRONIC THEOPHYLLINE TOXICITY

Patients with acute-on-chronic theophylline toxicity present with the same clinical manifestations as those with acute toxicity, but toxicity develops at lower levels. If not diagnosed by the history, acute-on-chronic toxicity is suspected in patients taking theophylline who develop multifocal atrial tachycardias, hypotension, or hypokalemia. The diagnosis is confirmed by an elevated theophylline level. Seizures occur with the same frequency as in acute presentations, but can occur at concentrations <30 mg/L. Significant toxicity is likely with concentrations >60 mg/L in acute-on-chronic and chronic patients, as opposed to >100 mg/L for acute overdoses. Worst case estimates can be calculated as for acute toxicity, with the addition of 20 mg/L to represent the chronic maintenance level.

Management is similar to that of acute toxic overdose. The only variation occurs with the use of elimination-enhancing treatment. The end point of multiple-dose activated charcoal is 30 mg/L, not 20 mg/L, if theophylline therapy remains indicated. Hemodialysis and charcoal hemoperfusion are indicated prophylactically in patients with theophylline concentrations >100 mg/L in an acute or acute-on-chronic overdose.

CHRONIC THEOPHYLLINE TOXICITY

Patients with chronic theophylline toxicity do not present with gastrointestinal bleeding, multifocal atrial tachycardias, hypotension, or hypokalemia due to theophylline toxicity. These findings in a patient on chronic theophylline therapy imply another diagnosis. All remaining toxic manifestations of theophylline occur in chronic patients but, importantly, at much lower serum levels. Severe toxic symptoms are often the presenting complaint.

Seizures in chronic patients present as either 1 to 3 partial complex or generalized tonic-clonic seizures. Status epilepticus is associated with more significant morbidity and mortality. There are no known predisposing factors for seizures in chronic toxicity. Seizures have been reported in chronic patients with theophylline concentrations >20 mg/L, and the incidence increases significantly with serum concentrations >60 mg/L. Age >60 years is the sole prognostic factor for chronic toxicities. Although there are no definitive supportive data, it is thought that serum theophylline concentrations >60 mg/L in a chronic presentation is associated with an increased incidence of significant morbidity or mortality.

Increased morbidity and mortality in the chronic presentation are more likely with drug-disease state etiologies than with drug-drug or drug-diet interactions.

Gastric decontamination is not indicated for the chronic patient. For theophylline concentrations >30 mg/L, oral activated charcoal at 25 g every 2 hours is initiated and continued until concentrations are <30 mg/L or gastrointestinal complications occur. Either hemodialysis or charcoal hemoperfusion is indicated in the chronic patient when serum theophylline concentration is >60 mg/L, especially in patients >60 years of age, although there are fewer data supporting this recommendation than there are for acute ingestions and concentrations >100 mg/L. Electrolyte disturbances are treated conventionally in the chronic overdose patient.

BIBLIOGRAPHY

Cooling DS: Theophylline toxicity. *J Emerg Med* 11:415–425, 1993.

Kempf J, Rusterholtz T, Ber C, et al: Hemodynamic study as guideline for the use of beta blockers in acute theophylline poisoning. *Intensive Care Med* 22:585–587, 1996.

Osborn HH, Henry G, Wax P, et al: Theophylline toxicity in a premature neonate—elimination kinetics of exchange transfusion. *J Toxicol Clin Toxicol* 4:639–644, 1993.

Polak M, Rolon MA, Chouchana A, et al: Theophylline intoxication mimicking diabetic ketoacidosis. *Diabetes Metab* 25:513–516, 1999.

Paloucek FP: Theophylline toxicokinetics. *J Pharm Pract* 6:57–62, 1993.

Sessler CN: Theophylline toxicity and overdose: Predisposing factors, clinical features, and outcome of 116 consecutive cases. *Am J Med* 88:567–576, 1990.

Shannon M: Predictors of major toxicity after theophylline overdose. *Ann Intern Med* 119:1161–1167, 1993.

Shannon M: Effect of acute versus chronic intoxication on clinical features of theophylline poisoning in children. *J Pediatr* 121:125–130, 1992.

Shannon MW: Comparative efficacy of hemodialysis and hemoperfusion in severe theophylline intoxication. *Acad Emerg Med* 4:674–678, 1997.

Shannon MW: Life-threatening events after theophylline overdose. *Arch Intern Med* 159:989–994, 1999.

108

Lethal Toxins
in Small Doses

Leon Gussow

HIGH-YIELD FACTS

- Camphor is present in many over-the counter liniments and cold preparations. As little as 1 g has been reported to cause death in an 18-month-old child.

- Clinical symptoms of camphor toxicity, which occur rapidly with onset 5 to 120 minutes after ingestion, typically begin with a feeling of generalized warmth progressing to pharyngeal and epigastric burning, followed by mental status changes. Muscle twitching and fasciculations may herald the onset of seizures, which have also been reported to occur suddenly, without preceding symptoms.

- Management of ingestion of camphor consists of supportive care and gastric decontamination. Seizures are managed with benzodiazepines or phenobarbital.

- Asymptomatic patients should be observed for 8 hours after ingestion of camphor prior to discharge from the emergency department.

- Benzocaine is present in many local anesthetics, including first aid ointments and infant teething formulas. Benzocaine is metabolized to aniline and nitrosobenzene, both of which can cause methemoglobinemia, especially in infants <4 months of age, who are deficient in methemoglobin reductase.

- Clinical signs and symptoms of benzocaine toxicity begin 30 minutes to 6 hours after ingestion, with tachycardia, tachypnea, and a characteristic cyanosis that does not respond to oxygen. Treatment of toxicity consists of gastric emptying, general support, and in selected cases the administration of the antidote, methylene blue, which is indicated for methemoglobin levels >30 percent and symptoms of respiratory distress or altered mental status.

- Lomotil is an antidiarrheal preparation that combines an opiate (diphenoxylate) with an anticholinergic (atropine). After ingestion, respiratory depression can recur as late as 24 hours and there appears to be no correlation between dose ingested and severity of symptoms. Therefore any child with known or suspected ingestion of any amount of Lomotil is admitted and monitored for at least 24 hours, no matter what the initial clinical condition.

- Chloroquine, an antimalarial agent, is a powerful rapidly-acting cardiotoxin capable of causing sudden cardiorespiratory collapse. The interval between ingestion and cardiac arrest is often <2 hours.

- Methyl salicylate is a concentrated liquid that is absorbed quickly and can produce early-onset severe salicylate toxicity. Ingestion of <1 teaspoon has been fatal in a child.

The majority of toxic exposures in pediatric patients do not result in serious side effects. Those that do generally result from toxic drugs that are taken in clearly excessive amounts. There are a number of prescription and over-the-counter preparations that can have extreme toxicity when taken in surprisingly small amounts. Familiarity with these is essential for the emergency department physician.

CAMPHOR

Camphor is present in many over-the-counter liniments and cold preparations. Campho-Phenique is 10.80 percent camphor, Ben-Gay Children's Rub contains 5 percent, and Vicks Vaporub 4.18 percent. Camphor has long been used as an antipruritic, rubefacient, and antiseptic. A common source of serious toxicity in the past has been camphorated oil, which was sometimes mistaken for castor oil and administered to children in high doses. Fortunately this product is no longer available.

Camphor is an aromatic cyclic terpene with a ketone group. It has a strong, unmistakable odor and a pungent taste that some children find appealing. It is highly lipophilic, and is a rapidly acting neurotoxin, producing both CNS excitation and depression. As little as 1 g has been reported to cause death in an 18-month-old child. Major toxicity has not been reported for ingestions <30 mg/kg and is rare in ingestions <50 mg/kg. Ingestions of <1 teaspoon of topical liniments or cold preparations should not cause toxicity.

Clinical symptoms begin rapidly, with onset 5 to 120 minutes after ingestion. Initially, a feeling of generalized warmth progresses to pharyngeal and epigastric burning. Mental status changes can follow, with confusion, restlessness, delirium, and hallucinations. Muscle twitching and fasciculations may herald the onset of seizures, which have also been reported to occur suddenly, without preceding symptoms. The epileptogenic potential of camphor was demonstrated in 1919 by a researcher who administered camphorated oil at a dose of 3 to 4.5 g to 20 children between 1 and 4 years of age. All the children developed symptoms and most developed seizures.

Management of ingestion of camphor consists of supportive care and gastric decontamination. Gastric lavage is the preferred method if it can be accomplished within 1 hour of ingestion. The use of ipecac is discouraged due to the potential for the ingestion to provoke seizures. Lavage is followed by the administration of activated charcoal. Seizures are managed with benzodiazepines. The drug of choice for status epilepticus is phenobarbital. Asymptomatic patients should be observed for 8 hours after ingestion prior to discharge from the emergency department.

BENZOCAINE

Benzocaine is present in many local anesthetics, including first aid ointments and infant teething formulas. Baby Orajel contains 7.5 percent benzocaine, Baby Orajel Nighttime Formula 10 percent, and Americaine Topical Anesthetic First Aid Ointment 20 percent. Exposure can be from oral ingestion or dermal absorption. Benzocaine is metabolized to aniline and nitrosobenzene, both of which can cause methemoglobinemia, especially in infants <4 months of age, who are deficient in methemoglobin reductase. Methemoglobinemia has occurred in an infant after an ingestion of 100 mg of benzocaine, the amount in one-quarter teaspoon of Baby Orajel. Recently, reports have appeared in the medical literature of male infants developing methemoglobinemia from EMLA cream (lidocaine/prilocaine) utilized for analgesia during circumcision.

Clinical signs and symptoms begin 30 minutes to 6 hours after ingestion, with tachycardia, tachypnea, and a characteristic cyanosis that does not respond to oxygen. In more severe exposures, agitation, hypoxia, metabolic acidosis, lethargy, stupor, and coma may supervene. Seizures can occur.

Treatment of toxicity consists of gastric emptying, general support, and in selected cases the administration of antidote. Gastric emptying is indicated in patients presenting within approximately 30 minutes of ingestion who have ingested more than one-quarter teaspoon of a benzocaine-containing substance. Gastric lavage is the preferred method. Ipecac-induced emesis is contraindicated. After gastric emptying, activated charcoal is administered along with a cathartic.

The antidote for patients with methemoglobinemia is methylene blue. Indications for use include methemoglobin levels >30 percent and symptoms of respiratory distress or altered mental status. The dose is repeated in 1 to 2 hours if symptoms persist. Isolated cyanosis is not an indication for methylene blue, since it often occurs at low methemoglobin levels, is usually well tolerated, and resolves spontaneously. There is a further discussion of the use of methylene blue in Chap. 98.

LOMOTIL

Lomotil is an antidiarrheal preparation that combines an opiate (diphenoxylate) with an anticholinergic (atropine). Several unique properties make Lomotil poisoning extremely dangerous in the pediatric population and a common cause of death. Respiratory depression can recur as late as 24 hours after ingestion, and there appears to be no correlation between the dose ingested and the severity of symptoms. Therefore any child with known or suspected ingestion of any amount of Lomotil is admitted and monitored for at least 24 hours, no matter what the initial clinical condition.

Each tablet or 5 mL of liquid Lomotil contains 2.5 mg diphenoxylate hydrochloride and 0.025 mg atropine sulfate. Difenoxine is the major metabolite of diphenoxylate and is both more active and longer-acting (half-life, 12 to 14 hours) than its parent drug. This metabolite is probably responsible for the recurrent respiratory depression often seen in these overdoses.

Ingestions of $\frac{1}{2}$ to 2 tablets have been reported to cause toxic signs and symptoms. The lowest reported fatal dose is 1.2 mg/kg. Both atropine and diphenoxylate are rapidly absorbed from the gastrointestinal tract, but since the anticholinergic effect from atropine can delay gastric emptying, intact tablets have been recovered on lavage as long as 27 hours after ingestion.

Although patients often present with a confusing mix of opioid and anticholinergic signs and symptoms, opioid effects are always seen in overdose and often predominate. Atropine symptoms can occur before, during, or after opioid manifestations, or may not occur at all. Initial manifestations of Lomotil overdose in children include drowsiness, lethargy or excitement, dyspnea, irritability, miosis, hypotonia or rigidity, and urinary retention. In severe cases the patient may present with coma, respiratory depression, hypoxia, and seizures. Symptoms may not be related to the dose ingested, and can recur as late as 24 hours after ingestion. Death is often accompanied by cerebral edema.

Treatment of Lomotil poisoning includes admission of all patients and close monitoring for a minimum of 24 hours. Syrup of ipecac is contraindicated, since CNS depression may supervene and induced emesis will delay the administration of activated charcoal. In any patient with CNS or respiratory depression, gastric lavage is indicated even if many hours have passed since ingestion. Multiple-dose activated charcoal (1 g/kg every 4 hours) is recommended because difenoxine undergoes enterohepatic recycling. A cathartic can be given with the first dose of charcoal, but is not repeated with every dose. A Foley catheter may be needed to relieve urinary retention. Excessive hydration should be avoided to minimize the risk of cerebral edema. Respiratory depression and coma are treated with intravenous naloxone (0.1 mg/kg), which may have to be repeated frequently. A maintenance dose of naloxone can be given, starting with two-thirds of the bolus dose that initially produced the desired response administered each hour, titrated to clinical condition. When naloxone is given, anticholinergic symptoms may emerge.

CHLOROQUINE

Chloroquine is a powerful rapidly-acting cardiotoxin capable of causing sudden cardiorespiratory collapse. The interval between ingestion and cardiac arrest is often <2 hours. Chloroquine is used for the treatment and prophylaxis of malaria, and also to treat certain connective tissue diseases. Even a slightly supratherapeutic dose can be toxic in a child, and deaths have been associated with ingestions of 0.75 to 1 g.

Chloroquine causes myocardial depression and vasodilation, producing sudden profound hypotension. Automaticity and conductivity of heart muscle is also decreased, resulting in bradycardia and ventricular escape rhythms. The electrocardiogram can show sinus bradycardia, widened QRS, prolonged intraventricular con-

duction time, T wave changes, ST depression, prolonged QT, complete heart block, ventricular tachycardia, or ventricular fibrillation. Neurotoxicity secondary to chloroquine often presents as drowsiness and lethargy, followed by excitability. Dysphagia, facial paresthesias, tremor, slurred speech, hyporeflexia, seizures, and coma can occur.

Treatment is largely supportive. The physician should be prepared to treat sudden cardiac or respiratory arrest. Intubation, ventilation, defibrillation, and cardiac pacing may be required. Blood pressure is maintained with intravenous fluids and pressors. Class IA antiarrhythmics (quinidine, procainamide, disopyramide) are contraindicated. Induction of emesis should be avoided; gastric lavage is the preferred method of gastric emptying. Activated charcoal (1 g/kg) and a cathartic should be given by mouth or via orogastric tube. Recent evidence suggests that early mechanical ventilation with high-dose diazepam and epinephrine may be life-saving in severe cases. A poison control center should be consulted for any case of significant chloroquine ingestion.

METHYL SALICYLATE

Methyl salicylate is a concentrated liquid that is absorbed quickly and can produce early-onset severe salicylate toxicity. It is found in many topical liniments (Ben Gay, Icy Hot Balm), and in oil of wintergreen food flavoring. One teaspoon of oil of wintergreen contains 7 g of salicylate (equivalent to 21 aspirin tablets). Ingestion of <1 teaspoon has killed a child, therefore any ingestion of these preparations is potentially serious. Clinical presentation and treatment of this overdose is similar to that of other types of salicylate poisoning.

BIBLIOGRAPHY

Couper RT: Methemoglobinemia secondary to topical lignocain/prilocaine in a circumcised neonate. *J Paediatr Child Health* 36:406, 2000.

Gouin S, Patel H: Unusual cause of seizure. *Pediatr Emerg Care* 12;298, 1996.

Koren G: Medications which can kill a toddler with one tablet or teaspoonful. *Clin Toxicol* 31:407–413, 1993.

Liebelt EL, Shannon MW: Small doses, big problems: A selected review of highly toxic common medications. *Pediatr Emerg Care* 9:292–297, 1993.

McCarron MM, Challoner KR, Thompson GA: Diphenoxylate-atropine (Lomotil) overdose in children: An update (report of eight cases and review of the literature). *Pediatrics* 87:694–700, 1991.

Phelan WJ: Camphor poisoning: Over-the-counter dangers. *Pediatrics* 57:428–430, 1976.

Potter JL, Hillman JV: Benzocaine-induced methemoglobinemia. *JACEP* 8:26–27, 1979.

Riou B, Barriot P, Rimailho A, et al: Treatment of severe chloroquine poisoning. *N Engl J Med* 318:1–6, 1988.

Siegel E, Wason S: Camphor toxicity. *Pediatr Clin North Am* 33:375–379, 1986.

Townes PL, Geertsma MA, White MR: Benzocaine-induced methemoglobinemia. *Am J Dis Child* 131:697–698, 1977.

109

Human and Animal Bites

David A. Townes

HIGH-YIELD FACTS

- Bite wounds account for approximately 1 percent of emergency department visits each year in the United States.

- The majority of bite wounds occur in children.

- It is important to obtain a thorough history and perform a complete examination of these injuries.

- Wound infection is the greatest potential complication of these injuries.

- Thorough wound cleaning including adequate irrigation is the best method to prevent wound infection.

- Antibiotic treatment should be directed at the most likely infective agent.

- *Pasteurella* species are a common infective agent in both dog and cat bite wounds.

- *Eikenella corrodens* is a common infective agent in human bite wounds.

- Rabies and tetanus prophylaxis should be considered in animal bite injuries.

- Bite wounds treated on an outpatient basis should be reevaluated within 48 hours.

An estimated 2 million bite wounds are reported each year in the United States. The actual number is undoubtedly higher. Bite wounds account for approximately 1 percent of all emergency department visits and result in numerous hospitalizations. More than half of these injuries occur in children. Dog bites account for the majority (75 to 90 percent), followed by cat bites (10 percent), with the remainder divided between a variety of animal species. Boys tend to be bitten more often than girls, and these injuries are clustered in the summer months. Due to the frequency of these injuries and the potential morbidity associated with them, it is important that the physician working in the emergency department be familiar with their management.

HISTORY AND PHYSICAL EXAMINATION

Proper management of bite wounds begins with a thorough history and physical examination. It is important to obtain a complete history of the injury, including what type of animal caused the wound and the age of the wound. One must also elicit host factors that may affect wound healing. Especially important is a history of diabetes, peripheral vascular disease, chronic use of glucocorticoids, or other immunocompromised states.

The physical examination should include a full examination and exploration of the wound. The type of wound (laceration, crush, or puncture) and the extent of involvement of deep structures must be determined. If the wound occurs over a joint, the joint should be examined through the full range of motion. When appropriate, radiographs should be obtained to look for fractures, foreign bodies, and air in the joint or soft tissues. One should keep in mind that the canine jaw can generate forces up to 450 pounds per square inch. In children this force may be sufficient to penetrate the cranium. Computed tomography of the head should be considered in bite wounds to the scalp. Careful attention should be paid to signs of infection, including erythema, swelling, discharge, lymphadenopathy, or pain on passive range of motion.

WOUND CARE

The most common complication associated with bite wounds is wound infection. Numerous studies have been performed to determine the rate of infection of bite wounds. These have demonstrated infection rates as high as 30 percent for dog bites, 50 percent for cat bites, and 60 percent for human bites. This is in comparison to an infection rate of approximately 15 percent for other wounds. It is therefore important to make every effort to minimize the risk of infection. One of the best methods of reducing the risk of infection is adequate irrigation of the wound. An acceptable method is to irrigate the wound with 1 to 2 L of normal saline through a 19- or 20-gauge vascular catheter. This will provide enough pressure to dislodge and wash away bacteria without inoculating organisms or further disrupting deeper tissues. The wound should be debrided as needed.

The decision to close the wound depends on its age, type, and location. Under no circumstances should a wound that appears infected be closed. In most cases, bite wounds on the hand should be left open because of the high potential for morbidity if these wounds become infected. Dog bites may be safely closed if they are not located on the hands. Cat bites, which are usually puncture wounds, should not be closed because they cannot be adequately cleaned. The question of whether puncture wounds should be extended to better irrigate them remains controversial and should be decided on an individual basis. Cat bites that are lacerations rather than puncture wounds may be closed if they are not on the hands. In general, wounds that are more than 8 to 12 hours old should be left open. Potentially disfiguring bite wounds on the face may be closed even when more than 12 hours old; however, these patients must be followed very carefully for evidence of infection. Surgical consultation should be obtained if there is a question concerning the management of these wounds.

The decision to close any bite wound must be made after adequate exploration and cleaning of the wound. All bite wounds treated on an outpatient basis should be reevaluated within 48 hours.

ANTIBIOTICS

Wounds that have evidence of infection should be treated with antibiotics. The use of antibiotics in prophylaxis remains controversial. The type of animal, location of the wound, and host factors must be considered. Wounds on the hands and feet should be treated with antibiotics, while those on the face and scalp are less likely to become infected and do not need prophylactic antibiotic coverage. In general, bite wounds caused by cats and humans should be treated prophylactically, while those caused by dogs and rodents may not need treatment with antibiotics. If the decision to treat with prophylactic antibiotics is made, the initial treatment should be for 3 days. If at the end of this time there is no evidence of infection, the wound is very unlikely to become infected and the antibiotics may be discontinued.

In general, the organisms responsible for bite wound infections are from the animal's oral flora rather than the host's skin flora. Over 200 different organisms have been identified in bite wounds. About one-third of wound infections demonstrate multiple organisms. One study of dog and cat bite wound infections demonstrated a median of five bacterial isolates per wound culture. The predominant organism in any bite wound will depend on the type of animal causing the wound. Dog bites tend to become infected with *Staphylococcus aureus, Streptococcus* species, and *Pasteurella canis,* but *Pseudomonas* species, *Enterobacter cloacae,* and many others have been identified. Cat bites are likely to become infected with *Pasteurella multocida.* In a recent study of infected wounds, *Pasteurella* species were the most common organisms isolated in both dog and cat bite wounds. These organisms cause a rapidly developing infection with signs and symptoms apparent in less than 24 hours. Delay in these findings for more than 24 hours should lead the physician to consider other etiologic agents such as *Staphylococcus* or *Streptococcus* species. Human saliva contains 10^8 bacteria per mL, with over 40 species represented. Human bite wounds tend to become infected with *Staphylococcus aureus, Streptococcus* species, and *Eikenella corrodens. Pasteurella* species are unlikely infectious agents in human bite wounds.

Antibiotic coverage should be directed at the most likely infective organism. In the case of dog and cat bites *Staphylococcus* and *Streptococcus* species may be covered by dicloxacillin or a first-generation cephalosporin. *Pasteurella* species are covered by penicillin, ampicillin, amoxicillin, amoxicillin/clavulanic acid, second- and third-generation cephalosporins, doxycycline, trimethoprim-sulfamethoxazole, clarithromycin, and azithromycin. In vitro, antistaphylococcal penicillins, first-generation cephalosporins, clindamycin, and erythromycin are less active against *Pasteurella* species. Empiric therapy for dog and cat bites should include a beta-lactam antibiotic and a beta-lactamase inhibitor, a second-generation cephalosporin with anaerobic activity, or a combination of penicillin and a first-generation cephalosporin. For human bite wounds, *Eikenella corrodens* is covered by penicillin or amoxicillin/clavulanic acid, and dicloxacillin can be used to cover *Staphylococcus* and *Streptococcus.* It may be necessary to use a two-antibiotic regimen for human bite wounds.

RABIES PROPHYLAXIS

Rabies infection should be considered in animal bite injuries. Rabies is a viral infection transmitted in the saliva of infected animals. It is caused by the rhabdovirus group and may lead to encephalomyelitis. The disease is almost universally fatal. Only 55 cases have been reported in the United States since 1960, but it continues to be a substantial problem in certain parts of the world.

In determining the need for rabies prophylaxis, the physician must consider the type of animal causing the injury and the prevalence of rabies in the region. If rabies is not suspected, no treatment is indicated. In the case of dogs, cats, and ferrets, the animal should be captured and quarantined for 10 days. If the animal remains healthy, no treatment is necessary. If the animal becomes ill or if rabies is suspected, the animal should be sacrificed and the brain examined for evidence of rabies. If the animal is infected the child should be immediately vaccinated. Most other carnivores including skunks, raccoons, and foxes should be considered infected unless proven negative by laboratory testing. Livestock, large rodents, lagomorphs, and other mammals should be considered on an individual case basis. If the animal cannot be located, decisions regarding prophylaxis must be based on the prevalence of rabies in the area and the species of biting animal. Local animal control authorities may be helpful in obtaining this information. Postexposure prophylaxis is indicated for bite, scratch, or mucous membrane exposure to a bat if the animal cannot be collected and tested. Postexposure prophylaxis may be indicated in cases in which contact is likely to have occurred but is not documented. This includes a child sleeping in a room where a bat is found.

Postexposure prophylaxis includes the administration of one of the available vaccines and human rabies immune globulin. The vaccine, such as human diploid cell vaccine (HDCV), is given in five 1-mL intramuscular injections on days 0, 3, 7, 14, and 28. It should be administered in the deltoid or anterolateral thigh. It should not be administered in the gluteal area. Human rabies immune globulin (HRIG) is dosed at 20 IU/kg. If feasible, the entire volume should be infiltrated into the wound and the surrounding area. Any remaining volume should be administered at a site remote from the vaccine administration. HRIG is not indicated in people who have been previously vaccinated. The same syringe should not be used to administer the vaccine and the HRIG.

TETANUS PROPHYLAXIS

Tetanus immunoprophylaxis should also be considered. Refer to Chap. 23 for guidelines.

CONCLUSION

Proper treatment of bite wounds includes a history, physical examination, exploration, and thorough cleaning of the wound, including adequate irrigation. In general, older wounds, puncture wounds, and those on the hands should be left open. It is essential that any wound suspected of being infected be treated with antibiotics. The choice of antibiotic should be based on the most likely infective agents. The need for antibiotic prophylaxis should be determined on a case-by-case basis. Rabies and tetanus prophylaxis must also be considered. Bite wounds treated on an outpatient basis should be reevaluated within 48 hours. Through careful and complete assessment and treatment of these wounds, the physician can optimize patient outcome.

BIBLIOGRAPHY

Dire DJ: Emergency management of dog and cat wounds. *Emerg Med Clin North Am* 10:719, 1992.

Edwards MS: Infections due to human and animal bites, in Geigin RD, Cherry JD (eds): *Textbook of Pediatric Infectious Diseases,* 4th ed. Philadelphia: Saunders, 1998, pp 2841–2855.

Human Rabies Prevention—United States, 1999. Recommendations of the Advisory Committee on Immunization Practices (ACIP). *MMWR* 48:1-21, 1999.

Jackson SC: Mammalian bites, in Surpure JS (ed): *Synopsis of Pediatric Emergency Care.* Boston: Andover Medical, 1993, pp 393–401.

Talan DA, Citron DM, Abrahamian FM, et al: Bacteriologic analysis of infected dog and cat bites. *N Engl J Med* 340: 85–92, 1999.

Trott A: Bite wounds, in Trott A (ed): *Wounds and Laceration: Emergency Care and Closure,* 2nd ed. St. Louis: Mosby-Year Book, 1997, pp 265–284.

Wilkerson JA: Clinical updates in wilderness medicine—rabies update. *Wilderness Environ Med* 11:31–39, 2000.

110

Snake Envenomations

Timothy Erickson
Bruce E. Herman
Mary Jo A. Bowman

HIGH-YIELD FACTS

- Pit vipers (crotalids) account for the majority of envenomations in children.
- Pit viper envenomations result in hematotoxicity while coral snakes (Eliapidae) cause neurotoxicity.
- Prehospital management of snakebites includes immobilization of the bitten extremity, minimization of physical activity, fluid administration, and rapid transport to the nearest health care facility.
- Because of their small body weight, infants and young children are relatively more vulnerable to severe envenomation.
- In addition to supportive care, Crotalidae antivenin is the fundamental treatment of pit viper envenomation.

Snake bites usually occur when people venture into the snake's natural habitat, but bites have been reported among religious sects that handle snakes, as well as in pet owners and zoo workers. Families of venomous snakes indigenous to the United States include the Crotalidae (pit vipers) and Elapidae (coral snakes). The pit vipers account for over 95 percent of all envenomations and are divided into the genuses *Crotalus* (rattlesnakes), *Agkistrodon* (cottonmouths and copperheads), and *Sistrusus* (pygmy rattlesnakes and massasaugas). According to the 1999 annual report of the American Association of Poison Control Centers (AAPCC), 228 children under 20 years of age were bitten by rattlesnakes, 160 by copperheads, 29 by cottonmouths, 12 by coral snakes, and 24 by exotic poisonous snakes. No deaths were reported. These statistics reflect the low case fatality rate associated with snake envenomations. Table 110-1 lists the poisonous snakes that are indigenous to the United States.

PIT VIPERS

Anatomy

A few anatomic characteristics differentiate venomous pit vipers from nonpoisonous snakes. Pit vipers classically possess a triangular or arrow-shaped head, whereas nonpoisonous snakes have a smooth, tapered body and narrow head. Crotalids have facial pits between the nostril and eye that serve as heat and vibration sensors, enabling the snake to locate prey. While nonpoisonous snakes typically possess round pupils, pit vipers have vertical or elliptical pupils. Members of the genus *Crotalus* are further characterized by tail rattles.

Pathophysiology

Since snakes are defensive animals and rarely attack, they will remain immobile or even attempt to retreat if given the opportunity. Bites most commonly occur in small children who are paralyzed with fear or in individuals who harass the snake. Because of their small body weight, infants and young children are relatively more vulnerable to severe envenomation. The severity of envenomation also depends on the location of the bite. Bites on the head or trunk are more severe than extremity bites. Bites on the upper extremities are most common and potentially more dangerous than those on the lower extremities, whereas lower extremity bites may result in delayed clinical signs of toxicity. Direct envenomation into an artery or vein is associated with a much higher mortality rate.

The venom itself is a complex mixture of enzymes that primarily function to immobilize, kill, and digest the snake's prey. Proteolytic enzymes cause muscle and subcutaneous necrosis due to a trypsin-like action. Hyaluronidase decreases the viscosity of connective tissue, phospholipase provokes histamine release from mast cells, and thrombin-like amino acid esterases act as defibrinating anticoagulants. The major toxic effects occur within the surrounding tissue, blood vessels, and blood components.

Clinical Presentation

Local cutaneous changes classically include 1 or 2 puncture marks with pain and swelling at the site, while nonvenomous snakes usually leave a horseshoe-shaped imprint of multiple teeth marks. If the envenomation is severe, swelling and edema may involve the entire extremity within an hour. Ecchymosis, hemorrhagic vesicles, and petechiae may appear within several hours.

Table 110-1. Indigenous Poisonous Snakes of the United States

Southeast
  Eastern coral snake (*Micrurus fulvius fulvius*)
  Cottonmouths and copperheads (*Agkistrodon* spp.)
  Timber rattlesnake (*Crotalus horridus*)
  Eastern diamondback rattlesnake (*C. adamamteus*)
  Massasauga pygmy rattlesnake (*Sistrurus miliarius*)
East/Northeast
  Cottonmouths and copperheads (*Agkistrodon* spp.)
  Timber rattlesnake (*C. horridus*)
  Eastern massasauga (*S. catenatus*)
Mideast/Midwest/Central
  Cottonmouths and copperheads (*Agkistrodon* spp.)
  Timber rattlesnake (*C. horridus*)
  Western prairie rattlesnake (*C. viridus*)
  Eastern massasauga (*S. catenatus*)
  Massasauga pygmy rattlesnake (*S. miliarius*)
Southwest/West
  Cottonmouths and copperheads (*Agkistrodon* spp.)
  Western coral snake (*M. fulvius tenere*)
  Western diamondback rattlesnake (*C. atrox*)
  Western prairie rattlesnake (*C. viridus*)
  Great basin rattlesnake (*C. viridus lutosus*)
  Sidewinder rattlesnake (*C. cerastes*)
  Mojave rattlesnake (*C. scutulatus*)
  Timber rattlesnake (*C. horridus*)
  Rock rattlesnake (*C. lepidus*)
  Black-tailed rattlesnake (*S. molossus*)
  Twin-spotted rattlesnake (*C. pricet*)
  Red diamond rattlesnake (*C. ruber*)
  Speckled rattlesnake (*C. mitchelli*)
  Tiger rattlesnake (*C. tigris*)

Systemic signs and symptoms include paresthesias of the scalp, periorbital fasciculations, weakness, diaphoresis, nausea, dizziness, and a minty or metallic taste in the mouth. Severe bites can result in coagulopathies and disseminated intravascular coagulation (DIC). Rapid hypotension and shock, with pulmonary edema and renal and cardiac dysfunction, can also result, particularly if the victim suffers a direct intravenous envenomation.

Management

The victim's extremity should be immobilized and physical activity minimized. To maintain renal flow and intravascular volume, oral fluids are vigorously administered. Overaggressive first aid measures can actually be dangerous. Incision and suction of the bite wound with the mouth may result in tissue damage or infection. Mechanical suction devices exist and have been anecdotally reported to remove up to one-third of the venom if used immediately after envenomation, but no well-designed human clinical trials exist that support their use. Cryotherapy can lead to further wound necrosis and is not currently recommended. Electric shock therapy was highly publicized as a first aid treatment of snakebites, but again case reports and animal studies have not documented any improvement with this technique.

Wounds are graded as

- Minimal, with local cutaneous swelling and tenderness at the bite site
- Moderate, with significant extremity swelling and evidence of systemic toxicity
- Severe, with obvious systemic findings, unstable vital signs, and laboratory evidence of coagulopathy

Useful laboratory tests include complete blood count, platelet count, prothrombin time, partial thromboplastin time, fibrin split products, electrolytes, renal functions, creatine phosphokinase, blood type, and cross-matched blood products.

The patient's tetanus prophylaxis should be updated if needed, and broad-spectrum antibiotics administered in moderate or severe envenomations. The progression of extremity edema and swelling should be carefully monitored. If evidence of compartment syndrome exists in the involved extremity, an orthopedic consultation and fasciotomy may be indicated. In reality, the likelihood of true compartment syndrome resulting from snakebites is low, and is greatly minimized with proper and timely management.

In addition to supportive care, Crotalidae antivenin is the fundamental treatment for pit viper envenomation. The antivenin is a high-affinity antibody that binds to the venom proteins and enhances elimination. It is effective against envenomations from rattlesnakes, cottonmouths, copperheads, fer-de-lance, cantiles, and South American bushmasters. The amount of antivenin administered depends on the severity of the envenomation. Antivenin is packaged in vials containing 10 mL. In general, if the envenomation is rated as minimal, 5 vials are routinely administered; in moderate cases, 10 vials are used; and in severe cases 15 to 20 vials are administered. The amount of antivenin administered can also vary depending on the species and geographic distribution of the snake. In comparison with adults, pediatric patients are given proportionately more antivenin, since children receive a greater amount of venom per kilogram of body weight. Antivenin is most efficacious if given within 4 to 6 hours of the bite. It is of less value if delayed for 8 hours, and is of questionable value after 24 hours. Prior to any antivenin administration, skin testing is done with dilute horse serum given subcutaneously (this is usually included in the antivenin kit). However, skin testing is often inconsistent and can produce false-negative and -positive results. In the setting of a severe envenomation, patients with positive skin reactions can still receive the antivenin, although close monitoring for anaphylaxis and pretreatment with diphenhydramine and glucocorticoids, as well as a readily available supply of epinephrine are critical.

Complications of the antivenin therapy include anaphylaxis and serum sickness. Serum sickness, a flu-like syndrome with fever, malaise, arthralgias, lymphadenopathy, rash, pruritus, and urticaria, usually develops 10 to 20 days after antivenin administration, with symptoms proportionate to the number of vials given. It is generally self-limited and effectively treated with antihistamines and a short course of glucocorticoids. A new affinity-purified ovine FAB antibody fragment antivenin that may minimize hypersensitivity reactions is currently being tested in clinical trials.

Disposition

The prognosis following pit viper envenomation is generally good, with an overall mortality rate of <1 percent if the antivenin is given in adequate amounts without delay. Even when the antivenin is withheld due to severe allergic reactions, the morbidity and mortality are low. If a pediatric patient only has a suspected bite, develops no signs or symptoms of envenomation during 6 to 12 hours of observation, and has normal laboratory studies, the child can be discharged. Exceptions to this rule are bites from the Mojave rattlesnake, which can cause delayed neurological and respiratory depression several hours after envenomation. If the child exhibits moderate to severe envenomation, has evidence of coagulopathy, or requires antivenin administration, admission to an intensive care unit is indicated.

CORAL SNAKES

Two members of the coral snake family (Elapidea) are indigenous to the United States. The western coral snake *(Micrurus euryxanthus)* is found in Arizona and New Mexico and the eastern coral snake *(Micrurus fulvius*

fulvius) is found in the Carolinas and the Gulf states. A mnemonic quote to help distinguish the coral snakes from nonpoisonous snakes in the United States is "red on yellow, kill a fellow; red on black, venom lack," which refers to order of the colored bands that run vertically down the body of the coral snake. Coral snakes account for only 1 to 2 percent of annual snakebites in the United States.

Clinical Presentation

The venom of the coral snake is primarily neurotoxic. The bite site will initially exhibit local cutaneous edema, swelling, and tenderness. However, there have been reports of envenomation without evidence of actual tooth marks. Within several hours the patient may experience paresthesias, vomiting, weakness, diplopia, fasciculations, confusion, and occasionally respiratory depression. Convulsions have been observed in smaller children. The fatality rate from eastern coral snake bites is as high as 10 percent.

Management

Coral snake bites are treated aggressively, since a significant bite can lead to neurological and respiratory depression within 24 hours. Antivenin is administered early in the treatment course. The coral snake antivenin is effective against bites of the eastern coral snake, but not against western coral snake bites. Fortunately the venom of the western coral snake is less toxic than that of its eastern counterpart. Three to five vials of the antivenin are generally recommended following skin testing. As with the *Crotalid* antivenin, adverse side effects include anaphylaxis and serum sickness.

Disposition

Any child who has sustained a documented bite from a coral snake is admitted to the intensive care unit for airway management and appropriate antivenin administration for a 24- to 48-hour period.

EXOTIC SNAKES

Several bites occur each year from nonindigenous snakes. Physicians encountering victims of exotic snake envenomation may receive assistance in treatment by calling the local zoo's herpetologist or regional poison control center. The general approach is local wound care, supportive treatment, and specific antivenin therapy, if available.

BIBLIOGRAPHY

Chippaux JP: Snake bites: Appraisal of the global situation. *Bull World Heath Org* 76:515–524, 1998.

Clark RF, Williams SR, Nordt SP, Boyer-Hassen LV: Successful treatment of crotalid-induced neurotoxicity with new polyvalent FAB antivenom. *Ann Emerg Med* 30:54–57, 1997.

Cruz NS, Albarez RG: Rattlesnake bite complications in children. *Pediatr Emerg Care* 10:30, 1994.

Dart RC, McNally J: Efficacy, safety and use of snake antivenoms in the United States. *Ann Emerg Med* 37:181–188, 2001.

Holstege CP, Miller A, Wermuth M, et al: Crotalid envenomation. *Crit Care Clin* 13:889–921, 1997.

Lawrence WT, Giannopoulos A, Hansen A: Pit viper bites: Rational management in locales in which copperheads and cottonmouths predominate. *Ann Plastic Surg* 36:276–285, 1996.

Litovitz TL, Schwartz-Klein W, White S, et al: 1999 Annual report of the American Association of Poison Control Centers toxic exposures surveillance system *Am J Emerg Med* 18(5):517–574, 2000.

Norris RL, Bush SP: North American venomous reptile bites, in Auerbach PS (ed): *Wilderness Medicine: Management of Wilderness Emergencies,* 4th ed. St. Louis: Mosby, 2001, pp 896–926.

Sing KA, Erickson TB, Aks SE, et al: Eastern massassauga rattlesnake envenomations in an urban wilderness. *J Wild Med* 5:77, 1994.

Whitley RE: Conservative treatment of copperhead snakebites without antivenin. *J Trauma* 41:219–221, 1996.

111

Spider and Arthropod Bites

Timothy Erickson
Bruce E. Herman
Mary Jo A. Bowman

HIGH-YIELD FACTS

- Black widow spider bites result in painful muscle spasms secondary to neurotoxicity, that are responsive to antivenin.
- Brown recluse spider bites result in hematotoxicity and manifest locally as skin necrosis.
- Scorpion stings cause severe localized pain with occasional systemic effects in children.
- Hymenoptera stings can result in severe anaphylactic reactions.
- Fire ant stings can cause painful localized skin reactions.

At least 50 to 60 species of spiders found in the United States are known to bite humans, although in most cases the diagnosis is not suspected and no treatment is necessary. Only the black widow and brown recluse spiders are known to cause significant wounds, and rarely death. According to the annual report of the American Association of Poison Control Centers (AAPCC), in 1999 589 children under 20 years of age suffered bites from black widow spiders, while 535 were envenomated by brown recluse spiders. During this period, one pediatric death was reported secondary to a brown recluse spider envenomation in a 6-year-old child.

BLACK WIDOW SPIDERS

Anatomy

Black widow spiders of the genus *Latrodectus* are found throughout the temperate and tropical zones of the earth. *Latrodectus mactans,* the black widow spider of North America, is a shiny black spider with eight eyes, eight legs, fangs, and poison glands, with a characteristic red hourglass mark on the ventral surface of the abdomen.

Pathophysiology

Black widow spiders are web-spinning, trapping spiders that normally bite only as a feeding or defense mechanism; however, on occasion the female may devour her male counterpart following the mating ritual. From a toxicological viewpoint, only the female is venomous to humans. The jaws and poison glands of the male are too small to be considered dangerous.

In the early decades of the 20th century, bites about the genitals were common because of the widespread use of outhouses. With the advent of indoor plumbing and electricity in rural areas, the frequency of envenomation has decreased, and currently the most common bite site is the hand. Bites normally occur when the spiders are distributed in the vicinity of homes in such objects as garden tools, old clothing, and woodpiles.

Latrodectus venom is a potent toxin. Physiologically, the venom of the black widow facilitates exocytosis of synaptic vesicles and the release of the neurotransmitters norepinephrine, gamma-aminobutyric acid, and acetylcholine. The toxin also causes degeneration of motor endplates, resulting in denervation. The venom destabilizes nerve cell membranes by opening ion channels, causing a massive influx of calcium into the cell, which results in hypocalcemia.

Clinical Presentation

Latrodectus bites produce a characteristic syndrome. The bite itself typically produces a pinprick or burning sensation and frequently goes unnoticed. Within the first few hours, the bite site may develop redness, cyanosis, urticaria, or a characteristic halo-shaped target lesion. This is followed by more generalized symptoms consisting of pain in the regional lymph nodes, chest, abdomen, and lower back. The pain classically descends down the lower extremities, with burning of the soles of the feet. Abdominal rigidity along with vomiting is often severe enough to be mistaken for a surgical emergency. Flexor spasm of the limbs will cause the patient to assume a fetal position while writhing in pain. Patients may also demonstrate hypertension, sweating, salivation, dyspnea with increased bronchosecretions, and convulsions. If untreated, symptoms may last for up to 7 days, with persistent muscle weakness and pain for several weeks. Although uncommon, death can result from respiratory or cardiac failure, with overall mortality rates of <5 percent.

Management

For local pain relief, early application of ice to the bitten area may be effective. Tetanus prophylaxis should be updated, but antibiotics are not routinely indicated unless there is evidence of wound infection. For pain control, opiates are useful, but are often suboptimal, particularly if administered orally. A parenteral opiate such as morphine is recommended. Muscle relaxants such as diazepam have been commonly administered, and these provide some, but usually limited, pain relief. Because of the relative hypocalcemia induced by black widow spider bites, many recommend 10 percent calcium gluconate at 1 to 2 mL/kg up to 10 mL/dose, given slowly with careful cardiac monitoring as the first-line treatment in symptomatic patients. However, many of the reports regarding the use of calcium have been anecdotal, and more recent studies refute its effectiveness. These studies strongly recommend administration of *Latrodectus*-specific antivenin for severe envenomations. The antivenin is available in Australia and Arizona, where these envenomations most commonly occur. Since the antivenin is derived from horse serum, the patient should be skin tested by injecting a 1:10 dilution subcutaneously to test for anaphylactic reactions prior to administration of a full dose of the antivenin. The use of *Latrodectus*-specific antivenin is restricted to patients with severe envenomation and no allergic contraindications and in whom opioids and benzodiazepines are ineffective. Patients who should receive the antivenin early include the very young and the elderly as well as those with hypertensive and cardiac disease. The antivenin provides relief within 1 to 2 hours and readministration is rarely indicated. Patients receiving the antivenin may experience flu-like symptoms or serum sickness 1 to 3 weeks following treatment. This entity is generally self-limited and responsive to antihistamines and steroids.

Disposition

Any symptomatic pediatric patient who has suffered a bite from a black widow spider is admitted for observation and pain control. If there is cardiopulmonary compromise or convulsions, the child is admitted to the intensive care unit for stabilization and antivenin administration.

BROWN RECLUSE SPIDERS

Anatomy

The brown recluse spider, *Loxosceles reclusa,* is a brown to fawn-colored spider, 1 to 5 cm in length, with a characteristic violin or fiddle-shaped marking on the dorsal cephalothorax (it is nicknamed the fiddleback spider). They have long, slender legs and have six eyes instead of the eight typical of most spiders.

Pathophysiology

These spiders are very reclusive nocturnal hunters. Their webs are scant and ill-defined, and these creatures only bite humans when threatened. Envenomations typically occur during the months of April through October, at night, while the victim rummages through an old closet or attic, puts on a shoe, or uses a blanket containing a trapped spider. Humans are most commonly bitten on the extremities.

The venom of the *Loxosceles* spider is more potent than that of the rattlesnake and can cause extensive skin necrosis. The venom acts directly on the cell wall, causing immediate injury and cell death. It contains the calcium-dependent enzyme sphingomyelinase D, which along with C-reactive protein has a direct lytic effect on red blood cells. Following cell wall damage, an intravascular coagulation process causes a cascade of clotting abnormalities and local polymorphonuclear leukocyte infiltration, culminating in a necrotic ulcer.

Clinical Presentation

The clinical response of loxoscelism ranges from a cutaneous irritation (necrotic arachnidism) to a life-threatening systemic reaction. Signs and symptoms of envenomation are most often localized to the bite area. Normally, there is little pain at the time of the bite. Within a few hours the patient experiences itching, swelling, erythema, and tenderness over the bite site. Classically, erythema surrounds a dull blue-grey macule circumscribed by a ring or halo of pallor. This color difference is important in identifying necrotic arachnidism. Gradually, within 3 to 4 days, the wound forms a necrotic base with a central black eschar. Within 7 to 14 days the wound develops a full necrotic ulceration.

The systemic reaction, which is much less common than the cutaneous reaction, is associated with higher morbidity. The reaction rarely correlates with the severity of the cutaneous lesion. Within 24 to 72 hours following the envenomation, the patient experiences fever, chills, myalgias, and arthralgias. If the systemic reaction is severe, the patient may suffer coagulopathies, disseminated intravascular coagulation (DIC), convulsions, renal failure, and hemolytic anemia, heralded by the passage of dark urine.

Of note is the increased incidence of a spider from a separate genus, most commonly called the hobo spider, which is geographically distributed throughout the northwestern United States. As with the brown recluse, bites of this spider have been documented to result in a similar, but milder, form of necrotic arachnidism.

Management

The proper management of envenomation by the brown recluse spider depends on whether the reaction is local or systemic. Since it is difficult to predict which type of wound will eventually progress to a disfiguring necrotic ulcer, the wound should be cleaned, tetanus immunization updated, and the involved extremity immobilized to reduce pain and swelling. Early application of ice to the bite area lessens the local wound reaction, whereas heat will exacerbate the symptoms. Antibiotic treatment is indicated only in secondary wound infections. Antihistamines may prove beneficial, particularly in children. Many experts advocate the use of a polymorphonuclear leukocyte inhibitor such as dapsone to diminish the amount of scarring and subsequent surgical complications. Its use is controversial and it has not been proven effective in any large study with human or animal control cases. Because of limited human studies and the potential for dapsone to induce methemoglobinemia, cautious administration is recommended in the pediatric population. Although supported in the early literature, early excisional treatment can cause complications such as recurrent wound breakdown and hand dysfunction. A better approach is to wait until the necrotic process has subsided (usually within several weeks) and perform secondary closure with skin grafting as indicated.

The systemic effects of brown recluse spider envenomation can be life threatening and should be treated aggressively. Although not proven in clinical trials, glucocorticoids may provide a protective effect on the red blood cell (RBC) membrane, thus slowing the hemolysis. The patient must be monitored closely for the development of DIC. Transfusion of RBCs and platelets may be necessary. Urine alkalinization with bicarbonate may lessen renal damage if the patient is experiencing acute hemolysis. Although it is not commercially available in the United States, there is ongoing research with a brown recluse antivenin.

Disposition

Patients with a rapidly expanding lesion or necrotic area with evidence of hemolysis are hospitalized. Patients who are asymptomatic following a period of observation in the emergency department and have normal baseline laboratory data may be discharged home with close outpatient follow-up and wound care within 24 to 48 hours.

TARANTULAS

Tarantulas are widely feared because they are the largest of all spiders. Found in the deserts of the western United States, these large, hairy spiders are relatively harmless. They are extremely shy and bite only when vigorously provoked or roughly handled. Their bite produces only local pain and edema. Treatment consists of local wound care and tetanus prophylaxis. Of more concern are the hairs on their abdomen, which when flicked off in defense are capable of producing urticaria and pruritus that may persist for several weeks. Treatment includes antihistamines and topical glucocorticoids.

SCORPIONS

Worldwide, scorpions are responsible for thousands of deaths annually. In the United States there have been no reported deaths from scorpion stings in more than 25 years. Nevertheless, they remain a public health concern throughout the South and Southwest. The scorpion has a pair of anterior legs with pinchers, a segmented body, and a long, mobile tail equipped with a stinger. While members of the genera *Hadrurus, Vejovis,* and *Uroctonus* are capable of inflicting painful wounds, only the southwestern desert scorpion *(Centruroides exilicauda,* formerly *C. sculpturatus)* poses a serious health threat in the United States. Also called bark scorpions because they cling to the bottom of fallen brush and trees, they are brownish in color, vary in length from 1 to 6 cm, and are most active at night. The chitin shell of this scorpion will fluoresce under an ultraviolet or Wood's lamp, aiding in identification. *Centruroides* venoms cause spontaneous depolarization of nerves of both the sympathetic and parasympathetic nervous systems.

Unless the scorpion is identified, the diagnosis is based on clinical symptoms. Most victims will have only local pain, tenderness, and tingling; however, young children and those who suffer more serious envenomations may manifest the venom effects as overstimulation of the sympathetic, parasympathetic, and central nervous systems. Elevation of all the vital signs usually occurs within an hour of envenomation, and tachydysrhythmias may develop during this time. Dysconjugate, "roving" eye movements are very common in children, along with other neurological findings, including muscle fasciculations, weakness, agitation, and opisthotonos. Less common findings are ataxia, respiratory distress, and seizures.

The treatment of *Centruroides* envenomations is supportive. Cool compresses and analgesics are used for the local symptoms and pain. Wound care and tetanus prophylaxis are indicated. Tachydysrhythmias and hypertension may be treated with intravenous beta blockers, such as esmolol or labetalol. Benzodiazepines may be helpful for agitation and muscle spasms. Advanced life support and airway control are essential for more severe envenomations. A hyperimmune goat serum antivenin has been used with success for more severe envenomations with potentially life-threatening symptoms; however, it is available only in Arizona. Consultation for treatment is available through the Arizona Poison Control System.

HYMENOPTERA

The order Hymenoptera includes bees, vespids (hornets and wasps), and fire ants. These insects cause one-third of all reported envenomations in the United Sates and an estimated 50 to 150 annual deaths. While Hymenoptera venoms possess intrinsic toxicity, it is their ability to sensitize the victim and cause subsequent anaphylactic reactions that makes them so lethal.

Bees and Vespids

Honeybees *(Apis mellifera)* are fuzzy insects with alternating black and tan body stripes. Not intrinsically aggressive, they usually sting defensively when stepped on. Like that of other Hymenoptera, the honeybee's stinger is a modified ovipositor (only females sting) that is connected to a venom sac.

African "killer" bees *(Apis mellifera scutellata)* were imported into Brazil during the 1960s in order to improve honey production. Over the years, they migrated north into Central America. Recently they have been sighted in the United States in areas with winter temperatures above 60°F, such as Texas, Arizona, New Mex-

ico, and southern California. They are very aggressive, attack in swarms, and death has occurred as a result of the large amount of venom injected.

The most common hornets in the United States are the yellow jackets *(Vespa pennsylvanica).* They are usually seen around garbage cans, beverage containers, and various foods. They are extremely aggressive and sting with little provocation. Wasps *(Polistes annularis,* the paper wasp) have thin, smooth bodies and a formidable sting. They build their nests in the eaves of buildings. These vespids are carnivorous, able to use their smooth stingers multiple times, unlike honeybees, which lose their stingers after a single sting.

Hymenoptera venoms contain enzymes that directly affect vascular tone and permeability. Although their enzymes are similar, there is little immunologic cross-reactivity between bee and vespid venoms. While a bee sting may not sensitize a person to yellow jacket venom, a yellow jacket sting would more likely sensitize one to wasp venom.

Sting reactions are usually classified as local, toxic, or systemic. Local reactions result from the vasoactive effects of the venom and are generally mild. There is variable edema and erythema associated with pain at the sting site.

If present, the embedded stinger should be removed manually. Previous sources recommended cautiously scraping the stinger off with lateral pressure, rather than grasping it, in order to avoid compression of the venom sac resulting in further release of venom. However, recent studies have demonstrated that this is erroneous, because the venom has likely been completely released within seconds of envenomation. Treatment is symptomatic, with ice or cold compresses and an antihistamine. In more severe local reactions, there is a more sustained inflammatory response; the swelling may spread to the entire extremity and persist for several days. A short course of prednisone (1 mg/kg/d for 5 days) may decrease the duration of symptoms. Toxic reactions reflect the effects of multiple stings (usually over 25 to 50 stings). Gastrointestinal symptoms are the principal features; urticaria and bronchospasm are not usually present. Treatment is supportive.

Systemic reactions occur in approximately 1 percent of Hymenoptera stings. They range from mild, non–life-threatening cutaneous reactions to classic anaphylactic shock. These reactions are generally IgE-mediated and reflect previous sensitization. However, 50 to 75 percent of patients who die from insect stings have no prior history of hypersensitivity. Sensitivity develops after a sting when venom-specific IgE antibodies are produced in reaction to antigens in the venom, and the antibodies then bind to tissue mast cells and circulating basophils. With a subsequent sting, the venom antigens bind with the venom-specific IgE antibodies on the surface of these target cells. Sensitivity causes degranulation and the release of mediators of anaphylaxis, such as histamine and products of the arachidonic acid cascade, which leads to systemic symptoms. The majority (7 percent) of systemic reactions in children consist of generalized urticaria, pruritus, or angioedema. More severe reactions are manifested as bronchospasm, laryngeal edema, and hypotensive shock secondary to massive vasodilation.

In all but the mildest of systemic reactions, the mainstay of treatment is epinephrine. Epinephrine counteracts the bronchospastic and vasodilatory effects of histamine. Epinephrine can be given as a subcutaneous injection (0.01 mL/kg of 1:1000 solution). In more severe reactions, the intravenous or endotracheal route is preferred (0.1 mL/kg of 1:10,000 solution). The dose may be repeated at 15-minute intervals as needed. Early intubation is indicated if there is evidence of severe laryngeal edema or stridor, because airway obstruction is the leading cause of death in anaphylaxis. Antihistamines should be given early, but not as a substitute for epinephrine. An H_2-receptor blocker (e.g., cimetidine or ranitidine), in addition to an H_1-receptor blocker (diphenhydramine), may aid in inhibiting the vasodilatory effects of histamine. Adjunctive therapy for bronchospasm might include inhaled β_2 agonists (e.g., albuterol) and intravenous aminophylline. When hypotension is present, vigorous isotonic fluid resuscitation should be instituted. Glucocorticoids should be given for their anti-inflammatory effects as well as their effect of preventing the late-phase response. A delayed serum sickness–like reaction may appear 10 to 14 days following the initial sting. This immune complex disorder may be treated with a short course of prednisone.

Essential to the treatment of any systemic reaction is the prevention of future reactions. Patients who have had a systemic reaction should be instructed to wear protective clothing and avoid Hymenoptera-infested habitats. Portable epinephrine kits are available. They should be prescribed prior to the patient leaving the emergency department. The patient should be urged to carry the kit at all times and to use epinephrine for any systemic symptoms. Even if symptoms are mild, the patient should still seek emergency care. The patient should also be instructed to wear a medical alert tag.

Venom immunotherapy desensitization is very effective in preventing further systemic reactions, with 95 to 100 percent protection after 3 months of treatment. Referral to an allergist is indicated for any child who has life-threatening respiratory symptoms (e.g., stridor or wheezing) or hypotension. Children less than 16 years old who have only urticaria or angioedema do not require venom immunotherapy. Only 10 percent of these children will have systemic reactions with subsequent stings.

Imported Fire Ants

Two species of fire ants have been imported into the United States: the red fire ant *(Solenopsis invicta)* and the black fire ant *(Solenopsis richteri),* of which *S. invicta* is the predominant species. They were "imported" aboard ships from South America during World War II and subsequently spread throughout the Southeast. They are presently found in 13 southern states, from Florida to Texas, their geographic range apparently limited by soil, temperature, and moisture.

S. invicta are 2 to 5 mm in size and red in color. They live in colonies and build large mounds up to 3 feet in diameter, which are interconnected by underground tunnels up to 80 feet long. These mounds are found most commonly in yards, playgrounds, and open fields. Fire ants are aggressive insects with no natural enemies. They are social insects and tend to attack in swarms, with multiple stings the norm. In endemic areas, nearly 50 percent of the exposed population is stung each year. Stings are more common among children and occur most frequently on their ankles and feet during the summer months.

Fire ants sting in a two-phase process. The ant first bites the victim with powerful mandibles, then, if undisturbed, will arch the body and swivel around the attached mandibles to sting the victim repeatedly with the stinger. This produces a characteristic circular pattern of papules/stings around two central punctures.

Fire ant venoms produce a sharp, burning sensation; hence the name. The venoms have cytotoxic, bactericidal, insecticidal, and hemolytic properties. They also activate the complement pathway and promote histamine release. Fire ant venoms are immunogenic and result in sensitization of the sting victim and the risk of future anaphylaxis.

Clinical manifestations reflect the venom's effects and are predominantly local dermatologic reactions. The initial bites and stings cause burning pain associated with circular wheals or papules around the central hemorrhagic punctures. The wheal-and-flare reactions resolve within 1 hour, but then develop into sterile pustules within 24 hours. The pustules slough off over 48 to 72 hours, leaving shallow ulcerated lesions. The pustules are intensely pruritic and often become contaminated after the victim scratches the lesions. These secondary infections are usually minor but may cause considerable morbidity. No intervention has been shown to prevent or resolve the pustules, and treatment consists of local conservative measures: application of ice or cool compresses for symptomatic relief and gentle, frequent cleansing of the affected areas to prevent secondary infections. An oral antihistamine may be helpful for the pruritus.

Between 15 and 50 percent of victims develop more severe local reactions, characterized by an exaggerated wheal-and-flare response followed by the development of erythema, edema, and induration >5 cm in diameter. These lesions are intensely pruritic, may resemble cellulitis, and persist for 24 to 72 hours before subsiding. Topical glucocorticoid ointments, local anesthetic creams, and oral antihistamines may be useful for the itching associated with these reactions.

Anaphylactic reactions have been estimated to occur after as many as 1 percent of fire ant stings. Anaphylaxis may occur several hours after a sting and is known to occur more frequently in children than in adults.

Immunotherapy may be appropriate for persons with severe hypersensitivity to fire ant venom or those who have had a previous anaphylactic reaction to a fire ant sting. The efficacy of immunotherapy has been variable, but it has been reported to provide as high as 98 percent protection.

BIBLIOGRAPHY

Clark RF, Wethern-Kestner S, Vance MV, et al: Clinical presentation and treatment of black widow spider envenomation: A review of 163 cases. *Ann Emerg Med* 21:782–787, 1992.

Cohen PR: Imported fire ant stings: Clinical manifestations and treatment. *Pediatr Dermatol* 9:44, 1992.

Erickson T, Hryhorczuk DO, Lipscomb J, et al: Brown recluse spider bites in an urban wilderness. *J Wild Med* 1:258–264, 1990.

Kim KT, Oguro J: Update on the status of Africanized honeybees in the western United States. *West J Med* 170:220–222, 1999.

Litovitz TL, Schwartz-Klein W, White S, et al: 1999 Annual report of the American Association of Poison Control Centers toxic exposures surveillance system. *Am J Emerg Med* 18:517–574, 2000.

Lovecchio F, Welch S, Klemmens J, et al: Incidence of immediate and delayed hypersensitivity to centruroides antivenin. *Ann Emerg Med* 34: 615–619, 1999.

Minton S, Bechtel B, Erickson T: North American arthropod envenomation and parasitism, in Auerbach PS (ed): *Wilderness Medicine,* 4th ed. St. Louis: Mosby, 2001, pp 863–887.

Philips S, Kohn M, Baker D, et al: Therapy of brown spider envenomation: A controlled trial of HBO, dapsone and cryoheptadine. *Ann Emerg Med* 25:363–368, 1995.

Sofer S, Shahak E, Gieron M: Scorpion envenomation and antivenin therapy. *J Pediatr* 124:973–978, 1994.

Vetter RS, Visscher PK, Camizine S: Mass envenomation by honey bees and wasps. *West J Med* 170:223–227, 1999.

112

Marine Envenomations

Timothy Erickson
Bruce E. Herman
Mary Jo A. Bowman

HIGH-YIELD FACTS

> - Hot water soaks are recommended for sting ray, scorpion fish, echinoderm, and catfish stings.
> - Alter the pH with weak acids such as vinegar to neutralize coelenterate and jellyfish envenomations.
> - For most marine stings, local wound care, irrigation, tetanus immunization, wound exploration for foreign bodies, and broad-spectrum antibiotic coverage are indicated.
> - Antivenins are available for stonefish, box jellyfish, and sea snake envenomations.

COELENTERATES

Coelenterates include jellyfish, sea anemones, and corals. They envenomate through organelles called nematocysts, which contain venom-coated threads that are found in specialized epithelial cells on the tentacles. Upon contact or when encountering a change in osmolality, these threads are injected through the epidermis to the nerve- and vascular-rich dermis. Both living and dead coelenterates can envenomate, as can fragmented tentacles and "unfired" nematocysts on the skin. Venoms vary, but generally contain histamine and enzymes capable of causing systemic as well as predominant local tissue effects. Jellyfish stings are the most common marine envenomations, with an estimated 500,000 annual stings occurring in the Chesapeake Bay and 250,000 in Florida.

One of the more feared jellyfish is the Portuguese man-of-war (*Physalia physalis*). This jellyfish is most commonly found in the Gulf of Mexico and off the Florida coasts between July and September. The tentacles can be up to 30 meters in length and envenomation causes char-

acteristic linear, spiral, painful urticarial lesions. The pain occurs almost instantly, peaks within a few hours, and persists for many more. Systemic symptoms may include nausea, vomiting, muscle cramps, diaphoresis, weakness, hemolysis, and rarely, vascular collapse and death. The most deadly and venomous coelenterate is the box jelly-fish (or sea wasp) of Australia. Death can occur within minutes of envenomation. If the victim can be rescued from the water, an antivenin is available.

The most commonly encountered jellyfish is the sea nettle (*Chrysacra quinquecirrha*), which is widely distributed in temperate and tropical waters. Sea nettles cause predominantly local effects consisting of painful urticarial lesions. Treatment includes reassurance of the patient and immobilization of the injured part. Ice may provide some analgesia. The area is rinsed with sterile saline or seawater to maintain isosmolar conditions and wash off unfired nematocysts. Fresh water is not used because it is hypoosmolar and will activate unfired nematocysts. To inactivate nematocysts remaining on the skin, vinegar (5 percent acetic acid solution) is recommended. The inactivated nematocysts are then removed by gentle scraping or shaving. One can also use the edge of a credit card, piece of driftwood, or clam shell. Analgesics and antihistamines are helpful. Tetanus immunization is indicated, but prophylactic antibiotics are not.

Sea anemones and corals are sessile creatures that cause local urticarial reactions upon contact. Contact with hard corals may cause lacerations that are treated with vigorous local wound care, tetanus prophylaxis, and a broad-spectrum antibiotic.

VENOMOUS FISH

There are over 250 species of venomous fish, consisting mostly of shallow water reef or inshore fish. Stingrays are the most commonly encountered venomous fish, with more than 2000 stings reported annually. Eleven species of stingrays are found in United States coastal waters. They are flat, round-bodied fishes that burrow underneath the sand in shallow waters. When startled or stepped on, the stingray thrusts its spiny tail upward and forward, driving its venom-laden stinging apparatus into the foot or lower extremity of the victim. As the sting is withdrawn, the sheath surrounding it ruptures and the venom is released. Parts of the sheath may be torn away and remain in the wound. The venom is short acting, heat-labile, and causes varying degrees of neurological and cardiovascular disturbance. Intense pain out of proportion to the injury is the initial finding, peaking within

1 hour but lasting up to 48 hours. Signs and symptoms are usually limited to the injured area, but weakness, nausea, anxiety, and syncope in response to the severe pain have been reported. Treatment of the wound includes irrigation with sterile saline or seawater to dilute the venom and remove sheath fragments. The injured part is immersed in hot water, no warmer than 113°F, for 30 to 90 minutes to inactivate the heat-labile venom. Analgesics are usually required. Because of the penetrating nature of the envenomation, wounds are debrided and left open. Tetanus immunization is updated and broad-spectrum prophylactic antibiotics such as trimethoprim-sulfamethoxazole (TMP-SMX), ciprofloxacin, or a third-generation cephalosporin are administered.

Varieties of scorpion fish include zebrafish *(Pterois),* lionfish, scorpion fish *(Scorpaena),* and stonefish *(Synanceja),* in increasing order of venom toxicity. Although more common in tropical waters of the Indo-Pacific, these fish are found in the shallow water reefs of the Florida Keys, Gulf of Mexico, southern California, and Hawaii. Envenomations occur from spines on their dorsal or pelvic fins and are often associated with lacerations. The venoms are heat-labile and cause immediate intense pain that peaks within 60 to 90 minutes and persists for up to 12 hours. Local erythema or blanching, edema, and paresthesias may persist for weeks. Systemic findings include nausea and vomiting, weakness, dizziness, and respiratory distress. Treatment is immersion of the affected limb in hot water (113°F) for 30 to 90 minutes, or until pain is relieved. Wounds are irrigated with sterile saline, explored, and cleaned of debris. The wound is left open and treated with prophylactic antibiotics (TMP-SMX, ciprofloxacin, or a third-generation cephalo-sporin) in addition to tetanus prophylaxis.

Stonefish envenomations occur less frequently. Although similar to those of the other scorpion fish, their clinical manifestations are more severe. Stonefish venom, a potent neurotoxin, can cause dyspnea, hypotension, and cardiovascular collapse within 1 hour and death within 6 hours. They can also cause local necrosis and severe pain that may persist for days. Local treatment of stonefish stings is the same as that for envenomations of other scorpion fish, with special attention given to maintaining cardiovascular support and administration of a specific stonefish antivenin, available in Australia.

Catfish

More than 1000 species of catfish are found in both fresh and salt water. Stings occur from spines contained within an integumentary sheath on their dorsal or pec-

toral fins. The hands and forearms of fishermen are the most common sites. The heat-labile venoms contain dermatonecrotic, vasoconstrictive, and other bioactive agents and produce symptoms similar to those of mild stingray envenomations. A stinging, burning, throbbing sensation occurs immediately and usually resolves within 60 to 90 minutes, but will occasionally last up to 48 hours. Treatment is immediate immersion in hot water (no warmer than 113°F) for pain relief. Catfish spines may penetrate the skin and break off, and the spines can be seen on radiographs. The wound should be explored and debrided and any retained catfish spines should be removed. The puncture wound should be left open and treated with prophylactic broad-spectrum antibiotics, in addition to tetanus prophylaxis.

ECHINODERMS

Echinoderms are spiny invertebrates that include sea urchins, starfish, sand dollars, and sea cucumbers. Of these, sea urchins are the only ones that regularly cause medically significant envenomations. They are slow moving, colorful bottom dwellers found at various ocean depths. The spines can be up to one foot long in the needle-spined urchin *(Diadema).* They can puncture the skin when picked up or stepped on, break off, and be retained. Their venom can cause local pain that may persist for days. Treatment is immediate immersion in hot water (no warmer than 113°F), careful removal of pedicellariae and radiopaque spines, and vigorous local wound care. Tetanus immunization and broad-spectrum antibiotic prophylaxis are indicated.

SEA SNAKES

Sea snakes are encountered throughout the Indo-Pacific region. They are among the deadliest snakes in the world, and will bite with little provocation. Envenomations result in severe neurotoxicity with rapid muscular and respiratory paralysis. If the patient can be rescued from the water, respiratory support is often required. An antivenin is commercially available.

BIBLIOGRAPHY

Aldred B, Erickson T, Lipscomb J, et al: Lionfish stings in an urban wilderness. *J Wilderness Environ Med* 4:291–296, 1994.

Auerbach P: Envenomation by aquatic animals, in Auerbach PS (ed): *Wilderness Medicine,* 4th ed. St. Louis: Mosby, 2001, pp 1450–1487.

Brown CK, Shepherd SM: Marine trauma, envenomations and intoxications. *Emerg Med Clinic North Am* 10:385, 1992.

Exton D, Moran PJ, Williamson J: Phylum Echinodermata, in Williamson JA, Fenner PJ, Burnett JW, et al (eds): *Venomous and Poisonous Marine Animals.* Sydney: University of South Wales, 1999, pp 312–326.

Fenner PJ, Williamson JA: Worldwide deaths and severe envenomation from jellyfish stings. *Med J Aust* 165:658, 1996.

Tomaszewski C: Aquatic envenomations, in Ford M, DeLaney K, Ling L, et al (eds): *Clinical Toxicology.* Philadelphia: Saunders, 2001, pp 970–984.

113

Near Drowning

Gary R. Strange
Simon Ros

HIGH-YIELD FACTS

- Drowning is the second most common cause of nonintentional death in children and adolescents. Unfenced swimming pools represent a major risk for children <5 years of age and approximately 50 percent of adolescent drownings are associated with the use of alcohol.

- Fluid aspiration occurs in 90 percent of drowning victims, but it is unusual for large quantities of water to be aspirated. Laryngospasm prevents aspiration in 10 percent of cases, resulting in "dry" drowning.

- Hypothermia appears to exert a protective effect on drowning victims, especially when rapidly induced. The diving reflex, which results in preferential shunting of blood to the brain and the heart, has been suggested as an additional contributing factor to intact survival following extended submersion in very cold water ($\leq 40°F$).

- Early initiation of cardiopulmonary resuscitation in a submersion victim is of paramount importance. As cardiopulmonary resuscitation in the water is not effective, the patient must be extricated as soon as possible, maintaining cervical spine precautions throughout.

- All patients are placed on a cardiac monitor and pulse oximeter, and 100 percent oxygen is administered by mask or endotracheal tube. Patients who have an arterial P_{O_2} <50 mmHg or P_{CO_2} >50 mmHg while on 100 percent oxygen are intubated.

- Death or long-term disability from pulmonary complications is rare and some 95 percent of victims will lead lives that are relatively unaltered. Poor prognostic indicators include prolonged submersion in non-icy water, ventricular fibrillation as the initial rhythm, and absence of a perfusing rhythm on arrival in the emergency department.

- Asymptomatic patients with normal arterial blood gases and chest radiographs may be discharged after a 6-hour period of observation. All other patients are admitted to the hospital.

The most widely accepted definitions for submersion injuries are

- Drowning: to die from suffocation in water.

- Near drowning: to survive, at least temporarily, after suffocation by submersion in water.

- Secondary drowning: delayed death (>24 hours after submersion) due to rapid deterioration of respiratory status. Secondary drowning occurs in approximately 5 percent of near drowning patients.

- Immersion syndrome: sudden death following contact with icy-cold water.

Drowning is the second most common cause of non-intentional death in children and adolescents, second only to motor vehicle crashes. Drowning is responsible for approximately 8000 fatalities in the United States each year. Two age groups in the pediatric population are especially at risk for submersion injuries: children under 5 years of age and adolescents.

Some 40 percent of childhood drownings occur in toddlers and young children who typically die in tubs or pools. Unfenced swimming pools represent a major risk for children <5 years of age. Adolescents usually drown in ponds, lakes, rivers, and the ocean. Approximately 50 percent of adolescent drownings are associated with the use of alcohol. Submersion injuries are more common in males than females in all age groups, with the male:female ratio being 3:1 among young children and 6:1 in adolescents. Patients of any age with the autosomal dominant long QT syndrome (Romano-Ward syndrome) may experience unexplained fainting, near drowning, unusual seizures, and sudden death.

The primary injury following submersion occurs in the lung. Hypoxemia, the result of the pulmonary dysfunction, is then the cause of secondary injuries, especially to the brain and heart, where cerebral edema and myocardial failure may develop. Although uncommon, coagulopathies or renal failure may also ensue.

Submersion-induced hypoxemia affects several additional organs. Cardiac dysrhythmias, including asystole, ventricular fibrillation, and bradycardia may occur in submersion victims. Central nervous system abnormalities, including mental status changes, are frequently present in anoxic patients. An ischemic injury to the kidney may result in acute tubular necrosis. Patients may become anuric, oliguric, or polyuric, and renal failure may develop in severe cases.

Fluid aspiration occurs in 90 percent of drowning victims, but it is unusual for large quantities of water to be aspirated. Laryngospasm prevents aspiration in 10 percent of cases, resulting in "dry" drowning. Life-threatening electrolyte abnormalities occur only when the amount of fluid aspirated exceeds 22 mL/kg. Autopsy studies have demonstrated that such quantities of water are aspirated by only 15 percent of drowning victims. Treatment of severe electrolyte disturbances is rarely required.

When significant aspiration occurs, the pathophysiology of lung injury is dependent on the characteristics of the aspirated fluid. Aspiration of fresh water inactivates surfactant and damages the alveolar basement membrane. The loss of surfactant's surface tension activity results in alveolar collapse and a ventilation-perfusion mismatch. The hypotonic water is rapidly absorbed into the pulmonary circulation. Aspiration of hypertonic seawater results in the movement of intravascular fluid into the alveoli, with subsequent edema and shunting.

Hypothermia appears to exert a protective effect on drowning victims, especially when rapidly induced. Low body temperature decreases oxygen requirements, thus enabling organs to survive without oxygen for prolonged periods of time. The diving reflex, which results in preferential shunting of blood to the brain and the heart, has been suggested as an additional contributing factor to intact survival following extended submersion in very cold water ($\leq 40°F$). Hypothermia is discussed in detail in Chap. 115.

MANAGEMENT

Prehospital Care

Early initiation of cardiopulmonary resuscitation in a submersion victim is of paramount importance. As cardiopulmonary resuscitation in the water is not effective, the patient must be extricated as soon as possible. In view of the possibility of neck injury, cervical spine precautions are maintained throughout the patient's management.

Once the patient is on a firm surface, attention is directed to evaluating the ABCs and providing resuscitation as indicated. Oxygen is administered to all patients. Airway maintenance and copious secretions are among the indications for endotracheal intubation. Postural drainage maneuvers are not recommended and may delay cardiopulmonary resuscitation. Cardiac monitoring is begun as soon as possible. Wet clothing is removed to minimize heat loss. Prolonged delay in transport in order to obtain IV access must be avoided. All submersion victims are taken to a hospital for evaluation regardless of their clinical condition following initial stabilization.

Hospital Management

The first step in the hospital management of the submersion victim is the reevaluation of the ABCs. All patients are placed on a cardiac monitor and pulse oximeter and 100 percent oxygen is administered by mask or endotracheal tube. Persistent hypoxemia suggests the need for continuous positive airway pressure (CPAP) or positive end-expiratory pressure (PEEP). Patients who have an arterial Po_2 <50 mmHg or Pco_2 >50 mmHg while on 100 percent oxygen are intubated. Apnea, unstable airway, and prevention of aspiration are other indications for intubation. A chest radiograph and an arterial blood gas are obtained as soon as possible.

Bronchospasm in submersion victims is treated with selective beta agonists such as albuterol. Glucocorticoids and prophylactic antibiotics have not been proven to be of benefit.

Occult injury is common in drowning victims, especially injuries to the head and neck as a result of falls or diving accidents. Emergent cervical spine radiography and computed tomography of the head is indicated in all patients with suspected head and neck injury.

Toxicologic studies should be considered in all victims of submersion. There is a very high correlation between submersion injury and alcohol intoxication in adolescents.

In small children, the potential for intentional abuse or neglect must be considered.

A nasogastric tube is inserted in all submersion victims in order to prevent gastric dilation. Intravenous access must be established promptly and poor perfusion treated with intravenous fluids. Repeated boluses of normal saline or Ringer's lactate (20 mL/kg) are administered until the patient's circulation is stable. Pressor agents, such as dopamine or dobutamine, are used if fluid volume management is ineffective. A Foley catheter is inserted to monitor urine output.

Hypothermia may not be detected unless a rectal temperature is obtained along with the rest of the vital signs. Hypothermia is managed by preventing additional heat loss (through use of heat lamps and the removal of wet clothes) and by core rewarming. Hypothermia merits lengthier resuscitative efforts in view of the reports of persons who survived following prolonged submersion in icy water.

The management of patients with suspected hypoxic cerebral injury includes hyperventilation, head elevation (in the absence of cervical spine injury), furosemide, and muscle relaxants. The use of intracranial pressure monitoring, dexamethasone, mannitol, and high-dose barbiturates are no longer recommended. Hypoxic seizures are controlled with intravenous diazepam (0.3 mg/kg) and phenytoin (20 mg/kg).

PROGNOSIS

The prognosis of near-drowning patients is determined by the severity of the anoxic brain injury and is generally good. Death or long-term disability from pulmonary complications is rare and some 95 percent will lead lives that are relatively unchanged.

The prognostic factors for survival following near drowning have been extensively studied. Early institution of resuscitative efforts and the presence of spontaneous respirations and heartbeat upon presentation to the emergency department are the best predictors of intact neurological survival in drowning victims. Poor prognostic indicators include prolonged submersion in non-icy water, ventricular fibrillation as the initial rhythm, and absence of a perfusing rhythm on arrival in the emergency department. Signs of increased intracranial pressure are consistent with devastating neurological insult and there is no evidence that intracranial pressure monitoring and aggressive treatment alter the outcome.

DISPOSITION

Asymptomatic patients with normal arterial blood gases and chest radiography may be discharged after a 6-hour period of observation. All other patients are admitted to the hospital. Near-drowning victims must not be discharged from the emergency department without observation because of the possibility of delayed pulmonary complications.

BIBLIOGRAPHY

Allen WC: The long-QT syndrome. *N Engl J Med* 342(7): 514–515, 2000.

Causey AL, Tilelli JA, Swanson ME: Predicting discharge in uncomplicated near drowning. *Am J Emerg Med* 18(1):9–11, 2000.

Gheen KM: Near drowning and cold water submersion. *Semin Pediatr Surg* 10(1):26–27, 2001.

Modell JH, Graves SA, Ketover A: Clinical course of 91 consecutive near drowning victims. *Chest* 70:231, 1976.

Pearn J: Successful cardiopulmonary resuscitation outcome reviews. *Resuscitation* 47(3):311–316, 2000.

Quan L: Near drowning. *Pediatr Rev* 20(8):255–259, 1999.

Sachdeva RC: Near drowning. *Crit Care Clin* 15(2):281–296, 1999.

Smith GS, Brenner RA: The changing risks of drowning for adolescents in the U.S. and effective control strategies. *Adolesc Med* 6(2):153–170, 1995.

Zuckerman GB, Conway EE Jr: Drowning and near drowning: A pediatric epidemic. *Pediatr Ann* 29(6):360–366, 2000.

Zuckerman GB, Gregory PM, Santos-Damiani SM: Predictors of death and neurologic impairment in pediatric submersion injuries: The pediatric risk of mortality score. *Arch Pediatr Adolesc Med* 152(2):134–140, 1998.

114

Burns and Electrical Injuries

Gary R. Strange
Barbara Pawel

HIGH-YIELD FACTS

- Scalding is the most common mechanism of thermal injury in the pediatric population. Scalding most commonly results when children <3 years of age reach and tip over hot liquids that are in containers on a stove or counter.

- By far the most lethal cause of burns in children is the house fire, accounting for 45 percent of burn-related deaths. Smoke inhalation and inhalation of other toxic gases also contribute to the morbidity and mortality of the house fire.

- The intentional inflicting of burns to a child is, unfortunately, a common form of abuse. Every burn injury in a child should be evaluated for the potential for abuse or neglect.

- The most common cause of death during the first hour after a burn injury is respiratory impairment. Inhalation injury produces upper airway edema, which can proceed with alarming speed to complete airway obstruction.

- With burns and electrical injury, myoglobin in the urine may result from muscle damage and is indicated by a positive dip test for blood in the absence of red blood cells on the microscopic examination. When myoglobinuria is suspected, aggressive hydration is initiated and potent diuretics, such as furosemide and mannitol, are considered in efforts to maintain high urine flow and prevent tubular necrosis.

- The Parkland formula, a widely accepted formula used to guide fluid resuscitation in burns, recommends isotonic crystalloid to a total amount of 4 mL/kg/%BSA over the first 24 hours, with half of this amount administered over the first 8 hours. Maintenance fluid requirements must be added to the fluid amounts calculated by the Parkland formula.

- It must be remembered that burn fluid calculations provide only an estimation of fluid requirements. Sufficient fluid should be administered to maintain a urine flow of 1 to 1.5 mL/kg/h.

- Room-temperature solutions are sufficient for local wound care. The application of ice or cold solutions is contraindicated due to the possibility of developing hypothermia in extensively burned patients and to the addition of cold injury to the burned surface.

- Very young children often bite on electrical cords, sustaining severe orofacial injuries that are often full-thickness, involving the lips and oral commissure. These burns are initially bloodless and painless, but, as the eschar separates in 2 to 3 weeks, severe bleeding can occur from arterial damage.

- The usual fluid replacement formulas utilized for burn patients underestimate fluid requirements in electrical burn patients. Fluids should maintain a urine output of 1 to 2 mL/kg/h.

BURNS

Thermal injuries are the second most common cause of death in children in the United States. These injuries account for approximately 30,000 hospitalizations and over 3000 deaths annually. Young children have a higher mortality rate from burns than older children and adults, but, with modern advances in treatment, mortality rates have improved significantly. In a recently reported series covering the years from 1991 through 1997, the mortality rate for children with 60 to 100 percent total body surface area (TBSA) burns was only 14 percent. There were no deaths in infants younger than 4 years of age. Sequelae remain significant, however, including respiratory compromise, sepsis, renal failure, vascular compromise, and functional impairment secondary to scarring.

Causes

The severity of a thermal burn is determined by the temperature exposed to and duration of contact. Scalding is the most common mechanism of thermal injury in the pediatric population. Scalding most commonly results when children <3 years of age reach and tip over hot liquids that are in containers on a stove or counter. Partial-thickness burns usually result (Fig. 114-1). Prevention through educating caretakers of the need to turn pot handles so that the child cannot reach them is effective. Bathtub scalds are another common mechanism. These can be prevented by setting hot water temperature at ≤120°F.

Flash injuries result from the ignition of volatile substances. Even though the heat generated is very high, the time of exposure is usually low and only partial-thickness burns result.

Contact of clothing with a flame may result in the ignition of fabrics. This is a common mechanism of burns in children over the age of 2 years who play with matches or other flammable material. Resulting burns may be either full or partial thickness. Flame retardant fabrics, especially for pajamas and nightgowns, are now in common use and have reduced the incidence and severity of injury from "catching on fire."

By far the most lethal cause of burns in children is the house fire, accounting for 45 percent of burn-related deaths. The type of burn varies from minor partial thickness injuries to full-thickness, total-body burns. Smoke inhalation and inhalation of other toxic gases (see Chaps. 87 and 90) also contribute to the morbidity and mortality of the house fire. Much has been done to reduce these injuries through the use of smoke detectors and fire safety instructional programs. Yet house fires continue to take the lives of far too many children every year, especially in the northern tier of the United States and in lower socioeconomic populations.

The intentional inflicting of burns to a child is, unfortunately, a common form of abuse. Every burn injury in a child should be evaluated for the potential for abuse or neglect. For further discussion, see Chap. 118.

Pathophysiology

The center of a burn is an area of coagulation necrosis and vascular thrombosis. There is intense vasoconstriction, caused by the release of vasoactive substance from injured cells, that may lead to ischemia and secondary injury. Surrounding this area are concentric areas of stasis and hyperemia. Later, there is vasodilation and development of gaps between endothelial cells. Vascular permeability is increased and both protein and fluid shift from the vascular to the interstitial space. Tissue edema results and, with major burns, there may be hypoperfusion of tissues, leading to shock. The area of coagulation necrosis provides an excellent medium for the growth of bacteria.

Burns are described in terms of location, depth, and body surface area involved. Location is an important determinant of disposition. Burns of the hands, feet, and perineum should always be considered serious, and all significant burns in these locations should initially be managed in the hospital, preferably in a burn center. Depth of the burn is estimated by clinical criteria, which are used to classify the burn by degrees.

- First-degree burns involve only the epidermis. The skin is erythematous but there are no blisters. Sensation is preserved. A common example is sunburn. First-degree burns heal within 1 week and require only symptomatic treatment.

- Second-degree burns are partial-thickness burns that involve the dermis to a variable degree. The dermal appendages are always preserved and provide a

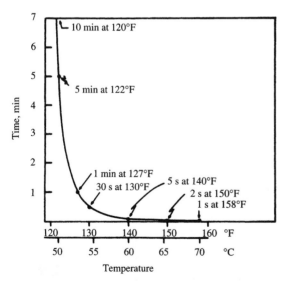

Fig. 114-1. Duration of exposure to hot water to cause full-thickness epidermal burns of skin at various water temperatures.(Reproduced with permission from Katcher ML: Scald burns from hot tap water. *JAMA* 246:1219, 1981. Modified from Moritz AR, Henriques FC Jr: Studies of thermal injury. *Am J Pathol* 23:695, 1947. Copyright 1981, American Medical Association.)

source for regeneration. Second-degree burns are characterized by the presence of marked edema, erythema, blistering, and weeping from the wound. There is usually marked tenderness to palpation. Deep partial-thickness burns may be difficult to distinguish from full-thickness burns. The most common causes of second-degree burns are exposure to hot liquids and flames. Healing requires 2 to 3 weeks.

- Third-degree burns are full-thickness injuries. The dermis and dermal appendages are destroyed. The skin appears whitish or leathery. The surface is dry and nontender to palpation. Third-degree burns result when there is prolonged exposure to fire or hot liquids.

- Fourth-degree burns are burns that extend into deep tissues, such as muscle, fascia, nerves, tendons, vessels, and bone.

The body surface area (BSA) involved is also important in determining treatment and disposition. The percentage surface area involved in the burn is estimated by the "rule of nines" in adults, but in children, the proportion of body surface area, made up by anatomic parts, especially the head, varies considerably with age (Fig. 114-2).

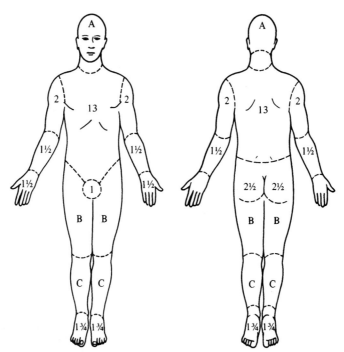

Relative Percentages of Areas Affected by Growth (Age in Years)

	0	1	5	10	15	Adult
A: half of head	$9\frac{1}{2}$	$8\frac{1}{2}$	$6\frac{1}{2}$	$5\frac{1}{2}$	$4\frac{1}{2}$	$3\frac{1}{2}$
B: half of thigh	$2\frac{3}{4}$	$3\frac{1}{4}$	4	$4\frac{1}{4}$	$4\frac{1}{2}$	$4\frac{3}{4}$
C: half of leg	$2\frac{1}{2}$	$2\frac{1}{2}$	$2\frac{3}{4}$	3	$3\frac{1}{4}$	$3\frac{1}{2}$

Second degree _____ and

Third degree _____ =

Total percent burned ____

Fig. 114-2. Classic Lund and Browder chart. (Reproduced with permission from Dimick AR: Burns, in Tintinalli JE, Kelen GD, Stapczynski JS (eds): *Emergency Medicine,* 5th ed. New York: McGraw-Hill, 2000.)

Diagnostic Evaluation

History and Physical Examination

The history of the events leading to the burn may be helpful in assessing the degree of injury and the likelihood of other injuries, such as smoke inhalation and blunt trauma. Concomitant medical problems, medications, allergies, and tetanus immunization status should be ascertained.

Primary Survey

The airway is assessed immediately on presentation. The most common cause of death during the first hour after a burn injury is respiratory impairment. Inhalation injury produces upper airway edema, which can proceed with alarming speed to complete airway obstruction. As edema develops, successful intubation becomes increasingly difficult. Therefore, intubation is indicated early in the emergency department course of patients who have signs of upper airway involvement (Table 114-1).

Humidified oxygen is used to maintain oxygenation. Positive end-expiratory pressure (PEEP) or continuous positive airway pressure (CPAP) may be useful to improve oxygenation when there is pulmonary involvement. Bronchospasm is treated with β-adrenergic agonists. Close monitoring of oxygen saturation by pulse oximetry, supplemented by arterial blood gases, is indicated.

Patients with >15 percent BSA burns require a large-bore intravenous line for isotonic fluid administration. A second line is advisable for extensive burns and is essential if there are signs of cardiovascular instability.

Secondary Survey

After stabilization, a thorough physical examination is needed to assess the burn injury completely and to evaluate for concomitant injury.

Table 114-1. Indications for Early Intubation in Burn Patients

---

Stridor
Hoarseness
Rales
Wheezing
Singed nasal hairs
Carbonized sputum
Cyanosis
Altered mental status

Particular attention to the vascular status of extremities is imperative. Circumferential burns may result in vascular compromise and require escharotomy to prevent limb loss. Limb ischemia is indicated by poor or absent pulses, paresthesias, severe pain, or by poor or absent flow on Doppler evaluation. If present, the patient should undergo prompt escharotomy to release the constricting pressure. Cuts are made laterally on both sides of the constricted structure and carried only to the depth required to see the edges of the wound separate.

Circumferential burns to the thorax may result in respiratory embarrassment, as indicated by poor chest expansion and declining oxygen saturation. Lateral thoracic escharotomy may be life-saving in this situation.

Laboratory Evaluation

A complete blood count is indicated to establish baseline characteristics. The hematocrit will often be elevated secondary to fluid loss, and the white blood cell count is often elevated as a result of an acute-phase reaction. Later in the course, elevation of the white blood cell count is an indicator of infection, which must be diagnosed early and treated aggressively. Serum electrolytes will often reveal an elevated potassium level due to the breakdown of cells, and depressed bicarbonate level due to metabolic acidosis resulting from fluid loss and hypovolemic shock. Renal function tests (blood urea nitrogen and creatinine) are used to assess renal and overall tissue perfusion. On urinalysis, the urine-specific gravity is helpful in assessing the hydration status. The presence of myoglobin is important to detect, since acute tubular necrosis can result. Myoglobin is indicated by a positive dip test for blood in the absence of red blood cells on the microscopic examination. When myoglobinuria is suspected, aggressive hydration is initiated and potent diuretics, such as furosemide and mannitol, are considered in efforts to maintain high urine flow and prevent tubular necrosis. Baseline clotting studies are indicated. Typing and crossmatching for blood is indicated if there is associated trauma or if surgical intervention, such as grafting, is considered. Pulse oximetry, arterial blood gases, and chest radiography are indicated in the management of the patient with airway involvement or with vascular instability. Carboxyhemoglobin level is indicated in all burns that occur in a closed space and for all patients with impaired consciousness (see Chap. 87).

Management

After assurance of airway integrity, the primary guiding principle in burn management is the restoration or maintenance of tissue perfusion. Fluid resuscitation in burns has been the subject of considerable controversy; however, the Parkland formula has gained wide acceptance. Using this formula, isotonic crystalloid, 4 mL/kg/%BSA, is administered over the first 24 hours. Half is administered over the first 8 hours and the remainder over 16 hours. Maintenance fluid requirements must be added to the fluid amounts calculated by the Parkland formula (see Chap. 51).

It must be remembered that burn fluid calculations provide only an estimation of fluid requirements. Sufficient fluid should be administered to maintain a urine flow of 1 to 1.5 mL/kg/h. Patients in shock require aggressive fluid resuscitation and may require hemodynamic monitoring as a guide (see Chap. 3).

Initial wound care consists of sterile saline–soaked dressings. Room-temperature solutions are sufficient; the application of ice or cold solutions is contraindicated due to the possibility of developing hypothermia in extensively burned patients and to the addition of cold injury to the burned surface. The burned surface can be cleaned with povidone-iodine solution and debris and devitalized tissue removed. If the patient is to be transferred to a burn unit, care should be taken to be in compliance with the burn unit protocol. Often, this will include simply covering the burn wound surface with dry sterile sheets after initial cleaning. Most burn units will not want the surface covered with any kind of ointment or cream, since this will impair their assessment of the patient.

Burns that are managed on an outpatient basis will require a bulky sterile dressing. Several biosynthetic dressings are currently available for use on small, superficial partial-thickness burns, but they are expensive and have not been conclusively shown to expedite healing or to improve outcomes.

It must also be remembered that burns are often extremely painful. Once the patient is hemodynamically stabilized, consideration for analgesia with a potent narcotic analgesic, such as morphine, 0.1 to 0.2 mg/kg IV, is indicated. This dose can be repeated at 15 minutes intervals as needed, while monitoring the adequacy of respirations (rate and oxygen saturation), blood pressure, and mental status. Intramuscular, subcutaneous, and oral routes of administration are not appropriate for significant burns due to fluid shifts and the potential for development of gastric stasis.

Tetanus prophylaxis should be considered for all burns. Guidelines are given in Chap. 23. All jewelry on or distal to the burned area and any other constricting items should be removed immediately on presentation.

Minor burns (Table 114-2) can be soaked in sterile saline, cleaned gently with povidone-iodine solution, and dressed with a topical antibiotic preparation. Silver

Table 114-2. Guidelines for Burn Triage and Disposition

Outpatient Management
Partial-thickness burn—less than 10% body surface
Full-thickness burn—less than 2% body surface

Inpatient Management
Hospital (other than burn center)
   Partial-thickness burn—less than 25% body surface
   Full-thickness burn—less than 15% body surface
   Partial-thickness burn—face, hands, feet, perineum
   Questionable burn wound depth or extent
   Chemical burn, minor
   Significant coexisting illness or trauma
   Inadequate family support
   Suspected abuse
   Fire in an enclosed space

Burn center
   Partial-thickness burn—more than 25% body surface
   Full-thickness burn—more than 15% body surface
   Full-thickness burn—face, hands, feet, perineum
   Respiratory tract injury
   Associated major trauma
   Major chemical and electrical burns

Reproduced with permission from Burns: Thermal and electrical trauma, in Strange GR (ed): *APLS: The Pediatric Emergency Medicine Course.* Elk Grove Village, IL: American Academy of Pediatrics and Dallas: American College of Emergency Physicians, 1998, p 108.

sulfadiazine is commonly used. Management on an outpatient basis should include periodic reevaluation until healing is clearly under way without evidence of infection. The treatment of blisters remains controversial. In outpatient management, it is reasonable to leave stable blisters intact. Flaccid blisters and those already broken should be debrided carefully and the surface covered with antibiotic cream and a sterile dressing.

Disposition

Criteria for outpatient management, admission, and transfer to a burn center are outlined in Table 114-2.

ELECTRICAL INJURIES

The first recorded death from electricity occurred in France in 1879. In 1881, Samuel W. Smith's accidental death from a DC generator terminal was witnessed in Buffalo, New York; it led to the use of electrocution as a method of capital punishment. Clinical investigations of electrical injury became prominent after the first legal electrocution in the 1890s.

With increasing use, knowledge of the physics and principles of injury causation have increased. The number of electrical injuries has also increased. There are approximately 1300 deaths per year from electrical injury and four times as many nonfatal injuries. The majority of victims are male. Those most commonly injured include individuals who work with electricity, home hobbyists, and children. Two groups of children are at increased risk: exploring toddlers (12 to 24 months) who chew on extension cords, and adventuresome adolescents. In toddlers, most injuries are due to appliance cords or extension cords, with fewer due to wall outlets. Adolescents often use the outdoors fearlessly as a proving ground, incurring injuries from climbing utility poles and trees and trespassing into transformer substations, resulting in more high-voltage injuries.

Electrophysiology

The factors that determine the extent of electrical injuries are voltage, current (amperage), resistance, current type, duration, and pathway.

Voltage is a measurement of the electrical "pressure" in a system. Injuries are divided into low (<1000 V) and high (>1000 V) voltage. The latter usually produces greater tissue destruction.

Amperage is a measure of the rate of flow of electrons. There is a direct relationship between current and damage. The margin between the household amperage (0.001 to 0.01 A) and that capable of causing respiratory arrest (0.02 to 0.05 A) and ventricular fibrillation (0.05 to 0.10 A) is narrow.

Resistance is a measure of the difficulty of electron flow. Resistance is measured in ohms and is related to voltage and current by Ohm's law:

$$\text{current (amperes)} = \frac{\text{voltage (volts)}}{\text{resistance (ohms)}}$$

Specific tissues have defined resistances. Resistance increases in the following order: nerve < blood < muscle < skin < tendon < fat < bone. The skin is the primary resistor to electric current. Its resistance is affected by thickness, age, moisture, and cleanliness. This explains more serious injuries in bathtub accidents or when a person is sweating. In general, skin with high resistance will sustain greater thermal damage at the site of contact but impede the intensity of current. Skin with lower resistance will have less local thermal damage and greater internal damage. Heat-generated tissue injury is inversely

proportional to the square area of the conductor through which it passes. The most severe injuries occur in extremities due to high internal resistance and small cross-sectional diameter. Damage to internal organs is less frequent due to low tissue resistance and the large cross-sectional diameter of the torso.

Current type is either alternating or direct. Alternating current is much more dangerous than direct current at the same voltage. Household circuits (110/220 V) operate at 60 cycles per second (cps), a frequency at which neuromuscular function remains refractory indefinitely, leading to tetany. These tetanic muscle contractions "freeze" the victim to the current course, increasing the duration of contact and the amount of tissue destruction. In addition, alternating current is often associated with local diaphoresis, which further reduces skin resistance.

Increased *duration* results in increased damage.

The *current pathway* will determine the nature of injuries and complications. Once surface resistance is overcome, low-voltage current follows the path of least resistance. High-voltage current follows a direct course to ground, regardless of tissue type and resistance.

Certain common pathways of current flow are related to specific types of morbidity and mortality.

- Hand-to-hand flow: carries a 60 percent mortality rate due to spinal cord transection at C4-8, myocardial injury, and tetanic muscle contractions of the thorax, resulting in suffocation.

- Hand-to-foot flow: carries a 20 percent mortality rate from cardiac arrhythmias.

- Foot-to-foot flow: generally not associated with fatalities.

- Current passing through the head: likely to produce brain and brain stem damage.

- Current passing through the thorax: likely to produce cardiorespiratory arrest.

Types of Injuries

Electrical injuries are often classified under burns but are more closely related to crush injuries. Victims of electrical injury may have very little external damage while sustaining serious underlying tissue damage.

Skin and Underlying Tissues

Entry and exit burns are found commonly in all nonwater-related electrical injuries. The most common entry points are the hands and skull. The most common exit points are the heels. The different types of burns are as follows.

- Contact burns. These result from direct contact with an electrical source.

- Localized arc burns. The victim becomes part of a circuit as the current arcs to him or her from a high-voltage line. These often generate temperatures up to 2500°C and are accompanied by extensive deep tissue damage.

- Flash burns. A current courses outside of the body from a contact point to the ground. An example is lightning injury.

- Flame-type burns. These are secondary to ignition of clothes or flammable chemicals in the environment and are often extensive.

Very young children often bite on electrical cords, sustaining severe orofacial injuries. Burns are often fullthickness, involving the lips and oral commissure. These burns are initially bloodless and painless. As the eschar separates in 2 to 3 weeks, severe bleeding can occur from damage to the labial, facial, or even carotid arteries. There can be mandibular damage, devitalization of teeth, and microstomia from extensive scarring.

Subcutaneous tissues, muscle, nerves, and blood vessels suffer thermal damage. Skeletal muscle damage is produced by heat or electrical breakdown of cell membranes. Tissue that may initially appear viable may later prove to have been ischemic.

Cardiovascular System

Current passing directly through the heart can induce ventricular fibrillation. Lightning injury will frequently induce asystole. A wide variety of arrhythmias can occur, including supraventricular tachycardia, extrasystoles, right bundle branch block, and complete heart block. The most common electrocardiographic (ECG) abnormalities are sinus tachycardia and nonspecific ST-T changes. Most rhythm disturbances are temporary and rhythms return to normal. Myocardial infarction and ventricular perforation have been reported.

Vascular injuries include thrombosis, vasculitis with necrosis of large vessels, vasospasm, and late aneurysm formation. Maximal decrease in blood flow will occur in the first 36 hours. Strong peripheral pulses do not guarantee vascular integrity.

Kidney

Acute renal failure may occur from myoglobin released by extensively damaged muscle and hemoglobin from hemolysis. Kidney damage may also occur from blunt trauma, hypoxic ischemic injury, cardiac arrest, and hypovolemia. Oliguria, albuminuria, hemoglobinuria, and renal casts may be seen transiently.

Neurologic Effects

Immediate central nervous system effects include loss of consciousness, agitation, amnesia, deafness, seizures, visual disturbance, and sensory complaints. Vascular damage may result in epidural, subdural, or intraventricular hemorrhage. Within several days, the syndrome of inappropriate antidiuretic hormone secretion (SIADH) may lead to cerebral edema and herniation. Peripheral nerve injury, from vascular damage, thermal effect, or direct action of current, may occur and be progressive. A variety of autonomic disturbances also occur. Late involvement of the spinal cord may produce ascending paralysis, amyotrophic lateral sclerosis, transverse myelitis, or incomplete cord transection.

Eyes

Cataracts can be seen in any electrical injury involving the head or neck.

Gastrointestinal Tract

Passage of current through the abdominal wall can cause Curling's ulcers in the stomach or duodenum. Other injuries described include evisceration, stomach and intestinal perforation, esophageal stricture, and electrocoagulation of the liver and pancreas.

Skeletal System

Blunt trauma or tetanic muscle contractions can cause fractures or dislocations. Amputation of an extremity is necessary in 35 to 60 percent of survivors due to extensive underlying injuries. Infections frequently occur in gangrenous tissue. Prevalent organisms include *Staphylococcus, Pseudomonas,* and *Clostridium* spp.

Psychological Sequelae

Victims often display depression, flashbacks, and general psychosocial dysfunction.

Management

Prehospital Care

Extrication is extremely dangerous until the power source is disconnected. Victims should be treated as multiple blunt trauma patients, with special attention given to spinal immobilization. Attention is first paid to the ABCs (airway, breathing, circulation), with standard protocols for arrest victims followed. Aggressive fluid therapy is essential to sustain circulation and begin diluting myoglobin. Transport to a health care facility should not be delayed.

Emergency Department Care

Any victim of electrical injury should be approached in the same way as a victim of blunt trauma with a crush injury. The greatest threats to life include cardiac arrhythmias, renal failure from myoglobin and hemoglobin precipitants, and hyperkalemia from massive muscle breakdown. A thorough search for entry and exit wounds and hidden skeletal injuries is necessary. Laboratory tests should include arterial blood gases, blood count, serum electrolytes, blood urea nitrogen, glucose, creatinine, creatine kinase (CK), blood type and crossmatch, and urinalysis for myoglobin. Radiographs of the cervical spine, chest, and pelvis may be done, in addition to areas dictated by physical examination. Baseline ECG and cardiac monitoring is not indicated for children exposed to household current (120 to 240 V) unless there was loss of consciousness, tetany, wet skin, transthoracic current flow, or the event was unwitnessed. Although CK-MB (muscle brain) isoenzyme elevations can be seen, they may be from damaged skeletal muscle. If the ECG is consistent with cardiac injury, further evaluation with echocardiography or nuclear scanning may be necessary.

The usual fluid replacement formulas utilized for burn patients underestimate fluid requirements in electrical burn patients. Fluids should maintain a urine output of 1 to 2 mL/kg/h. Accurate measurement requires Foley catheter placement. Alkalinization of the urine with bicarbonate and administration of mannitol or furosemide may be needed to treat myoglobinuria. These therapies should be approached cautiously if coexisting head trauma is possible. Overzealous use of bicarbonate can result in metabolic alkalosis or hypernatremia. Any unexplained coma, lateralizing signs, or change in mental status necessitates cranial computed tomography (CT).

Extensive muscle damage frequently requires fasciotomy. Debridement is best left to a burn surgeon. Tetanus prophylaxis should be evaluated and given as needed in the emergency department.

Nasogastric intubation may be required and antacids and cimetidine should be administered.

Consultations may be required, depending on the severity and type of injury. All children with oral injuries require plastic surgery or dental consults. Neurosurgical, ophthalmologic, and ear-nose-throat consults may also be necessary. Transfer to a burn center may be indicated.

Infection remains the most common cause of death after electrical injury. Despite aggressive debridement and decompression, digit or limb loss may be unavoidable.

Recommendations for admission are varied. It is generally agreed that admission is not required for nontransthoracic low-voltage injuries in the asymptomatic child without ECG abnormalities. All other patients require admission and close observation. A multidisciplinary approach, including medical, psychiatric, and social services, is required.

Prevention

Physicians can play an important role in prevention by educating patients and their families. The following advice should be given.

- Extension cords should be in good repair and not used to replace or avoid conduit wiring.
- Unused outlets should be covered with dummy plugs.
- Electrical appliances must be kept away from sinks and bathtubs.
- Electrically operated toys should be age-appropriate. Use of such toys should be supervised by adults.
- Older children and adolescents can benefit from school safety programs that address the dangers of power lines and transformer substations.

LIGHTNING INJURIES

Familiarity with the basic physics of lightning will facilitate the prompt recognition and proper treatment of lightning injuries. As Benjamin Franklin demonstrated, using a kite and key, lightning is an electrical event, and electrical charges are contained in thunderclouds.

Lightning is responsible for greater mortality in the United States than any other natural phenomenon. The incidence of injury corresponds with those months in which thunderstorms are most abundant (i.e., June, July, and August). Due to lack of standardization, statistics on lightning-related injuries and deaths are difficult to interpret and vary widely. Estimates from 77 to >600 deaths in the United States per year have been reported. The mortality rate of lightning-related injury approaches

30 percent, with 75 percent of survivors left with permanent sequelae.

Physics

Lightning is produced by the development of an electrical potential between a cumulonimbus cloud (thundercloud) and the ground. Within a cloud, rising warm air meets cooler air with vapor condensing. This generates an electrical potential, with positive charges in the upper cloud layers and negative charges in the lower cloud layers. Subsequently, the usually negatively charged ground becomes positively charged. This difference in electrical potential must be greater than air resistance to create a lightning bolt. Lightning discharge can be intracloud (most common), cloud-to-cloud (rare), ground-to-cloud (i.e., skyscrapers, mountains), or cloud-to-ground. The last is associated with injuries.

Mechanism of Injury

There are several mechanisms by which lightning can cause injury.

- Direct strike. This is the most serious form of lightning injury. The likelihood of direct strike is increased when the person is carrying or wearing metal objects, such as golf clubs, umbrellas, or hairpins.
- Side flash or "splash." In this form of lightning injury, the victim is near an object that is struck, with object resistance greater than air resistance between the object and the person.
- Ground current. In ground-current injury, lightning strikes the ground close to a victim, with the result that the ground current passes through the victim. When the victim stands with feet apart, a potential difference between the feet allows current to flow through the body to the ground (stride potential or step current).
- Thermal flash. Temperatures between 8000 and 30,000°C of short duration (0.001 to 0.010 seconds) can cause burns. These are generally not as severe as household or industrial electrical burns.
- Blunt injury. The cylindrical shock wave emanating from the axis of the lightning channel can cause perforation of the tympanic membrane or damage to internal organs. This shock wave can also throw a victim, causing secondary blunt injury.

Substantial differences in lightning-strike properties account for variability in the type and severity of injury.

Lightning acts as a direct-current countershock, with higher voltage and amperage than seen in high-voltage electrical accidents. The extremely short duration of lightning shock accounts for the small amount of skin damage usually seen. Most of the lightning energy flows around the outside of the body, with less energy actually flowing through the victim.

Types of Injuries

Skin

Skin damage is decreased by the short duration of contact and by lower skin resistance from rain or sweat. Entry wounds, exit wounds, and deep muscle damage are rare. Major types of burns include the following:

- Feathering burns. These are arborescent, spidery, erythematous streaks that are pathognomonic of lightning injury. They appear up to several hours after injury and disappear within 24 hours.
- Linear burns. Linear burns are partial-thickness burns in areas of high sweat concentration.
- Punctate burns. These are multiple, discrete, circular burns in groups. They can be full or partial thickness.
- Thermal burns. Heating of metal objects or ignition of clothing can cause secondary thermal burns.

More than 60 percent of patients have multiple burns, whereas approximately 10 percent are not burned at all.

Cardiopulmonary Effects

Asystole can result from the massive direct-current countershock produced by a lightning strike. Respiratory arrest may occur from effects on the medullary respiratory center. Although the heart usually resumes an organized rhythm spontaneously, prolonged respiratory arrest leads to hypoxia and ventricular fibrillation. Myocardial infarction occurs secondary to hypoxia or direct cardiac damage and has been reported as late as 30 days after injury in adults. Congestive heart failure, cardiac contusions, and rupture have also been reported.

Electrocardiographic changes include nonspecific ST-T changes, T-wave changes, axis shift, QT prolongation, and ST-segment elevation. These often resolve gradually. Lung injuries reported include pulmonary contusion, hemorrhage, pneumothorax, pulmonary edema, and aspiration secondary to altered mental status.

Vascular Effects

Arterial spasm and vasomotor instability result in cool, mottled, pulseless extremities. This usually resolves in several hours.

Neurologic Effects

Transient loss of consciousness, retrograde amnesia, transient paralysis, and paresthesias are common. Keraunoparalysis (from the Greek keraunos, meaning lightning) is a flaccid paralysis accompanied by vasomotor changes, which may last up to 24 hours. Other possible neurologic findings include seizures, skull fractures, intracerebral hemorrhages and hematomas, elevated intracranial pressure, cerebellar ataxia, Horner's syndrome, SIADH, and peripheral nerve damage. Cerebral edema may occur late. Direct or blunt injury to the spinal cord should always be ruled out, especially if symptoms do not resolve.

Kidneys

Myoglobinuria is rare; however, hypovolemia and prolonged cardiac arrest can lead to acute tubular necrosis. The kidneys may also be damaged by direct blunt trauma from a shock wave or other object.

Eyes

Cataracts are the most common injury and may develop immediately or over a prolonged period. Some resolve spontaneously. Fixed and dilated pupils are often seen after lightning strike and are not a prognostic factor. Other eye injuries reported include uveitis, hyphema, vitreous hemorrhage, retinal detachment, and optic atrophy.

Ears

Tympanic membrane rupture is common. Other complications include hearing loss, tinnitus, vertigo, and nystagmus.

Gastrointestinal Tract

Gastric dilatation is common. Hematoma or perforations can occur secondary to blunt trauma.

Psychological Sequelae

Anxiety, sleep disturbances, nocturnal enuresis, depression, and hysteria-related phenomena have all been reported.

Management

Prehospital Care

Lightning injury victims should be approached as blunt multiple trauma patients with attention to advanced life-support protocols and cervical spine protection. Due to the unusual findings of transient fixed and dilated pupils from autonomic abnormalities and transient asystole with prolonged apnea, standard triage procedures should be ignored. Victims who appear to be dead should be treated aggressively. If the history of lightning strike is unclear, protocols for altered mental status should be followed (i.e., glucose, naloxone). Bystanders may be helpful in providing history.

It should be noted that, contrary to popular belief, lightning can strike twice in the same area. Emergency personnel should exhibit caution if the threat of lightning strike still exists at the time of their arrival.

Emergency Department Care

Treatment follows the same guidelines as for all severely injured patients. Amnesia suffered by the victim and lack of available bystanders may limit history taking. Clues that may lead to the diagnosis of lightning strike include recent thunderstorm, outdoor occurrence, clothing disintegration, typical arborescent burn pattern, tympanic membrane injury, and magnetization of metallic objects on the victim's body. A complete physical examination, with priority to ABCs and cervical spine control, is indicated. A thorough search for blunt trauma injuries is necessary, as are baseline ECG and continued cardiac monitoring. Any arrythmia should be treated by standard protocols. Routine laboratory tests include complete blood count, creatine phosphokinase with isoenzymes, renal function tests, and urinalysis for myoglobin. The patient's status may necessitate arterial blood gas, serum chemistries, and blood type and crossmatch. Urine and blood should be sent for toxicology. Radiographs are done as indicated but include cranial CT in all unconscious patients.

Fluid resuscitation must be approached cautiously; central monitoring lines may be helpful.

Burns should be treated by protocol. Fasciotomy is rarely indicated, as the mottled, pulseless extremity associated with lightning injury often improves over several hours. Eye and ear examinations should not be overlooked. Careful attention to tetanus prophylaxis is necessary.

Disposition

Some authorities suggest admission for all victims of lightning injuries. Others suggest admission for all except those children with a completely normal examination, normal laboratory tests, and ECG, plus adequate home supervision and close follow-up care. Appropriate consultation and documentation is necessary.

Sequelae

Long-term sequelae may include paralysis, dysesthesia, and disturbances in mood, affect, and memory. Supportive psychotherapy may be necessary.

BIBLIOGRAPHY

Bailey B, Gaudreault P, Thivierge RL, et al: Cardiac monitoring of children with household electrical injuries. *Ann Emerg Med* 25:612–617, 1995.

Cooper MA, Andrews CJ, Holle RL, et al: Lightning injuries, in Auerbach PS: *Wilderness Medicine,* 4th ed. St. Louis: Mosby, 2001, pp 73–110.

Garcia CT, Smith GA, Cohen DM, et al: Electrical injuries in a pediatric emergency department. *Ann Emerg Med* 26:604–608, 1995.

Niazi ZV, Salzberg CA: Thermal, electrical and chemical injury to the face and neck in children. *Facial Plast Surg* 7:185–193, 1999.

Rabban JT, Blair JA, Rosen CL, et al: Mechanisms of pediatric electrical injury: New implications for product safety and injury prevention. *Arch Pediatr Adolesc Med* 151:696–700, 1997.

Sheridan RL, Remensnyder JP, Snitzer JJ, et al: Current expectations for survival in pediatric burns. *Arch Pediatr Adolesc Med* 154:245–249, 2000.

Smith ML: Pediatric burns: Management of thermal, electrical and chemical burns and burn-like dermatologic conditions. *Pediatr Ann* 29:367–378, 2000.

Stewart C: Emergency care of pediatric burns. *Pediatr Emerg Med Rep* 5:101–112, 2001.

Yowler CJ, Fratianne RB: Current status of burn resuscitation. *Clin Plast Surg* 27:1–10, 2000.

Zubair M, Besner GE: Pediatric electrical burns: Management strategies. *Burns* 23:413–420, 1997.

115

Heat and Cold Illness

Gary R. Strange

HIGH-YIELD FACTS

- Acclimatization to a hot, humid environment allows the individual to perform harder and longer without developing heat illness. Full acclimatization takes 3 to 4 weeks, during which the individual must limit exertion.

- Heat exhaustion is a syndrome of dizziness, postural hypotension, nausea, vomiting, headache, weakness, and, occasionally, syncope, which may be associated with normal temperature or moderate temperature elevation (39 to 41.1°C). It tends to occur in unacclimatized individuals.

- Heat stroke is the most severe form of heat illness, with reported mortality between 17 and 80 percent. Patients with heat stroke present with disorientation, seizures, or coma.

- Heat stroke is an immediately life-threatening entity and must be treated vigorously. After assessment and stabilization of the airway, breathing, and circulation, cooling should be instituted immediately, usually by spraying the skin with room-temperature water and directing an electric fan onto the patient's skin.

- Since the effects of heat stroke are widespread throughout essentially every system of the body and the differential diagnosis is broad, extensive diagnostic evaluation is indicated.

- Age is an important factor in determining the susceptibility to hypothermia and the morbidity and mortality associated with it. Neonates are at high risk for developing hypothermia due to their large surface area compared with body mass and the relative paucity of subcutaneous tissue.

- The core temperature defines the presence and severity of hypothermia. Most

thermometers for routine clinical use will record a temperature down to only 34.4°C. Special glass or electronic thermometers are required for accurate measurement of temperatures in hypothermic patients.

- Shivering will often be present in the older child or adolescent but ceases by the time the temperature reaches 31°C. The skin is typically cold, firm, pale, or mottled, and localized damage due to frostbite may be present.

- In moderate to severe cases of hypothermia, active rewarming is started as soon as possible (Fig. 115-3). Heated, humidified oxygen, and intravenous fluids heated to 40°C have been shown to be safe and efficacious and are used from the beginning.

- Extracorporeal rewarming is the most rapid method of rewarming and is indicated in hypothermic cardiac arrest and with patients who present with completely frozen extremities. Using this technique, young, otherwise healthy people have survived deep hypothermia with no or minimal cerebral impairment.

HEAT ILLNESS

The spectrum of heat illness varies from mild, self-limited problems, such as heat cramps, to major, life-threatening problems, such as heat stroke. The annual average number of deaths from heat illness in the United States for 1979 through 1996 was 381. Infants are predisposed to the development of heat illness due to their poorly developed thermoregulatory systems. Older children and adolescents are susceptible to heat illness when they exercise vigorously under hot, humid conditions. Adolescent zeal for competitive athletics, coupled with an often-held belief among the young in their invulnerability, can lead to serious heat illness. Heat illness is the second leading cause of death in athletes, after head and spinal injuries. Drug-related heat illness (see Table 79-1) is also seen with increasing incidence in the adolescent population. Other factors associated with the development of heat illness in pediatric patients are obesity, dehydration, excessive clothing and bundling, and infections. An especially tragic situation, which is entirely preventable through parental education, is the development of heat illness in small children left in closed cars on hot days. Children with cystic fibrosis (see Chap. 31) are prone to develop a form of heat illness characterized by excessive electrolyte loss with sweating. Any patient who has had a previous episode of heat stroke is markedly predisposed to recurrence.

Acclimatization to a hot, humid environment allows the individual to perform harder and longer without developing heat illness. Full acclimatization takes 3 to 4 weeks, during which the individual must limit exertion. Children take longer to acclimatize than adults. The process involves alterations in sodium and water balance, which are mediated by aldosterone. When a person is acclimatized, increased aldosterone secretion leads to sodium retention and expansion of extracellular fluid volume.

Pathophysiology

At rest, the body generates enough heat to raise the body temperature by about 1°C/h. Heavy exertion can increase heat production to 12 times this level. When the ambient temperature exceeds the body temperature, there is a net heat gain from the environment. The body can dissipate heat by four mechanisms:

- radiation
- conduction
- convection
- evaporation

Vasodilatation can increase peripheral blood flow and heat loss from radiation by a factor of 20. Wind currents or fanning increase dissipation by convection. Conduction occurs when there is direct contact with a cooler environment. Immersion in cool water produces an increase in heat dissipation by a factor of 32. Evaporation of sweat from the skin is a major heat-dissipation mechanism, especially in conditioned athletes. This source of heat loss is relatively ineffective, however, when the relative humidity exceeds 85 percent.

Types of Heat Illness

Heat Cramps

With heavy exertion, the muscles that are working hardest may begin to go into spasm. This can occur regardless of whether exercise is performed in the heat or the cold. The cause has long been described as dilutional hyponatremia, which usually occurs in conditioned athletes who replace fluid losses with water. However, there is no clear evidence that dilutional hyponatremia is the actual cause. The body temperature remains normal and

there is associated sweating. There are no central nervous system signs.

Heat Exhaustion

Heat exhaustion is a syndrome of dizziness, postural hypotension, nausea, vomiting, headache, weakness, and, occasionally, syncope, which may be associated with normal temperature or moderate temperature elevation (39 to 41.1°C). It tends to occur in unacclimatized individuals. The skin is usually wet from profuse sweating. The associated morbidity is low.

The cause of heat exhaustion may be either salt or water depletion. Salt depletion occurs when fluid losses are replaced by water or other hypotonic solutions and hyponatremia results. Severe hyponatremia results in significant mental status changes or seizures. Water depletion occurs when victims are unable to replace fluid losses, resulting in hypernatremic dehydration. This can occur in infants or mentally retarded children, who cannot communicate their thirst.

Heat Stroke

Heat stroke is the most severe form of heat illness, with reported mortality between 17 and 80 percent. Patients with heat stroke present with disorientation, seizures, or coma. Classic heat stroke is typically seen in the elderly and develops over a period of days. The skin is usually hot and dry. With exertional heat stroke, which is much more likely in the pediatric population, the skin may be dry or sweating may continue. The temperature ranges from 41.1 to 42.2°C. There is no clear scientific evidence to indicate that heat stroke results from fluid and electrolyte abnormalities. Although dehydration is no doubt a predisposing condition, other predisposing factors that are poorly understood seem to be necessary for heat stroke to occur.

Complications are common, leading to the high mortality rate. These include neurologic dysfunction (100 percent), moderate to severe renal insufficiency (53 percent), disseminated intravascular coagulation (45 percent), and adult respiratory distress syndrome (10 percent). Evidence of concomitant infection is also common (57 percent). Rhabdomyolysis occurs in up to 25 percent of patients with exertional heat stroke. In-hospital mortality is reported at 21 percent, and 33 percent of patients have moderate to severe functional impairment at the time of hospital discharge. In follow-up, the functional impairment was found to persist at 1 year. Whereas the outcome may be somewhat better for the young, otherwise healthy individual, mortality and morbidity are unquestionably significant.

Management

Heat cramps are treated by removing the patient to a cool environment and providing rest and oral electrolyte solutions. Salt tablets may cause gastrointestinal cramping and are not recommended. A solution of 1 tsp table salt in 500 mL water can be used if no prepared solutions are available.

Heat exhaustion is also treated by removal to a cool environment and providing rest. Intravenous rehydration is recommended, starting with 20 mL/kg of normal saline over 30 minutes and continuing rehydration as outlined in Chap. 51. If hypernatremic dehydration is suspected on clinical or laboratory grounds, slower replacement is indicated.

Victims of heat exhaustion may require observation in the hospital. However, if all symptoms have resolved during emergency department treatment and observation, the patient may be released to continue rest and rehydration in a cool environment.

On the other hand, heat stroke is an immediately life-threatening entity and must be treated vigorously. After assessment and stabilization of the airway, breathing, and circulation, cooling should be instituted immediately. Spraying the skin with room-temperature water and directing an electric fan onto the patient's skin will usually result in rapid reduction of the core temperature. Ice packs may be used in the groin and axilla, but ice water applied widely to the skin may cause vasoconstriction and impair the dissipation of heat. Submersion in cold water is very effective in lowering the temperature but makes other resuscitative efforts practically impossible. Invasive lavage to lower the body temperature has not been adequately studied and is not currently recommended. Antipyretics are also ineffective. Core temperature should be monitored continuously during treatment and active cooling should continue until the core temperature falls to 39°C.

Diazepam, 0.2 to 0.3 mg/kg/dose IV, may be required to prevent shivering.

Intravenous fluids are required and should initially be given as isotonic crystalloid at a rate of 20 mL/kg over the first hour. Central venous or pulmonary artery catheters are frequently needed for adequate monitoring of fluid resuscitation.

Since the effects of heat stroke are widespread throughout essentially every system of the body and the differential diagnosis is broad (Table 115-1), extensive diagnostic evaluation is indicated. Arterial blood gases are helpful in evaluating oxygenation, ventilation, and acid-base status. Changes in body temperature alter blood gas values, but whether corrections in the values are helpful before treatment decisions are made is controversial.

The complete blood count will usually show an elevated white blood cell count. Counts >20,000/mm^3 and elevated band counts are more consistent with an underlying infection and should prompt a complete septic work-up. Hemoglobin and hematocrit values are usually elevated due to dehydration. Electrolyte studies may reveal abnormal sodium levels. Elevated potassium levels may indicate the development of rhabdomyolysis. Renal function tests may initially be elevated due to dehydration and may rise later, as renal failure develops. Urinalysis will often show a high specific gravity as a reflection of the hydration status. If the urine is positive for hemoglobin in the absence of red blood cells on the microscopic evaluation, rhabdomyolysis should be suspected. Liver enzymes may be elevated, since the liver is very sensitive to heat stress. Transaminase levels peak in 24 to 48 hours and correlate well with the severity of injury. Very high levels (aspartate transaminase >1000 IU) are predictive of severe illness and complications. Serum glucose levels are variable but should be monitored to assess the need for replacement or control. Coagulation studies are needed to detect the development of disseminated intravascular coagulation. Cultures are an integral part of the sepsis work-up, which is essential to rule out an infectious etiology or concomitant infection.

Radiologic studies will usually include a chest radiograph as part of the sepsis work-up. Computed tomographic scanning of the brain is indicated to rule out intracranial pathology, especially if the mental status does not promptly improve with lowering of the temperature.

An electrocardiogram is indicated to evaluate for myocardial ischemia, which can result from severe cardiovascular stress.

After evaluation and stabilization, patients with heat stroke are admitted to an intensive care setting for continued monitoring and aggressive treatment.

COLD ILLNESS

Hypothermia is defined as a core temperature of <35°C. A low body temperature may develop as a result of exposure to low ambient temperature or may be secondary to a disease process (Table 115-2).

Table 115-1. Differential Diagnosis of Heat Stroke: Symptom Complex—Altered Mental Status, Hyperthermia

Potential Diagnosis	Pertinent History	Pertinent Findings on Physical Examination	Pertinent Laboratory Data
Encephalitis and meningitis	Fever Prodromal illness Severe headache Chills	Temperature Neck stiffness Kernig and Brudzinski signs positive	Lumbar puncture: elevated WBCs, positive Gram's stain, cultures
Malaria	Exposure Travel history Previous history	Fever pattern Confusion	Peripheral blood smear
Typhoid fever, typhus	Exposure Travel history	Fever pattern	Titers: Well-Felix reaction, complement fixation
Sepsis	Fever Age extreme Immunocompromised	Fever Confusion Coma Focal infection	Chest X-ray WBC: elevated Cultures: blood, urine, spinal fluid
Hypothalamic hemorrhage	Hypertension Anticoagulant therapy	Coma Fever Focal neurologic findings	Brain CT: hemorrhage
Thyroid storm	Pre-existing hyperthyroidism Risk factors Stress Surgery Trauma Infection Failure to take antithyroid medication	Goiter Tachycardia Seizures Hypotension	Thyroid function studies: T_3 and T_4
Malignant hyperthermia	Inhalation anesthetic Succinylcholine	Muscle fasciculation	Arterial blood gases: acidosis Electrolytes: hyperkalemia hypermagnesemia
Heat stroke	Risk factors Exposure to heat load Exercise	Hot, flushed skin Confusion Agitation Seizures Tachycardia Hypotension Vomiting Diarrhea Muscle tenderness	AST: elevated WBC: elevated Electrolytes: hyper- or hypo- kalemia, hyponatremia, hypocalcemia, hypophosphatemia Arterial blood gases: metabolic acidosis Urine: myoglobin Clotting factors: decreased Blood glucose: variable

Reproduced with permission from Barreca RS: Heat illness, in Hamilton GC, Sanders AB, Strange GR, Trott AT (eds): *Emergency Medicine: An Approach to Clinical Problem-Solving.* Philadelphia, Saunders, 1991, p 402.

Table 115-2. Causes of Hypothermia in Infants and Children

Environmental factors
  Exposure
  Near drowning
Infections
  Meningitis
  Encephalitis
  Sepsis
  Pneumonia
Metabolic and endocrine factors
  Hypoglycemia
  Diabetic ketoacidosis
  Hypopituitarism
  Myxedema
  Addison's disease
  Uremia
  Malnutrition
Toxicologic factors
  Alcohol
  Anesthetic agents
  Barbiturates
  Carbon monoxide
  Cyclic antidepressants
  Narcotics
  Phenothiazines
CNS disorders
  Degenerative diseases
  Head trauma
  Spinal cord trauma
  Subarachnoid hemorrhage
  Cerebrovascular accidents
  Intracranial neoplasm
Vascular factors
  Shock
  Pulmonary embolism
  Gastrointestinal hemorrhage
Dermatologic factors
  Burns
  Erythrodermas
Iatrogenic factors
  Cold fluid factors
  Exposure during treatment or postdelivery
  Prolonged extrications

Age is an important factor in determining the susceptibility to hypothermia and the morbidity and mortality associated with it. Neonates are at high risk for developing hypothermia due to their large surface area compared with body mass and the relative paucity of subcutaneous tissue.

They have also been postulated to have poorly developed thermoregulatory systems. The evaporation of warm amniotic fluid from the skin of the newborn is a major source of heat loss that must be guarded against in all cases. Throughout infancy and young childhood, children remain susceptible to hypothermia with exposure to cold, although less so with advancing age. Most cases of accidental hypothermia in older children and adolescents are associated with near drowning in cold water. However, in recent years, there has been an increase in exposure-related hypothermia in older children and adolescents; this is believed to be associated with the increased popularity of winter sports. Inexperience and lack of caution, which are common among adolescents, increase the likelihood of their becoming victims of hypothermia.

Pathophysiology

Normal body temperature varies over a narrow 1°C range. Exposure to cold stimulates skin receptors, resulting in peripheral vasoconstriction and conservation of heat. As the temperature of the blood declines, the preoptic anterior hypothalamus is stimulated. Heat production is then increased by shivering and by metabolic and endocrine means of thermogenesis, primarily mediated by thyroid and adrenal secretions (Fig. 115-1). Shivering can increase heat production by 4 to 5 times. Behavioral responses, such as seeking a warm environment or putting on protective clothing, are major preventive mechanisms that are entirely absent in the infant. Shivering is also absent in neonates, making them entirely dependent on care from others, vasoconstriction, and heat generated by lipolysis.

Heat is lost from the body by four mechanisms:

- Radiation accounts for 55 to 65 percent of heat loss. Radiation losses are reduced by insulation (clothing, subcutaneous fat) and by reduction in skin blood flow (vasoconstriction).

- Conduction is not a major route of heat loss under normal conditions, but conductive heat loss increases 5 times in the presence of wet clothing and 25 to 30 times with submersion in cold water.

- Convection heat losses are greatly increased by wind currents and bodily movement. The wind-chill effect significantly increases the likelihood of hypothermia developing at a given temperature.

- Evaporation accounts for 20 to 25 percent of heat loss, primarily via respiration and insensible water loss from the skin. When the skin is wet, evaporative losses are increased. Wet newborns are especially vulnerable to heat loss by evaporation.

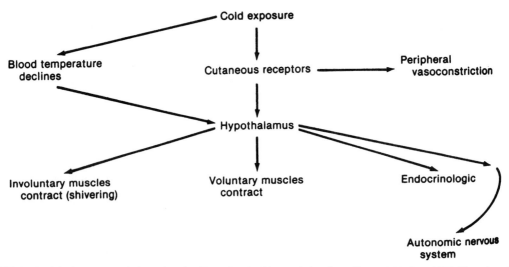

Fig. 115-1. Physiologic responses in hypothermia. (Reproduced with permission from Cooper MA, Danzl DF: Hypothermia, in Hamilton GC, Sanders AB, Strange GR, Trott AT (eds): *Emergency Medicine: An Approach to Clinical Problem-Solving*. Philadelphia, Saunders, 1991, p 410.)

Essentially every part of the body is affected by hypothermia (Table 115-3). The most prominent effects are seen in the cardiovascular, central nervous, respiratory, renal, and gastrointestinal systems.

Cardiovascular Effects

After an initial tachycardia, the heart rate falls as temperature falls. Mean arterial pressure also falls progressively, along with cardiac output. Atrial dysrhythmias commonly appear at temperatures below 32°C but are usually considered innocent because the ventricular response is slow. Ventricular ectopy is seen with temperatures <30°C and the risk of ventricular fibrillation is greatly increased. A J wave (Osborn wave) may be present at the junction of the QRS complex and ST segment (Fig. 115-2).

Central Nervous System Effects

Brain enzymes are less functional with declining temperature, resulting in a linear decrease in cerebral metabolism. Cerebral perfusion is maintained until autoregulation fails at about 25°C. At 20°C, the electroencephalogram shows a flat line.

Respiratory Effects

Cold initially stimulates the respiratory drive, but, as temperature falls, a progressive decline in minute venti-

lation supervenes. Bronchorrhea, due to the local effect of cold air, can be severe, simulating pulmonary edema.

Renal Effects

Vasoconstriction in the extremities results in an initial central hypervolemia. The kidney responds rapidly, producing a large "cold diuresis" of dilute glomerular filtrate. Ethanol and immersion in cold water increase this early diuresis.

Gastrointestinal Effects

Gastrointestinal motility is decreased and gastric dilatation, ileus, constipation, and poor rectal tone commonly result. Inflammatory changes in the pancreas are also often found.

Diagnosis

The diagnosis of hypothermia may be obvious when a history of exposure is known. However, hypothermia may develop insidiously due to causes other than exposure or to exposure in relatively warm environments.

The hypothermic patient is often not able to give an adequate history, and other sources of information should be sought. Family, friends, police, and paramedics are all valuable sources of information.

Once hypothermia is known or suspected, a history of exposure is sought, including the circumstances, location,

Table 115-3. Pathophysiologic Changes During Hypothermia

Centigrade Temperature	Farenheit Temperature	Findings
37.6	99.6	Normal rectal temperature
37	98.6	Normal oral temperature
35	95.0	Maximal shivering
		Increased metabolic rate
33	91.4	Apathy
		Ataxia
		Anmesia
		Dysarthria
31	87.8	Decreased level of consciousness
		Bradycardia
		Hypotension
		Bradypnea
		Shivering stops
29	85.2	Dysrhythmias
		Insulin not effective
		Dilated pupils
		Poikilothermia
27	80.6	Areflexia
		No response to pain
		Comatose
25	77	Cerebral blood flow one-third normal
		Cardiac output one-half normal
		Significant hypotension
23	73.4	No corneal reflex
		Maximal ventricular fibrillation risk
19	66.2	Asystole
		Flat electroencephalogram
15	59.2	Lowest temperature survived from accidental hypothermia in an infant
9	48.2	Lowest temperature survived from therapeutic hypothermia

Reproduced with permission from Cooper MA, Danzl DF: Hypothermia, in Hamilton GC, Sanders AB, Strange GR, Trott AT (eds): *Emergency Medicine: An Approach to Clinical Problem-Solving.* Philadelphia, Saunders, 1991, p 415.

and ambient temperature, the length of exposure, and presence or absence of submersion or wet skin and clothing.

If significant exposure is unlikely, an extensive history is required to search for clues for other causes of hypothermia (see Table 115-1).

The key physical findings in patients with hypothermia, and the temperature level at which they occur, are depicted in Table 115-3. The core temperature defines the presence and severity of hypothermia. Most thermometers for routine clinical use will record a temperature down to only 34.4°C. Special glass or electronic thermometers are required for accurate measurement of temperatures in hypothermic patients. Continuous monitoring of rectal, esophageal, or tympanic temperature is very useful during treatment.

Shivering will often be present in the older child or adolescent but ceases by the time the temperature reaches 31°C. The skin is typically cold, firm, pale, or mottled. Localized damage due to frostbite may be present.

Early neurologic signs of hypothermia include confusion, apathy, poor judgment, slurred speech, and ataxia. Coma usually supervenes by the time the temperature reaches 27°C. Focal neurologic defects may be present. The Glasgow Coma Scale can serve as a useful quantitative means of following the patient's response to treatment, but it is not as useful with the nonverbal infant.

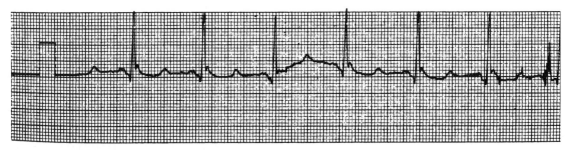

Fig. 115-2. Example of a J wave in a hypothermic patient. (Reproduced with permission from Cooper MA, Danzl DF: Hypothermia, in Hamilton GC, Sanders AB, Strange GR, Trott AT (eds): *Emergency Medicine: An Approach to Clinical Problem-Solving.* Philadelphia, Saunders, 1991, p 411.)

Since hypothermia affects multiple systems, other pathology can be masked. Signs of trauma, toxic ingestion, and endocrine disturbance should be sought, and the complete physical examination must be repeated at intervals during treatment to discover clues to problems that were initially masked by the hypothermia.

For patients with hypothermia not related to exposure and in those exposure-related individuals who present with temperatures <32°C, extensive diagnostic testing is indicated.

Arterial Blood Gases

These are useful for evaluation of oxygenation, ventilation, and acid-base status. In hypothermia, there is decreased tissue perfusion and the oxyhemoglobin dissociation curve is shifted to the left. Although some authorities have recommended correcting blood gas results for body temperature, correction can lead to false elevation of PO_2 and subsequent under-treatment. Metabolic acidosis is usually present and the buffering capacity of the blood is markedly reduced.

Complete Blood Count

Hematocrit increases 2 percent for each 1°C drop in temperature. Hemoglobin may be decreased due to blood loss or chronic illness. The white blood count is reduced by sequestration and bone marrow depression. Even in the presence of severe infection, leukocytosis may not be seen.

Serum Electrolytes

To assess the need for intervention, serum electrolytes should be monitored during the rewarming process.

There are no consistent effects of hypothermia on electrolyte concentrations, but hypokalemia is the most common finding.

Renal Function Tests

These tests are useful for establishing baseline renal function but are poor indicators of fluid status in hypothermia. Acute tubular necrosis may develop after rewarming.

Serum Glucose Concentration

This value may be elevated due to catecholamine effect and insulin inactivity below 30°C. Persistently elevated levels suggest pancreatitis or diabetic ketoacidosis (DKA). Hypoglycemia may develop due to inadequate glycogen stores in neonates and malnourished children.

Clotting Studies

Studies of prothrombin time and partial thromboplastin time, as well as platelet count and fibrinogen level, are indicated in cases of moderate to severe hypothermia. Cold induces thrombocytopenia and prolongs clotting times. Persistent changes after rewarming suggest the development of disseminated intravascular coagulation.

Pancreatic Enzymes

Amylase and lipase may be elevated and, due to the unreliability of the abdominal examination, may be the only indicators of the development of pancreatitis. Pancreatitis in hypothermia is associated with poor outcome.

Toxicologic Studies

These are frequently indicated to detect causative or predisposing agents.

Urinalysis

Urine study will demonstrate a low specific gravity due to cold diuresis. There are no other consistent findings.

Cultures of Urine, Sputum, and Blood

Cultures of body fluids are indicated in all cases of moderate to severe hypothermia. Cultures from other body sites may also be indicated on the basis of the history and physical findings. Sepsis is a common cause of hypothermia in the infant and may also develop as a complication of hypothermia due to other causes.

Radiologic Imaging

These studies will include a chest radiograph in all cases of significant hypothermia. Pulmonary edema may develop during rewarming and aspiration is relatively common. Cervical spine films may be indicated if there is suspicion of trauma. Cranial computed tomographic scanning may be indicated in the setting of trauma or to search for other etiologic factors, especially when mental status does not clear along with rewarming.

Electrocardiography

This procedure is indicated for all patients with a core temperature <32°C to detect dysrhythmias or evidence of myocardial ischemia. The J wave (see Fig. 115-2) is usually seen when the temperature falls below 32°C.

Prehospital Care

A high index of suspicion is required to diagnose hypothermia in the field. Prehospital providers should presume hypothermia in situations where exposure, even at moderate temperatures, has occurred.

Great caution is needed to prevent hypothermia or to initiate its early treatment in neonates. The neonate should immediately be dried and wrapped in warm blankets. Alternatively, the neonate can be placed against the body of the mother and then covered.

For other potentially hypothermic patients, wet clothing should be removed, and dry blankets applied. When prolonged extrications are required, hypothermia is par-

ticularly likely to develop. Protection should be provided whenever possible. Resuscitation fluids should be warmed whenever possible.

Ventilation should be supported as indicated and oxygenation maintained. Heated, humidified oxygen, if available, may minimize further core temperature loss and significantly add to other rewarming techniques. Cardiac monitoring is indicated to detect dysrhythmias. Because pulse and respiratory rates may be very slow in hypothermia, assessment for breathing and pulselessness is carried out over a 30- to 45-second period. If the patient is not breathing, ventilation is started immediately, using warmed humidified oxygen whenever possible. If there is no pulse, chest compressions are started immediately. Do not withhold basic life support while the patient is being rewarmed.

Emergency Department Management

The initial approach to the patient with hypothermia is the same as that for any seriously ill patient, with evaluation and stabilization of the airway, breathing, and circulation before moving to other aspects of treatment. Obtunded patients without protective airway reflexes require endotracheal intubation after preoxygenation. Endrotracheal intubation should be done as atraumatically as possible, but should not be withheld for fear of precipitating ventricular fibrillation. Intravenous lines are started and fluid resuscitation is guided by vital signs, urinary output, and pulmonary status. Cardiac monitoring is initiated. In addition, continuous monitoring of rectal, esophageal, or tympanic temperature is very helpful during treatment. A urinary catheter and a nasogastric tube are inserted. A bedside glucose determination is done to assess the need for glucose supplementation. If narcotic intoxication is a possibility, naloxone, 2 mg IV, is administered.

Cardiopulmonary resuscitation is begun, is started in the pulseless patient, and interventions are guided by cardiac monitor findings. The cold myocardium may be resistant to defibrillation and to pharmacologic agents. If the initial three defibrillation attempts fail to establish a rhythm, CPR is resumed and the patient is rewarmed to 30°C before defibrillation is repeated. Many patients spontaneously convert to an organized rhythm at a core temperature of 32 to 35°C. During hypothermia, protein binding of drugs is increased, and most drugs will be ineffective in normal doses. Pharmacologic attempts to alter the pulse or blood pressure are to be avoided because drugs can accumulate in the peripheral circulation and subsequently lead to toxicity as rewarming occurs. It is important to remember that infants and children who have sustained prolonged hypothermic cardiac arrest have recovered with little or no neurologic impairment. In general, resuscitative efforts should continue until the hypothermic child is warmed to at least 30°C.

In moderate to severe cases of hypothermia, active rewarming is started as soon as possible (Fig. 115-3). Heated, humidified oxygen and intravenous fluids heated to 40°C have been shown to be safe and efficacious and are used from the beginning. Further heat loss is prevented by using radiant warmers for neonates and infants. The older child and adolescent should be covered with dry blankets. Active external rewarming, as with hot packs and electric blankets, can be dangerous. The rewarming of cold extremities can result in the mobilization of cold peripheral blood to the central circulation, resulting in core-temperature after-drop. Immersion in warm baths makes monitoring and resuscitation difficult. Cold, vasoconstricted skin is also very susceptible to thermal injury. Because of these concerns, active core rewarming is used in most cases of moderate to severe hypothermia.

In addition to heated humidified oxygen and heated intravenous fluids, active core rewarming can be accomplished by irrigation of the stomach, bladder, and colon. Heat transfer by these techniques is somewhat limited. Rapid rewarming by irrigation of the mediastinum or pleural cavity via a thoracostomy tube is effective but very invasive. Peritoneal lavage with heated fluid (40 to 45°C) is probably a more effective method of active core rewarming. Extracorporeal rewarming is the most rapid method and is indicated in hypothermic cardiac arrest and with patients who present with completely frozen extremities. Using this technique, young, otherwise healthy people have survived deep hypothermia with no or minimal cerebral impairment.

Forced air rewarming has recently been described as effective, noninvasive, and not associated with an after-drop phenomenon. Another noninvasive means of rewarming involves applying subatmospheric pressure to the hand and forearm, along with heat. This technique is described as immediately resulting in subcutaneous vasodilatation and rapid heat acquisition, rapidly eliminating shivering and resulting in subjective improvement. Further studies of these techniques are needed.

Previously healthy patients who are only mildly hypothermic (35 to 33°C) will usually reheat themselves safely if they are placed in a warm environment and given dry insulating coverings (passive external rewarming).

Beyond the neonatal period, sepsis is the most common cause of hypothermia in infants. All hypothermic patients should have a thorough evaluation to search for a source of infection and should have broad-spectrum antibiotics initiated early. An animoglycoside combined with ampicillin or a third-generation cephalosporin is generally recommended.

Cold Water Drowning

A special consideration in pediatric hypothermia is near drowning in cold water. This entity is discussed in Chap. 113.

Frostbite

Another special consideration is frostbite, which may occur in conjunction with hypothermia or as an isolated localized injury. Once primarily a military problem, frostbite is now more prevalent in the civilian population as a result of occupational and recreational exposures.

Predisposing Factors

Factors predisposing to the development of frostbite fall into four categories:

- Environmental factors
  - Wind
  - Contact with metal objects
  - Poor insulation by clothing
  - Wet clothing
  - Tight clothing
  - Clothing permeable to wind
  - Lack of covering for cold-sensitive parts, such as the face and hands
- Individual factors
  - Poor fitness
  - Fatigue
  - Dehydration
  - Prior cold injury
  - Acute or chronic illness
  - Poor peripheral circulation
- Behavioral factors
  - Alcohol intoxication
  - Very young age with lack of awareness of behavior
  - Adolescent recklessness with feelings of invulnerability
  - Psychiatric disturbances
- Occasion-linked factors
  - Mountain-climbing
  - Cross-country skiing
  - Accidents

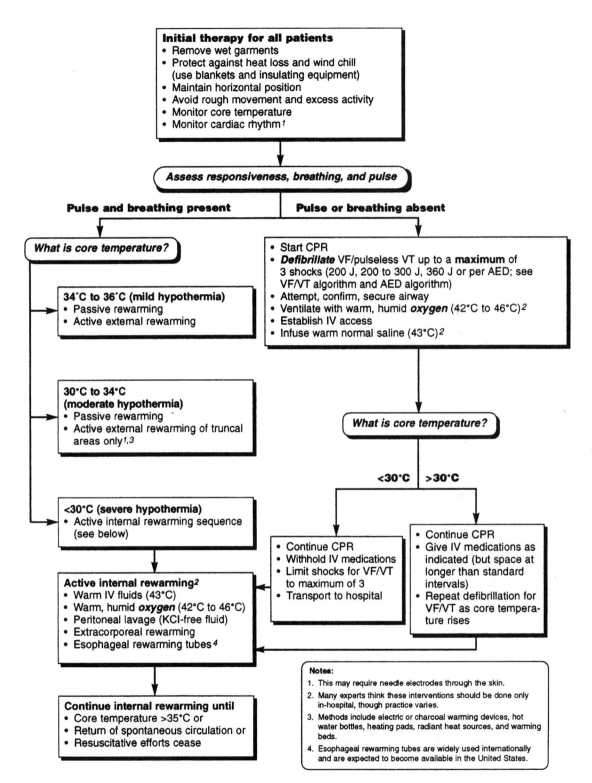

Fig. 115-3. Hypothermia treatment algorithm. (Reproduced with permission from International Liaison Committee on Resuscitation: Hypothermia. *Circulation* 102:I229–I232, 2000.) Permission pending.

Pathophysiology

Research into the pathophysiology of frostbite has shown marked similarities in inflammatory processes to those seen with burns and ischemia and reperfusion injuries. Localized hypothermia is described in terms similar to those used for burns. First-degree frostbite is limited to the superficial epidermis. Erythema and edema occur and resolve without sequelae. Second-degree frostbite results in deeper epidermal involvement and presents with large, clear bullae. Third-degree injury consists of full-thickness skin injury.

Treatment

The treatment of frostbite is rapid rewarming. The preferred technique is immersion of the affected part in circulating warm water (40 to 42°C). Narcotic analgesics are often required to control pain during rewarming. A number of adjunctive therapies, such as vasodilators, thrombolytics, hyperbaric oxygen, and sympathectomy, have been recommended, but firm evidence for their effectiveness is not yet available.

It is very difficult to determine tissue viability after significant hypothermic injury. Debridement of nonviable tissue is best delayed for several days to weeks to preserve as much tissue as possible. However, recent improvements in radiologic assessment of tissue viability have led to the possibility of earlier surgery and more rapid rehabilitation times.

Topical aloe vera cream and ibuprofen may be used for outpatient treatment after rewarming. More extensively injured patients will require continued inpatient treatment and pain control.

Rewarmed body parts are highly susceptible to refreezing, leading to even greater tissue loss. If exposure is anticipated, it is better not to rewarm the tissue.

Frostbite often results in sequelae that are persistent and may be permanent.

Disposition

Most patients with hypothermia will require hospitalization for further treatment and evaluation. Those patients with a core temperature of <32°C will require cardiac monitoring. Profoundly hypothermic patients with cardiac arrest and those with completely frozen extremities are candidates for extracorporeal rewarming and may require transfer to a tertiary care facility with this capability.

Patients with mild accidental hypothermia (35 to 32°C) may be rewarmed and discharged to a safe environment if there is no evidence of underlying disease.

Prevention

When used prior to the initiation of cold weather activities, proper planning can prevent most injuries. The first step is to be aware of cold risks. While little true acclimatization to the cold probably occurs, there is some value to practicing tasks that are to be performed in the cold and building up endurance before beginning a major cold activity. Good nutrition and hydration are helpful in resisting the stresses of cold weather activity. Sufficient clothing, either in layers or made of good insulating materials, is essential. Spare clothing is also essential, since it may be necessary to change into dry clothing if clothing becomes wet. Going slowly and avoiding exhaustion or excessive sweating is also helpful. Alcohol and tobacco should be strictly avoided, as should contact with metallic objects.

BIBLIOGRAPHY

Heat Illness

American Academy of Pediatrics Committee on Sports Medicine and Fitness: Climatic heat stress and the exercising child and adolescent. *Pediatrics* 106:158–159, 2000.

Backer HD, Shopes E, Collins SL, Barkan H: Exertional heat illness and hyponatremia in hikers. *Am J Emerg Med* 17:532–539, 1999.

Centers for Disease Control and Prevention: Heat-related illnesses and deaths—Missouri, 1998, and United States, 1979–1996. *MMWR Morb Mortal Wkly Rep* 48:469–473, 1999.

Dematte JE, O'Mara K, Buescher J, et al: Near-fatal heat stroke during the 1995 heat wave in Chicago. *Ann Intern Med* 129:173–181, 1998.

Noakes TD: Fluid and electrolyte disturbances in heat illness. *Int J Sports Med* 19(suppl 2):S146–S149, 1998.

Cold Illness

Kornberger E, Schwarz B, Lindner KH, et al: Forced air surface rewarming in patients with severe accidental hypothermia. *Resuscitation* 41:105–111, 1999.

Murphy JV, Banwell PE, Roberts AH, et al: Frostbite: Pathogenesis and treatment. *J Trauma* 48:171–178, 2000.

Soreide E, Grahn DA, Brock-Utne JG, et al: A non-invasive means to effectively restore normothermia in cold stressed individuals: A preliminary report. *J Emerg Med* 17:725–730, 1999.

Walpoth BH, Walpoth-Aslan BN, Mattle HP, et al: Outcome of survivors of accidental deep hypothermia and circulatory arrest treated with extracorporeal blood warming. *N Engl J Med* 337:1500–1505, 1997.

Weinberg AD: The role of inhalation rewarming in the early management of hypothermia. *Resuscitation* 36:101–104, 1998.

116

High-Altitude Illness and Dysbaric Injuries

Ira J. Blumen

HIGH-YIELD FACTS

- High-altitude illness most often affects young and otherwise healthy individuals, and there is a broad spectrum of disease. It progresses from the mildest form of acute mountain sickness (AMS) into the potentially life-threatening forms as high-altitude pulmonary edema (HAPE) and high-altitude cerebral edema (HACE).

- A slow graded ascent is the key to acclimatization. In the ideal setting, the first night's sleep occurs at <8000 ft, with the first day spent at rest.

- Pharmacologic agents may also be beneficial adjuncts to acclimatization. Acetazolamide (Diamox) has been shown to be very effective when staging is not possible or with individuals who are at an increased risk of high-altitude illness.

- Although normal acclimatization inhibits antidiuretic hormone (ADH) and aldosterone, resulting in a high-altitude–induced diuresis, the opposite is seen with AMS. Aldosterone, ADH, and renin-angiotensin increase, resulting in fluid retention and a leakage from the vascular space to the extravascular space.

- HACE is the most severe, life-threatening form of high-altitude illness. HACE is uncommon, affecting <1 to 2 percent of individuals who ascend without acclimatization.

- Definitive treatment of HACE is descent. High-flow oxygen is indicated as soon as symptoms are recognized, and dexamethasone, at an initial dose of 1 to 2 mg/kg orally or intramuscularly, can produce dramatic improvement.

- HAPE is a life-threatening manifestation of high-altitude illness and represents a unique form of noncardiogenic pulmonary edema. It is estimated that HAPE affects 0.5 to 15 percent of those who ascend rapidly to high altitudes and is the leading cause of high-altitude death other than trauma.

- An air embolism is the most serious dysbaric injury and requires aggressive care, which includes 100 percent oxygen, intravenous fluids, and hyperbaric treatment. Patients are placed in the Trendelenburg or left lateral decubitus position to minimize the passage of air emboli to the brain.

- Since nitrogen is not metabolized, it remains dissolved until the nitrogen gas pressure in the lungs decreases and the nitrogen can be removed. During a slow ascent, as the surrounding pressure decreases, the nitrogen that is absorbed into the tissues is released into the blood and the alveoli, but if the ascent is too quick, nitrogen levels do not have the opportunity to equalize among the tissues, blood, and alveoli, which results in the gas coming out of solution and forming gas bubbles in the blood or tissue.

- The treatment of choice for most air emboli and decompression illnesses is hyperbaric (recompression) therapy. This is initiated as soon as possible, ideally within 6 hours of the onset of symptoms.

HIGH-ALTITUDE ILLNESS

Episodes of high-altitude illness have been documented for thousands of years, but these were relatively rare entities until the advent of modern travel. The increasing popularity of various recreational activities has led individuals to try to go faster and higher than ever before. Hot air balloons, gliders, hiking, mountain climbing, biking, and skiing are among the various sports that predispose individuals to high-altitude illness. With modern modalities of travel, the incidence of high-altitude illness will continue to rise.

High-altitude illness most often affects young and otherwise healthy individuals. There is a broad spectrum of disease, progressing from the mildest form of acute mountain sickness (AMS) to the potentially life-threatening forms of high-altitude pulmonary edema (HAPE) and high-altitude cerebral edema (HACE). Symptoms of high-altitude illness may develop within hours or days after ascent. In contrast, hypoxemia occurs within minutes to hours and results in the initiation of the cascade of physiologic events that lead to AMS, HAPE, and HACE.

There are three major factors that influence the incidence, onset, and severity of high-altitude illness:

- Rate of ascent
- Altitude achieved
- Length of stay

Varying severity of high-altitude illness will occur when any of these factors, or a combination of them, exceeds the individual's ability to adapt to the new environment. Children, because of their physiologic differences, are at greater risk for developing both AMS and HAPE. The highest incidence of AMS occurs between the ages of 1 and 20 years. The severity of symptoms decreases with increasing age.

High altitude is generally considered to be ≥8000 ft (2439 m). At this altitude, arterial oxygen saturation falls below 90 percent (Pao_2 60 percent). Acclimatization is necessary to prevent illness. Although severe altitude illness is uncommon below 8000 ft, medically compromised individuals may become symptomatic at *moderate altitude* (5000 to 8000 ft). At *extreme altitude,* which is generally greater than 18,000 ft (approximately 5500 m), acclimatization is not possible and altitude illness is inevitable.

The Atmosphere and Physical Gas Laws

An understanding of the physical gas laws and the composition of the atmosphere is necessary to explain the occurrence of high-altitude illness. The atmosphere is a collection of gases with uniform percentage up to an altitude of approximately 70,000 ft. The largest percentage is nitrogen (78.08 percent), followed by oxygen (20.95 percent). At any given altitude the force exerted can be represented as the barometric pressure or atmospheric pressure (Table 116-1).

Boyle's law states that the volume of a given mass of gas will vary inversely with its pressure ($P_1V_1 = P_2V_2$; where P_1 = initial pressure, P_2 = final pressure, V_1 = initial volume, and V_2 = final volume). As an individual ascends, barometric pressure decreases and the volume of gas within an enclosed space expands. As the individual descends, the reverse is true.

Dalton's law of partial pressure describes the pressure exerted by gases at various altitudes. It states that the total pressure of a mixture of gases is the sum of the partial pressures of all the gases in the mixture. At sea level barometric pressure is 760 mmHg, and the percentage of oxygen in the atmosphere is equal to 20.95 percent. Therefore, the partial pressure of oxygen (Po_2) at sea level is Po_2 = 20.95 percent x 760 mmHg = 159.22 mmHg.

As altitude increases and pressure decreases, gas expansion causes the available oxygen to decrease. At 10,000 ft, where the barometric pressure is 523 mmHg, the percentage of oxygen *remains* 20.95 percent, but the partial pressure of oxygen will decrease to approximately 110 mmHg and the alveolar Po_2 will drop to 60 mmHg.

Physiologic Response

Several different responses are seen at high altitude. The response to hypoxia is the most significant. It includes increased cerebrospinal fluid (CSF) pressure, fluid retention, fluid shifts, and impaired gas exchange. Although no one is exempt from the effects of hypoxia, the onset and severity of symptoms will vary with individuals. The factors that influence an individual's threshold for hypoxia include physical activity, sleep, physical fitness, metabolic rate, diet, nutrition, emotions, and fatigue. Alcohol ingestion and smoking act as respiratory depressants and will exacerbate the effects of hypoxia. Exposure to temperature extremes will increase a person's metabolic rate, increasing oxygen requirements and reducing the hypoxic threshold.

The body responds with both immediate and chronic physiologic adaptations to the hypoxic environment. Through acclimatization, a series of physiologic adjustments works to restore the tissue oxygen pressure to near its sea level value. Successful acclimatization will vary between individuals and cannot be predicted by physical conditioning, examination, or testing.

A slow, graded ascent is the key to acclimatization. In the ideal setting, the first night's sleep occurs at <8000 ft, with the first day spent at rest. If the altitude of the desired climb is between 10,000 and 14,000 ft, then the daily ascent is limited to 1000 ft. Beyond 14,000 ft, 2 days should be taken for each 1000 ft ascent. Climbing to higher elevations during the day and descending to a lower altitude to sleep is one option to prevent AMS and facilitate acclimatization.

Pharmacologic agents may also be beneficial adjuncts to acclimatization. Acetazolamide (Diamox) has been shown to be very effective when staging is not possible or with individuals who are at an increased risk of high-altitude illness. Dexamethasone may also be effective

Table 116-1. Effects of Altitude

Altitude (in ft)	Barometric Pressure mmHg	Barometric Pressure PSI	Po$_2$ (mmHg)	Pao$_2$ (mmHg)	Paco$_2$ (mmHg)	Temp (F°)	Volume Ratio	O$_2$ Sat %
0	760	14.70	159.2	103.0	40.0	59.0	1.0	98
1000	733	14.17	153.6	98.2	39.4	55.4		
2000	706	13.67	147.9	93.8	39.0	51.8		
3000	681	13.17	142.7	89.5	38.4	48.4		
4000	656	12.69	137.4	85.1	38.0	44.8		
5000	632	12.23	132.5	81.0	37.4	41.2	1.2	
6000	609	11.78	127.6	76.8	37.0	37.6		
7000	586	11.34	122.8	72.8	36.4	34.0		
8000	565	10.92	118.4	68.9	36.0	30.4	1.3	93
9000	542	10.51	113.5	65.0	35.4	27.0		
10,000	523	10.11	109.6	61.2	35.0	23.4	1.5	87
11,000	503	9.72	105.4	57.8	34.4	19.8		
12,000	483	9.35	101.2	54.3	33.8	16.2		
13,000	465	8.98	97.4	51.0	33.2	12.6		
14,000	447	8.63	93.6	47.9	32.6	9.1		
15,000	429	8.29	89.9	45.0	32.0	5.5	1.8	84
16,000	412	7.97	86.3	42.0	31.4	1.9		
17,000	396	7.65	83.0	40.0	31.0	−1.7		
18,000	380	7.34	79.6	37.8	30.4	−5.2		72
19,000	364	7.04	76.3	35.9	30.0	−8.7		
20,000	349	6.75	73.1	34.3	29.4	−12.3	2.2	66
30,000	228	4.36	47.3			−47.9	3.3	
40,000	141	2.72	29.5			−62.7	5.4	
50,000	87	1.68	18.2			−62.7	8.7	

Source: Modified from Blumen IB, Abernethy MK, Dunne MJ, in Hageman JR, Fetcho S (eds): *Critical Care Clinics, Transport of the Critically Ill,* vol 8. Philadelphia: WB Saunders, 1992.

in preventing AMS, but it is generally reserved for treatment.

Respiratory System

As an individual ascends, the hypoxic ventilatory response (HVR) will attempt to compensate for the decrease in arterial Po$_2$ through an increase in the ventilatory rate. An inadequate HVR, resulting in relative hypoventilation, has been suggested as the etiology for AMS and HAPE. Individuals with low tidal volume and children are less able to respond to the hypoxic insult and therefore are more prone to AMS. HVR is genetically predetermined. It can be influenced by caffeine, alcohol, and numerous medications. Chronic hypoxia from chronic heart or lung problems desensitizes this effect.

The threshold for increased ventilation is approximately 4000 to 5000 ft elevation. At an altitude of 8000 ft, an arterial oxygenation saturation of 93 percent is experienced. The maximum response occurs at 22,000 ft, at which point the minute volume will be nearly doubled.

The initial maximal effect of the HVR occurs at approximately 6 to 8 hours after arrival to altitude. A decline in the partial pressure of inspiratory oxygen (Pio$_2$) results in an increase in ventilation, and Paco$_2$ will decrease accordingly. The falling Paco$_2$ causes a mild respiratory alkalosis and a shift of the oxyhemoglobin dissociation curve to the left. The result is increased binding of oxygen with hemoglobin for transport to the tissues. More importantly, the respiratory alkalosis provides negative feedback to the medulla, restricting the hypoxic ventilatory response. Further response is dependent on the renal excretion of bicarbonate, within 24 to 48 hours, to compensate for this respiratory alkalosis. Ventilation will slowly increase as the pH returns to normal. With no further ascent, this response can take 4 to 6 days. As an individual continues to higher elevation, subsequent acclimatization will be directed by the declining arterial P_{CO_2}.

Hypoxia and cold stressors will act as significant vasoconstrictors of the pulmonary vascular bed, resulting in an elevation of the pulmonary arterial pressure and an increased workload on the right side of the heart. The degree of pulmonary hypertension in response to a global hypoxia is thought to play an important role in the development of HAPE.

Cardiovascular System

The cardiovascular system is relatively resistant to hypoxia compared with the respiratory and central nervous systems. The cardiovascular system response to hypoxia may be observed in two phases. The heart rate will begin to increase at an altitude of 4000 ft. There will also be a slight increase in blood pressure secondary to increased catecholamines and selective vasoconstriction. These increase the cardiac output. As acclimatization occurs, the heart rate will return to normal. If the individual fails to acclimatize, the heart rate will remain elevated, and the increase in cardiac activity will require more oxygen. The already hypoxic myocardium will respond with a decrease in heart rate, hypotension, and arrhythmias.

Hematopoietic System

The hematopoietic response to high altitude is a critical element in an individual's ability to acclimatize. Within hours of ascent, erythropoietin output is increased in response to the hypoxia. In approximately 4 to 5 days, there will be an increase in circulating red blood cells. This increase in red cell mass persists for 1 to 2 months after return to lower altitudes. At extreme altitudes this hematopoietic response is detrimental. Oxygen transport is impeded by the increased blood viscosity, hemoconcentration, and increased red blood cell mass.

Increased 2,3-diphosphoglycerate (2,3-DPG) within the red blood cells is another hematopoietic response to hypoxemia. This shifts the oxyhemoglobin disassociation curve to the right, facilitating the release of oxygen from the blood to the tissues. With acclimatization, this shift to the right offsets the leftward shift of the oxyhemoglobin dissociation curve caused by hyperventilation and respiratory alkalosis.

Central Nervous System

Cerebral hypoxia begins when the P_{O_2} falls to 50 to 60 mmHg. The potent vasodilatory effects of hypoxia will overcome hypocapneic vasoconstriction and result in an increased cerebral blood flow. This response, which increases oxygen delivered to the brain, also increases intracranial pressure and can lead to HACE.

Renal System

Respiratory alkalosis stimulates renal excretion of bicarbonate, producing a metabolic acidosis to compensate for the respiratory alkalosis. As the pH equalizes, ventilation may continue to increase. This ventilatory acclimatization subsides after 4 to 6 days at altitude.

During ascent, central blood volume will increase secondary to peripheral vasoconstriction. Antidiuretic hormone (ADH) and aldosterone are inhibited, resulting in a diuresis, decreased plasma volume, and hemoconcentration. Individuals without this diuretic response are at greater risk for fluid retention and high-altitude illness.

Acute Mountain Sickness

AMS is the most common and mildest form of high-altitude illness. Up to 25 percent of individuals traveling to 8000 ft will become symptomatic, although nearly everyone who rapidly ascends to 11,000 ft will develop AMS.

The onset of AMS may be hastened by decreased vital capacity, increased CSF pressure, proteinuria, fluid retention, recent weight gain, or relative hypoventilation. It is postulated that children are more susceptible to AMS, as they are more sensitive to cerebral hypoxemia. Physical fitness does not impact on susceptibility to AMS.

Pathophysiology

Although normal acclimatization inhibits ADH and aldosterone, resulting in a high-altitude-induced diuresis, the opposite is seen with AMS. Aldosterone, ADH, and renin-angiotensin increase, resulting in fluid retention and a leakage from the vascular space to the extravascular space.

There are two theories for the development of cerebral edema in AMS. The first theory is cytotoxic edema, which is induced by a deficiency in the ATP-dependent sodium pump caused by a hypoxic cellular injury, leading to an accumulation of intracellular fluid. The second is vasogenic edema. In this situation, hypoxia causes cerebral vasodilation, which in turn increases cerebral blood flow, capillary perfusion, and leakage through the blood-brain barrier.

Clinical Presentation

The onset of AMS symptoms is usually within 4 to 8 hours of a rapid ascent, but it can be delayed for up to 4 days. Symptoms develop following strenuous activity or sleeping at high altitude. In most cases, symptoms peak in 24 to 48 hours and resolve by the third or fourth day. If the individual proceeds to a higher altitude after the onset of AMS, symptoms may last considerably longer.

The clinical presentation of AMS includes the following symptoms, in order of prevalence:

- Headache
- Sleep disturbance
- Fatigue
- Shortness of breath
- Dizziness
- Anorexia
- Nausea
- Vomiting

AMS should be considered the etiology in any individual at altitude who develops at least three of these symptoms. Headache occurs in approximately two-thirds of individuals with AMS. It is throbbing in nature and worse after exercise, at night or on awakening. Nausea and vomiting are common in children. Other symptoms associated with AMS include oliguria, mild peripheral edema, weakness, lassitude, malaise, irritability, decreased concentration, poor judgment, palpitations, deep inner chill, and a dull pain in the posterolateral chest wall.

On physical examination, vital signs may be normal or slightly elevated. Fluid retention is exhibited as fine rales or peripheral edema. Retinal hemorrhages may also be seen.

Sleep disturbance and periods of sleep apnea are common. Under normal sea level conditions there is a mild decrease in oxygen saturation during sleep. This becomes more pronounced at altitude. While sleeping, the increased respiratory rate that accompanies high-altitude exposure causes a mild respiratory alkalosis that inhibits the respiratory drive, resulting in hypoventilation and periods of apnea. Brief episodes of hyperventilation occur next, increasing oxygen saturation while exacerbating the hypocapnia and further inhibiting ventilation. These episodes of periodic breathing (Cheyne-Stokes respirations), with apnea lasting up to 90 seconds, continue through the night, increasing the hypoxia associated with being at altitude.

The differential diagnosis of these symptoms includes an alcohol hangover, exhaustion, dehydration, and a viral syndrome. In addition, respiratory and central nervous system infections, exhaustion, hypothermia, gastritis, and carbon monoxide poisoning should be considered. However, if the symptoms occur shortly after arrival to altitude, they must be considered AMS until proved otherwise.

Treatment

Treatment is initially directed toward prevention. Symptoms of AMS are most often mild and self-limiting, lasting only a few days. Once symptoms do occur, activity should be minimized, with no higher ascent until signs and symptoms have resolved. Proceeding to a lower altitude is indicated for any individual who shows no signs of improvement within 1 to 2 days or worsens. Immediate descent is indicated if ataxia, decreased level of consciousness, confusion, dyspnea at rest, rales, or cyanosis are present. A descent of 1000 to 3000 ft is recommended. In some situations, as little as a 500-ft descent may result in improvement.

If descent is not an option, the use of supplementary oxygen will relieve most of the signs and symptoms of AMS. During sleep, 1 to 2 L/min can be of significant benefit.

A Gamow bag is a portable fabric hyperbaric bag that has been shown to relieve the central effects of AMS. Using a foot pump, it can be pressurized in excess of 100 torr for the physiologic equivalent of a 4000- to 5000-ft descent.

Symptomatic treatment for the headache is with acetaminophen, which will have no impact on the hypoxic ventilatory response. Victims of AMS are to refrain from using narcotics, which depress this response. Prochlorperazine, given for nausea and vomiting, is also effective in *increasing* the respiratory drive. The dosage of prochlorperazine for children >10 kg in weight, or older than 2 years, is 0.1 to 0.15 mg/kg/dose IM, PO, or PR.

The carbonic anhydrase inhibitor acetazolamide may be used in the treatment or prophylaxis of AMS. It decreases the reabsorption of bicarbonate, forcing a renal bicarbonate diuresis and resulting in a mild metabolic acidosis. This increases the ventilation rate and arterial Po_2. Low-dose acetazolamide is a particularly effective respiratory stimulant in the treatment of sleep apnea. The pediatric dosage for acetazolamide is 5 to 10 mg/kg/day, given every 12 hours. Side effects include peripheral paresthesia, nausea, vomiting, polyuria, spoiling the taste of carbonated beverages, drowsiness, and confusion. Acetazolamide is contraindicated for those with sulfur sensitivities. When acetazolamide is used for prophylaxis, it should be started 48 hours before ascent and continued for at least 48 hours after arriving at the highest altitude. The dosage for older children and adults is 250 mg PO q8 to 12h. When used to treat AMS, improvement is generally seen within 12 to 24 hours.

Dexamethasone is also used to treat AMS, although its mechanism of action is unknown. Dexamethasone minimizes the symptoms of AMS but does not impact acclimatization. Its use is reserved for those with sulfur allergies or intolerance to acetazolamide. A loading dose of 4 mg PO or IM is given, and improvement is generally noted within 2 to 6 hours. If there is no improvement after descent, a maintenance dose of 1 to 1.5 mg/kg/day (not to exceed 16 mg/day) divided q4 to 6h should be initiated for 5 days. The dose is then tapered for 5 days before it is discontinued. Rebound AMS may occur if the dexamethasone is discontinued at altitude.

Prevention

Prevention of AMS through acclimatization is not always possible for vacationing climbers, skiers, and other sport enthusiasts. Prevention includes a slow graded ascent and a diet high in carbohydrates, low in salt, and with adequate fluid intake. Alcohol and tobacco are to be avoided.

High-Altitude Cerebral Edema

HACE is the most severe, life-threatening form of high-altitude illness. HACE is uncommon, affecting <1 to 2 percent of individuals who ascend without acclimatization. It is rare below altitudes of 12,000 ft, but has resulted in death at elevations as low as 8200 ft. A common problem is the difficulty in differentiating between AMS and early HACE.

Pathophysiology

HACE is thought to be associated with cytotoxic edema, vasogenic edema, or a combination of these two processes that cause cerebral edema. The time of onset for HACE would support the cytotoxic edema theory, whereas the response of HACE to corticosteroids would support the vasogenic edema theory.

Clinical Presentation

HACE commonly begins with the symptoms of AMS and progresses to diffuse neurologic dysfunction. Onset of severe symptoms is 1 to 3 days after ascent to altitude, but early signs of AMS may rapidly deteriorate to severe HACE in as few as 12 hours. Evidence of HAPE may also be present.

Severe headaches, nausea, vomiting, and altered mental status are common symptoms associated with HACE. Truncal ataxia is the cardinal sign. This alone warrants immediate descent. If not recognized, HACE will proceed to include confusion, slurred speech, diplopia, hallucinations, seizures, impaired judgment, cranial nerve palsies (third and sixth), abnormal reflexes, paresthesias, decreased level of consciousness, coma, and finally death. A 60 percent mortality is associated with HACE once coma is present.

The differential diagnosis includes head injury, subarachnoid hemorrhage, meningitis, encephalitis, carbon monoxide poisoning, transient ischemic attack, and cerebrovascular accident. Patients who become symptomatic at high altitude warrant a complete evaluation to rule out other etiologies.

Treatment

Definitive treatment of HACE is descent, and as quickly as possible. High-flow oxygen is indicated as soon as symptoms are recognized. Dexamethasone can produce dramatic improvement. An initial dose of 1 to 2 mg/kg PO or IM (maximum dose 8 mg) is given followed by a maintenance dose of 1 to 1.5 mg/kg/day (not to exceed 16 mg/day) divided q4 to 6h for 5 days. The dose is then tapered for 5 days before it is discontinued. Acetazolamide has not been shown to be effective in the treatment of HACE. Hyperbaric therapy with the Gamow bag has been reported to be useful in mild HACE and may be life-saving if descent is impossible.

For severe cases, intubation and hyperventilation are indicated to decrease intracranial pressure. Furosemide and mannitol are second-line treatments.

Acute episodes of HACE may result in long-term neurologic deficits. Coma may persist for days. Persistent ataxia, impaired judgment, and behavioral changes have been reported to last as long as 1 year. For this reason, it is essential that any evidence of HACE be recognized and treated early and that other etiologies be ruled out if symptoms persist.

The key to prevention of HACE is acclimatization. However, cases of HACE have been reported in individuals who have limited their ascent to 1000 ft a day.

High-Altitude Pulmonary Edema

HAPE is a life-threatening manifestation of high-altitude illness and represents a unique form of noncardiogenic pulmonary edema. It is estimated that HAPE affects 0.5 to 15 percent of those who ascend rapidly to high altitudes. Other than trauma, it is the most common cause of death at altitude. HAPE rarely occurs below 8000 ft and is more commonly associated with altitudes greater than 14,500 ft. At altitudes between 8000 and 10,000 ft, HAPE may develop after strenuous activity, whereas at higher elevations it may occur at rest.

HAPE is exacerbated by rapid ascent, cold stressors, a past history of HAPE, excessive exertion, and an inability to acclimatize. History of a recent upper respiratory tract infection has also been thought to be contributory.

Children and young adults are more susceptible to HAPE. Individuals younger than 20 years may be 10 to 13 times more prone to develop HAPE. Children are also more susceptible to a special form of this high-altitude illness identified as *reentry HAPE*. This occurs in individuals who are living at higher altitudes and return to the set elevation after spending as little as 24 hours at lower altitude.

Pathophysiology

HAPE can affect individuals without prior history of cardiac or pulmonary disease. Pulmonary vasoconstriction secondary to the hypoxic stimuli elevates pulmonary artery pressures. The pulmonary hypertension is exacerbated by increased blood volume secondary to peripheral vasoconstriction and fluid retention. The end result is a noncardiogenic pulmonary edema.

Individuals with an elevated pulmonary artery pressure or with a blunted hypoxic ventilatory response have been shown to be at increased risk for HAPE. This is thought to be the reason why children and infants with pulmonary arterial hypertrophy are more prone to the development of HAPE. Congenital absence of a pulmonary artery may also predispose an individual to HAPE. It should be noted that not all individuals with pulmonary hypertension will develop HAPE.

Clinical Presentation

The onset of HAPE usually occurs within 1 to 4 days after ascent to altitude, most commonly during the second night at altitude. However, initial symptoms may develop within hours following ascent.

Early in the course the victim will develop a dry cough, fatigue, and dyspnea on exertion. Symptoms of AMS often accompany these initial signs. A few localized rales may be audible in the right middle lobe auscultated over the right axilla. Rales increase with exercise.

As HAPE progresses, the patient will have a productive clear cough, orthopnea, weakness, and altered mental status. This intensifies to severe dyspnea at rest, a cardinal sign of HAPE. The patient may be tachycardic, tachypneic, and febrile to 102°F. Rales become bilateral. Peripheral cyanosis advances to central cyanosis if treatment is not initiated. Dyspnea at rest, while at altitude, is HAPE until proved otherwise.

A chest radiograph reveals bilateral fluffy asymmetric infiltrates and dilated pulmonary arteries. Cardiomegaly, a butterfly pattern of infiltrates, and Kerley-B lines, commonly seen in cardiogenic pulmonary edema, are not seen in HAPE. An electrocardiogram (ECG) may show sinus tachycardia, right ventricular strain, right axis deviation, P-wave abnormalities, prominent R waves in the right chest leads, and S waves in the left chest leads.

Without treatment, florid pulmonary edema and respiratory failure will develop. Dysfunction of the central nervous system will ensue, leading to coma and death.

The differential diagnosis includes pneumonia, congestive heart failure, high-altitude bronchitis, pharyngitis, asthma, neurogenic pulmonary edema, pulmonary embolism, and adult respiratory distress syndrome. Hyperviscosity from dehydration and increased red blood cell mass results in a hypercoagulable state, which may play a role in the development of HAPE.

Treatment

As with any form of high-altitude illness, immediate descent may be life-saving and is not to be delayed. There is a delicate balance, however, between rapid descent and the amount of energy the victim expends to descend quickly. Individuals may deteriorate from overexertion as they proceed to a lower altitude. Therefore, care must be taken to minimize the effort while maximizing the effect. A descent of 1000 to 2000 ft is usually adequate for symptomatic relief.

In addition to rapid descent, bed rest, supplemental oxygen, and keeping the patient warm are necessary.

Physical activity and exposure to cold increase the catecholamine response, which increases pulmonary pressure. Supplemental oxygen effectively lowers pulmonary arterial pressure, which raises arterial oxygen saturation. As a result, heart rate and respiratory rate will decrease. High-flow oxygen at 6 to 8 L/min by mask is administered to anyone with significant symptoms. It may be possible to reverse symptoms with oxygen alone (without descent) over a period of 2 to 3 days.

An end-expiratory airway pressure (EPAP) mask that can deliver 5 to 10 cm H_2O of end-expiratory pressure can be used to improve oxygen delivery. When oxygen is not available and descent is not possible, the portable Gamow bag may be used for hyperbaric treatment and has been shown to be effective in patients with HAPE.

Pharmacologic agents play a limited role in the treatment of HAPE. Acetazolamide may be useful in the prevention of HAPE. Although furosemide has been shown to be helpful, caution must be used due to the prevalence of hypovolemia and dehydration. Nifedipine has been shown to decrease pulmonary arterial pressure. Again, caution must be exercised in the use of a potentially hypovolemic dehydrated patient.

Rapid improvement and resolution of symptoms usually follow descent to a lower altitude. If oxygen saturation is <90 percent, hospitalization is indicated. In very severe cases of HAPE, intubation and ventilation with positive end-expiratory pressure may be needed.

The overall mortality of HAPE is 11 percent. Without treatment (descent or supplemental oxygen), the mortality increases to 44 percent.

An episode of HAPE is not a contraindication to further attempts to reach altitude. However, there is a higher incidence for recurrent symptoms with subsequent ascents.

Altitude-Related Syndromes

High-Altitude Retinal Hemorrhage

It is estimated that 50 percent of individuals who ascend to 16,000 ft and 100 percent of those who ascend to 21,000 ft will develop high-altitude retinal hemorrhage (HARH) within 2 to 3 days after arrival to altitude.

HARH presents with tortuous dilation of the retinal arteries and veins, retinal hemorrhages, and papilledema. The hemorrhages are most often throughout the fundus but spare the macula. It is painless and usually asymptomatic, with no visual disturbances noted. If the macula is involved, the victim may complain of cloudy or blurred vision. In these situations, descending to a lower altitude is indicated.

In most cases, HARH is self-limiting and usually resolves spontaneously within 2 to 3 weeks after descent. If the macula was involved, visual changes may be permanent.

HARH may occur alone or in the presence of AMS, HAPE, or HACE. The incidence of HARH increases with strenuous activity and with a history of previous HARH.

Chronic Mountain Sickness

Chronic mountain sickness (CMS), also referred to as Monge's disease, is a rare complication of high-altitude illness. Some individuals will fail to acclimatize despite prolonged exposure or living at high altitude. Symptoms are similar to those of AMS and include headache, dyspnea, sleep disturbance, and fatigue.

CMS is associated with an inadequate hypoxic ventilatory response, resulting in persistent hypoxia and excessive erythropoietin production. Polycythemia follows, with the hematocrit often greater than 60. Congestive heart failure is seen.

Treatment for CMS includes descent to a lower altitude, oxygen, phlebotomy, and the use of respiratory stimulants such as acetazolamide.

Ultraviolet Keratitis

Snow blindness is caused by increased ultraviolet (UV) light exposure at higher altitudes secondary to the loss of the protective atmosphere and fewer pollutants. For every 1000 ft of ascent, UV exposure will increase by 5 percent.

Patients develop a foreign body sensation or severe pain approximately 12 hours after exposure. They may also have periorbital edema, excessive tearing, photophobia, and conjunctival erythema. Treatment is with oral analgesics to alleviate the severe discomfort. Symptoms resolve within 24 hours. Sunglasses with polaroid lenses and side blinders are preventative.

High-Altitude Pharyngitis and Bronchitis

High-altitude bronchitis and pharyngitis are common at altitudes >8000 ft, secondary to the excessive inhalation of dry, cold air that causes drying and cracking of the upper airway mucous membranes. Symptoms include a dry, hacking, and often painful cough.

Symptoms are prevented or minimized by ensuring adequate hydration and salivation. Throat lozenges and hard candy help to maintain oral secretions. Inhaled steam, gargling, and oral fluids will also keep the mucous membranes moist. A cloth worn over the mouth and nose helps to warm the inspired air and trap moisture. Antibiotics are not helpful, whereas analgesics may be beneficial.

Preexisting Pulmonary Disease

Any pulmonary disease that affects breathing at sea level has the potential to cause further complications at high altitude. Supplemental oxygen may be necessary for any child with known hypoxemia, sleep disorder, or pulmonary hypertension. Neither asthma nor bronchospasm is known to be aggravated by high-altitude exposure. However, exposure to cold, dry air could worsen these problems.

Sickle Cell Disease

Patients with sickle cell disease are at increased risk for vasoocclusive crisis and hypoxemia over 5000 to 6500 ft. Patients with sickle cell trait are without risk for vasoocclusive crisis but are at increased risks for splenic infarction at increased altitudes. Patients with sickle cell disease are advised to use supplemental oxygen at elevations >5000 ft. Nonnarcotic analgesics and hydration are also indicated.

Pregnancy

Pregnancy is not a contraindication for women to participate in reasonable activities at reasonable altitude levels. There is no increase in complications, maternal or neonatal, associated with short-term exposure to high altitude. However, women who live at high altitude have been shown to have a higher incidence of low-birth-weight babies, maternal hypertension, and neonatal hyperbilirubinemia.

Peripheral Edema

Peripheral edema is a common complication at higher altitudes. Swelling of the face and distal extremities is most often noted and is more common in females. Although such edema responds spontaneously within 1 to 2 days, it should raise the suspicion of AMS.

Other Complications

Other syndromes associated with ascent to high altitude include altitude syncope and migraine headaches. Arterial or venous thrombosis (both peripheral and central) may develop secondary to increased viscosity, causing transient ischemic attacks. Central nervous system tumors may be unmasked as a result of increased brain volume from the increased intracranial pressures. Seizures may be secondary to the hypoxia.

Summary

Each year larger numbers of individuals head toward higher elevations. As a result, physicians who practice in or near high-altitude regions must be familiar with the signs, symptoms, and management of altitude illnesses (Table 116-2). Poor judgment and inadequate trainingon the part of the victim should be anticipated. Adults who travel with children need to know that children are more susceptible to high-altitude illness and to watch for symptoms.

In the high-altitude setting, any onset of symptoms that could represent high-altitude illness should be taken seriously. The mild symptoms of AMS can easily and quickly progress to the potentially deadly HACE or HAPE if not recognized, diagnosed, and treated promptly.

DYSBARIC INJURIES

Dysbaric injuries may be the result of several distinct events that expose an individual to a change in barometric pressure. The first possible etiology is an altitude-related event, which can be illustrated by the rapid ascent or descent during airplane transport or sudden cabin decompression at an altitude >25,000 ft. The second type of dysbaric injury results from an underwater diving accident. A third dysbarism is caused by a blast injury that produces an *overpressure* effect. This section primarily discusses dysbaric diving injuries and, to a lesser extent, aviation-related dysbarisms. Blast injuries are beyond the scope of this chapter.

Scuba (self-contained underwater breathing apparatus) diving was developed in the mid-1940s and currently allows the sport diver to descend to depths >100 ft. There are an estimated 8.5 million certified scuba divers in the United States. In 1999 alone, >800,000 divers worldwide completed formal training and certification. Candidates must be at least 16 years old for full certification. However, certification is not required to dive. It is the untrained or poorly trained individual who is at greater risk for injury. Scuba diving requires absolute adherence to safety rules and a modicum of common sense. In general, children younger than 12 years should not engage in scuba diving.

Several terms are often used when discussing this topic. *Dysbarisms* represents the general topic of

Table 116-2. An Overview of High-Altitude Illness

	Acute Mountain Sickness (AMS)	High-Altitude Cerebral Edema (HACE)	High-Altitude Pulmonary Edema (HAPE)
Altitude	Rare below 8000 ft Affects nearly everyone who rapidly ascends to 11,000	Rare below 12,000 ft	Rare below 8000 ft More commonly associated with altitudes >14,500 ft
Onset	Within 4–8 hours of a rapid ascent but can be as long as 4 days Peaks within 24–48 hr Usually resolves by the third or fourth day	Most often within 1–3 days after ascent to altitude	Usually within 1–4 days after ascent to altitude Most common during the second night at altitude
Symptoms	Most common: headache, sleep disturbance, fatigue, shortness of breath, dizziness, anorexia, nausea, vomiting, oliguria Other symptoms: mild peripheral edema, weakness, lassitude, malaise, irritability, decreased concentration, poor judgment, palpitations, deep inner chill, dull pain in the posterolateral chest wall	Severe headaches, nausea, vomiting, altered mental status Cardinal sign: truncal ataxia Will proceed to include confusion, slurred speech, diplopia, hallucinations, seizures, impaired judgment, cranial nerve palsies (third and sixth), abnormal reflexes, paresthesia, decreased level of consciousness, coma, death	Initial symptoms: dry cough, fatigue, dyspnea on exertion, few rales Symptoms of AMS may be present As symptoms progress: productive clear cough, orthopnea, weakness, altered mental status, tachycardia, tachypnea, fever, increased rales, cyanosis Cardinal sign: severe dyspnea at rest
Treatment	Rest Increase fluids No higher ascent until symptoms have resolved Proceed to a lower altitude if no improvement within 1–2 days or if symptoms worsen Supplemental oxygen, if available Symptomatic relief for headache, nausea Immediate descent is indicated for ataxia, decreased level of consciousness, confusion, dyspnea at rest, rales, or cyanosis Acetazolamide: adult, 250 mg bid; pediatric, 5–10 mg/kg/day bid Consider dexamethasone, 4 mg PO/IM	Immediate descent High-flow oxygen Dexamethasone: Initial dose of 8 mg IV Followed by 1–1.5 mg/kg/d divided qid to a maximum dose of 4 mg/dose Rest Hyperbaric therapy if descent is not possible	Mild to moderate HAPE: Bed rest Supplemental oxygen Observe closely Severe HAPE: Immediate descent Minimal exertion High-flow oxygen Furosemide Nifedipine Hyperbaric therapy if descent is not possible

(Continues)

Table 116-2. (*continued*) An Overview of High-Altitude Illness

	Acute Mountain Sickness (AMS)	High-Altitude Cerebral Edema (HACE)	High-Altitude Pulmonary Edema (HAPE)
Prevention	Acclimatization: slow graded ascent; first night's sleep should be at an altitude no greater than 8000 ft and the first day should be spent at rest; daily climb should then be limited to 1000 ft if the altitude is between 10,000 and 14,000 ft; beyond 14,000 climbers should take 2 days for each 1000-ft ascent. Avoid alcohol, sedatives, smoking		
	Acetazolamide: start 48 hr before ascent and continue for at least 48 hr after arriving at the highest altitude; pediatric, 5–10 mg/kg/day bid; adult, 250 mg bid	Acetazolamide efficacy is unproved	Acetazolamide may be helpful, but efficacy is unproved Watch for early signs of HAPE and, if present, stop ascent

Source: Courtesy of Ira Blumen, MD, Section of Emergency Medicine, Department of Medicine, University of Chicago.

pressure-related injuries. *Barotrauma,* the most common diving injury, refers to the injuries that are a direct result of the mechanical effects of a pressure differential. The complications related to the partial pressure of gases and dissolved gases are called *decompression sickness.*

Physical Gas Laws

Dysbarisms can best be explained through the physical gas laws and an understanding of pressure equivalents that cause these injuries. The amount of pressure exerted by air at sea level and at different altitudes or depths can be described several different ways, as shown in Table 116-3.

Individuals and objects under water are exposed to progressively greater pressure due to the weight of the water. Small changes in the underwater depth result in large atmospheric pressure and volume changes. This is significantly different from the pressure and volume variation noted in air above sea level. *Boyle's law,* as previously described, explains this relationship.

Under water, the largest proportionate change in the volume of a gas is seen close to the water surface. An air-filled cavity that is 33 ft below the water surface will double when it reaches the surface. In comparison, a volume of gas at sea level will need to rise to an altitude of 18,000 ft to double in volume.

Dalton's law of partial pressure, as previously presented, describes the pressure exerted by gases at various depths or altitudes. Each gas will exert a pressure

equal to its proportion of the total gaseous mixture ($P_{total} = P_1 + P_2 + P_3 . . . P_n$). Table 116-4 depicts the gaseous composition of the atmosphere at sea level and the corresponding partial pressures.

Henry's law states that the quantity of gas dissolved in a liquid is proportional to the partial pressure of the gas in contact with the liquid. The partial pressure of a gas and the solubility of the gas determine the amount of gas that will dissolve into a liquid. This law will help explain the increased absorption of nitrogen during descent.

Pathophysiology

The clinical findings of dysbaric injuries may be immediate or delayed in onset up to 36 hours. Most will occur during descent or in close proximity to ascent. A delayed presentation is possible, however, which may make diagnosis difficult.

There are three mechanisms for dysbaric injuries. The first follows Boyle's law for trapped gas and changes in ambient pressure. The second follows Henry's law when gas dissolved in blood is released. The third deals with abnormal tissue concentrations of various gases.

Barotrauma: Dysbarisms From Trapped Gases

Barotrauma is the direct result of a pressure difference between the body's air-filled cavities, which are subject

Table 116-3. Effect of Altitude or Depth on Air Pressure

Altitude (in ft) or Depth (in ft of sea water [FSW])	Absolute Pressure (ATA)	Torr	PSI	Volume Ratio
Altitude				
40,000	0.19	141	2.72	5.39
30,000	0.30	228	4.36	3.33
20,000	0.46	349	6.75	2.18
10,000	0.69	523	10.11	1.45
5000	0.83	632	12.23	1.20
1000	0.97	733	14.17	1.04
Sea level	1	760	14.7	1
Depth				
33	2	1,520	29.4	0.50
66	3	2,280	44.1	0.33
99	4	3,040	58.8	0.25
132	5	3,800	73.5	0.20
165	6	4,560	88.2	0.17
198	7	5,320	102.9	0.14

Source: Courtesy of Ira Blumen, MD, Section of Emergency Medicine, Department of Medicine, University of Chicago.

to the effects of Boyle's law, and the surrounding environment. While the individual is scuba diving, most symptoms will develop during a descent. On descent, a negative pressure develops within enclosed air spaces relative to the ambient surrounding pressure. If air is unable to enter these structures, equalization does not take place, and the air-filled cavities collapse. If the cavity is a rigid structure and unable to collapse, the negative pressure may result in fluid being displaced from the blood vessels of the surrounding mucosa into the intravascular space. The resulting injury pattern can include pain, hemorrhage, edema, vascular engorgement, and tissue damage.

If air is unable to escape on ascent, an expansion of gas within these enclosed air spaces causes a positive pressure to develop. This may result in the rupture of such spaces or the compression of adjacent structures.

Many of the symptoms of barotrauma in the human body result in a "squeeze" phenomenon. These trapped gas disorders are differentiated by the gas-filled part of the body that is affected.

Barotitis

Barometric pressure changes can result in disturbances of the external, middle, and inner ear. The tympanic membrane (TM) separates the middle ear from the outer ear. The eustachian tube usually functions as a one-way valve allowing gas to escape but not return to the middle ear.

Barotitis media is the most common diving-related barotrauma and involves the middle ear, commonly referred to as *barotitis media, middle ear squeeze,* or *ear block.* Equalization via the eustachian tube will occur when there is a pressure differential of approximately 15 to 20 mmHg. The diver becomes symptomatic if equalization is unsuccessful and the pressure differential reaches or approaches 100 mmHg.

Middle ear squeeze commonly develops on descent between 10 and 20 ft below the surface. The symptoms include a fullness in the ears, severe pain, tinnitus, vertigo, nausea, disorientation, and transient, conductive hearing loss. Up to 10 percent of divers may have no pain during descent but will become symptomatic after the dive. If the diver is unable to equalize the pressure and continues to descend, symptoms may be exacerbated and the tympanic membrane may rupture and bleed. With perforation, the caloric stimulation of cold water entering the middle ear can cause vertigo, nausea, and disorientation.

The physical examination may reveal erythema or retraction of the tympanic membrane, blood behind the TM, a ruptured TM, or a bloody nasal discharge.

Treatment for middle ear squeeze should be directed toward its prevention, before pain develops. Scuba divers

Table 116-4. Atmospheric Composition

	% of Gas in Atmosphere	Barometric Pressure (mmHg)
Oxygen	20.95	159.22
Nitrogen	78.08	593.41
Other gases	<1	<7.6
Total	100	760

should attempt to clear their ears every 2 to 3 ft during descent. Under normal situations, pressure in the middle ear is equalized without incident. The eustachian tube can be actively opened, allowing equalization with the middle ear by using positive pressure originating from the nasopharynx, or by using the jaw muscles.

Middle ear pressure can be equalized by swallowing, yawning, or performing the Valsalva maneuver. The Frenzel maneuver, another suggested treatment for barotitis, is performed by forcing closed the glottis and mouth while contracting the superior pharyngeal constrictors and the muscles of the floor of the mouth.

Equalization may be compromised if the eustachian tube is obstructed by swelling of the mucosa, the presence of polyps, previous trauma, allergies, upper respiratory infection, a sinus problem, or smoking. To decrease the incidence of ear discomfort and injury to the TM, a predive treatment of a topical vasoconstrictor nasal spray (oxymetazoline hydrochloride, 0.05 percent) may be beneficial when used about 15 minutes before beginning a dive. The recommended pediatric dosage for ages 6 and up is 2 to 3 sprays in each nostril. Oxymetazoline hydrochloride is not recommended for children younger than 6 years. Pseudoephedrine may also be considered as a predive treatment. For ages 6 to 12, the recommended dose is 30 mg PO. For children older than 12 years old, the adult dose of 60 mg PO may be used. If pain persists after the dive, analgesics may be used. If a predive decongestant was not used, it may be considered at this time.

Any patient with barotitis media is to be instructed to refrain from diving until all signs and symptoms have resolved. Erythema generally resolves within 1 to 3 days, whereas it will take 2 to 4 weeks when there is blood behind the TM. A perforated TM must heal before any further diving is attempted. A 10-day course of oral antibiotics and otic suspension is indicated if there is a perforation of the TM. ENT follow-up is given upon discharge from the emergency department.

Barotrauma can occur during either descent *or* ascent. If air is unable to escape the middle ear through the eustachian tube during ascent, a diver may develop symptoms of *reverse ear squeeze*.

Alternobaric vertigo may develop during descent, but it is more common during ascent. A sudden change in middle ear pressure or asymmetrical middle ear pressure may result in decreased perfusion, affecting vestibular function. Symptoms include transient vertigo, tinnitus, nausea, vomiting, and fullness in the affected ear. Symptoms last minutes to several hours after the completion of a dive. Decongestants, antiemetics, and medication for vertigo are recommended.

Barotitis externa occurs when the external auditory canal, which is normally a patent air-filled cavity that communicates with the surrounding environment, is occluded during descent. At the initiation of descent, the air would normally be replaced by water. If the external canal is obstructed, the enclosed air space will be subject to the increased ambient pressure, resulting in an *external ear squeeze* or *barotitis externa.*

Obstruction can be caused by cerumen, ear plugs, or other foreign bodies. A diver may experience pain with or without bloody otorrhea.

Barotitis interna or *inner ear squeeze* is uncommon but may result in permanent injury to the structures of the inner ear. It often follows a vigorous Valsalva maneuver.

In addition to sudden sensorineural hearing loss, symptoms include severe pain or pressure, vertigo, tinnitus, ataxia, nausea, vomiting, diaphoresis, and nystagmus. These patients must be seen emergently. The potential for recovery within a few months is very good in most patients treated conservatively. Others, however, may require surgical intervention.

Altitude-Related Barotitis

Barotitis media is the most common barotrauma of air travel. During ascent to altitude, gas will normally escape through the eustachian tube every 500 to 1000 ft to equalize pressures. As altitude decreases, the gas within the middle ear will contract. As with diving, equalization may be accomplished by yawning, swallowing, or performing the Valsalva maneuver. Children who are asleep should be awakened 5 minutes before descent and instructed to swallow more frequently. For infants, a bottle should be given during takeoff and landing. Although this may reduce the likelihood of barotitis media, it may increase the incidence of gastrointestinal distress after takeoff from swallowed air.

Barosinusitis

Normally, air can pass in and out of the sinus cavities without difficulty. However, if a person has a cold or sinus infection, air may be trapped and will be subject to the barometric pressure changes.

Failure of the air-filled frontal or maxillary sinuses to equilibrate results in pain or pressure above, behind, or below the eyes, which is commonly referred to as *sinus squeeze*. Pain may persist for hours and may be accompanied by a bloody nasal discharge. The ethmoidand sphenoid sinuses rarely contribute to this type of barotrauma.

The treatment for barosinusitis is similar to the treatment of barotitis media. The most effective treatment involves the use of a vasoconstrictor nasal spray before initiating a dive or before starting a descent from altitude in an airplane. Antibiotics should be started and continued for 14 to 21 days.

Reverse sinus squeeze is felt during a diving ascent when an obstruction of the sinuses results in excessive pressure. A sharp pain will be felt in the affected sinus. Numbness may be felt along the infraorbital nerve if the maxillary sinus is affected. The diver should descend to a greater depth, relieving some of the discomfort, and then ascend at a slower rate.

Barodentalgia

Barodentalgia or *tooth squeeze* is often associated with recent dental extraction, dental fillings, periodontal infection, periodontal abscess, or tooth decay. Although this is a rare problem, individuals with preexisting dental or periodontal disease are more susceptible to this barotrauma. Treatment is directed toward preventative dental care and pain control. Following dental procedures, a minimum of 24 hours is advised before initiating a scuba dive.

Face Mask Squeeze

During descent, the increased ambient pressure will tend to exert increasing pressure against the air-filled face mask of a scuba diver. The diver may develop facial or eye pain, subconjunctival hemorrhages, subconjunctival edema, epistaxis, and periorbital edema. Face mask squeeze is commonly prevented by using a mask that allows for additional small amounts of air to be blown into the mask from the nose. Relief is symptomatic.

Aerogastralgia

Under normal circumstances, the stomach and intestines contain approximately 1 quart of gas. Ingesting carbon-ated beverage, chewing gum (and swallowing air), eating large meals, and preexisting gastrointestinal problems increase the amount of gas in the intestines. Gas expansion will cause discomfort, abdominal pain, belching, flatulence, nausea, vomiting, shortness of breath, or hyperventilation. Symptoms are prevented or relieved by belching or passing flatus. Wearing clothes that are loose and nonrestrictive is also of benefit.

Although aerogastralgia is rarely a serious problem, significant distention of the abdominal contents may result in venous pooling and syncope. In addition, tachycardia, hypotension, and syncope may result from a vasovagal response to severe pain. Gastric rupture has been reported.

Pulmonary Over-Pressurization Syndrome

Pulmonary over-pressurization syndrome (POPS) is an example of the positive-pressure barotrauma that can be seen during ascent. The alveoli become overinflated and can rupture, causing a pneumothorax. Ruptured pulmonary veins allow air emboli to enter the systemic circulation. These can occur if the scuba diver fails to exhale adequately on ascent, or in the presence of predisposing lung disease.

Air Embolism

An air embolism is the most serious dysbaric injury. Due to the buoyancy of air and the fact that scuba divers are usually upright during ascent, the brain is most commonly affected. The onset of symptoms is immediately on ascent, or within 10 to 20 minutes of surfacing. Neurologic symptoms that develop later than this are more likely to be due to decompression sickness.

These victims require aggressive care, which includes 100 percent oxygen, intravenous fluids, and hyperbaric treatment. They are placed in the Trendelenburg or left lateral decubitus position to minimize the passage of air emboli to the brain.

Air emboli affect the heart if they embolize to the coronary circulation, causing coronary artery occlusion, dysrhythmias, shock, and cardiac arrest. Although these complications are rare compared with other dysbaric injuries, they represent a significant risk to the victim.

Arterial air embolization to the brain is more common than to the heart or spinal cord. Neurologic symptoms are similar to those of a stroke and include numbness, dizziness, headaches, weakness, visual field deficits, confusion, behavioral changes, amnesia, paralysis, vertigo, blindness, aphasia, deafness, sensory deficit, seizures, focal deficits, and loss of consciousness. Due to the variety of neurologic presentations, a careful medical evaluation is warranted for the onset of any neurologic symptoms during or within a short time after the conclusion of a dive.

Pneumothorax and Emphysema

The patient with a confirmed or suspected pneumothorax, pneumopericardium, pneumomediastinum, or subcutaneous emphysema should not be exposed to any further barometric pressure changes. This is a significant problem if a pneumothorax develops during a dive. On ascent, a simple pneumothorax may progress to a tension pneumothorax, shock, and loss of consciousness. These complications may also occur during air transport in an unpressurized aircraft. Treatment of a scuba diving pneumothorax is no different than the treatment of other traumatic or nontraumatic pneumothoraxes. Hyperbaric (recompression) treatment is avoided since it can convert a simple pneumothorax to a tension pneumothorax. If hyperbaric treatment will be necessary, chest tubes must be placed before initiating recompression.

Decompression Sickness: Dysbarisms from Evolved Gases

Henry's law explains the formation of gas bubbles that separate from solution. Gases coming out of solution result in *decompression sickness.*

A diver breathing compressed air is exposed to nitrogen, oxygen, and carbon dioxide. Approximately 4/5 of the air is nitrogen. Oxygen is metabolized, and the carbon dioxide is expelled. Under normal circumstances additional nitrogen gas will not be absorbed by the body during inhalation. However, when the body is exposed to a varying ambient pressure, uptake or removal of nitrogen gas from the blood occurs.

As ambient pressure increases, the positive-pressure gradient between the alveoli and the blood will result in more nitrogen being dissolved. As a dive progresses, the gas in the blood will equilibrate quickly with the gas in the alveoli. Nitrogen gas, however, is almost five times more soluble in fat. It will take longer to saturate these tissues. Therefore, the body will absorb more nitrogen gas at a rate that is dependent on the depth and duration of the dive. The longer and deeper the dive, the more nitrogen gas will be accumulated within the body.

Since nitrogen is not metabolized, it remains dissolved until the nitrogen gas pressure in the lungs decreases and the nitrogen can be removed. During a slow ascent, as the surrounding pressure decreases, the nitrogen that is absorbed into the tissues is released into the blood and the alveoli. If the ascent is too quick, nitrogen levels do not have the opportunity to equalize among the tissues, blood, and alveoli. The pressure outside the body will drop significantly below the sum of the partial pressures of the gases inside the body. This results in the gas coming out of solution and the formation of gas bubbles in the blood or tissue. Due to the increased dissolved nitrogen, it has a disproportionately higher partial pressure. Therefore, a significant difference in partial pressure occurs. It is the release of these nitrogen bubbles from solution that results in decompression sickness.

Diving tables are often used by scuba divers as a tool to minimize the risk of developing a decompression sickness. However, even if the dive tables are carefully followed, additional factors could precipitate a decompression sickness, such as increased physical activity during a dive, cold temperatures, obesity, alcohol ingestion, previous dives with inadequate surface time to equilibrate, and flying within 12 hours of a dive.

Decompression sickness can be classified as follows:

- Type I, which typically involves extravascular gas bubbles and causes joint pain, skin rashes, and lymphedema
- Type II, which is caused by intravascular nitrogen gas emboli. The presentation may be very similar to that of air emboli. Children are more prone to type II injuries.

The term *bends* is often used to identify any form of decompression sickness. When used correctly, however, the term refers to the musculoskeletal syndrome involving the joints, which is a very common dysbarism. The bends occurs in up to 75 percent of all decompression injuries and is caused by the release of nitrogen gas bubbles from the blood into the tissues surrounding the joint.

Symptoms usually develop within 6 to 12 hours after the conclusion of a dive. A sharp, throbbing, or dull achy pain is a common presentation. There may also be associated numbness or tingling (paresthesia). The pain commonly is diffuse in its origin but will become more localized as the intensity increases. The joints most often affected are the knees, shoulder, and elbows.

Symptomatic relief may be obtained by splinting the extremity or by applying pressure over the affected joint. Massaging or moving the affected extremity often exacerbates the pain associated with the bends.

The physical examination is usually unremarkable. On occasion, crepitus, edema, or tenderness are noted.

The decompression illness that affects the pulmonary system is referred to as the *chokes.* It is caused by arterial or venous nitrogen gas embolization that obstructs the pulmonary vasculature. The symptoms may begin immediately after a dive but often take up to 12 hours to develop. They last between 12 and 48 hours but can progress to a rapid deterioration.

The classic triad of symptoms includes shortness of breath, cough, and substernal chest pain or chest tightness. The shortness of breath is described as a feeling of suffocation. The individual becomes tachycardiac and tachypneic. There is a nonproductive, often uncontrollable paroxysmal cough, which is exacerbated by deep inspiration. The chest pain is most frequently appreciated with deep inspiration, increased activity, and smoking. There is no radiation of the pain to the neck, arms, or abdomen.

Neurologic Decompression Sickness

Nitrogen gas embolism is the most serious decompression sickness. Venous gas emboli can result in venous obstruction, and arterial gas emboli can cause ischemia as a result of arterial obstruction or induced vasospasm.

As with air embolus, the brain is most commonly affected. The onset of symptoms, however, will usually be delayed, with symptoms developing within 1 to 6 hours after a dive is concluded. These victims require aggressive care, which includes 100 percent oxygen, intravenous fluids, and hyperbaric treatment. They are placed in the Trendelenburg or left lateral decubitus position to minimize the embolization to the brain.

Cerebral decompression injuries are more common with altitude-related decompression than with diving injuries. The symptoms are also similar to those of the air embolus. Common symptoms are headaches, visual field deficits, scintillating scotoma, confusion, behavioral changes, restlessness, amnesia, paralysis, blindness, deafness, hallucinations, sensory deficit, and seizures. Children primarily present with abnormal behavior, disorientation, and memory loss.

The headache that develops is often dull and pulsating in nature. It may be unilateral and is often on the opposite side of the visual field deficits or scotoma. The mild to moderate pain will usually last for several hours.

Scotoma may be peripherally or centrally located but often appear to move peripherally. They are appreciated with the eyes opened or closed and are unilateral or bilateral, singular or multiple. They appear as visual distortions or as colored lines that are horizontal or V-shaped.

Spinal cord complications are seen more often than cerebral decompression injuries as a result of diving ac-

cidents. An air embolism affects the spinal cord by blocking the venous return in the epidural vertebral venous system. This results in back pain, numbness in the extremities, weakness, paralysis, and urinary retention.

Decompression Shock

Decompression shock may be secondary to hypovolemia or due to vasovagal responses. Hypovolemia is caused by fluid loss and third spacing. The patient may become agitated, restless, cool to the touch, tachycardic, tachypneic, and finally hypotensive. If vasovagal symptoms dominate initially, the victim may present with diaphoresis, nausea, vomiting, bradycardia, light-headedness, and hypotension.

Aggressive and timely management with intravenous fluids, 100 percent oxygen, and recompression therapy should be initiated as quickly as possible.

Cutaneous Decompression Sickness

The extravascular release of nitrogen gas bubbles from the blood usually results in benign dysbarisms. Rashes, with or without pruritus, can present with any of the following patterns: scarlatiniform, mottling (cutis marmorata), and erysipeloid.

The release of nitrogen gas bubbles can cause subcutaneous emphysema, often involving the neck and other sites. When the neck is involved, the victim's voice may be altered, and the individual may complain of difficulty breathing or swallowing.

Treatment of individuals with subcutaneous emphysema begins with 100 percent oxygen. The patient is then carefully examined for more serious dysbarisms and admitted.

Treatment of Decompression Sickness and Air Embolus

The morbidity and mortality for dysbaric injuries depends on the severity of the injury, rapid identification of the illness, and timely access to appropriate medical care. When the "system" works, the recovery rate is as high as 90 percent.

The treatment of choice for most air emboli and decompression illnesses is hyperbaric (recompression) therapy. This is initiated as soon as possible, ideally within 6 hours of the onset of symptoms. In some cases, hyperbaric therapy has been effective for patients who are not treated until 10 to 14 days after the onset of their symptoms.

The goal is to reduce the size of the liberated gas bubbles, facilitate the reabsorption of these air bubbles, prevent the formation of new bubbles, and improve oxygenation. Before hyperbaric treatment is initiated, certain procedures should be followed. Endotracheal tube cuffs and Foley catheter balloons should be filled with saline rather than air. It is essential to identify any pneumothorax and insert a chest tube prior to recompression.

The initiation of hyperbaric treatment is similar for types I and II decompression injuries. Victims are taken to a "depth" of 60 ft (FSW), which is equal to 2.8 atmospheres. Supplemental oxygen at an FIO_2 of 100 percent is provided at 20-minute intervals, alternating with room air. The hyperbaric pressure will be reduced at a rate of 1 ft a minute to equal a depth of 30 ft for a period of time and then slowly brought back to "sea level."

Victims of an arterial air embolus will commonly be brought to an initial hyperbaric depth of 165 ft (6 atmospheres). After 30 minutes, the patient will be brought slowly "up" to a depth of 60, and then 30, ft before returning to the normal ambient pressure.

In addition to hyperbaric therapy, patients should be dried off immediately and kept warm to prevent hypothermia. A urine output should be maintained in the pediatric patient between 1 and 2 mL/kg/hr. Intravenous fluids that are in plastic bags should be used instead of glass bottles.

Special precautions should also be taken for victims who must be transported by helicopter or airplane. In some cases, even the slightest elevation, which results in exposure to a decreased ambient pressure, may compromise the victim by causing further gas expansion. Helicopter transports should be done at as low an altitude as possible (less than 1000 ft), while ensuring the safety of the transport. Airplane transport should be conducted in aircraft that are capable of being pressurized to sea level.

Victims of type I decompression sickness are advised to abstain from any further scuba diving for at least 4 to 6 weeks, and type II victims must wait at least 4 to 6 months. An air embolism or a second occurrence of any type II complications is serious enough to cease diving on a permanent basis.

Dysbarisms Caused by Abnormal Gas Concentration

Scuba diving is made possible through the use of compressed air tanks. As a diver descends, ambient pressure will increase causing a proportionate increase in the partial pressure of the compressed gases (Dalton's law). As a result, the partial pressure of the inhaled gas will increase at greater depths. The increased partial pressure of nitrogen represents the greatest concern to scuba divers. These symptoms are referred to as nitrogen narcosis.

Nitrogen Narcosis

The inhalation of nitrogen gas at elevated partial pressures may cause an interference with nerve conduction. As a result, nitrogen narcosis can produce a narcotic or intoxicating effect during a dive. Symptoms can include euphoria, uncontrollable laughter, impaired judgment, memory loss, light-headedness, hallucinations, loss of coordination, and impaired reflexes.

The signs of nitrogen narcosis may become evident at depths beyond 80 ft. It is estimated that every 50 ft of depth during a dive can result in symptoms roughly equal to one martini on an empty stomach.

The greatest risk of nitrogen narcosis is drowning. With any evidence or suspicion of confusion, disorientation, or altered mental status, the dive should be terminated. The affected diver should be escorted slowly to the surface by a second diver. No other treatment is required.

Summary

An understanding and awareness of the clinical signs and symptoms of dysbaric injuries is important for all emergency physicians. The diverse clinical findings of barotrauma and decompression illness may begin immediately upon ascent from a dive or can be delayed for days. A patient may present to the emergency department directly from the dive site, making the diagnosis evident. However, a patient may present up to 36 hours later after traveling hundreds or thousands of miles in returning home from a vacation.

Some patients will require only supportive care and can be safely discharged. Other patients, who may have limited complaints or physical findings, will require careful monitoring or aggressive and time-critical treatment. The increasing popularity of scuba diving makes it essential for the emergency physician to be able to differentiate the benign from the potentially serious dysbaric injuries.

For assistance with scuba diving-related injuries, contact:
Divers Alert Network (DAN)
24-Hour Diving Emergencies: 919-684-8111 or
1-919-684-4DAN (collect)

Information Line: 1-800-446.2671 or 1-919-684-2948, Mon-Fri, 9 AM to 5 PM (EST)
Http://www.diversalertnetwork.org/

BIBLIOGRAPHY

High-Altitude Illness

Carpenter TC, Niermeyer S, Durmowicz AG: Altitude-related illness in children. *Curr Probl Pediatr* 28:177–198, 1998.

DeHart RL (ed): *Fundamentals of Aerospace Medicine,* 2d ed. Baltimore, MD: Williams & Wilkins; 1996.

Hackett PH, Roach RC: High altitude medicine, in Auerbach P (ed): *Wilderness Medicine.* St. Louis, Mosby, 2001.

Tso R: High altitude illness. *Emerg Med Clin North Am* 10:231, 1992.

Dysbaric Injuries

Bennett P, Elliott, D (eds): *The Physiology and Medicine of Diving,* 4th ed. Philadelphia: WB Saunders, 1993.

Bove A, Davis J (eds): *Diving Medicine,* 3d ed. Philadelphia: WB Saunders, 1997.

Hardy KR: Diving-related emergencies. *Emerg Med Clin North Am* 15:223, 1997.

Kizer K: Scuba diving and dysbarisms, in Auerbach P (eds): *Wilderness Medicine, Management of Wilderness and Environmental Emergencies.* St. Louis, MO: Mosby, 1995.

117

Radiation Emergencies

Ira J. Blumen

HIGH-YIELD FACTS

- Ionizing radiation is named for its ability to interact with matter, converting atoms to ions as a result of their gain or loss of electrons. Ionizing radiation is more dangerous than nonionizing radiation because such reactions lead to breaks in both DNA and RNA, damaging important biologic functions at the cellular metabolic level.

- The clinical effects of radiation exposure are related to the type of radiation involved, the amount of radiation, and the nature of the exposure (continuous or intermittent). In addition, the harmful effects of ionizing radiation may be affected by the total time of the exposure, the distance from the radiation source, and the presence of any shielding (amount and type).

- There are two categories of radiation injuries with which the emergency physician should be familiar:
  - *exposure* injury, which generally represents no threat to emergency care providers
  - *contamination,* which may represent a risk to emergency personnel

- Radiation injury should be considered in the differential diagnosis for any patient who presents with a painless "burn'" but who does not remember a thermal or chemical insult.

- *Acute radiation syndrome* may develop following a whole-body exposure of 100 rad or more that occurs over a relatively short period of time. Organ systems with rapidly dividing cells (bone marrow, gastrointestinal tract) are the most vulnerable to radiation injury.

- Although the effect of radiation on the hematopoietic system is characterized by pancytopenia, the absolute lymphocyte count represents the best way to estimate exposure hematologically. Leukocyte counts may be elevated initially due to demargination, but the lymphocyte portion of the differential will quickly start to decrease.

- Total-body irradiation with >1000 rad results in a neurovascular syndrome since, at such high radiation levels, even cells that are relatively resistant to injury are damaged. Ataxia and confusion quickly develop and there is direct vascular damage, with resultant circulatory collapse. The patient usually expires within hours.

- In the presence of contamination, if the patient's condition permits, decontamination should begin in the prehospital setting, which will reduce the potential spread of radioactive material and decrease the potential contamination of hospital workers or other rescuers. Fortunately, if appropriate management steps are taken, the radiation-contaminated patient should present little danger to hospital staff, even if decontamination was incomplete prior to arrival at the hospital.

- While both prehospital and hospital workers may be at risk, it is the prehospital personnel and other rescuers, who respond to the site of a radiation accident, who are more often exposed to significant radiation. A threshold of 5000 mrem (5 rem) should be the exposure limit, except to save a life. A once-in-a-lifetime exposure to 100,000 mrem (100 rem) to save a life has been established by the National Council on Radiation Protection as acceptable and will not result in any undue morbidity.

- The Joint Commission on Accreditation of Healthcare Organizations (JCAHO) requires each emergency department to have a radiation accident plan. In the event of a medically significant radiation accident, a well-prepared and practiced plan will supply emergency care providers with an appropriate knowledge base, management protocols, and additional resources that can be called upon.

In May 2000, an Egyptian man found a shiny metal object along the roadside near his hometown. He took it home, where he lived with his wife, four children, and a sister. The object was placed on a cabinet near the front door and the father and his 9-year-old son frequently rubbed the object, believing it was a precious metal to be shined. One month later, the 9-year-old son died in a local hospital. Doctors diagnosed the boy with bone-marrow failure and skin inflammation. Within 2 weeks, the father and a daughter also died and the rest of the family was hospitalized, all with the same signs.

The evidence suggested radiation sickness and was investigated by government authorities. The "precious metal" turned out to be iridium-192, a β-χ emitter, used like a portable radiography machine to check the quality of welds and perform other industrial scans.

In addition to exposing this family, several hundred family associates, who gathered on a regular basis outside the home, were also exposed. Fortunately, the rest of the family recovered from their radiation-related illnesses.

Radiation accidents involving discarded medical and industrial sources get little attention compared to problems at nuclear power plants or weapons facilities. Unfortunately, these accidents occur around the world with surprising regularity and, in some instances, prove deadly.

According to the Radiation Emergency Assistance Center/Training Site (REAC/TS) Radiation Accident Registry, between 1944 and 2001, there have been 416 accidents worldwide. These accidents resulted in significant radiation exposure to 3011 individuals and in 129 deaths (Table 117-1).

Despite the relatively rare incidence of medically significant pediatric radiation accidents, our dependence on nuclear energy makes it necessary for today's emergency physician to understand its potential for disaster. Most obvious are the threats of sophisticated nuclear weaponry to individuals of all ages. However, the near disaster of Three Mile Island in Pennsylvania in 1979 and the Chernobyl Nuclear Power Station catastrophe in the former Soviet Union in 1986 serve as potent reminders of the severe underlying hazards to children and adults, even in peaceful nuclear energy utilization. A more probable predicament, however, is an isolated or limited exposure in a medical, industrial, or research accident, or during the transport of radionucleotides. Basic preparation for radiation emergencies is not difficult, but a thorough understanding of the pathophysiology and clinical presentation is a must in order to handle all aspects of these complex problems successfully.

Radiation accidents do not differentiate between children and adults. Therefore, all individuals are susceptible to radiation injury if the exposure is of significant dose and duration. Especially sensitive are cells that divide rapidly and that are found in the gastrointestinal tract and the hematopoietic system. This preference for rapidly dividing cells may make young children more susceptible to the clinical effects of a radiation exposure.

TYPES OF RADIATION

Radiation is a general term used to describe energy that is emitted from a source. The term encompasses the broad-wavelength microwave and extends through the ultra-high-frequency gamma rays. A *radioactive* substance, referred to as a *radioisotope* or *radionucleotide,* gives off radiation. A person exposed to external or remote radiation has been *irradiated* but does not become radioactive. The victim may give off radiation only if there was external or internal *contamination* caused by the presence of radioactive particles (α and β).

Radiation can be classified as either *ionizing* or *nonionizing.* In addition, radiation can be described either as

Table 117-1. Major Radiation Accidents: Human Experience—1944 to March, 2001

	United States	Non-United States	Total	(FSU Data[a])
Number of Accidents	247	169	416	(137)
Number of Persons Involved	1354	132,405	133,759	(507)
Significant Exposures[b]	795	2216	3011	(278)
Fatalities[c]	30	99	129	(35)

[a]DOE/NRC dose criteria.
[b]Includes eight nonradiation deaths.
[c]Not included in totals due to incomplete FSU (Former Soviet Union) Registry Data.
Source: DOE/REAC/TS Radiation Accident Registry, Oak Ridge, TN, 2001.

nonparticulate (electromagnetic) or *particulate.* Electromagnetic radiation has no mass and no charge. It occurs in waveforms and is described by wavelengths. Examples of this nonparticulate/electromagnetic radiation can be found in both the ionizing and nonionizing radiation classifications. In contrast, particulate radiation has mass and can either be charged or uncharged ionizing radiation.

Ionizing Radiation

Ionizing radiation is named for its ability to interact with matter. Atoms will convert to ions as a result of their gain or loss of electrons. Ionizing radiation is more dangerous than nonionizing radiation because such reactions lead to breaks in both DNA and RNA, damaging important biologic functions at the cellular metabolic level. Anomalies may be passed on to subsequent offspring or they may result in cell death or the inability to replicate. Ionized radiation has a high frequency, a short wavelength, and a billion times more energy than nonionizing radiation. Common sources of ionizing radiation are nuclear reactors, nuclear weapons, radioactive material, and radiography equipment. Material identified by the label *radioactive* produces ionizing radiation.

Types of ionizing radiation include α-particles, β-particles, and neutrons, which represent particulate radiation; and X-rays and gamma-rays, which are nonparticulate forms of radiation.

Gamma rays have the highest energy content of the nonparticulate and massless radiations. Their photon radiation originates in the atomic nucleus. They can penetrate deep into the tissue, depositing energy and interacting with the various layers they penetrate. Constant low-level exposure through cosmic radiation is a usual source. Gamma radiation is a common cause of acute radiation syndrome due to radioisotope decay and radiation from linear accelerators. A lead shield 1 to 2 inches in depth or thick concrete would provide satisfactory protection from χ-rays.

X-rays have the next highest energy content of the nonparticulate, massless radiations. Unlike the χ-ray, which is produced within the nucleus of the atom, X-rays originate from outside the nucleus and are emitted by excited electrons. Like the χ-ray, X-rays can also penetrate tissue and deposit energy deep within the cells. Their usual source is medical or industrial in nature.

Alpha particles are composed of 2 protons and 2 neutrons and possess a 2^+ electrical charge. They originate from the nucleus of the atom and, being relatively heavy radioactive emissions, can travel only inches from their source. In general, they cannot penetrate paper or epidermis because of their mass and size and are rarely harmful. Examples include plutonium, uranium, and radium.

Beta particles have a small mass, composed of a single electron emitted from the atom's nucleus, and possess a 1^- charge. They can disperse only a few feet from their source and penetrate tissues only a small amount (up to 8 mm), primarily causing thermal injuries. Clothing alone can often provide adequate protection from beta particles. Despite their inability to penetrate the skin to any significant depth, both alpha particles and beta particles can be harmful if they are ingested or inhaled or if wounds are contaminated by these particles. The common research isotope tritium is an example, as is carbon[14] and phosphorous.

Neutrons are the third type of particulate radiation. Without an electrical charge, they ionize by colliding with atomic nuclei within cells and tissues. They possess strong power to penetrate and represent the only form of radiation that can make previously stable atoms within the body radioactive. They can be more damaging than X-rays or gamma rays and are responsible for radioactive fallout. Nuclear reactors, nuclear weapons, and nuclear accelerators are common sources of neutron radiation. Specialized concrete is necessary to provide shielding from neutron radiation.

Nonionizing Radiation

Nonionizing radiation is relatively low energy in nature and does not result in acute radiation injuries or contamination. The adverse effects to humans are limited to local heat production.

In order of decreasing energy content, the nonionizing forms of radiation include ultraviolet rays, visible light, infrared radiation, microwaves, and radio waves. These forms of nonionizing radiation also represent many of the electromagnetic radiations. Their energy content is less than that of gamma rays and X-rays, making them a less threatening form of radiation (Table 117-2).

MEASURING RADIATION

Although radiation cannot be sensed by the human body, it can be detected and quantified by dosimeters or Geiger-Meuller tubes at levels far below those that result in any biologic significance.

There are several units of measurement used in relation to radiation: *roentgen* is the unit of measurement used during the production of X-rays that measure the ion pairs produced in a given volume of air; *dose*

Table 117-2. Types of Radiation

Nonionizing
  Nonparticulate and electromagnetic[a]
    Ultraviolet rays
    Visible rays
    Infrared rays
    Microwaves
    Radio waves
Ionizing
  Nonparticulate and electromagnetic
    No mass
    No charge
    Penetrating
    Examples[a]
      Gamma rays
      X-rays
  Particulate
    Has mass
    Uncharged and penetrating
      Neutrons
      More damaging than X-rays or gamma rays
      No electrical charge
    Charged and nonpenetrating
      Alpha rays
        2 Protons
        2 Neutrons
        2+ Charge
      Beta rays
        1 Electron
        1− Charge

[a]In order of decreasing energy content.

represents the amount of energy deposited by radiation per unit of mass; and the *rad* (roentgen absorbed dose) is the basic unit of measurement. A rad can be defined as a unit of absorbed dose of radiant energy that is equal to 100 erg of energy deposited per gram of absorbing material. The gray (Gy) represents the standard international (SI) unit for dose, and

$$1 \text{ Gy} = 100 \text{ rad}$$
$$1 \text{ cGy} = 1 \text{ rad}$$

Units of *rem* (roentgen equivalent in man) represent a calculated radiation unit of dose equivalent. The absorbed dose (rad) is multiplied by a factor to account for the relative biologic effectiveness (RBE) of the various types of radiation:

$$\text{rem} = \text{rad} \times \text{RBE}$$

The *sievert* (Sv) is the SI unit for dose equivalent, where

$$1 \text{ Sv} = 100 \text{ rem}$$
$$1 \text{ cSv} = 1 \text{ rem}$$

Generally, the terms *rem* and *mrem* (millirem) are used when they refer to the exposure of biologic systems. For β-particles, X-rays, and χ-rays, the RBE = 1. Therefore, for these sources of radiation, 1 rad = 1 rem and 1 Gy = 1 Sv.

RADIATION EXPOSURE

The clinical impact of radiation exposure depends on several factors. These factors are also important to properly coordinate the safety of both prehospital and hospital providers who may respond to a radiation incident.

The clinical effects of radiation exposure are related to the type of radiation involved, the amount of radiation, and the nature of the exposure (continuous or intermittent). In addition, the harmful effects of ionizing radiation may be affected by the total time of the exposure, the distance from the radiation source, and the presence of any shielding (amount and type).

A radiation exposure over a prolonged period of time is less likely to be harmful to an individual than the same dose over a shorter time period. For example, an exposure of 100 rem in 1 second will be more harmful than an exposure of 100 rem over 1 year.

There is an inverse square relationship between distance from a radiation source and the resultant exposure, making increased distance an effective means to reduce the amount of exposure. An exposure can be reduced by a factor of 4 simply by doubling the distance from the radiation source. Tripling the distance will decrease the exposure by a factor of 9.

Shielding may be an effective method to reduce radiation exposure when one is dealing with low-energy radiation (X-rays). When dealing with medium- or high-energy radiation, shielding may become impractical due to the amount of lead or concrete that would be necessary.

There are natural and technological radiation sources to which children and adults are commonly exposed. Natural background radiation may represent an exposure between 300 and 360 mrem per year. Radon accounts for the largest amount of this natural radiation (approximately 200 mrem/year), whereas air (5 mrem/year), ground (10 mrem/year), food (25 mrem/year), building material (35 mrem/year), natural background (35 mrem/year), and medical sources (50 mrem/year) account for the balance.

Technological sources of radiation may represent a wide range of exposures to individuals. Color television may result in an exposure of 1 mrem/year; a round-trip, coast-to-coast jet flight may result in a 2 to 5 mrem exposure; and a chest x-ray causes an exposure between 5 and 10 mrem. The common radiation exposure to a patient during angiography may be 1000 mrem. As technology changes and new technologies are developed, we are likely to encounter additional sources of radiation in varying amounts.

RADIATION INJURIES

There are two categories of radiation injuries with which the emergency physician should be familiar. The first type is an *exposure* injury, which generally represents no threat to emergency care providers. *Contamination,* the second type of radiation injury, may represent a potential risk to emergency personnel.

Exposure

Exposure radiation injuries can be classified into two categories. A person may be the victim of a *localized radiation injury* or may have suffered a *whole-body exposure.*

Localized Radiation Injuries

A large dose of radiation exposure to a small part of the body will result in a local radiation injury. These injuries often occur over months or even years, but they may occur over a shorter amount of time.

Localized radiation injuries most commonly affect the upper extremities, with the buttocks and thighs representing the next most common sites. Typically, these injuries occur in the occupational setting. In addition, adults and children may unknowingly come into contact with a radiation source by handling an unknown object and putting it into their pockets. Localized radiation accidents may also result from an inadvertent exposure to an intense radiation beam.

The dose of radiation that can result in a local radiation injury varies greatly. Larger doses are often better tolerated than a whole-body exposure. Accidental exposures from radioactive sources with a surface dose of nearly 20,000 rad/min have been reported to have caused localized radiation injuries.

The initial clinical picture of a localized radiation injury depicts a thermal injury to the skin. While thermal burns develop soon after an exposure, erythema from a local radiation injury is delayed. Radiation injury should be considered in the differential diagnosis for any patient who presents with a painless "burn" but who does not remember a thermal or chemical insult.

Prolonged radiation exposure causes blood vessel fibrosis, leading to tissue necrosis. The outcome will be determined by the degree of blood vessel and tissue damage. Classification of these localized injuries can be divided into four types, differentiated by increasing epidermal and dermal injury. They are summarized in Table 117-3.

Whole-Body Exposure

Acute radiation syndrome may develop following a whole-body exposure of 100 rad or more that occurs over a relatively short period of time. Organ systems with rapidly dividing cells (bone marrow, gastrointestinal tract) are the most vulnerable to radiation injury. With greater doses of radiation, however, all organ systems may become involved, including the central nervous system.

Estimating the exposure (in rads) of a whole-body radiation victim may be difficult when the patient presents to the emergency department. Dosimeters and Geiger counters are not standard equipment in many emergency departments and are often of little help in determining the total radiation dose or duration of exposure. A mechanical dosimetry monitoring device worn by the victim during the time of exposure would be helpful but is rarely available. Instead, the emergency physician's history and physical, along with baseline laboratory values, are essential in estimating the whole-body exposure. This technique is referred to as biologic dosimetry. For this purpose, the primary indicators include the time of onset of symptoms and depression of absolute lymphocyte count. The earlier signs and symptoms develop, the higher the dose and the worse the prognosis. Table 117-4 identifies characteristic signs and symptoms with the radiation dose that can be anticipated following a whole-body exposure.

A progressive sequence of signs and symptoms following a whole-body exposure can be divided into four stages.

- *prodromal stage*
- *latent stage*
- *manifest illness stage*
- *recovery stage*

Table 117-3. Localized Radiation Injuries

Type	Presentation	Exposure	Comments
Type I	Erythema only	600–1000 rad	Similar to a first-degree thermal burn. Erythema may be delayed up to 2–3 weeks. A dose of 300 rad can result in a delayed hair loss (epilation). Dry desquamation or scaling may occur.
Type II	Transepidermal injury or wet desquamation	1000–2000 rad	Similar in severity to a second-degree partial-thickness thermal burn
Type III	Dermal radionecrosis	>2000 rad	Severe pain with or without paresthesia. Resembles a severe chemical or scalding burn. Skin grafting may be necessary.
Type IV	Chronic radiation dermatitis	Recurrent exposure over several years	Can result in an eczematous appearance of the skin. Ulcerations and carcinoma are not uncommon.

An individual's susceptibility and the dose of radiation, dose rate, and dose distribution, will dictate the onset, duration, and character of symptoms in a predictable representation. The prodromal stage can begin within minutes to hours after exposure and is dose-dependent. The most common symptoms of this stage include nausea, vomiting, and fatigue. Exposure to <100 rad rarely causes symptoms and patients who do not exhibit nausea or vomiting within 6 hours of a radiation accident are unlikely to have been subject to a significant whole-body exposure. Prodromal markers beginning within 6 hours suggest an exposure in excess of 100 rad. Higher doses will result in a more rapid onset of these initial signs and symptoms, probably due to acute tissue injury and the subsequent release of vasoactive substances, including histamine and bradykinin.

Table 117-4. Biological Dosimetry

Indicator	Total-Body Dose	Comments
Nausea and vomiting		
Onset within 6 h	>100 rad (1 Gy)	Prodromal stage represents a good clinical and biologic indicator to estimate whole-body exposure
Onset within 4 h	>200 rad (2 Gy)	
Onset within 2 h	>400 rad (4 Gy)	
Onset within 1 h	>1000 rad (10 Gy)	
Lymphocyte count at 48 h		
>1200/mm^3	100–200 rad (1–2 Gy)	Prognosis: good
300–1200/mm^3	200–400 rad (2–4 Gy)	Prognosis: fair
<300/mm^3	>400 rad (4 Gy)	Prognosis: poor
Diarrhea	>400 rad (4 Gy)	
Erythema of the skin	>600 rad (6 Gy)	Delayed onset
CNS symptoms (disorientation, ataxia, seizures, coma)	>1000 rad (10 Gy)	Rule out trauma; Death within days

A lower-dose exposure will yield a resolution of the prodromal symptoms over a period of days to weeks, during the latent stage. Progressively higher radiation doses will prolong the prodromal stage while limiting the latent period until a point is reached when it appears that the prodromal stage proceeds directly to the manifest illness stage without any resolution of the prodromal symptoms.

During the manifest illness stage, specific organ symptoms develop and the patient is at the greatest risk for infection and bleeding. Three syndromes may develop during this stage, depending on the total amount of radiation exposure: the hematopoietic syndrome (220 to 600 rad), the gastrointestinal syndrome (600 to 1000 rad), and the neurovascular syndrome (>1000 rad).

Although the effect of radiation on the hematopoietic system is characterized by pancytopenia, the absolute lymphocyte count represents the best way to estimate exposure hematologically. Leukocyte counts may be elevated initially due to demargination, but the lymphocyte portion of the differential will quickly start to decrease. A 48-hour check will suggest the severity of the exposure. A lymphocyte count >1200/mm^3 indicates a 100- to 200-rad exposure and most often a good prognosis. An absolute lymphocyte count of 300 to 1200/mm^3 suggests a 200- to 400-rad exposure, which promises a fair outcome. Exposure to >400 rad is marked by a poor prognosis and is expected with counts < 300/mm^3. Pancytopenia may develop after a latent period lasting a few days to 3 weeks. The patient will subsequently suffer from dyspnea, malaise, purpura, bleeding, and opportunistic infection (Fig. 117-1).

Gastrointestinal illness will be most evident with total-body exposures of 600 to 1000 rad. The prodromal phase is abrupt and is marked by severe vomiting and diarrhea. The latent stage may be quite short and is followed by continued GI symptoms, leading to relentless fluid loss, fever, and prostration. The radiosensitive

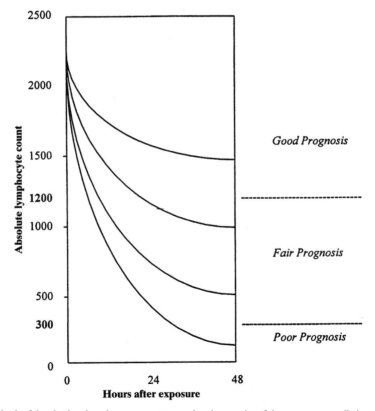

Fig. 117-1 A 48-h check of the absolute lymphocyte count suggesting the severity of the exposure to radiation. Good prognosis: a lymphocyte count greater than 1200/mm^3. 100- to 200-rad exposure. Fair prognosis: an absolute lymphocyte count of 300 to 1200/mm^3. 200- to 400-rad exposure. Poor prognosis: lymphocyte count below 300/mm^3. More than 400-rad exposure.

mucosal cells of the small bowel begin to slough, which, combined with the coexistent hematopoietic abnormalities, produces severe, bloody diarrhea. Even with intense supportive care, the patient rarely survives.

Total-body irradiation with >1000 rad results in a neurovascular syndrome. At such high radiation levels, even cells that are relatively resistant to injury are damaged. Ataxia and confusion quickly develop and there is direct vascular damage, with resultant circulatory collapse. The patient usually expires within hours.

Patients with lower levels of exposure, or those patients fortunate enough to respond to aggressive supportive management, will enter the recovery stage. Further management is guided by specific organ system insults. For these survivors, the long-term risks of exposure to ionizing radiation include cataracts, leukemia, and development of carcinomas. It should be noted that the median lethal dose of total-body irradiation is estimated at 400 rad (Table 117-5).

Contamination

Contamination is the second type of radiation accident. Radioactive particles, solid or liquid, may remain on the surface of the victim, resulting in an external contamination. Internal contamination may be the result of inhaled, ingested, or absorbed radioactive particles. Neutrons, α-particles, and β-particles are most commonly responsible for contamination. Unlike an exposure victim, the contaminated patient does represent an additional challenge and potential risk to hospital and prehospital personnel.

In most situations, if the patient's condition permits, decontamination should begin in the prehospital setting. This will reduce the potential spread of radioactive material and will decrease the potential contamination of hospital workers or other rescuers. Fortunately, if appropriate management steps are taken, the radiation-contaminated patient should present little danger to hospital staff, even if decontamination was incomplete prior to arrival at the hospital.

MANAGEMENT

General Concepts

It is important to realize that the general principles of patient care for radiation victims are no different than those for other medical problems. The initial assessment and management are directed toward the routine atten-

tion to the ABCs (airway, breathing, circulation). There are no acute, life-threatening complications of a survivable radiation injury that require immediate intervention. Emergency treatment should be supportive and directed toward the prevention of complications.

It will be important to determine, quickly, whether the patients are victims of a radiation exposure or a contamination. Radiation contamination requires that decontamination begin promptly after stabilization. The radiation exposure patient who is not contaminated represents no danger to the hospital staff or other patients. These victims can be managed in the emergency department and require no immediate intervention related to the radiation exposure.

At all times, there must be a proper balance between patient care and the personal safety of rescuers and health care workers. Appropriate measures must be taken by both prehospital and hospital personnel to minimize their risk of exposure while managing either life-threatening injuries or the decontamination of the patients they serve.

While both prehospital and hospital workers may be at risk, it is the prehospital personnel and other rescuers who respond to the site of a radiation accident, who are more often exposed to significant radiation. A threshold of 5000 mrem (5 rem) should be the exposure limit, except to save a life. A once-in-a-lifetime exposure to 100,000 mrem (100 rem) to save a life has been established by the National Council on Radiation Protection as acceptable and will not result in any undue morbidity.

Hospital personnel are at a very low risk of significant radiation exposure when treating victims of a radiation accident. Off-site medical personnel who treated victims of the Three Mile Island and Chernobyl accidents were exposed to radiation doses of <14 mrem.

Prehospital Management

The history obtained by prehospital personnel is of paramount importance in management decisions regarding radiation victims. When possible, rescuers must gather details regarding the exact type, location, and duration of exposure. For internal exposure, the route of entry, type, and quantity of radioactive material should be determined. If the incident has occurred in an industrial or laboratory setting, initial decontamination procedures may be instituted by on-site personnel according to established protocols before EMS personnel arrive. A quick response in decontamination will limit the exposure to the victim and decrease the amount of further contamination of both the ambulance and the emergency department. For unstable patients, the minimal action

Table 117-5. Whole-Body Exposure

Whole-Body Dose, rad	Characteristics
5	Asymptomatic; normal blood studies
15	Chromosome abnormality may be detectable
50–75	Asymptomatic; minor depression of platelets and white cell count may be detectable
75–100	Nausea, vomiting, fatigue in 10–15% of victims within 2 days
100–200	Prodrome: Mild nausea, vomiting, and fatigue; onset within 6 h, lasting 3–6 h
	Latent stage: >2 weeks
	Manifest illness stage:
	Lymphocyte count >1200/mm^3 at 48 h
	Transient sterility in men
	Recovery: Good prognosis with only symptomatic treatment
200–600	Prodrome: Nausea and vomiting within 2–4 h, last <24 h
	Latent stage: 1–3 weeks
	Manifest illness stage: Hematopoietic
	@ 200–400 rad: Lymphocyte count 300–1200/mm^3 at 48 h
	>400 rad: Lymphocyte count <300/mm^3 at 48 h
	Pancytopenia may develop after a latent period of up to 3 weeks: the patient will subsequently suffer from dyspnea, malaise, purpura, bleeding, and opportunistic infection
	Requires hospitalization, protective isolation, and support
	Upper dose range may require bone marrow transplantation within 7–10 days of exposure
	Recovery:
	@ 200–400 rad: Fair prognosis with supportive care and if the bone marrow damage was not irreversible
	@ 400 rad: Poor prognosis; lethal in approximately 50% of victims
600–1000	Prodrome: Severe nausea, vomiting, and diarrhea within 1–2 h, lasting >48 h
	Latent stage: 0–7 days
	Manifest illness stage: Gastrointestinal
	Recurrence of nausea and vomiting
	Fever, bloody diarrhea, dehydration, electrolyte imbalance, early sepsis, hemorrhage
	Leukocyte count drops to zero
	Recovery:
	Overall 90-100% mortality within 30 days
	Lower dose exposure with medical care has a 50% mortality
>1000	Prodrome: Nausea and vomiting within 1 h
	Latent stage: None
	Manifest illness stage: Neurovascular
	Dehydration, hypotension
	Disorientation, ataxia, confusion, seizures, coma
	Erythema and epilation (onset may be delayed)
	Recovery: 99–100% incidence of death within days
>5000	Prodrome: Almost immediate onset of nausea, vomiting
	Latent stage: None
	Manifest illness stage: Cardiovascular, GI, and CNS.
	Hypotension, ataxia, cerebral edema, seizures (rapid onset)
	Recovery: Death within 1–4 days

performed prior to rapid transport is the removal of contaminated clothing.

After transport of the patient to the hospital, EMS personnel and their vehicles must be inspected for the presence of radioactive contamination before they leave the facility. This must also be done at the scene for any ambulance and personnel who respond to the accident site and provide field assessment and stabilization without patient transport.

Emergency Department Management

Few hospitals will be called on to treat victims of life-threatening radiation accidents. The exceptions are hospitals in close proximity to nuclear power plants or in the event of a nuclear war. It is more likely, however, that hospitals will be called on to attend victims of a minor industrial accident or an accident involving the transportation of radioactive materials. The end result will be a patient with "routine injuries," whose treatment may be complicated by an inadvertent radiation exposure with or without low-level radioactive contamination.

Radiation Accident Plan

The Joint Commission on Accreditation of Healthcare Organizations (JCAHO) requires each emergency department to have a radiation accident plan. In the event of a medically significant radiation accident, a well-prepared and practiced plan will supply emergency care providers with an appropriate knowledge base, management protocols, and additional resources that can be called upon.

A major part of a well-prepared plan facilitates the identification of *significant* versus *perceived* radiation dangers. The incidence of significant radiation accidents may be rare for some hospitals, but the incidence of perceived radiation accidents may be much greater. A vehicular accident involving a truck or train carrying radioactive material near a school may send dozens (or hundreds) of anxious parents and their children to the emergency department. The staff of a well-prepared emergency department can assess the potential risks and, when appropriate, correct any misconceptions and ease the fears the general public may have.

A lack of experience, an incomplete knowledge base, and a significant degree of fear among health care providers often result in the mismanagement of radiation victims. Therefore, it is essential that an emergency department develop protocols for dealing with both the radiation exposure itself and the medical management of these victims.

The final component of an emergency department's resource plan for radiation emergencies is a list of "additional references." These resources include local, state, regional, and/or national agencies and their 24-hour telephone numbers that can be called for information or assistance. The U.S. Department of Energy also is available to coordinate a federal response and provide assistance through the Radiological Assistance Program (RAP). RAP provides advice and radiologic assistance to government agencies and to the private sector for incidents involving radioactive materials that pose a threat to the public health and safety or the environment. RAP can provide field deployable teams of health physics professionals equipped to conduct radiologic monitoring and assessment. RAP is managed at eight regional coordinating offices across the country (Fig. 117-2).

The Radiation Emergency Assistance Center/Training Site (REAC/TS) in Oak Ridge, Tennessee, is also available to provide treatment and medical consultation for injuries resulting from radiation exposure and contamination. REAC/TS can be contacted by calling 865-576-1005.

General Procedures

Early notification of estimated time of arrival (ETA) will allow the emergency department to implement its radiation accident plan and to advise EMS personnel on initial prehospital decontamination.

When exposed solely to irradiation from χ-rays, X-rays, β-particles and, frequently, neutrons, patients do not become radioactive. However, the radiation accident plan must assume that there will be external contamination. Table 117-6 outlines an example of many of the procedures and actions that should be addressed in the radiation accident plan.

Separate contaminated and clean treatment areas must be established. The floor of the contaminated treatment area and the ambulance receiving area must be covered with plastic or paper sheets to prevent the spread of contamination. Devices must be immediately available to monitor both the patients and personnel for any evidence of radioactive contamination.

All personnel in the treatment area must wear protective clothing. This includes gowns, caps, masks, shoe covers, double gloves, and personal monitoring devices (film badges). If airborne contaminants are suspected, respirators must be worn. In most cases, decontamination begins during the prehospital stage, significantly reducing the risk of exposure to emergency department staff. Despite this, fear of contamination may persist in poorly educated or ill-prepared hospital personnel.

Separate staff members are assigned to the clean and contaminated treatment areas. Medical staff is designated for triage and initial resuscitation, which must take place before decontamination.

A radiation control officer should be assigned to monitor the treatment area and everyone within. This officer is given a Geiger-Meuller counter for detecting β- and χ-radiation or a scintillation detector, which offers a higher sensitivity in detecting α-, β-, χ-, and neutron particles. This designated individual oversees the decontamination procedures, the routing of patients, and the movement of hospital personnel. This is important to ensure adequate decontamination and to prevent the unintentional spread of contamination.

Treatment protocols and priorities should be reviewed with assigned staff. Established mechanisms to minimize their exposure, while not compromising patient care, should be reinforced. Ideally, several medical personnel should be assigned to care for each contaminated patient. Individual exposure time can be decreased and a greater distance can be maintained from the patient when the health worker is not involved in direct decontamination or medical management. In cases of a highly radioactive contaminant or foreign body, a lead shield or apron is necessary to protect personnel. However, in most situations, lead aprons are not effective protection against the most common contaminant, the medium-energy gamma ray.

Patients enter the emergency department through a separate entrance where radiation detection equipment is in place. Patients on ambulance stretchers are transferred to clean hospital carts in the ambulance bay.

The ideal decontamination site is an isolated room designed with a closed drainage and ventilation system and fully equipped for a major resuscitation. In many hospitals, the morgue is the only available isolation room meeting these criteria. Resuscitation equipment and other emergency supplies must be relocated to this site when the radiation accident plan is activated.

Management of immediate life-threatening injuries remains the first priority for these patients. Following resuscitation, the radiation victim is carefully evaluated to determine if there is any surface contamination or if there is the possibility of inhaled or ingested radioactive material.

All burns and open wounds must also be evaluated for contamination. They must be irrigated with copious amounts of water and examined for foreign bodies. Highly contaminated foreign bodies, while rare, may represent the greatest single hazard to hospital personnel. These contaminants must be removed from the victim as safely and quickly as possible.

Radiation burns may be delayed in their presentation. They are managed in the same way as nonradiation-induced partial- and full-thickness burns. Extensive beta-particle burns often result in full-thickness injury and require skin grafting.

Individuals not directly involved in the evaluation or treatment of radiation victims must be kept away from the designated treatment areas. Personnel assigned to either the clean or contaminated treatment areas must remain there. If it becomes necessary to move between the treatment areas, it should be done only after appropriate monitoring for contamination. Once the decontamination process for all victims has been completed, all participating hospital personnel must be reevaluated and decontaminated as needed. Their protective garments must be removed before they leave the treatment area and disposed of properly.

A baseline complete blood count, differential, platelet count, and electrolytes on the radiation victim must be obtained. Patients who remain in the hospital should have blood for serial laboratory tests drawn at 12 and 24 hours. Patients who exhibit a decrease in absolute lymphocyte count will have to have a human leukocyte antigen (HL-A) typing performed in the event that a bone marrow transplant should become necessary.

If there is any evidence of infection, it should be treated in the same way as other infections. Neomycin has been recommended as a prophylactic antibiotic in cases of severe vomiting and diarrhea, whereas amphotericin B may be used as a prophylactic antifungal agent. The absolute indication for prophylactic antibiotics and antifungal agents without evidence of infection, remains controversial.

Not all radiation victims will require hospitalization, although, in general, exposures >100 rad may warrant inpatient care. If radiation victims exhibit severe vomiting, they should be admitted. Reverse isolation measures are used for all documented exposures of 200 to 1000 rem and for those patients with absolute lymphocyte counts <1200/mm^3 or 50 percent of the baseline value. For severely pancytopenic patients, bone marrow transplantation is often necessary within 7 to 10 days of exposure (Table 117-7).

In addition to the hematopoietic complications (infection and bleeding) that may be seen with whole-body radiation >200 to 600 rad, victims may develop significant fluid and electrolyte complications. Any indicated surgery must be performed without delay to avoid these additional problems.

Transfusion of selected blood products is based on the

Region	States	Regional Coordinating Office	Telephone
1	Connecticut Delaware Maine Maryland Massachusetts New Hampshire New Jersey New York Pennsylvania Rhode Island Vermont	Brookhaven Area Office Upton, NY 11973	516-282-2200 24 h
2	Arkansas Kentucky Louisiana Mississippi Missouri Tennessee Virginia West Virginia (Also Puerto Rico, Virgin Islands)	Oak Ridge Operations Office P.O. Box 2001 Oak Ridge, TN 34830	615-576-3131 24 h
3	Alabama Florida Georgia North Carolina South Carolina (Also Canal Zone)	Savannah River Operations Office P.O. Box A Aiken, SC 29808	803-725-3333 24 h
4	Arizona Kansas New Mexico Oklahoma Texas	Albuquerque Operations Office P.O. Box 5400 Albuquerque, NM 87115	505-845-4667 24 h
5	Illinois Indiana Iowa Michigan Minnesota Nebraska North Dakota Ohio South Dakota Wisconsin	Chicago Operations Office 9800 S. Cass Avenue Argonne, IL 60439	708-252-4800 Duty hours 708-252-5731 Off hours

Fig. 117-2. U. S. Department of Energy Radiological Assistance Program Regional Coordinating Offices.

Region	States	Regional Coordinating Office	Telephone
6	Colorado Idaho Montana Utah Wyoming	Idaho Operations Office P.O. Box 2108 Idaho Falls, ID 83401	208-526-1515 24 h
7	California Hawaii Nevada	San Francisco Operations Office 1333 Broadway Oakland, CA 94612	510-637-1794 24 h
8	Alaska Oregon Washington	Richland Operations Office 824 Jadwin Avenue Richland, WA 99352	509-373-3800 24 h

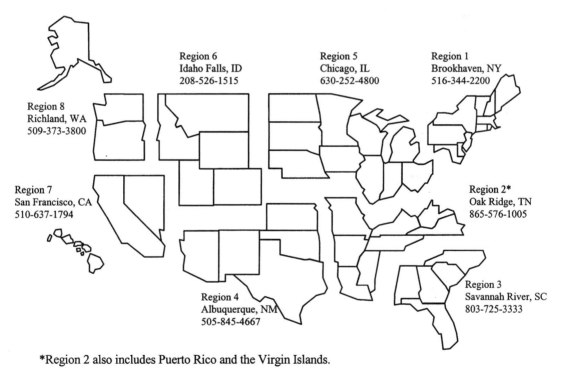

Region 6
Idaho Falls, ID
208-526-1515

Region 5
Chicago, IL
630-252-4800

Region 1
Brookhaven, NY
516-344-2200

Region 8
Richland, WA
509-373-3800

Region 7
San Francisco, CA
510-637-1794

Region 2*
Oak Ridge, TN
865-576-1005

Region 4
Albuquerque, NM
505-845-4667

Region 3
Savannah River, SC
803-725-3333

*Region 2 also includes Puerto Rico and the Virgin Islands.

Fig. 117-2. *Continued.*

individual hematologic derangement encountered and should follow the usual guidelines for their use.

External Contamination

External contamination often presents a logistical problem for hospital workers. However, an organized radiation accident plan should facilitate both the logistical and medical management of these patients.

Victims of radiation exposure who show no signs of injury and are otherwise healthy may be best served at designated decontaminated facilities. In general, hospital resources should be used for radiation victims who also require medical management.

Table 117-6. Radiation Accident Plan: Recommended Emergency Department Procedures

Emergency Department Preparation

Have appropriate contact with prehospital personnel to determine the following:

Type of radiation accident

Type, location, and duration of exposure

Type of injuries (trauma and radiation)

Number and condition of potential victims (contaminated and uncontaminated)

Prehospital decontamination

Radioactive material involved

Make the necessary preparation to receive, evaluate, and treat radiation victims:

Notify appropriate individuals as outlined in radiation accident plan.

Assure that adequate supplies and equipment are available for major resuscitation and decontamination.

Prepare the designated separate entrance (if possible) to the emergency department for radiation victims.

Establish separate contaminated and clean treatment areas that are clearly roped off.

Assign separate staff (physicians, nurses, technicians), if possible, to the clean and contaminated treatment areas.

Personnel assigned to either the clean or contaminated treatment areas must remain there.

If it becomes necessary to move within the treatment areas, it should be done only after appropriate monitoring for contamination.

Assign staff to triage victims.

Review treatment protocols and priorities with assigned staff.

Decontamination Area

Route from ambulance area to decontamination area, and floor of decontamination area, should be covered with plastic or paper secured with tape.

Light switches, door handles, cabinet handles, etc., should be covered with tape.

Assure that all staff are wearing film badges, and protective and disposable clothing prior to initiating decontamination:

Surgical pants and shirt

Surgical cap

Waterproof shoe covers (taped to surgical pants)

Surgical gown

Surgical gloves (taped to surgical gown sleeves)

Second pair of surgical gloves, not taped

Surgical mask (respirators should be worn if airborne contaminants are suspected)

Collect specimens for radiologic evaluation before and after decontamination.

All waste should be captured in sealed containers labeled "Radioactive Waste."

Use a drainage table if available.

Monitor patient for radiation contamination before and after decontamination procedures and record levels in patient's medical record.

Individuals not directly involved in the evaluation or treatment of radiation victims must be kept away from the designated treatment areas.

Patient Arrival

Triage officer and radiation safety officer should evaluate victims in ambulance upon arrival.

If victim is critically injured (inadequate airway, breathing, and/or circulation):

Proceed directly to decontamination area for initial resuscitation.

Clothes can be removed in decontamination area.

If victim is *not* critically injured and is contaminated:

Open wounds are covered initially and clothing removed in the ambulance.

Patient is transferred to a clean hospital cart in the ambulance bay.

Patient is taken to decontamination area.

(Continues)

Table 117-6. (*continued*) Radiation Accident Plan: Recommended Emergency Department Procedures

If victim is not contaminated:
    Clothes do not need to be removed in the ambulance.
    Patient is transferred to a clean hospital cart in the ambulance bay.
    Proceed to regular emergency department/trauma room as indicated.
Ambulance and EMS personnel:
    EMS personnel and their vehicles should be inspected for the presence of any radioactive contamination before leaving the facility.
    If contaminated, radiation safety officer should instruct for decontamination and further inspection prior to the ambulance returning to duty.

Patient Decontamination
Assure adequate airway, breathing, and circulation before proceeding with decontamination.
Open wounds should be covered initially while the patient's clothing is removed (if not already completed).
All the patient's clothing should be placed in clearly labeled plastic bags and patient reevaluated for contamination.
Collect cotton swab sample from ears, nares, mouth, and any open wounds:
    Place in labeled (patient name, site, time) glass containers.
Radiation safety officer and physician should assess for sites of possible contamination and proceed accordingly.
Obtain baseline laboratory tests.

Contaminated Open Wounds
    Open wound should be considered contaminated until proven otherwise.
    Decontamination of open wounds should precede the irrigation of intact skin surfaces.
    Protect uncontaminated surrounding areas by covering them with disposable adhesive surgical drapes.
    Irrigate for 3 min with copious amounts of water or normal saline.
    Sponges or cotton-tipped swabs should be used to further clean the orifices or wounds, as needed.
    Carefully assess for and remove any foreign bodies.
    Reevaluate for contamination and repeat the procedure as needed.
    If contamination persists:
        Wash with 3% hydrogen peroxide.
        Consider surgical debridement (save all tissue).
    Cover wounds following successful decontamination and proceed.

Contaminated Eyes
    Protect uncontaminated areas around eyes by covering them with plastic drapes.
    Irrigate eyes thoroughly with copious amounts of water or normal saline (proceed nose to temple).
    Reevaluate for contamination and repeat as needed.

Contaminated Ear Canals
    Irrigate ear canal gently with small amounts of water.
    Suction frequently.
    Reevaluate for contamination and repeat as needed.

Contaminated Nares and Mouth (Ingestion or Inhalation)
    If patient's condition permits, turn head to side.
    Irrigate gently with small amounts of water.
    Suction frequently.
    Prevent water from entering the stomach if possible.
    Sponges or cotton-tipped swabs can be used to further clean the orifices or wounds, as needed.
    Insert nasogastric tube into the stomach and monitor suctioned contents for contamination. If contaminated:
        Lavage with small amounts of water until clear of contamination.
    If inhalation or ingestion is considered, initiate other measures to eliminate, neutralize, or block further contamination:
        Ingestion: Activated charcoal, cathartics, specific chelating or blocking agents
        Inhalation: Bronchopulmonary lavage, specific blocking or chelating agents by nebulizer

(Continues)

Table 117-6. (*continued*) Radiation Accident Plan: Recommended Emergency Department Procedures

Contaminated Intact Skin

Decontaminate areas of the body with the highest radiation level.

If whole-body contamination:

Wash the entire body thoroughly with soap and copious amounts of water and rinse well.

Showering, if available, should be used *only* for patients with extensive body surface area contamination.

If localized contamination:

Protect uncontaminated areas by covering them with plastic drapes.

Wash the affected area thoroughly with soap and copious amounts of water and rinse well.

A scrub brush may be used, but *do not* abrade the skin.

Pay particular attention to skin folds, ears, and under fingernails.

Reevaluate for contamination and repeat the procedure as needed.

If contamination persists:

Wash with Lava soap or a mixture of half cornmeal and half laundry detergent. If this fails to remove contamination, proceed with bleach (full strength for small areas or diluted for large areas).

Contaminated Hair

Protect uncontaminated areas by covering them with plastic drapes.

Do not shave hair; if necessary hair can be cut, but avoid abrading the skin.

Wash the affected area thoroughly with soap and copious amounts of water and rinse well.

Reevaluate for contamination and repeat as needed.

Removal of Patient From Decontamination Area

Dry patient thoroughly.

Recollect cotton swab sample from ears, nares, mouth, and any open wounds.

Place in labeled (patient name, site, time of "postcontamination") glass containers.

Radiation safety officer should monitor swabs and patient for further contamination.

New floor covering should be placed from the door of the "clean" area to the patient.

Clean stretcher is brought in and patient is transferred by personnel not involved directly with decontamination.

Radiation safety officer monitors patient and stretcher as it leaves the decontamination area.

Patient proceeds to the clean treatment area for further medical evaluation and treatment.

Exit of Decontamination Personnel

All participating hospital personnel must be monitored and decontaminated, as needed.

Protective garments must be removed and disposed of properly.

Outer gloves are removed first, turning them inside out.

Remove tape from pants and sleeves.

Remove surgical gown, turning it inside out.

Remove surgical cap.

Remove surgical pants.

Remove first shoe cover.

Radiation safety officer monitors shoe for contamination.

If clean, this first foot steps into clean area.

Remove second shoe cover.

Radiation safety officer monitors second shoe for contamination.

If clean, second foot steps into clean area.

Inner pair of gloves is removed.

Monitor hand, feet, and entire body for final time.

Take a shower.

Table 117-7. Patient Disposition

Discharge criteria	Patient is asymptomatic
	Decontamination is complete
	CBC is normal
	Platelet count is normal
Admission criteria	Severe vomiting and diarrhea requiring IV therapy
	Absolute lymphocyte count at 48 h is <1200 mm^3 or $<50\%$ of baseline; requires reverse isolation
	Thrombocytopenia
	Evidence of CNS symptoms
	Multiple trauma or severe burns

The process of decontamination, or cleaning the patient of particulate radioactive debris, should be initiated as soon as possible following the event. Rescue personnel must wear protective clothing, including rubber gloves, shoe covers, masks, and film badges. This protective clothing does not reduce the exposure to penetrating radiation. Rather, it serves to prevent any radioactive particles from coming in contact with the personnel or their clothing and to facilitate cleanup and disposal.

Initially, any open wounds are covered and the patient's clothing is removed; all articles are placed in clearly labeled plastic bags. Up to 70 to 90 percent of external contamination can be eliminated by this action alone. Any open wound is considered contaminated until proven otherwise, and decontamination should precede the irrigation of intact skin surfaces. The skin is then washed with copious amounts of water and soap, with particular attention to skin folds, ears, and fingernails. The use of damp washcloths, rather than rinsing with running water, may be more practical for some emergency departments. The disposal of contaminated washcloths in plastic bags may be easier than the collection of contaminated wash water. All waste must be captured in sealed containers labeled "Radioactive Waste."

Shaving of the patient's hair is to be avoided, along with excessive rubbing of the skin. Both of these maneuvers cause an increased risk of transdermal uptake. Open, uncontaminated wounds are covered with sterile dressings, and contaminated wounds are then cleaned aggressively, similar to other dirty wounds.

Whenever possible, a dosimeter should be used to determine the completeness of the decontamination. The goal is to get the radiation level "as low as reasonably achievable"; this is commonly referred to as the ALARA principle. When dealing with an external contamination, it is important to prevent it from becoming an internal contamination.

Internal Contamination

Radioactive particles that are ingested or inhaled or that contaminate open wounds can cause significant cellular damage. These particles will continue to irradiate tissues until they are eliminated, neutralized, or blocked, or until they decay naturally. In general, there is a 1- to 2-hour window of time during which absorption of these particles occurs. Therefore, it is crucial that any interventions be performed during this period and as soon as possible.

At times, it may be difficult to determine the presence of an internal contaminant, especially if an external contaminant still clouds the picture. In addition, special treatment considerations will be determined by the type of radionucleotide involved. Therefore, it is extremely important to identify the offending agent as early as possible, so that the appropriate chelating or blocking agent may be used.

Ideally, chelating agents are administered within 1 hour of exposure. Chelating agents provide an ion-exchange matrix that binds metals. This prevents tissue uptake and promotes urinary excretion of a stable complex containing the radioactivity. Diethylenetriaminepentaacetic acid (DTPA) is an effective chelating agent for many heavy metals. A solution of DTPA is often found in hospital nuclear medicine departments, but this may be too dilute to be used as a chelating agent. Other examples of chelating agents are calcium di-sodium edetate (EDTA), succimer, and penicillamine. These are recommended when radioactive lead is the cause of an internal contamination.

A blocking agent reduces radioactive uptake by saturating the tissues with a nonradioactive element. Lugol's solution (potassium iodine) is a blocking agent that reduces the uptake of radioactive iodine (^{131}I) by the thyroid gland by as much as 90 percent if administered within 1 hour of exposure. If treatment is delayed until 6 hours after exposure, the uptake is reduced by approximately 50 percent. An exposure of 10 to 30 rem warrants the initiation of this treatment. If the diagnosis has not yet been confirmed, there is little harm in administering a first dose of potassium iodine. Stable potassium iodine (KI) is recommended at a dose of 390 mg PO.

A comprehensive list of radioactive agents and their respective treatments is beyond the scope of this text.

Detailed information can be obtained from REAC/TS or through many poison control centers.

Ingestion

Initial stabilization and decontamination of radiation ingestions are the same as those for "routine" ingestions. The goal is to prevent absorption and enhance elimination. Lavage and activated charcoal are used in the usual manner and cathartics may be used to shorten the GI transit time. All bodily excretions (lavage fluid, emesis, urine, feces) are saved and labeled for radioactive evaluation and proper disposal.

Inhalation

Acute inhalation of radionucleotides is much less common than chronic low-level exposure. An acute inhalation contamination can occur in the event of a radioactive accident in conjunction with a fire or explosion. Radioactive iodine, for example, is highly volatile and likely to be inhaled.

When an inhalation contamination is suspected, a moistened cotton-tipped applicator can be used to swab the nasal passages and check for radioactivity. Bronchopulmonary lavage is performed for removal of particulate matter. Specific-blocking agents and chelating agents can also be given by nebulizer.

Open Wounds

Wounds that undergo successful decontamination can be surgically closed. Wounds that remain contaminated despite aggressive irrigation are left open for 24 hours. Debridement of these wounds may become necessary for further decontamination. Contaminated surgical instruments must be replaced to prevent further wound contamination.

Amputation of contaminated extremities is rarely indicated. Two situations may warrant this aggressive management. In the first, the amount of persistent contamination is so high that severe radiation-induced necrosis is anticipated. In the second, the degree of traumatic injury is so severe that functional recovery is doubtful.

Exposure

Despite the significant illness and injury that can result from either a local radiation injury or whole-body exposure, an emergency physician can offer only limited treatment. Fluid resuscitation for severe vomiting and di-

arrhea, baseline laboratory values, the initiations of antibiotics for infection, and burn management may be all there is to do for the "exposure" patient in the emergency department. The patient will face the greatest risks and management problems several days to several weeks later, at the onset of the manifest illness stage.

In some cases, nothing will alter the patient's outcome. The mortality rate for victims with a whole-body exposure of >1000 rad is 99 to 100 percent. For triage purposes, these patients should be classified as expectant or impending. Death ensues from the complications affecting the hematopoietic system as well as the gastrointestinal and central nervous systems. Emergency department management should consist of appropriate sedation, analgesics, and supportive care.

Special Consideration

A nuclear explosion presents logistic and patient care issues that may be difficult to manage effectively. Medical resources may be quickly depleted depending on the number of victims and the magnitude of injuries. To further complicate the situation, routine communications equipment, electronic equipment, and computers may be rendered useless by the electromagnetic pulse generated by the nuclear blast.

Victims of a nuclear explosion will be subject to three types of injury patterns: first, mechanical trauma (blunt and penetrating) secondary to the blast effect of the explosion, which accounts for 50 percent of the released energy and, second, thermal injury from heat dissipation, which represents 35 percent of the energy release. The remaining 15 percent of the thermonuclear energy release will cause radiation injury, 10 percent from radioactive fallout and only 5 percent as a result of the immediate release of χ-rays and neutrons.

PROGNOSIS

The prognosis for survival and the concern for delayed complications, while important, are not of immediate concern to the emergency physician. The possibilities of leukemia, carcinoma, cataracts, accelerated aging, and secondary congenital defects are all issues that should be addressed at a later time, when personnel are available for counseling. Leukemia and delayed thyroid cancer and breast cancer are of significant concern in children <10 years of age. In utero, exposure to as little as 5 to 10 rad can be associated with mental retardation or a small head circumference.

Based on the presenting symptoms, patients can be classified into three major prognostic classifications: *survivor probable, survivor possible,* and *survivor improbable.*

Survivor Probable

This group includes individuals who are asymptomatic or who have minimal complaints that resolve within hours. Initial and subsequent leukocyte counts are not affected and estimated exposure is <200 rad (2 Gy). Following satisfactory decontamination, inpatient care is rarely needed.

Survivor Possible

This group consists of patients with relatively brief gastrointestinal sequelae, usually lasting <48 hours. After initial presentation and the latent period, patients develop characteristic pancytopenia. Estimated exposure for this group is between 200 and 800 rad (2 to 8 Gy). An exposure of 400 rad represents the median lethal dose.

Survival in this group is influenced by the aggressiveness of supportive therapy and hematologic intervention, antecedent health of the victim, and the response to bone marrow transplantation (when indicated).

Survivor Improbable

In these patients, the estimated whole-body exposure exceeds 800 rad (8 Gy). The prognosis is dismal despite aggressive supportive therapy and even the implementation of bone marrow transplantation. If severe nausea, vomiting, and diarrhea begin within 1 hour of exposure and CNS symptoms appear early, a relatively early death can be expected.

SUMMARY

Although a whole-body radiation disaster is uncommon even in the busiest emergency departments, today's nuclear-power society makes the potential for treating such a catastrophe a reality for all emergency physicians. Radiation accidents, however, continue to occur worldwide. The most probable scenario is the identification and management of local radiation exposures secondary to medical or industrial accidents. Despite efforts to educate people regarding the dangers of these sources of radiation, as the use and transport of radioisotopes in-crease, the possibility of accidents and human injury will continue to increase.

The medical response to radiation accidents continues to improve. Information is more readily available on how to recognize and treat these accidents, improving the chances for survival. The emergency physician may be presented with a child who has localized burns and is nauseous, vomiting, or lethargic. Laboratory results may show leukopenia and thrombocytopenia. Recognizing radiation exposure as a possible etiology for this illness is crucial. Failure to do so may result in continued exposure if the child unknowingly returns to the radioactive environment.

The overall prognosis of these injuries depends on the type and dose of exposure. Following initial resuscitation, decontamination, and supportive care of the radiation victim, little else can be done in the emergency department that will affect long-term survival. However, the emergency physician must be knowledgeable about the pathophysiology and clinical specifics of these complex injuries.

In dealing with a confirmed radiation accident, counseling must be made available to the pediatric patient and to the patient's family. In the event of a perceived radiation accident, reassurance and education are of the utmost importance. Addressing the psychological trauma of a confirmed or perceived radiation exposure may be the most difficult challenge for the emergency physician.

A radiation accident plan must be developed to provide the framework for education, procedures for implementation, and protocols for patient management. Adequate training and periodic drills by hospital personnel, in cooperation with local EMS agencies, are essential. This will minimize the potential risk to hospital and prehospital personnel and ensure appropriate treatment of the radiation victim.

BIBLIOGRAPHY

Aghababian RV: *Emergency Medical Response Plan for Radiation Accidents.* February 22, 1999. <http://www.bumc. bu.eduDepartments/PageMain.asp?Page=1880&Department-ID=286>

American Academy of Pediatrics: Risk of ionizing radiation exposure to children: A subject review. *Pediatrics* 101:717, 1998.

Berger ME, Ricks RC: Management of emergency care for radiation accident victims, in Miller KL (ed): *CRC Handbook of Management of Radiation Protection Programs,* 2d ed. Boca Raton, FL: CRC Press, 1992.

Fong G, Schrader DC: Radiation disasters and emergency department preparedness. *Emerg Med Clin North Am* 14: 349–370, 1996.

Guidance for Radiation Accident Management. Radiation Emergency Assistance Center/Training Site (REAC/TS), Oak Ridge Institute for Science and Education, Oak Ridge, TN <http://www.orau.gov/reacts/manage.htm>

Illinois Department of Nuclear Safety: *Evaluating and Treating Patients Accidentally Exposed to Radiation or Contaminated with Radioactive Materials.* Illinois Dept. of Nuclear Safety, Illinois, October, 1995.

Leonard RD, Ricks RC: Emergency department radiation accident protocol. *Ann Emerg Med* 9:462, 1980.

Mettler FA, Kelsey CA, Ricks RC (eds): *Medical Management of Radiation Accidents.* Boca Raton, FL: CRC Press, 1990.

Mettler FA and Williamson SL: Pediatric radiation injuries, in Behrman RE, Kliegman RM, Jenson HB(eds): *Nelson Textbook of Pediatrics,* 16th ed. Philadelphia: Saunders, 2000.

118

Child Maltreatment

Veena Ramaiah
Jill Glick

HIGH-YIELD FACTS

- The history is vital in distinguishing inflicted from noninflicted injury. The key component to making a diagnosis of physical abuse is the compatibility of the history and mechanism given by the caretaker to explain the injuries sustained.

- Cutaneous manifestations of physical abuse are the most common and most recognizable signs of maltreatment and include bruises, marks, bites, and burns. The presence of multiple cutaneous lesions in various stages of healing is highly suspicious for abuse.

- Overall, long bone fractures in children are less specific and less suspicious for child abuse. However, spiral fractures of the femur and humerus, in nonambulatory children, ARE very suspicious for abuse.

- Head injuries are the leading cause of death and morbidity from child maltreatment. The classic triad in inflicted traumatic head trauma consists of:

  - subdural hematoma

  - retinal hemorrhages

  - skeletal injury (most frequently rib fractures and metaphyseal corner fractures)

- Shaken baby syndrome or shaken impact syndrome occurs in children <2 years old.

Violent shaking causes a shearing acceleration and deceleration injury within the brain.

- The history is the key to establishing the diagnosis of sexual abuse. Sexually abused children can present to the emergency department with various complaints, including a disclosure of sexual abuse, abdominal or urogenital symptoms, genital injuries, sexual behavior inappropriate for the child's age, or medical reasons unrelated to abuse.

- There are two main visualization techniques for females being evaluated for abuse. The separation view involves separating the labia majora outward in both directions, while the traction view involves grasping the labia majora and pulling outward and downward to dilate the introitus and provide a clear view of the hymen, posterior fourchette, and anterior vagina.

- Forensic evidence is collected if the sexual abuse or assault occurred within 72 hours of the child's presentation to the emergency department. Collection of the underwear and linens for evidence improves recovery of forensic evidence.

- Neglect is the most common type of maltreatment reported. From the point of view of the emergency department, neglected children can be categorized as medical, supervisional, educational, physical, and nutritional neglect.

- In all 50 states, child protection laws require all professionals who interact with children to notify the state child protection services if there is a suspicion of child maltreatment. Suspicion is defined as having reasonable cause to believe a child may be harmed.

Child maltreatment is a serious and increasing source of morbidity and mortality for children. According to the most recent data, in 1998 approximately 3,154,000 children were reported to child protection agencies throughout the United States, and 1,009,000 were substantiated for maltreatment. Forty-seven out of 1000 children in the United States are investigated for suspected child maltreatment with 15 per 1000 children substantiated by child welfare or police investigations. Annually, it is estimated that 2000 children die in the United States due to homicide. Abuse is ranked as the third leading cause of homicide for children >1 year of age. The youngest are at the greatest risk to be abused, with 50 percent of maltreated children <5 years old. It is important to note that greater than 35 percent of children who die from fatal child abuse had contact with a child welfare system prior to their death. This highlights the need for medical professionals to provide appropriate evaluations, document clearly, and communicate the significance of these evaluations to police and child welfare investigators. As it is available at all times, the emergency department will always be one of the first places where abused and neglected children present for evaluation. Therefore, emergency health care professionals must have a working knowledge of the child welfare system within their community and have protocols in place to ensure the safety of children who present with signs or symptoms of abuse.

The spectrum of child maltreatment is broad and includes physical abuse (25 percent), sexual abuse (13 percent), emotional abuse, and neglect (50 percent). Neglect is further subdivided into medical, supervisional, educational, physical, nutritional, and fetal. There is a wide spectrum of presentation of child maltreatment, from clearly inflicted injuries to merely suspicious scenarios that warrant an interdisciplinary, forensically guided evaluation. This chapter delineates the types of child maltreatment most commonly seen in the emergency department, clarifies historical and physical indicators to differentiate noninflicted from inflicted injuries, describes modalities of detection, and discusses the legal obligations of health professionals regarding maltreatment. It is paramount that the emergency physician is trained to recognize signs of maltreatment and is prepared to initiate the appropriate work-up and referrals.

PHYSICAL ABUSE

Child physical abuse results when a caretaker inflicts an injury. Common manifestations include cutaneous lesions (bruises, marks, bites, burns), fractures, head injury, or visceral injury. In some cases, the patient may suffer an isolated injury. In many patients the abuse is recurrent and a diligent search will reveal multiple old injuries. The spectrum of injury ranges from acute, critical, or life-threatening to chronic, healed, or occult.

History

The history is vital in distinguishing inflicted from noninflicted injury. The key component to making a diagnosis of physical abuse is the compatibility of the history and mechanism given by the caretaker to explain the injuries sustained. The mechanism of injury must both explain the lesion and correlate with the developmental abilities of the child. For example, a toddler is capable of jumping off a couch and sustaining a lower extremity fracture, whereas an infant who cannot yet walk is very unlikely to sustain a similar injury. A detailed past medical and family history will reveal any disease entities that may mimic abusive injuries. Red flags include a changing or inconsistent history and an inappropriate delay in seeking care. A verbal child should be interviewed separately from the caretaker. Interview each caretaker separately, both for a more complete history and to discover any discrepancies. Interactions between the caretaker and the child can vary widely. It is also important to observe the interaction of the caretaker and the emergency department staff. Caretakers who are inappropriately hostile, threatening, or defensive may be trying to deflect the questioning away from the true cause of the child's injury. It is paramount that the examining physician, after completing a thorough history and physical examination, bases the level of suspicion upon the correlation between the injury and the history. Well-presenting parents of a child with retinal and intracranial hemorrhages should not deter the physician from reporting a case of suspected child abuse.

Physical Examination

The physical examination of the potentially abused child focuses on detecting both new and old injuries. The examination must be extremely thorough and requires the child to be completely undressed. If not, subtle injuries, such as faded scars or marks in protected areas, may be missed. The emergency department must have protocols for meticulous documentation of cutaneous injuries, including the use of body charts and photography. This is both to provide evidence for the investigation agencies and for recall during legal proceedings. Most criminal investigators have photodocumentation technicians who should be contacted to document cutaneous lesions for the police and states' attorney. Polaroid photographs are often inadequate to accurately depict cutaneous lesions. There is growing use of digital documentation by forensic pediatricians to provide immediately available, high-quality photographs. To date, there is no literature indicating the limitation of digitally obtained photodocumentation as evidence in court.

CUTANEOUS LESIONS

Cutaneous manifestations of physical abuse are the most common and most recognizable signs of maltreatment. These include bruises, marks, bites, and burns. When documenting these lesions, it is important to note the location, size, shape, and number. If possible, an estimation of age is also helpful. Multiple cutaneous lesions in various stages of healing are highly suspicious for abuse.

Bruises are common in active, healthy children. Noninflicted bruises tend to be on prominent bony areas, such as elbows/forearms, knees/shins, and forehead. Bruises in relatively protected areas of the body, such as eyes, cheeks, neck, trunk, genitals, and buttocks, are suspicious for abuse. The developmental age of the patient is important. Bruising in a nonambulatory child is suspicious for abuse. Once again, the history must be compatible with the injury.

Certain objects result in recognizable pattern marks. These include handprints, loop marks, linear marks from a belt or cord, circumferential marks from restraints, and geometric marks made by belt buckles, hangers, hairbrushes, and many other objects.

Determining the age of a bruise is both difficult and inaccurate. Studies have shown that color change and healing time vary with age of the patient, location on the body, and depth of injury. In a study by Langlois and Gresham documenting the visual aging of bruises, their conclusions were

1. A bruise with any yellow must be older than 18 hours.

2. Red, blue, and purple or black may occur anytime from 1 hour of bruising to resolution.

3. Red has no bearing on the age of the bruise, because red is present no matter what their ages.

4. Bruises of identical age and cause on the same person may not appear as the same color and may not change at the same rate.

Human bites are common inflicted injuries. In infants, they tend to occur around the genitalia or buttocks as punishment. In older children, they are random and associated with sexual abuse/assault. Human bite marks are oval or elliptical lesions caused by a crushing and sucking injury. Animal bites cause punctures and lacerations. Human bite marks should be photographed with a centimeter ruler placed in the field. An intercanine distance >3 cm is due to a bite by a person >8 to 9 years of age. To recover the perpetrator's DNA, swab the skin with saline moistened cotton, then label and store the swab in the refrigerator until it is transported to a forensic laboratory. A forensic dentist may be able to identify the perpetrator.

Approximately 30,000 children are hospitalized each year for burns, 10 to 20 percent of which are inflicted. Mortality from accidental burns is about 2 percent, whereas mortality from inflicted burns is about 30 percent. Inflicted burns include scald and immersion, flame, contact, electrical, and chemical, with immersion and contact the most common.

A child pulling a container filled with hot liquid from a counter-top or stove causes accidental scald burns. The pattern of these burns is typically arrow shaped, narrowing downward as the liquid runs off, with varying depth of the burn as the liquid cools, and separate satellite splash burns. An immersion burn caused by holding a child in hot water leaves a characteristic stocking or glove pattern on the extremities with well-demarcated edges, uniform burn depth, and few satellite splash lesions. The buttocks may be burned with central sparing where the buttocks are in contact with the tub. This is referred to as a "doughnut-shaped burn." Inflicted immersion burns are often seen as punishment for toilet training accidents.

Inflicted contact burns in children are usually patterned, uniform, and othen deep. In contrast, noninflicted contact burns are glancing and less uniform. The child's first response to withdraw from a hot object can make the burn less severe. Common objects used to burn children include cigarettes, irons, grids, hot plates, space heaters, and light bulbs. Less frequently, children are burned by flames, chemicals, and microwave ovens. Round lesions are often evaluated for cigarette burns. Intentionally inflicted cigarette burns are symmetric and deep, with central crater-like deformities. It is very important to distinguish these from impetiginous lesions that are very superficial when unroofed.

FRACTURES

Fractures commonly result from noninflicted injury, especially in active, healthy children. Estimates of fractures secondary to abuse vary from 10 to 15 percent. The vast majority of children who suffer inflicted skeletal trauma are <2 years of age. They present with crying, pain with movement, or decreased movement of the extremity. The mechanism of injury must be consistent with the type of fracture. Red flags include inappropriate delay in seeking medical care, multiple fractures in various stages of healing, and metaphyseal or rib fractures. Any child under the age of 2 with a fracture suspicious for abuse should have a complete skeletal survey to detect occult or healing fractures.

Skull fractures result from impact, either as a direct blow to the head or the head slamming against a hard surface. In noninflicted injury, motor vehicle collisions (MVC) and falls cause skull fractures. Isolated linear skull fractures have been well demonstrated in falls from heights less than 4 feet. Any child with a skull fracture found on x-ray must have a head CT to rule out intracranial injury. A fracture line in the region of the middle meningeal artery raises the concern for an epidural bleed. Multiple skull fractures warrant a thorough abuse evaluation unless caused by a witnessed/documented major noninflicted mechanism.

Due to the flexibility of the rib cage, rib fractures are rarely noninflicted. Most commonly, squeezing and pressure on the rib cage causes lateral and posterior fractures. They may be unilateral or bilateral, and are primarily seen in the setting of shaken baby/shaken impact syndrome. Rib fractures from a direct blow to the chest occur but are rare. Many studies indicate that rib fractures in children do not result from CPR.

Overall, long bone fractures in children are less specific and less suspicious for child abuse. However, spiral fractures of the femur and humerus in nonambulatory children ARE very suspicious for abuse. Spiral fractures result from rotational forces, whereas transverse fractures result from a direct blow or bending force to the bone. The most common morphology of inflicted lower extremity fracture is a transverse fracture. Metaphyseal corner fractures, also called bucket handle fractures, are highly suspicious for inflicted trauma. They occur when shaking or shearing acceleration and deceleration forces avulse metaphyseal fragments of bone attached to the tightly adherent periosteum. Similar to rib fractures, metaphyseal fractures are almost pathognomonic for inflicted trauma and are associated with inflicted head trauma.

The toddler's fracture deserves special mention. This is a nondisplaced spiral fracture of the lower tibia from noninflicted injury. It is caused by rotational stress on the tibia of a newly ambulating child. The history given may be as simple as a toddler ambulating and falling while twisting the lower leg. On physical examination, the child may present with a limp or leg pain with or without swelling. The fracture may be a subtle irregularity in the cortex on x-ray. If the fracture is transverse, comminuted, or moderately displaced without an adequate explanation, inflicted injury must be considered.

Osteogenesis imperfecta and rickets are skeletal disorders in the differential diagnosis of abuse that can be excluded by obtaining a detailed past medical, diet and family history, performing a thorough physical examination, noting the appearance of bone density on x-ray, and checking serum calcium, phosphorus, and alkaline phosphatase. Fibroblast studies for collagen abnormalities can be sent to special laboratories, if warranted by the history, family history, and physical examination. These tests are only 85 percent sensitive.

Correlating the age of fracture with the history is important in identifying suspected abuse. Acute injury causes soft tissue swelling and a fracture line visible on xray from 0–10 days. In some cases a clear fracture line is not visible and the injury is identified after callus formation. Callus is visible at 10–14 days and in infants as early as 7–10 days. These changes are seen in all the bones except the skull. Skull fractures cannot be dated. Rib fractures may be missed initially but detected on repeat x-ray after callus formation. Bone scan can diagnose an early fracture that is not apparent on x-ray, but cannot date the age of injury. With suspicious intracranial trauma and initial negative skeletal survey, if child protective concerns or criminal investigations require immediate diagnosis and evidence collection, a bone scan is warranted. Alternatively, a second skeletal survey can be done 2 weeks after the initial insult to look for the development of callus formation.

HEAD INJURY

Head injuries are the leading cause of death and morbidity from child maltreatment. Inflicted head injuries are caused by direct impact, shaking/shearing injury, or asphyxiation. Injuries range from scalp hematomas to skull fractures, intracranial hemorrhage, and cerebral edema. Presenting symptoms range from nonspecific vomiting and irritability to seizures and cardiorespiratory arrest.

Direct impact to the head causes scalp hematomas and skull fractures. Sometimes, intra-cranial hemorrhage occurs adjacent to the site of impact. In these situations, a thorough history is critical. For example, a 2-month-old with a large scalp hematoma and facial bruising after rolling off the bed is suspicious for abuse because infants that age cannot roll over. As noted previously, skull fractures are not uncommon after falls from <4 feet. Severe traumatic brain injury, however, is not explained by this mechanism. Epidural hematomas are well documented as the result of non-inflicted impact.

Shaken baby/shaken impact syndrome occurs in children <2 years old. Violent shaking causes a shearing acceleration and deceleration injury within the brain. The relatively large head and weak neck muscles in children contribute to the problem. The shearing results in subdural/subarachnoid hemorrhage, often with diffuse axonal injury and cerebral edema. There is ongoing debate whether an impact is required in addition to the shaking. Further research is needed to clarify the mechanisms involved in inflicted traumatic brain injury.

The classic triad in shaken baby/shaken impact syndrome consists of

- subdural hematoma
- retinal hemorrhages
- skeletal injury

The caretakers often give a history of minor trauma, no trauma, or injury inflicted by a sibling, all of which are inadequate explanations for this condition.

The skeletal injuries are most frequently rib fractures and metaphyseal corner fractures. The full triad is not required for diagnosis. However, skillful and thorough investigation by a child protection team and medical personnel with expertise in forensic evaluations is necessary in these less clear-cut scenarios. The physical examination may include cutaneous injury; however, classically, these infants have no evidence of external injury. They present with altered mental status or signs of increased intracranial pressure. After initial stabilization, a head CT scan revealing traumatic brain injury elucidates the diagnosis. Examination of the fundi in the emergency department is very important. A skeletal survey should be performed, but may be delayed if the patient is admitted. MRI is useful to differentiate between acute, subacute, and chronic hemorrhage. The prognosis in these children is poor, with a high incidence of adverse neurologic sequelae.

VISCERAL INJURY

Visceral injuries account for only 2 percent of inflicted injuries. However, they are the second leading cause of death from physical abuse. Solid organ injury is common in both inflicted and noninflicted trauma. On the other hand, hollow viscus injuries are more frequently the result of inflicted trauma, primarily a direct blow to the midepigastrium. Blunt trauma causes crushing of solid viscera, compression of hollow viscera against the vertebral column, or shearing of the posterior attachments or vascular supply of viscera. A common inflicted lesion is the duodenal hematoma, due to the duodenum's fixed position, close proximity to the vertebral column, and rich blood supply. The initial management, where the abdominal examination is obscured by either head trauma or a nonverbal patient, evaluation of the abdomen includes abdominal and pelvic CT scan.

EVALUATION AND MANAGEMENT

Evaluation of the child who is a suspected victim of physical abuse involves several steps. The history and physical examination are most important. Detailed descriptions of the history given are critical. Documentation of general appearance and all skin lesions, both related and unrelated to inflicted trauma, is mandatory. The laboratory evaluation varies according to the presentation. Any patient with significant bruising or hemorrhage should have a complete blood count, including platelets, PT, PTT, and bleeding time to evaluate a bleeding disorder. This is not necessary in children with patterned bruising (e.g., isolated loop marks). Patients less than 2 years old should undergo full skeletal surveys, particularly if they present with a suspicious fracture or traumatic brain injury. Any patient with altered mental status or signs of increased intracranial pressure must get a head CT once stabilized. Patients with abdominal complaints should have liver enzymes and amylase as well as a urinalysis and an abdominal CT, if clinically indicated. Patients with multiple fractures should have serum levels of calcium, phosphorus, and alkaline phosphatase to exclude underlying bone disease. In addition, children with severe cutaneous bruising should have a urinalysis for myoglobinuria.

The medical or surgical management is specific to the injury. In many cases, no treatment is required. If the injury is diagnosed as, or suspicious for, physical abuse, the child must be reported to the state child protection agency. The major decision for the emergency physician is the child's safety, and if admission for protection is required. This is difficult, and requires a detailed understanding of the patient's home situation and current practices by the regional child welfare system. It is extremely important to ensure the safety of the siblings of a traumatized child as well. Every emergency department physician should be familiar with the child protection services available for evaluations, consultation, or follow-up. These may consist of a single expert or a multidisciplinary team.

SEXUAL ABUSE

The most important factor in diagnosing sexual abuse is an awareness that sexual abuse occurs. It is estimated that 3 per 1000 children are sexually abused per year, although the true incidence is unknown. A 1985 national survey revealed that 27 percent of adult women and 16 percent of adult men reported having been sexually abused before age 18. In the vast majority of cases, the perpetrator is known to the child. Approximately 80 percent of the victims are females, but an increasing number of male victims are being identified.

The history is the key to establishing the diagnosis of sexual abuse. Sexually abused children can present to the emergency department with various complaints, including a disclosure of sexual abuse, abdominal or urogenital symptoms, genital injuries, sexual behavior inappropriate for the child's age, or medical reasons unrelated to abuse. Children are to be believed when they disclose a history of sexual abuse. Eliciting information of a sexual nature, especially from young children, can be a difficult and time-consuming process that requires special training and skills. It is difficult to perform in the emergency department. Ideally, the interview in the emergency department consists of a screening history that establishes suspicion of sexual abuse but does not provide a detailed account. Included are an evaluation for acute symptoms of trauma (e.g., bleeding, discharge, or lesions) and an assessment of victim safety (e.g., perpetrator access to the child). The screening history should be well documented, using direct quotations from the child whenever possible. The screening history questions must be open-ended and use the child's own words for anatomic body parts. The history is taken in a quiet room and performed in an unhurried manner. Whenever possible, the child is interviewed separately from the caregiver and other family members. The questioner's responses must be supportive and empathetic, without expressions of shock or unrealistic promises. Interview the family separately from the child to ascertain their knowledge of the abuse, as well as to assess the child's safety. A more in-depth forensic interview occurs outside of the emergency department by professionals trained to interview child victims of sexual abuse.

The physical examination leaves the genital and perianal examination for last. Document any signs of trauma. External inspection of the vaginal and perianal areas is usually sufficient. The prepubertal child is examined in the supine frog leg, supine knee chest, and prone knee chest positions whereas pubertal and postpubertal females are examined in lithotomy position. All males are examined supine or standing. Magnification with a colposcope, hand-held magnifying glass, or otoscope, aids in visualization of the genital area. Gross visualization with the aid of an adequate light source usually provides sufficient inspection in the emergency department. Prepubertal and pubertal females do not need a speculum examination unless there is concern of deeper trauma or foreign body. If a more detailed examination is needed, a professional who is trained in the management of intravaginal trauma should be consulted. The best examination may require the assistance of anesthesia.

There are two main visualization techniques for females, the separation and the traction views. The separation view involves separating the labia majora outward in both directions. The traction view involves grasping the labia majora and pulling outward and downward. This dilates the introitus and provides a clear view of the hymen, the posterior fourchette, and anterior vagina. Document any abnormalities including lesions, discharge, abrasions, bruises, and lacerations. Evaluate the shape, contour, opening, and state of the hymen in the 3 to 9 o'clock positions. Diameter of the hymenal opening has been shown to be extremely variable in both normal females and in victims of sexual abuse. Therefore, this measurement is not a sensitive or specific indicator of sexual abuse. However, it is necessary to document paucity of the hymen (posterior rim <1 mm) or absence of the hymen, both of which indicate prior penetration. Examine the perineum and inner thighs for bruising, abrasions, bites, and ejaculate. An abnormal finding must be verified in both positions in female patients. In the male child, document any signs of trauma around the penis, scrotum, and perianal area. It is important to be familiar with the descriptive terminology and the anatomy in sexual abuse evaluations.

Examine the perianal area of the prepubertal child in the supine knee chest position and document the presence of bruising, abrasions, lacerations, anal fissures, skin tags, or irregular skin folds. Document the sphincter tone. Assess the presence of stool in the rectal vault prior to documenting the appearance of the anus. Stool in the vault can cause the anus to dilate. Traction on the buttocks can falsely dilate the anus. Anal dilation more than 2 cm without traction is very suspicious for rectal penetration.

The most common finding in sexual abuse is a normal physical examination. In well over half of all sexual abuse cases, there are no signs of trauma. This is due to the nature of the sexual contact and the length of time between contact and disclosure. The most common forms of sexual abuse involve kissing, fondling, or other nonpenetrating contact. Children are often cajoled, bribed, or threatened into cooperating, so there may be minimal struggle. Children often disclose events days, weeks, or months after an incident. As genital injuries heal very quickly, little if any scar is left. For these reasons, it is crucial to realize that the lack of physical evidence does not rule out sexual abuse, particularly in the context of a clear disclosure.

Forensic evidence is collected if the sexual abuse or assault occurred within 72 hours of the child's presentation to the emergency department. Collection of the underwear and linens for evidence improves recovery of forensic evidence as seen in the study by Christian et al. The physician must assess which patients require culturing for sexually transmitted diseases. Many children do not fully disclose the extent of abuse, and an infection may be asymptomatic. Screening of sexually abused children has been positive for any STD only about 5 percent of the time. Therefore, many experts recommend that screening be reserved for the following situations:

- perpetrator with known STD or high STD risk
- multiple perpetrators
- patient or family preference
- postpubertal patients
- signs or symptoms of an STD
- STDs in siblings, other children, or adults in the household

If concerned about STDs, culture the throat, vagina or penis, and rectum for *Chlamydia trachomatis* and *Neisseria gonorrhoeae.* Enzyme-linked assays or DNA amplification tests are not used in the detection of chlamydial infections and gonorrhea because the potential for false positives renders them inadmissible in court. Blood should be drawn for serologic evaluation of syphilis and HIV. Vesicular lesions must be cultured to exclude herpes simplex. For patients with a vaginal discharge, send a wet mount to screen for *Trichomonas* or bacterial vaginosis. Patients with condylomata may require biopsy for papillomavirus. Documented infection with gonorrhea or syphilis outside of infancy is considered unequivocal evidence of abuse, whereas infection with *Chlamydia,* HSV, or *Trichomonas,* is highly suggestive of sexual abuse. Presence of HPV is controversial as evidence of sexual abuse since vertical transmission commonly occurs.

If sexual abuse is suspected, the physician is mandated to report the case to the child protection agency. In cases of sexual abuse, the police are also contacted. The history given by the child remains the most important aspect in the diagnosis of sexual abuse and, when taken by a trained examiner, can usually elucidate the exact nature of the abuse.

Disposition from the emergency department is usually made with the help of social services or the regional child protection services. The safety of the child is the most important consideration. A child should not be discharged home if there is concern by the physician that the child is at risk for reabuse. Follow-up referrals for psychological counseling for the child and family are recommended before discharge. If indicated, administer prophylactic therapy for sexually transmitted disease before discharge.

NEGLECT

Neglect is the most common type of maltreatment reported. Neglect is a broad term and encompasses a gray area involving multiple cultural and socioeconomic variables. From the point of view of the emergency department, neglected children can be categorized as medical, supervisional, educational, physical, and nutritional.

The spectrum of medical neglect ranges from the caretaker who refuses or denies treatment for serious acute illnesses, such as blood transfusion for shock, to the caretaker who does not seek basic care for his or her child. A common form of medical neglect occurs when a noncompliant caretaker presents repeatedly to the emergency department with multiple exacerbations of a chronic medical problem rather than seeking on-going scheduled care.

Supervisional neglect results in morbidity and mortality from potentially avoidable childhood "accidents." Unsupervised children fall out of windows, drown, ingest poisons, and sustain burns, asphyxiation, or other disastrous events. In motor vehicle accidents, children who have not been restrained in car seats or by seat belts may incur avoidable injuries. The emergency physician is in a position to provide injury prevention counseling and education to many of these caretakers.

Physical neglect is the lack of provision of adequate food, clothing, or shelter. Abandonment is the ultimate form of physical neglect. Typically, the child is left with a relative or babysitter. The emergency physician is often asked to examine the child for any acute medical problems before the child is placed in a safe environment.

Failure to thrive is the failure of an infant to grow and develop adequately. It may be secondary to organic or nonorganic causes, or a combination of both. Nonorganic failure to thrive, which is the absence of a medical disease causing the lack of growth, is a form of neglect. When an infant presents with an acute medical problem, an astute physician discovers failure to thrive by assessing the child's growth. It is important to document the child's birth weight, any known weights from other physician visits, a developmental history, and a careful feeding history. For example, eliciting that the caretaker is diluting the formula may explain poor growth from inadequate calories. Gastrointestinal symptoms are important to note. Vomiting may indicate an obstructive lesion, such as pyloric stenosis, or significant gastroesophageal reflux, whereas diarrhea can occur in malabsorption syndromes.

The physical examination of a child with failure to thrive reveals little subcutaneous tissue, prominent ribs, and hyper- or hypotonic muscle tone. Hydration status must be documented. The patient's height, weight, head circumference, and weight for height should be plotted on standardized growth charts. The weight is often disproportionately decreased compared with the height or head circumference. If the poor growth has been for an extended period of time, the child may be losing growth in length as well as weight. Head circumference is spared until extremely severe failure to thrive occurs. The laboratory evaluation of the child with failure to thrive includes, but is not limited to, a complete blood count, a urinalysis, and serum electrolytes. Further workup is determined by clinical indications.

Admission is warranted for failure to thrive. Neglect is confirmed when the patient gains weight on an appropriate diet in the hospital. Hospitalization also allows evaluation for an organic etiology and permits multidisciplinary involvement in educating and counseling the caretaker. The earlier failure to thrive is diagnosed, the less the impact on the child's long-term neurodevelopmental potential.

Management of the various causes of neglect must be individualized. With the exception of failure to thrive, many patients may be managed as outpatients. The physician is the advocate for the child. The physician must treat any specific medical problems, document carefully any physical signs of maltreatment, and notify the appropriate authorities if there is any suspicion of maltreatment. Quite often, forms of neglect are hard to document in the emergency department. A hospital child protection team will greatly enhance the ability to track these patients, and collaborate with regional child welfare teams after discharge.

The safety and well being of the child is of paramount importance. Occasionally, children need to be admitted both for medical reasons and for protection. Once in the hospital, if there is a child protection team, they can facilitate follow-up for suspected maltreatment. If the child is discharged from the emergency department to a parent, relative, or the state child protection worker, the emergency physician's concerns must be communicated to the child's physician. Emergency departments without specialized abuse services should refer these patients to an appropriate pediatric center.

CHILD PROTECTION SERVICES AND THE LEGAL SYSTEM

In all 50 states, child protection laws require all professionals who interact with children to notify the state child protection services if there is a suspicion of child maltreatment. Suspicion is defined as having reasonable cause to believe a child may be harmed. All health professionals working in the emergency department are mandated reporters. Failure to report suspicion could result in loss of license, malpractice suits, or possible felony charges. However, mandated reporters are protected from legal retribution by alleged abusers.

The physician has an obligation to inform the parents or caretakers of concerns about the child's well-being and to explain to them the mandated requirement to notify state child protection services. As an advocate for the child, the physician must refrain from angry or accusatory statements when talking with the family. An honest and direct approach to the parents is the best policy. It is important to remember that each day many people may interact with the child. The alleged perpetrator may not be immediately known or present.

The initial verbal report made by the physician to the appropriate agency is followed by a written report. If the perpetrator is a parent, family member, caretaker, or institutional caretaker, the state's child protection services are informed. If the identity of the perpetrator is known but he or she is not a caretaker, the police must be informed. Based on the local and state child protection system, each emergency department must establish protocols for reporting child maltreatment and determining a safe disposition for the child.

Once the report has been made, the child protection service worker has the responsibility of investigating the case. This worker will talk with the physician, other emergency department staff, the caretakers, and the child. The caseworker will determine if there is enough evidence to substantiate that child maltreatment has occurred. Further, the child protection worker determines the service plans for the family, oversees the safety of the home environment, and decides whether to take the case to juvenile or family court. If the case requires police involvement, they may interview the physician and emergency staff for evidence supporting an allegation of child abuse.

In juvenile or child protection court, the judge rules on whether a child is maltreated and adjudicates custody of the child. If the maltreatment has resulted in a homicide, physical abuse, or sexual abuse, the case may also go to criminal court. Health professionals in the emergency department may be subpoenaed to testify in court. The physician in court will be asked for factual findings from the emergency department evaluation. The physician should contact the hospital's legal department for support and guidance. Emergency physicians may be requested to formulate an opinion within a reasonable degree of medical certainty if a child has been abused. When available, the emergency physician should consult a child abuse specialist to aid in this assessment. It is in the best interest of the child that professional opinions are rendered carefully, so as not to either impeach oneself or be impeached during cross examination.

With the ever-increasing incidence of child maltreatment, the emergency physician must have the skills to identify, assess, and treat all forms of child abuse and neglect. Knowledge of the protocols and policies of the medical, legal, and social service systems are vital to ensure that children are discharged to safe environments with appropriate support and follow-up. Until society learns how to successfully prevent child maltreatment, emergency departments will continue to provide the medical and psychological assessment, support, and crisis intervention for children who have been maltreated.

BIBLIOGRAPHY

American Academy of Pediatrics Committee on Child Abuse and Neglect: Guideline for the evaluation of sexual abuse in children. *Pediatrics* 87:254, 1991.

Brodeur AE (ed): *Child Maltreatment: A Clinical Guide and Reference.* St. Louis: G.W. Medical Publishing, Inc., 1994.

Christian CW, Lavelle JM, De Jong AR, et al: Forensic evidence findings in prepubertal victims of sexual assault. *Pediatrics* 106:100–104, 2000.

Heger A, Emans SJ: *Evaluation of the Sexually Abused Child.* New York: Oxford University Press, 1992.

Kleinman PK: *Diagnostic Imaging of Child Abuse.* Baltimore: Williams & Wilkins, 1987.

Langlois NEI, Gresham GA: The aging of bruises: A review and study of the color change with time. *Forensic Sci Int* 50:227–238, 1991.

Ludwig S, Komberg AE (eds): *Child Abuse: A Medical Reference.* New York: Churchill Livingstone, 1992.

Reece RM (ed): *Child Abuse, Medical Diagnosis and Management.* Philadelphia: Lea & Febiger, 1994.

Wang C, Harding K: *Current Trends in Child Abuse Reporting and Fatalities: The Results of the 1998 Annual Fifty State Survey.* Publication of the National Center on Child Abuse Prevention Research, 1999.

119

Psychiatric Emergencies

Heather M. Prendergast
Tanya R. Anderson

HIGH-YIELD FACTS

- Attention to medical issues is the first priority when dealing with psychiatric patients.
- Evaluation of safety issues must occur early in the interview process.
- Considerations in restraining an agitated or aggressive patient include situational modifications, physical restraints, and chemical restraints.
- The suicidal or psychotic patient represents a true psychiatric emergency.
- Haloperidol and diphenhydramine are first-line agents for acute agitation.
- When evaluating a suicidal patient, important factors to consider include the lethality of the act, the true suicidal intent, and the family support system.
- Always screen patients for signs of depression or substance abuse.
- When faced with diagnostic or treatment dilemmas, a child psychiatry consultation is always appropriate.
- Acute dystonic reactions are treated with diphenhydramine or benztropine administered intramuscularly or intravenously.

Emergency department visits by children with social and emotional disorders have increased substantially in the last 10 years. Emergency physicians are expected to not only recognize and stabilize crisis situations, but also to facilitate the appropriate intervention and disposition. In the pediatric patient this can be a very challenging endeavor. It is important to be familiar with the most common emergencies and with approaches to assessment and disposition planning. In children on psychotropic medications, an additional layer of complexity is introduced into the clinical picture. This chapter highlights the principles of management of the pediatric psychiatric patient, with emphasis on the suicidal and psychotic child.

PRINCIPLES OF MANAGEMENT

An accurate psychiatric assessment of the pediatric patient will center on evaluating safety concerns and the need for hospitalization. In the majority of cases, decision making will be based on information obtained from multiple collateral sources.

The first priority is determining if in the current status the child poses a threat to self or others. Any issues regarding the medical stability of the patient must be addressed immediately. The management of the aggressive or violent child may require the use of physical or chemical restraints, but these measures should be viewed as a last resort. Children often have a positive response to simple situational interventions, such as placement of the child in a quiet room with minimal external stimulation; speaking with the child in a calm, reassuring tone; acknowledgment of the child's distress; and offering the child an opportunity to participate in the immediate decision making. If the child does not respond favorably and continues to pose a threat, the use of physical restraints may be required. For legal as well as ethical reasons, it is important that the physician and emergency department staff be familiar with the proper technique for applying physical restraints prior to use (Table 119-1). Chemical restraints are a third option available for use with agitated or aggressive patients. A careful assessment is necessary to make sure that there are no contraindications to sedation, and that there is no medical reason for the agitation.

A developmental approach to the assessment of the child is necessary for an accurate assessment. It may be necessary to modify the history-taking process in the younger or nonverbal child. Various modifications of interview techniques are customarily used in the office setting, but modified versions can be of benefit in the emergency setting as well. Effective techniques may involve drawing pictures, using toy figures, and communication through play.

For the older child, direct questioning is often the most effective technique. At the outset, it is important to convey a sense of understanding to the child and the caregivers in a nonjudgmental fashion. This will help to

Table 119-1. ABCDs of Physically Restraining a Child

A	Assistance in applying restraints. At least 4 members of the ED or security staff are needed
B	Be careful to avoid contact with bodily fluids
C	Communicate with the patient and family Constantly monitor the patient
D	Document reason for restraints, time placed, reassessments of the patient, and the time removed

establish rapport with all parties involved. Bringing a child for a psychiatric evaluation can be a distressing and embarrassing act for both child and parent. Addressing any perceived parental anxiety up front will facilitate a more informative exchange.

In the emergency setting, there are two vital components of the pediatric psychiatric interview: the *history* and the *mental status evaluation.* Information obtained during the history should include:

- Details of the current crisis situation
- Any apparent triggers
- Timeline
- Previous episodes
- Presence or absence of a psychiatric history
- Symptoms of depression
- Presence of suicidal or homicidal ideation
- The current home environment

In light of the fact that children rarely bring themselves to an emergency department, it is important to obtain collateral history from persons in contact with the child. These may include parents, caregivers, teachers, law enforcement agents, and siblings.

The mental status evaluation provides the physician with increased insight and augments the fact-finding process. Relevant information is gathered on a continuing basis during the interview, but there are specific components of the mental status examination that should be included at some point in the interview:

- Orientation
- Appearance
- Memory
- Cognition
- Relatedness
- Speech
- Affect

- Thought content
- Thought process

Of particular importance in the emergency patient is the ability to relate, the thought content, and thought process.

Time constraints may prevent conducting a full mental status examination. In these instances, assessment of danger to self or others is the primary goal of the emergency evaluation. Table 119-2 lists some important areas to address in evaluating the suicidal risk of a patient.

The decision to interview children and their parents together or separately needs to be assessed on an individual basis because there are benefits to both options. In general, children and adolescents more accurately report internal states, such as mood, while caregivers more accurately report external states that can be observed, such as behavior and aggression. It is generally recommended that children be interviewed separately from their parents if they can tolerate the separation. For the adolescent patient, it is important to acknowledge confidentiality concerns and to conduct a separate interview whenever possible.

The physician must perform a directed but thorough physical examination. The patient should receive a medical clearance. A careful search for signs or symptoms of poisoning, self-inflicting wounds, and abuse should be undertaken. It is not always necessary to obtain laboratory tests unless indicated by the history. However, most state psychiatric facilities require baseline chemistries including complete blood count, electrolytes, urine toxicology screen, and alcohol level.

By integrating all available information, the emergency physician should be able to arrive at a preliminary diagnosis and begin to explore treatment options. A child psychiatric consultation should be obtained whenever there is uncertainty about the assessment, safety, or diagnosis, or if there are treatment dilemmas. Often the treatment plans are best formulated in conjunction with a child psychiatry consultant and the family. It is important to be familiar with the indications for hospitalization (Table 119-3), as well as the resources available in the area.

The majority of psychiatric disorders are initially managed on an outpatient basis. The decision to hospitalize should be made on an individual basis and when possible in conjunction with a child psychiatry consultant.

THE SUICIDIAL PATIENT

The incidence of suicide among patients <18 years of age is increasing in epidemic proportions. It is a significant public health concern. Even more alarming is the

Table 119-2. Assessing Suicidal Risks in Children

Suicidal Fantasies or Actions
  Have you ever thought of hurting yourself?
  Have you ever threatened or attempted to hurt yourself?
  Have you ever wished to or threatened to commit suicide?
Consequences/Concepts of What Would Happen
  What did you think would happen if you tried to hurt or kill yourself?
  What did you want to have happen?
  Did you think you would die?
  Did you think you would have severe injuries?
Circumstances at the Time of the Child's Suicidal Behavior
  What was happening at the time you thought about killing yourself or tried to kill yourself?
  Was anyone else with you or near you when you thought about suicide or tried to kill yourself?
Previous Experiences With Suicidal Behavior
  Have you ever thought about killing yourself or tried to kill yourself before?
  Do you know of anyone who thought about, attempted, or committed suicide?
  How did this person carry out his or her suicidal ideas or action?
  When did this occur?
Motivations for Suicidal Behaviors
Open-ended questions:
  Why do you want to kill yourself?
  Why did you try to kill yourself?
Closed-ended questions (if patient does not provide enough information):
  Did you want to frighten someone?
  Did you want to get even with someone?
  Did you hear voices telling you to kill yourself?
  Did you wish someone would rescue you before you tried to hurt yourself?
Experiences and Concepts of Death
  What happens when people die?
  Can they come back again?
  Do they go to a better place?
  What will happen when you die?
Depression
  Do you cry a lot?
  Do you ever feel sad, upset, angry, or bad?
  Do you ever feel that you are not worthwhile?
  Do you have difficulty sleeping, eating, and concentrating on schoolwork?
  Do you blame yourself for things that happen?
Family and Environmental Situations
  Do you have difficulty in school?
  Do you worry that your parents will punish you for doing poorly in school?
  Do your parents fight a lot?
  Is anyone in your family sad, depressed, and very upset? Who?
  Does anyone in your family talk about suicide or try to kill themselves?

Source: Reproduced with permission from Pfeffer CR: *The Suicidal Child.* New York: Guilford, 1986.

Table 119-3. Indications for Hospitalization or Removal From Current Environment

- Danger to self
- Danger to others
- Family unable to care for the child
- Physical or sexual abuse
- Failure of outpatient treatment
- Need for stabilization on or adjustment of medication

progressive increase with age. Studies have found that by late adolescence, the rate of suicide attempts equals that of adults. In recent years, there has been considerable attention paid to this area. A number of risk factors have been identified:

- Presence of a psychiatric disorder
- Substance abuse
- Male gender
- High parental stress
- Presence of a firearm in the home
- Dysfunctional family relationships

Most adolescent suicidal behavior occurs within the context of a family disturbance or a perceived interpersonal loss. There is a high correlation with depression. A recent study identified increasing age, female gender, and weekday presentation during the school year as risk factors that demonstrated high correlation with suicide attempts. Another study found that racial minority status contributed additional risk. A postmortem study found that 90 percent of adolescent suicide victims had a psychiatric disorder. Another study found that 50 percent of adolescents who commit suicide have had contact with the health care system within 1 to 6 months prior to the event.

Assessment

The assessment of suicidal behavior or ideation requires understanding of the presence and degree of suicidal intent. While the distinction between suicidal attempts and gestures is made for epidemiological study, it is prudent for the emergency physician to regard all suicidal behavior as a suicidal attempt. The focus should be on the lethality of the act, the true suicidal intent of the child, and the family support system. Depending on the developmental stage, children have different perceptions of the concept of death (Table 119-4) and often miscalcu-

late the lethality of acts. Intent must be explored in a developmentally accurate manner. Children found to have true intent obviously are at high risk.

The basic principles of management of psychiatric patients presented above apply to the suicidal patient as well. There are certain areas that deserve special emphasis. The current home environment is carefully assessed with special attention given to whether there are adequate support mechanisms in place should the child be discharged from the emergency department. Because of the high correlation between depression and suicide, the interview should be structured to uncover signs or symptoms of depression, such as:

- Insomnia (or hypersomnia)
- Crying spells
- Poor appetite (or increased appetite)
- Fatigue
- Poor concentration
- Decreased attention to personal hygiene
- Flat effect
- Poor eye contact

It is important in the suicidal patient to be direct in your questioning in order to avoid misinterpreting thoughts or actions. The importance of collateral information cannot be overemphasized. Patients are often embarrassed by their actions and have a tendency to minimize or misrepresent the facts. Patients may also not be truthful with information regarding previous suicidal attempts.

Management

Any history of ingestion must be taken seriously and thoroughly investigated with appropriate toxicology screening. Most toxicology screens test for drugs of

Table 119-4. Developmental Concepts of Death

Concept of Death	Perception
Up to age 5	Death viewed as a reversible process
Ages 5 to 9	Death tends to be internalized; begins to understand the concept of irreversibility
Age 9 and older	Death viewed as irreversible, final

abuse. Specific drug screens should be requested if other agents are suspected. Agents commonly found in coingestions include alcohol, aspirin, and acetaminophen. A low threshold for seeking the presence of these substances should be maintained and levels ordered as indicated. Depending on the time of ingestion and presentation, the patient may be a candidate for gastric lavage or activated charcoal (see Chap. 79).

If the patient requires medical admission, it is important that an observer be placed with the patient for the duration of the medical portion of the hospital stay. Once the patient is medically cleared, a determination of the need for inpatient psychiatric hospitalization is made. Indications for inpatient psychiatric management include the following:

- Inability to maintain a no-suicide contract
- Active suicidal ideation (plan and intent)
- High intent or lethality of attempt
- Psychosis
- Previous history of suicide attempts
- Family incapable or unwilling to monitor and protect patient

THE PSYCHOTIC PATIENT

Psychosis is characterized by severe disturbances in mental functioning and may involve disruptions of cognition, perception, or reality testing. Psychotic patients often experience hallucinations and delusions and often feel threatened. Psychotic patients are actively attempting to regain control over their mental capacities and their resultant behavior underscores their extreme anxiety. These patients are high risk because of the self-endangering behaviors often exhibited. The prevalence appears to increase with age.

Assessment

Psychosis in the pediatric patient is divided into two groups depending upon etiology: organically-based causes and psychiatrically-based causes. It is important to identify patients belonging to the organic group, since the treatment options are different. In the younger child, the etiology is often organically based. Organic precipitants include:

- Central nervous system lesions
- Infections
- Trauma
- Hypoxia

- Toxins
- Vitamin deficiencies
- Metabolic disorders
- Endocrine disorders
- Rheumatic diseases
- Reye's syndrome
- Wilson's disease

Important diagnostic information can be obtained by reviewing the vital signs and through physical examination. A careful review of the medication list, including over-the-counter preparations, is mandatory and often yields helpful information. Indicated laboratory tests include:

- Complete blood count
- Serum electrolytes
- Serum calcium
- Drug screen
- Blood glucose
- Blood alcohol level

Additional laboratory tests may be ordered as directed by the medical history.

Once a search for organic causes has been undertaken, the physician can explore functional causes of psychosis. In childhood, functional causes include:

- Pervasive developmental disorders, such as autism
- Schizophrenia
- Posttraumatic stress disorder
- Mood disorders

Developmental level has a significant effect on symptom manifestations.

Regardless of the etiology, the presentation of the acutely psychotic patient tends to be quite uniform. Patients may be agitated and in a confused state. Thoughts may be bizarre, distorted, and disconnected from reality. There may be disturbances in memory, concentration, or mood. The child may show little insight or judgment. Acute disorientation, fluctuations in consciousness, disruption in intellectual functioning, and impairment in recent memory favor an organic etiology. A more insidious onset is consistent with a functional etiology.

Management

Management of a psychotic child is focused on behavioral control. Safety considerations are a priority. Children may develop psychotic symptoms when they are under stress. These episodes are often transient and non-recurring. It is important to alleviate a child's fear and anxiety. This requires use of supportive statements, specific instructions, and often repetition. Many patients will require physical or chemical restraints. First-line pharmacologic agents for agitation include:

- Diphenhydramine: 25 mg orally or intramuscularly
- Droperidol: 0.625 to 2.5 mg intramuscularly
- Haloperidol: ages 6 to 12 years: 1 to 3 mg/dose intramuscularly; over age 12: 2 to 5 mg/dose intramuscularly. Doses can be repeated every 30 minutes up to a maximum dose of 40 mg.

The latter agents are high-potency antipsychotics. In the psychotic patient, these agents are extremely effective, safe, and have a rapid onset. Side effects of neuroleptics include extrapyramidal symptoms, which respond to these anticholinergics:

- Benzotropine: 1 to 2 mg orally or intramuscularly
- Diphenhydramine: 25 mg orally or intramuscularly

Benzodiazepines should be avoided, especially when the etiology is not entirely clear. Benzodiazepines can lower the seizure threshold, may have a paradoxical effect, and can exacerbate underlying organic causes.

Schizophrenia

Childhood schizophrenia is a rare disorder characterized by impairment of basic mental functions. Children exhibit abnormalities in reality testing, perception, behavior, and social relatedness. The incidence of schizophrenia increases steadily after the onset of puberty. Early-onset schizophrenia occurs more often in males; however, incidence in males and females is equal by the adolescent period. Studies show that 39 percent of males and 23 percent of females developed their first psychotic episode by age 19. There is a higher incidence of new cases in families where one or more family members already carry the diagnosis. Previously autism was included as a subset of childhood schizophrenia. However, the current nomenclature in the fourth edition of the *Diagnostic and Statistical Manual* (DSM-IV) separates the pervasive developmental disorders from childhood schizophrenia.

Many of the symptoms exhibited are the direct result of the impaired thought content:

- Delusions
- Loose associations

- Catatonic states
- Inappropriate affect
- Auditory hallucinations (usually persecutory or commanding)

Psychotic patients may become dangerous when command hallucinations tell them to hurt self or others, when they exhibit poor impulse control, poor contact with reality, or poor decision making. In the younger child, delusions tend to be less complex and often are centered on simple childhood themes. They therefore tend to be less distressing to the child. A careful history often reveals a prodromal period. During this phase, patients begin to distance themselves from close friends and family. Frequently there is a decline in overall school performance and decreased attention to personal hygiene. It is not infrequent for a child to present to the ED with a first psychotic episode.

Admission must be considered when the conditions listed in Table 119-3 are met. Cooperative patients with good family support who do not meet those criteria can be referred for outpatient treatment. It is important to be familiar with the clinical spectrum of presentations since early intervention is paramount. Studies have shown that children with early-onset schizophrenia have a worse prognosis at least in part because of delay in diagnosis and treatment.

Mania

Manic episodes can be seen in late adolescence and are characterized by an expansive or irritable mood and a pattern of excessive indulgence. Patients exhibit inflated self-esteem, grandiosity, and erratic and disinhibited behaviors. They are prone to excessive spending, promiscuity, and reckless behavior. There is a decreased need for sleep, increased negative energy, exaggerated euphoria, racing thoughts, and pressured speech. Patients can experience delusions and sometimes become aggressive and combative. A careful history may reveal a period of depression preceding the current episode. In other cases, the manic episode is the first psychiatric presentation. There is often a family history of bipolar disorder. When evaluating a manic patient, it is important to keep a broad differential because many organic and psychiatric disorders can have similar presentations. Collateral history is very important in making an accurate assessment.

The mainstay of treatment for bipolar disorder is a mood stabilizer. Lithium and valproic acid are the most commonly prescribed. They may not be particularly useful in the emergency setting because of the time necessary to reach therapeutic levels. For this reason, patients may require hospitalization, often involuntarily. For the acutely agitated patient, low-dose neuroleptics may be required. Prior to admission, baseline laboratory tests should be obtained:

- Complete blood count
- Serum electrolytes
- Liver function tests
- Renal function tests
- Urine osmolality
- Pregnancy test (should be checked in all females of child-bearing age before giving any psychotropic medications because these agents are Class C drugs)

Lithium has a very narrow therapeutic range and requires monitoring of blood levels. If a patient is currently being treated with lithium, the lithium level should be checked. Therapeutic lithium levels are between 0.6 and 1.2 mEq/L, with toxicity occurring at levels of ≥1.5 mEq/L. Lithium toxicity is life threatening. The emergency physician must be aware of the symptoms of lithium toxicity:

- Nausea
- Vomiting
- Tremors
- Seizures
- Slurred speech
- Visual changes
- Mental status changes

Valproate is the other first-line agent for treatment of bipolar disorder in children and adolescents. Therapeutic concentrations are observed at serum levels of 50 to 100 ng/mL. Adverse effects include:

- Nausea
- Vomiting
- Pancreatitis
- Hepatotoxicity
- Leukopenia
- Thrombocytopenia
- Transient alopecia
- Sedation
- Nystagmus
- Gait abnormalities

Posttraumatic Stress Disorder

In 1980, posttraumatic stress disorder (PTSD) was officially recognized as a mental disorder occurring in children, adolescents, and adults. The symptoms exhibited vary according to the developmental stage of the child and the nature of the stressor. It is estimated that approximately 34 percent of urban youth have been exposed to neighborhood violence and are at risk for PTSD. At-risk children include:

- Those who have endured physical, sexual, or emotional abuse
- Those who have been threatened with serious injury
- Those who have witnessed violent acts

The exposure is internalized and manifested in several ways. Children continually relive the trauma through recurrent nightmares, flashbacks, and repetitive play involving aspects of the trauma. They exhibit intense distress during events that resemble the ordeal. Another possible response is to exhibit generalized numbness to certain stimuli and people. Children are frequently brought to the emergency department for signs of increased arousal, such as sleep difficulties, exaggerated startle response, irritability, problems concentrating, and generalized suspiciousness. PTSD is more likely to be the cause when the stress has been severe, there has been parental distress, and when there is temporal proximity to the traumatic event. Problems arise when children are not provided with a supportive and protective environment following traumatic events.

Most of the therapeutic interventions recommended for these children are trauma-focused and involve discussion of the trauma on some level. The role of the emergency physician is to recognize the risk factors and establish the connection with the history obtained. PTSD should be included in the differential of the confused and agitated patient. Patients should be screened for the presence of comorbid psychiatric disorders. Children require a lot of emotional support and it is important that their treatment in the emergency department is reflective of this. For the acutely agitated child, low-dose antipsychotics can be safely administered. Hospitalization may be required for patients unresponsive to medica-tion. Those patients discharged from the emergency department will need referral for counseling and family therapy.

THE SUBSTANCE ABUSER

Every year the number of children using drugs increases and the age at which the experimentation begins decreases. The Monitoring the Future Study found a very high incidence of drug use among high school seniors, of substances including marijuana, stimulants, cocaine, LSD, and heroin. There is a correlation between early substance abuse and the likelihood of dependency in adulthood. Almost 1 in 10 adolescents meet lifetime criteria for drug abuse or dependence. In July 2000 the American Academy of Pediatrics formed a Committee on Substance Abuse and developed guidelines for management and referral of substance abuse in pediatric patients. In order to intervene effectively, the emergency physician has to be familiar with the risk factors, stages of abuse, and treatment options (Table 119-5).

Assessment

Children are not likely to be forthcoming with information about substance abuse. Most often their presentation

in the emergency department is the result of either concerned caregivers or problems caused by the substance abuse. It is important to be direct in your questioning and speak in a calm, nonjudgmental tone. During the history it is very important to get a sense of the family environment. Two of the biggest risk factors for substance abuse are a substance-abusing parent or relative and frequent family conflicts. Other risk factors include lack of positive role models, negative peer influences, low self-esteem, and poor attention span. There is a high incidence of comorbid psychiatric disorders in substance abusers. There is likely to be a history of periods of social withdrawal, frequent mood changes, truancy, and altercations. As the drug use intensifies and the substances increase in potency, the behaviors become more dangerous. There may be history of sexual promiscuity, sexually transmitted diseases, motor vehicle crashes,

Table 119-5. Stages of Substance Abuse

Stage	Description
1	Potential for abuse
	Decreased impulse control
	Need for immediate gratification
	Availability of tobacco, drugs, alcohol, inhalants
	Need for peer acceptance
2	Experimentation: learning the euphoria
	Use of inhalants, tobacco, marijuana, and alcohol with friends
	Few consequences
	May increase to regular use
	Little change in behavior
3	Regular use: seeking the euphoria
	Use of other drugs, such as stimulants, LSD, sedatives
	Behavioral changes and some consequences
	Increased frequency of use
	Use alone
	Buying or stealing drugs
4	Regular use: preoccupation with the "high"
	Daily use of drugs
	Loss of control
	Multiple consequences and risk-taking
	Estrangement from family and "straight" friends
5	Burnout: use of drugs begins to feel normal
	Use of multiple substances; cross-addiction
	Guilt, withdrawal, shame, remorse, depression
	Physical and mental deterioration
	Increased risk-taking, self-destructive behavior, suicidal behavior

Source: Reproduced with permission from the American Academy of Pediatrics Committee on Substance Abuse: Indications for management and referral of patients involved in substance abuse. *Pediatrics* 106:143-148, 2000.

theft, weapons possession, and encounters with law enforcement.

During the physical examination, the physician should be alert for signs consistent with drug use or intoxication. Some important physical findings include:

- Needle marks
- Pinpoint pupils in opioid use
- Conjunctival congestion in marijuana use
- Nasal septal perforation in chronic cocaine users
- Excoriations from tactile hallucinations

Management

If the patient is found to have unstable vital signs, immediate action must be taken. Acute intoxications and withdrawal from some substances can be life threatening. This is especially true for alcohol and sedatives. The goal of emergency intervention is to normalize the vital signs. Benzodiazepines are utilized to prevent seizures and lessen the effects of delirium tremens. Although uncomfortable for the patient, withdrawal from opioids is not life threatening. The physician should have a low threshold for obtaining urine toxicology screens and blood alcohol levels.

Patients found to be acutely intoxicated but receptive to treatment should be referred or admitted for detoxification. It is mandatory that patients and their families be provided with information about and referrals to out-patient treatment centers. Arranging an intake prior to discharge from the emergency department increases the compliance rate. Inpatient treatment programs are usually reserved for those who have failed outpatient treatment.

PSYCHOTROPIC MEDICATIONS

Psychotropic medications should generally not be initiated in an emergency department. Referral to an outpatient child mental health clinic is usually necessary in order to obtain thorough evaluation, diagnosis, treatment planning, and appropriate follow-up care. The emergency physician may encounter patients who are already on psychotropic medications and therefore should be familiar with the most commonly prescribed agents (Table 119-6) and the most significant adverse effects.

Adverse Effects of Psychotropic Medications

Extrapyramidal side effects are secondary to blockage of the dopamine receptors and are characterized by movement abnormalities. Most often these symptoms occur early in the treatment phase. The exception is tardive dyskinesia, which occurs after prolonged use.

Acute dystonic reactions are the most frequently seen extrapyramidal side effects. Dystonic reactions are muscle spasms involving various muscle groups, typically in the limbs or trunk. Patients may also develop laryngeal dystonia and report a choking sensation. The airway must be carefully monitored and a means of securing the airway kept readily available. The laryngeal spasm appears to be relieved in the sleep state. The treatment involves intramuscular or intravenous diphenhydramine, followed by anticholinergic prophylaxis with a benzotropine. Psychiatric follow-up should be arranged so that changes in medications or doses can be considered.

Neuroleptic malignant syndrome is a life-threatening event. It is often, but not always, seen during the first

Table 119-6. Commonly Prescribed Psychotropics in Children and Adolescents

Trade Name	Generic Name	Typical Dose Range
Prozac	Fluoxetine	10–60 mg
Zoloft	Sertraline	25–150 mg
Paxil	Paroxetine	10–40 mg
Depakote	Divalproex sodium	Depends on blood level
Ritalin	Methylphenidate	10–60 mg in divided doses
Risperdal	Risperidone	1–10 mg
Haldol	Haloperidol	1–10 mg
Cogentin	Benztropine	0.5–2 mg
Zyprexa	Olanzapine	5–20 mg
Catapres	Clonidine	0.05–0.4 mg in divided doses

several weeks of treatment. There is a higher incidence with parenterally administered high potency antipsychotics. Presentation includes:

- Muscle rigidity
- Muscle breakdown
- High fevers
- Altered mental status
- Autonomic instability

Effective treatment requires aggressive fluid administration, cooling, discontinuation of the offending agent, and intensive care unit admission. See Chapter 100 for further discussion.

BIBLIOGRAPHY

American Academy of Pediatrics Committee on Substance Abuse: Indications for management and referral of patients involved in substance abuse. *Pediatrics* 106:143–148, 2000.

Feiguine R, Ross-Dolen M, Havens J: The New York Presbyterian Pediatric Crisis Service. *Psychiatr Q* 71:139–152, 2000.

Kaplan BJ, Sadock VA: *Kaplan and Sadock's Comprehensive Textbook of Psychiatry,* Vol. 1 and 2. Philadelphia: Lippincott Williams & Wilkins, 2000.

Halamandaris PV, Anderson TR: Children and adolescents in the psychiatric emergency setting. *Psychiatr Clin North Am* 22:865–874, 1999.

Labellarte M, Ginsburg G, Walkup J: The treatment of anxiety disorder in children and adolescents. *Biol Psychiatry* 46:1567–1578, 1999.

Olshaker JS, Browne B, Jerrard DA, et al: Medical clearance and screening of psychiatric patients in the emergency department. *Acad Emerg Med* 4:124–128, 1997.

Peterson B, Zhang H, Lucia S, et al: Risk factors for presenting problems in child psychiatric emergencies. *J Am Acad Child Adolesc Psychiatry* 35:1162–1173, 1996.

Sater N, Constantino J: Psychiatric emergencies in children with psychiatric conditions. *Pediatr Emerg Care* 14:42–50, 1998.

Schulz SC, Findling RL, Wise A, et al: Child and adolescent schizophrenia. *Psychiatr Clin North Am* 21:43–56, 1998.

Ulloa R, Birmaher B, David A, et al: Psychosis in a pediatric mood and anxiety disorders clinic: Phenomenology and correlates. *J Am Acad Child Adolesc Psychiatry* 39:337–345, 2000.

120

Pediatric Prehospital Care

Ronald A. Dieckmann
Robert W. Schafermeyer

HIGH-YIELD FACTS

- EMSC refers to an entire "EMS-EMSC continuum" of pediatric emergency, critical care, and trauma services.

- Diverse products from EMSC-funded projects are readily available on-line or through the federal EMSC Program.

- To encourage the expanded scope of inquiry into children and family issues, the EMSC program and NHTSA have jointly developed a pediatric survey to facilitate state review of children's issues.

- The leading causes of childhood death are both age- and geography-related. In some states, fires and burns are the leading causes in children under 5 years old, while in other states motor vehicle incidents or drowning are the leading causes.

- Pediatric life support programs for emergency physicians, pediatricians, nurses, and prehospital care providers have helped codify fundamental approaches to emergency pediatric care. National courses include Advanced Pediatric Life Support, Pediatric Advanced Life Support, the Emergency Nurses Pediatric Course (ENPC), and most recently the Pediatric Education for Prehospital Professionals (PEPP) Course.

- Prehospital professionals require special pediatric equipment and supplies for basic life support (BLS) and advanced life support (ALS) ambulances. Equipment and supplies must be logically organized, routinely checked, and readily available.

- Treatment policies or protocols are fundamental to pediatric prehospital care. Recently, the National Association of EMS Physicians developed pediatric field treatment protocols for prehospital professionals.

- *Minimum* voluntary requirements for community EDs that provide emergency care for children were endorsed by ACEP, AAP, and the federal EMSC program and published in 2001. The guidelines outline necessary resources for children's emergency care in all EDs and address stabilization and timely transfer of selected patients to specialized pediatric centers.

- Rehabilitation services for children are still poorly organized within EMS systems and represent an important area for future growth and development.

- Effective medical direction includes review and modification of treatment *and* nontreatment policies, procedures, and protocols for children. Medical direction entails both real time on-line (direct) elements, as well as off-line (indirect) elements.

Emergency medical services for children (EMSC) is now an important ingredient of American EMS systems. Originally, "EMSC" referred only to prehospital pediatric emergency care, but now the term EMSC refers to an entire EMS-EMSC continuum of pediatric emergency, critical care, and trauma services (Fig. 120-1). It includes children's and family services rendered at home, in the community, and primary physician's office, in the prehospital

Five components

Prevention
Medical home/primary physician
Prehospital system
ED and hospital
Rehabilitation

Clinical features

Prevention programs
Pediatric equipment
Pediatric treatment protocols and practice guidelines
Transportation
Emergency departments
Specialized pediatric centers
Pediatric rehabilitation

Operational features

EMS system adaptations for children
Communications
Medical direction
Human resources education
Data and information management
Public information and education
Research

Fig. 120-1 EMS-EMSC continuum

care system, in the emergency department (ED) and hospital, and in rehabilitation centers. EMSC is fully within the general EMS system and only works well when the general EMS system is effective.

The "EMS-EMSC continuum" requires unique clinical and operational features to develop, evaluate, and improve services focused primarily on children. Clinical features pertain to real-time elements in the delivery of emergency care; operational features pertain to administrative support and quality management of EMSC. *Clinical features* include prevention of illness and injury, pediatric equipment, pediatric treatment protocols, transportation, emergency departments, specialized pediatric centers, and pediatric rehabilitation. *Operational features* include EMS system adaptations for children, communications, medical direction and education, data and information management, public information and education, and research.

Children under the age of 18 years account for approximately 10 percent of patients transported by ambulance. In addition, a significant number of pediatric patients are secondarily transported to specialized pediatric centers for neonatology, psychiatric care, critical care, and trauma care. In the ED, about 30 percent of patients are children.

THE FEDERAL EMSC PROGRAM

EMSC had its birth in 1984, with passage of the Emergency Medical Services for Children (EMSC) Act. This act established funding for state and local pediatric components for EMS systems through the Maternal and Child Health Division within the Health Resources and Services Administration. It also established the Federal EMSC Program, which is now an active partner with the EMS Division of the National Highway Traffic Safety Administration (NHTSA) in improving emergency medical services for children. A new EMSC national resource center, an EMSC data center, and a huge resource library of EMSC products, original articles, national reports, and one textbook now provide the blueprints for integration of EMSC within state EMS systems.

Funding has supported an enormous array of innovative services and products for children and families, aimed at different components of the EMS-EMSC continuum. The diverse products of EMSC-funded projects, all readily available on-line or through the federal EMSC program, include the following examples:

- A national clearinghouse, the EMSC National Resource Center, in Washington, D.C. Its website (www.ems-c.org) provides detailed information on EMSC products, including the EMSC Five Year Plan.

- An EMSC data center, the National EMSC Data Analysis Resource Center (NEDARC), in Salt Lake City. The mission of NEDARC is to help EMS agencies develop their own capabilities to formulate and answer research questions, and to effectively convert available data into informative reports with appropriate statistical analyses (website: www.nedarc.med.utah.edu).

- A comprehensive booklet entitled "EMSC Model," published by the California EMS Authority, with nine different sets of EMSC guidelines and five sets of EMSC recommendations for integration of EMSC into state and local EMS systems.

- Model EMSC legislation. Many states have enacted EMSC bills to mandate and help fund EMSC within state EMS agencies. The American Academy of Pediatrics (AAP) has a template for EMSC legislation that can be easily modified for individual states (website: www.aap.org).

- A national standard curriculum (NSC) for emergency medical technician (EMT) basics, and most recently for EMT paramedics and EMT intermediates, sponsored by NHTSA and the

Maternal and Child Health Bureau (MCHB). These curricula outline comprehensive educational objectives for prehospital professionals (website: www.nhtsa.dot.gov/people/injury/ems).

EMSC IN STATE EMS SYSTEMS

One mechanism for highlighting EMSC within state EMS systems is through the ongoing NHTSA program for EMS system assessments. This standardized evaluation process provides an excellent opportunity for states to review their current EMSC capabilities and to plan and implement improvements. To encourage the expanded scope of inquiry into children and family issues, the EMSC program and NHTSA jointly developed a pediatric survey to facilitate review of children's issues (Appendix 1). The survey, a brief inventory of currently available products and services, focuses on statewide EMSC programs and activities.

EPIDEMIOLOGY

Studies of acute pediatric illnesses and injuries show that injuries account for half of pediatric ambulance transports and illnesses account for the other half (Table 120-1). A significant number of injuries are related to

Table 120-1. Epidemiology of Pediatric Illnesses and Injuries for ambulance transports

Injuries	Illnesses
Mechanism	*CNS*
Automobile incidents	Seizures
Occupant	Altered level of consciousness
Pedestrian	*Respiratory*
Bicyclist	Wheezing
Falls	Choking
Burns	Apnea
Frequency of	*Metabolic/toxic*
anatomic areas	Ingestions
of injury	Fever
Head	*Gastrointestinal*
Limbs/pelvis	Abdominal pain
Back	Vomiting
Chest	
Abdomen	

motor vehicle incidents. Important injury subtypes are occupant, pedestrian, and bicycle-versus-automobile events. Blunt injuries predominate and blunt trauma deaths continue to remain high in rural areas. Frequent prehospital illness problems include respiratory distress, seizures, and poisoning.

The leading causes of childhood death are both age- and geography-related. In some states, fires and burns are the leading causes of death in children <5 years of age. In other states motor vehicle incidents are the leading cause, and in some Sun Belt states, drowning is first. In rural areas motor vehicle incidents are the leading cause of death, but homicide and suicide are more common for urban males.

Important subpopulations of transported children include children with special health care needs (CSHCN) and psychiatric patients. Children with special health care needs are a diverse group of patients who frequently need out-of-hospital emergency assessment and treatment. This high-use group includes children with ongoing physical, developmental, or learning disabilities, and children with chronic medical conditions. Technology-assisted children are a subgroup of CSHCN who depend on medical devices for their survival. The American College of Emergency Physicians (ACEP) and the AAP have recently published an Emergency Information Form for CSHCN (Fig. 120-2). The form is intended for voluntary use by patients and families to facilitate prehospital and ED evaluation.

Identification and referral of children requiring specialized psychiatric services remains a vexing problem for EMSC personnel. Lack of funding and access are the principal problems.

PHYSICIAN AND EMS LEADERSHIP

Emergency physicians, pediatricians, and EMS experts have provided essential EMSC leadership. In 1991, the American Board of Emergency Medicine and the American Board of Pediatrics jointly created the pediatric emergency medicine board examination and formally established the subspecialty. Specialists in pediatric emergency medicine have driven much improvement in the organization and technology of EMSC, and in scientific understanding of the prevention, causes, pathophysiology, and management of critical illness and injury.

Pediatric life support programs for emergency physicians, pediatricians, nurses, and prehospital care providers have helped codify fundamental approaches to emergency pediatric care. National courses include the

Emergency Information Form for Children With Special Needs

		Date form completed By Whom	Revised	Initials
▦ American College of Emergency Physicians®	American Academy of Pediatrics		Revised	Initials

Name:	Birth date: Nickname:
Home Address:	Home/Work Phone:
Parent/Guardian:	Emergency Contact Names & Relationship:
Signature/Consent*:	
Primary Language:	Phone Number(s):

Physicians:

Primary Care Physician:	Emergency Phone:
	Fax:
Current Specialty Physician: Specialty:	Emergency Phone:
	Fax:
Current Specialty Physician: Specialty:	Emergency Phone:
	Fax:
Anticipated Primary ED:	Pharmacy:
Anticipated Tertiary Care Center:	

Diagnoses/Past Procedures/Physical Exam:

1. _____

Baseline physical findings: _____

2. _____

3. _____

Baseline vital signs: _____

4. _____

Synopsis:

Baseline neurological status: _____

*Consent for release of this form to health care providers

Fig. 120-1. The emergency information form for children with special needs.

Diagnoses/Past Procedures/Physical Exam continued:

Medications:

Significant baseline ancillary findings (lab, x-ray, ECG):

1.

2.

3.

4. Prostheses/Appliances/Advanced Technology Devices:

5.

6.

Management Data:

Allergies: Medications/Foods to be avoided   **and why:**

1.

2.

3.

Procedures to be avoided   **and why:**

1.

2.

3.

Immunizations

Dates						Dates					
DPT						Hep B					
OPV						Varicella					
MMR						TB status					
HIB						Other					

Antibiotic prophylaxis: Indication: Medication and dose:

Common Presenting Problems/Findings With Specific Suggested Managements

Problem   Suggested Diagnostic Studies   Treatment Considerations

Comments on child, family, or other specific medical issues:

Physician/Provider Signature: **Print Name:**

Advanced Pediatric Life Support: The Pediatric Emergency Medicine Course (APLS), sponsored by the American College of Emergency Physicians (ACEP) and American Academy of Pediatrics (AAP); the Pediatric Advanced Life Support (PALS) Course, sponsored by the American Heart Association and AAP; the Emergency Nurses Pediatric Course (ENPC), sponsored by the Emergency Nurses Association; and most recently the Pediatric Education for Prehospital Professionals (PEPP) Course, sponsored by the AAP.

CLINICAL COMPONENTS OF EMS-EMSC

Prevention

Pediatric emergency medicine specialists, emergency physicians, pediatricians, nurses, prehospital professionals, EMS experts, and others involved in the care of children have brought attention to reduction of injury and serious illness in children. Prehospital professionals have an important community role in prevention. They are frequently the first ones to identify a trend of injuries or illnesses. For example, recognition of an association of prone sleeping position and sudden infant death syndrome (SIDS) by prehospital professionals helped establish the successful public health program on SIDS prevention. Prehospital professionals are in an ideal position to identify the dangers to children in the community and the needs for preventive action. They can have a major impact on implementation of prevention programs by educating the public, and collaborating with legislative and regulatory officials.

Prehospital professionals, emergency nurses, and physicians have participated as educators and advocates in many injury and illness prevention programs and community strategies for patients and families (Table 120-2).

Pediatric Equipment

Prehospital professionals require special pediatric equipment and supplies for BLS and ALS ambulances (Tables 120-3 and 120-4). Equipment and supplies must be log-

Table 120-2. Examples of Common Injuries and Possible Prevention Strategies

Vehicle Trauma	Infant and child restraint seats
	Seat belts and air bags
	Pedestrian safety programs
	Motorcycle helmets
Cycling	Bicycle helmets
	Bicycle paths separate from motor vehicle traffic
Recreation	Appropriate safety padding and apparel
	Cyclist/skateboard/skater safety programs
	Soft, energy-absorbent playground surfaces
Drowning	Four-sided locked pool enclosures
	Pool alarms
	Immediate adult supervision
	Caretaker CPR training
	Swimming lessons
	Pool/beach safety instruction
	Personal flotation device
Poisoning and Household	Proper storage of chemicals and medications
	Child safety packaging
Burns	Proper maintenance and monitoring of electrical appliances and cords
	Fire/smoke detectors
	Proper placement of cookware on stovetop
Other	Discouragement of infant walker use
	Gated stairways
	Baby-sitter first aid training
	Child care worker first aid training

Table 120-3. Pediatric Basic Life Support Ambulance Equipment, Medications, and Supplies

1. Oropharyngeal airways: infant, child
2. Bag-valve resuscitator, child reservoir[a]
3. Clear masks for resuscitator: infant, child, adult
4. Nasal cannulas: child and adult sizes
5. Oxygen masks: child, adult
6. Blood pressure cuffs: infant, child, adult
7. Backboard
8. Cervical immobilization device[b]
9. Extremity splints
10. Burn dressings[c]
11. Sterile scissors or equivalent umbilical cord cutting device[d]
12. Thermal blanket
13. Portable suction unit[e]
14. Suction catheters: infant, child, adult
15. Tonsil suction tip
16. Bulb syringe
17. Obstetric pack
18. Car seat

[a]Ventilation bags used for resuscitation should be self-refilling without a pop-off valve. The child and adult bags are suitable for supporting adequate tidal volumes for the entire pediatric age range. A child bag is defined as one that has at least a 450-mL reservoir. An adult bag has at least a 1-L reservoir.
[b]A cervical immobilization device should be a soft device that can immobilize the neck of an infant, child, or adult. It may be towel rolls or a commercially available neck-cradling device. Cervical immobilization of a small infant can be achieved by use of towel rolls and tape rather than a cervical collar or sandbags. (Infants may need support under the shoulders to keep a neutral spine position.)
[c]Burn dressings may include commercially available packs and/or clean sheets and dressings.
[d]Sterile scissors or equivalent devices are for cutting the umbilical cord during childbirth and may be stocked separate from the obstetrical pack carried by the EMS provider to assure sterility.
[e]This may include a motorized suction device or a hand-driven device.

ically organized, routinely checked, and readily available. Unfortunately, many types of pediatric equipment, especially splints and backboards, are uncomfortable, overly rigid, or inflexibly sized for children and there is much opportunity for future innovation in pediatric product development.

Prehospital Treatment and Transportation

Safe and efficacious field treatment includes development and implementation of pediatric triage, transport, and treatment protocols. In some systems, the organization of pediatric emergency care, critical care, and trauma care includes protocols for bypass, for air transport, to direct the utilization of regional referral centers, and for air medical services.

Treatment policies or protocols are fundamental to pediatric prehospital care. Recently, the National Association of EMS Physicians developed pediatric field treatment protocols for prehospital professionals. They are available on-line (www.naemsp.org).

Emergency Departments

Emergency departments are key sources of children's emergency care. Often, caregivers take children directly to community EDs rather than to specialized pediatric centers (e.g., pediatric trauma centers, pediatric critical care centers). Managed care plans may also direct families to contracted community hospitals rather than to specialized pediatric centers. Automobile transport is especially common if the problem is acute illness rather than injury. Hence it is imperative that all hospital EDs in every community have the appropriate equipment, staff, and policies to provide appropriate care for children (Tables 120-5a, b).

Appendix 2 presents preparedness requirements for community EDs that provide children's emergency, trauma, and critical care. These are *minimum* voluntary requirements, published in 2001, and endorsed by ACEP, AAP, and a multidisciplinary task force sponsored by the federal EMSC Program. The guidelines outline necessary resources for children's emergency care in all EDs, and address stabilization and timely transfer of selected patients to specialized pediatric centers.

Specialized Pediatric Centers

Because of geographic distances, community size differences, and variable capabilities for treating children, sharing of specialized resources for children is essential to local and regional EMS systems. There are different schemes for facility selection (categorization, accreditation, and designation) of specialized pediatric hospitals for trauma, critical care, neonatology, and psychiatry. Several states such as California have spelled out specific facility requirements for neonatal, pediatric trauma, and pediatric critical care centers. While specialized centers are frequently children's hospitals, general hospitals may also provide such services. Some local EMS systems have a two-tiered plan for children, involving identification of hospitals with minimal ED capabilities and hospitals with specialized pediatric capabilities.

Table 120-4. Pediatric Advanced Life Support Ambulance Equipment, Medications, and Supplies

ALS units should have all the equipment listed on the BLS list plus the following additional items:

1. Monitor defibrillator[b]
2.[a] Laryngoscope with straight blades 0 through 4 and curved blades 2, 3, and 4
3.[a] Pediatric and adult size stylets for endotracheal tubes
4.[a] A pediatric Magill forceps
5.[a] Endotracheal tubes: uncuffed sizes 2.5 through 6.0 and cuffed 6.0 through 8.0
6. Arm boards: infant, child
7. Intravenous catheters 14–24 gauge
8. Microdrip and macrodrip IV devices[c]
9.[a] Intraosseous needles
10. Drug dose chart or tape[d]

[a]These items are required only if the skill to use them is part of the scope of practice of the local EMS providers.
[b]All defibrillators should be able to deliver 5 to 400 J. The addition of pediatric paddles may give the responding unit enhanced capabilities, but they may not be essential for units that rarely use this equipment. The defibrillator may be equipped with only adult paddles/pads or pediatric and adult paddles/pads. Units carrying only adult paddles/pads should ensure that providers are trained in the proper use of adult paddles in infants and children. When the defibrillator cannot deliver lower power, shock at lowest possible energy level.
[c]These may include burettes, microdrip tubing, or in-line volume controllers.
[d]This may include charts giving the drug doses in milliliters or milligrams per kilogram, with precalculated doses based on weight, or a tape that determines the proper dose based on the length of the patient.

Rehabilitation

Rehabilitation services for children are still poorly organized within EMS systems and represent an important area for future growth and development. However, these are crucial services for selected patients who sustain critical illnesses and injuries. Systematic identification of suitable rehabilitation services and facilities and implementation of referral procedures are key elements in the EMS-EMSC continuum.

OPERATIONAL COMPONENTS OF EMS-EMSC

EMS System

Development and maintenance of strong EMSC requires permanent state EMSC leadership within the state EMS system. Establishment of a state EMSC office may be legislated or implemented by state EMS regulation. EMSC advisory bodies and ongoing funding of state EMSC activities are important elements for oversight of children's services.

Medical Direction

Effective medical direction includes review and modification of treatment *and* nontreatment policies, proce-

dures, and protocols for children. Medical direction entails both real time on-line (direct) elements, as well as off-line (indirect) elements. On-line issues may include questions about treatment, field triage (Table 120-6), scene control, transport, destination, transport refusals, and consent.

Off-line medical direction includes prospective and retrospective components. Prospective medical direction includes development of treatment protocols, transport policies, procedural policies (e.g., intraosseous infusions, endotracheal intubation), destination policies, personnel education, data collection, and quality improvement programs. Retrospective components include reviews of run sheets, focused audits, and analyses of nontransport cases, deaths, and any unusual occurrences or untoward events, as well as medicolegal problems. Pediatricians are important collaborators in the off-line development and implementation of pediatric prehospital policies, procedures, and protocols.

Communications

The role of medical dispatchers in pediatric prehospital care has only recently been evaluated. Unfortunately, current training of dispatchers is highly variable. In advanced EMS systems, dispatchers may have an extensive role in prearrival instructions to scene bystanders and appropriate prioritization of vehicle dispatch. Dispatch-

Table 120-5a. Pediatric Medications for Emergency Departments

Resuscitation Medications	Other Drug Groups
Atropine	Activated charcoal
Adenosine	Analgesics
Calcium chloride	Antibiotics (parenteral)
Dextrose	Anticonvulsants
Epinephrine (1:1000, 1:10000)	Antidotes (common antidotes should be available), prostaglandin E_1[a]
Lidocaine	Antipyretics
Naloxone hydrochloride	Bronchodilators
Sodium bicarbonate (4.2%)	Corticosteroids
	Inotropic agents
	Neuromuscular blocking agents
	Oxygen
	Sedatives

[a] For less frequently used antidotes and medications, a procedure for obtaining them should be in place.

Source: Adapted from Committee on Pediatric Equipment and Supplies for Emergency Departments, National Emergency Medical Services for Children Resource Alliance: Guidelines for pediatric equipment and supplies for emergency departments. *Ann Emerg Med.* 31:54-57, 1998.

ers require special education in pediatric emergency care to appropriately evaluate calls for seriously injured or ill children. Some systems have documented dramatic successes where medical dispatchers have coached parents or bystanders through difficult circumstances, such as rescue breathing and chest compressions to a child in cardiopulmonary arrest.

Primary physicians must understand how to access emergency care in the community, how to provide emergency care in their offices, and how to educate their patients and families on the appropriate access to and utilization of 911. Some communities do not have a universal access 911 system, while others utilize a standard 911 system that only allows the dispatcher to ring back to that number. Many cities have now moved to enhanced 911, which allows the dispatcher to see the address and access other pertinent information about the location of the caller.

Education

Education of prehospital professionals is essential for optimal pediatric prehospital care. Both BLS and ALS services require unique pediatric adaptations to teach knowledge and skills. Because skills decay is rapid, continuing education is also essential to maintaining preparedness. Over the past several years, emphasis in EMT education has shifted from the diagnosis of disease to an assessment-based teaching format that includes cognitive, psychomotor, and attitudinal skills. Provision of supervised clinical time for practicing assessment skills with children is often especially useful. Appropriate clinical settings are EDs, pediatric wards, outpatient clinics, health departments, and pediatric offices.

The PEPP course was recently developed through a national consensus process orchestrated by the AAP. The course is a 2-day interactive, assessment-oriented, case-based continuing education program in pediatrics with both BLS and ALS versions that are fully consistent with the NSC curricula. The new PEPP has a 2000 PEPP textbook, a 2001 PEPP resource manual, a PEPP videotape, and a slide set on CD-ROM. The PEPP course has a website (www.PEPPsite.com) which allows ongoing on-line education and communication between the AAP, the national steering committee, and EMS professionals.

Data and Information Management

Information management and continuous quality improvement are important components of the EMS-EMSC continuum. This involves monitoring, evaluating, and modifying the education, patient care, and regional care protocols based on patient outcome. Information management mechanisms must identify not only performance problems, but also system deficiencies that affect children and families.

For EDs, clinical indicators are useful to evaluate the triage system and the care of the critically ill and injured

Table 120-5b. Pediatric Equipment and Supplies for Emergency Departments

Monitoring Equipment
- Cardiorespiratory monitor with strip recorder
- Defibrillator with pediatric and adult paddles (4.5 cm and 8 cm) or corresponding adhesive pads
- Pediatric and adult monitor electrodes
- Pulse oximeter with sensors and probe sizes for children
- Thermometer or rectal probe[a]
- Sphygmomanometer
- Doppler blood pressure device
- Blood pressure cuffs (neonatal, infant, child, and adult arm and thigh cuffs)
- Method to monitor endotracheal tube and placement[b]
- Stethoscope

Airway Management
- Portable oxygen regulators and canisters
- Clear oxygen masks (standard and nonrebreathing: neonatal, infant, child, and adult)
- Oropharyngeal airways (sizes 0–5)
- Nasopharyngeal airways (12F through 30F)
- Bag-valve-mask resuscitator, self-inflating (450 and 1000 mL sizes)
- Nasal cannulas (child and adult)
- Endotracheal tubes: uncuffed (2.5, 3.0, 3.5, 4.0, 4.5, 5.0, 5.5, and 6.0 mm) and cuffed (6.5, 7.0, 7.5, 8.0, and 9.0 mm)
- Stylets (infant, pediatric, and adult)
- Laryngoscope handle (pediatric and adult)
- Laryngoscope blades: straight or Miller (0, 1, 2, and 3) and Macintosh (2 and 3)
- Magill forceps (pediatric and adult)
- Nasogastric/feeding tubes (5F through 18F)
- Suction catheters: flexible (6F, 8F, 10F, 12F, 14F, and 16F)
- Yankauer suction tip
- Bulb syringe
- Chest tubes (8F through 40F)[c]
- Laryngeal mask airway (sizes 1, 1.5, 2, 2.5, 3, 4, and 5)

Vascular Access
- Butterfly needles (19–25 gauge)
- Catheter-over-needle devices (14–24 gauge)
- Rate limiting infusion device and tubing
- Intraosseous needles (may be satisfied by standard bone needle aspiration needles)
- Arm board
- Intravenous fluid and blood warmers[c]
- Umbilical vein catheters[c,e] (size 5F feeding tube may be used)
- Seldinger technique vascular access kit[c]

Miscellaneous
- Infant and standard scales
- Infant formula and oral rehydrating solutions[c]
- Heating source (may be met by infrared lamps or overhead warmer)[c]
- Towel rolls, blanket rolls, or equivalent
- Pediatric restraining devices
- Resuscitation board
- Sterile linen[f]
- Length-based resuscitation tape or precalculated drug or equipment list based on weight

(Continues)

Table 120-5b *(continued)*. Pediatric Equipment and Supplies for Emergency Departments

Specialized Pediatric Trays
- Tube thoracotomy with water seal drainage capability[b]
- Lumbar puncture
- Pediatric urinary catheters
- Obstetric pack
- Newborn kit[c]
- Umbilical vessel cannulation supplies[c]
- Venous cutdown[c]
- Needle cricothyrotomy tray
- Surgical airway kit (may include a tracheostomy tray or a surgical cricothyrotomy tray)[c]

Fracture Management
Cervical immobilization equipment[g]
Extremity splints[c]
Femur splints[c]

Medical Photography Capability

[a]Suitable for hypothermic and hyperthermic measurements with temperature capability from 25°C to 44°C.
[b]May be satisfied by a disposable CO_2 detector of appropriate size for infants and children. For children 5 years or older who are ≥20 kg in body weight, an esophageal detection bulb or syringe may be used additionally.
[c]Equipment that is essential but may be shared with the nursery, pediatric ward, or other inpatient service and is readily available to the ED.
[d]To regulate rate and volume.
[e]Ensure availability of pediatric sizes within the hospital.
[f]Available within hospital for burn care.
[g]Many types of cervical immobilization devices are available, including wedges and collars. The type of device chosen depends on local preferences and policies and procedures. Chosen device should be stocked in sizes to fit infants, children, adolescents, and adults. Use of sandbags to meet this requirement is discouraged, because they may cause injury if the patient has to be turned.

Source: Adapted from Committee on Pediatric Equipment and Supplies for Emergency Departments, National Emergency Medical Services for Children Resource Alliance: Guidelines for pediatric equipment and supplies for emergency departments. *Ann Emerg Med.* 31:54-57, 1998.

child. Continuous quality improvement requires selecting new targets to demonstrate improved quality of care and improved outcomes over time. Coding of external cause of injury (E-coding) will facilitate a better understanding of the cause of injury in the community and allow development of appropriate injury prevention programs.

Table 120-6. Examples of Field Treatment Protocols

Respiratory distress and failure
Airway obstruction
Bradycardia and tachycardia
Cardiopulmonary arrest
Trauma
Child maltreatment
Seizures
Toxic ingestions and exposures
Altered mental status and seizures
Newborn care

Public Information and Education

Public education is vital to the success of EMSC. While much of the public has a perception of EMS that is based on media stories and television programs, many caregivers still do not know how to use EMS. Many injured or seriously ill children still end up being transported to EDs by private vehicles. And many primary physicians do not know the procedures for accessing prehospital care for their patients or the capabilities of the system in their community. In a recent survey of 100 parents whose children attend day care, 66 percent stated that their private physician did not explain the EMS system to them.

Research

There are many opportunities for clinical pediatric research in the prehospital setting, but there are also significant difficulties. The setting is uncontrolled and many prehospital professionals are not motivated to participate. Also, prehospital databases are frequently inadequate and not easily linked to patient outcome information. Yet the prehospital setting offers a vast clinical laboratory for pediatric research and will in the future provide answers to critical unanswered questions. Physician leadership and funding are important features of productive EMSC research.

APPENDIX 1: PEDIATRIC SURVEY FOR STATEWIDE EMS SYSTEM REASSESSMENTS

A. Regulation and policy

1. Does your state have specific EMSC legislation?
2. Do you believe EMSC legislation is warranted?
3. Does the legislation provide for additional EMS funding for EMSC?
4. Has the legislation resulted in any measurable changes?
5. If your state does not have an EMSC bill, are you working on preparing such legislation?
6. Does your state have a permanent EMSC, or pediatric advisory committee or task force?
7. How are the EMSC advisory committee members selected?
8. If your state does not have an EMSC advisory committee, is there representation by a pediatric expert on your EMS advisory committee?

B. Resource management

1. Does your state have an EMS plan?
2. Does your state's EMS plan specifically address pediatrics?
3. If not, is there a separate state EMSC plan?
4. Does your state have an EMS administrator specifically assigned to EMSC? What percentage of his or her time is dedicated to EMSC?
5. What models or templates, if any, does your state use for planning, implementing, and evaluating EMSC standards, guidelines, and recommendations?

C. Human resources and training

1. Do you use the recommended pediatric content in the NHTSA-MCHB basic national standard curriculum (NSC) for EMT-B education?
2. If not, what curriculum is used? How many hours of pediatric education are required for EMT-Bs?
3. Do you intend to use the recommended pediatric content in the NHTSA-MCHB intermediate and advanced NSC for EMT-Is and EMT-Ps? If not, what curriculum will be used?

4. How many hours of pediatric education are required for EMT-Is and EMT-Ps?
5. How many hours, if any, of pediatric education are required for other out-of-hospital providers as part of their primary training curriculum for initial certification/licensure?
6. What curricula are used?
   a. Dispatchers
   b. First responders
   c. Mobile intensive care nurses
7. Does your state require pediatric continuing education (CE) courses for out-of-hospital providers? How many hours per year for each provider group? If not, how does your state assure that CE addresses children?
8. Does your state recommend or require any special pediatric life support course for either initial out-of-hospital provider education or CE [e.g., the Pediatric Education for Prehospital Professionals (PEPP) Course, the California Pediatric Airway Project, or PALS]?

D. Transportation

1. Do your BLS units have pediatric equipment which meets guidelines published in *Prehospital Emergency Care,* Vol. 1, No. 4, October 1997?
2. Do your ALS units have pediatric equipment which meets guidelines published in *Prehospital Emergency Care,* Vol. 1, No. 4, October 1997?

E. Facilities

1. Does your state have standards, guidelines, or recommendations for emergency department preparedness in pediatrics?
2. Is there a recommended system for categorization or selection of different levels of pediatric facilities?
3. Are pediatric capabilities of emergency departments in any of your local EMS systems verified, monitored, or evaluated? How?
4. Does your state have standards, guidelines, or recommendations for pediatric medical and trauma field triage protocols?
5. Does your state have standards, guidelines, or recommendations for interfacility consultation and/or secondary transfer of children to higher level centers?
6. Does your state have standards, guidelines, or recommendations for pediatric interfacility transport providers?
7. Does your state have standards, guidelines, or

recommendations, for pediatric critical care centers?

8. Does your state have standards, guidelines, or recommendations for pediatric rehabilitation?

9. Are there any standards, guidelines, or recommendations for transfer to or designation of pediatric rehabilitation facility(s) for your state?

F. Communication

1. Does your state recommend or have template examples of pediatric dispatch protocols?

2. If not, are there specific pediatric considerations within general dispatch protocols?

G. Public information, education, and prevention

1. Does your state recommend or require out-of-hospital providers to have specific education in childhood illness and injury prevention?

H. Medical direction

1. Does your state recommend or have template examples of out-of-hospital BLS and ALS pediatric field treatment protocols for use by local EMS agencies and providers? Which ones?

2. Does your state recommend or have template examples of out-of-hospital pediatric policies and procedures (e.g., consent, suspected abuse and neglect) for use by local EMS agencies and providers? Which ones?

3. Does your state allow or mandate the following out-of-hospital pediatric ALS field skills?
   a. Endotracheal intubation
   b. Administration of paralytic agents to facilitate endotracheal intubation
   c. Intraosseous infusion
   d. Rectal diazepam
   e. Needle thoracostomy

4. Is there a mechanism for concurrent and retrospective review of out-of-hospital pediatric care?

I. Trauma systems

1. Does your state have standards, guidelines, or recommendations for pediatric trauma centers or other designated pediatric trauma care facilities?

2. Does your state have standards, guidelines, or recommendations for pediatric trauma care within general trauma centers?

J. Evaluation

1. Does your state have an EMS data collection system that allows assessment of pediatric care by numbers, types of problems, field interventions, and ED outcomes?

2. Is there a specific pediatric component to your state's EMS quality improvement plan?

APPENDIX 2: PEDIATRIC PREPAREDNESS FOR COMMUNITY HOSPITAL EMERGENCY DEPARTMENTS

I. Guidelines for Administration and Coordination of the ED for the Care of Children

A. Physician Coordinator for Pediatric Emergency Medicine is appointed by the ED Medical Director

1. The Physician Coordinator has the following qualifications:

   a. The Physician Coordinator meets the qualifications for credentialing by the hospital as a specialist in emergency medicine, pediatric emergency medicine, or pediatrics.

   b. The Physician Coordinator has special interest, knowledge, and skill in emergency medical care of children as demonstrated by training, clinical experience, or focused continuing medical education.

   c. The Physician Coordinator may be a staff physician who is currently assigned other roles in the ED, such as the Medical Director of the ED, or may be shared through formal consultation agreements with professional resources from a hospital capable of providing definitive pediatric care.

2. The Physician Coordinator is responsible for the following:

   a. Assure adequate skill and knowledge of staff physicians in emergency care and resuscitation of infants and children.

   b. Oversee ED pediatric quality improvement (QI), performance improvement (PI), and clinical care protocols.

   c. Assist with development and periodic review of ED medications, equipment, supplies, policies, and procedures.

   d. Serve as liaison to appropriate in-hospital and out-of-hospital pediatric care committees in the community (if they exist).

   e. Serve as liaison to a definitive care hospital including a regional pediatric referral hospital and trauma center, EMS agencies, primary care providers, health insurers, and any other medical resources needed to integrate services for the continuum of care of the patient.

   f. Facilitate pediatric emergency education for ED health care providers and out-of-hospital providers affiliated with the ED.

B. A Nursing Coordinator for Pediatric Emergency Care is appointed.
1. The Nursing Coordinator has the following qualifications: The Nursing Coordinator demonstrates special interest, knowledge, and skill in emergency care and resuscitation of infants and children as demonstrated by training, clinical experience, or focused continuing nursing education.
2. The Nursing Coordinator is responsible for the following:
   a. Coordinate pediatric QI, PI, and clinical care protocols with the Physician Coordinator.
   b. Serve as liaison to appropriate in-hospital and out-of-hospital pediatric care committees.
   c. Serve as liaison to inpatient nursing as well as to a definitive care hospital, a regional pediatric referral hospital and trauma center, EMS agencies, primary care providers, health insurers, and any other medical resources needed to integrate services for the continuum of care of the patient.
   d. Facilitate ED nursing continuing education in pediatrics and provide orientation for new staff members.
   e. Provide assistance and support for pediatric education of out-of-hospital providers affiliated with the ED.
   f. Assist in development and periodic review of policies and procedures for pediatric care.
   g. Stock and monitor pediatric equipment and medication availability.

II. Guidelines for Physicians and Other Practitioners Staffing the ED

A. Physicians staffing the ED have the necessary skill, knowledge, and training to provide emergency evaluation and treatment of children of all ages who may be brought to the ED, consistent with the services provided by the hospital.
B. Nurses and other practitioners have the necessary skill, knowledge, and training to provide nursing care to children of all ages who may be brought to the ED, consistent with the services offered by the hospital.
C. Competency evaluations completed by the staff are age specific and include neonates, infants, children, and adolescents.

III. Quality Improvement Guidelines for the ED

A pediatric patient review process is integrated into the emergency department QI plan according to the following guidelines:
A. Components of the process interface with out-of-hospital, ED, trauma, inpatient pediatrics, pediatric critical care, and hospital-wide QI or PI activities.
B. Minimum components of the process include identifying indicators of good outcome, collecting and analyzing data to discover variances, defining a plan for improvement, and evaluating or measuring the success of the QI or PI process.
C. A clearly defined mechanism exists to monitor professional education and staffing.

IV. Guidelines for Policies, Procedures, and Protocols for the ED

A. Policies, procedures, and protocols for emergency care of children are developed and implemented, staff members should be educated accordingly, and they should be monitored for compliance and periodically updated. These should include, but are not limited to, the following (numbers 3 through 12 indicate policies, procedures, and protocols that may be integrated into ED policies and procedures with pediatric-specific components):
1. Child maltreatment (physical and sexual abuse, sexual assault, and neglect)
2. Consent (including situations in which a parent is not immediately available)
3. Death in the ED
4. Do not resuscitate (DNR) orders
5. Illness and injury triage
6. Sedation and analgesia
7. Immunization status
8. Mental health emergencies
9. Physical or chemical restraint of patients
10. Family issues, including
    a. Education of the patient, family, and regular caregivers
    b. Discharge planning and instruction
    c. Family presence during care
11. Communication with patient's primary health care provider
12. Transfers necessary for definitive care, according to the following guidelines:
    a. Transfer policies or procedures should include access to consultation (telephone or

telemedicine), transfer guidelines, interfacility transfer agreements, and a plan for return of the child back to his or her community as appropriate.

b. Transferring facility must ensure that the patient is stabilized before transport.

c. Transferring facility must transfer only patients who need a higher level of care, as per the Emergency Medical Treatment and Active Labor Act.

B. Hospitals may wish to adopt currently available clinical guidelines and protocols or develop their own.

V. Guidelines for Support Services for the ED

A. A transport plan is in place to deliver children safely and in a timely manner to the appropriate facility capable of providing definitive care. The following pediatric specialty referral resources are incorporated into the transport plan:
   1. Medical and surgical intensive care
   2. Trauma
   3. Reimplantation (replacement of severed digits or limbs)
   4. Burns
   5. Psychiatric emergencies
   6. Perinatal emergencies
   7. Child maltreatment (physical and sexual abuse and assault)

B. Radiology department has the skills and capability to provide imaging studies of children and has the equipment necessary to do so. The radiology capability of hospitals may vary from one institution to another; however, the radiology capability of a hospital must meet the needs of the children in the community it serves.

C. Laboratory has the skills and capability to perform laboratory tests for children of all ages, including obtaining samples, and has the availability of micro technique for small or limited sample size. The clinical laboratory capability must meet the needs of the children in the community it serves.

VI. Guidelines for Equipment, Supplies, and Medications for Children in the ED

A. Necessary medications, equipment, and supplies are listed in Tables 120-5a and 120-5b. Each hospital must develop a method for storage and provide accessibility of medications and equipment for children.

The method used must ensure that the health care practitioner can easily identify appropriate dosages of medication based on the patient's weight and choose appropriately sized equipment. Length-based systems or precalculated drug systems should be used to avoid calculation errors for medications delivered.

B. All equipment and supplies are listed in Table 120-5b and include age-appropriate and size-appropriate equipment for use for children of all ages and sizes from premature infants through adolescents.

C. Quality indicators ensure regular periodic review of drugs and equipment, monitoring of expiration dates of items, and replacement of used items.

BIBLIOGRAPHY

American Academy of Pediatrics, Committee on Pediatric Emergency Medicine: Guidelines for pediatric emergency care facilities. *Pediatrics* 96:526–537, 1995.

American Academy of Pediatrics, Committee on Pediatric Emergency Medicine, and American College of Emergency Physicians, Pediatric Committee: Care of children in the emergency department: Guidelines for preparedness: *Ann of Emerg Med* 37:423–427, 2001.

American College of Emergency Physicians: Emergency care guidelines. *Ann Emerg Med* 29:564–571, 1997.

Committee on Pediatric Equipment and Supplies for Emergency Departments, National Emergency Medical Services for Children Resource Alliance: Guidelines for pediatric equipment and supplies for emergency departments. *Ann Emerg Med* 31:54–57, 1998.

Dieckmann R, Brownstein D, Gausche-Hill M, American Academy of Pediatrics: *Textbook of Pediatric Education for Prehospital Professionals.* Sudbury, MA: Jones & Bartlett, 2000.

Foltin G, Tunik M, Cooper A, et al: *Teaching Resources for Instructors in Prehospital Pediatrics,* Version 2.0. New York: Center for Pediatric Emergency Medicine, 1998.

Gausche-Hill M, Brownstein D, Dieckmann R, American Academy of Pediatrics: *Resource Manual for Pediatric Education for Prehospital Professionals.* Sudbury, MA: Jones & Bartlett, 2001.

Institute of Medicine, Committee on Pediatric Emergency Medical Services: Durch JS, Lohr KN (eds): *Institute of Medicine Report: Emergency Medical Services for Children.* Washington, DC: National Academy Press, 1993.

National Emergency Medical Services for Children Resource Alliance, Committee on Pediatric Equipment and Supplies for Emergency: Guidelines for pediatric equipment and supplies for emergency departments. *Ann Emerg Med* 31:54–57, 1998.

U.S. Health Resources and Services Administration, Maternal and Child Health Bureau: *Five-Year Plan: Midcourse Review: Emergency Medical Services for Children, 1995-2000.* Washington, DC: Emergency Medical Services for Children, National Resource Center, 1997.

121

Interfacility Transport

Ira J. Blumen
Howard Rodenberg
Thomas J. Abramo

HIGH-YIELD FACTS

- Definitive management of some disease processes should be begun prior to transport. Especially when transport times are prolonged, early initiation of therapy can have a profound effect on outcome.
- The Emergency Medical Treatment and Labor Act (EMTALA) states that the referring hospital must examine, treat, and stabilize the patient with an emergency medical condition to the limits of its ability before transfer.
- A requirement of EMTALA is that hospitals with specialized facilities shall not refuse to accept appropriate transfers if they have the capacity to treat the individual.
- The condition of the patient, the distance to the receiving hospital, the cost, the availability of alternatives, and the weather all influence the choice of mode of transport.

The development of neonatal and pediatric intensive care units has significantly affected the morbidity and mortality of critically ill patients. Many of these patients are transported miles from one hospital to another, during which time life-saving monitoring and therapy must not be interrupted. The emergency physician must work with the receiving hospital to ensure that the transfer is effected in the safest and most expedient manner. The process of interfacility transport includes stabilizing the patient, identifying the need for transfer, selecting the most appropriate method of transport, communicating the pertinent information to the receiving hospital, and transporting the patient while maintaining appropriate monitoring and therapy.

STABILIZING THE PATIENT

Prior to transfer, a stable airway must be assured. Endotracheal intubation is required if the child is at risk of deteriorating and losing his or her airway en route. A pretransport arterial blood gas is usually needed to assess the adequacy of ventilation and oxygenation. A chest radiograph is useful to check on endotracheal tube placement and to rule out a pneumothorax, which, if present, can be converted into a tension pneumothorax with the use of positive pressure ventilation. If a pneumothorax is diagnosed, a tube thoracostomy is required prior to transport.

Adequate fluids or blood products should be administered to assure perfusion of vital tissues. Ongoing volume loss such as hemorrhage should be controlled prior to transport whenever possible. At times, active internal hemorrhage cannot be dealt with until the transfer is completed. In these cases, massive volume support may be required during transport.

Definitive management of some disease processes should be started prior to transport. For example, antibiotics should be started when infectious processes are involved. Early initiation of therapy can have a profound effect on outcome, especially when transport times are prolonged.

Endotracheal tubes, intravenous lines, and other life-saving equipment should be meticulously secured. Sedation alone or in combination with paralysis may be required to control the patient and to prevent dislodgment of the endotracheal tube, vascular access, Foley catheter, and other equipment.

REFERRING HOSPITAL RESPONSIBILITIES

Transfers are greatly facilitated when specific criteria and transfer agreements have been worked out beforehand. Such agreements should address the special medical services available at potential receiving facilities and admission criteria for each of these services. Transfer agreements with several hospitals may be necessary to cover the various specialty services that may be needed.

The decision to transfer must be in compliance with hospital guidelines and federal regulations laid out in the Consolidated Omnibus Budget Reconciliation Act (COBRA). Within this act is the Emergency Medical Treatment and Labor Act (EMTALA), which states that the referring hospital must examine, treat, and stabilize the patient with an emergency medical condition to the limits of its ability before transfer is considered appropriate.

The referring physician must determine the most appropriate receiving physician and hospital for the patient. A more distant institution may be considered more appropriate than a closer one if the referring institution has a specialized transport team able to perform advanced care during transport. Initial contact with the accepting physician should take place as early in the case as possible. Detailed institution- and patient-specific information must be relayed. Appropriate records and transfer forms that comply with EMTALA regulations must be completed and sent with the patient.

The referring physician should also discuss the rationale for transport with the family and explain the risks and benefits of transfer and the mode of transport to be used. Considerable time may be lost if a transfer is set in motion only to have the family refuse transfer or request a destination other than that selected by the medical team.

RECEIVING FACILITY RESPONSIBILITIES

A requirement of EMTALA is that hospitals with specialized facilities shall not refuse to accept appropriate transfers if they have the capacity to treat the individual. The receiving facility should have appropriate mechanisms in place to assure that referring hospitals can access their capabilities quickly. There should be a phone number available to contact a person at the receiving facility with the judgment, experience, and ability to facilitate the transfer.

The receiving physician may make further recommendations regarding evaluation and management. The receiving physician also should be aware of the availability of hospital resources for management of the case and the current availability of bed space for the patient. She or he should also be familiar with available transport options, and the referring and receiving physicians should agree on the mode of transport, the transport team's composition, and the equipment needed for the transport.

The receiving hospital should provide feedback to the referring institution regarding the condition of the child at the time of transfer, and updates on the child's condition during hospitalization.

MODE OF TRANSPORT

The condition of the patient, the distance to the receiving hospital, the cost, the availability of alternatives, and the weather conditions all influence the choice of mode of transport.

The ground ambulance is the vehicle most commonly used for pediatric and neonatal transport. Its advantages include a relatively large and stable working environment, resistance to most weather-related problems, and the ability to stop if a patient requires further resuscitation. It also provides a relatively quiet environment that allows for auscultation of the patient's chest and permits monitors to be heard. The greatest disadvantage is the time required for long transports.

Helicopters are increasingly used to transport critically ill patients between hospitals. The helicopter can quickly deliver a team and return the patient and team to the receiving hospital. Unfortunately, air travel may be prohibited by weather conditions. Noise and vibrations in helicopters make it difficult to auscultate and to hear monitor alarms. This environment may also have very limited working space and some procedures may be impossible to perform.

Fixed-wing aircraft are generally available and practical only for very long-distance transports. In many cases, the advantages of speed and a better working environment are offset by the dependence on an airport for landing, which then requires an additional vehicle for transport from the airport to the hospital.

According to EMTALA, the transfer must be effected by qualified personnel and requires the use of necessary and medically appropriate life-support measures during the transfer. Whenever possible, the individual needs of the patient should be matched by appropriate transport personnel and equipment. In many situations, however, the composition of the transport team is determined by staff availability and financial considerations. Critical care transport teams are usually composed of one registered nurse and one or more additional crew members, who may be physicians, paramedics, respiratory therapists, or other nurses. While many pediatric interfacility transports can be safely and efficiently handled by regular ambulance personnel, every effort should be made to determine when the assessment and procedural skills of other members of the critical care transport team will be required.

All patient transports require both direct and indirect physician medical control. Unless it is assumed by the accepting specialist or the medical director for the transport service, medical responsibility for the transfer remains with the referring physician until the patient arrives at the receiving facility. While the transferring physician may decrease his or her liability and accountability by consulting with the receiving physician, under

EMTALA the responsibility for appropriate transfer remains with the referring physician and hospital.

BIBLIOGRAPHY

American Academy of Pediatrics and American College of Obstetrics and Gynecology: *Guidelines for Perinatal Care,* 3d ed. Elk Grove Village, IL: American Academy of Pediatrics, 1992; and Washington, DC: American College of Obstetrics and Gynecology, 1992.

American Academy of Pediatrics Task Force on Interhospital Transport: *Guidelines for Air and Ground Transportation of Neonatal and Pediatric Patients.* Elk Grove Village, IL: American Academy of Pediatrics, 1993.

American College of Emergency Physicians: Appropriate interhospital patient transfer policy statement. *Ann Emerg Med* 22:768, 1993.

American College of Surgeons Committee on Trauma: *Hospital and Prehospital Resources for Optimal Care of the Injured Patient.* Chicago: American College of Surgeons, 1986.

Association of Air Medical Services: Position paper on the appropriate use of air medical services. *J Air Med Transport* 9:29–33, 1990.

Bitterman RA (ed): *Providing Emergency Care Under Federal Law: EMTALA.* Dallas: American College of Emergency Physicians, 2001.

Day S, McCloskey K, Orr R, et al: Pediatric interhospital critical care transport: Consensus of a national leadership conference. *Pediatrics* 88:696–704, 1991.

Frew S: *Patient Transfers: How to Comply With the Law.* Dallas: American College of Emergency Physicians, 1991.

McCloskey KA, Orr RA: Pediatric transport issues in emergency medicine. *Emerg Med Clin North Am* 9:475–489, 1991.

Venkataraman ST, Rubenstein JS, Orr RA: Interhospital transport: A pediatric perspective. Transport of the critically ill. *Crit Care Clin* 8(3), 1992.

122

Medicolegal Considerations

Steven Lelyveld

HIGH-YIELD FACTS

- There are two basic legal principles regarding consent in a pediatric emergency department:
  - In whom is ultimate responsibility vested?
  - What are the conditions by which that responsibility is breached?
- A competent adult, when given full information regarding benefits, risks, and alternatives to a proposed treatment, can give or deny consent to treat. For illnesses that are not life- or limb-threatening, a parent or legal guardian must give consent to treat.
- Implied consent to treat becomes operative when two conditions are met:
  - The patient lacks competence to make an independent decision. In the pediatric emergency department, with a few exceptions, this criterion is met by the state's definition of a minor and the lack of presence of a responsible adult.
  - A true emergency exists for which delay in treatment would endanger life or cause permanent disability to the patient.
- The *emancipated minor* may give consent to treat. This person is defined as below the stated statutory age, lives away from parents, is self-supporting and not subject to parental control and, in most states, the adolescent meets these criteria by being married, pregnant, or in the armed forces.

- An increasing number of states recognize a *mature minor*. While not fully emancipated, the adolescent can give consent if between the ages of 14 and 18 years, understands the risks, the physician believes the patient can make an informed decision, and the treatment does not involve serious risk of harm.
- Often, a child will present with an adult who is not a parent or, in the case of divorce, a noncustodial parent. The rules for implied consent apply to serious illness. The consent for less-serious problems should be obtained from the responsible adult "in locum parentis" and, when applicable, the mature minor. An attempt should be made to contact the parent or legal guardian.
- No parent has the right to refuse treatment if such refusal will result in harm to the child. The state's obligation to protect the child supersedes the parent's right to religious expression.
- Malpractice is based on liability stemming from negligence. The plaintiff must prove four things:
  - The physician had a *duty* to the plaintiff, based on a physician-patient relationship.
  - An applicable *standard of care* was violated.
  - An *injury* occurred that is compensable.
  - The violation of the standard of care *caused* the injury.
- The standard of care is defined as what a reasonable physician, with similar training and experience, practicing in a like setting, presented with the same type of patient, would be expected to do. It is not defined as what the best physician with the best resources can do.

- Most potential suits will not occur if patients feel that the physician truly cares about his or her health and is doing his or her best to help. Always explain your actions to those patients who can understand.

CONSENT

There are two basic legal principles regarding consent in a pediatric emergency department:

- In whom is ultimate responsibility vested?
- What are the conditions by which that responsibility is breached?

Although, on the surface, the issue of who can consent to treatment seems simple, there are some very specific legal guidelines that must be followed.

It is first necessary to dispel the myth that an insurance carrier can give or deny consent to treat. In the current health care environment, these contacts are purely for authorization for payment. They should not be used as an excuse to delay treatment of a true emergency.

Consent is either *direct* or *implied*. A competent adult, when given full information regarding benefits, risks, and alternatives to a proposed treatment, can give or deny consent to treat. Implied consent to treat becomes operative when two conditions are met:

- The patient lacks competence to make an independent decision. In the pediatric emergency department, with a few exceptions, this criterion is met by the state's definition of a minor and the lack of presence of a responsible adult.
- A true emergency exists, for which delay in treatment would endanger life or cause permanent disability to the patient.

For illnesses that are not life- or limb-threatening, a parent or legal guardian must give consent to treat. The adolescent, however, may not always present with this adult. The emergency physician must decide when it is appropriate to render care. Although each state has different laws on the subject, a common thread recurs.

The *emancipated minor* may give consent to treat. This person is defined as below the stated statutory age, lives away from parents, is self-supporting, and not subject to parental control. In most states, the adolescent meets these criteria by being married, pregnant, or in the armed forces.

An increasing number of states recognize a *mature minor*. While not fully emancipated, the adolescent can give consent if between the ages of 14 and 18 years, understands the risks, the physician believes the patient can make an informed decision, and the treatment does not involve serious risk of harm. While no suits have been successfully brought against a physician by the parent of such an adolescent, this area of law is in evolution. A number of states are drafting laws aimed at limiting the ability of minors to give medical consent, particularly in the area of reproductive health. The pediatric emergency physician must be familiar with these state and local variations.

Often, a child will present with an adult who is not a parent or, in the case of divorce, a noncustodial parent. The rules for implied consent apply to serious illness. The consent for less-serious problems should be obtained from the responsible adult "in locum parentis" and, when applicable, the mature minor. An attempt should be made to contact the parent or legal guardian. This attempt must be documented in the medical record.

Most states have laws dictating that parental consent need not be obtained for minors in detention facilities or foster homes. Consult your legal department for the state agency responsible for these wards of the state.

No parent has the right to refuse treatment if such refusal will result in harm to the child. The state's obligation to protect the child supersedes the parent's right to religious expression. These principles apply when a guardian refuses care for a victim of suspected child maltreatment. They also apply to those who refuse blood or common life-saving procedures to their child citing religious dictates. In such an instance, protective custody is temporarily taken. In a similar circumstance, unless emancipated, a child also cannot refuse care. In cases without significant threat, however, states are increasingly recognizing the older adolescent's right to privacy. A parent who brings a child for examination after the child has had consensual sex represents the major example of this dilemma. An examination for sexual activity cannot be forced on a reluctant patient.

MALPRACTICE

A major debate on the rights and obligations of patients, physicians, and health maintenance organizations is currently underway in the professional and lay press. There is never a guarantee of good outcome when dealing with human illness. Poor outcome, therefore, is not synonymous with malpractice.

Malpractice is based on liability stemming from negligence. The plaintiff must prove four things:

- The physician had a *duty* to the plaintiff based on a physician-patient relationship.
- An applicable *standard of care* was violated.
- An *injury* occurred that is compensable.
- The violation of the standard of care *caused* the injury.

The physician has a duty to the patient if the patient presents for care and the physician agrees to begin treating. As emergency physicians cannot refuse care, duty to treat is present for all patients presenting to an emergency department.

The standard of care is defined as what a reasonable physician, with similar training and experience, practicing in a like setting, presented with the same type of patient, would be expected to do. It is not defined as what the best physician with the best resources can do. A physician confronted with a patient in a small, local emergency department is not held to the standard of the specialist practicing in a fully equipped major medical center.

A compensable injury is generally permanent and easily preventable. Known complications of disease processes and treatment modalities, when explained to the patient, do not constitute compensable injuries. Injuries that fully resolve are compensable only to the extent of lost income and the patient's health care expenses.

To win in court, the plaintiff has to prove all four components, including the link between the physician's action and the result.

Most potential suits will not occur if patients feel that the physician truly cares about his or her health and is doing his or her best to help. Always explain your actions to those patients who can understand. Get consent to treat, but do not delay life- or limb-saving treatment to meet the demands of paperwork. Recognize that insurance carriers do not have the authority to prevent you from exercising your best judgment. Once care is rendered, carefully document all findings, actions, and communications with the patient or guardian as fully as possible. This aids health care workers who give subsequent treatment, and provides the best legal protection should a maloccurrence or malpractice become apparent months to years later.

BIBLIOGRAPHY

Annas GJ: Scientific evidence in the courtroom. *N Engl J Med* 330:1018, 1994.

Committee on Medical Liability: Guidelines for expert witness testimony in medical liability cases. *Pediatrics* 94:755, 1994.

Garner BA (ed): *Black's Law Dictionary,* 7th ed. St. Paul: West Publishing Company, 1999.

Sigman GS, O'Connor C: Exploration for physicians of the mature minor doctrine. *J Pediatr* 119:520–525, 1991.

Sullivan DJ: Minors and emergency medicine. *Emerg Med Clin North Am* 11:841, 1993.

123

Ethical Considerations

John D. Lantos

HIGH-YIELD FACTS

- In the emergency department (ED), as in other settings where treatment must be provided quickly for patients who may be unstable, standard medical treatment is generally considered to be best for children. If the child is in imminent danger of loss of life or limb, treatment should be provided, even over parental objections.

- Three major changes in the way medicine is practiced led to a reevaluation of the presumption that patients should be shielded from the truth.
  - Doctors now have a more complete knowledge about their patients than doctors did in the past.
  - Many modern therapies are initially worse than the diseases they treat.
  - The sophistication of clinical epidemiologic data creates choices among different therapies for the same condition.

- For young children, except in an emergency, parents or legal guardians must consent. For older children, parental consent may not be necessary for particular diseases, such as those related to reproductive health or for psychiatric conditions.

- It is nice to get informed consent in the ED; however, both physicians and parents are held to a higher standard, namely, to do what is best for the child. If physicians think that parents' failure to consent to a procedure places the child at imminent risk of harm, emergency protective custody is taken and the procedure is performed anyway.

- When the need for treatment is nonemergent, everything changes. Physicians still advocate for the child; however, rather than taking emergency protective custody and proceeding with treatment, the court is asked to take custody.

- In the United States, the Child Abuse Prevention and Treatment Act of 1974 defines abuse and neglect as "the physical and mental injury, sexual abuse, negligent treatment or maltreatment of a child under the age of 18 by a person who is responsible for the child's welfare under circumstances which indicate that the child's health and welfare are harmed or threatened thereby." Arguments about whether a particular act constitutes abuse may focus on the nature of the act itself, whether the act caused harm, whether there was or should have been prior recognition that the act would cause harm, and whether the caretaker might have prevented the harm.

- Cultural or religious differences may also play a role in evaluating what constitutes medical neglect. Christian Scientists, for example, may claim that it is appropriate not to take their sick children to a doctor, while courts may determine that such behavior constitutes neglect.

- Generally, the law requires reporting if someone "has reasons to believe that a child has been subjected to abuse." Such laws do not even attempt to quantify the degree of suspicion, the quality of the evidence, or the likelihood of abuse that must be present to compel a report.

In pediatrics generally, and pediatric emergency care more specifically, the central ethical issue is the relationship between physicians and parents in determining what is or is not in a child's best interest. Unlike competent adults, who may make decisions to accept or refuse treatment based on idiosyncratic personal preferences, decisions for children should be based on an assessment of what is or is not in the child's best interest.

This is not always easy. In the emergency department (ED), as in other settings where treatment must be provided quickly for patients who may be unstable, standard medical treatment is generally considered to be best for children. If the child is in imminent danger of loss of life or limb, treatment should be provided, even over parental objections. If treatment is medically indicated but might safely be delayed, physicians in the ED, as elsewhere, should notify child protection agencies to institute legal proceedings.

This general set of guidelines can lead to a number of specific problems. The current status of informed consent doctrine and specific problems that arise in the context of suspected child abuse are addressed in this chapter. With both of these issues, legal and moral standards have changed rapidly over the last 30 years. Therefore, the reasons for the changes, and some of the problems that such rapid social change creates, are discussed.

INFORMED CONSENT

Current standards for informed consent are more curious than is often realized. We take them for granted as both a moral and a legal imperative, even though they are a relatively recent development. From the time of Hippocrates until the late 20th century, doctors not only routinely withheld the truth from patients, but also vigorously defended the morality of their decisions to do so. The arguments for withholding the truth varied. Some were patient-centered, others focused on the physician, some were emotional, others economic; but none were apologetic. Given this historical record, recent moral sentiment dictating that patients ought to be told the truth represents one of those mysterious changes in morality that occur from time to time, whereby something that was once thought morally intolerable rather suddenly comes to be thought of as morally obligatory.

Three major changes in the way medicine is practiced led to a reevaluation of the presumption that patients should be shielded from the truth. First, doctors have a more complete knowledge about their patients than doctors did in the past. The capability to diagnose asymptomatic diseases creates new interpersonal situations that require reevaluations of ancient moral strictures.

Twentieth-century doctors are probably the first who are able to diagnose patients as being seriously ill when the patients feel perfectly healthy. This situation is common in oncology, where screening test results reveal early cancers in asymptomatic patients. It also occurs in other situations, such as screening for hypertension, tuberculosis, or glaucoma. If there is treatment available, the patient must be given the information that the doctor has in order to understand the necessity of treatment. This seemingly small change in medical diagnostics has profound implications for the doctor-patient relationship.

Patients who are diagnosed before they are sick are not really patients. They have not felt the physical symptoms that lead to the metaphysical dread and fear. People who are ill and suffering, who know pain, and perceive their own mortality, are in a different metaphysical state than healthy people. Literature by patients or about sickness suggests that they exaggerate their fears, crave reassurance, and eschew rationality. Denial, magical thinking, and a focus on the present rather than the future are all expected and, perhaps, desirable responses to news of serious illness. Traditional medical ethics, which encouraged hopeful evasion of difficult truths, acknowledged the psychological vulnerability of the patient in a way that modern bioethics does not.

The healthy patient with an abnormal screening test comes to the doctor not as a patient, in fear and hope, but as a healthy person, seeking the statistically likely reassurance that he or she is and will remain healthy. There is no question of denial or reassurance. Instead, the well person who must make a treatment decision may be able to weigh the risks and benefits of different treatment options rationally, as he or she might rationally evaluate choices on a menu or cars in a showroom.

A second reason for the change in approach to informed consent is that patients who feel healthy are routinely made quite sick in order to make them well again. To gain the cooperation of such patients, it is necessary to inform them about the anticipated side effects of treatment.

The age-old medical adage to do no harm has become essentially obsolete in modern medicine. Harm is done all the time in the hope of achieving a greater good. Often, treatments offer patients a diabolical choice among equally noxious options. These are the sorts of treatments that led judges to claim that doctors could no longer hide the facts from patients.

Two early malpractice cases involved these sorts of claims. In *Salgo v. Stanford* (1957), a 55-year-old man was left paralyzed after an aortogram. He sued the doctors for negligently failing to warn him of the risks of paralysis inherent in the procedure. Mr. Salgo's suit did not rely on proving that the doctors were negligent in performing the procedure. Instead, he claimed that if he had been told that there was a risk of paralysis, he would not have consented. In such situations, the judges thought, it was not justifiable to withhold information.

Similarly, in *Natason v. Kline* (1960), a patient suffered damage from radiation therapy that was given after a mastectomy to prevent recurrence of breast cancer. She later sued her doctor for not warning her about the effects that radiation therapy would have. Again, this was a situation in which a patient suffered a foreseeable side effect of a therapy that had not been negligently delivered.

These situations are not unique to modern medicine. One could argue that they existed in the days of bloodletting, amputation for gangrene, or the use of foxglove for dropsy. But they are more common and more predictable today and, thus, create an obligation for truth telling that may not have existed before.

This predictability is the basis for the third change in medicine that has altered the approach to informed consent. The sophistication of clinical epidemiologic data creates choices among different therapies for the same condition. Often, there is no single standard of care. To the extent that the effectiveness of treatments is studied, it is known with some precision how well they work. This database allows meaningful choices to be made among therapies for many diseases.

In many cases, knowledge about the risks and benefits of alternative treatments for a particular problem creates situations in which there is no longer one therapy that is clearly the "best" treatment. This is seen in all areas of medicine (e.g., the treatment of coronary artery diseases, breast cancer, or neonatal respiratory failure). There are a number of treatment options, each with its own risks and benefits. The existence of well-defined choices creates challenges for doctors and patients, both of whom want to know what is "best." Dispassionate evaluation of these situations shows that the term "best" is necessarily subjective. We must ask, best in terms of what? Since any determination of what is best must include both clinical data and the patient's values, the patient must be informed of the options.

All of these factors have created the need to provide patients with information. Nevertheless, in pediatrics generally, and especially in the pediatric ED, informed consent raises unique issues. First, it must be decided from whom to obtain consent. For young children, except in an emergency, parents or legal guardians must consent. In a true emergency (defined in most states as a situation in which there is an immediate threat of loss of life or limb), parental consent is not necessary and physicians must initiate treatment immediately. For older children, parental consent may not be necessary for particular diseases, such as those related to reproductive health or for psychiatric conditions. A patient <18 years of age is considered a minor in all states except Alabama, Nebraska, and Wyoming, where the age of maturity is considered to be 19 years. A minor is considered emancipated, and able to give consent, if he or she is married, pregnant, a parent, serving in the armed forces, or living apart from parents with financial independence. Some states have mature minor statutes, which apply to younger patients who demonstrate decisional capacity and may be able to give informed consent or decline treatment despite their parents' wishes.

From the viewpoint of ethics as opposed to law, the very requirement of obtaining consent from parents raises a unique dilemma.

Both doctors and parents have an objective to act in the child's interest. When treatment is recommended, it is because the physician feels it is in the child's interest. Parents' right to refuse recommended treatment in this situation must be limited. And yet we ask for their consent. Why?

This contradictory approach is best illustrated by consent to lumbar puncture. The risks and benefits of lumbar puncture must be explained to parents, who are then asked to consent. If they have concerns about the risks, they are given more information to address their concerns. If they still refuse, however, the lumbar puncture is done anyway if the physician thinks that it is really necessary. Drug testing is a different issue; it is not uncommon for parents to bring a minor to the emergency department and ask for a toxicology examination. The American Academy of Pediatrics opposes involuntary screening unless the minor is felt to lack decisional capacity or there exists "strong medical indications or legal requirements to do so." This situation exposes the potential conflicts arising between minors and their parents regarding issues of consent and confidentiality. The American College of Emergency Physicians (ACEP) considers confidentiality an "important but not absolute principle," citing treatment of minors as a "problem area."

In other words, it is nice to get informed consent in the ED. However, both physicians and parents are held to a higher standard, namely, to do what is best for the child. If physicians think that parents' failure to consent to a procedure places the child at imminent risk of harm, emergency protective custody is taken and the procedure is performed anyway. In such situations, informed consent is more a matter of public relations than of law. The legal requirement is to act in the child's best interest, and physicians and parents are both held to that obligation.

When the need for treatment is nonemergent, everything changes. Physicians still advocate for the child. However, rather than taking emergency protective custody and proceeding with treatment, the court is asked to take custody. A hearing then establishes whether the parents' or the physicians' views should prevail. Such an approach is also necessary in another common ED problem, the reporting of child abuse.

CHILD ABUSE

All physicians have a legal obligation to notify state child protection agencies of suspected abuse. When notified, these agencies initiate investigations that may result in legal action against parents and the removal of children from their homes. Parents may have their custodial rights terminated and may face criminal charges. The entire process of diagnosis and intervention for child abuse is accepted as both necessary and morally compelling.

As in the case of informed consent, however, this seeming consensus of moral sentiment hides a mystery. Until this century, what we now consider to be child abuse was largely unrecognized, was not illegal, and may not even have been considered immoral. Instead, it was not only permissible to abuse children physically but it was considered necessary for the children's own moral edification. Thus, "spare the rod and spoil the child." Parents and teachers had absolute authority over their children's lives. They could and did physically and sexually abuse children with an impunity so complete that such acts were seldom even recognized or acknowledged.

Our current approaches to child abuse reflect a sea of change in our moral view of the family. Until the 20th century, families were seen as small utilitarian moral universes. Parents (in most cases, fathers) could use children (and their wives) as they saw fit. Children had no independent moral rights. The movement to recognize and prevent child abuse and to punish abusers reflects a partial empowerment of the child. Such changes in moral sentiment raise important questions about the timelessness of moral principles. Either child abuse was always wrong but not recognized as wrong, suggesting that our moral sensitivities are improving over time, or child abuse became wrong only recently, suggesting that moral values are not timeless and immutable but transient and constantly evolving.

It seems unlikely that moral principles have changed or that people have become either more or less moral over the centuries. Instead, current responses to children reflect attempts to craft social and legal policies that best reflect our views of how children should be raised. Just as we have crafted policies to curtail certain activities regarding children, we have opted to condone other activities, such as sexual activity during early teenage years; exposure to violence in television, movies, and daily life; and child rearing in tiny nuclear or single-parent families, which would have been seen as morally problematic in the past. These changes could be viewed as experiments in social policy, testing whether particular policies enable or inhibit the development of communities or cultures embodying our moral ideals.

Premodern moral assumptions continue to exist today, hidden below the surface of an apparent moral consensus. Both physical and sexual abuse of children are still common. In most instances, such abuse is never reported or discovered. Furthermore, studies reveal that older doctors are less likely than younger doctors to report child abuse and males are less likely to report it than females.

There are a number of reasons why people might not report child abuse, even though they believe it to be wrong. Child abuse may be ignored because people have difficulty defining and recognizing it. It may go undiscovered because adults are reluctant to become involved and do not report it. Or, professionals may feel reluctant to threaten what they perceive as a therapeutic relationship with the parents. When abuse is reported, health professionals and legal agencies must weigh the relative risks and benefits of preserving the family against those of removing the child from the family. At each stage of this process, discrete ethical issues arise.

Definitions of abuse are notoriously variable, circular, or designed to leave room for interpretation on a case-by-case basis. In the United States, the Child Abuse Prevention and Treatment Act of 1974 defines abuse and neglect as "the physical and mental injury, sexual abuse, negligent treatment or maltreatment of a child under the age of 18 by a person who is responsible for the child's welfare under circumstances which indicate that the child's health and welfare are harmed or threatened thereby." State definitions based on this law vary. Arguments about whether a particular act constitutes abuse may focus on the nature of the act itself, whether the act caused harm, whether there was or should have been prior recognition that the act would cause harm, and whether the caretaker might have prevented the harm.

In both physical and sexual abuse, different individuals or communities distinguish acceptable from unacceptable behaviors using different criteria. In physical abuse, a distinction must be made between acceptable forms of discipline or punishment and abuse. Definitions must specify whether abuse should be defined in terms of particular actions or particular effects. Consider two children who are pushed roughly to the ground by an adult. One falls against a carpeted floor, the other hits a protruding cupboard door. The second sustains a skull fracture, the first is uninjured. If an act must cause harm to be abuse, then the second child was clearly abused while the first may not have been. Acts that leave no physical marks are harder to classify as abuse. It is generally harder to sustain criminal convictions or obtain civil sanctions in such cases, even though the children may sustain as much or more psychological harm as they would due to actions that cause physical signs of abuse.

In sexual abuse, definitional problems may arise. Child sexual abuse is generally intrafamilial and falls under the rubric of incest. While prohibitions against incest are universal, different cultures define incest to include or exclude different activities.

Parent-child nudity, communal sleeping arrangements, and tolerance for masturbation and peer sex play in children coexist with stringent incest taboos. Mothers in many cultures use genital manipulation to soothe and pleasure infants. Some cultures prescribe the deflowering of pubertal girls by an adult male or by the father.

Exotic cultural differences may be mirrored by different beliefs in our own culture. Some parents may sleep with their children, bathe with them, or take pictures of the children naked on the beach. In some jurisdictions, these activities may be defined as illegal or morally inappropriate.

Cultural or religious differences may also play a role in evaluating what constitutes medical neglect. Christian Scientists, for example, may claim that it is appropriate not to take their sick children to a doctor, while courts may determine that such behavior constitutes neglect. Some Native Americans believe that organ transplantation is prohibited and so may refuse life-sustaining treatment for their children in liver failure. Similarly, Jehovah's Witnesses will refuse consent for blood transfusions for their children, even if such transfusions would preserve life. In situations like these, judgments must be made about the relative importance of respecting religious and cultural diversity on the one hand and protecting the interests of vulnerable children on the other.

In addition to cultural differences in defining what behaviors are or are not permissible, serious moral problems arise when we attempt to determine whether, in any particular case, a behavior that is clearly not permissible has, in fact, occurred. Court cases may turn on the rules governing the collecting and presentation of evidence. Even in adult rape cases, victims have difficulty convincing juries that they have been raped. Such difficulties are compounded in child abuse cases, where young children cannot testify convincingly on their own behalf.

In summary, both physical and sexual abuse of children exist along a spectrum, from obvious cruelty and exploitation, to grayer areas of corporal punishment or sexual game playing. The strong moral arguments against egregious abuse of children often lose strength as the definition of abuse expands along a spectrum that includes activities which may be considered morally praiseworthy, morally acceptable, morally forgivable, or immoral but noncriminal.

Given these definitional vagaries, it is no surprise that most laws are vague in defining the reporting requirements. Generally, they require reporting if someone "has reasons to believe that a child has been subjected to abuse." Such laws do not even attempt to quantify the degree of suspicion, the quality of the evidence, or the likelihood of abuse that must be present to compel a report. In crafting such laws, it seems that the goal was to protect people who report abuse by allowing broad latitude to individuals in defining what they mean by a "suspicion" of abuse. Even with such vague and permissive requirements, evidence suggests that abuse is underreported, rather than overreported.

Reticence to report suspected child abuse may be based on the sociology of health care delivery, on respect for confidentiality in the doctor-parent relationship, on unwillingness to stigmatize parents when there is doubt about the actual occurrence of abuse, or on a desire to preserve the therapeutic relationship with parents or to avoid the perception that professionals are parents' enemies.

Physicians in private practice are paid by the parents of the children for whom they provide care. They often develop long-term relationships with both parents and children. In such situations, relationships must be based on mutual trust. Physicians may give parents the benefit of the doubt regarding injuries that may be associated with abuse. They may also be fearful that child abuse reports will be bad for business. These factors may partially explain why reports of abuse are more likely to come from hospital emergency departments than from private doctors' offices.

In addition to economic considerations, moral aspects of the doctor-patient relationship may impede reporting. Generally, doctors promise confidentiality to parents. The moral reasons for confidentiality are compelling. Parents must confide in doctors and may need to give them information that would be embarrassing or damaging were it known by others. However, this promise of confidentiality may conflict with a physician's concern about the child's best interest. Although the law requires doctors to report suspected child abuse, reporting is, in fact, quite sporadic and inconsistent. None of the studies documenting inconsistent reporting disentangle the economic, moral, and legal considerations that lead doctors and other child welfare professionals to report or not report abuse.

Reticence to report may also result from a lack of faith in the efficacy of interventions. Intervention for children who have suffered abuse is not straightforward. It requires a delicate balance between trying to protect the child, to help the parents, and to preserve the family. Parents who abuse children have often been abused themselves and have a higher incidence of psychiatric problems. Many parents regret their actions, desire psychiatric help, and comply with treatment programs. However, 5 to 30 percent of abused children who stay in their families are subjected to further episodes of abuse. Currently, there are no reliable indicators of which parents will continue to abuse their children and which are likely to respond to therapy. Furthermore, any data that might address this issue will necessarily be probabilistic. Thus, decisions about the value of such data in an individual case will incorporate normative values about the degree of risk appropriate for a particular child facing a particular custody decision.

Relatively few cases of child abuse lead to criminal prosecutions. Punishment of alleged offenders seems morally unassailable. However, given the ambiguities in the definition of abuse and in the reporting of abuse, there is an arbitrary quality to punishment that offends commonsense notions of justice. Evidence of abuse is generally not sufficient to establish the guilt of the alleged perpetrator with 100 percent certainty. Therefore, such punishment seems more random and symbolic than obligatory and just. Debates about the appropriateness of punishment must take place in the context of debate about the morality of incarceration or the potential for rehabilitation in other criminal situations.

An apparent consensus about child abuse masks profound disagreements about the proper boundaries of family privacy, parental obligations, and governmental responsibility to oversee the care and nurturing of children. These disagreements are reflected in difficulties in defining child abuse, in enforcing compliance with mandatory reporting requirements, and in evaluating the effects of interventions. Thus, while the law requires that child abuse be reported if it is suspected, health professionals can create their own index of suspicion. Some providers may report ambiguous cases, whereas others rarely report suspected abuse at all.

CONCLUSION

This chapter focuses on two of the principal nondeath-related ethical dilemmas that arise in the ED: obtaining informed consent and dealing with suspected child abuse or neglect. In each case, the physician is required to determine what is best for a child while trying to maintain a therapeutic alliance with the child's parents. In both situations, there are relatively straightforward cases in which parents are clearly not acting in the child's interests and where the pediatric emergency physician may assert moral and legal authority over the child's medical care. More often, however, ambiguous cases arise in which it is unclear whether the parents are acting appropriately in caring for their children. There are no simple formulas for dealing with these cases. Instead, an understanding of the evolution of current law and public policy may help guide physicians as they develop a personal set of moral guidelines to respond to these situations.

BIBLIOGRAPHY

Badger LW: Reporting of child abuse: Influence of characteristics of physician, practice and community. *South Med J* 1989;82:281.

Goodwin JM: Obstacles to policy making about incest: Some cautionary folktales, in Wyatt GD, Powell GJ (eds): *Lasting Effects of Child Sexual Abuse.* Newbury Park, London: Sage Publications, 1988, pp 21–37.

Jacobstein CR, Baren JM: Emergency treatment of minors. *Emerg Med Clin North Am* 1999;17:341–352.

Katz J: *The Silent World of Doctor and Patient.* New York: Free Press, 1984.

Kean RN, Dukes RL: Effects of witness characteristics on the perception and reportage of child abuse. *Child Abuse Negl* 1991;15:423.

Murphy RF: *The Body Silent.* New York: Norton, 1991, pp 24–25.

Peters JMD: Criminal prosecution of child abuse: recent trends. *Pediatr Ann* 1989;18:505–508.

Radbill SX: A history of child abuse and infanticide, in Helfer RE, Kempe CH (eds): *The Battered Child.* Chicago: University of Chicago Press, 1974, pp 3–21.

INDEX

Page numbers followed by the letters *f* and *t* indicate figures and tables, respectively.